# Manual of ORTHOPEDICS

# Manual of
# ORTHOPEDICS

**NANCY E. HILT,** R.N., B.S.N., M.S.N.

Clinical Specialist in Pediatric Orthopedics and
Nursing Supervisor, Children's Rehabilitation Center,
University of Virginia Medical Center;
Instructor, Department of Orthopaedics and Rehabilitation,
School of Medicine, University of Virginia;
Clinical Instructor, School of Nursing,
University of Virginia, Charlottesville, Virginia

**SHIRLEY B. COGBURN,** R.N., B.S.N.

Outpatient Nursing Coordinator, Children's Rehabilitation Center,
University of Virginia Medical Center, Charlottesville, Virginia;
formerly Nurse Clinician, Division of Orthopaedics,
Emory University Hospital, Atlanta, Georgia

*with 772 illustrations, including 183 in color*

# The C. V. Mosby Company

ST. LOUIS • TORONTO • LONDON    1980

Printed in the United States of America

The C. V. Mosby Company
11830 Westline Industrial Drive, St. Louis, Missouri 63141


**Library of Congress Cataloging in Publication Data**
Main entry under title:

Manual of orthopedics.

  Bibliography: p.
  Includes index.
    1. Orthopedia.   I. Hilt, Nancy E., 1943-
II. Cogburn, Shirley Berry, 1934-
RD731.M28        617′.3        78-31732
ISBN 0-8016-2198-4


C/VH/VH  9  8  7  6  5  4  3  2  1      02/D/234

# Contributors

**ANDREWS, LARRY F., B.S., R.P.T.**

Supervisor of Physical Therapy, Division of Orthopaedics, Emory University Hospital and Clinic, Atlanta, Georgia

**BRANDON, MARSHA, R.N., B.S., M.S.N.**

Assistant Professor, Department of Adult Nursing, School of Nursing, Medical College of Georgia, Augusta, Georgia

**CAMPBELL, A. LAURA, R.N., B.S., M.N.**

Clinical Nurse Specialist, Child and Adolescent Consultation Services, Grady Memorial Hospital, Atlanta, Georgia

**CROSS, PAMELA S., R.N., B.S.N., M.S.**

Assistant Professor, Nell Hodgson Woodruff School of Nursing, Emory University, Atlanta, Georgia

**DUNN, BARBARA H., R.N., M.S.N., P.N.P.**

Assistant Professor, Maternal-Child Nursing, Pediatric Nurse Practitioner Program, Virginia Commonwealth University, Medical College of Virginia, School of Nursing, Richmond, Virginia; formerly, Clinical Specialist and Nursing Supervisor, Children's Rehabilitation Center, University of Virginia Medical Center, Charlottesville, Virginia

**GETZ, PATSY A., R.N., B.S.N., M.N.**

Clinical Nursing Specialist, Rehabilitation, Center for Rehabilitation Medicine, Emory University Hospital, Atlanta, Georgia

**GRYTH, BEVERLY A., B.S., R.P.T.**

Supervisor, Department of Physical Therapy, Children's Rehabilitation Center, University of Virginia Medical Center, Charlottesville, Virginia

**HAKALA, MICHAEL W., M.D.**

Co-Medical Director, Children's Rehabilitation Center, University of Virginia Medical Center; Assistant Professor, Departments of Orthopaedics and Rehabilitation and Pediatrics, School of Medicine, University of Virginia, Charlottesville, Virginia

**HOGAN, GROVER B.**

Chairman, Department of Medical Illustrations, Emory University, Atlanta, Georgia

**JACKSON, JOSEPH T.**

Medical Photographer, Department of Medical Illustrations, Emory University, Atlanta, Georgia

**KERR, AVICE, R.N., B.A.**

Medical-Legal Consultant, Downey, California

**LANDRUM, D. FRANK, B.S.**

Supervisor, Inpatient Services, Pharmacy Department, Emory University Hospital, Atlanta, Georgia

**LYNE, E. DENNIS, M.D.**

Chief, Division of Pediatric Orthopaedic Surgery and Director, Multidisciplinary Clinic, Henry Ford Hospital, Detroit, Michigan

**MARTIN, MARGARET M., R.N., B.S.N.**

Infection Control Coordinator, Emory University Hospital, Atlanta, Georgia

**MOORE, PAMELA J., B.S., Ph.D.**

Assistant Professor, Department of Anatomy, School of Medicine, Medical College of Georgia, Augusta, Georgia

**SCHMITT, E. WILLIAM, Jr., M.D.**

Assistant Professor, Division of Orthopaedics, School of Medicine, Emory University; Chief of Orthopaedics, Henrietta Egleston Hospital for Children, Atlanta, Georgia

**SULTENFUSS, SYLVIA REUTER, R.N., B.A., M.S.N.**

Mental Health Consultant, Clinical Nursing Specialist, Emory University Hospital, Atlanta, Georgia

**VEDDER, KATHRYN N., M.D.**

Attending Physician, Department of Pediatrics, and Director, Protective Services Team, Cook County Hospital; Assistant Professor of Pediatrics, Abraham Lincoln School of Medicine and University of Illinois, Chicago, Illinois

**VOGTLE, LAURA K., B.S., O.T.R.**

Supervisor, Department of Occupational Therapy, Children's
Rehabilitation Center, University of Virginia Medical Center,
Charlottesville, Virginia

**WALLACE, KATHLEEN G., R.N., B.S.N., M.N.**

Assistant Professor, Nell Hodgson Woodruff School of
Nursing, Emory University, Atlanta, Georgia

A little knowledge that acts is worth infinitely more than much knowledge that is idle.

*Kahlil Gibran*

This edition of *Manual of Orthopedics*
is *respectfully* and *lovingly* dedicated to those who
have supported us the most
throughout its evolution and preparation . . .
*our families.*

To Sharon and Jim,
Jeff, Berry, Mark, and Mother

# Preface

The specialty of orthopedics has an extremely broad scope. Many allied health disciplines, as well as medical and nursing personnel, take an active role in the diagnosis, care, and treatment of patients with orthopedic problems. Numerous texts have been written to establish foundational knowledge for each of the individual participants in this care, but few attempts have been made to provide a multidisciplinary or interdisciplinary approach in one volume. The initial concept and design of the *Manual of Orthopedics* was an attempt to fulfill that need. We feel that it is extremely advantageous for *all* personnel involved with the care of these patients to have a much broader scope of knowledge than may be obtained only within their specialty area. Although we believe this book will be useful to students, it was designed primarily as a reference source for practitioners in medicine, nursing, occupational therapy, physical therapy, and other allied health disciplines.

The broad scope of information and nature of its content offered several options for organization. The organizational approach chosen logically follows the steps that may be encountered with a patient's introduction into the health care system for evaluation, diagnosis, and treatment. Within the parameters of available space and time, we have made every attempt in this first edition to be as comprehensive as possible and have utilized for research purposes what are considered to be known authorities in various areas. As is true with any major undertaking, we found it impossible in some areas to provide the depth of material that may be desired. For these areas it is suggested that the reader refer to the bibliographic material provided to assist in location of follow-up information if required.

Certain aspects of care of the orthopedic patient were difficult to classify according to our accepted outline. The approaches selected may be controversial but specifically reflect our personal philosophies. Two such areas are those of pain evaluation and infection control; both were felt to be separate entities and should be treated as individual treatment modalities. For these reasons both have been included in the section on treatment alternatives. Consistent presentation of content throughout the entire manual was difficult. Some areas, such as those on diseases and disorders, lend themselves well to consistency, while others do not. These areas utilize an approach that would best present the individual content. Other such areas may be reflected throughout the outline. Much information has been summarized in tabular form to provide maximum information as concisely as possible. Many line drawings and photographs have been used to illustrate content. An extensive glossary has been provided to facilitate quick reference and clarification. Individual referencing was not used for areas of common knowledge.

We wish to gratefully acknowledge those individuals without whose support, encouragement, and patience we could not have continued, much less completed, this endeavor. Through the sharing of their knowledge the contributors have broadened the scope of the manuscript. Without the obvious very fine skills and artistic ability of Grover Hogan and Joe Jackson, the effort would, at best, have been inadequate. For their relentless patience, tolerance, and very special sense of humor, a source of continued comfort to us, we owe a special thank you!

We are grateful to those who reviewed the manuscript, Patricia Alt, R.N., and Dr. Michael Sussman, and are very appreciative of their comments and recommendations. Many additional individuals were responsible for reviewing selected portions of the galley and page proofs: Jayleane Bell, R.N.; Ann Brinckerhoff, R.N., M.S.N.; Robyn Brooke, R.N., B.S.N.; Susan Burgess, R.N., B.S.N.; Margaret Burns, R.N., B.S.N.; Amanda Casberg; Anne Creech, R.N., M.N.; Jad Davis; Martha

ix

Davis, Ph.D.; Chris Ferguson, R.N.; Donna Goodling, R.N.; Linda Guhlow, R.N., M.S.N.; Annette Johnson, R.N.; Jan Knapstein, R.N., B.S.N.; Peppy Linden; Rita McGowan, R.N.; Bev Mirmelstein, R.N.; Nance Nuckols, R.N., B.S.N.; Beth Paine, R.N., B.S.N.; Irma Stewart, R.N.; Angie Tillman, L.P.N.; Kate Walsh, R.N., B.S.N.; Nancy Whitman, R.N., M.S.N.; and Mary Yeager, R.N., M.S.N. To these special people we are grateful for their willingness to assist us.

We wish to thank the administration of Emory University Hospital for the use of their facilities for photographic purposes. Dr. Cosmo Hahn and Dr. Brit Gay, from their respective Departments of Radiology at Emory University Hospital and Henrietta Egleston Hospital for Children, were extremely helpful in the selection of the radiographic films, all of which were used courtesy of these hospitals. We are indebted to those who provided typographic services under some rather difficult deadlines: Jad Davis, Genevieve Fiorente, B. J. Morris, and Audrey Thompson. We thank Bruce Baldwin, Administrator of the Children's Rehabilitation Center, for the continued support received in a variety of ways.

A very special gratitude is felt for several individuals for their continually offered support and encouragement at times when it seemed to be needed the most: Helen Ripple, Director of Nursing, University of Virginia Medical Center; Mary Yeager, Assistant Director of Pediatric Nursing, University of Virginia Medical Center; and Dr. Sharon Hostler, Co-Medical Director, University of Virginia Medical Center. Their support and encouragement was especially meaningful to us in the transition of new positions; the understanding of dual commitments under such circumstances was always evident and apparent.

Although many people have assisted in the completion of this manuscript, a project that has taken twice as long to prepare and been twice as comprehensive as initially intended, a very special group of individuals has composed a support system without which we could not have functioned. To those individuals—our nursing staff members and co-workers, our friends, and families—we can only offer our continued love and friendship. Although the time and attention each missed during the past few years because of the manuscript are irretrievable, it is hoped that somehow knowledge of their instrumental role in our accomplishment will create a degree of pride and satisfaction.

We respectfully submit this endeavor to those who are dedicated to the provision of quality health care, with the sincere hope that it will be useful in fulfilling its objectives.

**Nancy E. Hilt**
**Shirley B. Cogburn**

# Contents

**14 Lower extremity and hip, 266**

NANCY E. HILT
SHIRLEY B. COGBURN

**15 Cervical and spinal diseases and disorders, 310**

NANCY E. HILT
SHIRLEY B. COGBURN

**16 Trauma, 332**

NANCY E. HILT

**17 Joint diseases and disorders, 354**

NANCY E. HILT
SHIRLEY B. COGBURN

# PART ONE

# Anatomy and physiology

# 1

# Skeletal system

PAMELA J. MOORE

The skeletal system forms the supporting framework of the body and its appendages. Two hundred six bones and their intervening cartilages contribute to this moving and supportive mass of specialized connective tissue. Like other types of connective tissue, bone and cartilage consist predominantly of intercellular substance, called *matrix,* and relatively few living cells. The intercellular substance of bone is calcified due to the presence of calcium phosphate and calcium carbonate crystals. This impregnation of salts is responsible for the hard or osseous nature of bone.

The skeletal system has several important functions. First, it supports the soft tissue of the body and gives it form and shape. Second, the arrangement of bones allows them to act as levers, facilitating movement when the overlying muscles contract. Third, the system affords protection to the important underlying organs of the body. Fourth, the system is responsible for blood cell production, or *hematopoiesis.* And fifth, the chemical nature of bone allows it to store necessary minerals, especially calcium and phosphorus, for body use.

## TYPES OF BONES

Most bones are classified according to their shape: *long, short, flat,* and *irregular.* Long bones are found in the extremities and consist of a shaft with two expanded ends (e.g., tibia, femur, humerus). They are curved to give more strength and are composed predominantly of compact bone.

Short bones are cube shaped and consist mainly of spongy bone with a compact bone shell (e.g., carpal and tarsal bones).

Flat bones are thin and composed of two plates of compact bone with an intervening layer of spongy bone (e.g., cranial bones, ribs, scapula, ilium). These bones give a great deal of protection and have a large surface area for muscle attachment.

Irregular bones are of various shapes and do not fit into any of the previous three groups. The composition of these bones varies from mostly compact to a compact bony shell surrounding a spongy bony center (e.g., some skull bones and vertebrae).

Other bones are not classified by shape. Sesamoid bones are free-floating bones usually found in tendons or joint capsules. The patella is the largest of these, but small ones are found in the tendons of the hands and feet.

Wormian bones are specially classified. These are small clusters of bones found between the joints of some cranial bones (e.g., parietal sutures).

## BONE ANATOMY

All bones have some basic structures in common (Fig. 1-1). All are covered by a dense connective tissue layer called the *periosteum.* This layer's inner

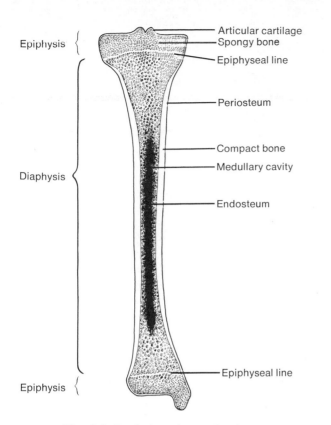

Epiphysis

Diaphysis

Epiphysis

Articular cartilage
Spongy bone
Epiphyseal line

Periosteum

Compact bone
Medullary cavity

Endosteum

Epiphyseal line

**Fig. 1-1.** Basic long bone structure.

aspect contains *osteoblasts,* cells that have the ability to produce more bone. Periosteum also carries blood vessels, lymphatics, and nerves to bone and is therefore essential for bone nutrition, growth, and repair. Inside bone is a generative membrane called the *endosteum.* This membrane is composed of osteoblasts and lines the space within the bone called the *medullary* or *marrow cavity.*

Long bones consist of a *shaft, diaphysis,* and expanded ends called *epiphyses.* Both epiphyses are covered by a thin layer of hyaline cartilage or articular cartilage where the bone forms a joint with another bone. Long bones are somewhat hollow with a rather extensive marrow cavity.

## BONE FORMATION AND GROWTH

Bone forms in the body by the process of *ossification.* There are two types of ossification, or growth, which begin in the embryo. The first is *intramembranous* ossification. This type of bone forms on or within a fibrous membrane framework. The bone formed from this type of ossification is spongy or cancellous in nature. It is generally found in flat, irregular, and short bones and in the epiphyses of long bones. This process begins with the clustering of mesenchymal cells in a fibrous membrane.

These mesenchymal cells become *osteoblasts* and begin to secrete an intercellular substance. This intercellular substance is composed of a collagenous fiber network or matrix in which calcium salts are deposited. This deposition of calcium salts is called *calcification.* A cluster of osteoblasts completely surrounded by a matrix is called a *trabecula.* As trabeculae form, they eventually fuse, and osteoblasts become entrapped in spaces called *lacunae* and lose their ability to form a matrix. These trapped cells are now called *osteocytes.* Osteoblasts are still present on the surface of trabeculae. In this spongy type of bone the trabeculae never fuse into a solid sheet; instead, spaces remain and become filled with bone marrow. The fibrous membrane that surrounds the growing bone mass becomes the *periosteum.* The ossified area is now true spongy bone. As maturation continues, the surface of spongy bone is reconstructed into solid, dense, compact bone. This type of bone, found in the skull, with a spongy center and compact inner and outer layers, is called *diploë bone.*

The second type of ossification is *endochondral* (Fig. 1-2) and refers to bone formation within hyaline cartilage. Endochondral ossification occurs in the diaphyses on long bones. This type of bone is compact or dense and totally replaces its cartilaginous model.

A change in pH begins the sequence of events leading to endochondral ossification, or calcification of the cartilaginous framework. In the middle of the diaphysis, chondrocytes and their lacunae hypertrophy, and calcium phosphate is deposited at the expense of the cartilaginous matrix, forming calcified spicules of cartilage. The surrounding perichondrium is activated, and mesenchymal cells become osteoblasts and perichondrium becomes periosteum. The osteoblasts begin to form bone on the outer surface, and a periosteal bone collar appears around the middiaphysis. This is the first true bone.

Blood vessels, carrying osteoblasts with them, grow from the periosteum into cavities of the diaphyses formed by the enlargement and confluence of lacunae left by dying chondrocytes. These spaces will eventually become the marrow cavity. The transformed periosteum will eventually send blood vessels into the epiphyses also. Osteoblasts lay down bone on the surface of the spicules of calcified cartilage; therefore these spicules or trabeculae are composed of calcified cartilage with a true bone covering. Eventually true bone will replace the calcified cartilage. As endochondral ossification proceeds, the cartilaginous model grows in length at the epiphyses. Secondary ossification centers will arise

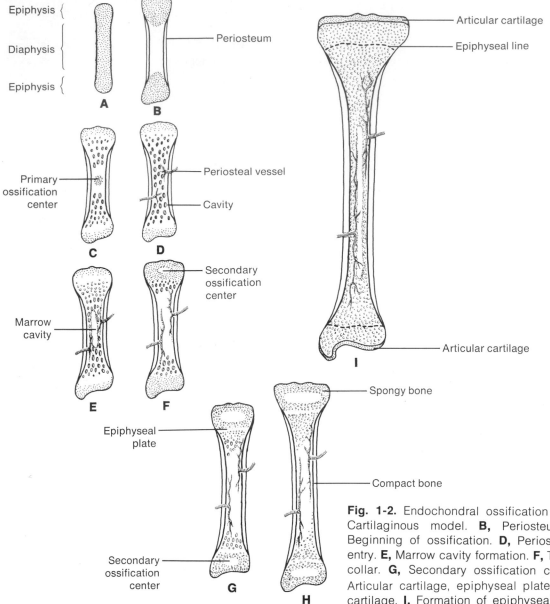

Epiphysis {

Diaphysis {

Epiphysis {

Periosteum

Primary ossification center

Periosteal vessel

Cavity

Marrow cavity

Secondary ossification center

Epiphyseal plate

Secondary ossification center

Articular cartilage

Epiphyseal line

Articular cartilage

Spongy bone

Compact bone

A   B   C   D   E   F   G   H   I

**Fig. 1-2.** Endochondral ossification of long bone. **A,** Cartilaginous model. **B,** Periosteum formation. **C,** Beginning of ossification. **D,** Periosteal blood vessel entry. **E,** Marrow cavity formation. **F,** Thickening of bone collar. **G,** Secondary ossification centers formed. **H,** Articular cartilage, epiphyseal plates, and remains of cartilage. **I,** Formation of epiphyseal line. Basic bone formation complete.

later at the proximal epiphyses, and spongy bone will develop there. The distal epiphyses begin to ossify after birth. Hyaline cartilage remains on the outsides of the epiphyses as articular cartilage. A plate of cartilage also remains in the area between the epiphysis and diaphysis. This area of cartilage allows bone to increase in length until early adulthood. Growth in diameter occurs by apposition, with osteoblasts from the periosteum adding osseous tissue, while specialized cells called osteoclasts destroy bone surrounding the marrow cavity. This causes the bone to get wider but not heavier.

Bone growth in length usually has ceased by age 17 years, when the epiphyseal plate of cartilage calcifies and is replaced by bone. Bones formed by endochondral and intramembranous ossification remodel themselves continuously, with old bone being destroyed and new bone being formed. This remodeling and replacement varies in different parts of the body according to body needs, injury, and wear. Factors influencing these processes are diet, mineral and vitamin concentration, and hormone levels. Thyrocalcitonin from the thyroid gland decreases blood calcium and causes its deposition in bone, while parathyroid hormone increases blood calcium levels by removing calcium from bone.

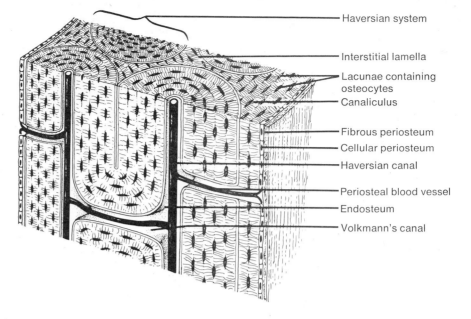

Haversian system
Interstitial lamella
Lacunae containing osteocytes
Canaliculus
Fibrous periosteum
Cellular periosteum
Haversian canal
Periosteal blood vessel
Endosteum
Volkmann's canal

**Fig. 1-3.** Cross and longitudinal sections of compact bone indicating specific histologic features.

## BONE HISTOLOGY AND COMPOSITION

The central medullary cavity of bone contains *bone marrow*. Active bone marrow is found in the medullary cavity of long bones, the spongy portion of vertebral bodies, the sternum, the ribs, and the flat bones of the pelvis. The activity and cellular composition of bone marrow varies with age. At birth all bone marrow is red, being composed of the cellular precursors of red blood cells and the granulocytic series of white blood cells. As an individual matures, many of the red blood cell precursors are replaced by adipose cells. This is now called yellow marrow. Yellow marrow has the ability to return to the red type if needed. The major functions of bone marrow are blood cell formation and phagocytosis of broken-down bone elements.

The periosteum, or covering connective tissue containing osteoblasts, blood vessels, lymphatics, and nerves, is common to all bone, as is the endosteum, or lining. Connective tissue fibers, or Sharpey's fibers, anchor the periosteum to the bone. Compact bone has a microscopically definitive morphology. Even though this type of bone is initially trabecular, it eventually forms into distinct structural units called *osteons* or *haversian systems* (Fig. 1-3). The haversian systems are composed of concentric lamellae. Connecting interstitial lamellae also are seen, which are remnants of old haversian systems that are being remodeled. In each osteon there is a central haversian canal carrying blood vessels and lined with endosteum. Volkmann's canals are seen traversing the osteons, carrying blood vessels from the periosteum to the central canals.

Osteocytes are seen trapped in lacunae found around the lamellae. Canaliculi extend from all lacunae and form vast interconnections of the lacunae with the central canals. These canaliculi allow the passage of nutrient material to the osteocytes. The intercellular matrix of compact bone is formed by osteoblasts. Once these cells become trapped they become osteocytes, and the osteocytes maintain the matrix. As mentioned, the composition of the matrix is mainly organic collagen with deposits of calcium salts (phosphate, carbonate, and fluoride), magnesium, and sodium. There is a constant turnover of these elements to maintain normal blood levels of these minerals.

The blood supply of bone comes from periosteal vessels, which send branches via Volkmann's canals to haversian systems. Large nutrient arteries also enter the diaphyses and pass into the medullary cavity. Innervation of bone is usually to the periosteal level only.

## SURFACE MARKINGS

A close look at bone reveals various kinds of bone markings (grooves, lines, and elevations). Their structure usually indicates their function. Long bones have rounded ends that form joints. Roughened areas usually indicate some attachment of muscle, ligament, or tendon. Common bone markings include the following:

### HOLES OR DEPRESSIONS

**foramen** rounded opening through bone for passage of blood vessels, nerves, or ligaments.

**ANTERIOR**

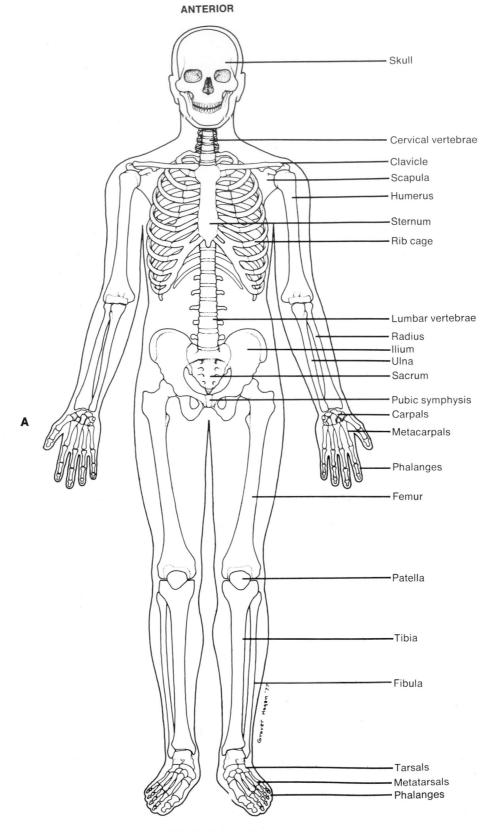

A

Skull

Cervical vertebrae

Clavicle

Scapula

Humerus

Sternum

Rib cage

Lumbar vertebrae

Radius

Ilium

Ulna

Sacrum

Pubic symphysis

Carpals

Metacarpals

Phalanges

Femur

Patella

Tibia

Fibula

Tarsals

Metatarsals

Phalanges

**Fig. 1-4.** Articulated skeleton.

POSTERIOR

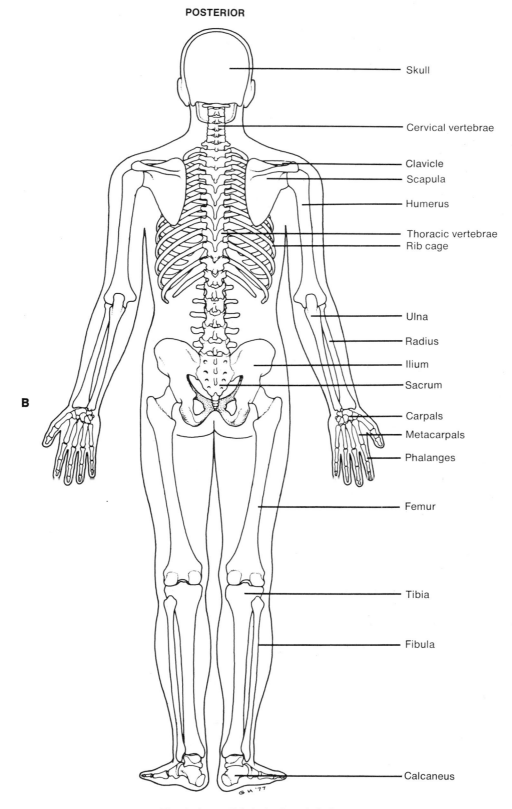

Skull

Cervical vertebrae

Clavicle

Scapula

Humerus

Thoracic vertebrae

Rib cage

Ulna

Radius

Ilium

Sacrum

Carpals

Metacarpals

Phalanges

Femur

Tibia

Fibula

Calcaneus

B

**Fig. 1-4, cont'd.** Articulated skeleton.

**fissure** slitlike opening in bone through which blood vessels, nerves, and ligaments pass.

**meatus (canal)** tubelike passage running through a bone.

**fossa** depression in a bone.

**groove** long, shallow depression in a bone.

**sinus** cavity or space within a bone.

**process** prominent, rough projection.

### PROCESSES FOUND AT JOINTS

**condyle** convex projection for articulation with another bone.

**head** rounded, expanded end beyond a constricted portion called a neck.

**facet** small, flat, shallow surface.

### PROCESSES FOR TENDON AND LIGAMENT ATTACHMENT

**tubercle** small rounded process.

**tuberosity** large, rounded, roughened process.

**spine (spinous process)** sharp, slender projection.

**trochanter** large, blunt projection found only on femur.

**crest** prominent ridge on a bone.

**line** less prominent ridge than a crest.

**epicondyle** roughened process above a condyle.

### SKELETAL SYSTEM

The skeletal system (Fig. 1-4) is divided into *axial* and *appendicular* portions. The appendicular division includes those bones forming the freely moving appendages of the upper and lower extremities and the bones of the shoulder and pelvic girdles. The axial skeleton consists of those bones found in the midline of the body. There are typically 80 bones in the axial skeleton and 126 bones in the appendicular division. They are grouped as follows:

**Axial skeleton**

| | |
|---|---:|
| Skull | |
|   Cranium | 8 |
|   Face | 14 |
| Hyoid | 1 |
| Vertebral column | 26 |
| Thorax | |
|   Ribs | 24 |
|   Sternum | 1 |
| Ossicles of ear | 6 |
| | 80 |

**Appendicular skeleton**

| | |
|---|---:|
| Shoulder girdle | |
|   Scapula | 2 |
|   Clavicle | 2 |
| Upper extremity | |
|   Humerus | 2 |
|   Radius | 2 |
|   Ulna | 2 |
|   Carpus | 16 |
|   Metacarpal bones | 10 |
|   Phalanges | 28 |
| Pelvic girdle | |
|   Innominate, coxa, hip | 2 |
| Lower extremity | |
|   Femur | 2 |
|   Tibia | 2 |
|   Fibula | 2 |
|   Patella | 2 |
|   Tarsus | 14 |
|   Metatarsals | 10 |
|   Phalanges | 28 |
| | 126 |

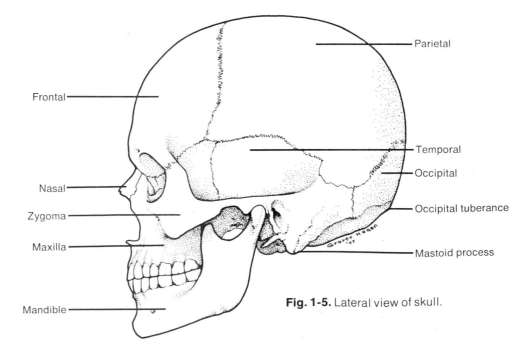

**Fig. 1-5.** Lateral view of skull.

## Axial skeleton

**Skull.** The skull, which is composed of 22 bones, rests on the cranial end of the vertebral column. The eight cranial bones enclose and protect the brain. These bones are of greatest importance in orthopedics because many neck and back muscles attach to some of them. These major bones and their prominent markings are seen in Fig. 1-5. The 14 facial bones are not discussed because they rarely are involved in orthopedics in the context of this book.

**Vertebral column.** The vertebral column forms the flexible longitudinal axis of the skeleton. It is composed of a series of bones called *vertebrae*. The average adult column is about 28 inches long with three planes of movement: forward, backward, and lateral. The functions of the column are to enclose and protect the spinal cord, to support the head, and to give attachment for ribs and muscles of the back. Intervertebral foramina are openings between the vertebrae that allow for the passage of spinal nerves from the cord. There are 26 or 27 vertebrae in the adult, depending on the amount of fusion, with the following distribution: seven cervical, twelve thoracic, five lumbar, and one sacral (formed by fusion of five), and one or two coccygeal (formed by fusion of four or five). The vertebrae are separated from each other by fibrocartilaginous pads called intervertebral discs. These discs help make the intervertebral joints strong and more pliable.

Viewed laterally, there are four alternately concave and convex curves in the column (Fig. 1-6, B). These curves increase the strength of the column, help absorb shocks to the column, help maintain balance and position, and protect the column from fracture. The fetus and the newborn have only one curve, which is concave anteriorly. At about 3 months of age the cervical curvature, which is convex anteriorly, develops as the infant begins to lift his head. The lumbar curvature, also convex anteriorly, develops when the child stands and puts weight on the column. Therefore the thoracic and sacral curves are primary in that they are concave anteriorly as in the newborn, while the cervical and lumbar curves are secondary.

Three conditions that involve exaggerated curvature of the column are *scoliosis,* left to right curvature; *kyphosis,* exaggerated anterior concavity (hunchback); and *lordosis,* exaggerated lumbar curvature (swayback).

All the vertebrae of the spinal column have a similar structure. However, vertebrae from different areas have different shapes, sizes, and articular surfaces. A typical vertebra has a thick, anteriorly located, disc-shaped body. This heavy structure has great weight-bearing ability. The superior and inferior surfaces of the body are roughened by the attachment of the intervertebral discs.

Extending posteriorly from the body is a neural arch composed of bilateral pedicles united posteriorly by a lamina of bone. These structures surround a space called the vertebral foramen. The continuous vertebral foramina of the vertebrae form the vertebral canal through which the spinal cord passes.

Several processes are found on the neural arch. Bilateral transverse processes extend from the point of union of the pedicles with the lamina. A single spinous process extends posteriorly and inferiorly from the lamina. Bilateral, superior, and inferior articular processes are present for articulation with the adjacent superior and inferior vertebrae, respectively.

There are seven cervical vertebrae. Generally the bodies of these vertebrae are smaller and the arches are larger than those seen in the thoracic vertebrae. Vertebrae C-2 through C-6 have bifid spinous processes, and all of the cervical vertebrae have transverse foramina in the transverse processes that allow for passage of the vertebral arteries, veins, and nerves.

The first cervical vertebra, the atlas, supports the head. It is circular, with no body and no spinous process. Its superior articular processes articulate with the occipital condyles, which permits nodding of the head. The inferior articular processes articulate with the second cervical vertebra, the axis. This vertebra has a body with an upward projection called the dens or odontoid process, which articulates through the atlas ring, forming a pivot joint that allows side-to-side movement (as in expressing "no"). Vertebrae C-2 through C-6 are considered typical. Vertebra C-7 is typical except that its spinous process is not bifid and it can be palpated at the base of the neck.

The twelve thoracic vertebrae are stronger than the cervical group. Their bodies are heavier and their transverse processes are longer. Their spinous processes project downward, and all but vertebrae T-11 and T-12 have facets for articulation with ribs.

The five lumbar vertebrae are the largest and strongest of the vertebrae, and their spinous processes are heavy and blunt. Their superior articular processes project medially instead of superiorly, and the inferior articular processes are directed laterally instead of inferiorly. The placement of these processes tends to stabilize the articulations of the lumbar vertebrae.

The sacrum, formed by the fusion of five vertebrae, is the foundation of the pelvic girdle. It is concave anteriorly and placed posteriorly between the two hip bones. Anteriorly, four transverse lines indicating where fusion occurred are visible, as are four pairs of pelvic foramina. On the dorsal aspect of the sacrum are medial and lateral sacral crests and four pairs of dorsal foramina. An extension of the vertebral canal, the sacral canal, extends into the sacrum.

The coccyx, formed by the fusion of four or five vertebrae, articulates with the sacrum and is a vestige of a tail.

**Thorax.** The chest, or thorax (Fig. 1-7, *A*), is supported by a bony cage composed of the ribs, sternum, costal cartilages, and thoracic vertebral bodies. It is narrow superiorly and wide inferiorly. It encloses and protects the organs of the thoracic cavity and supports the bony structure of the shoulder girdle and upper extremity.

The sternum is about 6 inches long and forms the midline anterior thoracic wall. It is composed of three fused parts: a superior triangular manubrium, which articulates with the clavicle and the first two ribs; a middle piece, the body, which articulates with ribs 2 through 10; and an inferior xiphoid

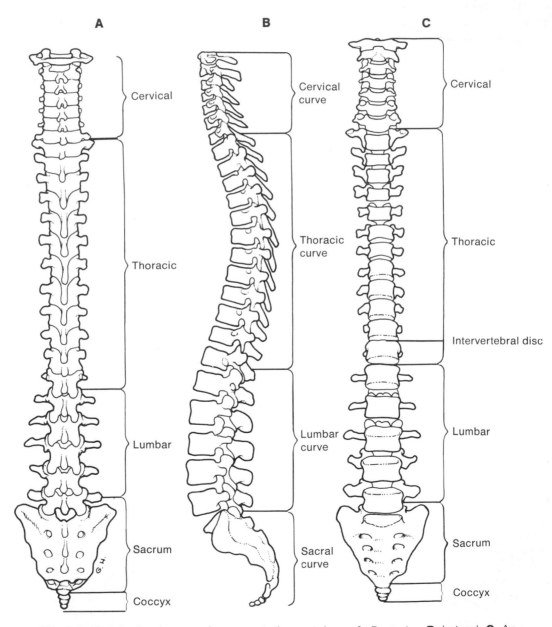

**Fig. 1-6.** Vertebral column and representative vertebrae. **A,** Posterior. **B,** Lateral. **C,** Anterior.

process that has no rib attachment but does give abdominal muscle attachment.

There are twelve pairs of ribs, which increase in length from 1 to 7 and decrease in length from 8 to 12. Ribs 1 through 7 attach directly to the sternum by means of costal cartilage and are called true ribs. Ribs 8 through 12 do not attach to the sternum and are called false ribs. However, ribs 8 through 10

attach to each other by means of adjoining cartilage and then attach to the seventh costal cartilage. Ribs 11 and 12 do not attach to those above them, so are considered to be floating ribs.

The head of each rib articulates posteriorly with a facet on a vertebral body. The neck of a rib is the constricted portion just below the head, and just below the neck is a tubercle that articulates with the

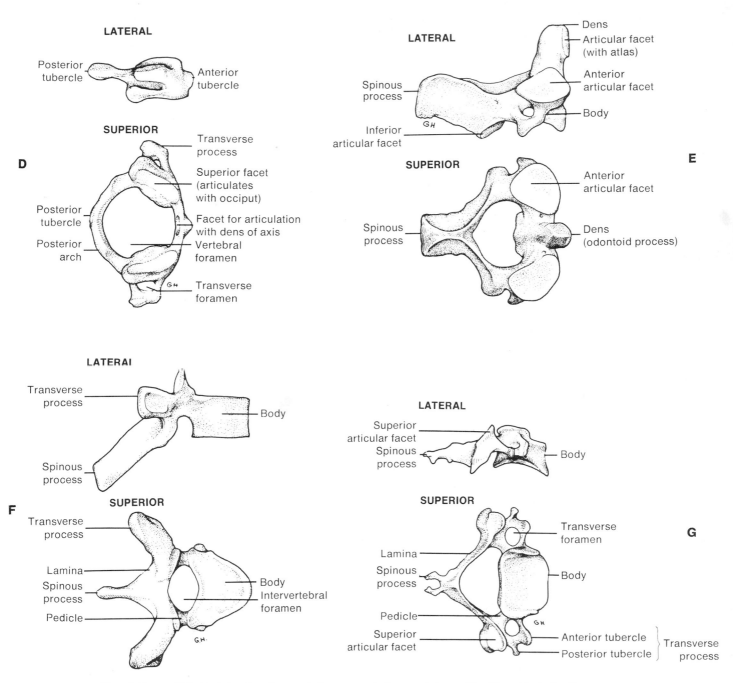

**Fig. 1-6, cont'd.** Vertebral column and representative vertebrae. **D,** Atlas. **E,** Axis. **F,** Seventh cervical. **G,** Typical cervical.

*Continued.*

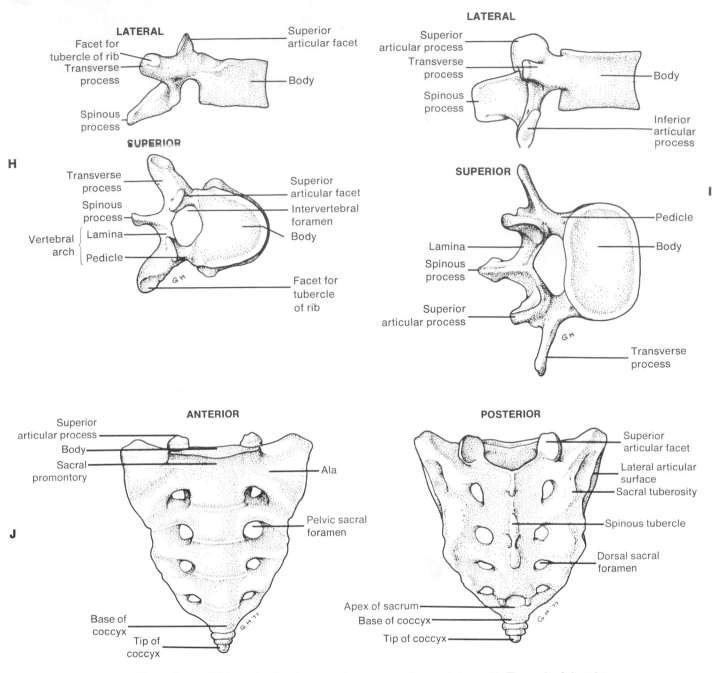

**Fig. 1-6, cont'd.** Vertebral column and representative vertebrae. **H,** Thoracic. **I,** Lumbar. **J,** Sacrum and coccyx.

transverse process of a vertebra. The body of the rib extends anteriorly, forming a crescent as it approaches the ventral side of the body. On the inner surface of each rib is a costal groove that allows for passage of the intercostal nerves and vessels. Ribs 2 through 9 articulate with the bodies of two adjacent vertebrae. Ribs 1 and 10 through 12 articulate only with their respective vertebral bodies. Ribs 11 and 12 have no articulations with vertebral tubercles or transverse processes. The spaces between the ribs are called intercostal spaces.

### Appendicular skeleton

**Shoulder girdle.** Each shoulder girdle consists of a clavicle and a scapula. The two shoulder girdles act as the points of attachment of the upper extremi-

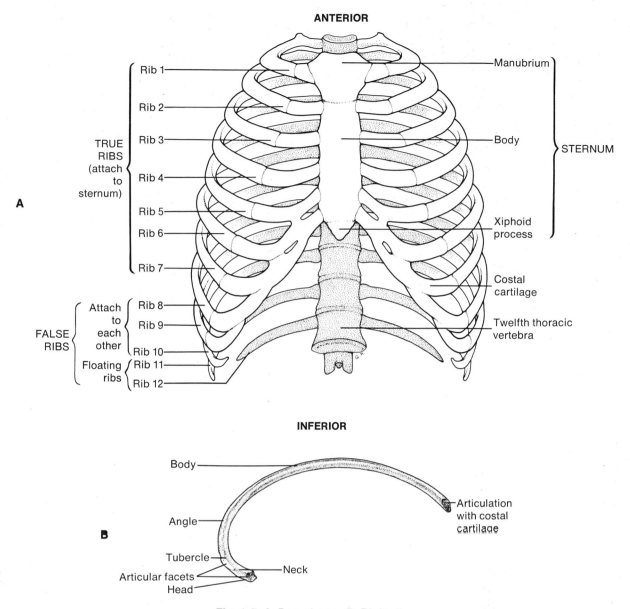

**ANTERIOR**

Rib 1 — Manubrium
Rib 2
Rib 3 — Body
TRUE RIBS (attach to sternum)
Rib 4
Rib 5
Rib 6 — Xiphoid process
Rib 7
FALSE RIBS — Attach to each other — Rib 8 — Costal cartilage
Rib 9 — Twelfth thoracic vertebra
Rib 10
Floating ribs — Rib 11
Rib 12

STERNUM

**A**

**INFERIOR**

Body
Angle
Tubercle
Articular facets — Neck
Head
Articulation with costal cartilage

**B**

**Fig. 1-7. A,** Bony thorax. **B,** Right rib.

ties to the axial skeleton. These girdles have no articulation with the vertebral column. The clavicle, or collarbone (Fig. 1-8, *A*), forms the anterior portion of the girdle and articulates in the anterior midline with the sternum and laterally with the acromium process of the scapula forming the acromioclavicular joint. A conoid tubercle is found on the inferior surface of the lateral end of the clavicle and serves as attachment for a ligament.

The scapula, or shoulder blade (Fig. 1-8, *B*), is a large, flat, triangular bone located at the level between the second and seventh ribs in the dorsal part of the thorax. Superior, vertebral, and axillary borders are prominent. A sharp spine projects diago-

nally across the upper third of the posterior surface of the flat body of the bone. The lateral extension of the spine is the acromium process, which articulates with the clavicle. Below the acromium is the glenoid cavity, which forms an articulation with the head of the humerus. At the lateral end of the superior border is an anterior projection, the coracoid process, which serves for muscle attachment. On the posterior surface of the scapula above and below the spine are the supraspinatus and infraspinatus fossae.

**Upper extremity.** The humerus, or upper arm bone (Fig. 1-9), articulates by its rounded head with the glenoid cavity of the scapula. The proximal end

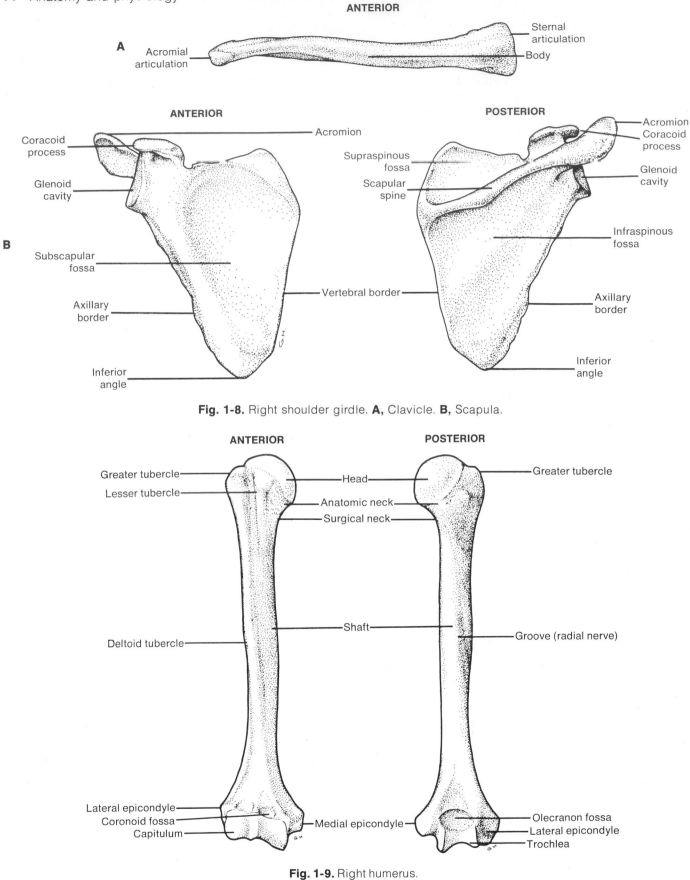

**Fig. 1-8.** Right shoulder girdle. **A,** Clavicle. **B,** Scapula.

**Fig. 1-9.** Right humerus.

of the bone has several distinct markings. Just below the head is a groove called the anatomic neck. The greater tubercle is a lateral projection below the neck, and the lesser tubercle is another anterior projection just below the neck. An intertubercular groove passes between the two tubercles. Below these tubercles the humerus narrows into a surgical neck, and it is in this area that the humerus commonly fractures. The humerus has a deltoid tuberosity on the anterolateral surface of the rounded shaft. At this midpoint the shaft begins to flatten into its broad distal end. On the posterior surface of the shaft is the radial groove through which the radial nerve passes. There are two projections from the medial and lateral margins of the lower end of the humerus, the medial and lateral epicondyles. The lower end of the humerus has two flattened areas, a lateral capitulum that articulates with the radius and a medial trochlea that articulates with the ulna. Above the trochlea on the anterior surface of the humerus is a depression, the coronoid fossa, which receives the coronoid process of the ulna when it flexes onto the humerus. Above the capitulum is the radial fossa, which receives the head of the radius when the forearm is flexed. On the posterior end of the humerus is a deep olecranon fossa, which receives the olecranon process of the ulna when it is extended.

The ulna (Fig. 1-10) is the medially placed bone of the forearm on the little finger side. Its olecranon process at the proximal end can be palpated at the elbow. The coronoid process is smaller and is inferior to the olecranon process. The smooth area between these two processes is the trochlear notch, which articulates with the trochlea of the humerus. The head of the ulna is at its distal end, and from it extends a projection, the styloid process, which is palpable at the wrist.

The radius (Fig. 1-10) is the bone of the forearm on the thumb side. Its proximally located head articulates with the capitulum of the humerus and the radial notch of the ulna. On its medial aspect is the radial tuberosity to which the biceps muscle attaches. The distal end of the radius has an ulnar notch for articulation with the ulna and a prominent styloid process. The broadened distal end of the radius articulates with the lunate and scaphoid bones of the wrist.

The wrist, or carpus (Fig. 1-11), is composed of two transverse rows of small carpal bones. In the anatomic position, palms facing outward, the proximal row, medial to lateral, consists of the pisiform,

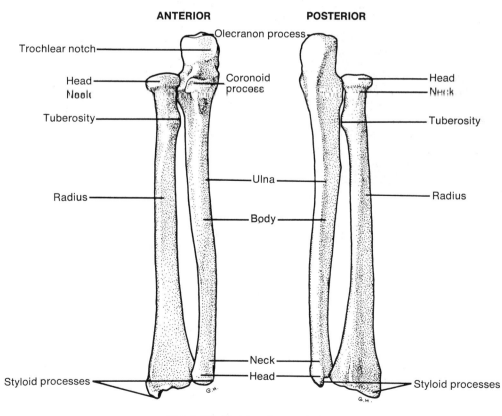

**Fig. 1-10.** Right radius and ulna.

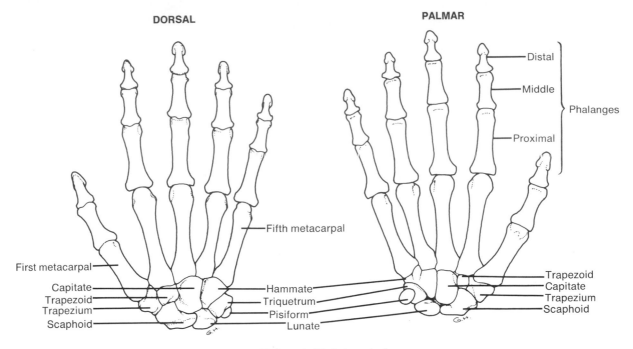

**DORSAL**

**PALMAR**

Distal

Middle

Phalanges

Proximal

Fifth metacarpal

First metacarpal

Capitate
Trapezoid
Trapezium
Scaphoid

Hammate
Triquetrum
Pisiform
Lunate

Trapezoid
Capitate
Trapezium
Scaphoid

**Fig. 1-11.** Right hand.

triquetral, lunate, and scaphoid bones. The distal row contains the hamate, capitate, trapezoid, and trapezium bones.

The distal row of carpal bones articulates with the bones that constitute the palm of the hand, the five metacarpals. Each of these consists of a proximal base, a shaft, and a distal head. The numbering of the metacarpals, 1 to 5, begins at the thumb, or lateral side. The heads articulate with the proximal phalanges of each finger.

The phalanges, the bones of the digits or fingers, number 14 on each hand. Each digit except the thumb has a proximal, a middle, and a distal phalanx. The thumb has only two, one proximal and one distal. The proximal phalanges articulate with the metacarpals and the middle phalanges. The middle phalanges articulate with the proximal and distal phalanges. The distal phalanges articulate with the middle phalanges only.

**Pelvic girdle.** The pelvic girdle is composed of two *coxae,* or hip bones. These two bones unite anteriorly at the pubic symphysis, and posteriorly both attach to the lateral aspect of the sacrum. The pelvic girdle functions to support and stabilize the lower extremities and protects the organs that lie in the pelvis.

Each hip bone is formed by the fusion of three bones: the ischium, the ilium, and the pubis (Fig. 1-12). The pelvis includes the two hip bones, the sacrum, and the coccyx. The pelvis is divided into a greater (false) and a lesser (true) pelvis by an oblique plane passing from the prominence of the sacrum through the pectineal lines and to the superior margin of the pubis. The greater pelvis is the flaring posterior portion above the narrow bony ring called the brim of the pelvis. The greater pelvis is composed of the superior portion of the sacrum and the two ilia. The lesser pelvis lies below the pelvic brim and is composed of the lower portions of the ilia and sacrum and the coccyx, ischia, and pubes. The lesser pelvis has a superior inlet and an outlet, which lie between the tip of the coccyx, the pubes, and the ischial tuberosities. Between the outlet and the inlet is the true pelvic cavity. The measurement of these pelvic areas is important to the physician who must determine whether there is sufficient room for a fetus to pass through the pelvis at birth.

The large upper flaring portion of the hip bone is the ilium. The superior border of the ilium, the iliac crest, ends anteriorly as the anterior superior iliac spine and posteriorly as the posterior superior iliac spine. Beneath both these spines are anterior and posterior inferior iliac spines, respectively. Muscles of the abdominal wall attach to these spines. Beneath the posterior inferior spine is the greater sciatic notch. The inner surface of the ilium is the iliac fossa, where muscles attach, and posterior to the fossa is the iliac tuberosity, at which the sacroiliac ligament attaches. On the outer surface of the ilium are three distinct lines, posterior, anterior,

**LATERAL**

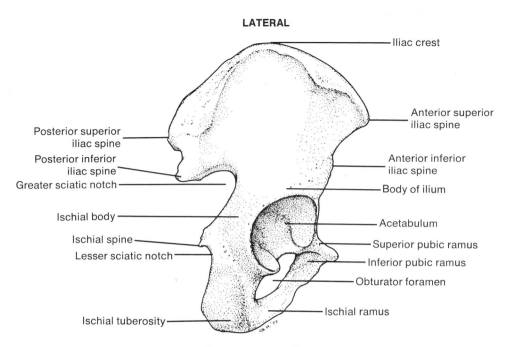

Iliac crest

Posterior superior
iliac spine

Posterior inferior
iliac spine

Greater sciatic notch

Ischial body

Ischial spine

Lesser sciatic notch

Ischial tuberosity

Anterior superior
iliac spine

Anterior inferior
iliac spine

Body of ilium

Acetabulum

Superior pubic ramus

Inferior pubic ramus

Obturator foramen

Ischial ramus

**Fig. 1-12.** Right hip.

and inferior, at which the gluteal muscles attach.

The ischium is the lowest and strongest portion of the hip bone. Posteriorly below the greater sciatic notch is the ischial spine; below this spine is the lesser sciatic notch; and below the notch, the prominent ischial tuberosity. The ramus of the ischium extends forward from the tuberosity and body of the ischium to unite with the pubis.

The pubis consists of a body and two rami, one on each side, that form the anterior portions of the coxae. The bodies unite anteriorly at the symphysis pubis. The rami of the pubis and ischium surround a large obturator foramen. At the point of the lateral fusion of the ilium, ischium, and pubis just above the obturator foramen is the acetabulum. This fusion forms a socket into which the head of the femur fits.

**Lower extremity.** The thigh, or upper portion of the lower extremity, receives its support from the femur (Fig. 1-13). This is the longest, heaviest, and strongest bone of the body and extends from the hip to the tibia. It receives and supports the entire weight of the trunk. It articulates proximally with the acetabulum of the coxal bone and inferiorly with the patella, or kneecap, and the tibia.

The rounded smooth head projects superiorly and medially for articulation with the hip bone. Below the head the constricted neck passes for about 5 cm. This long neck allows free movement of the femur. At the top of the shaft on the posterior as-

pect are a large superolateral greater trochanter and an inferolateral lesser trochanter. These trochanters are the attachment areas of gluteal and some thigh muscles. Between the trochanters are an anterior intertrochanteric line and a posterior intertrochanteric crest. The shaft of the femur bows, directing the distal end more medially. A roughened vertical ridge, the linea aspera femoris, runs down the posterior surface of the shaft.

Distally the shaft broadens into rounded, smooth, medial and lateral condyles, which articulate with the tibia. Above the condyles are roughened medial and lateral epicondyles. The condylar surfaces expand anteriorly in the midline to form an articular surface for the patella. Above the medial epicondyle is the adductor tubercle, and on the posterior surface between the condyles is the intercondylar fossa, which receives the intercondylar eminence of the tibia when it flexes onto the femur.

The patella, or kneecap (Fig. 1-14), is a triangular sesamoid bone found on the anterior aspect of the knee joint embedded in the tendon of the quadriceps femoris muscle. It articulates with the condyles of the femur but not with the tibia. It is held in position by ligaments and muscles and is surrounded by many bursae. The base is broad and located superiorly. The apex points inferiorly.

The tibia, or shinbone (Fig. 1-15), is the larger and more medially placed bone of the leg. It articulates proximally with the femur and fibula and dis-

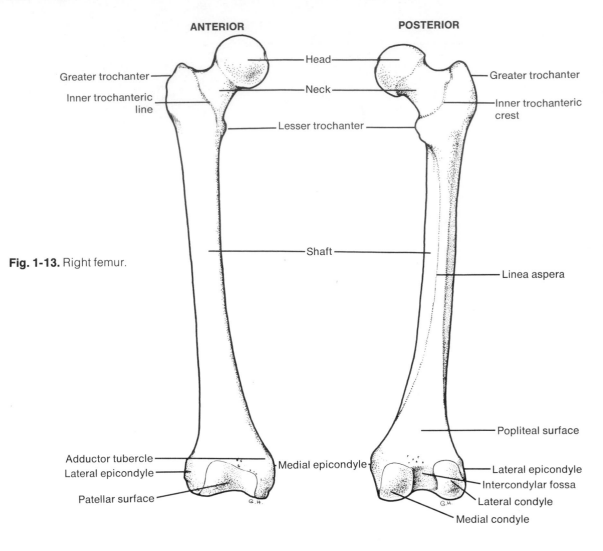

**ANTERIOR**          **POSTERIOR**

Greater trochanter —
Inner trochanteric line —
— Head —
— Neck —
— Greater trochanter
— Inner trochanteric crest
— Lesser trochanter —
— Shaft —

**Fig. 1-13.** Right femur.

— Linea aspera

— Popliteal surface

Adductor tubercle —
Lateral epicondyle —
Patellar surface —
— Medial epicondyle
— Lateral epicondyle
— Intercondylar fossa
— Lateral condyle
— Medial condyle

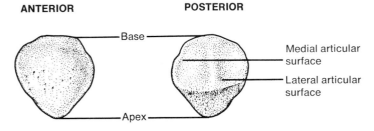

**ANTERIOR**          **POSTERIOR**

— Base —
— Apex —

Medial articular surface
Lateral articular surface

**Fig. 1-14.** Right patella.

tally with the fibula and talus. On the proximal end are smooth, concave, medial and lateral condyles, which articulate with the condyles of the femur. Between the condyles is the intercondylar eminence, which projects upward. Anterior and posterior to the eminence are the intercondylar fossae. On the anterosuperior surface below the condyles is a raised, roughened tibial tuberosity. Below the tuberosity the shaft narrows, and a sharp anterior margin can be felt through the skin. The posterosuperior border has a prominent popliteal line, and below this line the posterior surface of the shaft flattens out. The distal end of the tibia is extended medially as the medial malleolus and notched laterally as the fibular notch for articulation with the fibula.

The fibula (Fig. 1-15) is a long, narrow bone lateral to the tibia. Its proximal expanded head articulates with the tibia. Its distal end extends as the lateral malleolus, which articulates with the talus. The lower medial portion of the fibula also articulates with the fibular notch of the tibia.

The bones of the foot include the tarsals, metatarsals, and phalanges (Fig. 1-16). Of the seven tarsals, or ankle bones, the talus is the most superior. It articulates superiorly with the fibula and tibia and inferiorly with the largest tarsal bone, the calcaneus or heel bone. The Achilles tendon attaches to the

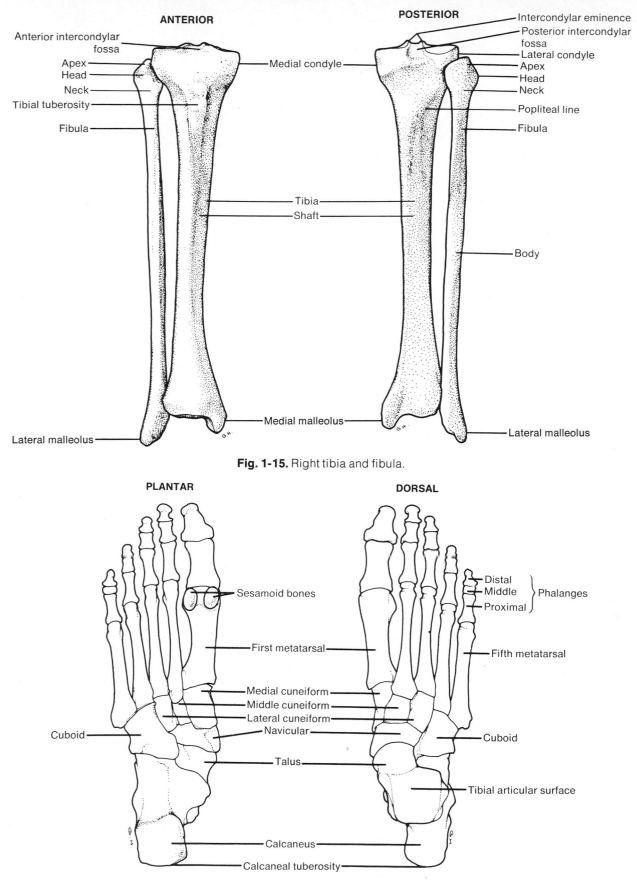

**ANTERIOR**

Anterior intercondylar fossa

Apex
Head
Neck
Tibial tuberosity

Fibula

Medial condyle

Tibia
Shaft

Medial malleolus

Lateral malleolus

**POSTERIOR**

Intercondylar eminence
Posterior intercondylar fossa
Lateral condyle
Apex
Head
Neck
Popliteal line

Fibula

Body

Lateral malleolus

**Fig. 1-15.** Right tibia and fibula.

**PLANTAR**

Sesamoid bones

First metatarsal

Medial cuneiform
Middle cuneiform
Lateral cuneiform
Navicular

Cuboid

Talus

Calcaneus

Calcaneal tuberosity

**DORSAL**

Distal
Middle    } Phalanges
Proximal

Fifth metatarsal

Cuboid

Tibial articular surface

**Fig. 1-16.** Right foot.

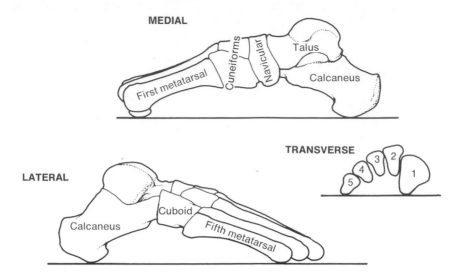

**Fig. 1-17.** Arches of foot.

posterior surface of the calcaneus. The talus receives all the body weight and transmits a large portion of it to the calcaneus and the rest of it to the more anterior tarsals. Anterior to the talus on the medial aspect of the foot is the navicular bone, and anterior to the navicular are the medial, intermediate, and lateral cuneiform bones. Lateral to the cuneiforms and navicular bone and anterior to the calcaneus is the cuboid bone. Tendons and an extensive ligamentous network hold all these bones together.

Anterior to the tarsals are the metatarsal bones, numbered 1 through 5 from the medial to lateral aspect of the foot. The proximal bases of the metatarsals articulate with the cuneiforms and cuboid bone, while the distal heads articulate with the proximal phalanges of each digit. Like the hand, digits 2 through 5 have proximal, middle, and distal phalanges, while the great toe, or digit 1, has only proximal and distal phalanges.

The foot is designed to support weight, and the bones are arranged to form a lengthwise and a crosswise arch (Fig. 1-17). The arches are not rigid but are elastic and springy due to ligaments and tendons that bind the bones together. The longitudinal arch has medial and lateral portions. The calcaneus forms the posterior base of these arches, while the bases of the metatarsals form the anterior base. The medial portion of the longitudinal arch is quite high and consists of the calcaneus rising to the talus, which then descends to the navicular bone, the cuneiforms, and the three medial metatarsals. The lateral portion of the long arch is lower and consists of the calcaneus, cuboid bone, and the two most lateral metatarsals. The transverse arch is formed by the calcaneus, navicular and cuboid bones, cuneiforms, and proximal bases of the metatarsals.

The arches have several functions: to distribute the weight of the body over the entire foot, to provide rigidity and strength to the foot as a lever, to provide a protected space for vessels and nerves of the sole of the foot, and to provide a resilient spring for shock absorption.

The support of the arches is by ligaments, tendons, and muscles. The tendon of the anterior tibial muscle braces and supports the talus from above, while the tendons of the short peroneal and third peroneal muscles insert into the convexity of the tarsal arch and pull it upward. Tendons of the long peroneal and long flexor muscles meet and cross the sole of the foot to form a sling on which the arch rests when the muscles contract. The tendon of the posterior tibial muscle binds together the tarsal bones and keeps them from separating when weight is put on the foot as in walking. The integrity of these arches depends on the shape of the bones, the strength and position of the intrinsic ligaments, and the tone of the leg muscles whose tendons insert into the foot.

The most important ligaments of the arches are: (1) the long plantar ligament, passing from the calcaneus to the cuboid to the lateral three metatarsals, and (2) the "spring," or plantar calcaneonavicular, supporting the head of the talus and passing from the calcaneus to the navicular bone. Flatfoot results if this ligament is torn. It is very elastic and receives support from the tendon of the posterior tibial muscle.

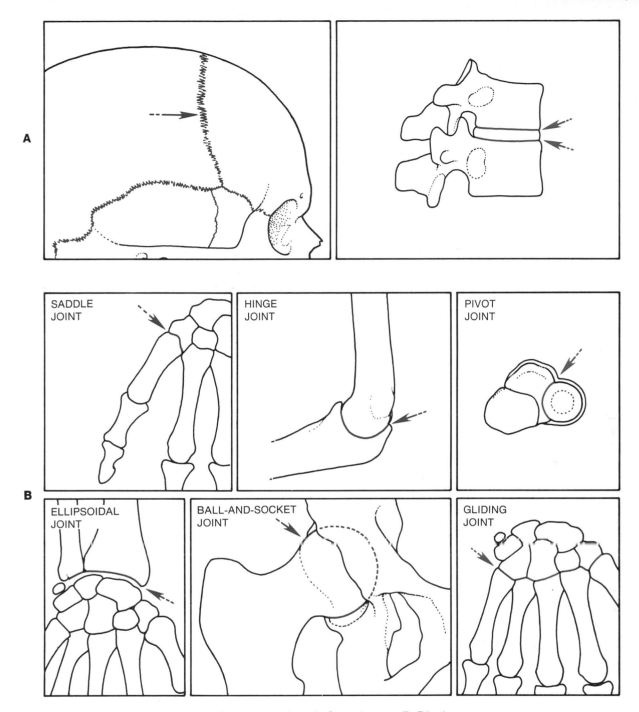

**Fig. 1-18.** Composite joints. **A,** Synarthroses. **B,** Diarthroses.

## ARTICULATION OF JOINTS

A joint is a junction between two or more bones. The classic junction is enclosed by a fibrous joint capsule held together by ligaments and stabilized by tendons. Fibrous bands, or retinaculae, are also found around some joints, giving additional strength.

Joints are classified by the degree of movement allowed at the articulation. *Synarthroses* (Fig. 1-18, *A*) are joints that allow little or no movement. They have no joint cavity, and there is fibrous tissue or bone growth between the articulating surfaces. A fibrous joint, or *syndesmosis*, exists when tissue between the bones is continuous with the perios-

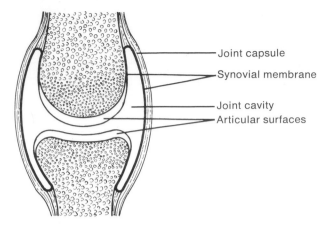

- Joint capsule
- Synovial membrane
- Joint cavity
- Articular surfaces

**Fig. 1-19.** Typical structure of diarthrotic joint.

teum, allowing no movement (e.g., sutures of the skull).

There are two *amphiarthrotic,* or slightly movable, types of joints, both having cartilage between the bones. A *synchondrosis* has hyaline cartilage growing between two articulating surfaces, as seen at the epiphyseal plate between the epiphysis and diaphysis. This cartilage is eventually replaced by bone. A *symphysis* has bone surfaces separated by fibrocartilage, as seen between vertebral bodies and at the pubic symphysis. The fibrocartilage remains throughout life and is not replaced by bone.

*Diarthroses* (Figs. 1-18, *B,* and 1-19) are freely movable joints. They are surrounded by a fibrous joint capsule and lined on all but the articular surfaces with an epithelium called synovium, which secretes a synovial fluid that is rich in mucins, especially hyaluronic acid. In synovial fluid the hyaluronic acid is highly polymerized, accounting for its viscosity and lubricating quality. Many monocytes, macrophages, and other blood leukocytes are found in synovial fluid. Proteins such as albumin and some fats are also found in this fluid. Synovial fluid bathes the joint to reduce friction of the articulating surfaces. The articular surfaces of the bones forming the joint are covered with hyaline articular cartilage. The joint may be divided by an articular disc or meniscus, whose periphery is continuous with the fibrous capsule, while its free surfaces are covered with synovium.

The degree of movement at a synovial joint depends on the shape of the bones forming the joint, the tautness of the ligaments of the capsule, and the position and action of muscles whose tendons cross or enter the joint.

There are six major types of diarthrotic joints:
1. *Hinge,* or *ginglymoid.* In this type of joint one surface is concave and one surface is convex. Movement is generally flexion or extension. Examples are the knee, elbow, and ankle joints.
2. *Pivot,* or *trochoid.* In this joint an articulating surface rotates around a peg or projection, and movement rotates on one axis. Examples include the rotation of the atlas on the axis and the proximal articulation of the radius on the ulna.
3. *Ball-and-socket,* or *endarthrodial.* This joint is the most versatile and has a head that fits into a concave socket. Flexion, extension, and circumduction are the three planes of movement allowed. The hip and shoulder joints are examples.
4. *Gliding,* or *arthrodial.* Both articular surfaces are flat in this joint with no axis of movement. Many of the carpal bones form this type of joint, as do the sacrum and ilium.
5. *Ellipsoidal,* or *condyloid.* In this joint an oval condyle fits into an elliptical cavity. Movement is in two planes that are perpendicular to each other. Extension, flexion, adduction, abduction, and circumduction are allowed, as in the movement of the radius on the carpal bones.
6. *Saddle.* In this joint a saddle-shaped bone fits onto a convex surface of another bone, allowing for the same movements as the condyloid joint but allowing no axial rotation. The articulation of the first metacarpal with the trapezium forms this kind of joint.

## BURSAE

Bursae are small sacs lined with synovial membranes and are found between structures that move against each other, such as between skin and bone, tendon and bone, muscle and bone, and ligament and bone. Bursae reduce friction between these moving parts and act as cushions to relieve pressure. Tendon sheaths are modified bursae that surround long tendons of some muscles such as those of the wrists and ankles. The synovial lined sheaths facilitate tendon movements.

## MAJOR JOINTS
### Shoulder

The shoulder joint (Fig. 1-20, *A*), a ball-and-socket joint, is formed by the articulation of the head of the humerus with the glenoid cavity of the scapula. Extension, flexion, abduction, adduction,

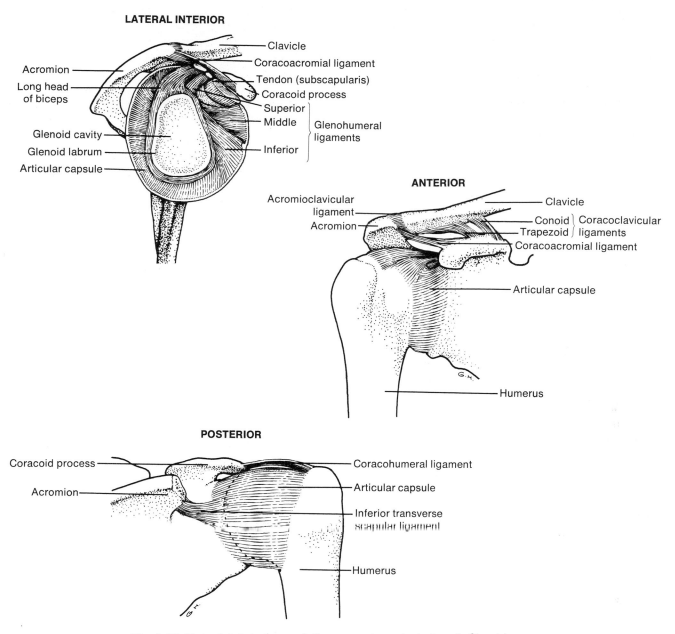

**LATERAL INTERIOR**

- Clavicle
- Coracoacromial ligament
- Acromion
- Tendon (subscapularis)
- Long head of biceps
- Coracoid process
- Superior
- Middle } Glenohumeral ligaments
- Glenoid cavity
- Glenoid labrum
- Inferior
- Articular capsule

**A**

**ANTERIOR**

- Acromioclavicular ligament
- Clavicle
- Acromion
- Conoid } Coracoclavicular ligaments
- Trapezoid
- Coracoacromial ligament
- Articular capsule
- Humerus

**POSTERIOR**

- Coracoid process
- Coracohumeral ligament
- Acromion
- Articular capsule
- Inferior transverse scapular ligament
- Humerus

**Fig. 1-20.** Major joints in terms of disease and surgical sites. **A,** Shoulder.

*Continued.*

and circumduction are allowed at this joint. The joint is heavily covered by muscles and tendons and protected by the corocoid process and acromium of the scapula, the clavicle, and the coracoacromial ligament. A rather loose fibrous capsule allowing free movement surrounds the joint, and a synovial membrane lines the capsule. A shoulder cuff of muscles including the supraspinatus, infraspinatus, teres minor, and subscapularis reinforces the articular capsule. The joint is weak inferiorly in the axillary region, and dislocation often occurs downward.

**Elbow**

The articulations of the humerus with the ulna, the humerus with the radius, and the proximal ends of the radius with the ulna collectively form the elbow joint (Fig. 1-20, *B*). All articulations are surrounded by an articular capsule with a common synovial membrane within. Fat pads are commonly found in the olecranon, radial, and coronoid fossae. A lateral radial collateral ligament and a medial ulnar collateral ligament stabilize the joint. Several bursae are located in close proximity to the joint, but none of them communicate with the synovial cavity. This joint is a common site of synovial inflammation, or synovitis.

### Sacroiliac

The sacroiliac (Fig. 1-20, *C*) transmits body weight to the lower extremity by way of the bony

pelvis. The joint has a fibrous capsule and is lined with synovium. Motion is prevented by strong ligaments that cover the joint capsule.

### Hip

The hip (Fig. 1-20, *D*), a ball-and-socket joint, is formed by the articulation of the head of the femur

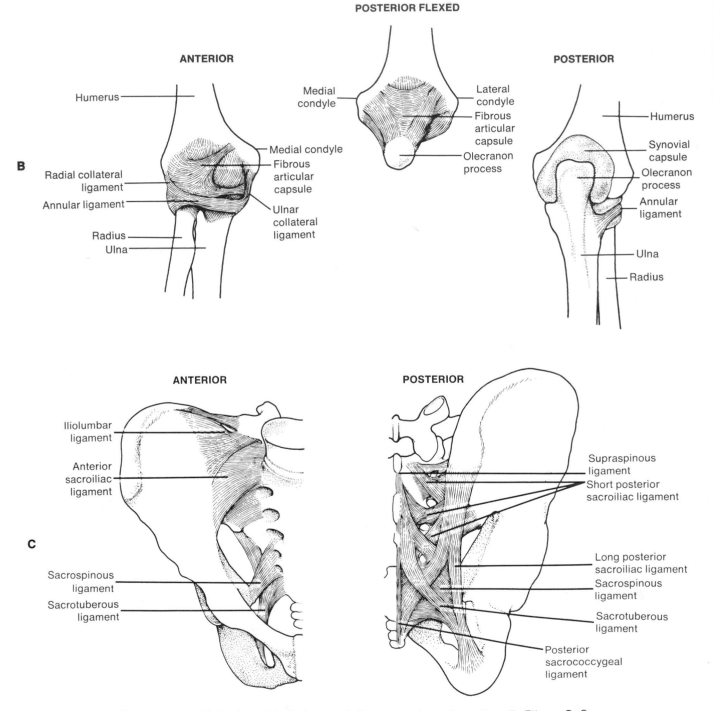

**Fig. 1-20, cont'd.** Major joints in terms of disease and surgical sites. **B,** Elbow. **C,** Sacroiliac.

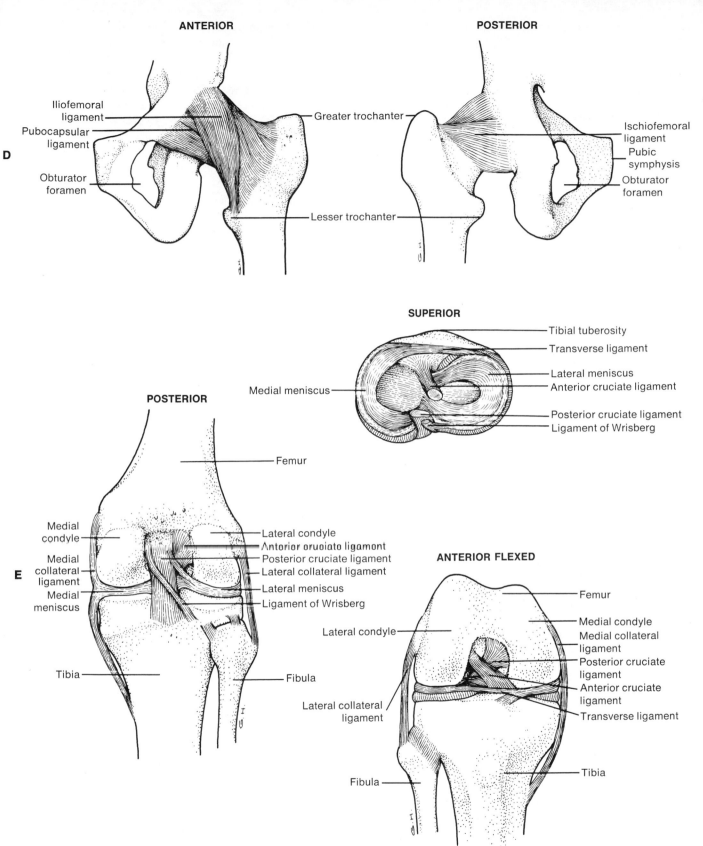

**ANTERIOR**

Iliofemoral ligament

Pubocapsular ligament

**D**

Obturator foramen

Greater trochanter

Lesser trochanter

**POSTERIOR**

Ischiofemoral ligament

Pubic symphysis

Obturator foramen

**SUPERIOR**

Tibial tuberosity

Transverse ligament

Lateral meniscus

Anterior cruciate ligament

Posterior cruciate ligament

Ligament of Wrisberg

Medial meniscus

**POSTERIOR**

Femur

Medial condyle

Medial collateral ligament

Medial meniscus

**E**

Tibia

Lateral condyle

Anterior cruciate ligament

Posterior cruciate ligament

Lateral collateral ligament

Lateral meniscus

Ligament of Wrisberg

Fibula

**ANTERIOR FLEXED**

Femur

Medial condyle

Medial collateral ligament

Posterior cruciate ligament

Anterior cruciate ligament

Transverse ligament

Lateral condyle

Lateral collateral ligament

Fibula

Tibia

**Fig. 1-20, cont'd.** Major joints in terms of disease and surgical sites. **D,** Hip. **E,** Knee.

into the acetabulum of the coxal bone. This stable, strong joint bears weight and allows a great deal of movement. The socket is deep in the anteroposterior direction and is deepened further by a fibrocartilaginous rim, the glenoid labrum. This rim stabilizes the position of the head of the femur. The labrum is incomplete inferiorly but is held together by a transverse ligament. The capsule is strong and thick and extends from the acetabulum to the intertrochanteric line of the femur. The weak points of the capsule are located posteriorly and inferiorly. A Y-shaped iliofemoral ligament strengthens the joint anteriorly and prevents hyperextension. Pubofemoral and ischiofemoral ligaments reinforce the joint anteriorly and posteriorly. The intracapsular ligamentum teres loosely attaches the head of the femur at the fovea to the acetabulum and serves as a channel for vasculature to pass to the head of the femur. Extension, flexion, abduction, adduction, and moderate circumduction are allowed at this joint.

### Knee

The knee joint (Fig. 1-20, *E*) is a typical diarthrotic joint of particular concern to the orthopedic surgeon. Basically it is a hinge joint that allows flexion and extension, but it also allows some glide as the joint approaches complete extension, or the locked position. Muscles, ligaments, and tendons surround the joint. Anteriorly the tendon of the quadriceps femoris covers the joint and attaches to the tibial tuberosity. The patella lies within this tendon and articulates with the femur. Below the patella this tendon is called the patellar tendon, and it prevents hyperflexion of the knee. Posteriorly the two heads of the gastrocnemius arise from the femoral condyles, wrap around from the sides of the femur, and pass posteriorly and inferiorly. The medial tibial collateral ligament, extending from the medial epicondyle of the femur to the medial condyle of the tibia, gives strength to the medial aspect of the joint. Laterally the fibular collateral ligament passes from the lateral femoral epicondyle to the head of the fibula.

Anteroposterior support of the joint is provided by the cruciate ligaments. The anterior cruciate ligament passes from the intercondylar eminence of the tibia to the medial surface of the lateral femoral condyle. The posterior cruciate ligament extends from the posterior portion of the intercondyloid fossa of the tibia to the posterior part of the lateral meniscus and the medial femoral condyle. Both cruciate ligaments lie outside the synovial cavity of the joint.

The knee joint has two articular discs, or menisci, between the articular surfaces of the femur and tibia. These medial and lateral menisci are wedge-shaped crescents of fibrocartilage. Their thick outer edges are attached to the fibrous joint capsule, and their thin inner edges are unattached. The function of the menisci is to provide lateral support to this joint that bears so much weight and is subjected to so much wear and tear.

The inside of the joint capsule is lined with synovial membrane, which secretes synovial fluid. The synovium does not cover the articular hyaline cartilage but does bathe the menisci. The synovial fluid of this joint prevents extreme wear and tear, but often injuries to ligaments or menisci cause an inflammatory response of the synovium (synovitis), causing increased production of synovial fluid.

## DIFFERENCES IN MALE AND FEMALE SKELETONS

The bones found in male skeletons are usually heavier and larger, and the articular ends are thicker than the shafts. The markings on these bones are much more distinct than those of the female.

In the female the pelvis is wider and more shallow with a distinct flaring of the ilia and broadening of the hips. The pelvic inlet is oval in the female and round and narrow in the male. In the female the sacrum is shorter, wider, and less curved, the coccyx is more movable, the ischial spines and tuberosities turn outward, the pubic arch is obtuse, and the ligaments holding the pelvis together are more stretchable than those of the male.

### BIBLIOGRAPHY

Anthony, C. P., and Thibodeau, G. A.: Textbook of anatomy and physiology, ed. 10, St. Louis, 1979, The C. V. Mosby Co.
Goss, C. M., editor: Gray's anatomy, Philadelphia, 1966, Lea & Febiger.
Grant, J. C. B.: Grant's atlas, Baltimore, 1972, The Williams & Wilkins Co.
Greisheimer, E. M., and Wiedeman, M.: Physiology and anatomy, Philadelphia, 1972, J. B. Lippincott Co.
Ham, A. W.: Histology, Philadelphia, 1974, J. B. Lippincott Co.
Pansky, B.: Dynamic anatomy and physiology, New York, 1975, Macmillan, Inc.
Tortora, G. J., and Anagnostakos, N. P.: Principles of anatomy and physiology, San Francisco, 1975, Canfield Press, Harper & Row, Publishers.
Stedman's medical dictionary, ed. 21, Baltimore, 1966, The Williams & Wilkins Co.

# 2

# Muscular and associated neurologic systems

**PAMELA J. MOORE**

Bones and the various joints they form are discussed in Chapter 1. Even though bones and joints form a framework and lever system, they are not capable of movement by themselves. Movement of parts of the body is made possible by the contraction of muscles. Muscle constitutes about half of our body weight and is a very complex type of tissue displaying some specialized characteristics. All muscle tissue is irritable, elastic, extensible, and contractile. Muscle also has some special functions. Muscle tissue is responsible not only for movement of body and limbs but also for passage of blood through vessels, food through the gastrointestinal tract, urine from the kidney to outside of the body, and air in and out of the lungs. Muscle is also responsible for the maintenance of body posture and for the production of heat through chemical reactions within muscle cells.

## CLASSIFICATION OF MUSCLE

There are three kinds of muscle: *skeletal, cardiac,* and *smooth* (Fig. 2-1). These types are classified further by microscopic appearance, location, and nervous control. Microscopically, skeletal muscle has striations, or bands, crossing each fiber at regular intervals; it is located in close apposition to bones and is voluntary because it is under conscious nervous control.

Cardiac muscle composes the heart and a portion of the proximal walls of the great vessels. It also appears striated when viewed with the microscope. It is involuntary because its contractions cannot consciously be controlled.

Smooth muscle has no striations and is found primarily in the walls of viscera and vasculature. Its contractions move materials through hollow organs and control the intrinsic eye muscles. It, too, is involuntary.

## MUSCLE HISTOLOGY

All muscle cells have some basic structures in common. A muscle cell is called a *fiber,* and its cell membrane is known as a *sarcolemma.* The cytoplasm within the cell is known as *sarcoplasm.* All muscle fibers have one or more nuclei, the number depending on the type of muscle. The smooth endoplasmic reticulum of muscle fibers is called sarcoplasmic reticulum. Mitochondria are prominent in muscle fibers. Contractile elements, those proteinaceous units responsible for contraction, differ in their arrangement in the muscle types. Threadlike structures that are about 1 $\mu$m in diameter are found in the sarcoplasm. These are myofibrils and are composed of even smaller units called myofilaments. The thin myofilaments are composed of the protein actin, and the thick myofilaments are composed of the protein myosin. Attached to the actin filaments are other proteins, the troponin-tropomyosin complex. The myosin filaments possess cross bridges of a heavy form of the myosin, meromyosin.

In skeletal muscle the fibers are long (10 to 100 $\mu$m) and cylindrical and are arranged in groups or bundles. The fibers are multinucleated with the nuclei peripherally located. Striations, or the band-

27

ing appearance (Fig. 2-2), are due to a definitive arrangement of myofibrils. The dark bands include thick and thin myofilaments, while the light bands include mainly thin myofilaments. This arrangement of myofilaments is responsible for the contractile capability of skeletal muscle. As seen in Fig. 2-2, *B,* the A band is dark and is composed of thick myosin filaments overlapping the ends of thin actin filaments. The H zone is a small light zone in the middle of the A band composed of myosin alone; no actin extends into this zone. This zone is visible only when the fiber is relaxed. A dark M line may be seen within the H zone. This is caused by an alignment of thickened areas of myosin filaments.

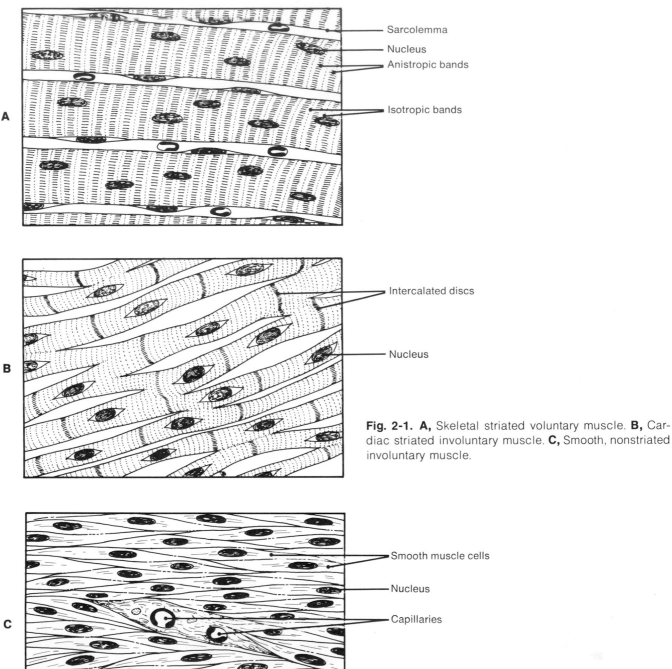

**Fig. 2-1. A,** Skeletal striated voluntary muscle. **B,** Cardiac striated involuntary muscle. **C,** Smooth, nonstriated involuntary muscle.

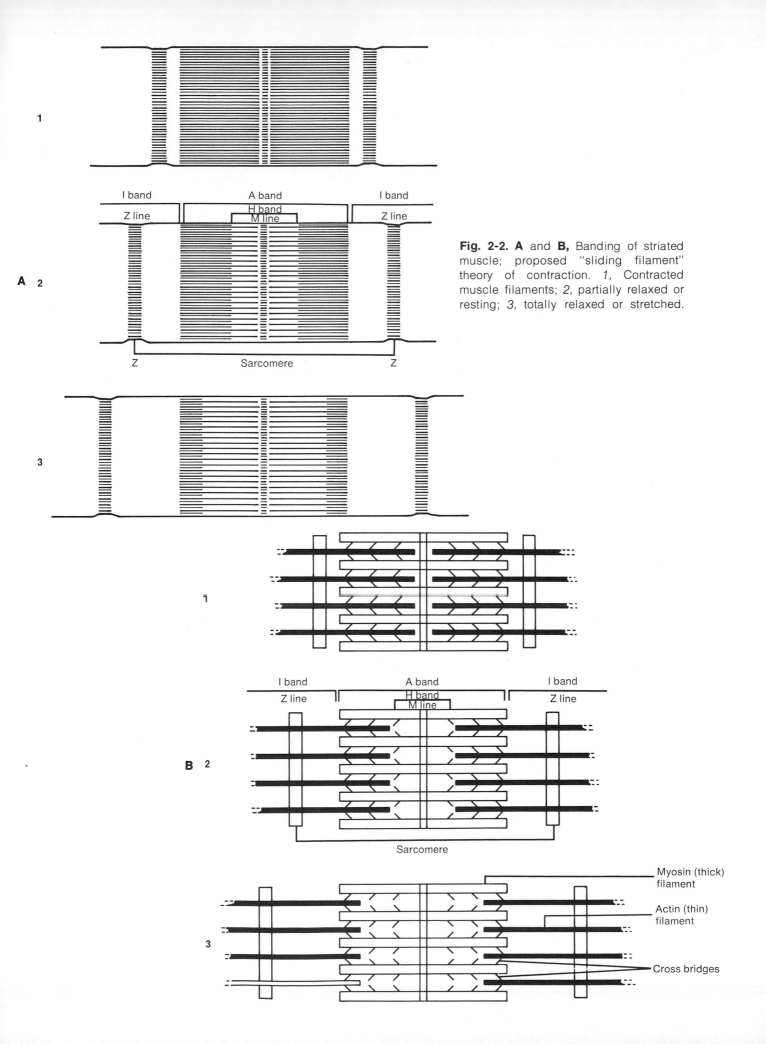

**Fig. 2-2. A** and **B,** Banding of striated muscle; proposed "sliding filament" theory of contraction. *1,* Contracted muscle filaments; *2,* partially relaxed or resting; *3,* totally relaxed or stretched.

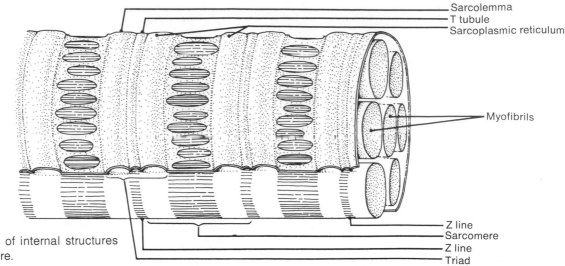

**Fig. 2-3.** Relationship of internal structures to Z lines and sarcomere.

Adjacent to the A band is the light I band. It is composed of thin actin filaments only. A Z line or disc is a thickened area in the middle of the I band.

This interdigitation of the myofilaments into distinct bands allows sliding of the myofilaments onto one another during contraction. The functional contractile unit of muscle is a *sarcomere* and is that area of myofilament that extends from one Z line to the next. Each myofibril has several sarcomeres lining up in registry. Note in Fig. 2-2, *B,* that the A bands are wider than the I bands. These alternating light and dark bands give skeletal and cardiac muscle their striated appearance.

Unique to striated muscle is the T system of tubules, so called because specialized tubules extend transversely from the sarcolemma at the Z lines (Fig. 2-3). These T tubules are in fact invaginations of the sarcolemma.

The sarcoplasmic reticulum also has a unique arrangement in the muscle sarcoplasm. The sarcoplasmic reticulum is separate from the T tubules, but its sacs end blindly at the end of each sarcomere directly adjacent to the Z line with its T tubule. The reticulum sacs extend in a parallel arrangement between the myofilaments. (At the Z line, then, is a triad of tubules composed of a central T tubule with the terminal cisternae of sarcoplasmic reticulum of adjacent sarcomeres on either side of the T tubule.) This close approximation of the tubular system to the myofilaments is important in muscle contraction.

## CONNECTIVE TISSUE COMPONENTS OF MUSCLE

Muscle fibers, bundles of fibers, and whole muscles are held together by connective tissue (Fig. 2-4). Skeletal muscles are held together by extensions of the deep fascia. The epimysium envelops the entire muscle and sends extensions into the muscle that divide it into bundles, or fasciculi. The connective tissue around the fasciculi is the perimysium, and the connective tissue that extends and surrounds each fiber is the endomysium. Skeletal muscles often taper at their ends into fibrous bands of connective tissue called tendons. These tendons attach the muscle to bone. A broad flat tendon is called an aponeurosis.

## MUSCLE SHAPE, SIZE, AND FIBER ARRANGEMENT

The shapes of muscles vary with their function. They may be broad, narrow, long, short, triangular, or irregular. Some are in sheets, while others are in bulky masses. Muscle fibers also vary in arrangement. Fibers may run parallel to each other, may converge to a narrow attachment, or may be curved or arranged obliquely in pennate or bipennate fashion. The strength of a muscle relates directly to the fiber arrangement. The bipennate form permits the strongest contraction.

## VASCULAR SUPPLY

A good vascular supply for muscle is absolutely necessary for good muscle function. Nutrients and oxygen must reach the muscle fibers to provide proper energy for contraction. Proper venous drainage is also necessary for removal of cellular waste. In most instances two veins accompany each artery. Vessels travel to muscle through the connective tissue layers that hold the muscle together. At the endomysium level, vasculature is of capillary size.

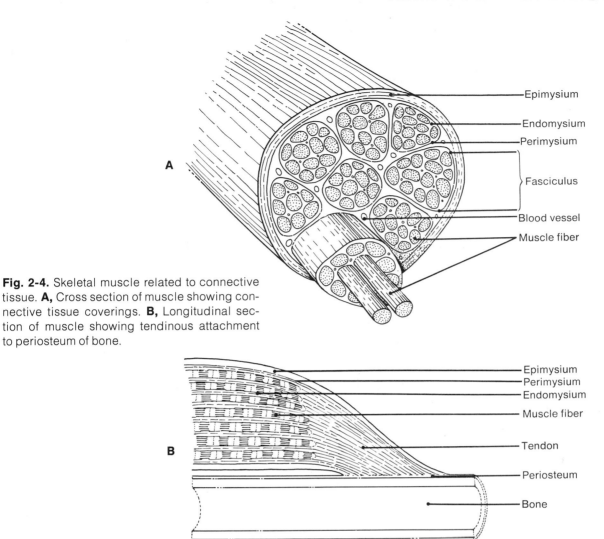

**Fig. 2-4.** Skeletal muscle related to connective tissue. **A,** Cross section of muscle showing connective tissue coverings. **B,** Longitudinal section of muscle showing tendinous attachment to periosteum of bone.

## INNERVATION

Sufficient innervation is also a requirement for muscle action. Nerve cells, or *neurons,* are composed of cell bodies and processes. *Dendrites* are the processes that receive stimuli and transport them to the cell body, while *axons* are the processes that take the stimuli away from the cell body. The cell membrane of a neuron is called the *neurilemma.* Those neurons responsible for sensing stimuli are sensory neurons, and those responsible for eliciting activity are motor neurons.

A nerve is a collection of neuronal processes and does not include the cell bodies of neurons. Nerves usually travel with the vasculature on their way to muscle cells, and each muscle fiber has contact with at least one nerve fiber or axonal process. Innervation to muscle is through spinal or cranial nerves. Fig. 2-5 demonstrates the anatomy of a typical spinal nerve as well as the route of an impulse from the

sensory receptor to the muscular effector. Cranial nerves have a similar structure except that many of their sensory neurons are in ganglia outside the brain and their motor neurons are within the substance of the brain. The association of stimuli of cranial nerves occurs within the brain instead of in the cord, and their divisions also differ from those of the spinal nerves.

There are 31 pairs of spinal nerves, each attached to the cord by anterior (ventral) and posterior (dorsal) roots. The dorsal root has an enlargement called the dorsal root ganglion, which houses the cell bodies of sensory neurons. The dorsal root is composed of the ganglion and, outside the ganglion, the processes of the sensory neurons. The ventral root contains the axonal processes of motor neurons whose cell bodies are located in the ventral gray matter of the spinal cord. The two roots unite at the intervertebral foramen and become a nerve

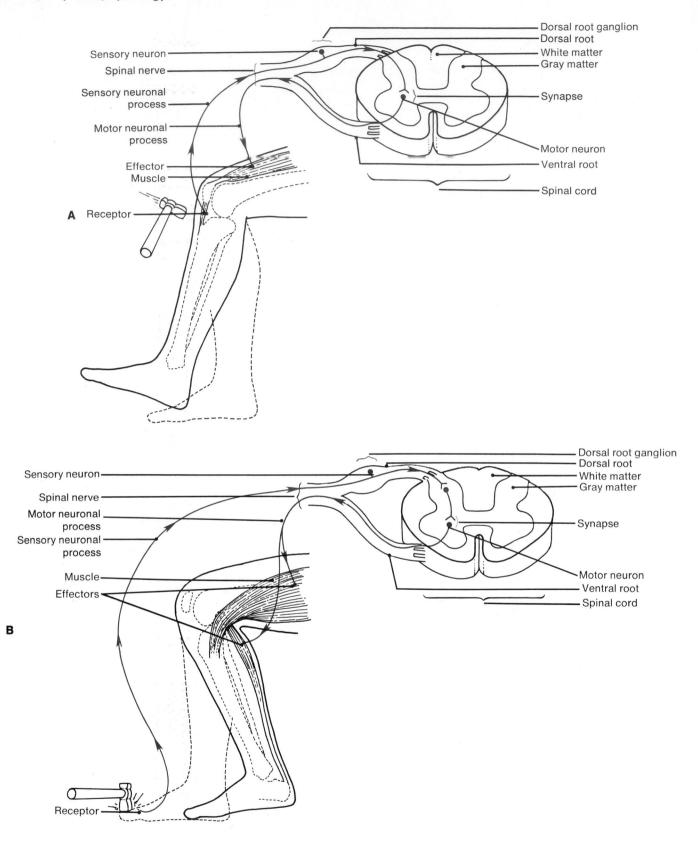

**Fig. 2-5.** Typical spinal nerve reflex arcs. **A,** Monosynaptic. **B,** Bisynaptic. This illustrates sensation at receptor site and passage of impulse along spinal nerve to effector (muscle) site.

carrying sensory and motor fibers. Immediately the nerve divides again into anterior and posterior divisions, the former supplying the anterior part of the body and limbs and the latter supplying the muscles and skin of the back.

The dendritic end of a sensory neuron is called a receptor. The receptor picks up stimuli and transports them to the sensory neuron cell body and on to the axon of the sensory neuron. This axon then passes into the spinal cord and ends there in close approximation to either an association neuron or a motor neuron. (If an association neuron is involved it will receive the impulse and pass it on eventually to a motor neuron.) For simplicity's sake, assume that the sensory axon terminates close to the motor neuron cell body. Motor neurons have very short dendrites, so they are very close to and surround the motor cell body. The sensory axons never quite touch either the dendrite or the cell body of the motor neuron. Instead there is a gap between the two, and the stimulus must cross this gap, or synapse, before it can pass on to the motor neuron. The term *synapsis* means an area of connection. An axon ends in little footlike processes called telodendria, which have small rounded expansions called synaptic knobs. At the electron microscopic level one can see small rounded synaptic vesicles at the inner edges of the synaptic knob. Within the vesicles is a chemical transmitter. The nature of this chemical transmitter is dependent on the location of the synapse in the nervous system. When a nerve impulse reaches these vesicles it causes the vesicles to burst and release the transmitter into the synaptic area. The chemical then makes contact with the next neuron's dendrites or cell body and stimulates the membrane of that neuron to propagate the impulse on down its own membrane.

The motor neuron's axon carries an impulse to the muscle or gland it will innervate; thus the motor neuron is called the effector. The way these neurons effect muscle activity and cause contraction is discussed later. Tables 2-1 and 2-2 of the cranial and spinal nerves clarify the areas innervated by these nerves.

## CONTRACTION OF SKELETAL MUSCLE

Since the contraction of skeletal muscle is easily observed, it is used as a model for discussion of contraction. However, both cardiac and smooth muscle have the same basic requirements and the same basic methods of contractions.

In order for muscle to contract, energy must be present. The energy source for muscle contraction is adenosine triphosphate (ATP). Stimulation of a muscle fiber triggers ATP breakdown, which releases energy by breaking a high-energy phosphate bond and yielding adenosine diphosphate (ADP) and phosphate (P). ATP is usually attached to the actin filaments, but excesses are stored on the myosin filaments. When space on myosin for storage is depleted, the high-energy phosphate bonds can be stored as creatine phosphate (CP). This phosphate store is quite accessible during strenuous activity when energy is needed.

There are, then, two direct sources of energy for muscle contraction:
1. Hydrolysis of ATP:
$$\text{ATP} \xrightarrow{\text{H}_2\text{O}} \text{ADP} + \text{P} + \text{energy}$$
2. Transferral of high-energy phosphate bonds:
$$\text{ADP} + \text{CP} \rightarrow \text{ATP} + \text{creatine}$$

**Table 2-1.** Cranial nerves

| Number | Name | Type | Location | Function |
|---|---|---|---|---|
| I | Olfactory | Sensory | Receptors arise in nasal mucosa; fibers terminate in olfactory bulbs | Sense of smell |
| II | Optic | Sensory | Receptors in retina and terminations in thalamus and midbrain (superior colliculus) | Vision |
| III | Oculomotor | Sensory | Extrinsic eye muscles except superior oblique and lateral rectus; location of cell bodies and termination unknown | Proprioception (muscle sense) |
| | | Motor | Cell bodies in midbrain and terminations in extrinsic eye muscles except superior oblique and lateral rectus; ciliary ganglia to ciliary and iris muscles | Eye movements, regulation of pupil size and accommodation |

*Continued.*

**Table 2-1.** Cranial nerves—cont'd

| Number | Name | Type | Location | Function |
|--------|------|------|----------|----------|
| IV | Trochlear | Sensory | Cell bodies and termination unknown; receptors in superior oblique | Proprioception |
| | | Motor | Cell bodies in midbrain; terminations in superior oblique muscle of eye | Eye movement |
| V | Trigeminal | Sensory | Receptors in skin, teeth and head; cell bodies in gasserian ganglion; terminations in pons | Sensation to head and face; muscle sense |
| | | Motor | Cell bodies in pons; terminations in muscles of mastication | Chewing |
| VI | Abducens | Sensory | Cell body location unknown; receptors in lateral rectus muscle of eye | Proprioception |
| | | Motor | Cell bodies in pons; termination in lateral rectus muscle of eye | Abduction of eye |
| VII | Facial | Sensory | Receptors in taste buds of anterior two thirds of tongue; cell bodies in geniculate ganglion | Taste |
| | | Motor | Cell bodies in pons; terminations in muscles of facial expression | Facial expression |
| VIII | Acoustic | | | |
| | Vestibular division | Sensory | Receptors in utricle, saccule, and semicircular canals; cell bodies in vestibular ganglion; terminations in pons and medulla | Equilibrium |
| | Cochlear division | Sensory | Receptors in organ of Corti in cochlear duct; cell bodies in spiral ganglion; terminations in pons and medulla | Hearing |
| IX | Glossopharyngeal | Sensory | Receptors in pharynx and taste buds of posterior third of tongue and carotid sinus and body; cell bodies in jugular and petrous ganglia; terminations in medulla | Taste and tongue sensations; reflex control of blood pressure and respiration |
| | | Motor | Cell bodies in medulla; terminations in muscles of pharynx and otic ganglion and on to parotid gland | Swallowing; saliva secretion |
| X | Vagus | Sensory | Receptors in larynx, pharynx, carotid body, thoracic and abdominal viscera; cell bodies in jugular and nodose ganglia; terminations in medulla and pons | Sensations of organs supplied |
| | | Motor | Cell bodies in medulla; termination in vagal ganglia in muscles of larynx, pharynx, thoracic and abdominal viscera | Movement of organs supplied; peristalsis; slows heart |
| XI | Spinal accessory | Sensory | Cell source unknown | Proprioception |
| | | Motor | Cell bodies in medulla; terminations in thoracic and abdominal viscera, pharynx, and larynx | Shoulder movements; head turning; visceral movement; voice production |
| XII | Hypoglossal | Sensory | Cell source unknown | Proprioception |
| | | Motor | Cell bodies in medulla; terminations in tongue muscles | Tongue movements |

**Table 2-2.** Plexuses of spinal nerves

| Spinal nerves | Plexus formed | Terminal branches of plexus | Parts of body supplied |
|---|---|---|---|
| $C_1$ $C_2$ $C_3$ $C_4$ | Cervical plexus | Lesser occipital ($C_2$)<br>Great auricular ($C_{2,3}$)<br>Transverse cervical ($C_{2,3}$)<br>Supraclavicular ($C_{3,4}$)<br>Phrenic ($C_{3-5}$) | Motor fibers to muscles and sensory fibers to skin of head, neck, and upper part of shoulders; motor fibers to diaphragm |
| $C_5$ $C_6$ $C_7$ $C_8$ $T_1$ | Brachial plexus | Musculocutaneous ($C_{5-7}$) | Motor fibers to anterior arm muscles and sensory fibers to skin of lateral forearm |
| | | Median ($C_{6-8}$, $T_1$) | Motor fibers to most of anterior muscles of forearm and some in palm; sensory fibers to skin on radial half of palm |
| | | Ulnar ($C_8$, $T_1$) | Motor fibers to anteromedial muscles of palm and sensory fibers to skin of ulnar side of hand |
| | | Radial ($C_{5-8}$, $T_1$) | Motor fibers to muscles on posterior aspect of arm and forearm and sensory fibers to skin of same regions and posterior surface of hand |
| $T_2$ $T_3$ $T_4$ $T_5$ $T_6$ $T_7$ $T_8$ $T_9$ $T_{10}$ $T_{11}$ $T_{12}$ | Anterior branches of these spinal nerves do not form a plexus but remain separate and travel between ribs as intercostal nerves | | Motor fibers to intercostal muscles and abdominal wall muscles and sensory fibers to skin overlying these muscles |
| $L_1$ $L_2$ $L_3$ $L_4$ | Lumbar plexus | Iliohypogastric ($T_{12}$, $L_1$) | Sensory fibers to anterior abdominal wall |
| | | Ilioinguinal ($L_1$) | Sensory fibers to anterior abdominal wall and external genitalia and motor fibers to muscles of anterior abdominal wall |
| | | Lateral femoral cutaneous ($L_{2,3}$) | Sensory fibers to lateral aspect of thigh |
| | | Femoral ($L_{2-4}$) | Motor fibers to muscles on anterior and lateral aspects of thigh and sensory fibers from skin on anteromedial aspects of thigh |
| | | Obturator ($L_{2-4}$) | Motor to anteromedial muscles of thigh |
| $L_4$ $L_5$ $S_1$ $S_2$ $S_3$ | Sacral plexus | Sciatic (two branches)<br>  Tibial ($L_{4,5}$, $S_{1-3}$) | Motor fibers to posterior muscles of thigh and muscles of calf of leg and sensory fibers to skin of calf and sole of foot |
| | | Common peroneal ($L_{4,5}$, $S_{1,2}$) | Motor fibers to dorsiflexor and evertor foot muscles and sensory fibers to top of foot |
| | | Superior and inferior gluteal ($L_{4,5}$, $S_1$ and $L_5$, $S_{1,2}$) | Motor fibers to gluteal muscles and tensor fascia latae |
| | | Posterior femoral cutaneous ($S_{1-3}$) | Sensory fibers to skin of buttocks, posterior thigh, and leg |
| | | Pudendal ($S_{2-4}$) | Motor fibers to muscles of anus and external genitalia; sensory fibers to skin around anus, scrotum, and labia majora |
| $S_4$ $S_5$ Coccygeal | Coccygeal plexus | Coccygeal nerve | Sensory fibers to skin in region of coccyx |

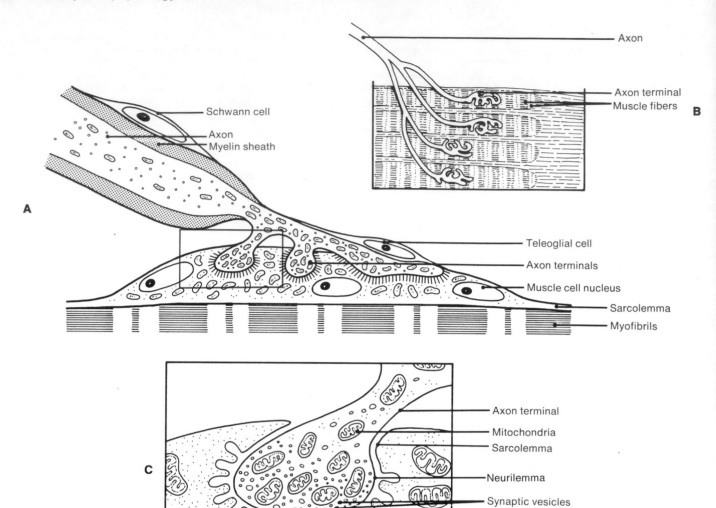

**Fig. 2-6.** Diagram of motor end-plate at light and electron microscopic levels. **A,** Motor end-plate on long axis of muscle fiber. **B,** Surface view of multiple end-plates from one nerve innervating several muscle fibers. **C,** High resolution of rectangle in **A.**

Ultimately energy for ATP and CP is from the catabolism of foodstuffs.

In order for muscle contraction to occur a stimulus must be applied to the muscle to provoke a contraction. The stimulus travels to muscle fibers through the axon of a neuron. As mentioned, the neurons that transmit impulses to muscle fibers are called motor neurons because they provoke movement. Many axons from many motor neurons travel together in a nerve, and when the nerve reaches the muscle the axons branch, and these branches make contact with individual muscle fibers. This area of contact is a myoneural junction or motor end-plate (Fig. 2-6) or neuromuscular junction.

## Myoneural junction

A myoneural junction is a specialized area for the transmission of a nerve impulse to a muscle fiber. In this area a naked nerve ending is applied to the muscle sarcolemma. The nerve cell membrane, or neurilemma, is called the presynaptic membrane, and the muscle cell membrane, or sarcolemma, is called the postsynaptic membrane. The area or gap between the axon and muscle cell is called a synapse, just as was the gap between two nerve cells. As with the neuronal-neuronal synapse, the axonal terminal is also in the form of synaptic knobs. These knobs sit in a cleft with sarcolemma folding around them. Synaptic vesicles filled with the neurotransmitter acetylcholine are in the knobs, and the acetylcholine is released into the synaptic cleft when a nerve impulse reaches them. This chemical affects receptor sites on the postsynaptic membrane and changes the membrane permeability at these receptor sites and thereby propagates or reestablishes the impulse or stimulus on the postsynaptic membrane.

## Strength of contraction

A sufficient number of impulses is needed for contraction; in other words, an "all or none" principle applies. There must be enough impulses to cause total contraction, or there will be no contraction at all. When there is sufficient stimulus to cause contraction, the threshold, or liminal level of contraction, has been reached. If the stimulus is too weak to provoke a contraction, it is subliminal, or subthreshold.

The strength of muscle contraction is dependent on several factors:
1. Initial length of muscle fibers
2. Metabolic condition of muscle fibers
3. Number of fibers activated and intensity and frequency of activation
4. Size of load put on the muscle; to a certain extent, the heavier the load the stronger the contraction

The strength of a contraction depends on the number of motor units involved; therefore there is a direct relationship between the amount of innervation of a muscle and the amount of force it can expend. The force of contraction also depends on the frequency of the nerve impulses. It should be noted that the fewer muscle fibers controlled by one axon, the more precise the movement of that muscle will be. Motor units also work alternately so that they do not get fatigued. The tension of a muscle also depends on the frequency of impulses and the number of motor units involved.

Muscle contraction requires energy and nerve impulses. The following discussion demonstrates how these two mechanisms work together.

## Molecular basis of contraction

The stimulus for muscle contraction is in the form of electrical energy or impulse, and this impulse travels along the neuron to the myoneural junction where it causes the release of the neurotransmitter and thereby reestablishes the stimulus on the muscle membrane. The stimulus then travels along the muscle membrane and spreads along the T tubules into the sarcoplasm. The T tubules then send an action message to the sarcoplasmic reticulum effecting the release of calcium from the sarcoplasmic re-

ticulum. The calcium ions ($Ca^{++}$) then combine with troponin on the actin filaments. Without calcium, troponin and tropomyosin form a complex within the actin filament that prohibits actin and myosin interaction. However, when calcium interacts with troponin this inhibition is negated, and actin and myosin now become attracted to each other.

This attraction of actin to myosin and then the movement of the actin filaments is known as the *sliding filament theory* (Fig. 2-2). With this attraction the thin actin filaments slide toward the center of the sarcomere and thereby obliterate the H zone. The attraction of actin is to the heavy, cross bridge portion of myosin known as meromyosin. At the time of the attraction there is a simultaneous release of energy at the cross bridges. The cross bridges rotate, facilitating the sliding of the filaments on each other. Pulling the actin filaments in from the ends of the sarcomere thickens the sarcomere and appears to thicken the Z line. This filament attraction and movement is the essence of muscle contraction. In relaxation the sarcomere returns to its resting length, and the filaments return to their original position. Relaxation occurs when there are no longer sufficient impulses to maintain the release of calcium into the sarcoplasm and its attachment to the actin.

## Impulse conduction

Both nerve and muscle fibers display the property of irritability. They both respond to stimuli, and the stimuli are conducted by neurons to muscle cells through an action potential (impulse) across a synapse at the myoneural junction. Nerve and muscle impulses revolve around one basic principle: the passive and active transport of ions across the cell membranes, particularly sodium ($Na^+$) and potassium ($K^+$).

Muscle cells rest when they are not receiving stimuli, but even at rest ions are being transported back and forth across the cell membrane. Ion concentrations on either side of the membrane are responsible for the membrane's ability to transmit an impulse. Sodium is not easily diffusible across a cell membrane, so it must be actively transported out of a cell by a sodium pump if it does diffuse in. Potassium diffuses easily, but a potassium pump also works to keep $K^+$ concentration inside the cell higher than outside. There are naturally many negative ions inside the cell. Generally a resting cell has more positive ions outside the cell (mainly $Na^+$) and more negative ions inside the cell. This charge difference on either side of a membrane is referred to as *resting potential;* and the membrane is considered to be polarized.

Following is a step-by-step synopsis of the movement of an impulse from a neuron and on to the muscle fiber and how this impulse travels down a membrane[2,p.187]:

1. A stimulus moves down a neuron.
2. Acetylcholine is released at the synapse.
3. Acetycholine affects receptor sites of the postsynaptic membrane, and if the stimulus is sufficient there is a change in the permeability of the polarized muscle cell membrane.
4. $Na^+$ diffuses into the muscle cell at the point of stimulation.
5. $K^+$ permeability stays the same.
6. As $Na^+$ moves in, the difference of electrical charge across the membrane decreases toward zero.
7. At zero the membrane is depolarized.
8. $Na^+$ continues to go into the cell and a membrane potential develops, but this time the inside is positive and the outside is negative at the stimulated area.
9. An action potential (impulse) is initiated once all these events occur.
10. The negatively charged point on the outside of the membrane sends out an electrical charge to the positive area next to it (still polarized).
11. This local current acts as a stimulus and causes the adjacent point to change its potential in the same way, that is, positive to negative.
12. Therefore the impulse is propagated on down the muscle cell membrane by a point-by-point electrical current.
13. As an impulse travels from one point on the membrane to the adjacent point, the previous point repolarizes and its resting potential is reestablished.
14. This is accomplished by another change in membrane permeability. The membrane now becomes permeable to $K^+$ and impermeable to $Na^+$. $K^+$ moves out of the cell and makes the outer surface more positive than the inner surface.
15. Recovery or restoration of ions to original position occurs by means of the $Na^+$ pump.
16. Resting potential is achieved again.

### Types of muscle contraction

Contraction of skeletal muscle may be of several types. The following listing is similar to that of Anthony and Thibodeau[1]:

1. An *isometric* contraction occurs when the ends of a muscle remain fixed; thus activity is noted by an increase in tension without a change in length. No movement is produced.
2. In *isotonic* muscle contraction one end of the muscle is attached to a light weight, which is lifted when the muscle shortens. Tension within the muscle remains the same, but the length changes.
3. A *twitch* is a momentary, spasmodic contraction of a muscle in response to a single stimulus. Twitches rarely occur in the body. For experimental purposes it can be demonstrated that a muscle's response to a stimulus is not immediate; there is a latent period after the stimulus is applied before contraction occurs. The contraction is then followed by relaxation.
4. *Tetanic* (tonic) contractions are longer lasting than twitches. They are produced by many successive impulses stimulating the muscle without relaxation between stimuli. They produce tautness in muscle fiber but not movement (e.g., maintenance of posture).
5. *Treppe* is a type of contraction in which a skeletal muscle contracts more forcefully after it has contracted several times. This phenomenon is used by athletes in warming-up exercises.
6. *Fibrillation* is an unusual type of contraction in which individual muscle fibers contract asynchronously. It is a sustained twitching of individual muscle fibers.
7. *Convulsions* are violent involuntary tetanic contractions of groups of muscles.

### ACTION OF SKELETAL MUSCLES

Skeletal muscles produce movement by pulling on bones and muscles that move a part but do not usually lie over that part. When speaking of muscle attachments, the bone attachment that remains stationary is the origin of the muscle, and the bone of attachment that moves is the insertion.

Skeletal muscles act in groups and not singly. A muscle that causes a desired action is known as a prime mover. With the contraction of a prime mover such as the biceps of the upper extremity, there is relaxation of a muscle with the opposite action, the antagonist, in this case the triceps. Muscles that assist the prime mover by having similar actions and facilitating the action of the prime mover are called synergists.

Muscles are named by several criteria such as location, origin, insertion, size, and shape. They are

*Text continued on p. 61.*

**Table 2-3.** Major muscles of the body

| Muscle | Origin | Insertion | Action | Innervation |
|---|---|---|---|---|
| **Muscles of facial expression** (Fig. 2-7) | | | | |
| Epicranius (scalp muscle) | | | | All facial muscles innervated by branches of facial nerve (VII) |
| Frontalis | Aponeurosis (galea aponeurotica) | Muscles of skin and eyebrows | Draws scalp and eyebrows upward; wrinkles forehead | |
| Occipitalis | Occipital bone | Galea aponeurotica | Draws scalp backward | |
| Orbicularis oculi (eye sphincter) | | | Generally closes eye tightly; wrinkles forehead vertically; draws lid medially | |
| Pars orbitalis | Medial palpebral ligament and medial wall of orbit | Near origin | Gives "crows feet" laterally with age | |
| Pars palpebralis (eyelids) | Medial palpebral ligament | Lateral palpebral ligament | Closes lids in blinking and sleeping; gentle closure | |
| Pars lacrimalis (behind lacrimal sac) | Posterior ridge of lacrimal bone | Joins palpebral portion | Keeps lids close to eyeball; causes squinting reaction, e.g., to light and wind | |
| Corrugator supercilii | Medial end of superciliary arch | Deep surface of skin above orbital arch | Draws eyebrows downward and medially; produces vertical wrinkles of forehead and frown | |
| Orbicularis oris (mouth sphincter) | Muscles surrounding mouth | Skin at lip rim and corners of mouth | Closes, purses, opens, inverts, and everts lips; shapes lips for speech | |
| Levator labii superioris | Lower margin of orbit; maxilla below infra-orbital foramen; some fibers from zygomatic bone | Orbicularis oris of upper lip | Elevates upper lip | |
| Levator labii superioris alaeque nasi | Frontal process of maxilla | Greater alar cartilage and skin of nose and orbicularis oris at corners of mouth | Raises angle of mouth; dilates nares | |
| Levator anguli oris | Canine fossa of maxilla | Muscles of lower lip at angle of mouth | Pulls down corners of mouth | |
| Zygomaticus minor | Malar surface of zygomatic bone | Muscles of upper lip (orbicularis oris) | Draws lip up and out | |
| Zygomaticus major | Zygomatic bone | Muscles at angle of mouth | Draws angle of mouth upward and backward as in laughing | |
| Risorius | Fascia of masseter muscle; passes superficial to platysma | Muscles and skin at corners of mouth | Retracts angle of mouth causing dimple or grin | |

Continued.

**Table 2-3.** Major muscles of the body—cont'd

| Muscle | Origin | Insertion | Action | Innervation |
|---|---|---|---|---|
| **Muscles of facial expression—cont'd** | | | | |
| Depressor labii inferioris | Oblique line or lower border of mandible | Skin of lower lip and orbicularis oris | Depresses lower lip | |
| Depressor anguli oris | Oblique line or lower border of mandible | Muscle at angle of mouth | Depresses angle of mouth | |
| Mentalis | Incisive fossa of mandible | Skin of chin | Raises and protrudes lower lip; wrinkles skin of chin as in pouting | |
| Buccinator | Outer surfaces of alveolar processes of maxilla above and mandible below | Orbicularis oris at angle of mouth | Compresses cheek; accessory muscle of mastication; retracts angle of mouth | |
| Procerus | Fascia over lower part of nasal bone and upper lateral nasal cartilage | Skin between eyebrows and frontalis muscle | Draws down medial angle of eyebrows causing transverse wrinkles on bridge of nose | |
| Nasalis | Maxilla below ala of nose | Lower margin of ala of nose and lower nasal septum | Dilates nasal aperture; lowers and compresses ala of nose | |
| Depressor septi | Incisive fossa of maxilla | Septum and back part of ala of nose | Draws ala downward, constricting aperture of nares | |
| Auricularis (anterior, posterior, superior) | Fascia in temporal region | Into auricle | Moves ear anteriorly, posteriorly, and inferiorly | |
| Platysma | Fascia over superior part of pectoralis major and deltoid muscles | Fascia of face, lower jaw, and corners of mouth | Wrinkles skin of neck and upper chest | |
| **Muscles of soft palate** | | | | |
| Levator veli palatini | Apex of petrous portion of temporal bone and medial lamina of auditory tube cartilage | Aponeurosis of soft palate | Raises soft palate | The tensor veli palatini is supplied by a branch of the trigeminal nerve (V); the other muscles of this group are supplied by the bulbar portion of accessory nerve (XI) through the pharyngeal plexus |
| Tensor veli palatini | Scaphoid fossa of medial pterygoid plate and cartilage of lateral wall of auditory tube | Aponeurosis of soft palate and posterior border of hard palate | Stretches soft palate | |
| Uvulae | Posterior nasal spine of palatine bones and palatine aponeurosis | Uvula | Shortens and raises uvula | |

2 Ocean Point
APT 207
Revere ma

| Muscle | Origin | Insertion | Action | Nerve supply |
|---|---|---|---|---|
| Palatoglossus | Anterior surface of soft palate | Side of tongue | Elevates and retracts tongue; draws soft palate inferiorly | |
| Palatopharyngeus | Soft palate | Posterior border of thyroid cartilage and aponeurosis of pharynx | Assists in elevation of larynx and pharynx; narrows fauces and shuts off nasopharynx | |
| **Muscles of tongue** *Extrinsic muscles* | | | | |
| Genioglossus (paired) | Superior mental spine of mandible | Undersurface of tongue | Depresses center of tongue; protrudes tongue; draws tongue tip back and down | All muscles of this group innervated by hypoglossal nerve (XII) except palatoglossus, which is innervated by spinal accessory nerve (XI) |
| Hyoglossus (paired) | Side of body and greater cornu of hyoid bone | Side of tongue | Retracts, flattens, and draws down sides of tongue | |
| Chondroglossus (paired) | Medial side and base of lesser cornu of hyoid | Side of tongue | Retracts tongue | |
| Styloglossus (paired) | Anterior and lateral surfaces of the styloid process of the temporal bone | Side and undersurface of tongue | Retracts and elevates entire tongue | |
| Palatoglossus (paired) | Anterior surface of soft palate | Side of tongue | Elevates and retracts tongue and draws soft palate inferiorly | |
| *Intrinsic muscles* Longitudinalis (superior and inferior), transversus, and verticalis linguae | | | Alters shape of tongue | |
| **Muscles of mastication** (Fig. 2-8) Temporalis | Temporal fossa and temporal fascia | Medial surface and anterior border of ramus and apex of coronoid process of mandible | Closes and retracts jaw | All innervated by mandibular division of trigeminal nerve (V) |
| Masseter | Zygomatic process of maxilla and inferior border of zygomatic arch | Superior half of ramus and lateral surface of coronoid process of mandible | Closes and protrudes jaw | |

*Continued.*

**Table 2-3.** Major muscles of the body—cont'd

| Muscle | Origin | Insertion | Action | Innervation |
|---|---|---|---|---|
| **Muscles of mastication—cont'd** | | | | |
| Pterygoideus medialis (internal) | Medial surface of lateral pterygoid plate, pyramidal surface of palatine bone, and tuberosity of maxilla | Inferior and posterior part of medial surface of ramus and angle of mandibular foramen | Raises mandible; closes jaw | |
| Pterygoideus lateralis (external) | Lateral surface of great wing of sphenoid and inferior and lateral surface of lateral pterygoid plate | Neck of condyle of mandible and articular disc of temperomandibular articulation | Opens jaw; protrudes jaw; moves mandible from side to side | |
| **Muscles of neck** | | | | |
| Sternocleido-mastoideus | By two heads from ventral surface of manubrium sterni and supero anterior surface of medial third of clavicle | Lateral surface of mastoid process | Each bends cervical vertebrae laterally, pulling head to shoulder of same side and rotates head pointing chin to opposite side; together they flex head, bringing chin to chest | Spinal accessory (XI) |
| **Suprahyoid** | | | | |
| Digastricus Anterior belly | Inner side of inferior border of mandible | Common tendon to greater cornu of hyoid bone | Draws hyoid bone forward; assists in opening jaw | Mylohyoid nerve off inferior alveolar branch of mandibular division of trigeminal nerve (V) |
| Posterior belly | Mastoid notch of temporal bone | Common tendon to greater cornu of hyoid bone | Draws hyoid bone upward and backward; assists in opening jaw | Branch of facial nerve (VII) |
| Stylohyoideus | Posterior and lateral surface of styloid process | Body of hyoid bone | Draws hyoid bone superiorly and posteriorly | Branch of facial nerve (VII) |
| Mylohyoideus | Whole length of mylohyoid line of mandible | Body of hyoid bone and median raphe separating bilateral muscles | Raises hyoid bone and tongue | Mylohyoid nerve off inferior alveolar branch of mandibular division of trigeminal nerve (V) |
| Geniohyoideus | Inferior mental spine | Anterior surface of body of hyoid bone | Draws hyoid bone and tongue anteriorly | Branch of first cervical nerve through hypoglossal nerve |

| Muscle | Origin | Insertion | Action | Nerve supply |
|---|---|---|---|---|
| **Infrahyoid (strap muscles)** | | | | |
| Sternohyoideus | Posterior surface of medial end of clavicle and manubrium sterni | Inferior border of body of hyoid bone | Draws hyoid bone inferiorly | Branch of ansa cervicalis (fibers from $C_1$ to $C_3$) |
| Sternothyroideus | Dorsal surface of manubrium, edge of cartilage of first rib | Lamina of thyroid cartilage | Draws thyroid cartilage caudally | Branch of ansa cervicalis (fibers of nerves $C_1$ to $C_3$ |
| Thyrohyoideus | Lamina of thyroid cartilage | Inferior border of greater cornu of hyoid bone | Draws hyoid bone inferiorly and thyroid cartilage superiorly | Fibers from nerves $C_1$ and $C_2$ through hypoglossal nerve |
| Omohyoideus | Central tendon from cranial border of scapula into inferior belly | By superior belly into hyoid bone | Draws hyoid bone caudally | Ansa cervicalis ($C_1$ to $C_3$) |
| **Anterior vertebral** | | | | |
| Longus colli | | | | |
| Superior oblique portion | Transverse processes of C-3 to C-5 vertebrae | Tubercle of anterior arch of atlas | Flexes neck and slightly rotates cervical vertebral column | Branches of nerves $C_2$ to $C_7$ |
| Inferior oblique portion | Bodies of T-1 to T-3 vertebrae | Transverse processes of C-5 and C-6 vertebrae | Same as superior oblique portion | |
| Vertical portion | Bodies of C-6 to C-8 and T-1 to T-3 vertebrae | Bodies of C-2 to C-4 vertebrae | Same as superior oblique portion | |
| Longus capitis | Transverse processes of C-3 to C-6 vertebrae | Superior surface of occipital bone | Flexes head | Branches of nerves $C_1$ to $C_3$ |
| Rectus capitis anterior | Lateral mass of atlas | Inferior surface of basilar part of occipital bone anterior to foramen magnum | Flexes head | Branch of loop between nerves $C_1$ and $C_2$ |
| Rectus capitis lateralis | Superior surface of transverse process of atlas | Inferior surface of jugular process of occipital bone | Bends head laterally | Branch of loop between nerves $C_1$ and $C_2$ |
| **Lateral vertebral** | | | | |
| Scalenus anterior | Transverse processes of C-3 to C-6 vertebrae | Scalene tubercle of first rib | Raises first rib; bends and rotates neck | Branches of lower cervical nerves |
| Scalenus medius | Transverse processes of C-3 to C-8 vertebrae | Cranial surface of first rib | Raises first rib; bends and rotates neck slightly | Branches of lower cervical nerves |
| Scalenus posterior | Transverse processes of last two or three cervical vertebrae | Outer surface of second rib | Raises second rib; bends and rotates neck slightly | Ventral primary division of last three cervical nerves |

*Continued.*

**Table 2-3.** Major muscles of the body—cont'd

| Muscle | Origin | Insertion | Action | Innervation |
|---|---|---|---|---|
| ***Pharyngeal*** | | | | |
| Constrictor pharyngeus inferior | Oblique line on lamina of thyroid cartilage | Fibrous raphe at posterior median line of pharynx | Narrows lower pharynx in swallowing | Pharyngeal plexus, external laryngeal, and recurrent laryngeal |
| Constrictor pharyngeus medius | Superior border of greater cornu of hyoid bone, lesser cornu, and stylohyoid ligament | Fibrous raphe at posterior median line of pharynx | Narrows pharynx in swallowing | Pharyngeal plexus |
| Constrictor pharyngeus superior | Medial pterygoid plate and hamulus, alveolar process of mandible | Median raphe and pharyngeal spine of basilar part of occipital bone | Narrows pharynx | Pharyngeal plexus |
| Stylopharyngeus | Styloid process | Constrictor muscles and posterior border of thyroid cartilage | Draws pharynx up and laterally | Glossopharyngeal nerve (IX) |
| Salpingopharyngeus | Inferior part of auditory tube | Palatopharyngeus | Draws lateral walls of pharynx upward and inward | Pharyngeal plexus |
| Palatopharyngeus | Soft palate | Posterior border of thyroid cartilage and sponeurosis of pharynx | Elevates pharynx and larynx | Pharyngeal plexus |
| ***Laryngeal (intrinsic)*** | | | | |
| Cricothyroideus | Front and lateral part of cricoid cartilage | Inferior cornu and lamina of thyroid cartilage | Produces tension and elongation of vocal folds by drawing cricoid cartilage upward and backward | Vagus (X) via superior laryngeal nerve; external laryngeal |
| Cricoarytenoideus posterior | Posterior surface of cricoid cartilage | Muscular process of arytenoid cartilage | Opens glottis | Recurrent laryngeal |
| Cricoarytenoideus lateralis | Cranial border of cricoid cartilage | Front of muscular process of arytenoid cartilage | Closes glottis | Recurrent laryngeal |
| Arytenoideus | Posterior and lateral surface of one arytenoid cartilage | Corresponding part of opposite cartilage | Closes glottis | Recurrent laryngeal |
| Thyroarytenoideus | Caudal half of thyroid cartilage and middle cricothyroid ligament | Base and anterior surface of arytenoid cartilage | Shortens and relaxes vocal cords | Recurrent laryngeal |

**Muscles of thorax** (Fig. 2-9)

| Muscle | Origin | Insertion | Action | Nerve |
|---|---|---|---|---|
| External intercostals (11) | Caudal border of rib | Cranial border of rib below | Draws ribs together; lifts ribs, increasing volume of thoracic cavity | Intercostal nerves $(T_1-T_{11})$ |
| Internal intercostals (11) | Ridge on inner surface of rib and costal cartilage | Cranial border of rib below | Draws adjacent ribs together; with quadratus lumborum lowers rib to decrease volume of thoracic cavity | Intercostal nerves $(T_1-T_{11})$ |
| Subcostals | Inner surface of rib near its angle | Inner surface of second or third rib below | See internal intercostals | Intercostal nerves |
| Transversus thoracis | Caudal third of inner surface of body of sternum, dorsal surface of xiphoid process, and sternal ends of costal cartilages of last three or four true ribs | Caudal borders of costal cartilages of ribs 2 through 6 | Draws ventral portion of ribs caudally, decreasing thoracic cavity | Branches of intercostal nerves |
| Levatores costarum | Ends of transverse processes of C-7 and T-2 to T-12 | Outer surface of rib caudal to vertebra from which it takes origin | Raises ribs; extends vertebral column, bends it laterally, and rotates it slightly toward opposite side | Branches of intercostal nerves |
| Serratus posterior superior | Ligamentum nuchae, spinous processes of C-7 and T-1 to T-2 or T-3 vertebrae | Cranial borders of ribs 2 through 5 | Raises ribs | Branches of ventral primary divisions of nerves $T_1$ to $T_4$ |
| Serratus posterior inferior | Spinous processes of T-10 to T-12 and L-1 to L-3 vertebrae | Inferior borders of last four ribs | Draws ribs to which it is attached outward and downward | Branches of ventral primary divisions of nerves $T_9$ to $T_{12}$ |
| Diaphragm | Circumference of thoracic inlet, xiphoid process, cartilage of last six ribs, lumbar vertebrae through crura | Central tendon | Draws central tendon downward increasing volume and decreasing pressure in thoracic cavity and decreasing volume and increasing pressure in abdomen | Phrenic nerve from cervical plexus; fibers from nerves $C_3$ to $C_5$ |

*Continued.*

**Table 2-3.** Major muscles of the body—cont'd

### Muscles of upper member
### Muscles that connect upper member to vertebral column (Fig. 2-10, A)

| Muscle | Origin | Insertion | Action | Innervation |
|---|---|---|---|---|
| Trapezius | External occipital protuberance, nuchal line and ligament, spinous processes of C-7 vertebra and all thoracic vertebrae | Posterior border of lateral third of clavicle, medial acromium | Rotates scapula, raises point of shoulder in full abduction and flexion of arms; adducts scapula; upper part draws scapula cranially and lower part draws it downward; one side draws head to same side and turns face to opposite side; together both sides draw head backward | Spinal accessory and ventral branches of nerves $C_3$ and $C_4$ |
| Latissimus dorsi | Lumbar aponeurosis, T-7 to T-12 and spinous processes of lumbar and sacral vertebrae, posterior part of iliac crest | Anterior surface of upper part of humerus, intertubercular groove | Extends, adducts, and rotates arm medially; draws shoulder backward and downward | Thoracodorsal nerves ($C_6$ to $C_8$) |
| Rhomboideus major | Spinous processes of T-2 to T-5 vertebrae and supraspinal ligament | Vertebral border of scapula at root of scapular spine | With rhomboideus minor, adducts scapula, drawing it up and medially to depress tip and rotating it | Dorsal scapular nerve off brachial plexus ($C_5$) |
| Rhomboideus minor | Inferior part of ligamentum nuchae and spinous processes of C-7 and T-1 vertebrae | Vertebral border of scapula at base of root of scapular spine above insertion of rhomboideus major | | Same as major |
| Levator scapulae | Transverse processes of atlas, axis, C-3 and C-4 vertebrae | Vertebral border of scapula between superior angle and root of scapular spine, above insertion of rhomboid muscles | Raises scapula and pulls it medially and rotates it to lower lateral angle | Branches of nerves $C_3$ and $C_4$ |

### Muscles that connect upper member to anterior and lateral thoracic walls (Fig. 2-10, B)

| Muscle | Origin | Insertion | Action | Innervation |
|---|---|---|---|---|
| Pectoralis major | Medial half of clavicle, ventral surface of sternum, cartilages of true ribs (2 to 6 especially), aponeurosis of external oblique | Crest of greater tubercle of humerus | Flexes, adducts, and rotates arm medially | Medial and lateral pectoral nerves from brachial plexus ($C_5$ to $C_8$ and $T_1$) |

| Muscle | Origin | Insertion | Action | Nerve supply |
|---|---|---|---|---|
| Pectoralis minor | Cranial margins and outer surfaces of ribs 3 to 5 near their cartilages | Medial border and superior surface of coracoid process of scapula | Pulls scapula ventrally and caudally rotates it to lower lateral angle | Medial pectoral nerves ($C_8$, $T_1$) |
| Subclavius | First rib and its cartilage | Inferior surface of clavicle | Draws shoulder ventrally and caudally | Nerve from lateral trunk of brachial plexus containing fifth and sixth cervical fibers |
| Serratus anterior | Outer surfaces of first eight or nine ribs and aponeuroses of intervening intercostal muscles | Vertebral border of scapula | Rotates scapula to raise tip of shoulder | Long thoracic nerves from brachial plexus ($C_5$ to $C_7$) |

## Muscles of shoulder (Fig. 2-11)

| Muscle | Origin | Insertion | Action | Nerve supply |
|---|---|---|---|---|
| Deltoid | Anterior border and superior surface of lateral third of clavicle, superior surface of acromium, posterior border of scapular spine | Deltoid prominence of humerus | Abducts arm; clavicular portion flexes arm; spinous portion extends arm; ventral portion rotates arm medially; dorsal portion rotates arm laterally | Axillary nerves of brachial plexus ($C_5$, $C_6$) |
| Subscapularis | Axillary border of scapula; subscapular fossa | Lesser tubercle of humerus and ventral capsule of joint | Rotates arm medially; draws humerus toward glenoid fossa giving strength to joint | Upper and lower subscapular nerves of brachial plexus ($C_5$, $C_6$) |
| Supraspinatus | Supraspinatus fossa | Greater tubercle of humerus | Abducts arm; weak lateral rotator and flexor | Branches of suprascapular nerve of brachial plexus ($C_5$) |
| Infraspinatus | Infraspinatus fossa | Greater tubercle of humerus | Rotates arm laterally | Suprascapular nerves of brachial plexus ($C_5$, $C_6$) |
| Teres minor | Dorsal surface of cranial two thirds of axillary border of scapula | Greater tubercle of humerus | Rotates arm laterally and weakly adducts it | Branch of axillary nerve ($C_5$) |
| Teres major | Dorsal surface of inferior angle of scapula | Crest of lesser tubercle of humerus | Adducts, extends, and rotates arm medially | Branch of lower subscapular nerve of brachial plexus ($C_5$, $C_6$) |

## Muscles of arm (Fig. 2-12)

| Muscle | Origin | Insertion | Action | Nerve supply |
|---|---|---|---|---|
| Coracobrachialis | Apex of corocoid process | Middle of medial surface and border of body of humerus | Flexes and adducts arm | Branch of musculocutaneous nerves ($C_6$, $C_7$) |

*Continued.*

**Table 2-3.** Major muscles of the body—cont'd

| Muscle | Origin | Insertion | Action | Innervation |
|---|---|---|---|---|
| **Muscles of arm—cont'd** | | | | |
| Biceps brachii | | | | |
| Short head | Corocoid process | Posterior portion of radial tuberosity | Flexes arm, flexes forearm, supinates hand | Branch of musculocutaneous nerves (C$_5$, C$_6$) |
| Long head | Supraglenoid tuberosity | | | |
| Brachialis | Distal half of anterior aspect of humerus | Tuberosity of ulna | Flexes forearm | Branch of musculocutaneous nerves (C$_5$, C$_6$) |
| Triceps brachii | | Posterior portion of olecranon process | Extends forearm; long head extends and adducts arm | Branch of radial nerves (C$_7$, C$_8$) |
| Long head | Infraglenoid tuberosity of scapula | | | |
| Lateral head | Posterior surface of body of humerus | | | |
| Medial head | Posterior surface of body of humerus | | | |
| **Muscles of forearm (palmar aspect)** (Fig. 2-13, A) | | | | |
| *Superficial* | | | | |
| Pronator teres | | | | |
| Humeral head | Proximal to medial epicondyle | Middle of lateral surface of body of radius | Pronates hand | Branch of median nerve (C$_6$, C$_7$) |
| Ulnar head | Medial side of coronoid process | | | |
| Flexor carpi radialis | Medial epicondyle of humerus | Base of second metacarpal | Flexes hand and helps abduct it | Branch of median nerve (C$_6$, C$_7$) |
| Palmaris longus | Medial epicondyle of humerus | Flexor retinaculum, palmar aponeurosis | Flexes hand | Branch of median nerve (C$_6$, C$_7$) |
| Flexor carpi ulnaris | | | | |
| Humeral head | Medial epicondyle of humerus | Pisiform bone, hamate and fifth metacarpal bones | Flexes and adducts hand | Branch of ulnar nerve (C$_8$, T$_1$) |
| Ulnar head | Medial margin of olecranon, posterior border of ulna | | | |
| Flexor digitorum superficialis | | | | |
| Humeral head | Medial epicondyle of humerus | Four split tendons passing on either side of profundus tendons into sides of second phalanx of each finger | Flexes second phalanx of each finger; flexes first phalanx and hand | Branches of median nerves (C$_7$, C$_8$, T$_1$) |
| Ulnar head | Medial coronoid process | | | |
| Radial head | Oblique line and middle third of lateral border of radius | | | |

*Deep*

| Muscle | Origin | Insertion | Action | Nerve |
|---|---|---|---|---|
| Flexor digitorum profundus | Proximal three fourths of volar and medial surfaces of body of ulna, coronoid process, dorsal border of ulna | Base of last phalanges | Flexes terminal phalanx of each finger; flexes other phalanges and to some extent the hand | Branches of median and ulnar nerve ($C_8$, $T_1$) |
| Flexor pollicis longus | Body of radius, interosseous membrane, coronoid process | Base of distal phalanx of thumb | Flexes second phalanx of thumb; flexes first phalanx; flexes and adducts metacarpals | Branch of palmar interosseous nerve of median nerve ($C_8$, $T_1$) |
| Pronator quadratus | Pronator ridge of ulna; distal fourth of ulna | Distal fourth of lateral border of radius | Pronates hand | Branch of palmar interosseous nerve of median ($C_8$, $T_1$) |

### Muscles of forearm (dorsal aspect) (Fig. 2-13, B)

*Superficial*

| Muscle | Origin | Insertion | Action | Nerve |
|---|---|---|---|---|
| Brachioradialis | Supracondylar ridge of humerus | Lateral side of base of radial styloid process | Flexes forearm | Branch of radial nerve ($C_5$, $C_6$) |
| Extensor carpi radialis longus | Distal third of lateral supracondylar ridge of humerus | Dorsal surface of base of second metacarpal on radial side | Extends and abducts hand | Branch of radial nerve ($C_6$, $C_7$) |
| Extensor carpi radialis brevis | Lateral epicondyle of humerus | Dorsal surface of base of third metacarpal on radial side | Extends and may abduct hand | Branch of radial nerve ($C_6$, $C_7$) |
| Extensor digitorum | Lateral epicondyle of humerus | Second and third phalanges of fingers | Extends phalanges and wrist | Branch of deep radial nerve ($C_6$ to $C_8$) |
| Extensor digiti minimi | Extensor tendon from intermuscular septum | Expansion of extensor digitorum tendon on dorsum of first phalanx of little finger | Extends little finger | Branch of deep radial nerve ($C_6$ to $C_8$) |
| Extensor carpi ulnaris | Lateral epicondyle of humerus | Tubercle on ulnar side of base of fifth metacarpal | Extends and adducts hand | Branch of deep radial nerve ($C_6$ to $C_8$) |
| Anconeus | Lateral epicondyle of humerus | Side of olecranon and body of ulna | Extends forearm | Branch of radial nerve ($C_7$, $C_8$) |

*Deep*

| Muscle | Origin | Insertion | Action | Nerve |
|---|---|---|---|---|
| Supinator | Lateral epicondyle of humerus | Lateral edge of radial tuberosity and oblique line of radius; dorsal and lateral surfaces of body of radius | Supinates hand | Branch of deep radial nerve ($C_6$) |
| Abductor pollicis longus | Lateral part of dorsal surface of body of ulna; dorsal surface of radius | Radial side of first metacarpal bone; slip to trapezium | Abducts thumb and wrist | Branch of deep radial nerve ($C_6$, $C_7$) |
| Extensor pollicis brevis | Dorsal surface of body of radius | Base of first phalanx of thumb | Extends first phalanx of thumb; abducts hand | Branch of deep radial nerve ($C_6$, $C_7$) |

*Continued.*

**Table 2-3.** Major muscles of the body—cont'd

| Muscle | Origin | Insertion | Action | Innervation |
|---|---|---|---|---|
| **Muscles of forearm (dorsal aspect)—cont'd** | | | | |
| Extensor pollicis longus | Lateral part of middle third of dorsal surface of body of ulna | Base of last phalanx of thumb | Extends second phalanx of thumb; abducts hand | Branch of deep radial nerve ($C_6$ to $C_8$) |
| Extensor indicis | Dorsal surface of body of ulna | Joins ulnar side of extensor digitorum tendon to index finger | Extends and partially adducts index finger | Branch of deep radial nerve ($C_6$ to $C_8$) |
| **Muscles of hand** | | | | |
| *Thenar* | | | | |
| Abductor pollicis brevis | Scaphoid tuberosity, transverse carpal ligament, trapezium | Radial side of base of first phalanx of thumb | Abducts thumb | Branch of median nerve ($C_6$, $C_7$) |
| Opponens pollicis | Trapezium and flexor retinaculum | Whole length of metacarpal of thumb on radial side | Abducts, flexes, rotates metacarpal of thumb | Branch of median nerve ($C_6$, $C_7$) |
| Flexor pollicis brevis Superficial portion | Trapezium | Radial side of base of proximal phalanx of thumb | Flexes and adducts thumb | Branch of median nerve ($C_6$, $C_7$) |
| Deep portion | Ulnar side of first metacarpal bone | Ulnar side of base of first phalanx | | Nerve from deep branch of ulnar nerve ($C_8$, $T_1$) |
| Adductor pollicis Oblique head | Capitate bone; bases of second and third metacarpals | Ulnar side of base of proximal phalanx of thumb; sesamoid bone in tendon | Adducts thumb; brings thumb toward palm | Branches of deep palmar branch of ulnar nerve ($C_8$, $T_1$) |
| Transverse head | Distal two thirds of palmar surface of third metacarpal | Ulnar side of base of first phalanx of thumb | | |
| *Hypothenar* | | | | |
| Palmaris brevis | Transverse carpal ligament; palmar aponeurosis | Skin on ulnar portion of hand | Draws skin on ulnar side of hand toward palm | Branch of ulnar nerve ($C_8$) |
| Abductor digiti minimi | Pisiform bone | Ulnar side of base of first phalanx of little finger | Abducts little finger and flexes proximal phalanx | Branch of ulnar nerve ($C_8$, $T_1$) |
| Flexor digiti minimi brevis | Hamulus of hamate bone | Ulnar side of base of first phalanx of little finger | Flexes little finger | Branch of ulnar nerve ($C_8$, $T_1$) |
| Opponens digiti minimi | Hamulus of hamate bone | Metacarpal bone of little finger on ulnar margin | Abducts, flexes, and rotates fifth metacarpal | Branch of ulnar nerve ($C_8$, $T_1$) |
| *Intermediate* | | | | |
| Lumbricalis manus First and second | Radial side and palmar surface of flexor tendons of index and middle fingers, respectively | Extensor expansion of each finger | Flexes metacarpophalangeal joints and extends two distal phalanges | First and second: digital branches of median ($C_6$, $C_7$) |

| Muscle | Origin | Insertion | Action | Nerve supply |
|---|---|---|---|---|
| Third | | Adjacent sides of tendons of middle and ring fingers | | Third and fourth: branches of deep palmar branch of ulnar ($C_8$) |
| Fourth | | Adjacent sides of tendons of ring and little fingers | | |
| **Interossei palmares (3)** | | | | |
| First | Ulnar side of second metacarpal | Ulnar side of index finger | Adducts fingers toward axis of middle finger and flexes first phalanx | Branches of deep palmar of ulnar ($C_8$, $T_1$) |
| Second and third | Radial side of fourth and fifth metacarpals | Radial side of ring and little fingers | | Branches of deep palmar of ulnar ($C_8$, $T_1$) |
| **Interossei dorsales manus (4)** | By two heads, each from the shafts of adjacent metacarpal bones | First phalanges and extensor expansion; first and second on radial side of index and middle finger; third and fourth on ulnar side of same fingers | Abducts all four fingers from axis of middle finger and flexes first phalanx | |
| **Muscles of abdomen** (Fig. 2-14) *Anterolateral* | | | | |
| External oblique | Inferior borders of lower eight ribs | Outer lip of iliac crest and linea alba | Compresses abdomen; together flex vertebral column laterally and rotate it | Branches of eighth to twelfth intercostals, iliohypogastric, and ilioinguinal nerves |
| Internal oblique | Iliac fascia, iliac crest, lumbar aponeurosis | Inferior borders of cartilages of last three or four ribs, linea alba | Same as external oblique | See external oblique |
| Cremaster | Internal oblique | Tubercle and crest of pubis and sheath of rectus abdominis | Draws testis up toward superficial inguinal ring | Genital branch of genitofemoral nerve |
| Transversus abdominis | Inner lip of iliac crest, thoracolumbar fascia, cartilages of last six ribs | Linea alba | Constricts abdomen | Branches of seventh to twelfth intercostal, iliohypogastric and ilioinguinal nerves |
| Rectus abdominis | Crest of pubis and ventral surface of symphysis pubis | Cartilages of fifth to seventh ribs | Flexes vertebral column, tenses anterior abdominal wall, compresses abdominal contents | Branches of seventh to twelfth intercostal nerves |
| Pyramidalis | Ventral surface of pubis and anterior pubis ligament | Linea alba | Tenses linea alba | Branch of nerve $T_{12}$ |

*Continued.*

**Table 2-3.** Major muscles of the body—cont'd

| Muscle | Origin | Insertion | Action | Innervation |
|---|---|---|---|---|
| **Muscles of abdomen—cont'd** | | | | |
| ***Posterior*** | | | | |
| Psoas major | Included with muscles of lower limb | | | |
| Psoas minor | | | | |
| Iliacus | | | | |
| Quadratus lumborum | | | | |
| **Muscles of pelvis** (Fig. 2-15) | | | | |
| Levator ani | Inner surface of superior ramus of pubis lateral to the symphysis; inner surface of ischial spine | Side of last two segments of coccyx, anococcygeal raphe, sphincter ani externis | Supports and slightly raises pelvic floor | Branches of pudendal plexus, fibers of nerves $S_4$ and sometimes $S_3$ and $S_5$ |
| Coccygeus | Spine of ischium and sarcospinous ligament | Margin of coccyx and side of last piece of sacrum | Draws coccyx ventrally | Branches of pudendal plexus containing fibers of nerves $S_4$ and $S_5$ |
| Obturator internus | Included with muscles of gluteal region | | | |
| Piriformis | | | | |
| **Muscles of perineum** | | | | |
| ***Urogenital muscles of male*** | | | | |
| *Superficial* | | | | |
| Transversus perinei superficialis | Inner and anterior part of ischial tuberosity | Central tendinous point of perineum | Simultaneous contraction of two fixes central tendinous point of perineum | Perineal branch of pudendal nerve |
| Bulbospongiosus (bulbocavernosus) | Central tendinous point of perineum and its ventral extension into median raphe | Encircles corpus spongiosum penis and joins fibers of other side and into body of corpus cavernosum penis | Serves to empty canal of urethra after bladder has expelled its contents; aids in erection of penis | Perineal branch of pudendal nerve |
| Ischiocavernosus | Inner surface of ishial tuberosity and from rami of ishium and pubis | Sides and undersurface of crura as they become body of penis | Compresses crus penis; retards return of blood through veins and maintains erect penis | Perineal branch of pudendal nerve |

| Muscle | Origin | Insertion | Action | Nerve |
|---|---|---|---|---|
| *Deep* | | | | |
| Transversus perinei profundus | Inferior rami of ischium | Tendinous raphe with its fellow of opposite side | Acts as sphincter, compressing membranous portion of urethra | Perineal branch of pudendal nerve |
| Sphincter urethrae | Junction of inferior rami of pubis and ischium and fascia of area | See transversus perinei profundus | See transversus perinei profundus | Perineal branch of pudendal nerve |
| ***Urogenital muscles of female*** | | | | |
| Transversus perinei superficialis | Inner ventral part of ischial tuberosity | Central tendinous point of perineum | Simultaneous contractions of two fixes central point of perineum | Perineal branch of pudendal nerve |
| Bulbocavernosus (bulbospongiosis) | Surrounds vaginal orifice; covers lateral parts of vestibular bulbs and attaches posteriorly to central tendinous point of perineum | Corpora cavernosus clitoridis | Diminishes orifice of vagina | Perineal branch of pudendal nerve |
| Ischiocavernosus | Inner surface of ischial tuberosity | Sides and undersurface of crus clitoridis | Compresses crus clitoridis; retards return of blood through veins, serving to maintain organ erect | Perineal branch of pudendal nerve |
| Transversus perinei profundus | Inferior rami of ischium | Sides of vagina | Compresses membranous portion of urethra | Perineal branch of pudendal nerve |
| Sphincter urethrae | Margin of inferior ramus of pubis | Muscle fibers on opposite side | See transversus perinei profundus | Perineal branch of pudendal nerve |
| **Muscles of back** (Fig. 2-16) | | | | |
| **Deep** | | | | |
| Splenius capitis | Spinous processes of C-7, T-1 to T-4; ligamentum nuchae | Occipital bone at superior nuchal line and mastoid process | Draws head and neck dorsally and laterally and rotates them; two sides together extend head and neck | Lateral branches of dorsal primary division of middle and lower cervical nerves |
| Splenius cervicis | Spinous processes of T-3 to T-6 | Posterior tubercles of transverse processes of C-1 to C-3 | See splenius capitis | See splenius capitis |
| Erector spinae Iliocostalis l. lumborum | Sacrospinalis tendon from middle crest of sacrum, spinous processes of lumbar and T-11 to T-12 vertebrae and sacrospinal ligament, posterior iliac crest | Inferior borders of angles of last six or seven ribs | Extends vertebral column and bends it to one side; draws ribs caudally | |

*Continued.*

**Table 2-3.** Major muscles of the body—cont'd

| Muscle | Origin | Insertion | Action | Innervation |
|---|---|---|---|---|
| **Muscles of back—cont'd** *Deep—cont'd* | | | | |
| I. thoracis | Upper borders of angles of lower six ribs | Cranial borders of angles of first six ribs and transverse process of C-7 vertebra | See I. lumborum | |
| I. cervicis | Angles of ribs 3 to 6 | Transverse processes of C4 to C-6 vertebrae | Extends vertebral column and bends it to one side | |
| Longissimus | | | | |
| L. thoracis | Continuation of sacrospinalis | Transverse processes of lumbar and thoracic vertebrae and processes of lower nine or ten ribs | Extends vertebral column and bends it to one side; draws ribs caudally | Branches of primary division of spinal nerves |
| L. cervicis | Transverse processes of T-4 to T-5 vertebrae | Transverse processes of C-2 to C-6 vertebrae | See L. thoracis | See L. thoracis |
| L. capitis | Transverse processes of upper T-4 to T-5 vertebrae and articular processes of C-5 to C-6 vertebrae | Posterior margin of mastoid process | Extends head; muscle on one side bends head to same side and rotates it | Branches of dorsal primary divisions of middle and lower cervical nerves |
| Spinalis | | | | |
| S. thoracis | Spinous processes of T-11 to T-12 and L-1 to L-2 | Spinous processes of T-4 to T-8 vertebrae | Extends vertebral column | Branches of dorsal primary divisions of spinal nerves |
| S. cervicis | Ligamentum nuchae, spinous process of C-7 vertebrae | Spinous process of axis | See S. thoracis | See S. thoracis |
| S. capitis | Inseparable from semispinalis capitis (see below) | | | |
| Semispinalis | | | | |
| S. thoracis | Transverse processes of T-6 to T-10 vertebrae | Spinous processes of T-1 to T-4 and C-7 to C-8 vertebrae | Extends vertebral column and rotates it toward opposite side | See S. thoracis |
| S. cervicis | Transverse processes of T-1 to T-5 or T-6 vertebrae | Cervical spinous processes from axis to C-5 vertebra | See S. thoracis | See S. thoracis |
| S. capitis | Transverse processes of T-1 to T-6 or T-7 and C-7 | Between superior and inferior nuchal lines of occipital bone | Extends head and rotates it toward opposite side | Branches of dorsal primary division of cervical nerves |
| Multifidi | Back of sacrum, aponeurosis of sacrospinalis, | Spinous processes of vertebrae | Extends vertebral column and rotates it toward opposite side | Branches of dorsal primary division of spinal nerves |

| Muscle | Origin | Insertion | Action | Nerve supply |
|---|---|---|---|---|
|  | posterior superior iliac spine; mammillary processes in lumbar region; all transverse processes; articular processes of C-5 to C-8 vertebrae |  |  |  |
| Rotatores | Transverse process of one vertebra | Base of spinous process of vertebra above | Extend vertebral column and rotate it toward opposite side | See multifidi |
| Interspinales | Spinous process to spinous process | Next spinous process | Extend vertebral column | See multifidi |
| Intertransversarii anteriores and posteriores | Anterior and posterior tubercles of transverse processes | To anterior and posterior tubercles of transverse processes of next vertebra | Bend vertebral column laterally | Branches of ventral primary divisions of spinal nerves |
| ***Suboccipital*** |  |  |  |  |
| Rectus capitis posterior major | Spinous process of axis | Lateral part of inferior nuchal line of occipital bone | Extends head and rotates it to same side | Branch of dorsal ramus of suboccipital nerve |
| Rectus capitis posterior minor | Tubercle of posterior arch of atlas | Medial part of inferior nuchal line of occipital bone | Extends head | Branch of dorsal primary division of suboccipital nerve |
| Obliquus capitis inferior | Spinous process of axis | Inferior dorsal part of transverse process of atlas | Rotates atlas, turning face to same side | See rectus capitis posterior minor |
| Obliquus capitis superior | Superior surface of transverse process of atlas | Occipital bone between superior and inferior nuchal lines | Extends head and bends it laterally | See rectus capitis posterior minor |
| **Muscles of lower member** (Fig. 2-17) |  |  |  |  |
| ***Iliac region*** |  |  |  |  |
| Psoas major | Transverse processes of lumbar vertebrae; sides of bodies and intervertebral discs of T-12 and all five lumbar vertebrae | Lesser trochanter of femur | Flexes thigh; flexes lumbar vertebral column and bends it laterally | Branches of lumbar plexus ($L_2$, $L_3$) |
| Psoas minor | Sides of bodies of T-12 and L-1 and intervertebral disc between | Pectineal line of ilium | Flexes pelvis and lumbar vertebral column | Branch of nerve ($L_1$) |
| Iliacus | Superior two thirds of iliac fossa, inner lip of iliac crest | Lateral side of tendon of psoas major | Flexes thigh | Branches of femoral nerve ($L_2$, $L_3$) |

*Continued.*

**Table 2-3.** Major muscles of the body—cont'd

| Muscle | Origin | Insertion | Action | Innervation |
|---|---|---|---|---|
| **Muscles of lower member—cont'd** | | | | |
| **Thigh** | | | | |
| *Anterior femoral* | | | | |
| Sartorius | Anterior superior iliac spine of ilium | Proximal part of medial surface of body of tibia | Flexes thigh and rotates it laterally; flexes leg and rotates it medially | Branches of femoral nerve ($L_2$, $L_3$) |
| Quadriceps femoris | | | | |
| Rectus femoris | Anterior inferior iliac spine; groove above rim of acetabulum | Base of patella | Entire quadriceps extends leg; rectus femoris flexes thigh also | Branches of femoral nerve ($L_2$ to $L_4$) |
| Vastus lateralis | Intertrochanteric line; greater trochanter; gluteal tuberosity | Lateral border of patella | Common quadriceps tendon to tibial tuberosity | |
| Vastus medialis | Intertrochanteric line; medial lip of linea aspera | Medial border of patella | | |
| Vastus intermedius | Front and lateral surfaces of body of femur; intermuscular septum | Deep border of patella | | |
| Articularis genus | Anterior surface of distal body of femur | Proximal part of synovial membrane of knee joint | Draws articular capsule proximally | Branch of nerve to vastus intermedius |
| *Medial femoral* | | | | |
| Gracilis | Inferior body of symphysis pubis and superior half of pubic arch | Medial surface of body of tibia distal to condyle | Adducts thigh; flexes leg and after flexion helps rotate leg medially | Branch of anterior division of obturator nerve ($L_3$, $L_4$) |
| Pectineus | Pectineal line of pubis | Line between lesser trochanter and linea aspera of femur | Adducts, flexes, and medially rotates thigh | Branch of femoral nerve ($L_2$, $L_3$, $L_4$) |
| Adductor longus | Anterior pubis at junction with symphysis | Linea aspera of femur | Adducts, flexes, and medially rotates thigh | Branch of anterior division of obturator nerve ($L_3$, $L_4$) |
| Adductor brevis | Inferior ramus of pubis | Line between lesser trochanter and linea aspera | Adducts, flexes, and medially rotates thigh | Branch of obturator nerve ($L_3$, $L_4$) |
| Adductor magnus | Inferior ramus of pubis, inferior ramus of ischium, tuberosity of ishium | Linea aspera and adductor tubercle | Adducts thigh; upper portion medially rotates and flexes thigh; lower portion extends and laterally rotates thigh | Branches of posterior division of obturator ($L_3$, $L_4$); branch of sciatic nerve |

| Muscle | Origin | Insertion | Action | Nerve |
|---|---|---|---|---|
| *Gluteal muscles* | | | | |
| Gluteus maximus | Posterior gluteal line of ilium and iliac crest; posterior surface of sacrum and side of coccyx | Iliotibial band of fascia lata and gluteal tuberosity of femur | Extends and laterally rotates thigh | Inferior gluteal nerve ($L_5$, $S_1$, $S_2$) |
| Gluteus medius | Outer surface of ilium between iliac crest and anterior and posterior gluteal lines | Greater trochanter of femur | Abducts and medially rotates thigh | Superior gluteal nerve ($L_4$, $L_5$, $S_1$) |
| Gluteus minimus | Outer surface of ilium between anterior and inferior gluteal lines | Anterior border of greater trochanter of femur | Abducts and medially rotates thigh and helps flex thigh | Branches of superior gluteal nerve ($L_4$, $L_5$, $S_1$) |
| Tensor fasciae latae | Iliac crest, anterior superior iliac spine | Iliotibial band | Flexes thigh and helps to rotate it medially | Branch of superior gluteal nerve ($L_4$, $L_5$, $S_1$) |
| Piriformis | Anterior sacrum | Superior border of greater trochanter of femur | Abducts and laterally rotates thigh; helps in extension | $S_1$ or $S_1$ and $S_2$ |
| Obturator internus | Internal surface of superior and inferior rami of pubis, ramus of ischium | Medial surfaces of greater trochanter | Laterally rotates thigh; extends and abducts thigh when flexed | Special nerve from sacral plexus ($L_5$, $S_1$, $S_2$) |
| Gemellus superior | Ischial spine | Greater trochanter | Rotates thigh laterally | Branch of nerve to obturator internus |
| Gemellus inferior | Ischial tuberosity | Greater trochanter | Rotates thigh laterally | Branch of nerve to quadratus femoris |
| Quadratus femoris | Ischial tuberosity | Intertrochanteric ridge distal to chest | Rotates thigh laterally | Special branch from sacral plexus ($L_4$, $L_5$, $S_1$) |
| Obturator externus | Pubic rami, ischial ramus | Trochanteric fossa of femur | Rotates thigh laterally | Branch of obturator nerve ($L_3$, $L_4$) |
| *Posterior femoral* | | | | |
| Biceps femoris | | | | |
| Long head | Ischial tuberosity | Lateral side of head of fibula | Flexes leg and after flexion rotates it laterally; long head extends thigh and rotates it laterally | Tibial portion of sciatic ($S_1$ to $S_3$) |
| Short head | Lateral lip of linea aspera | | | Branch from peroneal portion of sciatic ($L_5$, $S_1$, $S_2$) |

*Continued.*

**Table 2-3.** Major muscles of the body—cont'd

| Muscle | Origin | Insertion | Action | Innervation |
|---|---|---|---|---|
| **Muscles of lower member—cont'd** | | | | |
| ***Thigh—cont'd*** | | | | |
| Semitendinosus | Ischial tuberosity | Medial surface of body of tibia | Flexes leg and after flexion rotates it medially; extends thigh | Branches of tibial portion of sciatic ($L_5$, $S_1$, $S_2$) |
| Semimembranosus | Ischial tuberosity | Medial condyle of tibia, lateral condyle of femur | Flexes leg and rotates it medially after flexion; extends thigh | Branches of tibial portion of sciatic ($L_5$, $S_1$, $S_2$) |
| **Leg** (Fig. 2-18) | | | | |
| ***Anterior or extensor*** | | | | |
| Tibialis anterior | Lateral condyle and surface of tibia | Medial and plantar surface of first cuneiform and first metatarsal | Dorsiflexes, adducts, and inverts foot | Branch of deep peroneal nerve ($L_4$, $L_5$, $S_1$) |
| Extensor hallucis longus | Anterior surface of fibula and interosseous membrane | Base of distal phalanx of great toe | Extends proximal phalanx of great toe; dorsally flexes and supinates foot | Branch of deep peroneal nerve ($L_4$, $L_5$, $S_1$) |
| Extensor digitorum longus | Lateral tibial condyle; anterior surface of fibula body | Second and third phalanges of lesser four toes | Extends proximal phalanges of four small toes; dorsally flexes and pronates foot | Branches of deep peroneal nerve ($L_4$, $L_5$, $S_1$) |
| Peroneus tertius | Anterior distal third of fibula | Base of metatarsal of little toe | Dorsally flexes and pronates foot | Branch of deep peroneal nerve ($L_4$, $L_5$, $S_1$) |
| ***Posterior*** | | | | |
| Gastrocnemius | Medial and lateral condyles of femur | Calcaneus tendon with soleus | Plantar flexes foot | Branches of tibial nerve ($S_1$, $S_2$) |
| Soleus | Head of fibula and proximal third of posterior surface; medial border of tibia | Calcaneus tendon with gastrocnemius | Plantar flexes foot | Branches of tibial nerve ($S_1$, $S_2$) |
| Plantaris | Linear aspera of femur | Posterior part of calcaneus | Plantar flexes foot; flexes leg | Branch of tibial nerve ($L_4$, $L_5$, $S_1$) |
| Popliteus | Lateral condyle of femur | Popliteal line of tibia | Flexes leg and rotates it medially | Branch of tibial nerve ($L_4$, $L_5$, $S_1$) |
| Flexor hallucis longus | Inferior two thirds of body of fibula | Base of terminal phalanx of great toe | Flexes second phalanx of great toe; plantar flexes and supinates foot | Branch of tibial nerve ($L_5$, $S_1$, $S_2$) |

| Muscle | Origin | Insertion | Action | Nerve supply |
|---|---|---|---|---|
| Flexor digitorum longus | Posterior surface of body of tibia below popliteal line | Bases of distal phalanges of lesser four toes | Flexes terminal phalanges of four small toes; plantar flexes and supinates foot | Branch of tibial nerve ($L_5$, $S_1$) |
| Tibialis posterior | Posterior surface of body of tibia | Tuberosity of navicular bone, calcaneus, three cuneiforms, cuboid, second to fourth metatarsals | Supinates (adducts and inverts) foot; plantar flexes foot | Branch of tibial nerve ($L_5$, $S_1$) |
| *Lateral* | | | | |
| Peroneus longus | Head and lateral surface of fibula | Base of first metatarsal and lateral side of medial cuneiform | Pronates (abducts and everts); plantar flexes foot | Branch of superficial peroneal ($L_4$, $L_5$, $S_1$) |
| Peroneus brevis | Distal two thirds of lateral body of fibula | Tuberosity at base of fifth metatarsal | Pronates; plantar flexes foot | Branch of superficial peroneal ($L_4$, $L_5$, $S_1$) |
| **Foot** | | | | |
| *Dorsal* | | | | |
| Extensor digitorum brevis | Calcaneus | Base of proximal phalanx of great toe; tendons of extensor digitorum longus of second, third, and fourth toes | Extends proximal phalanges of great and adjacent three small toes | Branch of deep peroneal nerve ($L_5$, $S_1$) |
| *Plantar* | | | | |
| **FIRST LAYER** | | | | |
| Abductor hallucis | Tuberosity of calcaneus | Tibial side of base of first phalanx of great toe | Abducts great toe | Branch of medial plantar nerve ($L_4$, $L_5$) |
| Flexor digitorum brevis | Tuberosity of calcaneus | Second phalanges of four small toes | Flexes second phalanges of four small toes | Branch of medial plantar nerve ($L_4$, $L_5$) |
| Abductor digiti minimi | Tuberosity of calcaneus | Fibular side of base of first phalanx of little toe | Abducts small toe | Branch of lateral plantar nerve ($S_1$, $S_2$) |
| **SECOND LAYER** | | | | |
| Quadratus plantae | | | | |
| Medial head | Medial surface of calcaneus | Plantar surfaces of tendons of flexor digitorum longus | Flexes terminal phalanges of four small toes | Branch of lateral plantar nerve ($S_1$, $S_2$) |
| Lateral head | Lateral surface of calcaneus | | | |

*Continued.*

**Table 2-3.** Major muscles of the body—cont'd

| Muscle | Origin | Insertion | Action | Innervation |
|---|---|---|---|---|
| **Muscles of lower member—cont'd** | | | | |
| *Foot—cont'd* | | | | |
| Lumbricales (4) | Tendon of flexor digitorum longus | Expansion of tendons of extensor digitorum longus at first phalanges | Flex proximal phalanges and extend two distal phalanges of four small toes | Branch of medial plantar nerve ($L_4$, $L_5$); branches of lateral plantar nerve ($S_1$, $S_2$) |
| **THIRD LAYER** | | | | |
| Flexor hallucis brevis | Plantar surface of cuboid bone, lateral cuneiform | Adductor hallucis before its insertion | Flexes proximal phalanx of great toe | Branch of medial plantar nerve ($L_4$, $L_5$, $S_1$) |
| Adductor hallucis | | | | |
| Oblique head | Bases of second, third, and fourth metatarsal bones | Lateral side of base of proximal phalanx of great toe | Adducts great toe | Branch of lateral plantar nerve ($S_1$, $S_2$) |
| Transverse head | Plantar metatarsophalangeal ligaments of third, fourth, fifth toes | Lateral side of first phalanx of great toe | | |
| Flexor digiti minimi | Base of fifth metatarsal bone | Lateral side of first phalanx of fifth toe | Flexes proximal phalanx of small toe | Branch of lateral plantar nerve ($S_1$, $S_2$) |
| **FOURTH LAYER** | | | | |
| Interossei | | | | |
| Dorsal (4) | Bipenniform: two heads each from adjacent sides of metatarsal bones | Bases of first phalanges: 1 into medial side of second toe, 2-4 into lateral side of second, third, and fourth toes | Abduct toes from axis of second toe; flex proximal, extend distal phalanges | Branches of lateral plantar nerve ($S_1$, $S_2$) |
| Plantar (3) | Bases of medial sides of third, fourth, fifth metatarsal bones | Medial sides of bases of first phalanges of same toes | Adduct toes toward axis of second toe; flex proximal, extend distal phalanges | Branches of lateral plantar nerve ($S_1$, $S_2$) |

also named by their actions. The following are types of muscles and their actions:

**flexor** decreases the angle of a joint.
**extensor** increases the angle of a joint.
**adductor** moves a bone toward the midline of the body.
**abductor** moves a bone away from the midline of the body.
**rotator** moves a bone around its longitudinal axis.
**levator** causes an upward, superior movement.
**depressor** produces a downward, inferior movement.
**tensor** causes increased rigidity of a muscle or body part.
**sphincter** decreases the size of an opening.
**supinator** turns the palm outward (anteriorly).
**pronator** turns the palm inward (posteriorly).
**invertor** turns the sole of the foot inward (toward the midline).
**evertor** turns the sole of the foot outward (away from the midline).
**dorsiflexor** extends the ankle joint.
**plantar flexor** flexes the ankle joint.

## CARDIAC MUSCLE

Cardiac muscle differs histologically from skeletal muscle in several ways (Fig. 2-1, *B*). The nuclei of a cardiac muscle fiber are located centrally instead of peripherally, the cardiac fibers are short and branched instead of being long and tapered, and cardiac fibers have terminal specializations of their membranes, called intercalated discs. Cardiac muscle cells have the same basic arrangement of actin, myosin, and sarcoplasmic reticulum as do skeletal muscle fibers, and their T tubule systems are also similar. Cardiac muscle, however, is involuntary and normally contracts constantly, about 72 times per minute.

Cardiac muscle can contract without nervous stimulation, whereas skeletal muscle cannot. Instead cardiac muscle has its own specialized conduction system composed of specialized cardiac muscle cells and not neurons. This conduction system of the heart sends out electrical impulses that cause the heart to contract. Nervous stimulation from outside the heart only causes the conducting tissue to increase or decrease its rate of stimulation, thereby causing about 72 contractions per minute.

## SMOOTH MUSCLE

Like cardiac muscle, smooth muscle is involuntary. Smooth muscle fibers are long and spindle shaped with only one centrally located nucleus (Fig. 2-1, *C*). Their fibers contain the contractile elements of actin and myosin, but they do not appear striated because these elements are not

*Text continued on p. 76.*

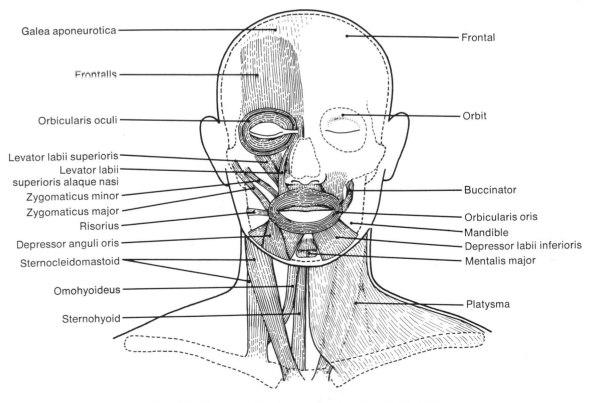

**Fig. 2-7.** Muscles of facial expression. See Table 2-3.

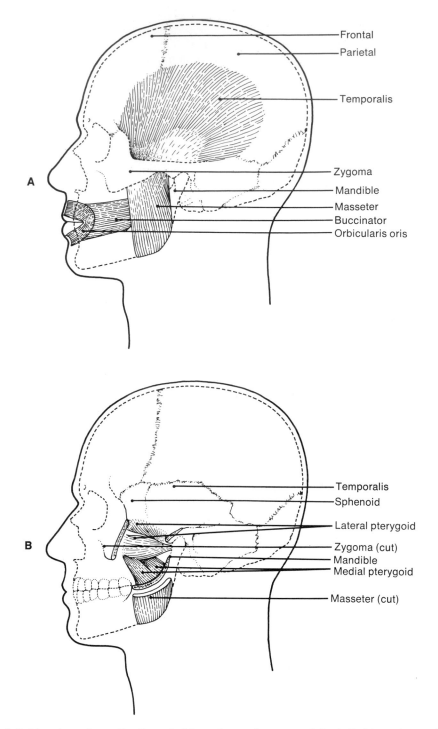

Frontal
Parietal

Temporalis

Zygoma
Mandible
Masseter
Buccinator
Orbicularis oris

Temporalis
Sphenoid

Lateral pterygoid

Zygoma (cut)
Mandible
Medial pterygoid

Masseter (cut)

**Fig. 2-8.** Muscles of mastication. **A,** Masseter and zygoma intact. **B,** Masseter and zygoma removed to show deeper structures. See Table 2-3.

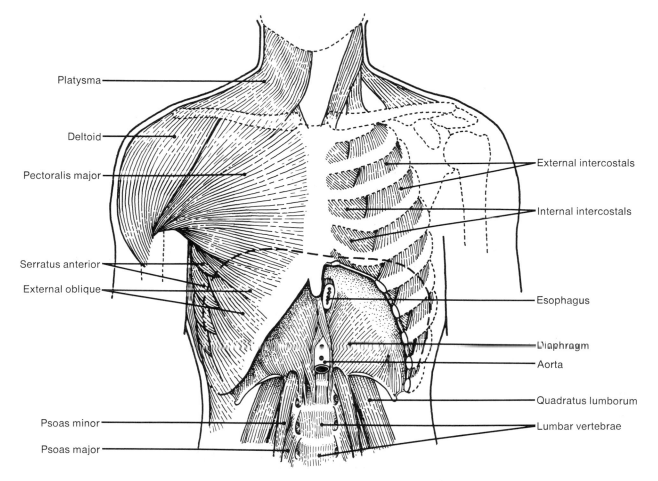

Platysma

Deltoid

Pectoralis major

Serratus anterior

External oblique

Psoas minor

Psoas major

External intercostals

Internal intercostals

Esophagus

Diaphragm

Aorta

Quadratus lumborum

Lumbar vertebrae

**Fig. 2-9.** Muscles of thorax. See Table 2-3.

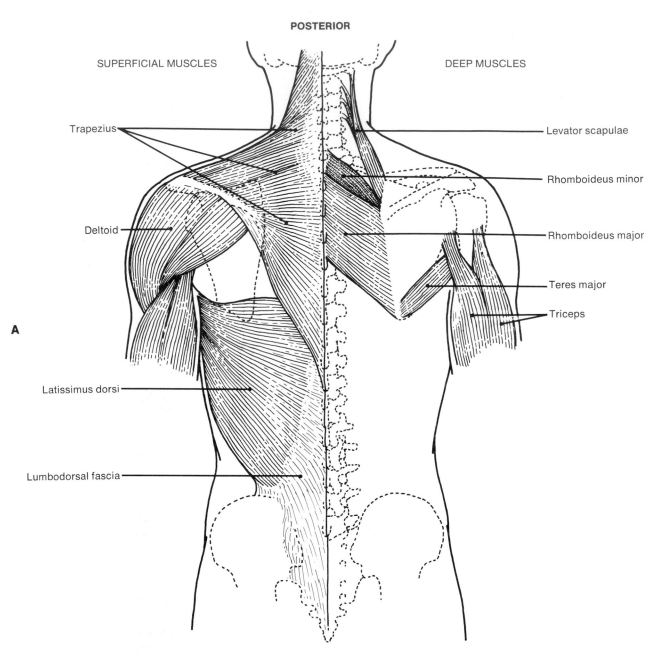

**POSTERIOR**

SUPERFICIAL MUSCLES

DEEP MUSCLES

Trapezius

Levator scapulae

Rhomboideus minor

Deltoid

Rhomboideus major

Teres major

Triceps

A

Latissimus dorsi

Lumbodorsal fascia

**Fig. 2-10. A,** Muscles that connect upper member to vertebral column. See Table 2-3.

**ANTERIOR**

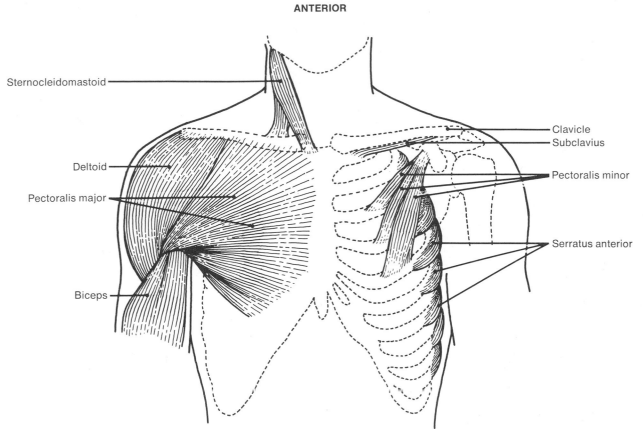

Sternocleidomastoid

Clavicle
Subclavius

Deltoid

Pectoralis minor

Pectoralis major

Serratus anterior

Biceps

B

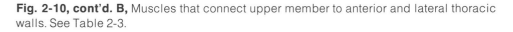

**Fig. 2-10, cont'd. B,** Muscles that connect upper member to anterior and lateral thoracic walls. See Table 2-3.

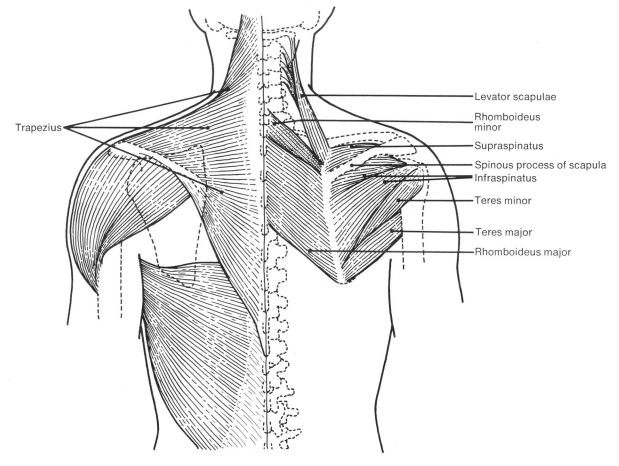

**Fig. 2-11.** Muscles of shoulder. See Table 2-3.

POSTERIOR                    ANTERIOR

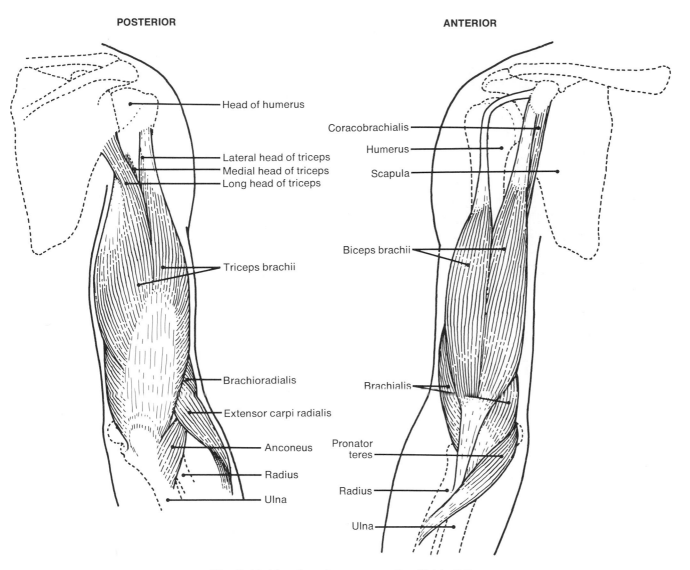

Head of humerus

Coracobrachialis

Humerus

Scapula

Lateral head of triceps
Medial head of triceps
Long head of triceps

Triceps brachii

Biceps brachii

Brachioradialis

Brachialis

Extensor carpi radialis

Anconeus

Pronator
teres

Radius

Radius

Ulna

Ulna

**Fig. 2-12.** Muscles of upper arm. See Table 2-3.

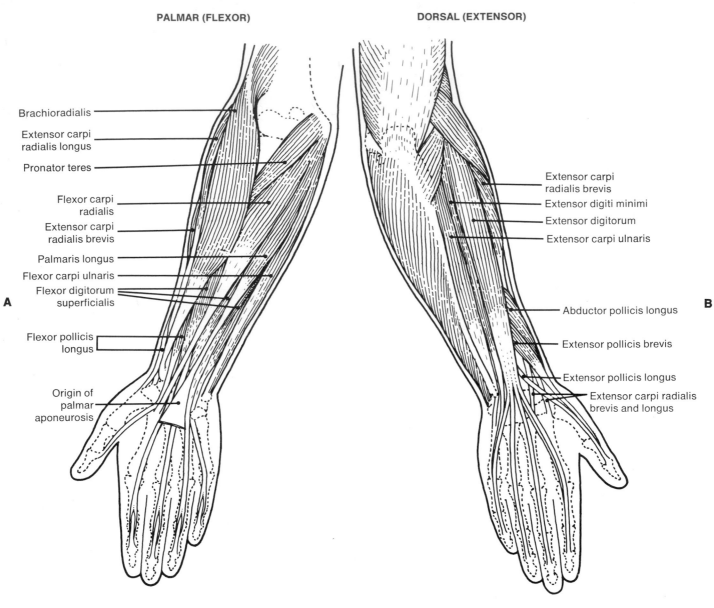

**PALMAR (FLEXOR)**

**DORSAL (EXTENSOR)**

Brachioradialis

Extensor carpi radialis longus

Pronator teres

Flexor carpi radialis

Extensor carpi radialis brevis

Palmaris longus

Flexor carpi ulnaris

Flexor digitorum superficialis

Flexor pollicis longus

Origin of palmar aponeurosis

**A**

Extensor carpi radialis brevis

Extensor digiti minimi

Extensor digitorum

Extensor carpi ulnaris

Abductor pollicis longus

Extensor pollicis brevis

Extensor pollicis longus

Extensor carpi radialis brevis and longus

**B**

**Fig. 2-13.** Muscles of forearm; muscles that move fingers. **A,** Anterior. **B,** Posterior. See Table 2-3.

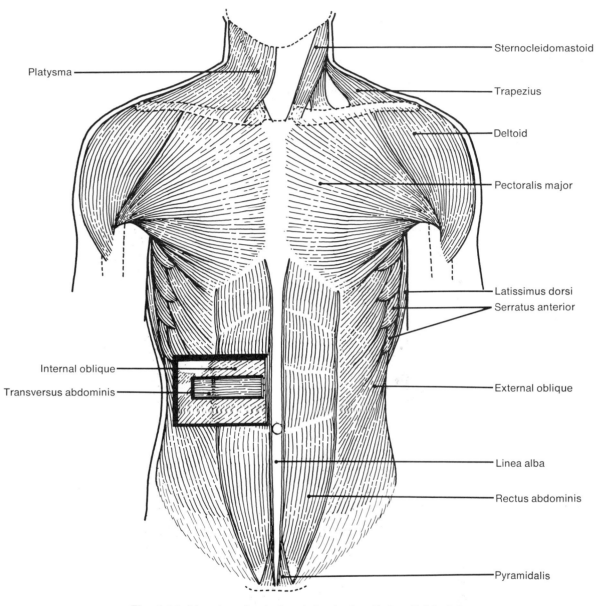

**Fig. 2-14.** Muscles of anterior abdominal wall. See Table 2-3.

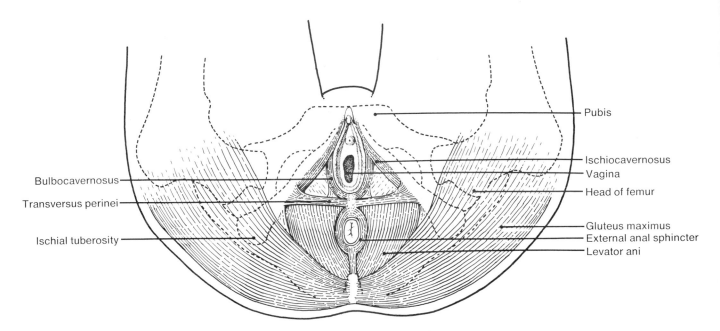

**Fig. 2-15.** Muscles of pelvic floor and perineum. See Table 2-3.

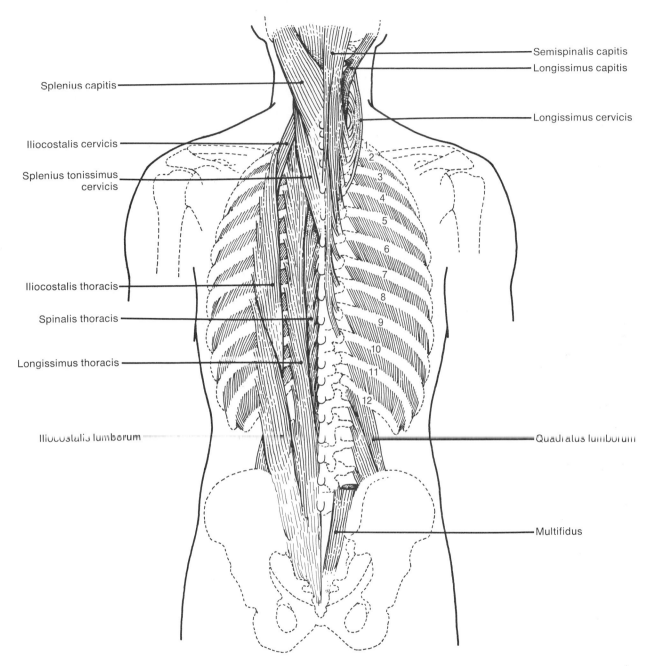

Splenius capitis

Iliocostalis cervicis

Splenius tonissimus cervicis

Iliocostalis thoracis

Spinalis thoracis

Longissimus thoracis

Iliocostalis lumborum

Semispinalis capitis
Longissimus capitis

Longissimus cervicis

Quadratus lumborum

Multifidus

**Fig. 2-16.** Muscles of back. See Table 2-3.

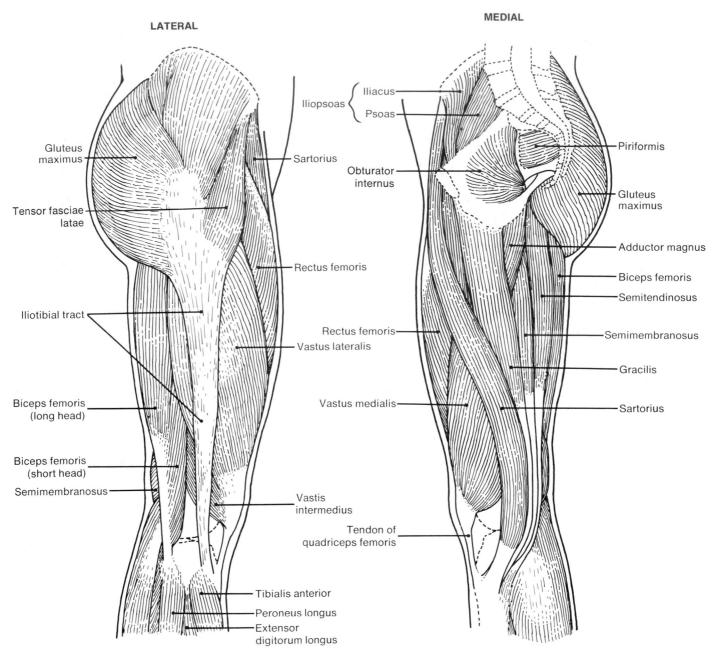

**Fig. 2-17.** Muscles of buttocks and thigh. See Table 2-3.

LATERAL

MEDIAL

Iliopsoas { Iliacus
Psoas

Gluteus maximus

Sartorius

Tensor fasciae latae

Obturator internus

Piriformis

Gluteus maximus

Rectus femoris

Adductor magnus

Iliotibial tract

Biceps femoris

Semitendinosus

Rectus femoris

Semimembranosus

Vastus lateralis

Gracilis

Biceps femoris (long head)

Sartorius

Vastus medialis

Biceps femoris (short head)

Semimembranosus

Vastis intermedius

Tendon of quadriceps femoris

Tibialis anterior

Peroneus longus

Extensor digitorum longus

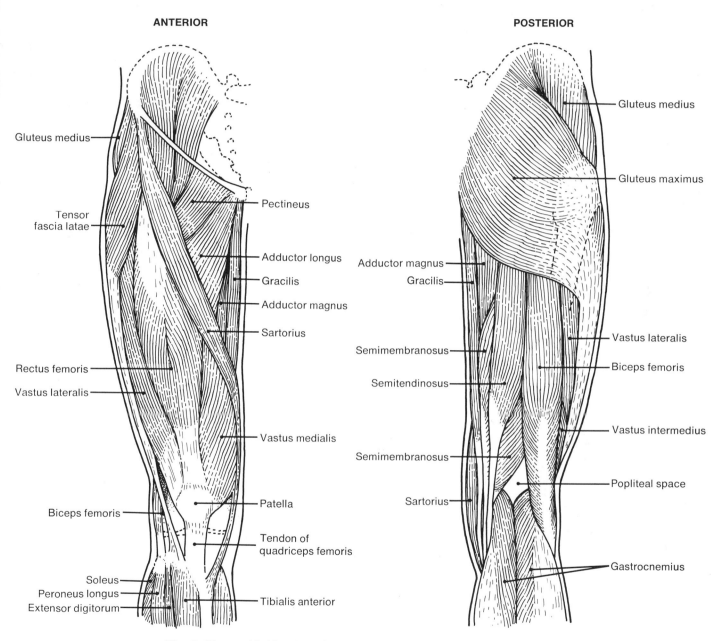

**ANTERIOR**

Gluteus medius

Tensor fascia latae

Rectus femoris

Vastus lateralis

Biceps femoris

Soleus
Peroneus longus
Extensor digitorum

Pectineus

Adductor longus

Gracilis

Adductor magnus

Sartorius

Vastus medialis

Patella

Tendon of quadriceps femoris

Tibialis anterior

**POSTERIOR**

Gluteus medius

Gluteus maximus

Adductor magnus
Gracilis

Semimembranosus

Semitendinosus

Semimembranosus

Sartorius

Vastus lateralis

Biceps femoris

Vastus intermedius

Popliteal space

Gastrocnemius

**Fig. 2-17, cont'd.** Muscles of buttocks and thigh. See Table 2-3.

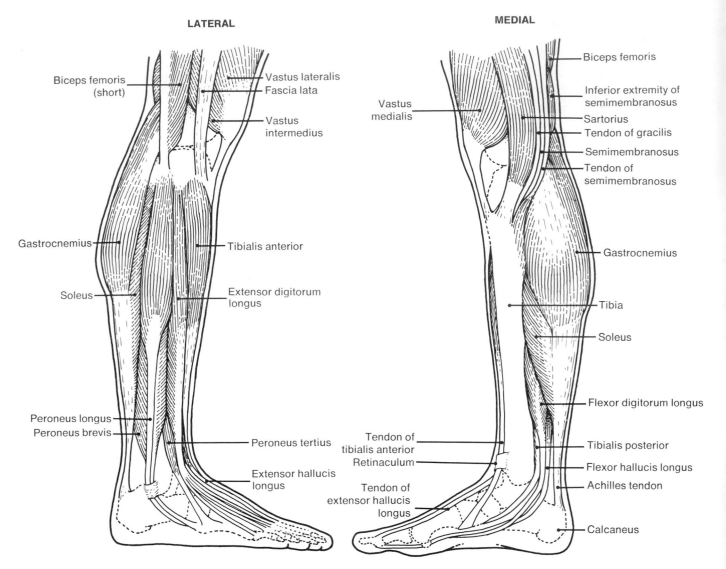

**LATERAL**

Biceps femoris (short)

Vastus lateralis

Fascia lata

Vastus intermedius

Gastrocnemius

Tibialis anterior

Soleus

Extensor digitorum longus

Peroneus longus

Peroneus brevis

Peroneus tertius

Extensor hallucis longus

**MEDIAL**

Biceps femoris

Inferior extremity of semimembranosus

Vastus medialis

Sartorius

Tendon of gracilis

Semimembranosus

Tendon of semimembranosus

Gastrocnemius

Tibia

Soleus

Flexor digitorum longus

Tendon of tibialis anterior

Retinaculum

Tibialis posterior

Flexor hallucis longus

Achilles tendon

Tendon of extensor hallucis longus

Calcaneus

**Fig. 2-18.** Muscles of lower leg. See Table 2-3.

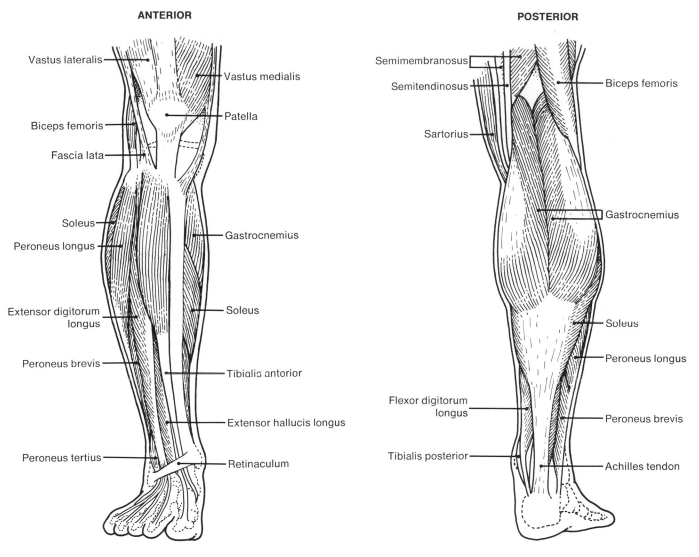

**ANTERIOR**

Vastus lateralis

Vastus medialis

Biceps femoris

Patella

Fascia lata

Soleus

Peroneus longus

Gastrocnemius

Extensor digitorum
longus

Soleus

Peroneus brevis

Tibialis anterior

Extensor hallucis longus

Peroneus tertius

Retinaculum

**POSTERIOR**

Semimembranosus

Semitendinosus

Biceps femoris

Sartorius

Gastrocnemius

Soleus

Peroneus longus

Flexor digitorum
longus

Peroneus brevis

Tibialis posterior

Achilles tendon

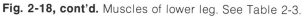

**Fig. 2-18, cont'd.** Muscles of lower leg. See Table 2-3.

arranged synchronously as they are in striated muscle. This unorganized arrangement of actin and myosin may be why smooth muscle contracts more slowly than skeletal muscle.

Smooth muscle is found in sheets in the walls of hollow organs such as the intestine. The fibers tend to be arranged in such a way that when a neuron stimulates one fiber the impulse travels over adjacent fibers in a wavelike fashion. Other types of smooth muscle have a single motor unit for each muscle fiber, causing more precise contraction as in the intrinsic muscles of the eye or the smooth muscle in the walls of blood vessels. Immediate and precise contraction of these muscles is more necessary than in the smooth muscle of the viscera.

## MAJOR MUSCLES

Table 2-3 lists the major muscles of the body with their origins, insertions, actions, and innervations (somewhat simplified for brevity).

**REFERENCES**

1. Anthony, C. P., and Thibodeau, G. A.: Textbook of anatomy and physiology, St. Louis, 1979, The C. V. Mosby Co.
2. Pansky, B.: Dynamic anatomy and physiology, New York, 1975, Macmillan, Inc.

**BIBLIOGRAPHY**

Anthony, C. P., and Thibodeau, G. A.: Textbook of anatomy and physiology, ed. 10, St. Louis, 1979, The C. V. Mosby Co.

Bloom, W., and Fawcett, D. W.: A textbook of histology, Philadelphia, 1975, W. B. Saunders Co.

Goss, C. M., editor: Gray's anatomy, Philadelphia, 1966, Lea & Febiger.

Greisheimer, E. M., and Wiedeman, M.: Physiology and anatomy, Philadelphia, 1972, J. B. Lippincott Co.

Ham, A. W.: Histology, Philadelphia, 1974, J. B. Lippincott Co.

Pansky, B.: Dynamic anatomy and physiology, New York, 1975, Macmillan, Inc.

Stedman's medical dictionary, ed. 21, Baltimore, 1966, The Williams & Wilkins Co.

Tortora, G. J., and Anagnostakos, N. P.: Principles of anatomy and physiology, San Francisco, Canfield Press, 1975, Harper & Row, Publishers.

# 3

## Processes of growth

NANCY E. HILT

*Growth* may be defined as the development or increase in size of living cells. Growth, as utilized in the context of this discussion, applies not only to the normal stages of growth associated with childhood and adolescence but also to the growth processes that affect the musculoskeletal system throughout life. The major objective here is to outline those specific processes associated with growth or with specific age groups. These processes are specifically related to diseases and disorders, the treatment of which may be determined or affected by portions of these processes.

Musculoskeletal growth is the primary determinant of one's size, height, and shape. In addition adipose tissue to some degree affects the general shape and size. The physiologic components of the musculoskeletal system that assist in this determination are not examined here because, unless they are related to diseases or disorders and their treatment, they are of little significance to those in the health care system involved with orthopedics. The specific processes reviewed have a direct or indirect relationship to treatment of diseases and disorders during the specific stages of life and include (1) *ossification process*, (2) *epiphyseal growth plate development*, and (3) *osteoporosis*. The relationship of the "remodeling" process of fractures during growth periods is discussed in Chapter 16.

## OSSIFICATION PROCESS

The *ossification process* may be defined as the formation of osseous cells from cartilaginous tissue. This is a normal physiologic process that begins during embryonic development and ceases at some time during the adolescent years. Evidence of the completion of the ossification process may be exhibited on radiographic examination by fusion of the epiphysis and the diaphysis of a longitudinal bone. This fusion is apparent at the area designated as the epiphyseal plate. Physiologic representation of the ossification process is shown in Fig. 1-2. Further details of the cellular process may be reviewed in Chapter 1.

Of specific importance here in relation to the ossification process and its effect on the development of diseases and disorders and their treatment are the following facts:

1. Until the ossification process is complete in any specific bone, a major portion of the bone, decreasing with growth, is composed of cartilaginous rather than osseous tissue.
2. The appearance of centers of ossification as well as the inevitable anticipated epiphyseal fusion are dependent on the specific bone and its location.
3. The rate of growth is relatively dependent on the normal physiologic process of ossification accompanied by normal epiphyseal growth plates.
4. The rate of ossification is similar in males and females during the first decade of life, but during the second decade it is accelerated in females.
5. The completion of ossification in females is approximately 2 years ahead of that in males (Fig. 3-1).

### Relationship to injury, diseases, and disorders and their treatment

The ossification process is not directly responsible for the inducement of a disease process, nor

*Text continued on p. 82.*

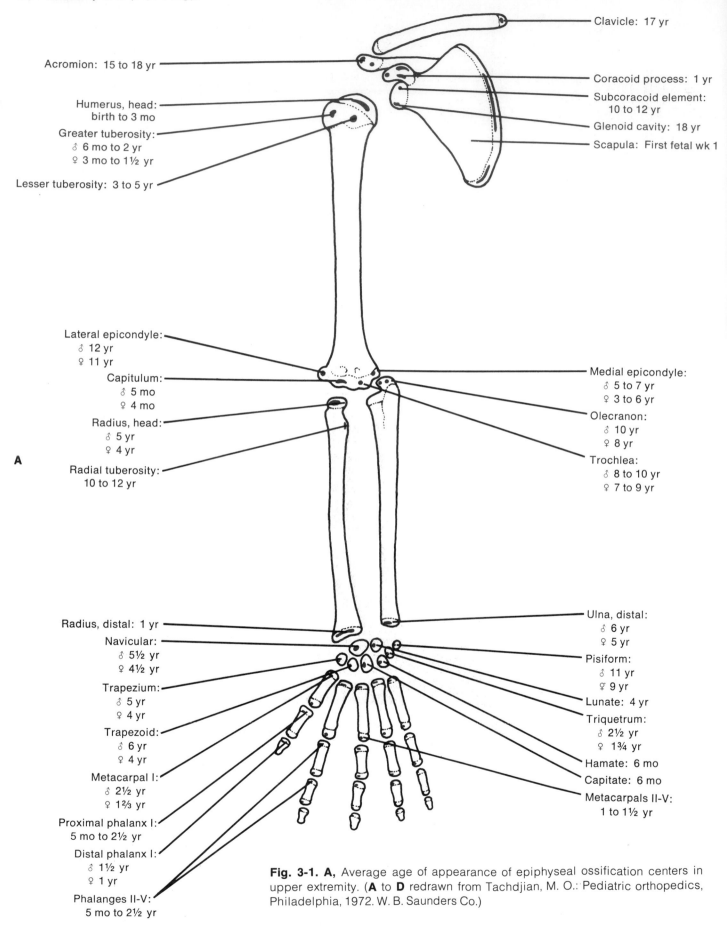

Clavicle: 17 yr

Acromion: 15 to 18 yr

Coracoid process: 1 yr

Subcoracoid element:
10 to 12 yr

Humerus, head:
birth to 3 mo

Glenoid cavity: 18 yr

Greater tuberosity:
♂ 6 mo to 2 yr
♀ 3 mo to 1½ yr

Scapula: First fetal wk 1

Lesser tuberosity: 3 to 5 yr

Lateral epicondyle:
♂ 12 yr
♀ 11 yr

Medial epicondyle:
♂ 5 to 7 yr
♀ 3 to 6 yr

Capitulum:
♂ 5 mo
♀ 4 mo

Olecranon:
♂ 10 yr
♀ 8 yr

Radius, head:
♂ 5 yr
♀ 4 yr

Trochlea:
♂ 8 to 10 yr
♀ 7 to 9 yr

**A**

Radial tuberosity:
10 to 12 yr

Ulna, distal:
♂ 6 yr
♀ 5 yr

Radius, distal: 1 yr

Navicular:
♂ 5½ yr
♀ 4½ yr

Pisiform:
♂ 11 yr
♀ 9 yr

Trapezium:
♂ 5 yr
♀ 4 yr

Lunate: 4 yr

Triquetrum:
♂ 2½ yr
♀ 1¾ yr

Trapezoid:
♂ 6 yr
♀ 4 yr

Hamate: 6 mo

Metacarpal I:
♂ 2½ yr
♀ 1⅔ yr

Capitate: 6 mo

Metacarpals II-V:
1 to 1½ yr

Proximal phalanx I:
5 mo to 2½ yr

Distal phalanx I:
♂ 1½ yr
♀ 1 yr

**Fig. 3-1. A,** Average age of appearance of epiphyseal ossification centers in upper extremity. (**A** to **D** redrawn from Tachdjian, M. O.: Pediatric orthopedics, Philadelphia, 1972. W. B. Saunders Co.)

Phalanges II-V:
5 mo to 2½ yr

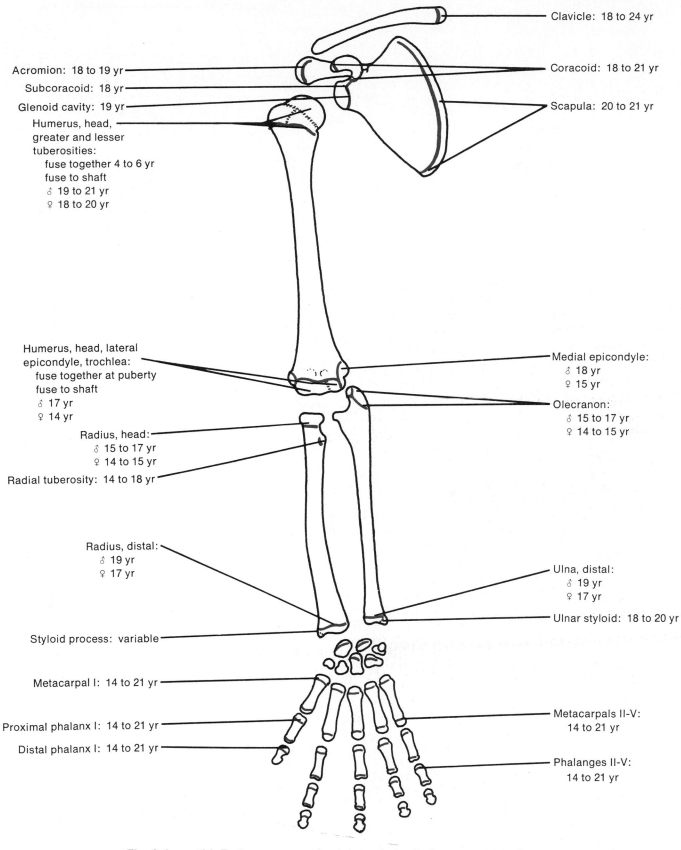

Clavicle: 18 to 24 yr

Coracoid: 18 to 21 yr

Acromion: 18 to 19 yr

Subcoracoid: 18 yr

Glenoid cavity: 19 yr

Scapula: 20 to 21 yr

Humerus, head,
greater and lesser
tuberosities:
    fuse together 4 to 6 yr
    fuse to shaft
        ♂ 19 to 21 yr
        ♀ 18 to 20 yr

**B**

Humerus, head, lateral
epicondyle, trochlea:
    fuse together at puberty
    fuse to shaft
        ♂ 17 yr
        ♀ 14 yr

Medial epicondyle:
    ♂ 18 yr
    ♀ 15 yr

Olecranon:
    ♂ 15 to 17 yr
    ♀ 14 to 15 yr

Radius, head:
    ♂ 15 to 17 yr
    ♀ 14 to 15 yr

Radial tuberosity: 14 to 18 yr

Radius, distal:
    ♂ 19 yr
    ♀ 17 yr

Ulna, distal:
    ♂ 19 yr
    ♀ 17 yr

Ulnar styloid: 18 to 20 yr

Styloid process: variable

Metacarpal I: 14 to 21 yr

Metacarpals II-V:
14 to 21 yr

Proximal phalanx I: 14 to 21 yr

Distal phalanx I: 14 to 21 yr

Phalanges II-V:
14 to 21 yr

**Fig. 3-1, cont'd. B,** Average age of epiphyseal closure in upper extremity.

*Continued.*

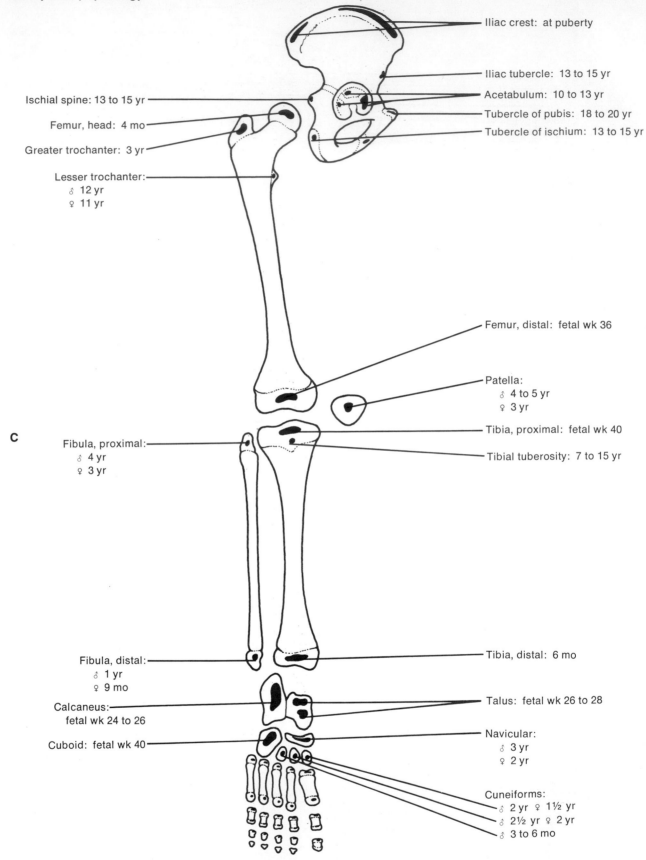

Iliac crest: at puberty

Iliac tubercle: 13 to 15 yr

Acetabulum: 10 to 13 yr

Ischial spine: 13 to 15 yr

Femur, head: 4 mo

Greater trochanter: 3 yr

Lesser trochanter:
♂ 12 yr
♀ 11 yr

Tubercle of pubis: 18 to 20 yr

Tubercle of ischium: 13 to 15 yr

Femur, distal: fetal wk 36

Patella:
♂ 4 to 5 yr
♀ 3 yr

Tibia, proximal: fetal wk 40

C

Fibula, proximal:
♂ 4 yr
♀ 3 yr

Tibial tuberosity: 7 to 15 yr

Fibula, distal:
♂ 1 yr
♀ 9 mo

Calcaneus:
fetal wk 24 to 26

Cuboid: fetal wk 40

Tibia, distal: 6 mo

Talus: fetal wk 26 to 28

Navicular:
♂ 3 yr
♀ 2 yr

Cuneiforms:
♂ 2 yr ♀ 1½ yr
♂ 2½ yr ♀ 2 yr
♂ 3 to 6 mo

**Fig. 3-1, cont'd. C,** Average age of appearance of centers of epiphyseal ossification in lower extremity.

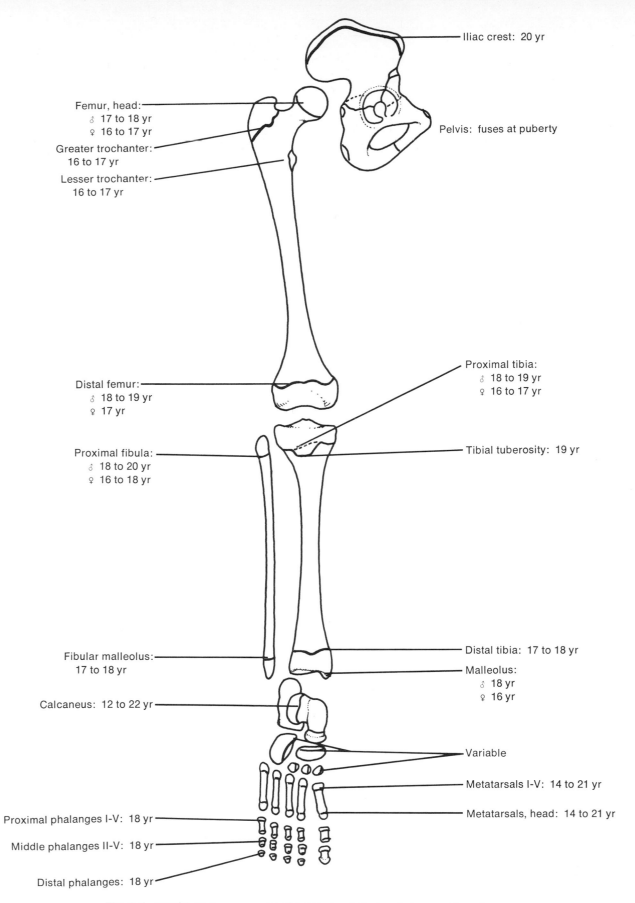

Iliac crest: 20 yr

Femur, head:
♂ 17 to 18 yr
♀ 16 to 17 yr

Greater trochanter:
16 to 17 yr

Lesser trochanter:
16 to 17 yr

Pelvis: fuses at puberty

Distal femur:
♂ 18 to 19 yr
♀ 17 yr

Proximal tibia:
♂ 18 to 19 yr
♀ 16 to 17 yr

D

Proximal fibula:
♂ 18 to 20 yr
♀ 16 to 18 yr

Tibial tuberosity: 19 yr

Fibular malleolus:
17 to 18 yr

Distal tibia: 17 to 18 yr

Malleolus:
♂ 18 yr
♀ 16 yr

Calcaneus: 12 to 22 yr

Variable

Metatarsals I-V: 14 to 21 yr

Proximal phalanges I-V: 18 yr

Metatarsals, head: 14 to 21 yr

Middle phalanges II-V: 18 yr

Distal phalanges: 18 yr

**Fig. 3-1, cont'd. D,** Average age of epiphyseal closure in lower extremity.

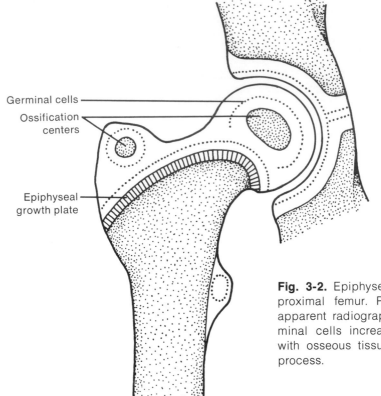

**Fig. 3-2.** Epiphyseal and ossification development of proximal femur. Primary centers of ossification are apparent radiographically at an early age, while germinal cells increasingly replace cartilaginous tissue with osseous tissue during the aging and maturation process.

Germinal cells

Ossification centers

Epiphyseal growth plate

does it directly influence deformities or disorders to any great degree. Rather, disease processes, traumatic injuries, and developmental anomalies may directly influence the ossification process. This most frequently occurs when the epiphyseal growth plate is directly involved during any stage of the growth process with traumatic injuries, neoplasms, or congenital or developmental anomalies. Such circumstances may delay the ossification process considerably and, with growth, be responsible for varying degrees of deformities.

The progression of the ossification process may be monitored quite well radiographically. Fig. 3-2 shows the normal progression of the ossification centers in the proximal femur. All ossification centers throughout the body may be monitored accordingly. Because the cartilaginous tissue, which composes a major portion of the end of the long bone and surrounds the ossification center, cannot be radiographically viewed, full visualization of the bone requires arthrography.

The ability to accurately visualize the ossification process through radiographic techniques is of great diagnostic value. In addition it provides a high degree of predictive reliability in attempts to project total growth of the skeletal system at the time of epiphyseal closure. This determination is sometimes critical to the ability of the orthopedic surgeon to make an appropriate and accurate choice in the anomalies and disorders where treatment alternatives are available. The most striking example is lower limb length discrepancies, in which predicted height at the completion of the ossification process determines whether the appropriate surgical intervention will involve lengthening or shortening procedures (see Chapter 14). In this case it also greatly influences the appropriate time of accomplishing the procedure to provide for the best and most accurate result. It should be noted that the ossification process and epiphyseal growth plate development are very closely related insofar as our ability to appropriately relate growth to treatment alternatives.

## EPIPHYSEAL GROWTH PLATE DEVELOPMENT

The epiphyseal growth plate is responsible for longitudinal bone growth. This plate is constructed of cartilaginous tissue and is situated in long bones between the diaphysis and the epiphysis. This cartilage or disc appears as the epiphyseal line when

**Table 3-1.** Major long bones: contribution of each growth plate to final length of shaft

| Bone | Proximal end (%) | Distal end (%) |
| --- | --- | --- |
| Humerus | 80 | 20 |
| Radius | 25 | 75 |
| Ulna | 20 | 80 |
| Femur | 30 | 70 |
| Tibia | 55 | 45 |
| Fibula | 60 | 40 |

From Rang, M.: The growth plate and its disorders, Baltimore, 1969, The Williams & Wilkins Co.

growth is completed and fusion has occurred. Growth plates exist in all bones that grow gradually and continually throughout the ossification process, although specific characteristics can be differentiated among bones.

The epiphyseal growth plates are normally associated with the long bones of the upper and lower extremities (Table 3-1). Those associated with the lower extremity are probably more crucial and of greater significance because they are subjected to the continual stress of weight bearing and assist more than any other growth plates in the ultimate determination of height. These specific growth plates are located between the epiphysis and the metaphysis of the long bones. The vertebrae have growth plates at each upper and lower surface. These growth plates physiologically fulfill the same function as those in the long bones, but no epiphysis is present. The innominate bone (triradiate cartilage) and the tibial tubercle have bipolar growth plates, that is, two growth plates next to each other. Smaller bones such as those found in the wrist and the foot have a spherical growth plate that surrounds the nucleus of the ossification center.[3,p.2]

There are two types of growth plates: those involved with the compression of weight bearing or surrounding muscles and those subjected to distraction by muscles or ligaments. Each contributes to a different type of growth within a specific bone: those involved with the compression forces of weight bearing and muscular actions contribute to the longitudinal growth of the bone (the length), and those subjected to distraction forces contribute to the general shape and proportion of the bone.[3,p.3]

Each growth plate contains several components that contribute to its viability as well as to its ability to maintain specific functions[3,p.3]:

**basic cells** responsible for growth within the plate and production of intercellular matrix; also involved in production of enzymes required for the ossification process.

**matrix** responsible for maintaining stability and strength of the growth plate; the physiologic processes responsible for growth occur within this medium; maintains an active role in new bone formation during ossification.

**vascular system within the growth plate** responsible for nutritional needs of the growth plate for active maintenance of the required physiologic processes.

**enzyme system** responsible for activation of the physiologic processes.

The ability of a specific growth plate to fulfill its functions is greatly dependent on (1) its vascular system, (2) mechanical forces on and about the growth plate, (3) growth of other bones adjacent to the epiphyseal plate, and (4) the presence or absence of abnormal physiologic factors that directly influence the specific growth plate.[3,pp.35-36] The degree to which any of these factors affect growth is greatly dependent on the location and function of the growth plate involved, although adjacent structures may be affected. Not only do local disturbances affect the general pattern of growth, but it is also greatly influenced by general nutrition, genetic aberrations, and the secretion of hormones.

It must be emphasized in clarification of terminology used to describe bone growth that the growth plate and not the epiphysis is responsible for the longitudinal growth of long bones. Long bones grow longitudinally and transversely (in diameter), both processes occurring concurrently.

## Relationship to injury, diseases, and disorders and their treatment

The most profound concern of any orthopedic surgeon in relation to the first two decades of life, which have been established as the primary years of growth, is that of injury or disease process affecting the combined processes of ossification and epiphyseal growth plate development. A wide range of diseases and disorders may affect growth to varying degrees. These diseases and disorders are categorized into three groups[3,p.37]:

*Group I:* diseases and disorders involving the growth plate that result from generalized disease entities

*Group II:* diseases and disorders of generalized growth plates throughout the body that result from lesions of musculoskeletal involvement only

*Group III:* diseases and disorders involving a single growth plate

Traumatic injuries result in and contribute to a major portion of growth plate diseases and disorders in group III. The effects of these diseases and disorders vary from minor or insignificant to severe in nature.

Etiologic factors contributing to the development of growth plate diseases and disorders include neoplasms, traumatic injuries, vascular insufficiency, nutritional aberrations, disturbances of the normal hormone balance, infections, genetic abnormalities producing congenital anomalies, and metabolic disturbances. Pathogenic alterations may produce several types of clinical features[3,pp.40-41]:

**local growth failure** anomalies and disorders resulting from errors in fetal development leading to partial or total absence of a bone or limb, trauma destructive to a portion of the growth plate, or generalized disease processes affecting a single growth plate.

**extremity lengthening** spontaneous lengthening after sepsis or fracture felt to be due to increased vascular nutrition to the area in response to trauma.

**eccentric growth** disorders following destruction of a portion of a growth plate when the undamaged portion continues to fulfill its functions, creating resulting deformities.

**epiphyseolysis** disorder resulting in shearing of the growth plate, usually due to trauma; does not disturb growth itself.

**swelling** enlargement of the growth plate due to generalized reaction to specific trauma or disease entities.

**exostosis** disorder of the growth plate resulting from disturbed growth function.

**faulty bone** fractures and bowing, especially of the long bones, resulting from faulty bone production by the growth plate; usually associated with a specific disease process such as osteogenesis imperfecta.

Although the effects of some of these diseases and disorders are manifested in adulthood, the disturbances occur during the growth phases. After closure of the epiphyseal growth plate, disturbances to the area will not have the overall effect about which we are so concerned in the child or adolescent. The specific disorders and deformities associated with epiphyseal growth plate destruction from various causes are shown in the following outlines. For specific data regarding injuries of the growth plate see Chapter 16.

### DISTURBANCES OF STATURE*

**I. Tall**
  A. Familial
    1. Physiologic: family or racial characteristics
    2. Pathologic: e.g., Marfan's syndrome, XYY

---

*Modified from Rang, M.: The growth plate and its disorders, Baltimore, 1969, The Williams & Wilkins Co.

  B. Overnutrition
  C. Hormonal
    1. Pituitary gigantism
    2. Precocious puberty (tall when young, but finally short)
    3. Decreased adrenal androgen secretion

**II. Short**
  A. Familial and congenital
    1. Physiologic: family or racial characteristics
    2. Pathologic
      a. Local growth plate disorders such as
        (1) Achondroplasia
        (2) Vitamin D–resistant rickets
        (3) Osteogenesis imperfecta
      b. Chromosomal
        (1) Down's syndrome (mongolism)
        (2) Turner's syndrome
      c. Intrauterine
        (1) Dysmaturity
  B. Undernutrition, malnutrition
    1. Starvation
    2. Protein deficiency (e.g., kwashiorkor)
    3. Malabsorption (e.g., celiac disease, fibrocystic disease)
  C. Hormonal
    1. Hypopituitary dwarfism
    2. Cretinism
    3. Excess cortisone
    4. Excess estrogen and adrenal androgen
  D. Cellular nutrition
    1. Hypoxia of congenital heart disease or anemia
    2. Renal disease
    3. Hepatic disease

### DISEASES AND DISORDERS MANIFESTED THROUGH POTENTIAL GROWTH PLATE DISTURBANCES[3]

**Group I** (systemic origin)
  A. Diseases and disorders of matrix
    1. Diaphyseal aclasia
    2. Hurler's syndrome
    3. Hypercalcemia
    4. Hypoparathyroidism
    5. Juvenile rheumatoid arthritis
    6. Leukemia
    7. Lupus erythematosis
    8. Marfan's syndrome
    9. Metaphyseal dysostosis
    10. Morquio's syndrome
    11. Osteogenesis imperfecta
    12. Osteopetrosis
    13. Renal osteodystrophy
    14. Rheumatoid arthritis
    15. Rickets
    16. Scurvy
  B. Chromosomal abnormalities
    1. Klinefelter's syndrome
    2. Turner's syndrome

C. Infections
  1. Congenital rubella
  2. Congenital syphilis
  3. Osteomyelitis variolosa
  4. Pyogenic osteomyelitis
  5. Tuberculosis of bone
  6. Vaccinia
  7. Varicella
D. Endocrine disturbances
E. Vitamin and nutritional deficiencies
  1. Malnutrition
F. Miscellaneous
  1. Hemaglobinopathy
  2. Phenylketonuria

**Group II** (general musculoskeletal origin)
A. Achondroplasia
B. Diaphyseal aclasia
C. Dyschondroplasia
D. Multiple epiphyseal dysplasia
E. Trevor's disease

**Group III** (local origin)
A. Diseases and disorders of part of growth plate
  1. Blount's disease
  2. Idiopathic scoliosis
  3. Madelung's deformity
  4. Tibia valga
  5. Tibia vara (adolescent form)
B. Injuries to growth plate
  1. Epiphyseal separation
  2. Fractures crossing growth plate
C. Poliomyelitis
D. Disorders of hip
  1. Congenital coxa vara
  2. Slipped capital femoral epiphysis

The effect of treatment of disorders resulting in growth plate abnormalities is greatly dependent on the specific cause and pathologic features involved. The topic is obviously much too broad to review in depth here. It should be emphasized, however, that early diagnosis of epiphyseal destruction and appropriate intervention are critical to the anticipated outcome. Assessment and evaluation of growth plate involvement for adequate judgment as to the treatment is multifaceted and extensive. Many factors such as age, sex, specific location of involved growth plate, skeletal age, and anticipated adult height are weighed heavily during this process. Specific treatment will be extremely individualized and is dependent on some of these factors as well as the degree of destruction present and anticipated. (The treatment of epiphyseal injuries is discussed in Chapter 16.) During surgical procedures, treatment of fractures, and other diseases and disorders involving children and adolescents, all efforts should be made to maintain the integrity of the growth plate.

## OSTEOPOROSIS

Osteoporosis is a normal physiologic function during the adult and elderly years resulting in increased porosity of the bone structure and cells due to gradual degeneration and a tendency to reabsorb cells faster than they are manufactured. The term *senile osteoporosis* may be used to attribute this natural and normal process to fractures or other symptomatology. Although the specific cause of this process is not known, it is felt that certain factors may assist in its acceleration: (1) limited exercise, (2) decreased concentration of blood estrogens, and (3) increased ratio of calcium to phosphorus in the blood.[1]

The increased porosity may be monitored by radiographic examination and appears as increased

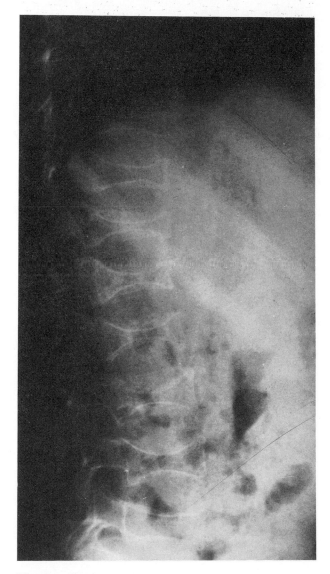

**Fig. 3-3.** Osteoporosis. Note marked collapse of vertebral bodies with biconcavity of discs.

bone density. It is most often general in nature, and despite the porosity adequate mineralization does exist. Additional features that may be noted as evidence of this process are (1) decrease in the total amount of bone, (2) trabeculae that appear thin, and (3) enlargement of marrow spaces.[2,pp.101-102] Radiographic evidence in addition to adequate history regarding diet and activity may assist in the determination of the progression of osteoporosis.

Osteoporosis is also a part of the *disuse phenomenon* related to immobilization and atrophy of musculature surrounding bone. This may be a significant factor in the elderly, who often decrease their level of activity. In any case, osteoporosis is a normal, anticipated process and is of significance only when symptoms arise.

### Relationship to injury, diseases, and disorders and their treatment

Osteoporosis of the senile form or disuse type often produces a pattern of symptomatology that includes pain induced by a specific activity such as lifting or bending. The pain is characteristically sudden in onset. When the vertebral column is involved, there may be decreased disc space apparent on radiographic examination (Fig. 3-3). Resulting deformities may ultimately lead to excessive kyphosis and loss of height. In addition osteoporosis is significant in either category when fractures result from the increased porosity, which causes the bones to be much more brittle than usual.

Specific preventive measures may be encouraged in working with both immobilized and elderly patients. Prevention of fractures may be adequately monitored and focused on through the careful handling of extremities during repositioning and other procedures. An elderly individual who shows any evidence of osteoporosis may be encouraged to be careful when ambulating on slippery surfaces or to use an ambulatory device to assist in providing stability and the prevention of fractures resulting from falls. The preventive aspects are mentioned in relation to complications resulting from osteoporosis; there is no known means to control or prevent the process itself.

The treatment of osteoporosis is not extensive beyond the preventive aspects unless symptomatology is present or a fracture has been incurred. In such cases the general health of the individual is extremely important to promote appropriate healing, although it is known that many of these persons heal very slowly. Encouragement of appropriate diet, increased calcium intake, and supplementary vitamin D may be advantageous. Appropriate treatment of the fracture through immobilization with cast or traction or through surgical intervention should be accomplished as usual but with anticipated increase in healing time.

### REFERENCES

1. Anthony, C. P., and Thibodeau, G. A.: Textbook of anatomy and physiology, ed. 10, St. Louis, 1979, The C. V. Mosby Co.
2. Brashear, H. R., Jr., and Raney, R. B., Sr.: Shands' handbook of orthopaedic surgery, ed. 9, St. Louis, 1978, The C. V. Mosby Co.
3. Rang, M.: The growth plate and its disorders, Baltimore, 1969, The Williams & Wilkins Co.

### BIBLIOGRAPHY

Adams, J. C.: Outline of orthopaedics, Baltimore, 1971, The Williams & Wilkins Co.

Aegertu, E., and Kirkpatrick, J.: Orthopedic diseases, Philadelphia, 1975, W. B. Saunders Co.

Anthony, C. P., and Thibodeau, G. A.: Textbook of anatomy and physiology, ed. 10, St. Louis, 1979, The C. V. Mosby Co.

Gardner, W., and Osburn, W.: Structure of the human body, Philadelphia, 1973, W. B. Saunders Co.

Gartland, J. J.: Fundamentals of orthopaedics, Philadelphia, 1974, W. B. Saunders Co.

Brashear, H. R., Jr., and Raney, R. B., Sr.: Shands' handbook of orthopaedic surgery, ed. 9, St. Louis, 1978, The C. V. Mosby Co.

Rang, M.: The growth plate and its disorders, Baltimore, 1969, The Williams & Wilkins Co.

Tachdjian, M. O.: Pediatric orthopedics, Philadelphia, 1962, W. B. Saunders Co.

# 4

# Motion

**LARRY F. ANDREWS**

*Motion* may be defined as a continuing change of place or position. To facilitate understanding of the process of motion, it may be divided into two areas: *kinematics* and *kinetics*.

## KINEMATICS

Kinematics has been defined as the geometry of motion without regard to forces acting to produce the motion. It deals with the description, measurement, and means of recording bodily motion. To comprehend its scope, it is helpful to view the three-dimensional system of motion. The body is divided into three perpendicular planes (Fig. 4-1), used as the basis for describing the motions that take place. The *cardinal sagittal*, often called the midsagittal plane, divides the body into left and right sides. The *cardinal frontal*, or vertical plane, divides the body into front and back. The third plane, the *cardinal horizontal*, or transverse plane, divides the body into upper and lower portions.[3,pp.1-2] Motions and their recordings are defined in one-plane relation-

ships. Natural motions, however, often occur in more than one plane.

It is not necessary to define anatomic position used as a basis for motion recording, since motions and parts are relative to segments and not to anatomic position. For example, the fingers move in relation to the midline of the hand and not the midline of the body. This concept is basic to the understanding of the dimensions of motion.

Terminology specific to the topic of motion and kinematics should be familiar to all health care personnel involved in patient care. The following are the most common motions:

**flexion** motion involving decrease of angle at a joint between two bones.
**extension** opposite of flexion; increase of the angle of the joint between two bones.
**adduction** motion in which a part moves toward a defined line (e.g., midline of the body).
**abduction** opposite of adduction; motion in which a part moves away from a defined line.
**internal rotation** transverse turning toward the anterior side of the body; inward rotation.
**external rotation** transverse turning toward the posterior side of the body; outward rotation.

Flexion and extension usually take place in the sagittal plane, abduction and adduction take place in the frontal plane, and internal and external rotation take place in the transverse plane.

## KINETICS

Kinetics deals with the forces that produce, arrest, or modify motions of the body.[3,p.13] Newton has described these motions through several laws. Two that apply here are his *first law of inertia*, which states that bodies at rest tend to remain at rest and that bodies in motion tend to remain in motion, and his *third law*, which states that action and reaction are equal in magnitude but opposite in direction. Muscle forces that act on the joints are applicable to Newton's laws. The reaction forces of muscles contribute to equilibrium and motion.

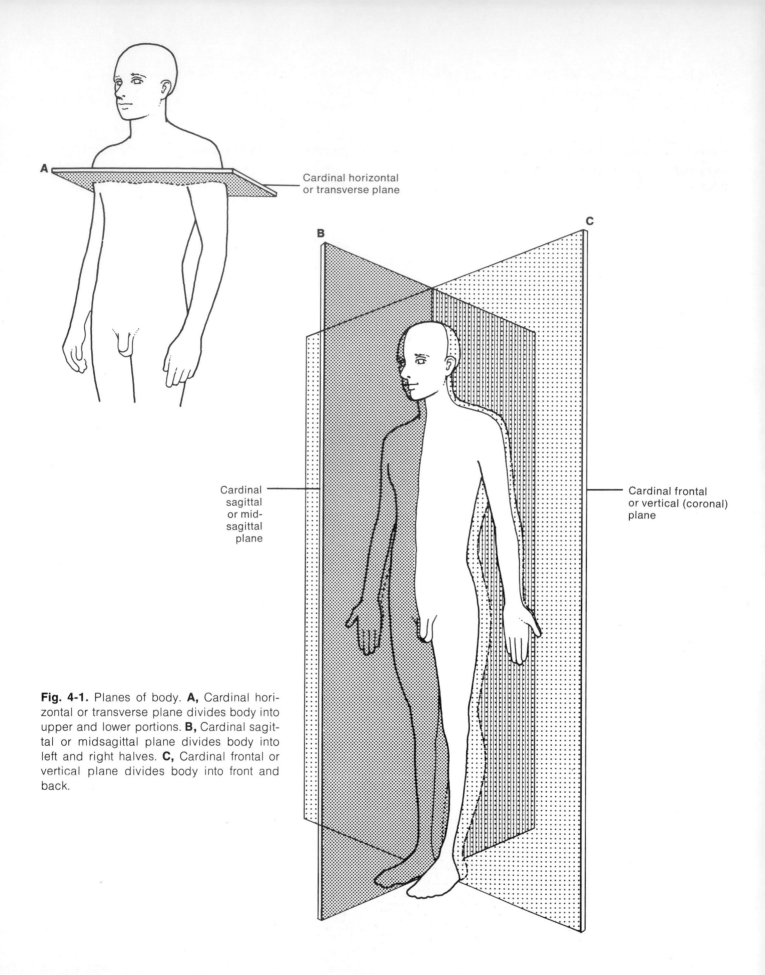

Cardinal horizontal
or transverse plane

Cardinal
sagittal
or mid-
sagittal
plane

Cardinal frontal
or vertical (coronal)
plane

**Fig. 4-1.** Planes of body. **A,** Cardinal horizontal or transverse plane divides body into upper and lower portions. **B,** Cardinal sagittal or midsagittal plane divides body into left and right halves. **C,** Cardinal frontal or vertical plane divides body into front and back.

Within the scope of understanding joints and their motion, it is necessary to deal briefly with leverage. A lever is a means by which a motion takes place more efficiently. There are four basic components to levers. The *fulcrum,* or center of motion, is the fixed point or axis on which the lever pivots. The *force arm* is the perpendicular distance from the fulcrum to the line of action of the force. The *weight arm,* or resistance arm, is the perpendicular distance from the fulcrum to the line of action of the weight. *Moment of force,* or torque, is the product of the force and its force arm or the product of the weight and the weight arm.

Levers are commonly divided into first, second, and third classes. First-class levers are represented by a seesaw with the fulcrum between the weight and the force (e.g., the hip).

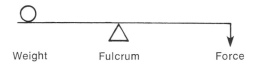

Weight      Fulcrum      Force

In second-class levers the weight lies between the fulcrum and the force. The force arm is always longer than the weight arm, and the mechanical advantage results for the force (e.g., a wheelbarrow). Second-class levers are rarely found in the body.

With third-class levers the force is between the fulcrum and the weight. Such levers are found at all joints of the upper and lower extremities (e.g., the biceps acting over the elbow joint).

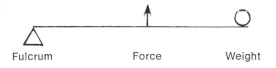

Fulcrum      Force      Weight

Levers are used for either force or speed. Third-class levers are used for speed. First-class levers may be used either to gain force or speed depending on the relative length of the force on the weight arm. The key to remember is that with a lever you either lose force and gain speed or you lose speed and gain force.

In solving problems of leverage in the body, the moment of force produced by the weight of the body part is a consideration. This can be determined if the center of gravity of the part is known, since the weight of the body is concentrated at the center of gravity. This is made simpler by the fact that the force of gravity is always vertical. Charts available in several references list the center of gravity of various body parts (e.g., Brunnstrom, S.: Clinical Kinesiology, Chapter 10).

Often in the body there are areas where two parallel forces equal in magnitude but opposite in direction act on different points away from each other. This is commonly called a force couple.

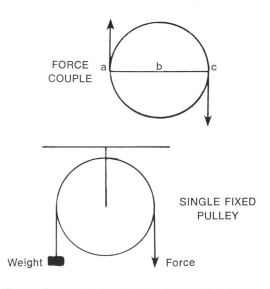

All rotations about a joint axis require the action of couples. Also represented in the body is the single fixed pulley. The line of action by single fixed pulley is upward and the force is downward. An example of this is the patellar tendon. The quadriceps normally changes its direction of pull as a result of interposed patella, but its leverage also improves.

Work equals force times distance. Energy may be expended without work being performed, such as in an isometric contraction. Fick computed the work capacity of the individual muscles of the extremities by comparing the work capacity of one muscle with that of another to obtain an approximate idea of the relative importance of each muscle for particular movement. For example, Fick's tables show that the internal rotator of the shoulder, the subscapularis, has about five times as much work capacity as the teres major.[3,pp.17-21,24,25,27,28]

In this chapter the joints of the body are examined, their motions are determined, their muscles and bony segments are listed, and they are recorded by measurement. It is important to remember that measurements should involve the comparison, if possible, of right and left sides of the body. For example, when measuring right knee flexion, the left knee should be measured also to help determine normal motion for the individual.

The *goniometer* is the instrument used to ensure that joint measurement is more accurate with each repetition of measurement recorded. The axis of measurement is perpendicular to the plane of motion, while the goniometer arm moves in the plane of motion. For example, the axis of motion for measurement of the cervical spine in flexion and extension is in the vertical plane, whereas the motion takes place in its perpendicular plane or its midsagittal plane. When measuring with the goniometer it is important to use the same points of reference each time you measure. Also, if the same person or persons consistently perform the measurements, they are more likely to be accurate.

## SPECIFIC JOINT MOTION
### Cervical spine

The major motions of the cervical spine are those of flexion and extension, lateral bending, and rotation (Fig. 4-2). Table 4-1 lists the muscles used in these motions.

Cervical motion is usually measured by comparison of right and left sides, as previously stated. Flexion and extension in the cervical spine are measured by placement of the goniometric axis at the level of the C-1 vertebral body with the stationary arm parallel with the coronal suture, or external auditory meatus. The stationary arm remains vertical, while the movement arm moves with the reference point as flexion and extension are recorded. Normal cervical flexion and extension combined are 90°. With lateral bending the superior nuchal line is used as the axis of motion. The midsagittal suture is used as the reference point for the stationary arm. As right and left flexion take place, the movement arm remains parallel with the suture and the stationary arm remains vertical.

Cervical rotation involves movements to the right and left, with placement of the axis of the goniometer where the coronal and sagittal sutures intersect. The stationary arm is parallel with the sagittal suture, or when viewed from the above the subject's head, the stationary arm remains perpendicular to the trunk, superimposed on the nose. The movement arm moves over the sagittal suture at combined range of approximately 120°.

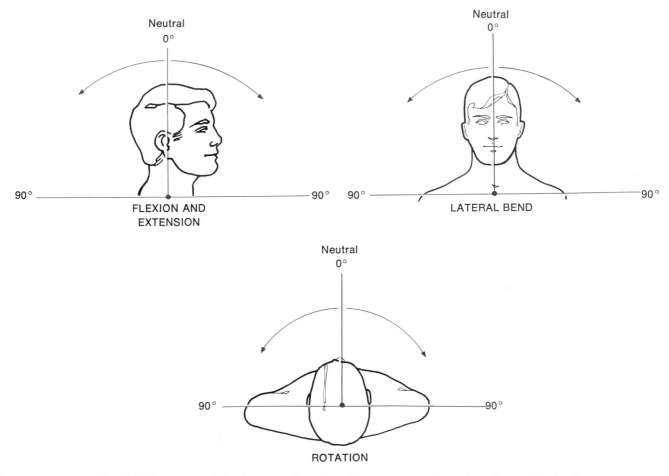

**Fig. 4-2.** Cervical vertebral range of motion. (Redrawn from Committee for the Study of Joint Motion: Joint motion: method of measuring and recording, Chicago, 1965, American Academy of Orthopaedic Surgeons.)

**Table 4-1.** Muscles used in specific motions

| Joint | Muscle(s) | Maximum degrees* |
|---|---|---|
| **Elbow** | | |
| Flexion | Biceps, brachialis, brachioradialis | 150 |
| Hyperextension | Triceps, anconeus (pectoralis major) | |
| **Forearm** | | |
| Pronation | Pronator teres, pronator quadratus | 80 |
| Supination | Biceps supinator (brachioradialis) | 80 |
| **Wrist** | | |
| Extension | Extensor digitorum communis with finger extension | 70 |
| | Extensor carpi ulnaris | |
| | Extensor carpi radialis brevis | |
| Flexion | Palmaris longus, flexor carpi radialis, flexor carpi ulnaris, flexor digitorum superficialis | 80 |
| Ulnar deviation | Extensor carpi ulnaris, flexor carpi ulnaris | 30 |
| Radial deviation | Extensor carpi radialis longus, flexor carpi radialis (abductor pollicis longus, extensor pollicis brevis) | 20 |
| **Thumb** | | |
| Abduction | Abductor pollicis longus, extensor pollicis brevis, abductor pollicis brevis | 70 |
| Flexion | | |
|   IP | Flexor pollicis longus | 80 |
|   MP | Flexor pollicis brevis, flexor pollicis longus | 50 |
|   MC | | 15 |
| Extension | | |
|   IP | Extensor pollicis longus (thenar muscles) | 20 |
|   MP | Extensor pollicis brevis, extensor pollicis | 0 |
|   MC | | |
| **Fingers** | | |
| Flexion | | |
|   Distal | Flexor digitorum profundus | 90 |
|   Middle | Flexor digitorum superficialis (2-5) | 100 |
|   Proximal | Lumbricales (with IP extended) | 90 |
| | Interossei (flexor digitorum superficialis assists) | |
| Extension | | |
|   Distal | Lumbricales, extensor digitorum superficialis | 0 |
|   Middle | Lumbricales, extensor digitorum superficialis | 0 |
|   Proximal | Extensor digitorum | 45 |
| Adduction | Interossei palmares (index, ring, little finger) | |
| Abduction | Interossei dorsales (2,3,4) | |
| | Abductor digiti minimi (5) | |
| **Shoulder** | | |
| Forward flexion | Deltoid (anterior and middle), supraspinatus (to 90°, clavicular pectoralis major coracobrachialis, biceps brachii) | 180 |
| Horizontal abduction | Deltoid pectoralis major | 135 |
| Extension | Latissimus doris, teres major, pectoralis major, posterior deltoid, long head triceps | 60 |
| Adduction | Latissimus dorsi, teres major, pectoralis major, posterior deltoid, long head triceps | 75 |
| Hyperextension | Posterior deltoid | |
| Abduction | Deltoid supraspinatus (long head triceps with external rotation) | 180 |

*Adapted from Committee on Joint Motion, American Academy of Orthopaedic Surgeons, 1965.

*Continued.*

**Table 4-1.** Muscles used in specific motions—cont'd

| Joint | Muscle(s) | Maximum degrees |
|---|---|---|
| **Shoulder—cont'd** | | |
| Rotation, arm at side | | |
|   Internal | Subscapularis, teres major, latissimus dorsi, pectoralis major, anterior deltoid | 80 |
|   External | Infraspinatus, teres minor, posterior deltoid | 60 |
| Rotation, arm in 90° abduction | | |
|   Internal | | 70 |
|   External | | 90 |
| **Hip** | | |
| Flexion | Iliopsoas, pectineus, tensor fasciae latae, sartorius, rectus femoris | 120 |
| Extension | Gluteus maximus, hamstrings, adductor magnus | 30 |
| Abduction | Gluteus medius and minimus, periformis | 45 |
| Adduction | Adductor magnus and longus, gracilis, brevis pectineus | 30 |
| Rotation in flexion | | |
|   Internal | Anteroposterior gluteus medius and minimus (in extension, adductors help) | 45 |
|   External | Piriformis, quadratus femoris, gemellus superior and inferior, obturator internus and externus | 45 |
| Rotation in abduction, 90° flexion | Dependent on age | 45-60 |
| **Knee** | | |
| Flexion | Hamstrings (gastrocnemius, gracilis, sartorius) | 135 |
| Extension | Quadriceps (tensor fasciae latae helps hold in extension) | 10 |
| Internal rotation of tibia | Medial hamstrings, gracilis, popliteus | |
| External rotation | Biceps femoris, tensor fasciae latae | |
| **Ankle** | | |
| Flexion (plantar) | Gastrocnemius, soleus | 50 |
| Hyperextension (dorsi) | Tibialis anterior | 20 |
| **Hind foot** (subtalar) | | |
| Inversion | Tibialis posterior | 5 |
| Eversion | Peroneus brevis and longus | 5 |
| **Forefoot** | | |
| Inversion | Tibialis posterior | 35 |
| Eversion | Peroneus longus and brevis | 15 |
| **Toes** | | |
| Great toe (interphalangeal) | | |
|   Flexion | Flexor hallucis longus | 90 |
|   Extension | Extensor hallucis longus | 0 |
| Great toe (proximal joint) | | |
|   Flexion | Flexor hallucis longus | 45 |
|   Extension | Extensor hallucis longus | 70 |
| Toes 2 to 5 | | |
|   Flexion (distal, middle, proximal) | Flexor digitorum longus and brevis | 60 35 40 |
|   Extension | Extensor digitorum longus and brevis | 40 |
| Lumbricales and interossei have similar function to that of hand | | |
| **Spine** | | |
| Cervical | | |
|   Flexion | Scalene (Bilateral rectus capitis, anterior longus capitis, longus colli) | 45 |

**Table 4-1.** Muscles used in specific motions — cont'd

| Joint | Muscle(s) | Maximum degrees |
|---|---|---|
| **Spine — cont'd** | | |
| Extension | Suboccipital, longissimus capitis, semispinalis capitis and cervicis | 45 |
| Lateral bending | Scalene, sternomastoid | 45 |
| Rotation | Sternomastoid | 60 |
| Thoracic and lumbar | | |
| Flexion | Rectus abdominis, obliques | 80 (4″) |
| Extension (hyper) | Erector spinae | 20-30 |
| Lateral bending | Quadratus lumborum | 35 |
| Rotation | External and internal obliques | 45 |

Limitations of the cervical spine in the extremely young often involve contracture of the sternocleidomastoid muscle. This is commonly called wryneck or torticollis. Often present at birth, it may be corrected either surgically or with passive stretching. Later in life ankylosis of the cervical spine involves degeneration of the discs, which may result in cervical limitations and pain.

### Lumbar dorsal spine

Lumbar dorsal mobility is a combined motion of the lumbar and thoracic spines involving flexion, extension, lateral bending, and rotation. Muscles involved in these actions are listed in Table 4-1. Flexion and extension of the lumbar spine may be measured by placement of the goniometric axis at the level of the hips, or lumbosacral junction. The stationary arm remains vertical, while the movement arm is parallel with the trunk. Forward bending may also be measured by recording the distance of the subject's fingers from the floor. Lateral bending may be measured by placement of the goniometric axis at the L-4 to L-5 level. The stationary arm is parallel with the posterior spinous processes and remains vertical, while the movement arm moves in reference to the spinous processes. Movement from the erect vertical position of the trunk to that of the extreme of extension is often called hyperextension and involves an extreme increase in what is commonly called swayback or lumbar lordosis. Stabilization of the pelvis is necessary to measure true motion of the lumbar spine.

The range of vertebral motion in the spine is determined by the resistance of the discs to distortion and the angular size of the articular surfaces between the processes. Motion is greatest in the lumbar region where the discs are thickest and joint surfaces are largest. Therefore motion at the L5 to S1 disc space is greatest, followed by the L4-5. Due to the anterior and posterior relationship of the facets and no restraint of ribs, flexion and extension of the spine take place mainly in the lumbar region. Rotation is theoretically possible but limited in the lumbar spine due to the tightening effect of the surrounding ligaments and annulous fibers of the disc; therefore an illustration of its recording is not given here.

Lumbar flexion (Fig. 4-3, *A*) primarily involves the hips. This can be demonstrated by the fact that spinal fusions usually do not affect significantly the mobility of forward bending. Forward bending usually involves motion of the hips and reversal of the lumbar lordosis. For example, forward flexion involves relaxation of the anterior longitudinal ligament and stretching of the supraspinal ligament, the flaval ligament, and the posterior longitudinal ligament. Extension stretches the anterior ligament, contracts the posterior spinal muscles, and relaxes the rectus abdominis muscle.

### Hip

The motions of the hip are flexion and extension, internal and external rotation in flexion and extension, and abduction and adduction. The muscles involved in hip motion are divided into four groups. The anterior muscles flex the hip; the lateral muscles abduct the hip; the posterior muscles extend the hip; and the medial muscles adduct the hip. The function of these muscles varies according to the amount of flexion in the hip. For example, the gluteal muscle may be a flexor if the hip is at 90° or an abductor when the hip is in extension.

Fig. 4-4 shows the motions of the hip. Measurement of hip flexion involves placement of the goniometer axis at the greater trochanter with the movement arm parallel to the shaft of the femur, using the greater trochanter and femoral epicondyle as the bony landmarks. The stationary arm remains

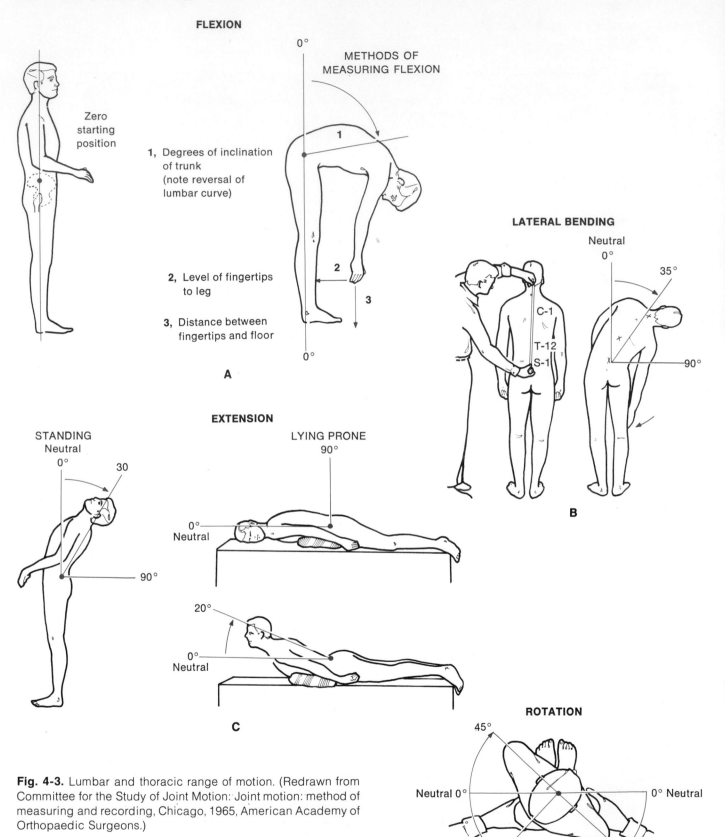

**FLEXION**

0°

METHODS OF
MEASURING FLEXION

**1,** Degrees of inclination
of trunk
(note reversal of
lumbar curve)

**2,** Level of fingertips
to leg

**3,** Distance between
fingertips and floor

0°

Zero
starting
position

A

**LATERAL BENDING**

Neutral
0°

35°

C-1

T-12

S-1

90°

B

**EXTENSION**

STANDING
Neutral
0°      30

90°

LYING PRONE
90°

0°
Neutral

20°

0°
Neutral

C

**ROTATION**

45°

Neutral 0°

0° Neutral

45°      45°

D

**Fig. 4-3.** Lumbar and thoracic range of motion. (Redrawn from
Committee for the Study of Joint Motion: Joint motion: method of
measuring and recording, Chicago, 1965, American Academy of
Orthopaedic Surgeons.)

**FLEXION**

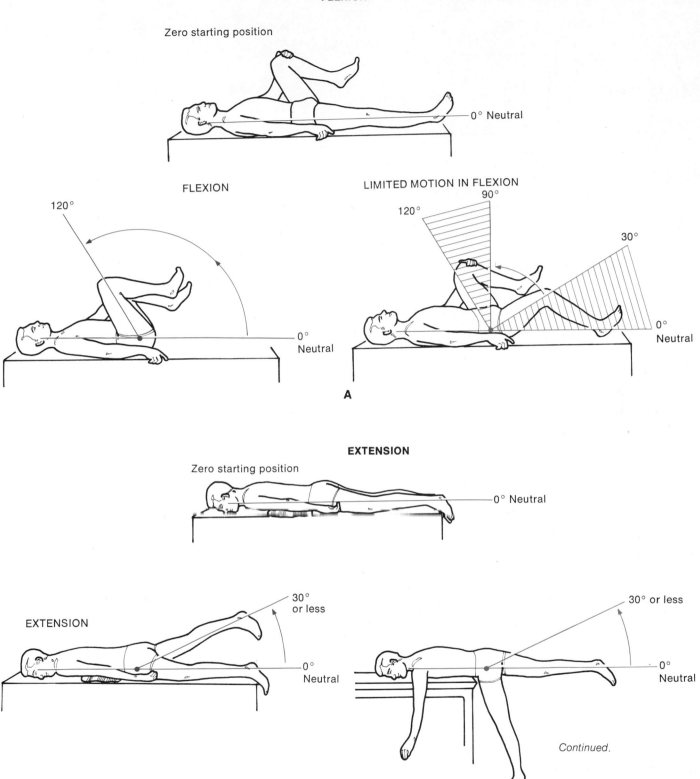

Zero starting position

0° Neutral

FLEXION

120°

0° Neutral

LIMITED MOTION IN FLEXION

90°

120°

30°

0° Neutral

**A**

**EXTENSION**

Zero starting position

0° Neutral

EXTENSION

30° or less

0° Neutral

30° or less

0° Neutral

*Continued.*

**B**

**Fig. 4-4.** Hip range of motion. (Redrawn from Committee for the Study of Joint Motion: Joint motion: method of measuring and recording, Chicago, 1965, American Academy of Orthopaedic Surgeons.)

**ROTATION**

ROTATION IN FLEXION

ROTATION IN EXTENSION

**Prone**

**Supine**

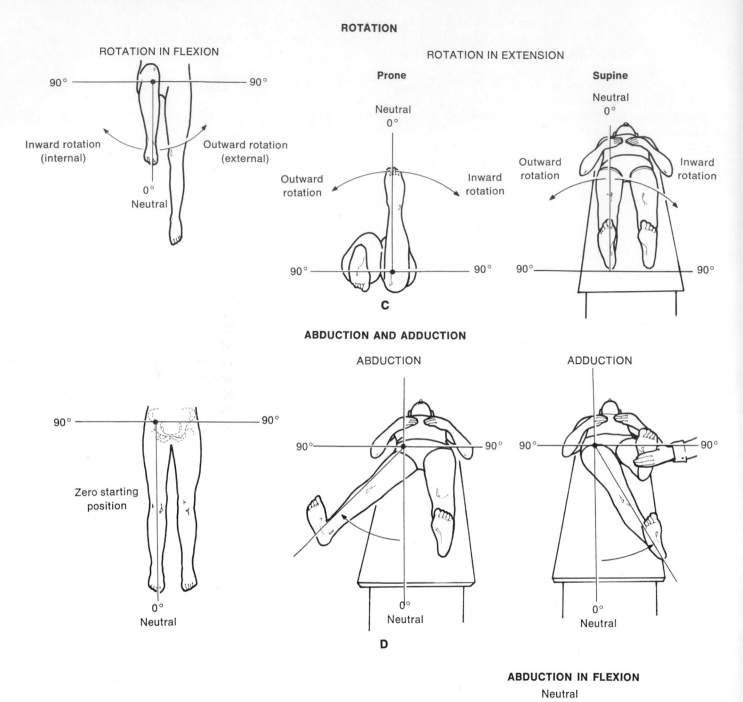

90°        90°

Inward rotation (internal)

Outward rotation (external)

0°
Neutral

Neutral
0°

Outward rotation

Inward rotation

90°       90°

**C**

Neutral
0°

Outward rotation

Inward rotation

90°       90°

**ABDUCTION AND ADDUCTION**

ABDUCTION

ADDUCTION

90°       90°

Zero starting position

0°
Neutral

90°       90°

0°
Neutral

90°       90°

0°
Neutral

**D**

**Fig. 4-4, cont'd.** Hip range of motion.

**ABDUCTION IN FLEXION**

Neutral
0°

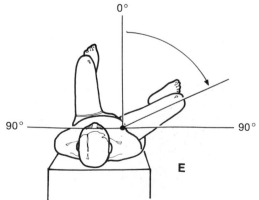

90°       90°

**E**

parallel with the trunk. The knee should be flexed to allow the hamstrings to relax. Extension of the hip involves the same bony landmarks. However, the patient is prone and the knee is extended to relax the rectus femoris muscle. Abduction and adduction of the hip are measured by placement of the goniometric axis on the anterior superior iliac spine. The stationary arm is parallel to the trunk, and the movement arm is parallel to the midshaft of the femur in line with the midpatella. In order to obtain a true measurement of adduction, the uninvolved hip is flexed to allow passage of the involved leg beyond the midline. It is wise to use two examiners when measuring hip abduction and adduction, one to perform the goniometric measurement and the other to stabilize the pelvis. An increase in lateral pelvic motion gives a false measurement.

Internal and external rotation may be measured with the hip in full extension or in 90° of flexion. In full extension the goniometric axis is placed parallel to the midshaft of the tibia or at midheel. The stationary arm remains vertical, while the movement arm moves with the midplantar surface of the foot. In flexion the patient is usually sitting. The axis is placed parallel to the midshaft of the femur. The stationary arm remains vertical, while the movement arm moves parallel with the midshaft of the tibia.

Two common tests involving musculature around the hip joint are the Thomas test and Trendelenburg's sign. The Thomas test is the test for tight hip flexion contractures (Fig. 4-4, A). With the patient supine, the uninvolved leg is flexed toward the chest until the lumbar spine is flat. The degree of hip flexion of the uninvolved leg is measured with the goniometer and recorded. The second test, which is very common in determining hip abductor weakness, is Trendelenburg's sign. The patient is asked to stand by the examiner, who places both hands on the iliac crest. The patient is then asked to lift the uninvolved leg while standing on the involved leg. If he has sufficient abductor strength, the hips will remain level. Thus the test results will be considered negative. If there is sufficient abductor weakness, the patient will compensate by learning over the involved leg. Thus the test results will be considered positive.

In his 1956 presidential address to the American Academy of Orthopaedic Surgeons, Blount stated the importance of the use of a cane in decreasing hip joint stress, and this may also be applied to reduction of hip abductor weakness. The upward pressure of the cane used in the upper extremity opposite the involved hip decreases the stress on the hip while also maintaining a level pelvic motion with stance phase of the involved extremity.[2,pp.695-708]

### Shoulder

Movement of the shoulder involves a combination of scapulohumeral motion about the axial skeleton. This motion is highly mobile, as illustrated in Fig. 4-5, A. Its motion takes place in three planes. The main motions of the shoulder are flexion and extension, abduction and adduction, external and internal rotation, and horizontal abduction and adduction. Fig. 4-5, B depicts the goniometric measurement of shoulder abduction and adduction. The goniometric axis is placed on the coracoid process. The stationary arm remains parallel to the trunk, while the movement arm is parallel to the midshaft of the humerus.

When measuring shoulder flexion (Fig. 4-5, B), the patient is supine. The goniometric axis is placed inferior to the tip of the acromion process on the lateral surface of the deltoid region of the shoulder. The stationary arm is parallel with the trunk, while the movement arm is parallel with the humerus. Extension or hyperextension is determined with the patient prone, using the same main reference points as in shoulder flexion. Internal and external rotation are measured with the patient supine. The humerus is in 90° of abduction, the elbow is flexed to 90°, and the axis is placed on the epicondyle; that is, it runs parallel with the midshaft of the humerus, and the movement arm is parallel with the midshaft of the forearm. The stationary arm remains vertical. External rotation may also be measured with the upper arm parallel to the trunk. When measuring shoulder motion the shoulders should be stabilized so that they remain level, or flat, as in the supine position. A good goniometric measurement often requires two examiners.

The most common limitation of shoulder motion involves a tear in the rotator cuff musculature and usually develops into further problems such as adhesive capsulitis. The classic "frozen shoulder syndrome" actually involves multiple problems, with the main limitations being lack of external rotation, shoulder flexion, and often internal rotation. A classic exercise in the area of the shoulder has been described by Codman (Codman's shoulder exercise or pendulum exercise[4,p.45]). It involves the mobilization of the humeral head and the glenoid fossae with maximum relaxation of the shoulder musculature. The patient leans forward (90°-90° position of trunk) while resting his head on the uninvolved upper extremity, which is placed on the back of a chair. The involved upper extremity is allowed to

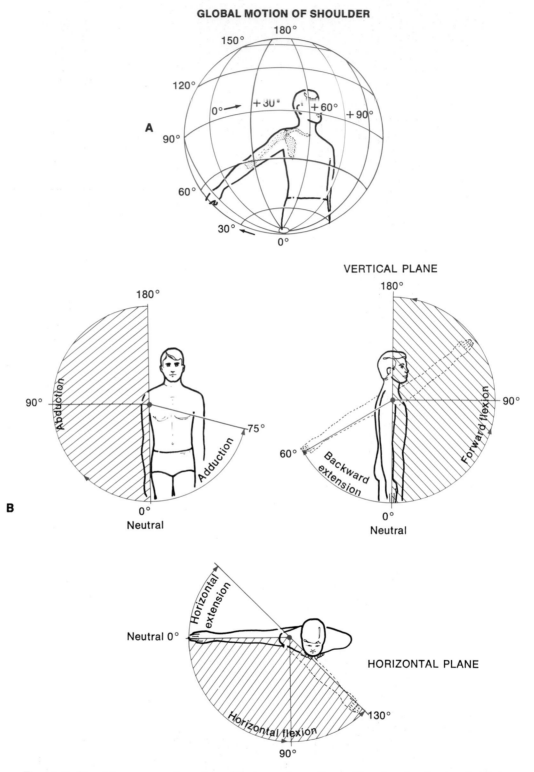

**Fig. 4-5.** Shoulder range of motion. (Redrawn from Committee for the Study of Joint Motion: Joint motion: method of measuring and recording, Chicago, 1965, American Academy of Orthopaedic Surgeons.)

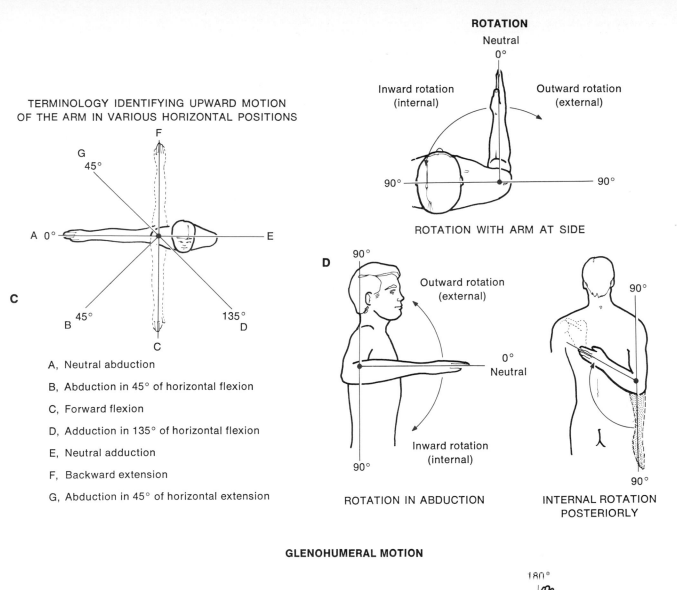

## TERMINOLOGY IDENTIFYING UPWARD MOTION OF THE ARM IN VARIOUS HORIZONTAL POSITIONS

A, Neutral abduction

B, Abduction in 45° of horizontal flexion

C, Forward flexion

D, Adduction in 135° of horizontal flexion

E, Neutral adduction

F, Backward extension

G, Abduction in 45° of horizontal extension

**ROTATION**

Neutral
0°

Inward rotation (internal)     Outward rotation (external)

90°     90°

ROTATION WITH ARM AT SIDE

**D**

90°

Outward rotation (external)

0° Neutral

Inward rotation (internal)

90°

ROTATION IN ABDUCTION

90°

90°

INTERNAL ROTATION POSTERIORLY

## GLENOHUMERAL MOTION

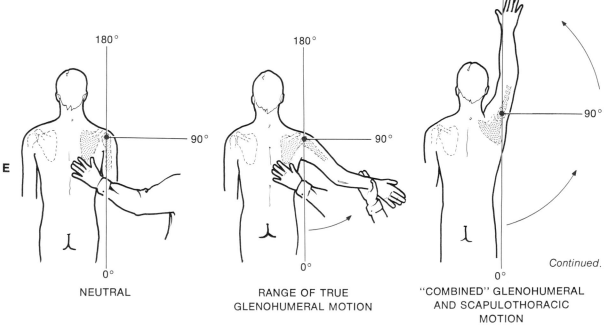

**E**

NEUTRAL

RANGE OF TRUE GLENOHUMERAL MOTION

"COMBINED" GLENOHUMERAL AND SCAPULOTHORACIC MOTION

*Continued.*

**Fig. 4-5, cont'd.** Shoulder range of motion.

**MOTION OF SHOULDER GIRDLE**

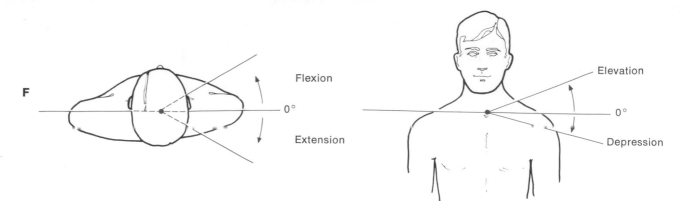

Fig. 4-5, cont'd. Shoulder range of motion.

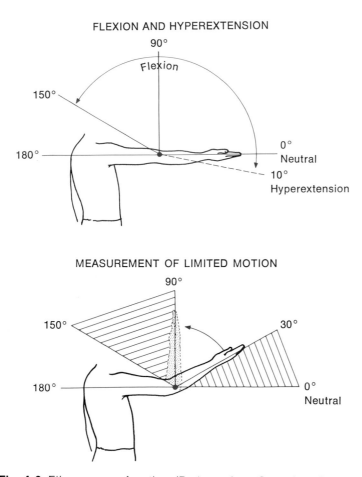

**Fig. 4-6.** Elbow range of motion. (Redrawn from Committee for the Study of Joint Motion: Joint motion: method of measuring and recording, Chicago, 1965, American Academy of Orthopaedic Surgeons.)

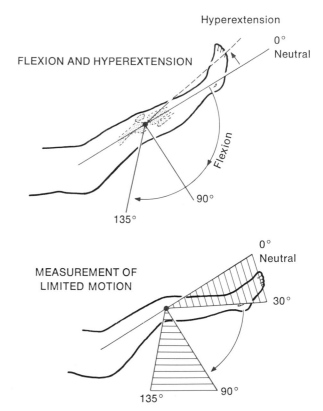

**Fig. 4-7.** Knee range of motion. (Redrawn from Committee for the Study of Joint Motion: Joint motion: method of measuring and recording, Chicago, 1965, American Academy of Orthopaedic Surgeons.)

dangle perpendicular to the trunk, and by moving the trunk backward or forward and from side to side the upper extremity begins to move, like a pendulum.

### Elbow

Elbow motion should be measured with the patient supine. The goniometric axis is placed at the lateral epicondyle of the humerus. The stationary arm is placed parallel to the humerus, with the movement arm parallel to the radius (Fig. 4-6).

The muscles and muscular actions of the elbow are listed in Table 4-1. It is interesting to note that the extensors and flexors of the forearm, along with the pronators and supinators, vary in strength dependent on their cross section. The larger its cross section, the more powerful the muscle. The biceps has the largest cross section, and it is the most effective as a supinator when the elbow is flexed at an angle of 90°. However, the effectiveness of the supinator muscle is not influenced by the elbow angle. At an angle of 90° the biceps is almost four times as effective as the supinator; when in extension it is only twice as effective. The pronator teres is the strongest of the pronators, and the triceps is the most powerful extensor of the elbow. Limitations of elbow mobility may be due to contractures, such as shortening of the biceps secondary to "frozen shoulder syndrome," spasticity due to stroke, brachial plexis injury, or other pathology.

### Knee

The knee is mainly involved in flexion and extension (Fig. 4-7). Rotation of the tibia on the femur also occurs, and this rotation is important in ambulation. Goniometric measurement of the knee is determined by placement of the stationary arm parallel with the lateral shaft of the femur, using the greater trochanter and lateral femoral condyles as reference points or bony landmarks. The movement arm is parallel with the shaft of the fibula, using the fibular head and lateral malleolus as the bony landmarks.

The main power muscles of knee mobility are the quadriceps and hamstrings. The most important muscles to be strengthened when the knee is damaged are the quadriceps. In determining good quadriceps contraction, palpation of the patella is necessary to determine its immobilization by the patellar tendon. Straight leg raising may be performed without a true significant quadriceps contraction, especially of the vastus medialis. Isometric quadriceps strengthening is beneficial in that it increases quadriceps strength in full extension with minimal de-

generation of the knee joint. One condition that may restrict knee motion and function is a torn meniscus. This is usually evidenced by locking or giving way of the knee. A controversy still continues as to the benefit of the meniscus in preventing degenerative arthritis between the femoral condyles and tibial plateaus. Injury often occurs on the athletic field but also may occur with the process of arthritis. At some time in the patient's life internal repair or implantation may be necessary to replace the worn out joint.

The knee is discussed here in its simplicity. However, the knee is a very complex joint, not only in its structure but in its mobility (see Chapter 1).

### Ankle and foot

The common motions of the ankle (Fig. 4-8) are those of plantar flexion and dorsiflexion, plantar flexion being approximately 2½ times that of dorsiflexion, and inversion (movement toward the midline of the body) and eversion (movement away from the midline) of the foot. The muscles involved in flexion and extension of the forefoot (metatarsals and phalanges) and the hindfoot (calcaneus and talus) are listed in Table 4-1. Motions of the distal portions of the foot, that is, the phalangeal joints (Fig. 4-9), are not discussed here as their measurement is similar to that of the phalanges of the hand.

Muscles involved around the ankle are divided into posterior, anterior, and lateral compartments. The posterior compartment muscles are involved with plantar flexion and inversion. The lateral compartment muscles, which are separated from the anterior and posterior compartments by intermuscular septum, are composed of the peroneal musculature. These muscles run laterally and are essential for protecting ankle stability, helping to prevent sprained ankle. The anterior compartment is made up principally of the tibialis anterior, which is so often involved in patients with cerebrovascular accident, anterior compartment syndrome, or peroneal nerve palsy. Goniometric measurement of the ankle involves use of the lateral and medial malleoli as axes. The stationary arm remains vertical or may be parallel to the midshaft of the fibula, while the movement arm remains parallel with the fifth metatarsal.

Limitations of the foot and ankle are usually involved in such conditions as cerebral palsy and hemiplegia or triplegia. If the tibialis anterior muscle is weak, the gastrocnemius and soleus muscles shorten, thus limiting the mobility of the ankle. Weakness of the tibialis anterior muscle also allows footdrop, common in the stroke patient, while

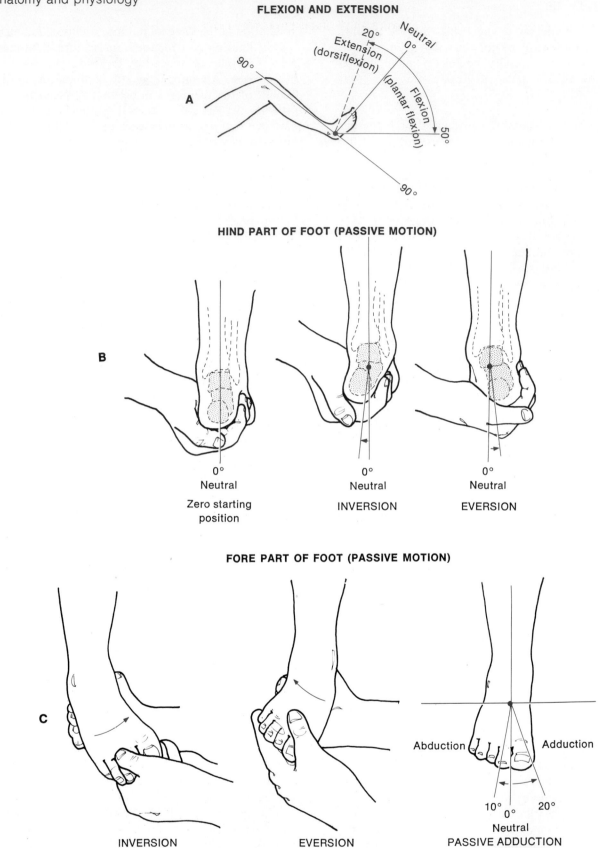

**Fig. 4-8.** Ankle range of motion.

## FORE PART OF FOOT (ACTIVE MOTION)

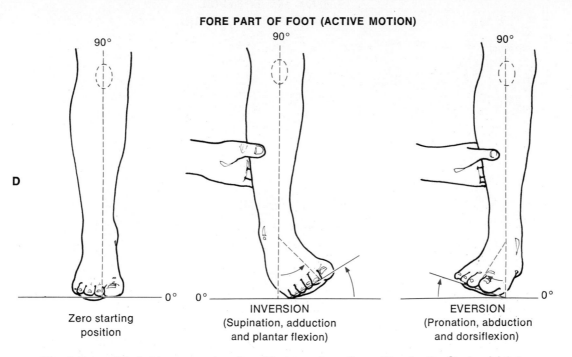

D

Zero starting
position

INVERSION
(Supination, adduction
and plantar flexion)

EVERSION
(Pronation, abduction
and dorsiflexion)

**Fig. 4-8, cont'd.** Ankle range of motion. (Redrawn from Committee for the Study of Joint Motion: Joint motion: method of measuring and recording, Chicago, 1965, American Academy of Orthopaedic Surgeons.)

## GREAT TOE

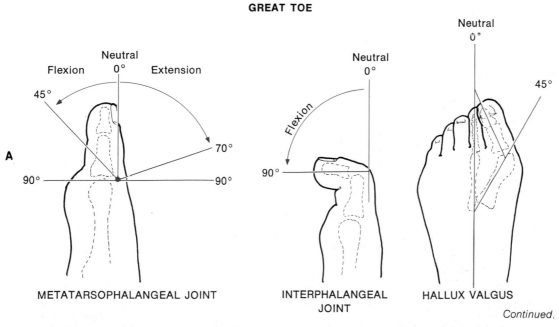

A

METATARSOPHALANGEAL JOINT

INTERPHALANGEAL
JOINT

HALLUX VALGUS

*Continued.*

**Fig. 4-9.** Toe range of motion. (Redrawn from Committee for the Study of Joint Motion: Joint motion: method of measuring and recording, Chicago, 1965, American Academy of Orthopaedic Surgeons.)

**TOES (SECOND TO FIFTH TOES)**

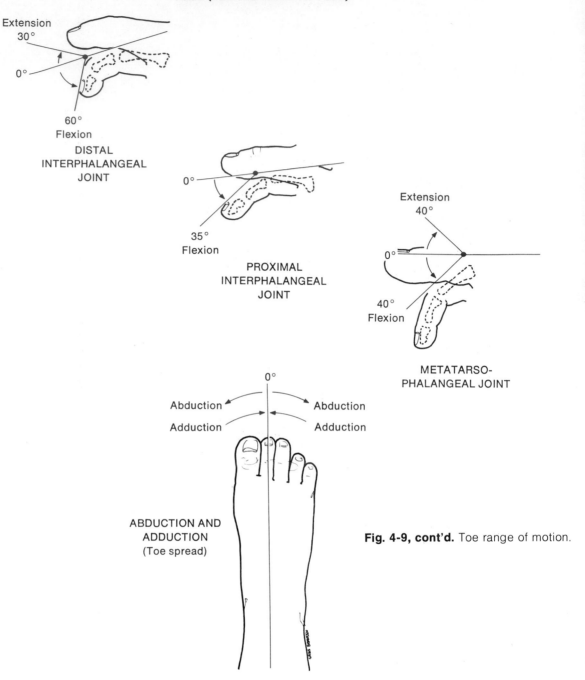

**Fig. 4-9, cont'd.** Toe range of motion.

weakness of the peroneal musculature allows the foot to become inverted or pronated. Weakness in the soleus muscle may result in genu recurvatum (abnormal hyperextensibility of the knee joint).

### Wrist and hand

The movements of the forearm are included with movements of the wrist and hand (Figs. 4-10 and 4-11). Movement of the radius over the ulna pro-

vides for the common forearm movements of pronation (palms down) and supination (palms up). These may be measured by placement of the goniometer vertically on the subject's closed fist. The palm should be in the neutral position, with the stationary arm placed vertical. The goniometer axis runs parallel to the shaft of the forearm. The movement arm remains parallel with the metacarpophalangeal joints in pronation and supination.

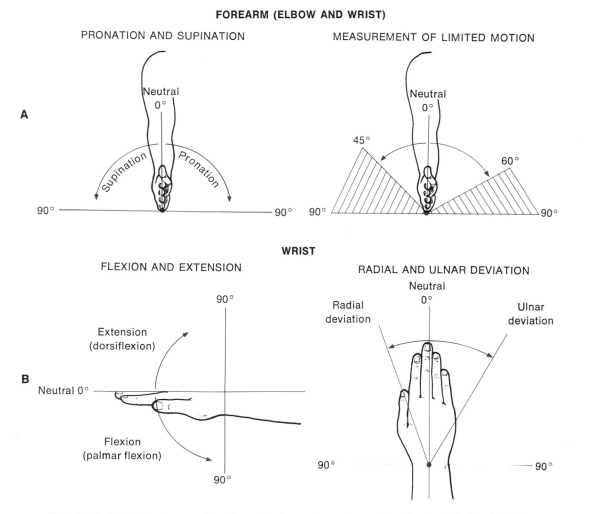

**FOREARM (ELBOW AND WRIST)**

PRONATION AND SUPINATION

MEASUREMENT OF LIMITED MOTION

Neutral 0°

Supination    Pronation

90°    90°

Neutral 0°

45°    60°

90°    90°

**WRIST**

FLEXION AND EXTENSION

90°

Extension (dorsiflexion)

Neutral 0°

Flexion (palmar flexion)

90°

RADIAL AND ULNAR DEVIATION

Neutral 0°

Radial deviation    Ulnar deviation

90°    90°

**Fig 4-10** Forearm range of motion. (Redrawn from Committee for the Study of Joint Motion: Joint motion: method of measuring and recording, Chicago, 1965, American Academy of Orthopaedic Surgeons.)

The motions at the wrist are mainly those of flexion and extension and ulnar and radial deviation. Flexion and extension may be measured by placement of the goniometric axis distal to the head of the ulna and using the medial shaft of the forearm for placement of the stationary arm. Placement of the movement arm is parallel with the metacarpal bone, usually the fifth metacarpal. Ulnar or radial deviation is side-to-side motion of the carpal bones in relationship to the ulnar and radial bones. Deviation to the thumb side is radial deviation; deviation to the little finger side is ulnar deviation. Normalcy of these motions is best determined for the individual by comparison of right with left sides. Both upper extremity radial and ulnar deviations may be limited or increased, as in rheumatoid arthritis.

Great detail may be taken to determine the exact motions of the metarcarpophalangeal (MP) and interphalangeal (IP) joints. A small goniometer may be used, parallel with the shaft of the metacarpal bones and parallel to the phalangeal bones, to determine MP flexion and extension. The goniometer may also be placed superior to the MP and IP joints to record motion. However, a gross method for determining this is done by asking the subject to make a tight fist while the distance from the tips of the distal phalanges to the proximal and distal palmar creases is measured. If the subject is able to touch the proximal palmar crease with the tips of the phalanges, normal MP and IP motion is attainable. If the tips of the phalanges touch the distal palmar crease, normal IP motion is attainable. This is a good test of joint measurement that may be done very quickly.

# HAND

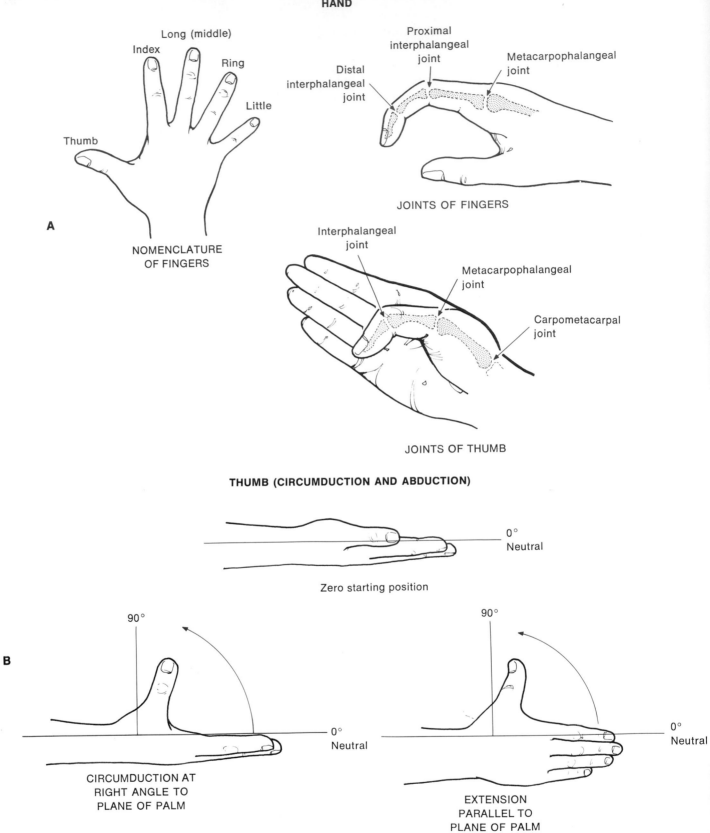

**NOMENCLATURE OF FINGERS**

Thumb
Index
Long (middle)
Ring
Little

**JOINTS OF FINGERS**

Distal interphalangeal joint
Proximal interphalangeal joint
Metacarpophalangeal joint

**JOINTS OF THUMB**

Interphalangeal joint
Metacarpophalangeal joint
Carpometacarpal joint

A

**THUMB (CIRCUMDUCTION AND ABDUCTION)**

0° Neutral

Zero starting position

B

90°
0° Neutral

**CIRCUMDUCTION AT RIGHT ANGLE TO PLANE OF PALM**

90°
0° Neutral

**EXTENSION PARALLEL TO PLANE OF PALM**

**Fig. 4-11.** Hand range of motion. (Redrawn from Committee for the Study of Joint Motion: Joint motion: method of measuring and recording, Chicago, 1965, American Academy of Orthopaedic Surgeons.)

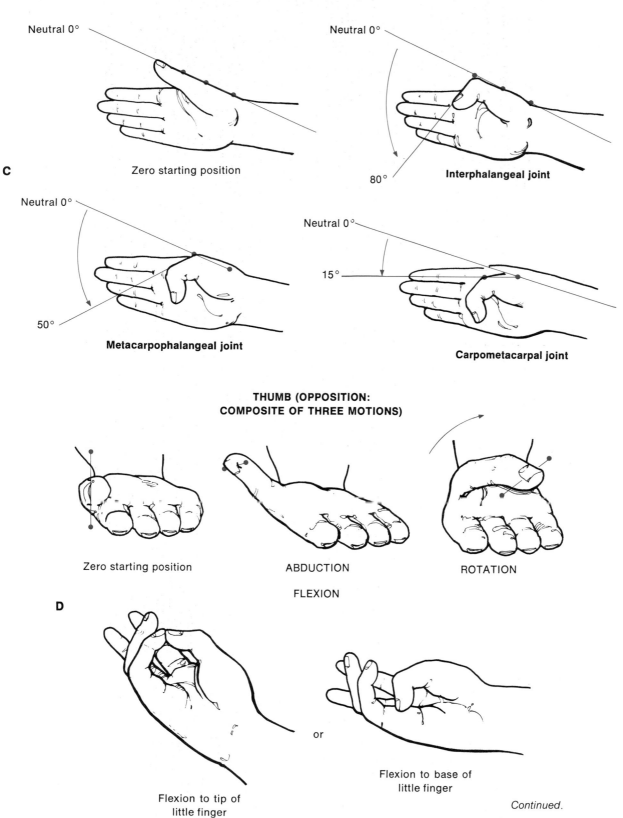

**THUMB (FLEXION)**

Neutral 0°

Zero starting position

Neutral 0°

80°

**Interphalangeal joint**

Neutral 0°

50°

**Metacarpophalangeal joint**

Neutral 0°

15°

**Carpometacarpal joint**

**C**

**THUMB (OPPOSITION:
COMPOSITE OF THREE MOTIONS)**

Zero starting position

ABDUCTION

ROTATION

FLEXION

**D**

Flexion to tip of
little finger

or

Flexion to base of
little finger

*Continued.*

**Fig. 4-11, cont'd.** Hand range of motion.

**FINGERS (FLEXION)**

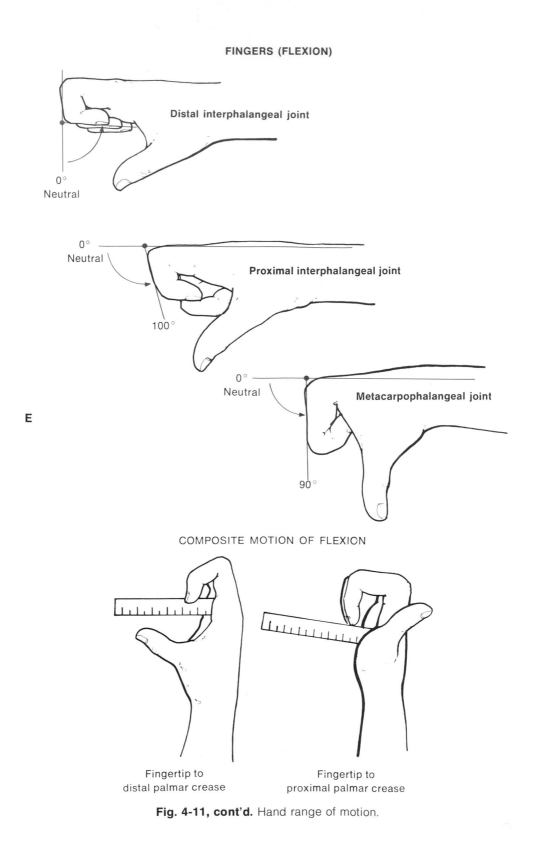

**Fig. 4-11, cont'd.** Hand range of motion.

**FINGERS
(EXTENSION, ABDUCTION, AND ADDUCTION)**

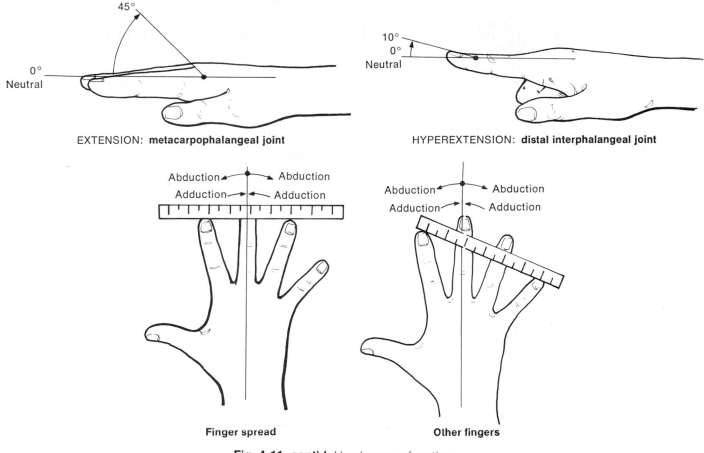

EXTENSION: **metacarpophalangeal joint**

HYPEREXTENSION: **distal interphalangeal joint**

**F**

Finger spread

Other fingers

**Fig. 4-11, cont'd.** Hand range of motion.

Although abduction and adduction of the fingers can also be recorded, they are not dealt with here at any length. The basic movements of the thumb are flexion and extension, adduction and abduction. Flexion and extension take place across the palm of the thumb. Abduction and adduction take place perpendicular to the palm of the thumb. The car-pometacarpal joint of the thumb is highly mobile because it has an independent saddle-shaped surface (see Chapter 1). The measurement of the thumb generally described is the movement of the metacarpal bone in relationship to the palm of the hand. Opposition of the thumb may also be recorded and is usually compared with the standards set by the ability of the individual to touch the distal phalanx of the thumb with the distal phalanx of the fifth finger. These motions are used for gross examination of the hand; more detailed testing may be done with a goniometer.

## LOCOMOTION

A chapter on motion would not be complete without a discussion of locomotion. It has been pointed out by Long[5,pp.1-10] that normal gait consists of a complex series of accelerations and decelerations with maximum forward translations of the center of gravity and minimal vertical and lateral oscillation. Pathologic gait is excessive motion or asymmetric movement of the body parts and center of gravity.

Before discussing locomotion it is necessary to define some basic terms:

**locomotion** movement from one place to another.
**gait** manner or style of walking, including rhythm and speed.
**bipedal gait** gait using both feet.
**plantigrade gait** gait characterized by walking on the sole of the foot with the heel touching the ground; occurs in the three-dimensional plane.

## Major determinants

Saunders, Inman, and Eberhardt[7] have divided locomotion into the following determinants or areas of analysis: pelvic rotation, pelvic tilt, knee and hip flexion, knee and ankle interaction, and lateral pelvic displacement. Observation of the abnormalities of these determinants provides insight into the assessment of pathologic gait.[7,pp.550-551]

Pelvic rotation involves alternate rotation to the right and left of the pelvis. This rotation is approximately 4° to either side of the central axis and occurs at each hip joint, which passes from relative internal to external rotation during the stance phase. If we describe normal locomotion as a progressive motion of sinusoidal movement, then the purpose of the pelvic rotation is to flatten somewhat the arc of passage of the center of gravity by elevating the extremities of that arc. In other words, the vertical displacement of the center of gravity of the body is kept at a minimum.

The second determinant is pelvic tilt. The pelvis tilts or lists downward relative to the horizontal plane on the side of the swinging limb; that is, the pelvis tilts downward relative to the horizontal plane on the side opposite that of the weight-bearing limb, producing a positive Trendelenburg's sign. This downward motion takes place at the hip joint, producing an equivalent adduction of the extremity in the stance phase and abduction of the extremity in the swing phase. Also to permit pelvic tilt, the knee joint of the non-weight-bearing limb flexes to allow clearance for the swing through of that limb. Again the effect is to decrease the summit of the arc of the center of gravity to conserve energy.

The third determinant is knee flexion in the stance phase. In this determinant the passage of the body weight takes place over the supporting extremity while the joint is undergoing flexion. This stance phase is referred to as the period of double knee lock: the knee first is locked into extension at heelstrike, then is unlocked, then is in full extension again during full weight bearing, and is once again unlocked by final flexion and initiation of the swing phase.[7,p.548] These three determinants of gait (pelvic rotation, pelvic tilt, and knee flexion) all act in the same direction by flattening the arc through which the center of gravity of the body is translated.[7,p.550]

The fourth and fifth determinants (foot and knee mechanisms) are concerned with smoothing out of the pathway of the center of gravity as the body moves forward at the point of intersection of its sinusoidal arcs. The knee and foot work simultaneously to lower the center of gravity. When the foot is at heel contact, it is dorsiflexed and the knee is fully extended, so that the extremity is at its maximum length and its center of gravity has reached its lower point of downward placement. Plantar flexion of the foot with the initiation of knee flexion maintains the center of gravity with its forward progression at approximately the same level, again minimizing the vertical displacement of the center of gravity.

Lateral displacement of the pelvis is the final determinant. It is produced by a horizontal shift of the pelvis or by relative hip adduction.

## Gait

Perry[7,p.14] describes classic gait in two phases: stance and swing. The stance phase begins at heel-strike and ends at toe-off.

Stance has been divided into five stages: *initial contact,* which is the moment when the foot touches the floor; *loading response,* which is when the limb reacts to the weight or with limb reaction as weight is accepted; *midstance,* which is the period of single-limb support with body advancement over the stationary foot; *terminal stance,* which is a continuation of single limb support during which the body moves forward on the supporting foot (double limb support is initiated during the latter part of this stage); and finally *preswing,* which is the transitional period of double-limb support during which the limb is rapidly unloaded and prepared for swing. Swing has been divided into three stages: *initial swing,* which is the lift and advancement of a limb from a trailing to a neutral position, the neutral position being the swing foot placed adjacent to the stance limb; *midswing,* described as limb advancement to achieve a vertical tibial position; and *terminal swing,* which is continued limb advancement toward full knee extension.

By using the two phases of stance and swing, in-depth analysis of the trunk, pelvis, hip, knee, ankle, and foot can be used to determine gait deviations.

## Muscles involved in gait analysis

It is necessary here to mention some of the main muscles involved in gait and at what time they are involved in the walking cycle. To minimize energy consumption and permit a reasonable propulsion speed, the most comfortable walking speed is close to 3 ft/sec. Energy expended appears to increase considerably as speeds in excess of 6 ft/sec are attained.[7,p.14]

Many studies have been done on the electromyographic (EMG) activity of muscles during gait. The following data are from Basmajian,[1,pp.317-325] who has carried out the most recent studies on

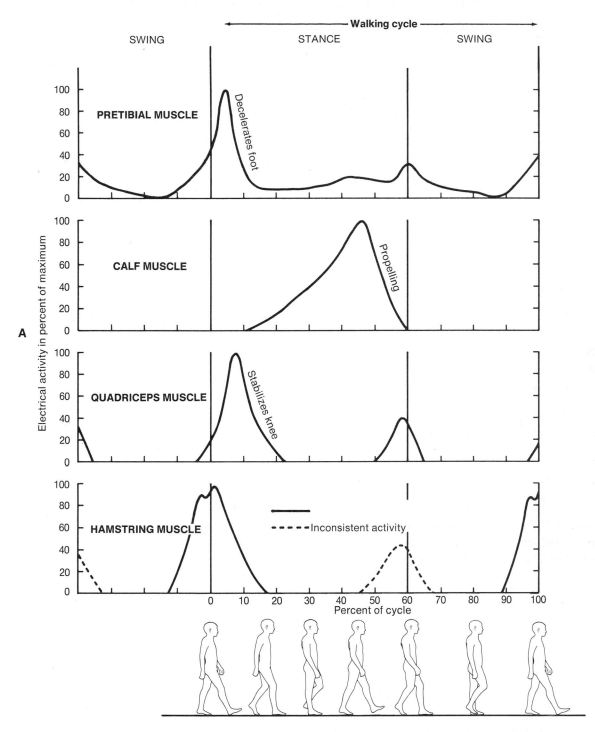

**Fig. 4-12.** Phasic action of major muscle groups during level walking. EMG studies, 10 men. (Adapted from Eberhart, H. D., Inman, V. T., and Bresler, B.: Human limbs and their substitutes, Washington, D.C., 1954, National Academy of Sciences. Reproduced with permission of the National Academy of Sciences.)

*Continued.*

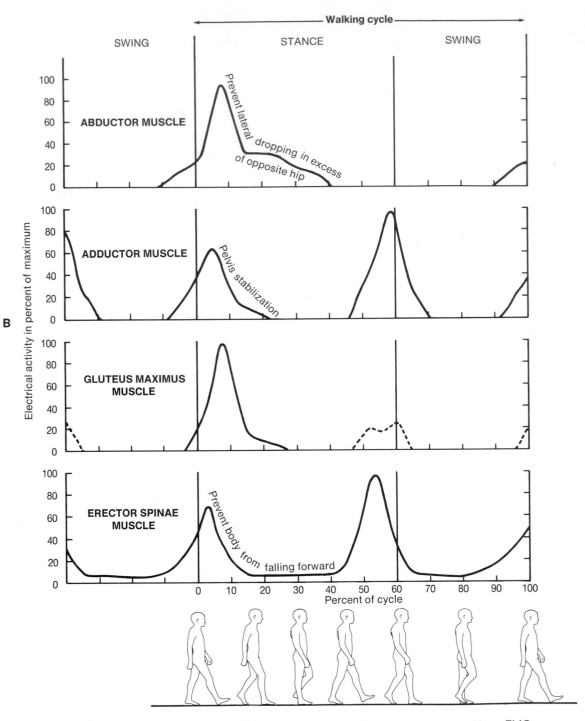

**Fig. 4-12, cont'd.** Phasic action of major muscles groups during level walking. EMG studies, 10 men.

EMG activity, and can be compared with the previous data of Inman and Eberhart (1953) (Fig. 4-12) and of Radcliff (1962). It is evident that Basmajian's studies allude to possibly a more precise recording of the activity of these muscles. However, it also shows that since the studies done in 1962 the basic peak activities of the muscles have not significantly changed.

**Tibialis anterior.** EMG activity of the tibialis anterior occurs at heelstrike of the stance phase, at which time the foot is inverted and dorsiflexed. It has been suggested that the tibialis anterior at this time counteracts forces applied to the heel by the ground. A more common proposal is that the muscle decelerates the foot at heelstrike by gradual lengthening or eccentric contraction. Basmajian's studies show that there is relatively no tibialis anterior activity in normal subjects at the time of midstance or heel-off. There is, however, a peak of EMG activity at toe-off, probably in response to necessity for the ankle to be dorsiflexed to allow the toes to clear the floor. In conclusion, the tibialis anterior is responsible for dorsiflexion during acceleration and for inversion of the foot during deceleration of the swing phase.

**Tibialis posterior.** During ordinary walking the tibialis posterior shows activity at midstance of the stance phase. This muscle is an inverter during non-weight-bearing movements of the foot, but it also has a role at midstance to restrain the foot from everting past the neutral position. This muscle has been considered to be a plantar flexor of the ankle. However, during level walking with an unaccustomed foot position, there is virtually no activity at heel-off.

**Flexor hallucis longus.** The flexor hallucis longus has its greatest activity at midstance when the entire body weight is concentrated on one foot.

**Peroneus longus.** The peroneus longus has its greatest activity during midstance. It has been shown that the peroneus longus and tibialis posterior work in unison to control the shift of the ankle from inversion during full foot to neutral at midstance. These two muscles also work together to control rotary movements at the ankle and foot during the midstance position.

**Abductor hallucis and flexor digitorum brevis.** The abductor hallucis and digitorum brevis work together during midstance and continue through toe-off. Some experts think that these muscles also help in support of the arches.

**Gluteus medius and minimus** (abductors). The anterior fibers of the gluteus medius and minimus perform moderate activity at heel contact that continues through to midstance; there is also a burst of activity at toe-off and another just before heel contact.

**Tensor fascia latae.** The tensor fascia latae is active during early stance, at which time it has a peak through midswing and another short and smaller peak during toe-off.

**Gluteus maximus.** The gluteus maximus was tested by Basmajian in its three portions (upper, middle, and lower). The upper and lower fibers were found to show a biphasic pattern with a small peak at heelstrike and one near the end of the swing phase; the middle fibers were found to show these same activities with the addition of a high peak just before toe-off.

**Hamstrings.** The hamstrings, which include the semitendinosus, semimembranosus, and biceps femoris, have their peaks mainly at heel contact and just before the end of 90% of the cycle. The semitendinosus muscle also has a third peak at midcycle.

**Sartorius and rectus femoris.** The sartorius has only one peak, immediately during toe-off. The rectus femoris may show two peaks but generally shows one peak along with the sartorius.

**Iliopsoas and iliacus.** These muscles act continuously through the walking cycle with some rise and fall. The highest peaks are during swing and midstance phases. The psoas muscle has a peak corresponding to that of the iliacus. However, it has a third peak at about midcycle.

**Adductors.** The adductor magnus acts continuously, resting only at midswing. The lower portion of the adductor magnus acts in conjunction with the hamstring. Activity of the adductor brevis varies with the speed of walking and occurs at 40% and 90% of the walking cycle. The adductor longus and gracilis have a peak activity at toe-off, with initial peaks at late stance and early swing phase.

**Quadriceps femoris.** This is probably the most noted muscle. Its main contractions occur as extension of the knee is completed, not during the early part of extension when motion of the limb is passive. It continues to act during the early part of the supporting phase, and activity occurs once again at the end of the supporting phase to fix the knee in extension.

## Gait deviations

Before concluding the discussion of locomotion it is necessary to speak briefly about pathologic gait deviations and to mention some of the key muscles involved (Table 4-2). After observing normal gait pattern and disciplining oneself to evaluate it, deviations from normal are easier to note. Long,[6,p.14] in

**Table 4-2.** Pathologic gait deviations

| Gait | Characteristics | Muscle(s) involved |
|---|---|---|
| Trendelenburg | Dropping of pelvis on unaffected side until heelstrike | Gluteus medius |
| | Dropping of pelvis on affected side at time of heelstrike | |
| | Apparent protrusion laterally of affected hip | |
| | Lateral deviation of trunk and pelvis toward affected side during stance phase of affected limb | |
| | Shortened step on unaffected side | |
| Compensated | Dropping of pelvis on unaffected side between heelstrike on affected side and heelstrike on unaffected side | |
| | Medial deviation of hip on affected side | |
| | Dipping of shoulder on affected side (no dipping is seen with uncompensated gait) | |
| | Bending of entire trunk downward and sideways over affected hip | |
| Dorsiflexor | Footdrop during swing phase | Dorsiflexors of ankle |
| | Excessive knee and hip flexion during swing phase | |
| | Slapping of sole of foot forcibly against ground with heelstrike | |
| Gastrocnemius | Dropping and lagging of pelvis on affected side at last moment of stance phase | Gastrocnemius |
| Triceps surae limp | Pelvis drops and lags on affected side | |
| Quadriceps | Limp affecting all phases of gait | Quadriceps |
| | Sudden forcible extension of knee at or preceding heelstrike | |
| | Smooth lurch immediately following heelstrike | |
| | Recurvatum knee pattern following heelstrike | |
| | With rapid walking, lag of foot after it leaves ground in swing phase, with tendency to swing upward about knee; lag of swing phase | |
| Hip flexor | Limp starting at push-off on affected side | Hip flexors |
| | Sudden backward throwing of trunk and pelvis as a limit, followed by pelvic flexion from push-off to midswing | |
| Hip extensor | Sudden backward throwing of trunk and pelvis just after heelstrike on affected side | Gluteus maximus |
| | Apparent forward protrusion of affected hip just after heelstrike on affected side | |
| | Slight elevation of affected hip at full weight bearing | |

his discussion of pathologic gait due to muscular weakness, describes pathologic gait as characterized by excessive or asymmetric movement of the body parts and of the center of gravity. The following is a short discussion of the gaits produced by isolated weaknesses or paralysis of certain muscle groups. Weaknesses usually are not isolated but occur in multiple, leading to combinations of gaits.

**Trendelenburg gait.** Perhaps the most common gait deviation seen in orthopedics is the gluteal, or Trendelenburg gait. In this gait there is a dropping of the pelvis on the unaffected side at the time of heelstrike on the affected side until heelstrike on the unaffected side and an apparent protrusion laterally of the affected hip. The lateral deviation of the entire trunk and pelvis toward the affected side occurs during the stance phase of the affected limb. The patient also shortens his step on the unaffected side.

It is thought that the uncompensated gluteal gait is more likely to be possible with moderate weakness of the medius. However, the more common compensated gluteal gait is seen clinically. This involves dropping of the pelvis on the unaffected side between the time of heelstrike on the affected side and heelstrike on the unaffected side, medial deviation of the hip on the affected side, and dropping of the entire trunk downward and sideways over the affected hip. A short step on the unaffected side occurs with both the uncompensated and compensated gluteal gait.

With a compensated gait, the trunk is forcibly thrown laterally; that is, on weight bearing (stance phase of the involved lower extremity), the trunk over that extremity is thrown laterally. This lateral movement is an attempt to put a large amount of weight above and outside the center of rotation of the affected hip. Also, the erector spinae and quadratus lumborum of the involved side function to lift the entire weight of the pelvis and opposite lower extremity off the floor to allow the uninvolved leg to clear during swing phase.

**Dorsiflexor gait.** The dorsiflexor gait is caused by weakness of the dorsiflexors of the ankle. Its characteristics are footdrop during the swing phase, with excessive knee and hip flexion to allow clearance of the involved extremity during swing phase, and finally a slapping of the sole of the foot forcibly against the ground with heelstrike due to the dorsiflexor's inability to decelerate the body weight as the heel strikes the floor. Therefore there is footdrop throughout the entire gait.

**Gastrocnemius gait.** Gastrocnemius gait is characterized by dropping of the pelvis on the affected side at the last moment of stance phase accompanied by lagging, or slowness of forward movement, of the pelvis.

**Triceps surae limp.** Triceps surae limp involves a deficiency in the elevating and propulsive factors of the affected side. Therefore, since the triceps surae is not functioning to keep the pelvis elevated, it drops, and since it is not functioning to keep the pelvis moving forward, the pelvis lags behind.

**Quadriceps gait.** In quadriceps gait there is a limp affecting all phases of gait; a sudden forcible extension of the knee at or preceding heelstrike, much as is characteristic of the above-the-knee amputee with a single-axis knee; a lurch immediately following heelstrike, driving the femur backward and the hip forward, or the recurvatum knee pattern; and finally, in rapid walking a lag of the foot just after it leaves the ground in the swing phase, with a tendency to swing upward about the knee. Due to its action as a buffer just after heelstrike, the weakness of the quadriceps does not allow knee flexion to occur in the walking cycle. Therefore the body throws the knee into *recurvatum*. The knee mechanism locks the hip against the posterior capsule of the hamstrings, providing a safe base for the center of gravity as the body approaches full weight bearing. In fast cadence there is a lag of the swing phase, which may not be present during slower gait patterns, due to the pendulum effect of the leg, and it is pointed out that acceleration of the normal foot in early swing phase reaches somewhere around 100 mph in rapid walking.

**Hip flexor gait.** The hip flexor gait has the characteristics of a limp starting at push-off on the affected side, a sudden backward throwing of the trunk and pelvis as a unit, followed by pelvic flexion within this unit, the whole deviation lasting from push-off to midswing. The hip flexors act primarily through swing phase. They act to provide the forward swing and to shorten the extremity so that it can pass between the pelvis and the ground. In order to help clear the ground, the weakened patient leans backward, stabilizing the pelvis against the trunk and causing relative extension of the pelvis and the femur. This allows the femur to ride back until the ligament of Bigelow (Y ligament, ligamentum iliofemorale) can be brought into action to provide fibrous reinforcement of the anterior portion of the hip joint and prevent hyperextension of the hip.

**Hip extensor gait.** Hip extensor (gluteus maximus) gait is characterized by sudden backward throwing of the trunk and pelvis just after heelstrike on the affected side and by apparent forward protrusion of the affected hip at the same time due to trunk motion and by tightly extending the knee in midstance. This results in slight elevation of the affected hip at full weight bearing as compared with the normal side. With normal standing posture the gluteus maximus is not necessary because the pelvis can be hyperextended to land on the ligament of Bigelow. However, if the center of gravity is forward, as in bending forward from the hip, active contraction of the gluteus maximus is necessary. Also, if the trunk is moving forward over one leg the major retarding force must be the maximus or hamstrings, which act to pull the pelvis backward. To keep the femur relatively extended and held tight against the ligament of Bigelow, the knee is held tightly in extension in the gluteus maximus gait.

## SUMMARY

This chapter introduces the basic principles essential to examination of motion in the clinical setting. These principles are initially explained in the areas of kinematics and kinetics as they apply to the human body and its motions. Understanding fundamental principles for description and measurement of body segments and impairments of their motions is necessary in patient evaluation and treatment.

## REFERENCES

1. Basmajian, J. V.: Muscles alive, ed. 3, Baltimore, 1974, The Williams & Wilkins Co.
2. Blount, W. P.: Don't throw away the cane, J. Bone Joint Surg. **38**(13):695-708, 1956.
3. Brunnstrom, S.: Clinical kinesiology, ed. 2, Philadelphia, 1968, F. A. Davis Co.
4. Calliet, R.: Shoulder pain, Philadelphia, 1966, F. A. Davis Co.

5. Long, C. II: New York, Institute of Physical Medicine and Rehabilitation.
6. Perry, J.: Principles of lower extremity bracing, Washington, D.C., 1970, American Physical Therapy Association.
7. Saunders, J. B., Inman, V. T., and Eberhart, H. D.: Major determinants in normal and pathological gait, J. Bone Joint Surg. 35:543-558, 1953.

## BIBLIOGRAPHY

Basmajian, J. V.; Muscles alive: their functions revealed by electromyography, ed. 3, Baltimore, 1974, The Williams & Wilkins Co.

Basmajian, J. V.: Primary anatomy, Baltimore, 1970, The Williams & Wilkins Co.

Basmajian, J. V., and McConaill, M. A.: Muscles and movements: a basis for human kinesiology, Baltimore, 1969, The Williams & Wilkins Co.

Blount, W. P.: Don't throw away the cane, J. Bone Joint Surg. 38(13):695-708, 1956.

Broer, M.: Efficiency of human movement, ed. 3, Philadelphia, 1973, W. B. Saunders Co.

Brunnstrom, S.: Clinical kinesiology, ed. 2, Philadelphia, 1968, F. A. Davis Co.

Calliet, R.: Shoulder pain, Philadelphia, 1966, F. A. Davis Co.

Hoppenfeld, S.: Physical examination of the spine and extremities, New York, 1976, Appleton-Century-Crofts.

Kelley, D. L.: Kinesiology: fundamentals of motion description, Englewood Cliffs, N.J., 1971, Prentice-Hall, Inc.

Kendall, H. O., Kendall, F. P., and Wadsworth, G. E.: Muscles: testing and function, ed. 2, Baltimore, 1971, The Williams & Wilkins Co.

Kindall: Guides to the evaluation of permanent impairment, Chicago, 1971, American Medical Association.

Long, C. II: New York, Institute of Physical Medicine and Rehabilitation.

O'Connell, A. L., and Gardner, E. B.: Understanding the scientific bases of human movement, Baltimore, 1972, The Williams & Wilkins Co.

Perry, J.: Principles of lower extremity bracing, Washington, D.C., 1970, APTA.

Saunders, J. B., Inman, V. T., and Eberhart, H. D.: Major determinants in normal and pathological gait, J. Bone Joint Surg. 35:543-558, 1953.

# PART TWO

# Assessment

# 5

# History and physical examination

BARBARA H. DUNN

MICHAEL W. HAKALA

It is a mistake to believe that there is such a thing as an "orthopedic" history and physical examination. Because of the complexity and interrelated nature of body systems, particularly components of the neuromusculoskeletal system, a complete history and physical examination should be done on all patients, with particular emphasis on systems involved with chief complaints.

The purpose of this chapter is to describe those components of a complete history and physical examination felt to be essential in assessment of the musculoskeletal system. Emphasis is on the normal and on description of possible variations from normal. For more detailed information regarding diagnostic evaluation of specific conditions, refer to Chapters 13 to 21.

## HISTORY TAKING

When the chief complaint is not musculoskeletal related, a satisfactory history can be obtained from the usual information elicited in the past medical history, review of systems, and family and social history. In children this should include prenatal, birth, and developmental history, with particular emphasis on motor development.

If the chief complaint is primarily musculoskeletal it will usually involve pain, loss of function, or change in appearance, and the following information should be obtained from the history[1,pp.9-11]:

1. *Injury (whether recent or old):* how, what, when, where occurred
2. *Onset of symptoms:* immediate, gradual, associated with particular activity, systemic symptomatology
3. *Pain:* location, character (dull, sharp, throbbing), severity, radiation, what relieved or aggravated by, daily variation, getting better or worse
4. *Deformity:* when any change first noted, character (associated with swelling, stiffness), disability, family history, previous treatment
5. *Paralysis:* time of onset, extent, progression or regression, sensory disturbances, disability, sphincter control, previous treatment
6. *Activities of daily living:* affected how or by what, independent or requires assistance

## MUSCULOSKELETAL EXAMINATION

The examination of the musculoskeletal system primarily involves two basic areas of anatomy, kinesiology, and biomechanics: statics and dynamics. In other words, it consists of a basic analysis of body structure and function. The examination includes the body as a whole and its individual units (upper extremities, trunk, and lower extremities) in both the supine and erect positions and analysis of body function while it is in motion (dynamics): gait, walking, running, climbing, crawling, stooping, bending, and so on.

In practice, the bones, joints, and muscles are examined simultaneously, with systems examined individually if an abnormality exists. Examination of the adult may usually proceed according to the examiner's preference and the patient's individual problem, while examination of the child will depend on age, condition, and cooperation. It is usually advisable when examining a child to begin with observation of gait or inspection of hands and feet, as these procedures are minimally threatening.

Basic examination of the musculoskeletal system involves observation and inspection, palpation, evaluation of range of motion, assessment of motor power, auscultation, and neurologic evaluation.

### I. Observation

A. Posture and gait. If ambulatory, patient is asked to stand for observation of posture and body outline from front, back, and sides; note body build (habitus) and facial appearance (facies). Ask patient to walk normally; note basic phases of gait (stance and swing, Fig. 5-1). In normal walking the body weight is supported by one lower extremity, while the other limb executes the movement of progression (except for a brief

STANCE PHASE

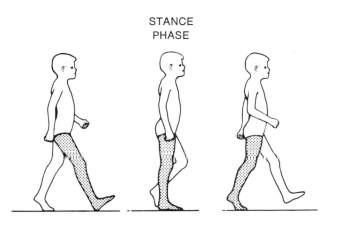

SWING PHASE

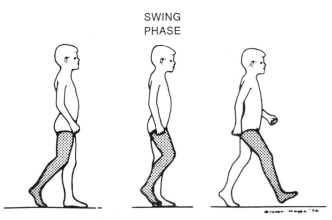

**Fig. 5-1.** Normal gait. (From Hilt, N. E., and Schmitt, E. W., Jr.: Pediatric orthopedic nursing, St. Louis, 1975, The C. V. Mosby Co.)

period of double support). Normal locomotion represents a heel-to-toe phase of support and progression with associated movements of the pelvis (rotation and tilt), hip (flexion), and knee (flexion) as well as swinging of the upper extremities.[3, pp. 4, 10, 24-37]

1. Observe walking, standing, sitting up, lying down.
2. Note position of body parts, usual posture, evidence of discomfort, muscle weakness or joint stiffness. Specific gait patterns are associated with various disease states.
3. Ask patient to walk on heels and on toes and to run. If disorders are suspected, ask to walk tandem (forward and backward), then to walk rapidly and stop suddenly.
4. Listen to walking: flopping (footdrop), dragging or scraping (spasticity), stomping (ataxia).
5. Observe gait with and without assistive devices (crutches, braces, walker).
6. Abnormal gait may be caused by muscle weakness, pain, structural deformities of the bones and joints, or neurologic disorders.

B. Symmetry of movement, alignment. Note coordination of movement; physiologic spinal curves; shoulders carried behind pelvis in lateral view; position of head, shoulders, gluteal and popliteal creases; iliac crest level, shoulders balanced over pelvis; deviation of truck to one side. Scoliosis: one hip higher or more prominent, flank asymmetry, level of shoulder, rib hump on forward bending. Lower extremities: center of gravity passes just anterior to first sacral vertebra.

C. Deformities. Shortenings, lengthenings, absence of a part; torsional or angular deformities (measured in degrees), type and site; severity; fixed deformity or passively or actively correctable; soft tissue, bone, or joint; produced by what; associated spasm, local tenderness or pain on motion; bony enlargement or joint swelling.

### II. Inspection

A. Soft tissues and muscles. Swelling, symmetry, atrophy.
B. Skin. Color, erythema, cyanosis, pigmentation, scratches, bruises, scars, lesions, rashes.
C. Bones and joints. Swelling, deformity, or bony enlargement.

### III. Palpation

A. Joints. Swelling; thickened synovial membrane, excessive fluid in joint (effusion); subcutaneous nodules; temperature; tenderness; joint stability.
B. Bones. Shape and outline; abnormal relationships between bones and joints.
C. Skin and muscles. Tone, turgor, elasticity; painful trigger points; muscle bulk; peripheral pulses.

### IV. Range of motion

A. Deviation from normal or limitation of motion;

instability or ankylosis; crepitation or grating; specify degree lacking full range, whether passive or active motion and plane of motion (flexion, extension, abduction, adduction, internal rotation, external rotation). Method of measurement and recording has been standardized by AAOS based on the zero neutral method (Cane and Roberts): motion measured in degrees of a circle with joint as its center, zero starting position defined (military position), and degrees of motion added in direction joint moves. May use goniometer until can gauge accurately. Visual representations of range of motion are given in Chapter 4.

  B. Normal range of motion in major joints:
    1. Neck
      a. Flexion 45°
      b. Extension 55°
      c. Rotation 70°
      d. Lateral flexion 40°
    2. Shoulder
      a. Flexion 180°
      b. Extension 50°
      c. Abduction 180°
      d. Adduction 50°
      e. External rotation 90°
      f. Internal rotation 90°
    3. Elbow
      a. Flexion 160°
      b. Extension 0°
    4. Wrist
      a. Flexion 90°
      b. Extension 70°
      c. Ulnar deviation 55°
      d. Radial deviation 20°
      e. Pronation 90°
      f. Supination 90°
    5. Trunk
      a. Flexion 75° to 90°
      b. Extension 30°
      c. Rotation 30°
      d. Lateral flexion 35°
    6. Hip
      a. Flexion 120°
      b. Extension 15°
      c. Adduction 45°
      d. Abduction 45°
      e. External rotation 40° to 45°
      f. Internal rotation 40° to 45°
    7. Knee
      a. Flexion 130°
      b. Extension 0°
    8. Ankle
      a. Plantar flexion 45°
      b. Dorsiflexion (extension) 20°
      c. Inversion 30°
      d. Eversion 20°

**V. Motor power**
  A. Active and passive, muscle development, tenderness, spasm, paralysis, tone, paresis, flaccidity, atrophy, fasciculations, rigidity, contractures.
  B. Muscle strength and power classified as static (passive: examiner performs) or kinetic (active: carry out against resistance).
  C. Note fatiguability, rate and coordination of movement, tremulousness, clumsiness, ability to perform skilled tasks. Weakness, diffuse (general) or localized, degree, character, cause, associated sensory changes.
  D. Muscles graded by objective grading system:
    1. 0/zero: no palpable contraction of muscle.
    2. 1/trace: palpable contraction of muscle; no motion of part that muscle should move.
    3. 2/poor: muscle moves part through its range but not against gravity.
    4. 3/fair: muscle carries part through its full range of motion against gravity but not against added resistance.

**Table 5-1.** Reflex maturation in the infant[3, pp. 25-37]

| Reflex | Method of eliciting | Normal reaction | When present |
|---|---|---|---|
| Crossed extension (Philippson's reflex) | Extend one lower extremity and apply pressure to sole of foot | Opposite leg flexes and adducts, then extends (may be toe fanning) | Birth to 6 mo |
| Placing | Support infant upright at waist and bring anterior tibia or dorsum of foot against table edge | Flexion of hip and dorsiflexion of ankle on side stimulated (places foot on table) | Birth to 6 mo |
| Stepping-walking | Support infant upright at waist with soles of feet pressing on table, gently move forward | Reciprocal flexion and extension of lower extremities (simulated walking) | Birth to 6-8 wk |
| Extensor thrust | With lower extremities flexed, apply pressure to soles of feet | Lower extremities extend (sometimes followed by flexion) | Birth to 2 mo |

**Table 5-1.** Reflex maturation in the infant — cont'd

| Reflex | Method of eliciting | Normal reaction | When present |
|---|---|---|---|
| Moro | With infant supine, give quick downward pull to blanket or crib sheet | Abduction and extension of all extremities with extension and fanning of digits followed by flexion and adduction of extremities and frequently crying | Birth to 4-6 mo |
| Palmar grasp | Examiner places finger or other object in infant's palm | Fingers flex and grasp object (*Note:* tactile stimulation over dorsum will open grasp) | Birth to 4-6 mo |
| Plantar | Apply digital pressure to plantar surface of foot, proximal to toes | Toes flex and grasp fingers | Birth to 10-12 mo |
| Trunk incurvation (Galant's reflex) | With infant prone, stimulate lateral lumbar area with finger | Trunk flexes toward side stimulated | Birth to 2 mo |
| Oral | | | |
| Suck | Introduce finger or nipple in infant's mouth | Vigorous sucking | Birth to 4 mo, awake |
| Root (search) | Stimulate circumoral with finger | Turns toward and searches for source of stimulus | 7 months, asleep |
| Positive support response (leg-straightening reflex) | Support infant upright and press soles of feet to table several times | When soles contact table, lower extremities and trunk extend | Birth to 4 mo |
| Righting reflexes | | | |
| Neck | With infant supine and midline, rotate head to one side and hold for about 10 sec | Body rotates as a whole toward side head turned to | Birth to 6 mo |
| Body | Same position as above | Body rotates cephalocaudally — head, then shoulders, trunk, and pelvis | 6 mo |
| Labyrinthine | Baby blindfolded | | |
| | Body held *prone* in space | Head extends | 1-2 mo |
| | Support body vertically in space, tilt from one side to the other. | When tilted right or left, head rights itself to vertical position with mouth horizontal | 6-8 mo, persists |
| Optical | Same maneuvers as labyrinthine with baby's eyes open | Same as labyrinthine | Same as labyrinthine |
| Tonic neck reflex (TNR) | | | |
| Asymmetric (ATNR) | With infant supine, rotate head to one side for 5-10 sec, then rotate to other side | Arm and leg on chin side extend, on occiput side flex (fencing position) | 2 to 4-6 mo |
| Symmetric (STNR) | Place infant prone in examiner's hand or over knee, alternately flex and extend neck | When neck flexes, arms flex and legs extend; neck extended, arms extend and legs flex | 6-12 mo |
| Landau | Body held prone in space over examiner's hand | Attempts to hold body parallel to floor (note hyper- or hypotonicity) | 3-6 mo to 2 yr |
| Parachute | Body supported prone in space, head moved suddenly toward floor (downward) | Immediate extension of arms and wrists | 6 mo, persists (present in all directions, 9-10 mo) |

5. 4/good: muscle lifts part against gravity and added resistance (minus and plus used to indicate variations in resistance).
6. 5/normal: normal strength.

**VI. Auscultation** (listening with ear or stethoscope)
A. Sounds arising from bones, joints, or muscle action: crepitus, grating, snapping, peripheral arteriovenous fistula. Conduction of sound slowed and diminished by fractures and joint effusions.

**VII. Neurologic evaluation**
A. Includes components of usual neurologic examination with emphasis on stance and gait, reflexes, and motor development in the child. Neurologic assessment of infants should also include eliciting primitive reflexes (Table 5-1). Absence or persistence of some of these reflexes generally indicates insult or delayed maturation of central nervous system, as seen with brain damage, cerebral palsy, prematurity, or developmental retardation.

## REGIONAL EXAMINATION

**I. Head and neck (patient sitting)**
A. Inspect
1. Neck for abnormal posture or deformity; lymphadenopathy, nodules, tophi (e.g., torticollis, spasm, gout).
B. Palpate
1. Temporomandibular joint for tenderness,

swelling, crepitance (e.g., rheumatoid arthritis).
2. Cervical spine, paravertebral and trapezius muscles for tenderness (diffuse or localized to trigger points).
C. Range of motion
1. Temporomandibular joint for mouth opening (e.g., rheumatoid arthritis).
2. Neck for flexion, extension, lateral flexion, and rotation.
3. Muscle power
a. Through normal range of motion of head and neck against resistance.

**II. Upper extremities (patient sitting)**
A. Inspect
1. Position and symmetry of shoulders and scapulae (e.g., Sprengel's deformity, scoliosis, winged scapulae).
2. Arms for torsion, deformity, shortening, or lengthening (e.g., cubitus varus or valgus).
3. Hands and wrists for atrophy, swelling, nodules, tophi, nail pitting, ulnar or radial deviation (e.g., arthritis, dislocated radial head, ganglion cysts).
4. Fingers for deformity (e.g., mallet, swan neck, boutonniere, trigger).
B. Palpate
1. Wrist joint and proximal and distal interphalangeal joints for swelling, bogginess, bony

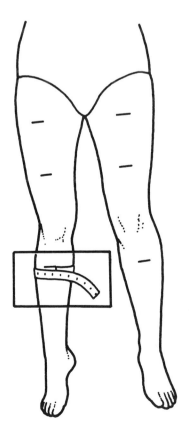

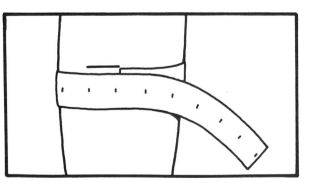

**Fig. 5-2.** Circumferential measurement of limb deficiency. Levels for measurement should first be marked, as indicated.

enlargement, tenderness, trigger points (e.g., arthritis).
2. Metacarpophalangeal joints (proximal to knuckles) for bogginess, swelling, tenderness.
3. Olecranon, lateral epicondyle of elbow for tenderness, swelling (e.g., tennis elbow, student's elbow).
4. Shoulder (rotation cuff) for diffuse or localized areas of tenderness.

C. Range of motion
1. Shoulder flexion, extension, adduction, abduction, external rotation, internal rotation.
2. Elbow flexion, extension, supination, pronation.
3. Wrist flexion, extension, ulnar and radial deviation.
4. Finger extension, flexion, hyperextension, abduction and adduction, opposition.

D. Muscle power
1. Through normal range of motion and against resistance. Test by muscle groups first; if weakness found, test individual muscles.

## III. Lower extremities (patient sitting, prone and supine, standing)

A. Inspect
1. Gluteal and popliteal creases; legs for atrophy (Fig. 5-2), calf contour, shortening or lengthening, torsion, angulation, bowing (e.g., genu varum or genu valgum, Fig. 5-3; in-toe or out-toe).
2. Knee for swelling, tenderness, deformity (e.g., Baker's cyst, patella alta).
3. Feet for deformities (e.g., corns, calluses, hallux valgus, metatarsus adductus, high arches, pes planus, syndactyly, polydactyly, claw toe, mallet toe, curly toes, overlapping toes), swelling, tenderness.

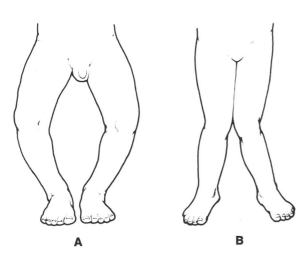

**Fig. 5-3. A,** Genu varum. **B,** Genu valgum. (From Hilt, N. E., and Schmitt, E. W., Jr.: Pediatric orthopedic nursing, St. Louis, 1975, The C. V. Mosby Co.)

B. Palpate
1. Patella for swelling, tenderness, stability.
2. Anterior ankle and metatarsophalangeal joints for swelling, tenderness (e.g., arthritis, bunion, gout). Individual metatarsophalangeal joints may be further evaluated by compressing the metatarsal heads in the sole of the foot.
3. Achilles tendon for nodules (e.g., rheumatoid arthritis), shortening (e.g., spasm), tenderness, or defects (complete or incomplete tears).

C. Range of motion
1. Ankle and foot dorsiflexion, plantar flexion, inversion and adduction (supination), and eversion and abduction (pronation).
2. Knee for flexion, extension, hyperextension, and mediolateral, anteroposterior, and rotatory stability.
3. Hip for flexion, extension, abduction, adduction, internal and external rotation (prone and supine). Note instability, clicks, or contracture.

D. Muscle power
1. Through normal range of motion and against resistance.

## IV. Spine (patient prone or sitting, standing)

A. Inspect
1. For sinuses, hair tufts, pigmentation, dimples, cysts, masses, malalignment of spinous processes, curvature (e.g., kyphosis, scoliosis, lordosis, buffalo hump).

B. Palpate
1. Spinous processes and paravertebral muscles for tenderness, swelling, increased or decreased muscle bulk, spasm.

C. Range of motion
1. Flexion, extension, lateral flexion, rotation.

D. Muscle power
1. Through normal range of motion and against examiner resistance.

## V. Gait (patient standing, walking)

A. Observe
1. Muscle weakness: gluteus medius lurch (Trendelenburg gait), gluteus maximus hyperextension, calcaneus gait, Penguin gait (muscular dystrophy), quadriceps paralysis.
2. Structural deformities: short-leg limp, ankylosed joint, antalgic gait.
3. Neurologic disorders: spastic gait (scraping or dragging), footdrop (steppage) gait (flopping), ataxic gait (stamping or slapping), dystrophic gait (Penguin).

## SUPPORTIVE DIAGNOSTIC MEASURES

Depending on the chief complaint or findings elicited during the general musculoskeletal examination, further assessment may be indicated (see Chapters 9 through 11 for more detail).

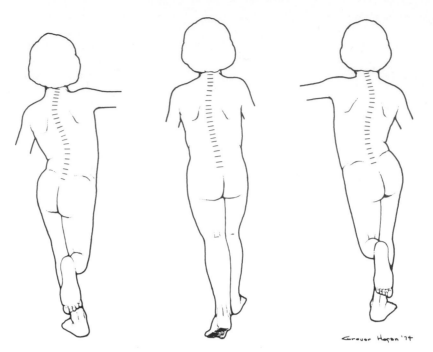

**Fig. 5-4.** Trendelenburg gait, often seen in child with congenital dislocation of hip. Note that child is unable to lift opposite side of pelvis during stance phase. In bilateral dislocation, as shown, child has waddling gait. (From Hilt, N. E., and Schmitt, E. W., Jr.: Pediatric orthopedic nursing, St. Louis, 1975, The C. V. Mosby Co.)

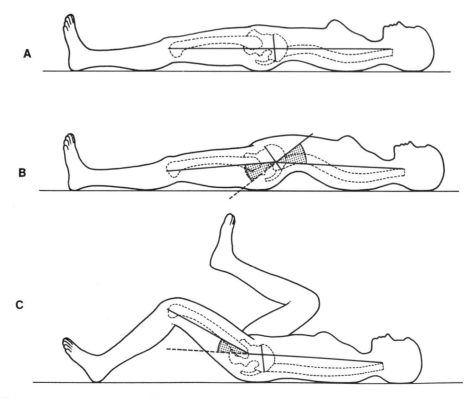

**Fig. 5-5.** A, Thomas' sign. **A,** Normal. **B,** Hip flexion contracture. **C,** Maximal hip and knee flexion, loss of lordosis, hip flexion contracture.

**I. Special tests or physical signs**
  A. Upper extremity
     1. Carpal tunnel syndrome: wrist flexing or sharp percussion of nerve will reproduce numbness or tingling along distribution of median nerve.
  B. Lower extremity
     1. Hip weakness or dislocation: Trendelenburg sign (Fig. 5-4), Thomas' sign (Fig. 5-5), Ober's sign (Fig. 5-6), Allis' (Galeazzi's) sign (Fig. 5-7, *A*), Ortolani maneuver (Fig. 5-7, *B*), Barlow's test, Gower's sign.
     2. Hip contracture: Thomas test, Ely test.
     3. Knee stability or injury: ballottement, bulge, MacMurray's test, anterior and posterior drawer tests, rotatory instability tests, pivot shift.
     4. Leg length discrepancy: measure actual versus apparent length (Fig. 5-8).
     5. Ankle sprain: forced inversion test.

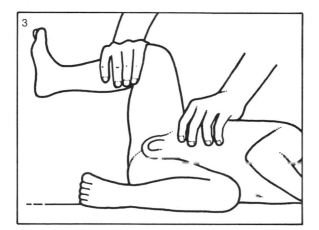

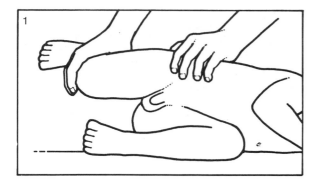

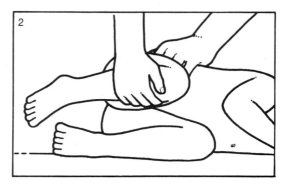

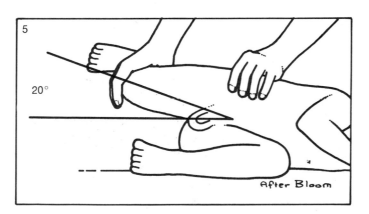

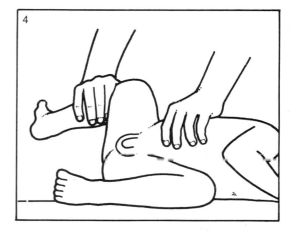

**Fig. 5-6.** Ober's sign for determination of degree of abduction contracture of hip.

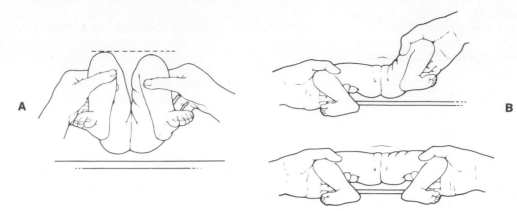

**Fig. 5-7. A,** Galeazzi's sign. **B,** Ortolani's sign. (From Hilt, N. E., and Schmitt, E. W., Jr.: Pediatric orthopedic nursing, St. Louis, 1975, The C. V. Mosby Co.)

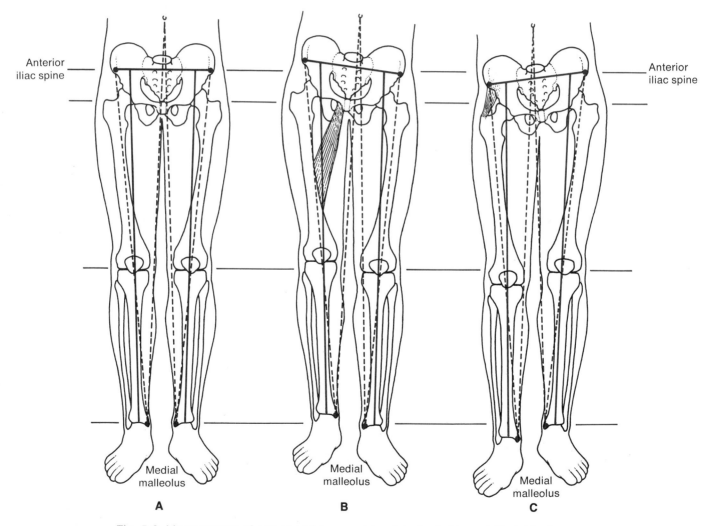

Anterior iliac spine

Anterior iliac spine

Medial malleolus

Medial malleolus

Medial malleolus

A              B              C

**Fig. 5-8.** Measurement of actual and apparent leg length. **A,** Normal. **B,** Adduction contracture with apparent shortening. **C,** Abduction contracture with apparent lengthening.

C. Spine
  1. Scoliosis, kyphosis, ankylosing spondylitis: forward bending test.
  2. Low back pain (sciatica), spinal irritation: straight leg raise (Lasègue's sign), tripod sign.
## II. Laboratory aids
A. Biochemical
  1. Cerebrospinal fluid: infection, degeneration, or neoplasm.
  2. Synovial fluid, muscle enzymes: aldolase, CPK.
  3. Mineral metabolism: calcium, phosphorus, alkaline phosphatase.
  4. Bacteriologic: smears, cultures.
  5. Rheumatologic: latex fixation, rheumatoid factor, HLA-27, antinuclear antibody.
  6. General: CBC, ESR, UA, serology.
B. Radiographic: routine roentgenograms, laminograms, scanograms, arthrograms, myelograms, arteriograms, bone scans, axial tomography.
C. Other: EMG and nerve conduction, biopsy.

## REFERENCES

1. American Orthopedic Association: Manual of orthopedic surgery, Chicago, 1972, The Association.
2. Tachjdian, M. O.: Pediatric orthopedics, vol. I, Philadelphia, 1972, W. B. Saunders Co.

## BIBLIOGRAPHY

American Orthopedic Association: Manual of orthopedic surgery, Chicago, 1972, The Association.
Salter, R. B.: Textbook of disorders and injuries of the musculoskeletal system, Baltimore, 1970, The Williams & Wilkins Co.
Tachdjian, M. O.: Pediatric orthopedics, vol. I, Philadelphia, 1972, W. B. Saunders Co.

# 6

# Nursing assessment

**PAMELA S. CROSS**

**KATHLEEN G. WALLACE**

As nursing becomes more and more specialized, patient care seems to become more and more fragmented. This indictment is perhaps justified. Nurses in a specialty often concentrate their energies on one area of the body, and therefore other patient problems assume less importance. In contrast, throughout their entire educational experience nurses are taught to think in terms of the whole patient as their concern and responsibility. Concern for the whole person should also guide the nurse in completing the orthopedic assessment.

## DEFINITION AND PROCESS

In the last 5 years much has been written about the nursing process as a whole. These texts have contributed to the nursing profession's beginning understanding of the assessment phase of the nursing process.

Fuerst, Wolf, and Weitzel[8,p.63] define the nursing assessment process as the collection of data to determine where a person is on the health-illness continuum. This statement implies that there is more to the assessment process than looking for pathologic problems. These authors suggest, as did F. McCain,[17] that the nurse should evaluate the individual's coping mechanisms, support systems, and abilities that may influence his movement toward health or illness. Just as the physician takes the time to complete a health history on each patient individually, so must the nurse. If individualized care is the goal of the nurse, then each patient must be assessed separately. Before beginning the nursing assessment, the nurse must prepare to perform this step of the nursing process. Yura and Walsh[25,p.72] support the idea that the depth of knowledge the nurse has affects the quality of judgment and eventually the conclusions drawn from the assessment. These authors further state that the nurse needs to have a background that includes knowledge of normal growth patterns and of major illnesses that affect each age group. The nurse must understand the signs, symptoms, onset, treatment, causes, and outcomes of these major illnesses. Assessment also depends on the nurse's experience. Clinical experience and expertise tend to alert the nurse to situations that are potentially serious and that may slow or impede the patient's recovery. Experience influences judgment, which affects when and how the nurse reacts to a problem.

Part of being able to assess the whole person is having a background not only in physical development and pathophysiology but also in the psychology of human beings. This psychological background should include knowledge of an individual's emotional responses to stress, illness, anxiety, and fear. The nurse must have understanding of defense mechanisms and the behavior these mechanisms may evoke.

Since nurses must operate in cultures that are at times very different from their own, they must have some background in sociology and anthropology. This social science background affords the nurse information on different family and life styles as well as different cultural attitudes and beliefs about health and illness.

The nurse with a solid and diverse background in the aforementioned disciplines is ready to begin the process of assessment. Fuerst, Wolf, and Weitzel[8,p.65] describe the assessment process succinctly, noting that it includes gathering data; comparing these data to a standard, norm, or average; stating the assessment; validating the nurse's final assessment; and evaluating the accuracy with which the assessment reflects the patient's position on the health-illness continuum.

## Observation

The process of assessment begins with the collection of data through observation. Observation is more than merely looking at some object or person; it implies perception of the intended object or person. In nursing it is necessary to train oneself to observe with special focus on physical and emotional problems. With astute observation the nursing history can be merely a validating tool for what the nurse has already noted through observation. Generally the nurse should note the environment; interactions the patient has with friends, family, and strangers; obvious problems; facial expressions and gestures; posture and gait; and if the medical diagnosis is known, the particular area of disease, if possible. Not only is observation accomplished through the eyes but also through the other senses as well. Hearing, smelling, and touching can be important adjuncts to the observation phase of assessment. Observation, like assessment, should continue throughout the time the patient requires nursing intervention.

## Nursing history

The next phase of the assessment process is taking a nursing history. Little and Carnevali describe the starting point of history taking as the nursing assessment transaction. They define it as a time-limited, focused interaction in which high-priority subjective and objective data regarding the patient's situation and resources and deficits in coping are elicited, observed, and recorded in both physiologic and psychological dimensions.[13,p.96] The tool that has been developed to add structure and consistency to the type of information gathered during the assessment transaction is the nursing history. The nursing history simply refers to the total information collected by the nurse during the admission interview with the patient. The nursing history provides a systematic format from which to develop a written record of information about a patient.

In many institutions the nursing history has been made a part of the client's permanent record. The format of the history may be that of a questionnaire or a checklist. Nursing care data about the patient as a person is collected as well as information that deals with the patient's specific health problems and needs. No universal nursing history format exists. Therefore a format can be developed to meet the requirements of each particular situation. It is important, however, that the format developed be evaluated from time to time and, where weaknesses are noted, revisions made.

## Interview

The structured interview is used to collect the data for the nursing history. The interview is defined as "a method of learning about people through purposeful, goal-directed communication."[15,p.28] Its purpose is to encourage the patient or significant other to express ideas, feelings, and facts that help identify immediate and long-range needs.

The interview usually takes place as soon as the nurse and patient meet.[25,p.85] Because time for the interview is limited, efficient use of time is mandatory. Although the nurse may use a standardized form to collect data, it is of utmost importance that the interview be conducted in a flexible manner. The nurse is challenged to obtain as much information as possible while at the same time allowing opportunity for the patient to express himself completely. Various communication techniques such as using open-ended questions and seeking clarification often afford this opportunity and facilitate communication. The setting in which the interview takes place should be conducive to an unhurried exchange of information. Data may be recorded during the interview.[15,p.24] Although some nurses feel that it makes the patient uncomfortable to have the nurse take notes during the interview, it has been found that the climate of trust increases when the patient can see what is being written.[13,p.105]

While the primary focus is on collection of data, a concomitant function is the initiation of the relationship between patient and nurse. During the interview the nurse has the opportunity to communicate concern and interest in the patient as a person, and a sense of trust and respect is often created.

The process of nursing assessment is only partially complete after the nursing history has been recorded. The comprehensiveness and quality of the information collected is of utmost importance, and it may be necessary to return to collect more information after the initial interview.

### Setting standards

After gathering the data, the nurse then compares them with a standard. For example, when the nurse is assessing the temperature of a patient, he or she immediately reflects on the normal temperature (37 C or 98.6 F), which is the standard. The nurse has compared the patient's temperature with a standard, in this case almost without realizing it. This phase of the assessment process is done many times during the course of total assessment of an individual, as there are many standards by which patients are evaluated. These standards may be physical, psychological, or sociological. For some areas of practice standards have not yet been developed, for example, in psychiatry. The actual parameters for judging disease states such as schizophrenia are not yet defined. As a result the nurse may be in the position of comparing the data with a standard that is solely founded on his or her knowledge and prior experiences.

### Nursing diagnosis

After comparing the data with a standard, a conclusion is drawn about what the nurse has observed. This conclusion should be written on the chart, nursing care plan, or nursing history form as appropriate. Included in the statement should be mention of the underlying problem that supports this conclusion. For example, the nurse would state, "The patient has 40° flexion of the right knee due to rheumatoid arthritis."

Validating the statement of conclusion of the as-

sessment process can be accomplished through a multitude of resources and methods. Nurses should and can consult with other nurses to validate the appropriateness of their conclusions. Reassessment or recalculation, use of texts, and consultation with other health professionals is appropriate. Finally, the nurse looks at the standard used to compare data. Was the data measurable? Was the standard appropriate for the patient? At the conclusion of the entire assessment process the nurse makes a statement of the problem, or a nursing diagnosis.

The nursing diagnosis is distinct from the medical diagnosis in that the nurse's objectives are different from those of the physician. The physician assesses the patient with the objective of "curing" the individual, correcting the disease process or problem, manipulating the physiologic status of the individual to effect a cure, or making the individual more comfortable with the disease. The nurse, on the other hand, uses assessment to promote efficiency and effectiveness in caring for the individual undergoing treatment or to assist a patient who wishes to help himself in performing some aspect of health care. In doing so the nurse strives to make the nursing diagnosis appropriate for the objectives of "caring" for a patient rather than "treating" the patient.

The accomplishment of this task is greatly dependent on the nurse's being able to make the conclusions from and about the assessment data very specific for nursing. Durand and Prince[7,p.57] suggest that in wording the nursing diagnosis the statement itself could be different from the medical diagnosis, except in an emergency perhaps. For example, if the patient's heart stopped, both the nurse and physician would make the same diagnosis. However, in other situations the nurse attempts to state the diagnosis in such a way that nursing interventions or prescriptions can be planned and implemented. An example for clarification is as follows:

**Medical diagnosis:** sciatica — Does not suggest nursing actions or care except in a very general way; it does suggest disease process and may imply treatment

**Nursing diagnosis:** back and leg pain unrelieved by traction and bed rest — Conclusion obtained from assessment data and on which intervention or prescription may be determined

The nursing diagnosis states the exact status of the patient. Interventions can be planned that are specific to the patient's needs. Notice also that a diagnosis simply of "pain" is not specific enough to begin care for the patient. The nursing diagnosis may also include a physiologic process as well as symptoms that require management.[7,p.56] An example might be "decreased peripheral blood circulation in legs." This states a physiologic problem that may be the result of various diseases but does not designate the medical diagnosis. Patients with these various diseases must have, at some point, similar nursing care plans and prescriptions designated or developed.

The purpose of making a nursing diagnosis or actually naming the problem is to permit nurses to begin working within a scientific framework. In addition it permits nurses to improve specific nursing care planning and well-designed nursing intervention.[7,p.58]

### Reassessment

When the nursing diagnosis has been established and the care or prescription initiated, the nurse must be prepared to reassess the patient as well as the diagnosis and prescriptions. The initial assessment is based on observation, interview, and the nursing history. The nursing history should allow for periodic reassessment so that change from baseline data can be demonstrated.

The patient and nurse should cooperate in developing a better understanding of the patient's problems and response to therapy. Reassessment can be continuous, it can be accomplished when emergency situations arise, or it can be planned and built into the structure of the nursing process. In any case there should be some time allotted for reassessment of the patient in order to better determine in which direction the patient is moving. The data gathered from reassessment will determine whether nursing therapies are assisting the patient toward health or whether nursing interventions need to be redesigned.

In order to clarify the process of nursing assessment it is schematically presented in Fig. 6-1. The nurse brings to the assessment process his or her background, education, and experience. To these are added information gathered during the nursing history. The nurse then formulates the nursing diagnosis based on observation, knowledge, judgment, standards, and patient input. If it is found that this diagnosis is invalid for any reason, the nurse then reassesses the problem and begins the process again.

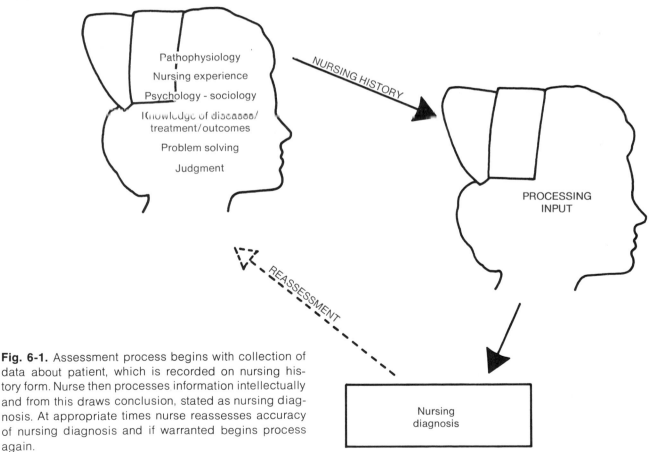

Pathophysiology

Nursing experience

Psychology - sociology

Knowledge of diseases/ treatment/outcomes

Problem solving

Judgment

NURSING HISTORY

PROCESSING INPUT

REASSESSMENT

Nursing diagnosis

**Fig. 6-1.** Assessment process begins with collection of data about patient, which is recorded on nursing history form. Nurse then processes information intellectually and from this draws conclusion, stated as nursing diagnosis. At appropriate times nurse reassesses accuracy of nursing diagnosis and if warranted begins process again.

## FRAMEWORK FOR ORTHOPEDIC NURSING ASSESSMENT

Thorough, systematic nursing assessment of a patient with an orthopedic need has several purposes and outcomes. First, it allows the nurse to become familiar with the long-term or chronic effects of the disease on the patient. When the nurse explores with the patient the ways in which he has learned to live with any limitations in function or activity and his feelings about this, the nurse gains an appreciation for the patient's ability to cope with the problem. The nurse also obtains information that will assist in assessing the patient's rehabilitation potential. Each patient should participate in his rehabilitation, but the degree to which he does, as well as the expected pace of recovery, can be determined most appropriately if it is based on individualized assessment of the particular patient.

Case finding, the discovery of previously undiagnosed disease or physical limitations, may occur during assessment. A knowledge base and familiarity with the expected incidence of certain orthopedic problems enables the nurse to anticipate their occurrence and refer patients for appropriate evaluation, diagnosis, and treatment.

Prevention of loss of function, incapacitating disabilities, or serious complications may be another outcome of the orthopedic nursing assessment. The earlier that problems are assessed and appropriate intervention delivered, the higher the level of recovery that might be expected.

## DISUSE PHENOMENA

In a well-known article on the effects of immobility on the human body, Olson stated that "motion is synonymous with life."[19,p.780] The human body depends on movement for a balance between building up and tearing down of some tissues. When working with any patient subjected to bed rest, it is essential to understand disuse phenomena. Disuse can effect psychosocial as well as physical changes in an individual, and often these changes are degenerative.

This knowledge of disuse is of particular concern and value to the orthopedic nurse. Most of the patients cared for within this specialty are confined to bed for varying periods. The patient who undergoes surgical spinal fusion or total hip replacement often requires bed rest. Policies at some institutions dictate bed rest for months after back surgery. In addition, immobilization of specific parts of the body may be necessary for extended periods. In all cases the results of disuse should be known by all nurses caring for these patients.

## Psychosocial

When assessing the psychologic concerns and needs of the patient, the nurse should consider his ability to cope with confinement and to some extent seclusion. Levine states that "the world is meaningful to the individual only as he experiences it."[11,p.96] Persons confined to bed are often deprived of interaction with the world around them and as a result experience decreased drives, motivations, expectations, and even abilities involved in learning and retaining what they have learned.[23,p.795] On the orthopedic unit a patient may be confined to bed for weeks, and the only interactions he may have are with the housekeeping staff, an aide, or a nurse who occasionally brings medication. None of these individuals tests his intellectual capacity or involves him in extensive conversation.

Downs[6,p.435] reported in her study that young, healthy individuals who were placed on bed rest for $2\frac{3}{4}$ hours reported disturbances of time and memory. These subjects also experienced olfactory, tactile, auditory, and visual hallucinations. How much more patients experience when they are confined to a private room with drugs, pain, and disease compounding sensory disturbance is only conjecture.

Emotional reactions of the patient are not so predictable. Reactions may include "apathy, withdrawal, frustrated anger, aggression, or regression."[6,p.435] Children react to treatment or illness more on how they feel at the moment than on any psychosociologic interpretation of illness. The nurse should be prepared to assess behavior that is indicative of the emotions described and explore the meaning behind these feelings.

In the United States there is much emphasis on middle-class or upper-middle-class youth, beauty, and upward social mobility. It is admirable to have many friends, attend social functions, and interact with interesting people. An individual confined to bed does not have this opportunity and therefore over long periods may see himself as not able to achieve these physical and social goals.

The individual may see himself as a useless person with his usual roles nonexistent or usurped by others. If a scar or physical deformity results from some surgical intervention, the person may see himself differently, as not whole, as degenerating, or his body image being less than he can tolerate. These feelings may set the stage for emotional outbursts, decreased motivation, and withdrawal.

In the world of decreased physical and social movement, the patient may become egocentric. Since he is less able to participate in decision making and has less control over his own life style, it may be difficult to see a larger world outside his room. As a result he may feel that he and his illness are the most important factors in his surroundings. He may expect others to be concerned about him to the point that he demands all their energy and time. This egocentricity may also take on the form of withdrawal. The patient is so involved in getting himself well that he cannot relate to others. He simply does not have the energy to invest in activities outside himself.

With continued disuse of intellectual functions, persons can become less efficient in terms of mental activity, that is, remembering, problem solving, and learning. As mentioned, it may become impossible for the individual to make decisions or draw conclusions. The nurse will want to assess carefully how much is reasonable to ask the patient in terms of problem solving. Although many nursing texts instruct nurses to give patients a choice, perhaps for some patients this is a disservice.

Wade[23,p.795] discussed another psychological change associated with disuse, that of distortion of time. Activities of most individuals revolve around the clock. People eat at a certain time, bathe at a certain time, work at a designated time. When an individual is confined to bed, all time seems to be altered. Work is no longer a part of the individual's day; bathing and eating are often dictated by others. The individual's landmarks in a day become confused, and day and night seem to run together. Wade wrote that the immobile individual has decreased sensory stimulation, and this further contributes to his confusion of time.

Obviously the person confined to bed in any setting cannot carry on work at the same level as before confinement. Students can study, businessmen can make telephone calls, but they cannot interact with the same impact when recumbent. It is very difficult to make a strong argument for or against anything when the individual is flat in bed. If the confinement lasts for an extended period, the individual may be forced to relinquish his job and thereby reinforce his powerlessness. Occupational changes can add increased physical and psychological stress. Physical stress can cause increased hormonal and gastric secretions, which can lead to gastric and blood pressure changes.[11,p.96] Psychological stress can make the individual less able to handle emotions that he is already handling tenuously.

Regardless of the length of confinement, the client may experience changes in life style. Rituals of eating, bathing, dressing, and socializing are altered to varying degrees. If he loses his job and the income it provides, he will suffer loss of some role identification. This also means he will be unable financially to care for himself and for others for whom he may be responsible.

Favorite activities such as sports, travel, and exercise may no longer be possible for the patient. All of these changes are serious psychological and social adjustments to be faced. The patient who will be in bed a day or two may not experience all of these situations and feelings but surely will face some to a limited degree.

When caring for children confined to bed for extended periods it is well to consider the emotional responses different age groups demonstrate to this restraint. Older children will most likely react to bed rest in a manner similar to that of an adult. The older child is usually capable of a certain degree of self-direction and industry in thought and activity level. In contrast, the very young child is dependent on those around him to assist in meeting his need for activity and interaction. Thus the young child will most likely respond more to the lack of physical contact and separation from parents than to bed rest itself.

### Physical

When addressing the problems of bed rest, the nurse needs to consider the multitudinous physical problems of an immobile patient. These problems have been discussed in many nursing texts, books devoted to the topic, and numerous journal articles; therefore this discussion is intended to give only enough information to help the orthopedic nurse assess the patient and perhaps anticipate potential problems.

**Skin.** Probably the first thing nurses think of when a patient is confined to bed is the possibility of skin breakdown. It is appropriate that the nurse consider this serious complication, as it is reported that the treatment of decubitus ulcers can result in additional hospital costs ranging from $2,000 to $10,000 for the patient.[21,p.283] This, of course, does not include the misery, scarring, and deformity also involved.

Decubitus ulcers can be produced by both low pressure (such as pressure exerted by the bed on skin) for long periods or high pressure (such as pressure exerted by one limb on another limb) for short periods.[9,p.350] Any pressure that causes collapse of superficial capillaries will lead to ischemia of the skin and eventual tissue necrosis. Pressure exerted on the skin by the bed has been measured by Lindan[12] and found to be slightly higher than capillary hydrostatic pressure. The nurse should consider assessing other factors that might lead to tissue trauma in the patient confined to bed, such as shearing forces, moisture, inadequate nutrition, friction, poor general hygiene, length of immobility, and presence of anemia. Of particular interest to the orthopedic nurse is that neurologically impaired patients may not feel pain as the first sign of ischemia, and therefore skin breakdown may occur more rapidly.

Some of the signs of skin ischemia the nurse should observe for are redness, pain, edema, and then skin breakdown. The elderly, because of possible poor nutrition, lack of movement, and general skin condition, are often more susceptible to skin breakdown. However, the young are just as susceptible if there is lack of movement. Tissue ischemia can occur in anyone in 1 to 2 hours.[5] (See Chapter 30 for additional information on decubiti.)

**Nutrition.** Adequate nutrition is essential for all age groups, regardless of their orthopedic status. When the patient is to undergo surgery or has an orthopedic injury, it is necessary that his diet contain the full requirements of vitamins D and C, calcium, and protein.

The protein requirement generally recommended for an adult is 0.36 g/lb.[1,p.752] Children and pregnant or lactating women require higher amounts. "At least one-third of the dietary protein of adults should be derived from complete protein foods; one-half to two-thirds of the child's protein should come from complete protein foods."[1,p.752]

Beland[1,p.752] notes that in patients who are undernourished, healing cannot take place as quickly, or in some cases not at all until nutrient requirements are met. Complete proteins can be found in meat, milk, cheese, and eggs. An adequate intake of protein for one day would include two or three cups of milk and two other servings of a complete protein for children and two or more cups of milk and two other servings of complete protein for adults.[24,p.304]

Vitamin C plays an important role in wound healing. It aids in the formation of collagen, which is essential in the repair of blood vessels and other tissues. Surgical patients can require as much as ten times the normal intake of vitamin C prior to surgery.[24,p.117] Since many orthopedic patients undergo surgery, it is important to assess this area of intake. Vitamin C is contained in citrus juices and fruits, tomatoes, potatoes, and cabbage. Vitamin C is not stored for extensive periods and therefore must be replenished on a regular basis. Adults usually require more vitamin C than children. Adequate intake for a healthy adult is one serving daily of a fruit or vegetable high in vitamin C.

Vitamin D plays a key role in bone repair following surgery. This vitamin enables the intestines to actively transport the calcium molecule from the food eaten to the bloodstream. Once the calcium transfer occurs, phosphorus absorption into the bloodstream follows the calcium molecule. Vitamin D continues to work by assisting in calcification of bones. Vitamin D also controls some factors in citrate metabolism. Citrate is responsible for mobilizing calcium from the bone and blood. Studies of metabolism of vitamin D indicate that children and pregnant or lactating women need 400 IU per day.[24,p.83] Adults generally receive enough vitamin D through sunshine, as vitamin D is synthesized on the skin when it is exposed to sunlight. Vitamin D can be found in small amounts in eggs and fish oils, and milk and margarine are often supplemented with vitamin D.

Nurses assessing orthopedic patients must also assess the volume of fluid taken in by the immobilized individual. Although kidney function is not altered by immobility, other systems (bones, muscles) undergo changes that may alter the concentration of certain products that the kidney must excrete. The recommended daily intake of fluids is between 2,100 and 2,800 ml for the average adult. Fluid intake for children is based on weight, from 67.5 ml/kg (2¼ oz/lb) for an infant to 22.5 ml/kg (¾ oz/lb) for a 13-year-old.[24,p.83] If the patient is perspiring heavily, has excess drainage, or has respiratory increases above normal, the fluid intake should be increased to recover the fluid lost through these mechanisms. While administering intravenous fluids or giving the patient water to drink will accomplish the goal of increased fluids, the nurse should attempt to get the patient to consume fluids that will supply some of the electrolytes and nutrients lost as well. In consideration of the immobilized patient's propensity to form calcium stones, some authors recommend that the patient drink cranberry juice, which may have some acidifying properties in the urine.[24,p.83]

Monitoring of the nutritional status for prevention of constipation is required for almost all patients confined to bed or who have decreased mobility. If assessment is continuous, minor alterations in diet will frequently prevent the use of laxatives, enemas, and other unnatural means of bowel control.

It is important for the nurse to utilize this type of information and note dietary deficiencies and likes and dislikes of each individual and then determine whether these requirements are met. Instruction of the patient, and family if necessary, is essential so that these necessary nutrients are consumed.

**Musculoskeletal.** Another important area of the nursing assessment is evaluation of the patient's strengths, weaknesses, and problems of the musculoskeletal system. Since patients on an orthopedic service require intervention within the musculoskeletal system, it is often necessary to keep one extremity or part immobilized while the patient or nurse exercises other parts of the body. Assessment of muscle motion and strength prior to bed rest, treatment, or intervention is essential.

One of the greatest problems associated with extended bed rest or limited activity of a part of the body is disuse atrophy, which may occur in both muscle and bone. An important concept for the nurse to remember is that stress applied to the bone or muscle is an important factor in maintaining its health and function. The body of a weight lifter is an example of what exercise and resistance do to muscle tone. During disuse the muscle loses size and strength. The result of this wasting is that the muscle is unable to carry out its important functions such as supporting the back or abdomen or limb function.

*Contractures.* Contractures are the result of constant flexion or extension of a body part. Usually they are the result of flexion, because patients flex knees and hips in order to relax muscles when in pain or when cold.[14,p.300] The amputee often flexes the affected limb for comfort or to decrease edema. As a result the individual often experiences joint stiffness, which may slow rehabilitation. If the joint is not moved, permanent stiffness may result. This can be corrected only by manipulation of the joint, and casting or surgical correction may be required. Special emphasis on assessment in terms of contractures should be placed on the patient with an amputation, back injury, or spinal cord injury. Although the nurse should be alert to the development of contractures with all patients on orthopedic units, preventive care with range-of-motion exercises should be maintained when possible.

*Constipation.* Decreased muscle strength in limbs often involves decreased strength of abdominal musculature required for adequate bowel elimination. This problem, compounded by the horizontal position, change in dietary habits, and other factors, may encourage the development of constipation. The nurse should also consider drugs such as narcotics and anesthetic agents that slow peristalsis and therefore may also aid in the development of this problem. In addition increased fluid loss or decreased fluid intake may contribute to constipation in the orthopedic patient. It is important for the nurse to assess the individual's elimination status during the initial assessment so that prevention of constipation may begin on admission and not when

the patient has developed an impaction or intestinal obstruction.

*Demineralization.* Along with muscle atrophy, disuse causes bone demineralization. As mentioned, calcium and phosphorus are dependent on vitamin D for absorption from the gut and movement into bone. The immobilized patient whose food intake may be decreased or restricted may experience bone demineralization. Browse[2,p.116] stated that loss of calcium is a natural phenomenon of bed rest. The increased activity of osteoclasts may be due to decreased blood flow to the bone. Muscle action is required to produce this blood flow, and therefore muscle action is necessary to prevent some demineralization. Disuse osteoporosis develops as a result of an imbalance between osteoblasts and osteoclasts. Both cells proliferate during bed rest; however, osteoclastic activity is greater. It seems that degeneration of bone matrix occurs prior to osteoclastic resorption. This degeneration causes the breakdown of the bony matrix and the resultant loss of minerals. Browse[2,p.117] describes the loss of calcium from the bones as a progressive problem through the sixth week of bed rest; the peak calcium loss is in the fifth and sixth weeks. The bone will attempt to compensate for osteoporosis by trying to increase the rate of bone formation, but this is not successful, and breakdown and demineralization continue.

The dangers of osteoporosis are pathologic fracture, softening of bones that can lead to deformity, and pain in joints due to calcium deposits. When calcium is released from the bone, it enters the bloodstream. The body handles this excess by depositing the calcium in the joints and in the kidney by trying to excrete large amounts of calcium in the urine. Unfortunately, often the kidney cannot keep pace with the calcium, and a rise in urine pH occurs and stones are formed by the precipitating mineral. These stones can block the ureter and cause kidney damage, glomerular degeneration, and acute pain. It is important for the nurse to know something about prior kidney problems (e.g., stone formation) and the length of bed rest. Recumbency also aids in the pooling of urine in the kidney, which may also precipitate renal calculi formation.

**Respiratory.** Another important consideration of patients who remain recumbent for long periods is the pooling of respiratory secretions. As soon as the individual lies down, secretions in the lungs tend to rest in the bronchioles unevenly, wetting the dependent side of the bronchioles and drying the other surfaces.[14,p.304] Browse[2,p.53] states that the diameter of the bronchioles decreases when the individual is

## DISUSE PHENOMENA

| Area of concern | Questions to be explored | Area of concern | Questions to be explored |
|---|---|---|---|
| Nutrition | | Respiratory—cont'd | |
| Vitamin D | Loss of exposure to sunshine? Sufficient consumption of eggs, fish, milk, margarine? | Hypostatic pneumonia—cont'd | assistive device be of help (e.g., blow glove, blow bottle, IPPB)? What does the chest x-ray film demonstrate? What does the chest sound like? Any identifiable rales? Rhonchi? History of smoking? Hydration status? Temperature? |
| Vitamin C | Sufficient consumption of fruits, juices, fresh fruits? | | |
| Fluids | Does the person consume 2,100 to 3,000 ml/day? Any unusual fluid loss? Types of fluids consumed? Skin turgor? Dry mouth? Thirst? | | |
| | | Atelectasis | Consider many of the above points and also the following. Has the patient received anesthetics recently? Analgesics? Alcohol or tobacco abuse? Restriction of movement? Temperature increase? |
| Bulk/roughage | Amount of whole-grain products, lettuce, celery, cabbage, fruits, vegetables consumed? | | |
| Protein | Amount of complete protein (eggs, milk, cheese, meat) consumed? | | |
| | | Gastrointestinal | |
| Likes/dislikes | What does the patient say he likes or dislikes? What does he eat besides that which is on the tray? How do likes/dislikes influence what he eats? | Constipation | Intake of roughage/bulk? Is there a history of laxative dependency? Has the person taken in food in the last couple of days? What was the date of the last bowel movement? Was this a normal evacuation for this patient? What is the fluid status? Length of immobility? Strength of abdominal musculature? Any drugs that alter peristalsis? |
| Musculoskeletal | | | |
| Contractures | Amount of exercise (range-of-motion, active, passive, resistive)? Walking? Immobile? How much self-care is the individual capable of? | | |
| Muscle weakness | Is it necessary for the client to perform isometric exercise? Range-of-motion exercise? Weight bearing? What is the nutritional status? What is the length of immobility? What part do drugs play in the weakness? | Impaction | What are the bowel sounds? Sometimes obstruction will produce hypermotile sounds above the obstruction and decreased sounds below the obstruction. How long has the patient been constipated? When was the last bowel movement? Is there passage of liquid fecal matter? Is there distention, abdominal cramping, pain? |
| Respiratory | | | |
| Hypostatic pneumonia | Does the patient have a history of pulmonary problems? Can the patient move independently? Does he require turning? How effective is his coughing and deep breathing? Would an | | |

## DISUSE PHENOMENA—cont'd

| Area of concern | Questions to be explored | Area of concern | Questions to be explored |
|---|---|---|---|
| Anorexia | Amount of fluid and food intake in 24-hour period? What is the patient's weight now as compared with admission or first encounter? Is there contributory anxiety, pain, fatigue, depression, fear? What are the patient's food likes/dislikes? Are drugs adding to anorexia? Are boredom and lack of exercise adding to the problem? | Psychosocial Decreased sensory input | How has the patient coped with confinement before? Is the person active or sedentary in usual daily activities? Are there areas where sensory input could be increased (e.g., TV, radio, visits)? What is the status of the patient's short-term and long-term memory? Is the patient hallucinating? |
| Cardiovascular Thrombus formation | Any recent damage (even minor) or injury to tissue or blood vessels? History of emboli? Concurrent signs of phlebitis? Positioning that might lead to undue pressure on vessels? Any areas of venous stasis (e.g., legs, pelvis)? Hydration status? Other disease states that may make the individual more prone to thrombus formation? Platelet count? Partial thromboplastin time? Prothrombin time? | Socioeconomic deprivation | To what degree have work patterns been interrupted? Could the patient reestablish these during bed rest? Is vocational rehabilitation necessary due to immobility? Who is supporting the individual or the family? What is the impact of the loss of the person's role since immobilization? What is the person's insurance coverage? What new roles must the patient assume since immobilized? What visitors come to see the patient? Could more be encouraged to see the patient? |
| Orthostatic hypotension | Length of bed rest? Types of activities during bed rest? Is it possible to use CircOlectric bed before ambulating patient? Drugs that may contribute to hypotension when the person is ambulated? | Stress | What is the extent of loss of the individual's favorite activities? What changes has the patient had to make in terms of roles, job, life style? What are the financial burdens imposed by immobility? What has the inactivity meant to the patient? How well has the individual handled stress in the past? Is there a history of ulcers? Nervous disorders? What is the major support system for this patient? |
| Valsalva maneuver | What is the patient's bowel status? Should stool softeners be used? How does the patient move in bed? Trapeze bar? Does the patient know the technique of exhaling during exertion? Was the patient cautioned against straining when defecating? | | |

supine, and this gives a thicker coating of mucus to the bronchioles in all directions. The result is inadequate operation of cilia to rid the tracheobronchial tree of mucus. The pooling then brings about stasis and creates a medium for bacterial growth. If the mucus is not removed, hypostatic pneumonia will result.

The orthopedic nurse should be aware that this is a particular problem because surgical intervention for these patients often requires long recovery periods. Dehydration, lack of fluids before surgery, atropine and other anticholinergic drugs, and narcotics all contribute to stasis of bronchial secretions. To compound the problem, patients are often restricted severely in their movements because of pain and the surgical procedure itself. The orthopedic nurse should perform a careful, continuing assessment of respiratory status prior to any surgical intervention. Assessment of the same nature is required for patients who undergo nonsurgical intervention such as traction and other forms of recumbent therapy.

Part of the assessment should include adequate monitoring of the types of beds and chairs available to the patient. These may further complicate the respiratory problem by limiting chest expansion and thus decreasing ventilation and removal of mucus from the tracheobronchial tree. Adequate respirations require that there is no pressure or resistive force against the chest wall.

**Cardiovascular.** Another problem of disuse of the body occurs within the cardiovascular system. Prolonged bed rest encourages venous stasis in the pelvis and lower extremities. Venous stasis in itself will not cause clot formation; however, if there is trauma and a resultant increase in platelets the likelihood of clot formation is great. Dehydration can also increase the likelihood of clot formation by increasing the viscosity of the blood. Surgery, trauma, and medical disorders such as cancer and myocardial infarction increase the individual's chance of developing a thrombus. Thus the nurse who cares for a patient with a multitude of problems must realize the increased chance for thrombus formation and pulmonary embolism. A careful nursing and medical history will provide the nurse with the necessary information, which might warrant additional assessment and attention to this problem.

Another factor that may predispose the orthopedic patient to thrombus formation is improper positioning. If the patient is improperly positioned on his side, the upper leg may exert pressure on the lower leg, causing damage to the veins. As a result platelets clump around the bruised vessels, a clot is formed, and a potential embolus threatens. Orthopedic nurses must be cognizant of the proper use of pillows and positioning of patients to alleviate this hazard.

Positioning problems may also arise if the patient is being treated for sciatica or other back problems and his legs are suspended in traction or raised to 90° of flexion at the knee and hip. The pressure exerted under the knee may promote damage to vessel walls and cause clot formation. This same problem may also be simulated if the extremity is improperly positioned or handled during cast application or while the plaster is setting or becoming hardened.

Contributing to the cardiovascular problems is the Valsalva maneuver. The orthopedic patient is particularly at risk due to high incidence of constipation. In performing the Valsalva maneuver the individual sets his thorax by taking in a deep breath, holding it, and exerting pressure. When he relaxes, blood rushes to the heart, overloading the cardiac system, and cardiac arrest may ensue. This too should be of special interest to the orthopedic nurse, for not only does it have application from the standpoint of assessing problems in reference to constipation but also in the use of the trapeze bar. An extremely high percentage of orthopedic patients use the trapeze to assist themselves in a variety of movements necessary to their daily routine. In lifting themselves they set the thorax. These individuals must be taught to exhale while they move and to allow others to assist them.

Orthostatic hypotension is often the cause of dizziness that patients experience when they stand after bed rest. The vertigo is caused by a decrease in the efficiency of the response of the neurovascular reflexes that push blood to the brain when the individual moves from sitting to standing or lying to sitting. Patients may even faint when first arising if they are not brought to the erect posture slowly. Use of a CircOlectric bed aids in maintaining this reflex. The nurse can gradually tilt the bed each day until the patient is ready to stand.

This discussion of bed rest is by no means exhaustive, but it provides a background for the orthopedic nurse on which to base a very significant part of the assessment. Implications may be drawn for the partially immobilized patient in a cast, traction, or orthosis. In all cases a sound theoretical and practical knowledge base will assist the nurse in making appropriate assessments and later judgments concerning nursing intervention.

Areas of concern in the immobilized patient are summarized in the box on pp. 136-137. Also in-

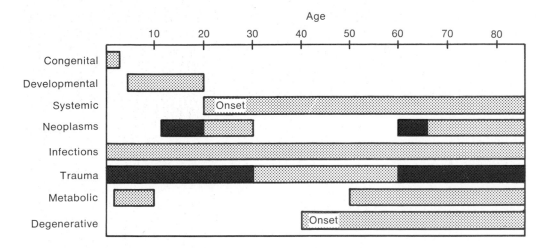

**Fig. 6-2.** Bar graph illustrating ages during which major categories of orthopedic defects may be expected to occur. Areas in red indicate age groups in which problem more frequently occurs.

cluded are some questions the nurse should explore when assessing various problems listed.

## ORTHOPEDIC PROBLEMS OVER LIFE CYCLE

Orthopedic problems occur in every age group, though certain conditions or disease states are identifiable in and may be limited to specific age groups (Fig. 6-2). Categorizing the main groups of orthopedic conditions provides the nurse with a framework from which to make a more informed assessment. An overview of these categories is presented here. For details of specific diseases injuries, and deformities see Part Four.

### Congenital

Some orthopedic deformities are present at birth. These defects may be the result of genetic variation or other influences affecting embryologic development. The types of congenital orthopedic deformities are almost limitless. Certain defects such as polydactyly may not require immediate treatment, but time is often an important factor in beginning treatment of many defects such as congenital dislocation of the hip and clubfoot.

Cerebral palsy is a congenital condition that may lead to orthopedic defects in childhood. The abnormal muscle function that is a result of cerebral palsy may require multiple surgical interventions to lengthen or release muscles and improve function. The orthopedic features may in some cases provide the differential diagnosis of this disease.

Other congenital defects may have associated orthopedic implications. Of those most frequently seen, variations of spina bifida and myelomeningocele probably carry the greatest number of implica-

tions. Many of these children are orthopedically evaluated for clubfeet, congenital dislocation of the hips, a variety of congenital and developmental spinal deformities, and orthotic prescriptions for gait training.

### Developmental

A number of bone and joint problems occur in childhood and adolescence. Many are self-limiting and require treatment only to prevent deformity while the condition runs its cycle. Legg-Perthes disease is most frequently seen in boys between the ages of 5 and 10 years.[10,p.369] Another common condition is slipped capital femoral epiphysis, most frequently found between the ages of 10 and 16 years and seen more often in boys.[20,p.818] Adolescent idiopathic scoliosis is seen more frequently in girls, occurring as early as 9 or 10 years of age and as late as 16 to 18 years or until growth ceases.[10,p.375]

### Systemic

A major orthopedic disease, rheumatoid arthritis is caused by sytemic factors. An estimated 5 million persons in the United States have this disease. While rheumatoid arthritis can occur at any age, it most commonly affects the young adult, with the usual age of onset between 20 and 40 years of age. This chronic systemic disease involves inflammatory changes throughout the body's connective tissues. The smaller, peripheral joints are most commonly involved.[14,p.1220]

### Neoplasms

Bone tumors may be benign or malignant. The benign type, such as osteochondroma and giant cell tumors, grow slowly and do not tend to destroy surrounding tissue or spread to other parts of the body. Malignant tumors such as osteogenic sarcoma, Ewing's sarcoma, and multiple myeloma grow rapidly and can spread to other parts of the body by way of the bloodstream. The occurrence of bone tumors is highest during adolescence, falls during young adulthood, and then begins to rise after the age of 60 years, when the incidence equals that during adolescence.[22,p.377]

### Infections

Bone and joint infections can occur in all age groups. Osteomyelitis is primarily a disease of children, with boys being affected more frequently than girls. In 80% to 90% of cases, *Staphylococcus aureus* is the responsible organism. Septic arthritis is another infection, with the hip joint as the site of highest incidence. Infants and children 1 or 2 years of age are most often affected, although it may occur in all age groups.[20,p.804]

### Trauma

Accidental injury to the musculoskeletal system occurs in every age group. Falls, sports injuries, automobile accidents, and occupational injuries are some of the major causes. Musculoskeletal injuries can range in severity from relatively minor soft-tissue injuries to severe crushing fractures. Age is a factor in predicting the incidence of orthopedic trauma, with the young and the elderly being at highest risk.

### Metabolic

Metabolic bone diseases occur for many diverse reasons and are often related to the nutritional or endocrine status of the patient. Rickets is a generalized disease of growing bone caused by inadequate calcification of bone matrix and evidenced by bone deformities.[20,p.860] Growth disorders and deformities of the bone may result from this disease. Primary osteoporosis is a common disease of bone metabolism in which the mass of bone is decreased. Both mineral and protein matrix components are reduced. This reduction in bone density occurs in approximately one fourth of all elderly persons, with the highest incidence in women between the ages of 50 and 70.[14,p.1237]

### Degenerative

The largest incidence of degenerative orthopedic changes is in the joints. Osteoarthritis is the most common joint degenerative disorder. Symptoms usually do not appear before age 40 years unless the involved joints have been subjected to trauma.

Almost all persons over age 45 have some form of osteoarthritis. The weight-bearing joints and terminal interphalangeal joints of the fingers are characteristically involved. Osteoarthritis progresses slowly, and although there is no cure for this disorder, joint function may be maintained more effectively than in other types of arthritis.[14,p.1229]

## ORTHOPEDIC NURSING ASSESSMENT

Orthopedic nursing assessment holds the nurse responsible for collecting specific information about the patient's musculoskeletal status. Several major areas should always be included and are discussed more specifically here. Data gathering in these areas is best done by direct observation whenever possible rather than relying wholly on the patient's subjective interpretation.

### Locomotion

In children the ability to move about follows a logical progression. The nurse must inquire about the child's ability to sit, crawl, stand, and walk. With older children and adults the nurse must collect data on their ability to move about independently. The nature and scope of any limitations must be described.

### Gait

When assessing gait the nurse looks for uniformity in body movement. Children up to age 3 or 4 years, however, have less uniform gait patterns, which should be taken into consideration. The toddler's legs frequently show bowing (tibial torsion) early in the ambulatory phase, along with flat feet, which are usually corrected without assistance by the time the child reaches preschool age. In the older child and adult the nurse looks for a balanced, smooth gait, with steps of equal length and toes and knees pointing straight ahead.

### Posture

Equal distribution of body weight is necessary for correct posture. When observing the patient in a standing position, the nurse draws an imaginary line of gravity and observes for any malalignment of body segments and a distorted weight-bearing line. The presence of lordosis, kyphosis, or scoliosis should be identified. However, the expected lumbar lordosis in toddlers and the increased dorsal kyphosis seen in the elderly should not be cause for concern.

### Assistive devices

All assistive devices such as canes, walkers, or crutches that the patient uses should be listed. The nurse needs to assess the way in which the patient is using any special device and his degree of independence. If a brace is worn, it should be determined whether the patient is able to apply it without assistance and under what conditions he is to wear the brace.

## Exercises

Often an exercise program is prescribed for patients with orthopedic conditions. The nurse must collect specific information about the type of exercise, whether active, passive or resistive, that the patient has been performing. The specific body parts to be exercised, the frequency and time of day exercises are usually done, the patient's understanding of the exercise program, and the progress noted as a result of the exercises should be recorded.

## Range of motion

Patients with orthopedic problems may have accompanying limitation in joint range of motion. When assessing the existing level of range of motion, attention must be given to the uninvolved extremities as well as the involved limb. If range of motion is limited, the specific joint affected and the degree of limitation should be recorded. Any pain or discomfort elicited in assessing a patient's range of motion should also be noted.

## Muscle strength and function

As with joint range of motion, the muscle strength and function of all extremities should be assessed. Although muscle function may be present, the muscle tone, strength, and endurance may vary. During later adulthood, as activity lessens, varying degrees of muscle weakness may occur. Requesting the patient to do some resistive range-of-motion exercises often gives an accurate indication of muscle strength. Any limitations noted should be recorded, showing the specific muscle affected and the degree of limitation.

## Previous history

Collecting pertinent data about a patient's previous orthopedic and other major health problems allows the nurse to make a more informed assessment of physiologic and emotional response to his current health need (see history form). Complications that occurred in response to previous surgeries or bed rest may be anticipated and a plan begun to prevent their recurrence.

## Activities of daily living

Specific limitations in physical functioning should be noted. The length of time the limitation has exist-ed, as well as any rehabilitative efforts toward relearning the activity, should also be recorded. Some of the activities to be assessed are the patient's ability to sit, bend, turn, get out of bed, walk, climb stairs, put on clothes, feed himself, and manage personal hygiene and care. Assessment of activities of daily living should assist in the process of planning care (box, p. 143). The goal of the care plan is to maintain the level of self-care of which the patient is capable.

## Skin

The skin should be insepcted frequently for signs of pressure or irritation. Assessment is best accomplished by utilizing the senses of sight, touch, and smell. Skin color, temperature, and abnormal swelling should be noted. When a cast is present the areas of skin in close proximity to it must be observed. A flashlight may be utilized to inspect the skin around and under the cast. When the patient's ability to change position is limited or restricted, the frequency and pattern of turning are assessed. Any special skin care practices or assistive devices used to maintain skin integrity should be listed and their value in maintaining skin integrity assessed by the patient and the nurse (box, p. 144).

## Pain

Because pain is subjective, nursing assessment that is as complete as possible will help to narrow the gap between the patient's experience and the nurse's understanding. Not only may orthopedic disorders cause pain, but pain may also result from some orthopedic treatment procedures. The cause of the pain and discomfort must be carefully assessed. The characteristics of pain to be assessed are location, duration, intensity, and pattern.

Generally severe musculoskeletal pain causes the patient to be restless and to change position frequently. At the same time he may attempt to protect the painful area by immobilizing the part. The nurse needs to consider that there is injury to both soft tissue and bone and that pain may originate from either or both.

The nurse should consult with the patient to discover ways in which he has previously experienced and coped with pain. If deemed appropriate, the nurse should encourage the patient in the use of these techniques. If these methods are detrimental to pain relief, the nurse should instruct the patient in new ways of coping with pain[16] (see Chapter 27).

## NURSING CARE PLAN FORM

Although not a part of the assessment process, the nursing care plan card file is included here to

*Text continued on p. 151.*

## ORTHOPEDIC NURSING HISTORY

Name _____ Age _____ Date _____

Address _____

Date of admission _____ Expected length of stay _____

Previous admissions: Yes _____ No _____ Date(s) _____

Medications taken today _____

Medications brought to hospital _____

Allergies _____

Previous blood transfusion reactions _____

Patient understanding of illness or reason for admission _____

_____

### Musculoskeletal assessment

Ambulatory _____ If no, assistive devices used: Wheelchair _____ Crutches _____

   Walker _____ Cane _____ Prosthetics _____ Other _____

Bedridden _____ Length of time _____

Gait problems _____

Posture: Normal _____ Lordosis _____ Kyphosis _____ Scoliosis _____

Previous history of bone or joint disease or trauma _____ Type and date(s) _____

_____

Full joint ROM _____ If no, circle affected joints on diagram.

Muscle strength/function limitations _____ If yes, locate specific areas of muscle weakness on diagram with a square.

Exercise program:
   Type _____
   Frequency _____

**Code**
○ = Joint limitations
□ = Muscle limitations
Describe degree of limitations

## Activities of daily living

|  | Independent | Limitations |
|---|---|---|
| Bed activities |  |  |
|   Turning |  |  |
|   OOB |  |  |
| Personal hygiene |  |  |
| Dressing |  |  |
| Eating |  |  |

## Sensory-neurologic assessment

|  | Yes | No |
|---|---|---|
| Orientation |  |  |
|   Time |  |  |
|   Place |  |  |
|   Person |  |  |

|  | No | Yes (describe) |
|---|---|---|
| Deficits |  |  |
|   Taste |  |  |
|   Touch |  |  |
|   Hearing |  |  |
|   Vision |  |  |
|   Speech |  |  |

Mental retardation _____ If yes, describe _____

Ability to understand verbal and written words _____
_____

Ability to read, write, and verbalize needs _____
_____

Pain _____

Discomfort occurring now _____

Previous experience with pain _____
_____

Usual methods for relieving pain _____
_____

Usual sleep pattern _____

Other neuromotor deficits _____ Type _____

## Neurovascular assessment

|  | Color | Temperature | Capillary filling | Edema | Numbness, tingling | Sensation | Motion |
|---|---|---|---|---|---|---|---|
| LUE |  |  |  |  |  |  |  |
| RUE |  |  |  |  |  |  |  |
| LLE |  |  |  |  |  |  |  |
| RLE |  |  |  |  |  |  |  |

**Code**
Color: pink, pale, cyanotic. Temperature: warm, cool, cold. Capillary filling: rapid, sluggish. Edema: present (specify degree), absent. Numbness, tingling: present, absent. Sensation: present (specify with or without stimuli), decreased, absent. Motion: present, decreased, absent.

*Continued.*

# ORTHOPEDIC NURSING HISTORY—cont'd

**Skin condition**

| | No | If yes, describe |
|---|---|---|
| Preexisting skin problems | | |
| Old scars | | |
| Ecchymosis | | |
| Reddened areas | | |
| Decubitus ulcers | | |

General skin condition _____

Special skin care patient requests _____

Turning required _____ Frequency _____

Need for special bed _____ Stryker _____ Foster _____ Circle _____

Need for protective devices _____ Air-water mattress _____ Foam pad _____

Sheepskin _____ Bedboard _____ Footboard _____ Other _____

**Genitourinary assessment**

Voiding habits: Frequency _____ At night _____

Current problems with voiding _____

Incontinence _____ If yes, describe current management _____

Catheter _____ Type _____ Date to be changed _____

LMP _____ Next menstrual period expected _____

Bladder training program instituted _____

Previous GU tract problems or surgery _____
(e.g., stones, infection)

**GI function**

Frequency of:

Bowel movements _____

Constipation _____

Incontinence _____

Indigestion _____

Medication used for above _____ If yes, list type and frequency _____

Previous GI tract problems or surgery _____

**Nutritional status**

Problems with dentition _____

Special mouth care _____

Present diet _____

Assess intake of vitamins C and D, calcium, protein over 24 hr:

Breakfast _____

Lunch _____

Dinner _____

Snacks _____

Food likes/dislikes _____

Food intolerances _____

**Nutritional status — cont'd**

Anorexia _____ Usual appetite _____

Fluids, usual amount/24 hr _____

Alcohol consumption _____

Height _____ Weight _____

**Cardiovascular function**

| | No | If yes, describe |
|---|---|---|
| Dizziness on ambulation | | |
| Previous heart problems | | |
| Previous circulatory problems | | |

Resting pulse _____ Resting BP _____

Bed rest anticipated _____ If yes, how long _____

   Number of weeks already on bed rest _____

**Respiratory function**

| | No | If yes, describe |
|---|---|---|
| Use of auxilliary respiratory muscles | | |
| Respiratory problems now | | |
| Previous respiratory problems | | |

Respiratory rate at rest _____ Smoker _____ If yes, packs per day
                                                            × no. of years _____

**Psychosocial assessment**

Marital status _____ Number and ages of children _____

Residence: Apartment _____ House _____ Rooming house _____ Other _____

Persons living at home _____

Socioeconomic status _____

Occupation _____

Insurance/hospitalization coverage: Adequate _____ Inadequate _____ None _____

Religious preference _____

Special interests or hobbies _____

_____

Life style: Very active _____ Active _____ Sedentary _____

Brief description of client during assessment: General appearance, mood, behavior, any feelings about himself that client mentions

Interviewed by _____

*Continued.*

## ORTHOPEDIC NURSING HISTORY—cont'd

### Patient problems

|  | Initial assessment | Reassessment | Reassessment |
|---|---|---|---|
| Date |  |  |  |
| Musculoskeletal |  |  |  |
| Sensorineural |  |  |  |
| Skin |  |  |  |
| Genitourinary tract |  |  |  |
| Gastrointestinal tract |  |  |  |
| Nutrition |  |  |  |
| Cardiovascular |  |  |  |
| Respiratory |  |  |  |
| Psychosocial |  |  |  |
| Other |  |  |  |

**Code**
A, actual
P, potential
R, resolved

Assessed by   _____   _____   _____

Form can be used to systematically define problems for which the orthopedic patient is at risk.

# NURSING CARE PLAN*

Name _____  Sex ____  Age ____  Birth date _____  Admission date _____

Hospital no. _____  X-ray no. _____  Phone no. _____  Visitors _____

Diagnosis _____

Surgery and date _____

Medical history _____

_____ Allergies _____

Social history _____  Religion _____

**Vital signs**

BP _____

TRP _____

Neurovascular _____

Wt _____ Scale _____

**Diet**

Type _____

Fluids _____

Positioning _____

Assistance _____

**Hygiene**

Bath _____

Back care _____

Special skin care _____

Shave _____

Shampoo _____

Mouth care _____

Denture care _____

**Elimination**

Bowel habits _____

Last bowel movement _____

Urinary habits _____

I and O _____

Foley _____
(Inserted/changed)

**Toilet**

Bedpan or urinal _____

Bedside commode _____

Commode _____

**Rest/sleep**

Naps _____

Pattern _____

**Ambulation**

Activity level ordered _____

Assistance needed _____

Assistive devices _____

Walker _____

Cane _____

Crutches _____ (Gait)

Wheelchair _____

Pair splint _____

Knee splint _____

Other _____

Weight bearing _____

No weight bearing _____

Touchdown _____

Weight to tolerance _____

Full weight bearing _____

**Bed positioning**

Bed type _____

Positioning allowed _____

HOB ↑ _____ degrees

FOB ↑ _____ degrees

Hip flexion to _____ degrees

**Turning**

L or R side only and back _____

Side-back-side _____

Prone _____

**Exercises**

Quadriceps sets _____ Gluteus sets _____

ROM _____ Extremities _____
(Schedule)

Deep breathe/cough _____

Dorsiflexion/ankle _____

R/L handweights _____

R/L hip and knee flexion _____

with pulley _____

R/L knee flexion and extension,

sitting _____

Other _____

_____

*Treatment and medication pages of Nursing Care Plan form may be combined on one two-sided page and used as insert between other two pages.

## NURSING CARE PLAN—cont'd

| Date | Treatments | | Date ordered | Diagnostic | |
|---|---|---|---|---|---|
| | Cast care | | | X-ray | |
| | | | | | |
| | | | | | |
| | | | | | |
| | Traction | | | Laboratory | |
| | | | | | |
| | | | | | |
| | Dressings | | | | |
| | | | | | |
| | | | | Other | |
| | Other | | | Consults | |
| | | | | | |
| | | | | | |

**Medications**

| Date started | Date expired | Standing | Time | Date started | Date expired | PRN |
|---|---|---|---|---|---|---|
| | | | | | | |
| | | | | | | |
| | | | | | | |
| | | | | | | |
| | | | | | | |
| | | | | | | |
| | | | | | | |

| Time and date given | Area | Skin tests | Time and date to be read | Miscellaneous |
|---|---|---|---|---|
| | | | | |
| | | | | |
| | | | | |
| | | | | |

Name _____  Primary nurse _____  Physician _____  Room no. _____

**NURSING CARE PLAN—cont'd**

| Date | Patient problems or needs | Interventions |
|------|---------------------------|---------------|
|      |                           |               |

demonstrate how the assessment process and the philosophies stated here can be utilized (form, pp. 147-150). The form was designed to be used expressly in an acute care orthopedic setting for both children and adults. It has been developed to accompany the Orthopedic Nursing History (p. 142-146).

## SUMMARY

Nursing assessment of the orthopedic patient is a complex process. The nurse may apply the principles presented here to inpatient or outpatient settings, pediatric or adult patients, during acute or rehabilitative phases of disease processes, and for admission, continuing, and discharge phases of assessment and planning. Thoughtful, organized collection of data is essential. Internalizing the data and drawing appropriate, informed conclusions is a demanding responsibility. Accepting this responsibility, as well as the legal implications and accountability that accompany it, requires that nurses constantly update their knowledge and improve their judgments.

## REFERENCES

1. Beland, I., and Passos, J.: Clinical nursing, New York, 1975, Macmillan, Inc.
2. Browse, N.: The physiology and pathology of bedrest, Springfield, Ill., 1965, Charles C Thomas, Publisher.
3. Byers, V.: Nursing observation, Dubuque, Ia., 1968, W. C. Brown Co., Publishers.
4. Carnevali, D., and Bruechner, S.: Immobilization: reassessment of a concept, Am. J. Nurs. 70(7):1502-1507, 1970.
5. Davis, L. A.: Comparison of healing decubitus ulcers treated with power spray. Unpublished master's thesis, 1976.
6. Downs, F.: Bedrest and sensory disturbances, Am. J. Nurs. 74(3):435, 1974.
7. Durand, M., and Prince, R.: Nursing diagnosis: process and decision, Nurs. Forum 5(4):56-58, 1966.
8. Fuerst, E., Wolff, L., and Weitzel, M.: Fundamentals of nursing, Philadelphia, 1974, J. B. Lippincott Co.
9. Husain, I.: An experimental study of some pressure effects on tissue, J. Pathol. Bacteriol. 66:350, 1953.
10. Larson, C. B., and Gould, M. L.: Orthopedic nursing, ed. 9, St. Louis, 1978, The C. V. Mosby Co.
11. Levine, M.: The pursuit of wholeness, Am. J. Nurs. 69(1):96, 1969.
12. Lindan, O.: Etiology of decubitus ulcers: an experimental study, Arch. Phys. Med. Rehab. 42:774-783, 1961.
13. Little, D., and Carnevali, D.: Nursing care planning, Philadelphia, 1976, J. B. Lippincott Co.
14. Luckman, J., and Sorensen, K.: Medical-surgical nursing, Philadelphia, 1974, W. B. Saunders Co.
15. Marriner, A.: The nursing process: a scientific approach to nursing care, ed. 2, St. Louis, 1979, The C. V. Mosby Co.
16. McCaffery, M., and Moss, F.: Nursing intervention for bodily pain, Am. J. Nurs. 67(6):1224-1227, 1967.
17. McCain, F.: Nursing by assessment, not intuition, Am. J. Nurs. 65(4):82-84, 1965.
18. Moidel, H., et al.: Nursing care of the patient with medical-surgical disorders, ed. 2, New York, 1976, McGraw-Hill Book Co.
19. Olson, E.: Hazards of immobility, Am. J. Nurs. 67(4):780-797, 1967.
20. Passo, S.: The musculoskeletal system. In Soipien, G., et al.: Comprehensive pediatric nursing, New York, 1975, McGraw-Hill Book Co.
21. Spence, W., Burk, R., and Row, J.: Gel support for prevention of decubitus ulcers, Arch. Phys. Med. Rehab. 48:283, 1967.
22. Statford, T.: Bone tumors. In Rubin, T., editor: Clinical oncology for medical students and physicians, New York, 1974, American Cancer Society.
23. Wade, M.: Psychosocial equilibrium. In Olson, E., editor: Hazards of immobility, Am. J. Nurs. 67(4):795, 1967.
24. Williams, S.: Nutrition and diet therapy, St. Louis, 1973, The C. V. Mosby Co.
25. Yura, H., and Walsh, M.: The nursing process, New York, 1973, Appleton-Century-Crofts.

## BIBLIOGRAPHY

Browse, N.: The physiology and pathology of bedrest, Springfield, Ill., 1965, Charles C Thomas, Publisher.
Carnevali, D., and Bruechner, S.: Immobilization: reassessment of a concept, Am. J. Nurs. 70(7):1502-1507, 1970.
Downs, F.: Bedrest and sensory disturbances, Am. J. Nurs. 74(3):435, 1974.
Durand, M., and Prince, R.: Nursing diagnosis: process and decision, Nurs. Forum 5(4):56-58, 1966.
Larson, C. B., and Gould, M. L.: Orthopedic nursing, ed. 9, St. Louis, 1978, The C. V. Mosby Co.
Little, D., and Carnevali, D.: Nursing care planning, Philadelphia, 1976, J. B. Lippincott Co.
Olson, E.: Hazards of immobility, Am. J. Nurs. 67(4):780-797, 1967.
Yura, H., and Walsh, M.: The nursing process, New York, 1973, Appleton-Century-Crofts.

# 7

# Sociopsychological assessment

**A. LAURA CAMPBELL**

**SYLVIA REUTER SULTENFUSS**

Perhaps the most significant factors in an individual's ability to adapt to illness and subsequently return to normal functioning are psychosocial variables such as pre-illness personality, coping behaviors, support systems, and patterns of social interaction. Any illness, regardless of severity, stimulates a change within the individual and his relationships with others. The concept of the individual as a physical, psychological, and social being requires a comprehensive assessment of these variables so that a corresponding comprehensive plan of intervention may be formulated and implemented.

In this chapter are presented principles of sociopsychological assessment from a foundation of crisis theory. The authors believe that an illness is significant stress to an individual and his family and that the adaptation to this stress requires a social and psychological process that is predictable, normal, and functional. The individual also experiences normal and predictable maturational crises, which influence the significance of the stress experienced. Both situational and maturational factors need to be considered in comprehensive assessment, corresponding comprehensive plan of intervention, and implementation of care provided.

## ADAPTATION: CRISIS THEORY IMPLICATIONS

Illness and hospitalization may precipitate a crisis situation for the individual and his family (Fig. 7-1). By definition, *crisis is a state of disequilibrium or imbalance that occurs when there is an incongruency between the problem-solving or coping skills of the individual, his family system, and the stressful event.* Illness and hospitalization present a danger to the individual's well-being, stimulate role changes, and interfere with normal patterns of relating. Whether illness develops into a crisis for the individual or his family depends on their perception of the event, available supports and resources, the number and intensity of stressors, and pre-illness

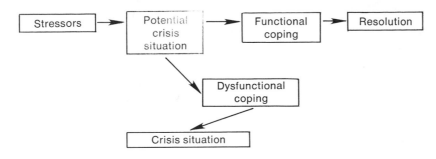

**Fig. 7-1.** Stressors on individual and family create potential crisis situation that requires mobilization of coping and problem-solving behaviors. If behaviors are adequate to meet needs of situation and stress is relieved, resolution will be acquired. If coping is inadequate to meet needs of situation, state of disequilibrium or crisis occurs.

problem-solving and coping behaviors. The failure of the individual and family to integrate the stressful event effectively and of problem-solving resources to meet the demands precipitated by the stressful event results in feelings of helplessness and ineffectiveness. This affectual state may lead to behavior disorganization and thus to a state of crisis. If the individual's coping behavior is functional, there will be mobilization toward and maintenance of physical and sociopsychological health; dysfunctional coping behaviors will interfere significantly with health mobilization and maintenance.

Stressors other than the illness itself influence the intensity and resolution of crisis. The illness or hospitalization may be considered a significant stressor to the individual and his family system. However, if other significant stressors occur simultaneously or during resolution of the illness crisis, crisis resolution will be delayed. A child may be hospitalized for corrective surgery for a congenital orthopedic problem. If during his hospitalization his mother dies or becomes seriously ill, the crisis situation becomes more complex and is intensified for both the child and his family.

It might be helpful to note here that some individuals and families appear to be in a constant state of crisis. In such cases the crisis state is part of a life style due to a general inadequacy and inability to function socially. Crises in these cases do not have a beginning, middle, and end but flow together, are compounded, and circular. The concepts of crisis theory and intervention do not adequately apply to individuals and families beset by multiple and chronic problems that produce a continuous high level of tension and disorganization.[7,pp.22-31]

Crisis may be categorized into two groups: the *anticipated, developmental, or maturational crisis,* and the *unanticipated, accidental, or situational crisis.* Crisis may be acute (short term) or chronic

(long term), intrapersonal or interpersonal, or a combination of the above. Defining the variables of a crisis situation is a complex task. Each crisis situation may contain numerous stressors and potential crisis states. A comprehensive evaluation of the crisis of illness includes correlating those stressors of a maturational and situational nature with those of an interpersonal and intrapersonal nature.

A crisis theory approach provides the assessor with an understanding of the expected behavioral responses to crisis and provides the intervener with problem-solving techniques to help the client or patient achieve a level of sociopsychological equilibrium the same as or better than the precrisis level.[1] The individual and family in crisis are vulnerable and susceptible to influence and support from others. One might view a crisis as a state for potentient achieve a level of sociopsychological equilibrium the same as or better than the precrisis level.[1]

## INTEGRATION OF SELF AND BODY IMAGE

Concept of self is a complex, interrelated phenomenon that includes conscious and unconscious feelings, attitudes, and perceptions about one's value, role, and body. The individual and his body are perceived as distinct and apart from all others and yet influenced by and interrelated with others. Self and body image are a psychological entity resulting from the integration of past experiences, social interactions, and current sensorimotor sensations. Perhaps the most significant determinant of self-concept and body image is the response of significant others and society to the individual. A healthy self-concept and realistic body image are derived from the integration of positive social reactions and images. Thus we become to a large extent what people tell us we are.

Each stage of life or change in the individual physically, socially, or psychologically is accompanied by a change in the self and body image of the individual. People invest emotionally in their bodies and their well-being and become anxious if there is an imagined or real change in the body and its integrity. A body image crisis occurs when there is failure to accept the body as it is and to adapt to it.

Recent literature on the relationship of stressful events to the generation of crisis suggests that it is change rather than stress that precipitates crisis. Duhl[3] has outlined five types of significant change or threat of change that present a critical adaptation situation for the individual and his family. Each type of change involves the individual's concept of self and body image and his relationship to his family system.

First is a change in a family member's view of his sociopsychological self. A man's confrontation with a physical disability resulting from an automobile accident requires a painful revision in his concept of self as a physically functional, independent person able to provide and care for himself and his family.

The second occurs when the affected individual experiences difficulty in integrating the changes in self and body image. Frequently major adjustments for all family members are necessary for effective adaptation. The physical disabilities resulting from the automobile accident may be perceived by the man as unacceptable. In rejecting and disapproving of himself, he may withdraw from his family in an attempt to protect them from "this burden, this unlovable person." Understanding this change in behavior and relating effectively to the man they love may be very difficult for family members.

The third precipitant of disequilibrium is changes in relevant social networks from the addition or loss of another family member such as through birth, divorce, death, or hospitalization. These changes require adaptation in the social interaction and role delineation of family members. Since the man who suffered physical debilitation from the automobile accident will be unable to resume his preaccident level of functioning and independence, family members may assume behaviors and role functioning that were previously his. The wife may work to provide financially for the family. Children may care for their father and perform home management tasks that were previously defined within parental roles.

Fourth, changes in the nonhuman environment such as confinement to a wheelchair or bed or a change of residence may present a crisis situation. Confinement after an automobile accident, whether permanent or temporary, may require structural adjustments in the home, specialized equipment, and provisions for physical care. Many of these adjustments will increase the financial burden on the family.

And fifth, a change in beliefs, values, and expectations may be threatening to the family. Adjustment of all family members will be necessary to incorporate a drastic revision in the aspirations and ideals of a single family member.

The individual with an orthopedic illness may experience or be threatened with all of the five types of change due to a congenital deformity or illness, accident, or degenerative process. Healthy adaptation will depend on the individual's and family's perception of the illness, the number and intensity of stressors confronting them, their modes of coping and communicating, and the internal and external resources available to them. Assessing the ability of the individual to adapt to illness would include identifying his concept of self and body, his relationship with others, and their perception of him.

## CRISIS INTERVENTION

Individuals and families in crisis are vulnerable and need help. They may be able to seek help independently or may need to be supported in seeking assistance. One purpose of the crisis approach is to provide the services of a helping agent who is skilled in problem-solving techniques. Those care providers in immediate proximity are logically in a position to recognize the needs of the individual in crisis and his family, assess their ability to cope with the situation, and identify resources available to them. These problem-solving techniques facilitate achieving the primary goal of crisis intervention, which is to restore the individual and family to the precrisis state of equilibrium or level of functioning.

The resolution of crisis is dependent on relearning, unlearning, or learning what is needed to solve the present crisis situation. Crisis resolution may involve removing the precipitating stressors, mobilizing previously developed coping skills, modifying or substituting for dysfunctional behaviors that interfere with health maintenance and mobilization, and learning new functional coping behaviors.

Crisis intervention requires a direct active involvement of the helping agent in assessing the variables of the life situation of the individual and family and in mobilizing the resources necessary to reduce the impact of the event. Crises, by definition, are self-limiting and of short duration, usually lasting from 4 to 6 weeks.[2] There will be variance in the resolution time factor based on the number and intensity of stressors affecting the crisis situation. During this time the individual and family are emotionally vulnerable and are thus ready for learning and growth. An active problem-solving process of intervention based on practical application most effectively utilizes the limited time factor and motivation of the individual and family. The problem-solving method includes assessment and definition of the problem situation, formulation of a plan of intervention, evaluation, and summarization to integrate and reinforce the experience and related learning.

The crisis intervention approach assumes a working relationship with shared responsibility between two or more individuals for the purpose of solving a problem that is precipitating an emotional state of disequilibrium.

### Stages in crisis resolution

The four stages of crisis, according to Fink,[5] are *shock, denial or defensive retreat, acknowledgement of reality,* and *adaptation.*

After a stressful event the individual initially feels shock, anxiety, numbness, and helplessness. Mild anxiety is necessary for learning and creativity. However, as the anxiety level increases, perception narrows and attention becomes more selective. With severe anxiety energy is directed toward surviving the psychological pain experienced. Perception may be distorted, and survival takes priority over everything else.

The defensive behaviors that result include denial, retreat from reality, fantasies about the body and its capabilities, euphoria, and rationalization. The individual is defending himself in a normal manner against feelings and a reality he is currently unable to resolve and integrate effectively.

During this phase of crisis a nonjudgmental, supportive environment communicates to the individual his uniqueness and importance and encourages the expression of feelings, fantasies, and fears. Sharing with the individual the normal process he is experiencing may minimize his feelings of losing control and of responding abnormally.

Acknowledgement of reality begins when the individual starts integrating the stressful event and its implications for change into his life style. This acknowledgement is difficult and is accompanied by feelings of depression, apathy, agitation, and bitterness. This stage may be perceived as a stage of grieving for the loss of a body structure, function, or role. Somatic symptoms such as anorexia, pain, nausea, and insomnia may serve as an outlet for feelings. Unresolved feelings about previous losses may interfere with the individual's ability to direct his energies toward adapting to the present loss. The individual may also anticipate rejection by and withdrawal of significant others. An accepting response from others reinforces a perception of self that is acceptable, and exploration of feelings promotes resolution of the crisis state.

Resolution or adaptation is the last phase. Some successful problem solving has occurred, and new coping behaviors have been tried. The crisis is seen in a more positive perspective. Along with a certain sense of mastery comes a new feeling of worth, relief, and commitment to life.

The phases of crisis resolution are not mutually exclusive, nor are the feelings final. Certain feelings and behaviors may be recurrent and may be revived with any threat or perceived threat related to the crisis situation.

In correlating the stages of crisis to the individual who may experience repeated hospitalizations related to the same orthopedic problem, it is important to recognize that each anticipated hospitalization may initiate the feelings, responses, and behaviors of the crisis state. It would be inaccurate to assume that because the individual and his family have experienced hospitalization before, or recognize and anticipate the need for repeated hospitalizations, they will not experience a state of crisis. With some orthopedic problems repeated hospitalizations may actually intensify the crisis state, especially when the illness is life threatening and death is a potential reality.

*Crisis theory and intervention are compatible with the concept of health assessment, management, and maintenance.* This framework is applicable to the individual and the family. Health care providers can anticipate, prepare for, and intervene effectively with the client and family who are experiencing an illness-related crisis by viewing the situation within a crisis theory framework. Stressors that can be readily anticipated and identified are those that relate to the illness and those that relate to the individual's maturational stage of development.

## ASSESSMENT AND INTERVENTION

Erikson[4] views life as a series of developmental crises, which he calls the eight stages of man. Each stage of development has its own *primary needs and conflicts, which are natural and predictable.* Fulfillment of needs and resolution of conflicts are attained through intrapersonal and interpersonal experiences during each stage of development. The primary needs and conflicts of each stage can be met and resolved to various degrees of adequacy based on (1) the extent to which the individual experiences primary need fulfillment in his experiences with self and others and (2) the extent to which he has reached resolution in previous stages. Adequate resolution of primary conflicts prepares the individual to cope more successfully with the same conflicts as they arise again throughout life. Developmental needs that are not met adequately, and thus conflicts that are not adequately resolved, persist and influence the individual's maturational and adaptational processes. For example, during infancy each individual faces the conflict of trust for the first time. The infant needs food, rest, comfort, and personal hygiene provided for him. When his needs are determined correctly and provided for consistently, he learns to trust his mother's ability to provide for his needs. As he matures he takes with him his experience that one other person can be trusted, and he has a better potential for future relationships with others.

If his needs are not determined and met consistently enough, the infant moves into toddlerhood without trusting when, how, or even if his needs will be met. Thus he will be more reluctant to begin autonomous skills. When this initial conflict of trust is not resolved, the individual in childhood, adolescence, and adulthood will show evidence of difficulty or inability in developing adequate trusting relationships with others. Though trust is first learned during infancy, people need and utilize trusting relationships throughout life.

The potential crises and *related conflicts* precipitated by illness are those of separation, threatened self and body image (physical appearance or function or both), and regression (movement back to a previous state). These conflicts are experienced during any stage of development by individuals confronted with illness or hospitalization. However, the crisis potential of the conflict is influenced by the individual's past experiences and coping patterns. The crisis potential is therefore of greatest significance during the stage of development where it relates more directly to the normal and primary conflict. In other words, when the individual has never experienced or adequately resolved the conflict previously, the potential for maladaptive behavior is greater. For example, a man confronted with a physical disability resulting from an automobile accident may significantly experience the stress of regression if his disability influences his ability to continue in his profession and thus provide for his family. However, he may have the potential for adaptation, as he has experienced feeling and being

productive as an individual. A school-age child whose primary conflict (industry versus inferiority) involves learning to be productive for the first time has a greater potential for developing lasting feelings of inferiority as a productive individual when faced with a physical disability and the resulting conflict of regression.

The authors believe that *the combined concepts of crisis theory and maturational process provide each member of the health care team with a solid basis for more accurate assessment of sociopsychological factors influencing the management and maintenance of acute and rehabilitative orthopedic care.* In assessing patient needs we have assumed that health care providers will utilize opportunities to observe (1) the patient's statement about himself, (2) how he relates to his environment and persons in his environment, and (3) how those persons relate to him. It is also assumed that health care providers utilize an empathetic approach, effective interviewing techniques, and teaching skills during their communications with patients and family members. Compiling and coordinating all health team members' observations and information about the patient and related illness stressors, maturational stressors, potential crisis, and supports available to the patient and family are necessary for an accurate and comprehensive assessment. Intervention approaches can be integrated into the formulation and implementation of the patient's treatment plan.

In the following discussion the potential crisis of an orthopedic illness is viewed in relation to the developmental needs and conflicts of the individual and the needs of family members. Intervention approaches described promote health mobilization and maintenance and minimize the impact of crisis.

### Infancy: birth to 1 year (Table 7-1)

**Psychosocial development.** Normally a child is born with a repertoire of abilities on which he, with the help of his family, begins to build immediately. He can move his limbs, cry, suck, hear, and see; however, he is totally dependent on others to meet most of his needs. His mother, having anticipated birth, has readied herself to meet his needs, and a process of mutual interaction begins.

According to Erikson,[5] it is the task of the infant to learn trust during his first year of life. The infant's ability to learn trust is dependent on his mother's interactions with him and her ability to meet his needs, both physically and emotionally. In having one major and consistent caretaker, the infant can learn what to expect and to recognize how and when comfort and need satisfaction are forthcom-

**Table 7-1.** Infant: birth to 1 year
**Psychologic conflict: trust versus mistrust**

| Age (mo) | Primary task | Potential crisis | Interventions |
|---|---|---|---|
| 1 | Babbles<br>Follows moving object with eyes | *Failure of attachment between mother and infant* | *Focus staff support on mother or staff who provide mother substitute* |
| 3 | Can control head<br>Smiles | Prolonged or frequent hospitalization decreases infant's contact with one consistent caretaker and decreases mother's feelings of responsibility or adequacy as a parent, which influence the extent of attachment between mother and child. | Encourage her to provide as much care for her infant as possible (holding, feeding, bathing, dressing, stroking, face-to-face visual contact, talking to infant) |
| 4 | Laughs<br>Reaches with arms | | Stay with the parent who is fearful as she provides care for child until she becomes comfortable providing what she can. |
| | | Immobilization further decreases quantity and quality of tactile comfort and stimulation needed for attachment and muscle development necessary for motor development later on. | Keep parents informed of diagnosis, prognosis, treatment plans, and effects these factors have on child's functioning. Parent's need time to assimilate information and adjust to impact of child's illness. |
| | | | Allow parents time to question and discuss child's diagnosis, prognosis, and treatment plan as well as feelings they have about child's problem. Provide a quiet setting. |
| | | | Teach and prepare parents for home care necessary and discuss their fears about home care. |
| | | | Provide financial and resource counseling for parents to reduce their anxieties about providing financially so that more energy may be used to maintain child emotionally and physically. |
| 6 | Sits alone<br>Is aware of strange situations<br>Begins making sounds | *Separation anxiety* | *Focus on mother-child relationship* |
| 7 | Bounces in standing position<br>Transfers toys from one hand to the other | | Encourage mother to provide as much comfort as she can, holding, touching, talking to, singing to, and spending time with her face in child's visual field. |
| 9 | Crawls<br>Says first words | | Encourage mother to provide mobiles, music boxes, hand toys, and items that are familiar or special to child. |
| 10 | Holds own bottle<br>Feeds self cookies<br>Pulls self up to stand | | |
| 12 | Walks with one hand held<br>Cooperates in dressing | | |

ing. This is a subtle and complex interaction between mother and infant and is critical for the infant's development of trust.

With the encouragement from this major relationship the infant begins to increase his skills and responses as he learns to respond to expectations of his mother. The infant is encouraged by the response he gets when he babbles, smiles, and kicks, and within the security of this encouragement he risks new skills of sitting, crawling, standing, and walking, trusting that he will be comforted when at first he is not successful with new skills. With increased age and security, the infant begins to develop this trust with his father and significant others.

Interferences in the mother-infant bond and inconsistencies in the infant's care impair the infant's learning to trust his accomplishments in developmental skills. Major and extended interferences cause the child to develop a sense of mistrust that may be irreversible. Less severe interferences may be compensated for by the infant with later reinforcement in his relationships.

**Family needs.** Before a child is born, parents have ideas of what they expect their child to be like. These ideas may include specific characteristics that they desire including sex, size, appearance, and activity level. If the child's conception was unexpected, unwanted, or occurred at a time of marital or personal crisis, unrealistic expectations may be focused on the birth of the infant. Normally from the time of birth parents begin to develop pride in their baby. The infant becomes a special extension of themselves, something they have produced. Their pride in the infant is fostered by intimate contact with the baby and by the attitudes of family members and others around them. Their pride in the infant helps parents adjust more readily to the differences between their prenatal expectations and the actual characteristics of their infant. The process of accepting the infant, getting to know him, and learning to meet his needs begins and develops into an interaction that is emotionally satisfying to both parents and infant. The infant thus meets the parent's needs to feel proud, to experience being needed, and to feel valued as adequate providers of the physical and emotional needs of the infant. As the infant grows and develops skills, the parents' needs continue to be met as they feel pride in their child's accomplishments.

**Potential crisis.** The birth of a handicapped child is difficult for any parent, as the loss of the anticipated normal child makes the process of parental adjustment to the new infant more complicated and prolonged. Parental depression over the loss of the anticipated normal child influences the intimate contact between mother and infant and thus the adequacy of stimulation given the new infant. The development of parental pride is delayed by the parents' need to work through their grief. Immediately after the birth, feelings may be exaggerated by the influence of the parents' prenatal feelings or expectations. Ambivalent feelings toward wanting a child may result in extreme guilt feelings or negative feelings toward the handicapped infant.

When a handicap is evident at birth, the parental adjustment to the reality of the defect and the care it requires influences the process of initial parental attachment to the infant. It may heighten feelings of protectiveness, or it may produce feelings of rejection, interfering with the development of a healthy mother-child bond.

A major factor that influences parental adjustment to the birth of an infant with a congenital handicap is the seriousness of the problem and the extent to which it is correctable. However, the birth of any infant who is "less than perfect" to his parents, regardless of how minute the defect may be, requires adjustment of some type. For parents of an infant born with one or more anomalies that will cause lifelong medical and functional problems, the process of adjustment is much more difficult and tends to be a continuous process of learning to cope with the effect it has on the child's life and on theirs. The potential for failure in the family's ability to adjust adequately and for an unhealthy parent-child relationship to develop is much greater.

An orthopedic problem that develops or is caused by traumatic injury in the first year of life presents a different potential crisis for the child and his family. The initial shock of the situation is felt by both infant and parent after their attachment has developed.

Parental adjustments to this situation are influenced by the circumstances of the problem, the seriousness of it, and the coping patterns of the family. Feelings of guilt, inadequacy as a parent, and fear are often seen. Guilt seems to be a particularly strong feeling when traumatic injuries occur, especially if one or both parents blame themselves or each other. Conflicts between parents tend to increase with the stress, and feelings of protectiveness may cause tension between parents and hospital staff.

At some point in the process of learning to cope with the child's medical problem, parents are likely to become angry. Most of this anger is related to their lack of control and inability to change the reality of having an ill child. Some parents may be able to focus their anger directly with comments such as, "Why did *my* child have to have this problem?" or, "I don't like having a deformed child." Others may displace their anger onto the staff providing care for the infant. It is important for personnel to be understanding of angry comments and not cut off or put down a parent's feelings. This is a normal part of the process of learning to cope with and accept the situation. Ambivalence is another feeling that staff may recognize in parents. This too can be worked through with most parents when the health care providers can tolerate and respond nonjudgmentally and even assist parents in understanding their feelings and expressions as normal and necessary. Involvement of the parents should be allowed and encouraged. This will help develop or build on the parent-child bond and assist in providing more consistency in the infant's total care after he returns home.

It is important to note here that some traumatic injuries in infancy are the result of child abuse. Most child abuse results from a parent's loss of control of feelings under stress and not as an intentional, purposeful act of harming the child. Abusing parents may be helped with their problems of control through appropriate counseling.

### Toddler: 1 to 3 years (Table 7-2)

**Psychosocial development.** During the toddler years, from age 1 to 3, a child's major task, according to Erikson, is to develop a sense of autonomy. One of the major behaviors involved in learning autonomy is the motor skill of learning to walk and thus being able to explore the environment. As the toddler acquires mobility, he gains the freedom to explore his environment with relative independence.

Language skills are another major development that assists in the achievement of autonomy. As language skills develop, the toddler is able to express needs and desires rather than depending on parents to anticipate his needs. He is able to relate his needs to other significant persons as well.

A third major development that influences autonomy is bowel and bladder training. As in learning to walk, the focus in bowel and bladder training is on learning to control one's body.

From the age of 6 months the infant gradually begins to see himself as separate from his mother. The toddler learns who he is in relation to his environment and how to master his own body. He begins to develop an awareness of himself and his body even though his body image and self-concept are not clearly formulated. Parents are particularly important during this time. Their attitudes toward the toddler and approval or disapproval of his behavior serve as a guide in his determining the extent of his exploration and how his explorations make him feel about himself. The toddler needs protection from real dangers but freedom to independently explore his environment and become autonomous. He feels good about himself as he gains more independence and receives warmth and praise for most of his accomplishments. He feels most safe and secure when his parents are close by to observe his successes and to comfort him when he at first does not succeed. Based on the trust in his parents that he developed in infancy, the toddler depends on their responses to him in building his own self-concept. If parents place too many restrictions on and provide disapproving responses to his explorations, he develops feelings of doubt and shame about himself as an individual.

**Family needs.** Toddlerhood is a difficult time for most parents, as the often stated "terrible twos" implies. It is a time of excitement and frustration. Normally parents are excited, encouraged, and proud when their child begins to take his first steps. As he becomes more accomplished at moving about on his own, however, they find it difficult to keep up with him and protect him from dangers of which he is not aware. Toilet training is another task of this age group that parents look forward to and encourage, but the process can be frustrating and time consuming.

The role of the parent changes as the toddler develops autonomy. The responsibility for the toddler's care still remains primarily that of the parents. It becomes more time consuming to provide that care as he struggles to do for himself under his parents' supervision. The toddler's "no" to the parents' offer of assistance as he decides he wants to explore or experiment with doing something for himself requires a different response from the parents. The balance between allowing the child independence to try experiences he is ready for and not allowing those he is not ready for is at times delicate.

During the toddler years parents often compare their child's abilities with those of every other toddler they know. This stimulates pride in what their child has done and concerns about the skills he has not accomplished.

Also during the toddler years the child begins to actively relate to his parents. The toddler will often run to mother with enthusiasm to see her or tell her something. For many parents this serves as a reward for their efforts and patience during this difficult phase.

**Potential crisis.** Toddlerhood is one of the most difficult times to be hospitalized. The toddler has learned to cope with strange places in the presence of his mother, but it is normal for him to protest her absence when he is in strange surroundings or with strange people. At the onset of hospitalization the toddler can sense his mother's anxiety and therefore needs her security even more. When mother is absent during the initial phase of hospitalization, he may cry frequently. Comfort from others may help for brief periods of time; however, the toddler remains insecure until his mother returns. When mother is present following any absence, he usually cries even more because he trusts her to remove his discomforts.

If the parents' presence is tremendously decreased or absent for any extended period of time, the toddler will begin to withdraw and regress from his behaviors of growth to behaviors that brought mother's security at an earlier age. Long and repeated absence can cause detachment and break down the trust that was built in infancy. Detachment may be difficult to identify because the child appears "good" (compliant and easy to manage). This state is followed by a period of despair (sadness and resistance to care and comfort provided) when the child's protest is not acknowledged and comforted.

The normal surge for independence is retarded during hospitalization by changes in the mother-toddler routines. The toddler will give up practicing skills of independence when the security of his

**Table 7-2.** Toddler: 1 to 3 years
**Psychologic conflict: autonomy versus shame and doubt**

| Age (yr) | Primary task | Potential crisis | Interventions |
|---|---|---|---|
| 1 | *Motor skills* <br> Walks <br> *Language skills* <br> Uses single words <br> *Social skills* <br> Responds to simple verbal request | *Separation anxiety* <br> Highest peak around 18 mo but a major issue throughout toddler years | *Emphasize mother-child relationship* <br> Encourage mother to provide as much time and comfort to her child as she can (holding, feeding, touching, bathing, diapering, visual contact, talking to him). <br> Encourage mother to play with her child and his familiar toys; if he cannot play himself, encourage mother to play with his toys for him within his visual field. <br> Encourage parents to let their child see them leave and tell him they will be back: <br> Allows child to trust that they will not leave without his knowing it. <br> Between 2½ and 3, toddler can understand when to expect them back if told in terms he understands (dinnertime, bedtime, when Sesame Street's on TV, when you wake up). <br> Help parents understand and allow tears both when they arrive after being away and when they leave again. This is their child's way of letting them know his distress about their having been away and their leaving again. |
| 2 | *Motor skills* <br> Runs <br> Climbs stairs with one hand held <br> *Language skills* <br> Three-word sentences <br> *Social skills* <br> Toilet training begins | | Provide comfort for toddler while his parents are away: <br> Comforting toddler while his parents leave lets him know he's not being left alone and can be used to reinforce that his parents will be back. <br> Support toddler's crying as a necessary expression of feeling. <br> Periodically provide contact and comfort during parents' absence and reinforce that they will be back. <br> Provide toddler with items from home with which he is familiar and provide security for him. <br> Talk with parents and help establish to the extent possible the child's home routines and items with which he is accustomed (night lights; own pajamas, cup, blanket, or toy; favorite foods; bedtime stories or prayers). <br> Provide consistency in staff care providers so that toddler can become familiar and more comfortable and trusting of those who care for him during parents' absence. <br> Provide financial and resource counseling for parents to reduce their anxieties about providing financially so that more energy may be used to maintain child emotionally and physically. |
| | | *Detachment* <br> Occurs when even regression to previously secure behaviors does not bring about enough comfort and security | Allow toddler regressive behaviors he initiates (i.e., behaviors that have provided him security before): <br> Return to use of a bottle (will give it up again when he feels more secure). |

| Age (yr) | Primary task | Potential crisis | Interventions |
|---|---|---|---|
| | | from others, particularly mother. | Thumb sucking may begin or increase. |
| | | Signs of detachment are: | Refusal to feed himself (provides more contact with mother or caretaker). |
| | | Toddler shows decreased efforts to be comforted and shows same response to comfort provided by familiar and unfamiliar people. | Loss of interest in toilet training if it has started. Independent efforts are stressful in insecure situations. |
| | | Shows a significant decrease in or stops crying even in response to painful, undesirable, or uncomfortable processes (e.g., injections, enemas). | Refusal to walk; would rather be held. Increase stimulation and comfort when detachment is observed (holding, rocking, touching, singing and talking to child). |
| | | Shows little interest in what happens to or around him. | Provide as minimal a number of caretakers as possible so that increased consistency in who provides stimulation is obtained. |
| | | Detachment usually occurs when child loses consistent mothering figures (e.g., mother does not visit and child has not had consistent staff providing care). | Consider consultation with child psychiatrist if child does not improve with increased consistency and stimulation. |
| | | *Immobilization* | Allow toddler to do those things he can and wants to do for himself (e.g., help feed himself) |
| | | Restricts toddler's ability to move about and be independent. Temper tantrums and fussiness are common in children who are frustrated by immobilization and restrictions. | Offer him choices where possible and appropriate (milk or juice for a snack, which toy he would like in bed with him). |
| | | | Help toddler understand that you know he can and likes to do specific things for himself and that you are helping him until he gets well enough to do for himself again. |
| | | | Provide as much active play in bed as possible and encourage parents to do the same. |
| | | | Help parents understand their child's fussiness and temper tantrums as his expression of frustration over not being able to actively move about as he wishes and his lack of understanding of why he cannot. |
| 3 | *Motor skills* Jumps Rides tricycle *Language skills* Uses plurals Knows body parts Knows sex and full name Can make needs known verbally *Social skills* Fantasy play begins | *Distortion of body image* Body image is beginning to form in late toddlerhood and can be threatened. Children are often fearful that their body part is gone when they cannot see it due to cast or bulky dressings. | Use of a doll and gauze can help toddler understand that his leg or arm, which he cannot see, is still there. Demonstrate with doll how the doll's leg or arm is still there when covered and uncovered. Allow child to play with the doll and gauze when possible. Use of preoperative play and explanations of what he will experience prior to surgery is helpful in decreasing older toddler's fear of surgery. Allow him to play with safe equipment that will be used in his care (syringe without needle, masks, disposable scrub cap, stethoscope). Usually helps to do this the day prior to surgery. |

mother's presence is threatened. Immobilization places further limits on his surge for independence.

Surgery and hospital procedures have their effect on the toddler. Body image is not yet clearly formulated, but he is beginning to focus on his body and its parts and on his ability to control and manipulate them. Incisions and bandages may be a focus of concern for him. Casts hide his body, or at least parts of it, from him and interfere with his recognition of it as his own. His body concept may be delayed in developing or distorted by surgical procedures, cast applications, or traction therapy.

Following brief hospitalization, the toddler will gradually resume seeking autonomy upon discharge and the return to the security of his home environment and routines. During long-term hospitalization autonomy will resume as he adjusts with his mother to the hospital situation. This will, of course, depend on the course of hospitalization and treatment as well as the mother's comfort with the situation. If routines and treatments are consistent, both the toddler and his mother will have less difficulty adjusting to a long stay in the hospital. Developmental progress that is not interfered with by treatment may continue to develop but most likely at a slower pace.

Discharge from a long hospitalization is often an exciting but anxious time for the parents, particularly when special care needs to be provided at home. Parental anxieties are often felt by the toddler. Parents can be reassuring to him with support from the hospital staff and personnel. Returning home becomes another adjustment process for both toddler and parent but is usually easier than adjustment to the hospital. Security at home needs to be reestablished before the toddler will resume his surge for autonomy. If parents become too overprotective, autonomy does not adequately develop, and the toddler begins to feel shame and to doubt himself.

### Preschool child: 3 to 6 years (Table 7-3)

**Psychosocial development.** During the preschool years, from 3 to 6, the psychological conflict of the child is between initiative and guilt. Having accomplished autonomy, the child begins to deal with who he is. His major focus is still on exploring, but now he is exploring his own body and finding pleasure in his genitalia. He begins to notice, question, and compare his likeness to or difference from others, including his parents, siblings, and playmates. He becomes intrigued by the parent of the opposite sex and later begins to model the parent of his own sex.

The preschooler is also exploring his environment more and people other than parents. With his developing language skills he can now share discoveries and ask questions about the things he does not understand. He uses play to reenact experiences, which helps him integrate new discoveries with what he already knows. He also uses play and fantasy to help him deal with anxiety and fear rather than depending on his parents to provide all of his comforting. When his exploring and learning are encouraged, questions answered, and discoveries acknowledged, the preschooler develops a sense of initiative. When he is punished for exploring his body and his questions and discoveries are not rewarded, he develops a sense of guilt about his body and himself.

**Family needs.** During the preschool years most parents begin to recognize that their child is no longer a baby. They observe their child's individual personality emerge. The preschooler does not require the physical care and constant supervision previously necessary. This can be an enjoyable time for parents as the developing personality discloses affective responses to them and their behaviors. Parents can see some of their own personality characteristics emerging in the child.

This stage of development also presents its difficulties to parents. There is a delicate balance between allowing the child's discoveries and expression of them and providing appropriate limits on behavior. Parents and others may be uncomfortable when the child shares his discoveries outside of the home. Yet too strict limits interefere with the child's developing initiative through exploring and sharing what he finds. The child seems always to be asking questions, which are often difficult to answer. Mocking behaviors may point out parents' undesirable as well as desirable traits, which often poses a problem to the parent. The preschooler's discoveries often emerge from experiences with persons other than the parents and may come up unexpectedly, making it difficult for the parents to know how to respond. Protecting the child and guiding him in dealing with the things he is learning is necessary, yet overprotecting him discourages his efforts to satisfy curiosity. The parents' role in their child's development is still paramount and requires their adjustment in providing for him in new and different ways.

**Potential crisis.** One of the greatest potential exaggerations that illness or hospitalization imposes on the preschooler is its effect on his perceptions of reward and punishment. When his behavior has been acceptable, he has received praise and devel-

**Table 7-3.** Preschooler: 3 to 6 years
**Psychologic conflict: initiative versus guilt**

| Age (yr) | Primary task | Potential crisis | Interventions |
|---|---|---|---|
| 3 | *Motor skills*<br>Become more refined<br>Alternates feet going up stairs without assistance<br>Buttons and unbuttons clothes<br>Puts on shoes<br>*Language skills*<br>Uses more complete sentences<br>Can tell simple stories<br>*Social skills*<br>Feeds self well<br>Able to leave mother for short periods without fear<br>Begins to play with others and learns to take turns | *Punishment distortion*<br>Hospitalization or treatment may be perceived as punishment, especially pain, immobilization, and isolation. | *Teach and prepare child and parents about his illness, hospitalization, and treatments.* Children have a tremendous curiosity and inquisitiveness, and including them in what is happening stimulates their initiative and decreases guilt.<br>Encourage parents to tell child about hospitalization prior to admission. With elective admissions, staff can start this process during preadmission clinic visits by explaining to parents and child what will take place in the hospital.<br>Allow child to play with safe hospital equipment used in care (e.g., medicine cups, tongue blades, syringes without needles, stethoscopes, isolation mask, cups). This decreases fear. |
| 4 | *Motor skills*<br>Stands and hops on one foot<br>Alternates feet going down stairs<br>Can copy a plus sign<br>*Language skills*<br>Begins to learn numbers, colors, shapes, and coins<br>*Social skills*<br>Washes own face<br>Brushes own teeth | | Inform child prior to process what treatment is, what it is for, and whether it will hurt. Be honest and use simple explanations. Drawing blood is a good example. Tell child you are going to take just a little bit of his blood to test it so that you can help him get well and that it will hurt a little.<br>Puppet and doll play with child can help him understand what he will experience after the procedure or surgery. Encourage child to take part in teaching by allowing him to play out with you what will happen or draw pictures about what will or has happened. |
| 5 | *Motor skills*<br>Learns to skip<br>Can copy a square<br>Can draw a simple person with head, body, and limbs<br>*Language skills*<br>Can tell long, detailed stories<br>Knows numbers, colors, shapes, and coins<br>*Social skills*<br>Can dress and undress self<br>Plays competitive games | | The use of body outline to draw damaged body organs or parts that cannot be seen helps child understand what is going to be fixed (e.g., broken bones and casting can be explained with dolls or drawing). Help child understand that even though he cannot see body part, it is inside the cast.<br>Asking child to explain treatments or procedures to you or for you to a parent helps staff know if child understands what is occurring and why.<br>Encourage child to take part in care as much as possible (e.g., brush own teeth, take part in bath and dressing).<br>Encourage parents to visit regularly and take part in their child's care.<br>Child learns to trust in parents' return when visiting is regular.<br>By taking part in child's teaching and care, parents let child know of their approval of and trust in what is happening to him.<br>Routines established at home are still important and when maintained during hospitalization help to decrease confusion for child. |
| | | *Body image fear or distortion*<br>Body image is fairly well formed by this age but can be threatened by hospitalization and treatment processes. Children this age are experiencing the Oedipal conflict, are curious about their body, and are aware of body differences between girls and boys.<br>*Castration fear* may be great. | Teaching child about his body and its damaged part and how it will be fixed decreases fear of other parts of body being hurt.<br>This intervention is helpful in decreasing body image threat and castration fear as well. A boy particularly needs to be prepared for urinary catheters and told that his penis is not going to be taken away or hurt. |

oped good feelings about what he has done and thus about himself. When his behavior has been unacceptable, he has experienced punishment. Feelings of shame and guilt about what he has done and thus about how he perceives himself result. By the time he reaches 3 to 4 years of age he has learned to correlate his behavior with the response he receives. Methods of punishment may vary. Spankings (physical pain), being sent to his room (isolation), having to sit out of activity (immobilization) all become indicators that he has behaved in an undesirable way. Hospitalization and illness seem like punishment, and he perceives them as punishment unless efforts are made to help him understand what has happened.

As the preschooler is focusing attention on his own body and its different parts, body image is also threatened and there is an existing potential crisis when hospitalization, treatment, or surgery is necessary. Castration fear is common in boys; at this age they have noticed that girls do not have a penis, but they do not understand why. It is common for preschool boys to perceive girls as having lost their penises, possibly due to punishment, and they fear the loss of theirs as well.

### School-age child: 6 to 12 years (Table 7-4)

**Psychosocial development.** During the school-age years the child begins to relate more extensively with his peers and compare himself with other children. Erikson identifies the primary conflict of this age as industry versus inferiority. The child begins to develop cognitive abilities and expends time and energy acquiring knowledge. Performance becomes a major focus of cognitive abilities and extends into the child's play. In his beginning relationships with peers, competitive games and rules assume major interest and importance. Performance becomes a focus in motor skills as well. The years from 6 to 12 are filled with opportunities for expanding relationships with others, both peers (classmates) and significant adults (teachers). New experiences such as scouting, field trips, and spending the night at a friend's house are available and intriguing.

When the child's cognitive abilities, motor skills, and expanding interests are encouraged and his performance is adequate, he develops a sense of industry and good feelings about himself as a productive individual. This increases his interest in school and peer activities. It is when the child's cognitive abilities, motor skills, and expanding interests are not encouraged or recognized by significant adults or are not adequately performed in relation to his peers that a sense of inferiority develops. The child

then feels a sense of failure as an individual. He loses interest in school and withdraws from play activities with peers.

**Family needs.** It is during the school-age years that the parents, though still very important, begin to share the spotlight in their child's eyes with other adults who have become significant to him at school. This can be a very pleasant time for parents as they share pride in their child's performance and encourage his expanding interest in school and peers. The child's personal care no longer requires close supervision, and the parents' role becomes more one of verbal influence.

Difficulties may arise for parents when their particular expectations of their child differ from the child's interests. For example, there is a conflict when the father wants his son to be an athlete but the child shows little interest in sports. Parents may find it difficult to adjust to their child's individuality and thus provide too little encouragement or fail to recognize the child's accomplishments. Parents may also have difficulty providing appropriate punishments and rewards when their child experiences difficulties in school or appropriate intervention when he has difficulty with peer relationships. Again, the parents' role has changed as the child has grown, and it provides a new challenge for them.

**Potential crisis.** Hospitalization presents less of a problem for the school-age child than for any other age. Separation from home, family, and school usually produces some fear, particularly if the hospitalization is prolonged, painful, or related to permanent physical disability. Body image continues to be threatened, particularly in terms of insults related to limitations on performance. Regression to a more dependent, parent-focused state may also be seen. However, with his interest in new experiences and ability to make new friends, the school-age child can adapt more easily to the hospital and treatment process if he is included in learning about his illness, the treatment process, hospital routines, and his care. It is also helpful if he is permitted continued contact through cards, letters, and visits with those who are significant to him.

Prolonged hospitalization presents the greatest potential crisis for the school-age child, especially if it is accompanied by pain, isolation, or immobilization. The hospital loses its fascination as a new experience when fears of failure in school and loss of friends become great. Visitors and mail are not likely to come as often, and classmates continue in school without him. Depression or a sense of inferiority may occur. Depression often is undetected in children, as their feelings are frequently expressed through behavior and play rather than verbally.

## Adolescent: 13 to 18 years (Table 7-5)

**Psychosocial development.** Adolescence is considered to be one of the most, if not the most, difficult stages of development. Erikson calls it the stage of identity versus role confusion.

With the onset of puberty and secondary sexual characteristics, the adolescent's bodily appearance is rapidly changing and again becomes a major focus of his attention. Though he is excited and interested in these changes, they are new and usually produce feelings of awkwardness and embarrassment until he becomes accustomed to them. Intense modesty results. Along with these changes in appearance, the adolescent is faced with new sexual sensations and beginning interest in the opposite sex. Much attention is focused on becoming a physically mature person and questioning one's femininity or masculinity and appeal to the opposite sex. Fears of not being attractive to the opposite sex and fantasies of love and appeal to the opposite sex are common and natural. Acceptance by peers of both sexes becomes important, and attention is focused on personal appearance, from concern over acne to clothing style. Dating begins and interpersonal relationships with peers of the same sex intensify. The development of a physically mature body and its concomitant feelings are not the only focus for the adolescent. With increasing cognitive and intuitive abilities, the adolescent faces new responsibilities and expectations from authority figures and begins to enjoy independent thoughts and actions. Peers become all-knowing as the adolescent begins to realize that his parents and significant authority figures do not know everything or have acceptable solutions to all his problems. He begins to rebel against his parents. He must begin to learn to work out his own problems and make decisions for himself. Thoughts and fantasies about one's adult life begin (e.g., college, trade school, work, marriage). The adolescent gradually develops more and more independence, while still essentially dependent on his parents, and prepares for adult life.

When the adolescent experiences acceptance of his developing body and appropriate encouragement in independent efforts from interpersonal relationships with significant others, he develops an adequate concept of himself as an individual and thus an identity. Role confusion, or an indefinite concept of one's self as an individual, occurs when he is unable to resolve struggles about who or what he is as a physical, sexual, and independent person.

**Family needs.** Adolescence is a difficult time for parents as well as children. Parenting the adolescent involves a delicate balance between allowing and accepting the youth's growing up and yet maintaining the limits and structure he needs, permitting the independence for which he is ready and not permitting the independence for which he is not ready, being flexible with some of his interests and requests and yet firm against others. Parents are still vitally important to the adolescent. He needs them to help deal with unsuccessful attempts at independent functioning, but his focus is movement away from parental care and control toward independent self-care and self-control. Parents may feel threatened by loss of control and restrict their youth's independence too severely. They may also feel rejected by his movement toward independence and thus set too few limitations.

Parenting involves not only helping their youth deal with his developing sexuality but also accepting it themselves. Parents who have had difficulty dealing with their own sexuality have even more difficulty dealing with their adolescent's sexuality. Parents may fear pregnancy in adolescent girls and therefore avoid preparing them for menarche. Parents who are uncomfortable talking about sexuality are not likely to deal with their youth's questions or concerns.

For parents who understand the adolescent's struggle and who have an adequate self-concept, this stage of development can be somewhat enjoyable as they watch their youth emerge from childhood toward adulthood and take pride in the adult he becomes. Adolescence provides a challenge to parents, for it requires them to examine their own life experiences and feelings as well as their adolescent's.

**Potential crisis.** Body image again becomes a potential crisis with hospitalization, illness, treatment, or surgery during the adolescent years. Whereas the preschooler is learning what his body parts are and gaining awareness of anatomic differences, the adolescent is dealing with changes in his body and gaining awareness of the import and purpose of his body's parts and functioning. Hospitalization or surgery produces fears of scars and disfigurement, which the adolescent sees as interfering with masculine or feminine attractiveness or sexual performance. When scarring and disfigurement are a reality, they become a focus for the youth and are applied to his concerns about sexual attractiveness and functioning. The influence this has on his developing concept of himself will depend to a great extent on the response he obtains

**Table 7-4.** School age: 6 to 12 years
**Psychologic conflict: industry versus inferiority**

| Age (yr) | Primary task | Potential crisis | Interventions |
|---|---|---|---|
| 6 to 7 | *Physical-motor skills*<br>Loses baby teeth<br>Increases in height<br>*Language skills*<br>Learns to read, spell, and write<br>*Social skills*<br>Gains interest in peers<br>Begins school<br>Games and rules become very important | Generally school-age children have less difficulty with hospitalization and illness than others. They can tolerate being away from home and parents more easily. They can enjoy meeting different adults and peers. They usually enjoy new experiences and learning about new things. | *Teach and prepare child about his illness, hospitalization, and treatment.*<br>Encourage his natural interest in learning through this process.<br>Teach proper technical terms for body parts, procedures, and equipment with explanation of treatment processes he will experience.<br>Include proper timetables as child is able to conceptualize time and can understand length of hospital course.<br>Provide him with safe hospital equipment to play with and inspect (e.g., syringes, stethoscopes [children enjoy hearing their own heartbeat and those of others], reflex hammer). |
| 8 | *Physical-motor skills*<br>Rides two-wheel bike well<br>*Language-intellectual skills*<br>Learns cursive writing<br>Begins understanding concrete operations (e.g., concepts of time, cause and effect; generalizations ability to reason)<br>*Social skills*<br>Morals and rules become even more important (fairness) | Prolonged hospitalization may decrease child's intrigue with new experiences and new people, particularly if accompanied by pain, immobilization, or isolation. This can contribute to the onset of depression or a sense of inferiority. | Encourage questions.<br>Use of dolls and body outlines can be helpful, as with preschoolers but with more specific and detailed explanations.<br>Inform child of rules and routines in the hospital and limits on behavior.<br>Provide financial and resource counseling for parents.<br>Encourage parents to visit regularly and to tell their child when they are leaving and when they will return.<br>Inform child of changes in treatment processes that have been explained (e.g., if hospitalization is to be longer than initially expected).<br>Encourage letters and cards between child and siblings and peers at school or in the neighborhood.<br>Encourage honesty about physical limitations that will prohibit activities in which others his age can participate. Encourage interest and activities in which he can participate.<br>Allow time for and encourage the child and parents separately to talk about their feelings about physical limitations of child, both limited and permanent.<br>Encourage child to take part in his care to the extent that he can. Help child keep up with schoolwork.<br>Provide tutoring to decrease fear of failure.<br>Allow choices whenever possible, especially when the child is immobilized and most dependent.<br>Provide and help parents provide diversional activities and projects that the child can be successful at. |

| Age (yr) | Primary task | Potential crisis | Interventions |
|---|---|---|---|
| 9 to 10 | *Physical-motor skills*<br>Female growth spurt may begin<br>*Language-intellectual skills*<br>Begins to learn to conceptualize using language and vocabulary; abstract thinking begins<br>*Social skills*<br>Relaxes severe emphasis on rules | *Depression*<br>Depression from loss of control and ability to exert skills and energy toward normal interests. Depression is often difficult to detect readily in childhood and may be exhibited by (1) too much compliance with hospital treatment process, (2) increased activity level, even if immobilized, (e.g., yelling, calling for the nurse constantly, defecating or urinating in bed consistently, exposing genitalia even when sheets and covers are provided). | *Encourage child to tell you about his feelings and to express them through play.*<br>Allow him time to talk, helping him identify what he is feeling.<br>Let him know what other children his age have expressed ("Most kids complain about having to stay in bed. I bet you don't like it either.") thus approving his feelings.<br>Encourage aggressive games and activities. Provide activities he can do and enjoy as well as accomplish, allowing him some choice of which activity he does each time. This encourages the too-compliant child's expression and helps direct the aggressive child's behavioral expression.<br>Offer as much choice as possible in daily routines and activities.<br>Specifically for aggressive behavior:<br>Be honest and specific with the child concerning unacceptable behavior.<br>Specify that it is the behavior that is disliked, not the child. |
| 11 to 12 | *Physical-motor skills*<br>Preadolescent growth spurt<br>Onset of menarche for some girls<br>Secondary sexual characteristics appear<br>*Language-intellectual skills*<br>Widened range of interest through language<br>*Social skills*<br>Increased interest in peers and body<br>Begins to oppose parental ideas | | Recognize behavior as indicator of child's feelings and offer alternative behaviors that help express his feelings (e.g., stooling in bed may indicate feelings of anger due to loss of control over body care and forced dependency on others; offering the child other activities such as aggressive games he can play as outlets for his anger may decrease stooling in bed).<br>Set limits on undesirable behaviors.<br>Use punishment you can provide (e.g., closing curtain around bed, turning off TV).<br>Length of punishment needs to be within the attention span to be effective (i.e., if child's attention span is 15 min, then punishment needs to be for 15 min or less to be effective).<br>Warn child that behavior must stop, and specify the punishment prior to use of punishment. This gives the child a chance to change his behavior without being punished.<br>Praise the child for desirable behaviors (e.g., asking for bedpan instead of stooling in bed). |

**Table 7-5.** Adolescent: 13 to 18 years
**Psychologic conflict: identity versus role confusion**

| Age (yr) | Primary task | Potential crisis | Interventions |
|---|---|---|---|
| 13 to 15 | *Physical-motor skills*<br>Secondary sexual characteristics develop more rapidly and body appearance changes<br>*Language-intellectual skills*<br>Increase in ability to think abstractly<br>*Social skills*<br>Interest in opposite sex begins | *Body image fears or distortions*<br>Body image concerns are normal for the adolescent as his body is changing with the development of secondary sexual characteristics. Surgical scars or disfigurement intensify fears of not being attractive and of not being able to attain sexual performance. | *Teach and prepare the adolescent about his physical problem, hospitalization, and treatment.*<br>Provide teaching time for the adolescent separately from parents. This allows him a chance to ask questions and discuss things he may not want to talk about in front of parents.<br>Use correct terminology for body parts.<br>Be specific about scars, what he will and will not be able to do.<br>Encourage questions and allow private time for him to ask them and discuss his concerns.<br>Provide privacy. Adolescents are not comfortable with their changing bodies and are easily embarrassed.<br>Provide roommates who are also adolescents.<br>Encourage personal hygiene and masculine or feminine interest (e.g., pretty nightgowns, model cars to build).<br>Encourage visits or contact with friends by phone or mail. This promotes feelings of acceptance by "all-important" friends in spite of his physical scars.<br>Recognize flirtatious and coy behaviors with staff of opposite sex as adolescent testing own sexuality. |
| 16 to 18 | *Physical-motor skills*<br>Fairly well-developed, physically mature body<br>*Language-intellectual skills*<br>Expanding fund of knowledge<br>*Social skills*<br>Gaining independence from parents (e.g., gets driver's license, plans toward moving away from parents)<br>Begins testing sexuality | *Dependence-independence struggles*<br>Teens normally are leaning to become more independent while still dependent on their parents and authority figures to not allow them more independence than they are ready to handle. Prolonged hospitalization and particularly immobilization curtails the mobility they have gained and forces them into a much more dependent situation. | Provide as much independence as possible:<br>Encourage teen to do as much of his own personal care as possible.<br>Allow choices whenever possible (e.g., help plan meals within the restrictions of diet and what is available).<br>Encourage and allow time for the adolescent to express feelings about having to be cared for.<br>Maintain school work, as this is one of the ways the adolescent works toward independence and develops intellectually commensurate with peers.<br>Explain rules and regulations to adolescent on admission and throughout hospitalization. This allows teen to know what to expect from hospital staff and to know what is expected from him.<br>Set limits on undesirable behavior in the hospital: Explain the "why" of the limit.<br>Offer alternative behaviors for the expression of feelings (e.g., adolescent who is angry because he cannot do things for himself may become aggressive with staff responsible for caring for him). Hitting staff is *not allowed*. Alternative behaviors for expression of anger may be talking with staff about how angry he is, hitting a pillow, or competitive games such as cards, board games.<br>Guard against allowing an adolescent more dependency than is necessary, such as requesting staff and parents to do things for him that he is capable of doing. |

from others including parents, significant others, and to some extent hospital personnel. The adolescent may withdraw from interactions with peers in the hospital and may exhibit decreased interest in personal hygiene and appearance. He also may become less modest and show everyone his disfigurement to test their reaction to him and his body. If his concerns and behaviors are not recognized and responded to openly, he may not develop an adequate concept of his body, attractiveness to the opposite sex, and potential for sexual performance.

Hospitalization adds additional stress to the adolescent's dependency-independency struggle. This presents another potential crisis, especially if hospitalization is prolonged. Anger because of forced dependency is normal and needs to be given appropriate outlets. Compliance or regression to a more dependent state than required due to physical limitations is an indicator that the adolescent has given up his drive to become independent and may view himself as incapable of ever being independent. When regression is allowed and accepted, he may develop a concept of himself as inadequate in providing for himself in adult life.

## Young adult: 18 to 25 years (Table 7-6)

**Psychosocial development.** The conflict in young adulthood is identified by Erikson as being between the achievement of intimacy and the experience of isolation. The newly won identity and independence of adolescence is now tested in terms of personal and career commitments. Intimacy includes not only sexual intimacy but also the ability to develop psychologic intimacy with another. A relationship of mutual intimacy is not possible unless the individual has a secure sense of identity and inner resources to share freely with another without fear of losing his own identity. Without a secure self-identity the individual will avoid interpersonal intimacy and isolate himself with defensive behaviors lacking in spontaneity and warmth and inability to give freely of self; he may inhibit further psychological growth by concentrating on sex without love or on social or intellectual status that avoids intimacy.

Intimacy also includes the concept of commitment and the strength to abide by that commitment. These commitments may involve interpersonal relationships as well as assumed responsibilities in career and educational endeavors. The successful achievement of maturity in young adulthood requires self-confidence and an ability to give to one's mate, employer, children, and home. When one does not receive commensurate with one's giving, insecurity, fears, and suspicions may result that in-

crease the difficulty of giving. Without the ability to give and to love, the individual becomes emotionally isolated, absorbed in self, and competitive and insecure in relationships.

**Potential crisis.** Most orthopedic problems occurring after childhood are of a traumatic or degenerative nature. If the problem is of a temporary nature such as a fractured arm or leg, there will be little or no interference with psychosocial development. However, those problems of a more permanent (spinal cord injury) or degenerative nature will have a significant effect on the psychosocial development of the individual because these problems require reassessment of self and adaptation to significant change in body image, activities, roles, and ability to maintain established commitments.

An orthopedic problem requiring long-term hospitalization or physical immobilization separates the individual from family, friends, and work relationships. This separation occurs at a time when the individual is beginning to establish intimacy and commitments in relationships and thus may intensify feelings of insecurity and isolation. Finding oneself in a dependent, receiving position at a time when one is testing ability to be interdependent and to give freely may stimulate feelings of inadequacy and guilt. Integrating a permanent or dramatic change in body image while attempting to formulate a secure self-identity within intimate relationships may result in depression and withdrawal from others. The young adult may become angry when his newly learned independence and freedom to direct his life are inhibited. Any threat to sexual image or performance is especially significant because of its role in the establishment of intimate relationships.

It is not uncommon for the young adult experiencing long-term or repeated hospitalizations due to a permanent, long-term, or degenerative orthopedic problem to transfer his desire for sexual intimacy and friendship to caretakers. This transfer is not surprising, since the caretakers provide frequent physical and social contacts. Often caretakers are in the same age group as the patient and are accustomed to and accepting of the patient's physical and social limitations. The patient is concerned about potential rejection from family and friends; therefore his transfer of affection and social investment is naturally directed to the caretakers whose attitudes appear safe and accepting. Consequently the hospital and staff may become the patient's primary community. The hospital community may be perceived as a testing and validating ground during the adaptation period, and the gained sense of security

**Table 7-6.** Young adult: 18 to 25 years
**Psychologic conflict: intimacy versus isolation**

| Primary task | Potential crisis | Interventions |
|---|---|---|
| Establish close relationships<br>Develop personal and career commitments<br>Develop independency and interdependency<br>Develop self-confidence, sense of security, and ability to give freely<br>Develop sense of ethics and morality | Social isolation due to physical limitations, withdrawal because of fears of acceptability, and inability to relate and perform as prior to problem.<br>Threatened self-image and body image and ability to perform as prior to problem may result in depression, aggressive behavior related to feelings of helplessness and forced dependency, exaggerated dependent behavior, refusal or reluctance to cooperate in treatment plan.<br>Physical and psychologic pain may result in increased immobility, drug dependency.<br>Financial inadequacy may result from ineffective health insurance coverage, limited pre-illness opportunity to establish financial security. | Recognize honestly patient's physical changes and limitations and consequent effect on functioning.<br>Encourage and give patient permission to talk about his feelings, identifying the normalcy and acceptability of these feelings. Bring up potential concerns the patient may not be talking about (e.g., "Many people who have experienced this injury have said they feel worthless. Do you share this feeling?"). Respond to expression of feelings nonjudgmentally.<br>Encourage patient and significant others to discuss together their feelings and concerns to minimize social isolation. Provide and encourage visits and phone and written contacts with family and friends.<br>Identify and reinforce strengths and abilities of patient (physical, psychosocial, intellectual) to enhance feelings of worth.<br>Whenever possible, allow patient to make decisions that do not interfere with health (e.g., diet, schedule, procedures).<br>If patient behavior significantly interferes with treatment, verbalize acceptance of his feelings and offer behavioral alternatives ("I know you're upset about being immobilized; perhaps you can get rid of some of your energy by punching the pillow").<br>Provide sensory stimulation and distracting activities for the immobilized and long-term patient.<br>Provide for dependency needs:<br>  Provide frequent social contacts by staff.<br>  Encourage patient to identify and participate in realistic behavioral activities. The young adult is likely to try to do more than is appropriate or realistic and then become frustrated as a result.<br>  Allow opportunities for patient to do for himself even if it is less efficient than doing it for him.<br>  Stay with patient while he is performing activities that may be difficult. Support and aid him if necessary.<br>Continually teach and inform patient (and those who may provide care after discharge) about physical status, treatment plan, and expectations. Encourage patient to participate in planning care to increase sense of control and minimize dependency.<br>For patients with permanent or long-term physical limitations, psychologic, sexual, and vocational counseling will aid in adaptation to significant change in self- and body image. Significant others are appropriately included in this counseling to assist them in supporting and adjusting to the patient more effectively.<br>Administer pain medication appropriate to minimize discomfort and to maximize mobility. Use and teach alternative pain relief measures (e.g., body rubs, distraction, self-relaxation techniques). Withdraw pain medication before discharge unless still necessary because of physical problem.<br>Provide financial and resource counseling for inpatient, intermediary, or home care status. |

and confidence may then be transferred to relationships outside the hospital setting. However, there may be great difficulty in transferring from an environment where disfigurement and mobilization limitations are common and acceptable to a world and community where social rejection and isolation are responses to the same body image changes.

**Goals of psychosocial intervention.** Approaches that support the young adult's ability to maintain a sense of control will minimize the threat to his newly achieved independence and subsequent responses of depression, aggression, and exaggerated dependency. Intervention must enhance the young adult's ability to perceive himself as a productive, worthwhile, and functional being. Maintaining social ties and relationships is important in minimizing potential isolation, already a conflict of this stage. This goal may be a difficult one to achieve with the young adult who has experienced a permanent injury that changes his ability to function and relate to others. The patient with a spinal cord injury, for example, must learn to accept his body, adjust to its functional changes, and learn new ways of relating effectively and productively for health adaptation. This may require extensive and comprehensive psychological, sexual, and vocational counseling with the patient and his significant others in addition to the necessary physical and medical therapy.

## Adult: 25 to 60 years (Table 7-7)

**Psychosocial development.** The task of adulthood is generativity. This task can be described in terms of caring, producing, creating, and in general having concern for the next generation. The accomplishment of this task is dependent on the successful resolution of past developmental conflicts. Adults who are not generative are bitter, bored, and appear dull, thus communicating the conflict of adulthood as generation versus stagnation.

Psychological maturity may or may not occur in adulthood, but even though physical well-being continues there is an inevitable gradual physiological decline. Physiological changes may go relatively unnoticed until a routine incident or task provokes anxiety and recognition that one is vulnerable and older. Noticing the first gray hair, being unable to perform usual physical tasks without tiring, being admonished by an adolescent child for being oldfashioned, each in its own way confronts and acknowledges the changes of aging. Hormonal changes make aging and its results keenly visible. Hormonal changes of the menopausal stage diminish clearly feminine traits and result in the loss of child-bearing potential. These physical changes may stimulate intrapersonal and interpersonal concerns about feminine identity and desirability. One's own vulnerability and finality also are acknowledged as illness and death afflict friends and relatives. It is evident that one of the maturational challenges of adulthood is the preparation for and integration of an altered body image.

Self-image and role relationships also undergo significant changes and thus require appropriate adaptation. The transition includes changing from creator and doer to ancestor and observer, from the guiding parent with authority to a role of limited influence or of intrusion. Once regarded with respect for knowledge and skills, the adult now may be simply tolerated.

Family relationships and structures change rapidly in adulthood. Children seek significant relationships outside the home and thus turn away from parents. Adolescent children begin to test and find conflict with parental values. Young adult offspring begin to commit themselves to relationships and future goals outside the home environment, and many move some distance from home.

Parents may find themselves threatened by the vitality of their youthful children or find themselves clinging fearfully to their children with painful anticipation of their leaving home.

In a culture that values youthfulness, the aging process presents a significant conflict to the adult, which may result in the expenditure of extensive time, energy, and money in learning how to appear and behave youthfully. Proving vitality, viability, and worth may become the focus of the adult's energy.

**Potential crisis.** Certainly a major event such as an illness or accident threatens established patterns and relationships. For the adult already experiencing conflict related to the aging process, with the accompanying recognition of vulnerability, finality, and role changes, an orthopedic illness is a major critical event.

Orthopedic problems common to the adult are those of a traumatic or degenerative nature. Either of these problems and the resulting physical implications and limitations may seem to confirm the physiologic decline of aging and feelings of worthlessness and loss. Depression, exaggerated dependency, and resentment may result.

Any orthopedic problem that requires a permanent or long-term change is especially critical to the adult who has firmly established roles and career activities. The potential for changing careers is limited because of age. (Many employers consider age and experience as major factors in employment.)

**Table 7-7.** Adult: 25 to 60 years
**Psychologic conflict: generation versus stagnation**

| Primary task | Potential crisis | Interventions |
|---|---|---|
| Creativity<br>Productivity<br>Parenting<br>Concern for next generation<br>Integrating biophysical changes of aging (e.g., menopause) | Illness and hospitalization may intensify difficulty integrating physical and psychosocial changes and losses, resulting in:<br>Depression, with feelings of low self-esteem and recognition of vulnerability and finality.<br>Bitterness and resentment communicated by demanding behavior and frequent requests and refusal or resistance to cooperating in treatment plan.<br>  This may be related to fears of loss, vulnerability, helplessness, and forced dependency<br>  Due to threatened or real change in role and career status.<br>Exaggerated dependent behavior resulting from fear and pain.<br>Social isolation due to physical limitations and withdrawal due to feelings of inadequacy and worthlessness.<br>Physical and psychologic pain may result in increased immobility or drug dependency.<br>Financial inadequacy may result from ineffective health insurance coverage, pre-illness financial status, or increased stress of present and long-term care situation. | Honestly recognize patient's physical condition and functional implications.<br>Encourage and give patient permission to verbalize feelings, identifying the normalcy and acceptability of these feelings. Bring up potential concerns patient may not be talking about (e.g., "Many people with such an injury wonder whether they will be able to function sexually. Do you have this concern?"). Respond to all feeling expression nonjudgmentally.<br>Identify and reinforce patient's strengths and support significant roles within family relationships as possible (e.g., a father can provide guidance and advice to children even when he is physically dependent).<br>Encourage patient participation in plans for and activities of care. Allow patient to make decisions that do not interfere with health (e.g., diet, schedule, procedures).<br>Maintain social and work relationships by providing opportunities for visits and phone and written contacts, as long as activities are not too stressful or tiring.<br>If patient behavior significantly interferes with treatment, verbalize acceptance of his feelings and offer behavioral alternatives.<br>Provide for dependency needs:<br>  Provide frequent social staff contacts.<br>  Encourage patient to participate in activities, while explaining their purpose.<br>  Provide opportunities for patient to do for himself even if less efficient than doing it for him.<br>  Stay with patient while he is performing independent activities that may be difficult. Support and aid as necessary.<br>Continually teach and inform patient (and those who may provide care after discharge) about physical status, treatment plan, and care to increase sense of control and minimize fears.<br>For patients with permanent or long-term problems, psychological, sexual, and vocational counseling will aid in adaptation. Significant others are appropriately included in counseling to enhance relationship with patient.<br>Administer pain medication to minimize discomfort and to maximize mobility. Use and teach alternative pain relief measures (e.g., body rubs, distraction, and self-relaxation techniques). Withdraw pain medication before discharge unless it is still necessary because of the physical problem.<br>Provide financial and resource counseling for inpatient, intermediary, or home care status. |

Flexibility, creativity, and productivity may be limited if the orthopedic problem significantly interferes with previous ability to perform. Intensive psychological and vocational counseling may be necessary to facilitate healthy adaptation.

An orthopedic problem in the adult also may increase the stress on changing family relationships and structures. Hospitalization or physical limitations may intensify the social isolation and related feelings already being experienced by the adult.

Any stress to the financial capability of the adult to provide effectively for the family will be major. Providing for children's needs (education, clothing, food, luxuries) is a primary functional role of the adult.

**Goals of psychosocial intervention.** Psychosocial intervention based on an awareness of the already difficult process of adaptation to aging and the recognition of the additional burden that results from the orthopedic problem is important for the adult. If the patient feels depressed, worthless, and inadequate prior to the illness or accident, he will then require integration and acceptance of aging as well as of the present situation. Maintaining the adult patient's ability to maintain a sense of control, ability to be productive, and role significance is primary in psychosocial intervention.

### Elderly adult: over 60 years (Table 7-8)

**Psychosocial development.** In a sense, with maturity or old age life has come full circle. In the last third of life the individual reviews his life, evaluates its meaning and direction, and looks to the future with a sense of trust, the first developmental task of the newborn infant. The individual who adapts successfully to this stage is able to accept his individual life and the people who are and have been significant to it. In accepting his life the individual is without remorse, bitterness, or sadness. The individual who feels that his life has come to an end and does not feel good about himself, his accomplishments, and his relationships will experience a sense of despair and disgust.

Although this final stage of development is perceived as a maturational stage with its normative changes, it is experienced in our culture as a significant crisis because it is seen only as a decline, accompanied by forced relinquishment of status, respect, role, recognition, and function. Most people are not prepared to be old, to lose their spouse and loved ones, or to become dependent. Consequently those natural aspects of the maturational process are perceived as unexpected and disastrous to self and body image, which intensifies the critical nature of the aging experience.

All human beings grow old. The physiologic degeneration of aging is a process that affects the physical, social, and psychological functioning of the individual. Neurologic changes result in sensory impairment. Farsightedness and narrowing of the visual field are common. Hearing declines, especially the acuity for high tones. Taste is blunted, which interferes with pleasureful eating. Organic brain changes may contribute to personality changes and problems with equilibrium.

Atrophy within the circulatory system may contribute to an increase in heart size, rigidity of heart valves, and an increase in blood pressure. Ventilation may be diminished due to limited chest wall elasticity. Tissue repair is retarded. In addition aging results in increased brittleness and shrinking of the bone structure. Skeletal muscles decrease in strength, and motor activity is retarded. The external body shows the affects of aging with even greater visibility. The skin becomes wrinkled, thin, and dry and contains brown pigmentation. The hair becomes gray, dry, and thin. Nails thicken. Teeth yellow.

If the changes resulting from the aging process occur and are integrated gradually into the individual's concept of self and functional activities, the potential crisis will be minimized.

Changes in social role and position also intensify the maturational crisis of aging. The elderly individual generally experiences a lowering of status in relation to productivity within career endeavors and family structure. The number of people with whom the older person interacts is likely to decrease as spouse and peers die and as the individual is unable to maintain his activity and mobility level. Financial concerns are primary for many elderly people. Their financial planning and savings may leave them inadequately prepared to support a style of living to which they were accustomed, and an illness at this time may overburden and drain financial capabilities.

**Potential crisis.** Common to the elderly are orthopedic problems of a traumatic (broken bones) or degenerative (arthritis) nature. Either problem intensifies the already predictable maturational stressors of pain, neuromuscular atrophy, and mobility retardation. The illness and subsequent hospitalization (often long term) exaggerate the elderly person's sense of isolation and worthlessness, fear of dependency, and inadequate financial capabilities.

Depression and exaggerated dependency behavior are common in the hospitalized elderly patient. Integrating this illness and its subsequent limitations may overwhelm an already tenuous adjustment. Feelings of fear, helplessness, and pain inten-

**Table 7-8.** Elderly adult: over 60 years
**Psychologic conflict: ego integrity versus despair**

| Primary task | Potential crisis | Interventions |
|---|---|---|
| Accept and integrate past life and present situation (including meaning and relationships) Adjust to biophysical changes and deteriorations Integrate role changes resulting from aging, retirement, living arrangements, health, and so on Integrate loss of loved ones | Illness and hospitalization may intensify difficult integrating physical and psychosocial losses and changes and may result in: Depression, with feelings of low self-esteem, anticipation of own death, and unresolved past losses. Bitterness and anger About having to continue living (many elderly have fantasies about reunion with loved ones and desire death) related to feelings of helplessness and fear. Reluctance or refusal to cooperate in treatment plan. Social isolation due to physical limitations, withdrawal because of fear of inadequacy, worthlessness. Exaggerated dependent behavior resulting from feelings of helplessness, fear, and pain. Disorientation due to sensory deprivation or sensory overload, perceptual limitations, change in environment or routine, drug therapy or immobilization. Financial inadequacy may result from ineffective health insurance coverage, preillness financial status, increased stress of present and long-term care situation. Physical and psychologic pain may result in increased immobility or drug dependency. | Recognize patient as an adult, not a child. Call by proper name (e.g., not "granny") to enhance sense of dignity and self-respect. Integrate age-related physical changes and limitations into rehabilitation plan. Individualize plan. Especially provide for sensory limitations (e.g., sight, hearing, touch). Provide for social and physical dependency needs, slowly encouraging movement toward realistic independent behaviors. Progress from doing for patient to doing with patient to patient doing for self to minimize complaints, demands, and dependent behavior. Provide frequent social contacts by staff. Provide predictability in daily activity schedule. Encourage patient to identify preferences. Tell patient what is expected and appropriate rationale. Encourage verbalization about the past, family, social relationships, hobbies, and successes to enhance sense of worth. Encourage verbalization of feelings (e.g., fear, anger, helplessness, hopelessness). Acknowledge normalcy and acceptability of feelings. Feelings may be released through physical activities. Provide familiarity in environment (e.g., pictures, own clothing) to enhance sense of identity and minimize disorientation. Allow patient to make decisions where possible (e.g., when to bathe, which arm for IV therapy) to maximize sense of control. Instruct patient and provide diet based on nutritional requirements for effective healing as well as integration of patient's likes and desires to enhance sense of control. Provide ongoing informal teaching focusing on conciseness, clarity, and repetitiveness. Progress from least complex important information and activities to more complex to increase probability of retention and successes. Repetition should be expected because of sensory interference and anxiety. Elderly may not feel comfortable asking questions. Anticipate probable questions and encourage questioning. Teach significant others care factors to provide for continuity and effectiveness of care after discharge. Encourage maintenance of social and family relationships through visits and phone and written contacts. Identify and support patient strengths; identify a social role within the hospital setting or home (e.g., creative hobbies, mothering, gardening). Minimize disorientation and confusion with use of touch, informing patient of time, place, and person regularly, evaluating effects of medication; at night use effective lighting, provide frequent staff checks, or have familiar person stay with patient. Maintain mobility to minimize neuromuscular atrophy and to aid in patient orientation. Provide financial and resource counseling for inpatient, intermediary, or home care status. Give pain medication to minimize discomfort and fear and maximize mobility. Use alternative pain relief measures (e.g., body rubs, distraction, self-relaxation techniques). Withdraw pain medication before discharge whenever possible. |

sify dependent needs. The illness may be perceived by the elderly adult as a confirmation of worthlessness and inability to be productive. He may resist the treatment program because of bitterness about having to continue living and "be a burden" to others. Some of these responses may even occur in the patient who is anticipating hospitalization for corrective surgery or therapy such as a hip replacement. Surgery, however, may be anticipated as an opportunity for increased mobilization, and thus a hopeful attitude may minimize fears of dependency and motivation may be high.

**Goals of psychosocial intervention.** Any approaches that maximize the elderly person's sense of worth and productivity will minimize sense of loss, isolation, and thus feelings of depression and bitterness. An individual who feels significant and worthwhile is motivated to participate more effectively in a treatment plan.

Also important to the elderly person is an adequate understanding of what he can expect from his environment and what is expected of him. One can anticipate that a health care setting will be foreign territory to him. He functions best in a familiar, predictable, and structured environment. Disorientation and fear may result if intervention does not provide effectively for these needs. The elderly person may also perceive care providers as threatening authority figures and thus may not ask questions freely or comfortably. Anticipating and encouraging questions is therapeutic. A health care setting must also provide for the elderly adult as a social being to minimize social isolation. Approaches that support the patient's self-identity, integrity, and respect are important. Providing opportunities for the elderly patient to visit and relate with family, friends, and others in the environment will maintain his perception of self as a social being and will maintain his role within the social structure and setting.

Significant in the care of the elderly is the recognition and integration of health problems in addition to the orthopedic problem, such as diabetes or heart disease. Care must be comprehensive in providing for individual needs related to the total health status. Counseling and intervention appropriate for potential nursing home or convalescent placement is an additional consideration. Frequently the elderly adult perceives such placement as personal rejection and isolation, and many have negative attitudes toward this established need.

## CONSULTATION FOR DYSFUNCTIONAL COPING

It is evident from the previous discussion that one can expect significant levels of psychologic dis-

turbance in the rehabilitation of patients. Disturbances in mood are very common, with varying degrees of anxiety, depression, anger, and resentment. These feelings may interfere with the patient's capacity to cooperate in the treatment plan, thus having an obvious impact on the progress of rehabilitation. Those behavioral responses that interfere significantly with health maintenance and mobilization are considered to be dysfunctional and thus appropriate for psychiatric intervention (Table 7-9). An example might be the patient in a body cast who becomes disoriented and paranoid, making it difficult for staff to provide personal care.

Direct psychiatric intervention is not always available, necessary, or even desirable. Many of the adaptive behaviors and feeling responses in crisis resolution are perceived by the care providers to be inappropriate and unmanageable and thus dysfunctional. In many instances psychiatric referral is initiated by the paramedical team member and is authenticated by the physician. Subsequent communications then occur between physician and psychiatrist, excluding the staff member(s) most knowledgeable and distressed about the problem. This form of consultation is of value in identifying discrete psychiatric problems and referring patients for additional treatment. However, it is not usually helpful to the paramedical staff caring for the patient during hospitalization. Only a small number of patients fall into this category. It is our belief that much of the management of emotional disturbance can be provided by the caretakers already involved with the patient, provided the support of skilled professional consultation is available to them. Professionals with consulting expertise include the psychiatrist, psychiatric nurse, psychologist, and psychiatric social worker. Most patient care settings have one or more of these resource persons available but have not utilized them effectively for the support of care providers.

Consultation in which efforts are directed toward helping the care providers in the management of difficult patient problems is referred to as patient-centered (mental health) or liason consultation (Table 7-9). In such a process the care provider(s) consults the professional with psychiatric expertise about a patient who is presenting a management problem. Usually the consultant does not see the patient but relies entirely on the staff for necessary information. The purpose of a patient interview (if deemed necessary) is to provide further information about issues that relate to the defined problem.

Working with the care providers, the consultant attempts to understand the nature and precipitants of the problems and to discuss management alterna-

**Table 7-9.** Consultation for dysfunctional coping

| Type of consultation | Purpose | When to refer | Referrent process | What to include in referral |
|---|---|---|---|---|
| Patient-centered | Direct assessment of overt psychiatric symptoms<br>Suggest medical management<br>Provide or refer for psychiatric treatment | Patient has overt psychiatric symptoms (poor reality testing)<br>Patient behavior is interfering with medical management plan and health<br>Patient has previous psychiatric history (present situation may exacerbate symptoms) | Written communication between physician and psychiatrist (usually) | Concise description of patient's physical diagnosis, history, present treatment plan, and present behavior<br>State requested role of consultant (drug therapy, behavioral management, follow up) |
| Liaison | Assist direct care providers in understanding nature of problem<br>Suggest management alternative<br>Consultant may share responsibility for aspects of patient care | Care provider feels distressed, angry, helpless about patient situation | Significant verbal communication between direct care providers and consultant with psychiatric expertise (psychiatrist, psychologist, nurse, social worker)<br>Written summary of consultant's assessment | Concise description of patient's physical history, present treatment plan<br>Detailed description of patient behavior, feelings, responses<br>Patient's social history<br>Description of staff response and intervention approaches<br>Identify opportunity for consultant to talk with care providers |

tives. The indication for referral for consultation by this method is a rising level of concern or distress by a staff member about some aspect of patient management. The distress usually takes the form of angry frustration, despair, and feelings of helplessness about the patient's condition and prognosis or a desire to avoid the patient. For example, patient-centered consultation might be indicated when the mother of a child hospitalized for a fractured bone received when hit by a car has been so critical of staff caring for the child that everyone wants to avoid him. Through talking with the staff the consultant may assist them in realizing that the mother's behavior is related to her own feelings of guilt and perception of herself as a "bad mother" for not watching the child closely enough. The consultant can also help staff develop intervention techniques to reduce the mother's negative feelings about her "mothering," which will probably decrease her criticism of staff care. This behavioral change on the part of the mother and the understanding and behavior change of the staff may result in a more effective relationship between mother and staff.

## SUMMARY

The word *crisis* is used to describe everything from day-to-day problems to international situations. It is a word that, because of its frequent use and abuse, may have lost much of its value.

In the context of this chapter crisis is determined by the inability of the individual and family to resolve the stressful event and resulting situation. There are many stressful events and situations that may precipitate a crisis and thus may be considered as "potential crises." However, it is the response to and the effect of the stressful event and situation on the individual and family system that determine whether a crisis occurs. Thus coping behavior that is dysfunctional creates a state of disequilibrium or crisis.

Maturational needs and conflicts, illness, and adaptational issues related to self and body image are considered to be stressors and thus potential crises. If the response to these stressors is dysfunctional and the situation is not resolved but is one of disequilibrium, it is defined as a crisis.

It is our philosophy that individuals *do* have the

ability to resolve their own potential or actual crisis situations. Resolution of potential crisis situations requires mobilization of functional coping and problem-solving behaviors. Resolution of crisis is dependent on relearning, unlearning dysfunctional coping patterns, or learning functional coping and problem-solving behaviors to solve the present crisis situation. Within the prevention or resolution of the crisis process, health care providers may be significant participants in supporting the individual's use of existing functional coping patterns or encouraging mobilization and learning of new and more effective problem-solving behaviors.

It is our intention that health care providers assess comprehensively the needs of the individual (maturational and situational), ability to cope with the stressful situation (existing functional coping behaviors), and the timing and extent to which outside intervention (crisis intervention) is necessary and appropriate for restoring the individual to a state of equilibrium (resolution).

## REFERENCES

1. Aguilera, D. C., and Messick, J. M.: Crisis intervention: theory and methodology, ed. 3, St. Louis, 1978, The C. V. Mosby Co.
2. Caplan, G.: Principles of preventive psychiatry, New York, 1964, Basic Books, Inc.
3. Duhl, F. J.: Grief. Paper presented before the Ohio League for Nursing Convention, Columbus, Ohio, 1964.
4. Erikson, E.: Identity, youth and crisis, New York, 1968, W. W. Norton Co.
5. Erikson, E.: Childhood and society, New York, 1964, W. W. Norton Co.
6. Fink, S.: Crisis and motivation: a theoretical model, Arch. Phys. Med. Rehabil. **48**:592-597, 1967.
7. Rapoport, L.: The state of crisis: some theoretical considerations. In Parad, H. J., editor: Crisis intervention: selected readings, New York, 1965, Family Services Association of America, pp. 22-31.

## BIBLIOGRAPHY

Apley, J., and MacKeith, R.: The child and his symptoms, ed. 2, Oxford, England, 1968, Blackwell Scientific Publications.
Arnoff, F.: Body image deterioration in paraplegia, J. Nerv. Mental Dis. **137**:88-92, 1963.
Arnold, H. M.: Elderly diabetic amputees, Am. J. Nurs. **69**:2646-2649, 1969.
Barrell, L. M.: Crisis intervention: partnership in problem solving, Nurs. Clin. North Am. **9**(1):5-16, March 1974.
Bart, M. M.: Perceptual deficits in hemiplegia, Am. J. Nurs. **70**:1026-1029, 1970.
Blaesing, S., and Brockhaus, J.: The development of body image in the child, Nurs. Clin. North Am. **7**(4):597-607, 1972.
Brown, F.: Knowledge of body image and nursing care of the patient with limb amputation, J. Psychiatr. Nurs. **2**:397-409, 1964.
Brown, M. M.: Psychodynamic nursing: a biosocial orientation, Philadelphia, 1972, W. B. Saunders Co.
Caine, D.: Psychological considerations affecting rehabilitation after amputation, Med. J. Aust. **2**:818-821, 1973.
Corbeil, M.: Nursing process for a patient with a body image disturbance, Nurs. Clin. North Am. **6**:155-163, March 1971.
Davidites, R.: The extended roles of the prepared professional psychiatric-mental health nurse in the general hospital setting. In Stokes, G., editor: The roles of psychiatric nurses in community mental health practice: a giant step, New York, 1969, Faculty Press, pp. 80-87.
Dempsey, M. O.: The development of body image in the adolescent, Nurs. Clin. North Am. **7**(4):609-615, 1972.
DiFabio, S.: Crisis: a complex process, Nurs. Clin. North Am. **9**(1):47-56, March 1974.
Fisher, S., and Cleveland, S.: Body image and personality, New York, 1968, Dover Publications.
Francis, G. M., and Munjas, B. A.: Manual of social-psychologic assessment, New York, 1976, Appleton-Century-Crofts.
Freeman, R. D.: Emotional reactions of handicapped children, Rehab. Lit. **28**:274-282, 1967.
Fujita, M. T.: The impact of illness or surgery on the body image of the child, Nurs. Clin. North Am. **7**(4):641-649, 1972.
Gordon, I. J.: Human development from birth through adolescence, New York, 1962, Harper & Row, Publishers.
Gruendemann, B. J.: The impact of surgery on body image, Nurs. Clin. North Am. **10**(4):635-643, December 1975.
Hall, J. E., and Weaver, B. R.: Nursing families in crisis, Philadelphia, 1974, J. B. Lippincott Co.
Holaday, B. J.: Achievement behavior in chronically ill children, Nurs. Res. **23**:25-30, 1974.
Hymovich, D. P.: Bobby: a very difficult little boy. Nursing 73 **3**:44-45, 1973.
Kolb, L. C.: Disturbances of body image. American handbook of psychiatry, vol. 1, New York, 1969, Basic Books, Inc.
Kolb, L. C., Psychology of amputee: phantom phenomena, body image and pain. Mayo Clin. Proc. **44**:586, 1952.
Kurtz, R.: Your body image: what it tells about you, Science Digest, 1969, pp. 52-55.
Lane, P. A.: A mother's confession: home care of a toddler in a hip spica cast — what it's really like, Am. J. Nurs. **71**(11):2141-2143, 1971.
Leonard, B. J.: Body image changes in chronic illness, Nurs. Clin. North Am. **7**(4):687-695, 1972.
Mann, S. A.: Coping with a child's fatal illness: a parent's dilemma, Nurs. Clin. North Am. **9**(1):81-87, 1974.

Mattsson, A.: The chronically ill child: a challenge to family adaptation, MCV Quarterly 8(3):171-175, 1972.

McDanniel, J. W.: Physical disability and human behavior, New York, 1970, Pergamon Press.

Millians, W. S.: Emotional and behavioral reactions of children and adolescents to handicaps and chronic illness. Unpublished paper.

Murray, R. L.: Body image development in adulthood, Nurs. Clin. North Am. 7(4):617-629, 1972.

Murray, R. L.: Principles of nursing intervention for the adult patient with body image changes, Nurs. Clin. North Am. 7(4):697-707, 1972.

Norris, C. M.: The professional nurse and body image: behavioral concepts and nursing intervention, Philadelphia, 1970, J. B. Lippincott Co. pp. 39-65.

Parad, H. J.: Crisis intervention: selected readings, New York, 1965, Family Service Association of America.

Petrillo, M., and Sanger S.: Emotional care of hospitalized children, Philadelphia, 1972, J. B. Lippincott Co.

Riddle, I.: Nursing intervention to promote body image integrity in children, Nurs. Clin. North Am. 7(4):651-661, 1972.

Rubin, R.: Body image and self esteem, Nurs. Outlook 16:20-23, 1968.

Schechter, M.: The orthopedically handicapped child: emotional reactions, Arch. Gen. Psych. 4:53-59, 1961.

Sutterly, D., and Donnelly, G.: Perspectives in human development, Philadelphia, 1973, J. B. Lippincott Co.

Trail, I. D., and Monke, J. V.: Psyche sequelae of surgical change in body structure, Nurs. Forum 2:14-23, 1963.

Williams, F. S.: Intervention in maturational crisis: nursing of families in crisis. Adapted with permission from *Perspectives in Psychiatric Care,* Vol. 9, No. 6.

Williams, F. S.: The crisis of hospitalization, Nurs. Clin. North Am. 9(1):37-45, 1974.

Wright, B.: Physical disability: a phychosocial approach, New York, 1960, Harper & Row, Publishers, Inc.

Zind, R. K.: Deterrents to crisis intervention in the hospital unit, Nurs. Clin. North Am. 9(1):27-36, 1974.

# 8

# Documentation

**AVICE KERR**

Documentation is an important step in the process of medical diagnosis, treatment, and care. All health care personnel are involved in documentation to varying degrees. The current emphasis on documentation is based on two factors: (1) *the increasing recognition that better records contribute to better patient care,* and (2) the need for corroborating evidence in legal cases.

Because the topic of documentation is vast, this chapter simply offers terminology and practical suggestions for use in documentation by physicians, therapists, and particularly, nurses.

## TERMINOLOGY

Reviewers soon learn that not everyone writes what he or she means. Some institutions have descriptive terms listed on the backs of forms, but with no definitions. Many on the staff may use the terms with only a vague idea of their exact meaning. Thus the information is inaccurate and meaningless. The following are some commonly used terms and their definitions.

### PAIN

**intensity**
    ± **slight** causes annoyance but no handicap.
    ± **mild**
    ±± **mild to moderate** can be tolerated for short periods; may at times limit activities that cause pain.
    ++ **moderate**
    +++ **moderately severe** causes decrease or cessation of activities that precipitate pain.
    ++++ **markedly severe** precludes any activity that precipitates pain; may preclude all activity.
**persistent** symptoms continue despite treatment or beyond expected time.
**paroxysmal** sudden, violent, usually recurring.
**sporadic** occasional, scattered, or isolated episodes.
**intermittent** occurring at intervals, stopping and starting.
**localized** occurring in a specific area.
**generalized** affecting many or all parts; not localized.

### SKIN

**hot** flushed.
**ruddy** reddish.
**pale** lacking color.
**cyanotic** bluish discoloration secondary to insufficient oxygenation.
**mottled** splotchy or dappled patches of color.
**jaundiced** skin or mucous membrane showing yellowish color due to bile pigment
**contusion** bruise caused by a blow.
**abrasion** skin scraped off.
**excoriation** skin peeled off as result of mechanical or chemical irritation.
**ulcer** lesion with inflamed base, usually caused by prolonged pressure.
**macular rash** unelevated spot.
**papular rash** small elevated, solid, usually red, circumscribed spots.
**pustular rash** small elevations filled with pus.

### BEHAVIOR

**alert** attentive, vigilant.
**oriented** aware of and adjusted to surroundings and circumstances.
**disoriented** confused about surroundings and circumstances.

# PHYSICAL EXAMINATION

Name _____

Age _____ Sex _____ Height _____ Weight _____

Temperature _____ Pulse _____ Respirations _____ Blood pressure _____

Appearance: Well nourished _____ Robust _____ Fair _____ Debilitated _____

Posture: Normal _____ Impaired _____ Antalgic _____

           Distance, fingertips to floor _____

Ambulation: Normal _____ Impaired _____ Difficult _____

           Needs assistance _____ Needs equipment _____ Painful _____

Gait: Stance _____ Swing _____ Heel walk _____ Toe walk _____

| **Range of motion** | **Sitting** | **Supine** |
|---|---|---|
| *Cervical* | | |
| Flexion | _____ | _____ |
| Extension | _____ | _____ |
| Left rotation | _____ | _____ |
| Right rotation | _____ | _____ |
| Left lateral flexion | _____ | _____ |
| Right lateral flexion | _____ | _____ |
| Left lateral bend | _____ | _____ |
| Right lateral bend | _____ | _____ |
| *Thoracolumbar* | | |
| Flexion | _____ | _____ |
| Extension | _____ | _____ |
| Left rotation | _____ | _____ |
| Right rotation | _____ | _____ |
| Left lateral flexion | _____ | _____ |
| Right lateral flexion | _____ | _____ |
| Circumduction | _____ | _____ |

## PHYSICAL EXAMINATION—cont'd

| | Pain | Tenderness | | Pain | Tenderness |
|---|---|---|---|---|---|
| Occipital | _____ | _____ | T-7 | _____ | _____ |
| C-1 | _____ | _____ | T-8 | _____ | _____ |
| C-2 | _____ | _____ | T-9 | _____ | _____ |
| C-3 | _____ | _____ | T-10 | _____ | _____ |
| C-4 | _____ | _____ | T-11 | _____ | _____ |
| C-5 | _____ | _____ | T-12 | _____ | _____ |
| C-6 | _____ | _____ | L-1 | _____ | _____ |
| C-7 | _____ | _____ | L-2 | _____ | _____ |
| C-8 | _____ | _____ | L-3 | _____ | _____ |
| T-1 | _____ | _____ | L-4 | _____ | _____ |
| T-2 | _____ | _____ | L-5 | _____ | _____ |
| T-3 | _____ | _____ | Sacrum | _____ | _____ |
| T-4 | _____ | _____ | Coccyx | _____ | _____ |
| T-5 | _____ | _____ | Right iliac | _____ | _____ |
| T-6 | _____ | _____ | Left iliac | _____ | _____ |

**Code**

Pain and tenderness:

± to +, minimal
+ to ±±, slight
++, moderate
+++, moderately severe
++++, severe

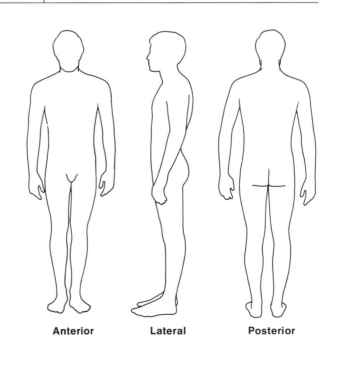

Anterior     Lateral     Posterior

**confused** disturbed mental state; clouding of consciousness, inaccurate or jumbled expression; bewildered, perplexed.
**anxious** fearful, greatly troubled, worried.
**apprehension** forboding; anticipation of adversity, dread.
**frightened** terrified, alarmed.
**calm** quiet, self-controlled, tranquil.
**irritable** readily excited to impatience or anger; easily exasperated.
**cooperative** participates in and with plan of care.
**lethargic** drowsy, sluggish, mildly stuporous.
**apathetic** showing little or no interest or emotion.
**demanding** insistent; requiring much attention.
**withdrawn** retreated; pulled away from contact.

## COMMUNICATION

**aphasia** impairment or loss of capacity to use words as symbols of ideas. Aphasia is organic secondary to central nervous system lesion, not a defect in mechanics of speaking.
**stammer** difficulty in uttering word or syllable, resulting in broken or inarticulate sounds. Stammering is markedly affected by emotion.
**stutter** Rapid involuntary repetition of a syllable, particularly initial sound. Rhythm of speech interrupted by blocks and spasms, resulting in repetition or prolongation of sounds or syllables. Stuttering is often an inherent speech defect.

## PHYSICIAN DOCUMENTATION
### Physical examination

Physical examination forms (box, pp. 180-181) are designed to obtain pertinent data organized so that all members of the health team have access to the information they need. Documentation in a haphazard fashion may mean that important information is missed by those who need it. Care must be taken to make examination entries accurate and consistent. Sometimes notes are written from sheer habit. For example, "PERLA, sclera clear. Right pupil dilated and reacts sluggishly to light." Obviously the person who wrote this was not thinking, or would have remembered that PERLA means that the pupils are equal and react normally to light and accommodation.

### Orthopedic history

Orthopedic histories may be taken by physicians or by orthopedic nurses. The physician may evaluate the findings while performing the examination, omitting unimportant items and recording only pertinent facts. The nurse must include all findings so that the physician has all the necessary information on which to base an evaluation. Data obtained in the orthopedic history include the following:

**I. Chief complaint**
  A. Onset
    1. If an accident, what forces were exerted on the body
    2. If gradual, describe in detail
  B. Associated complaints
**II. Past history**
  A. Birth defects, developmental problems
  B. Fractures, dislocations, sprains
  C. Joint problems
    1. Pain
    2. Swelling
    3. Limitation of motion
    4. Arthritis
      a. Osteoarthritis
      b. Rheumatoid
      c. Posttraumatic
      d. Gout
  D. Skeletal deformities
  E. Muscular weakness, atrophy, cramps, spasms
  F. Infections
    1. Bone
    2. Soft tissues
  G. Soft-tissue problems
    1. Swelling
    2. Ulcers
      a. Decubitus
      b. Diabetic
  H. Spinal problems
    1. Back problems, associated sciatica
    2. Neck problems, associated radiculitis
    3. Describe any severe episodes (how often, duration, associated with unusual activities)
**III. Neurologic**
  A. Motor
    1. Gait disturbance
    2. Incoordination of movement
  B. Sensory (Note areas involved)
    1. Anesthesia
    2. Diminished sensation
    3. Paresthesia (abnormal sensation such as tingling, prickling, "bugs crawling on skin")
  C. Pain
    1. Area involved
    2. Intensity (sharp, dull)
    3. Severity (mild, severe, agonizing)
    4. Character (aching, persistent, continuous, fixed distress, bumping, throbbing, burning, cramping, lancinating, stabbing, shocklike, tingling)
    5. When does pain occur
    6. Effect on sleep (Does it keep you from going to sleep? Do you go to sleep, then waken with pain? Do you waken in the morning stiff and sore?)
    7. What increases or decreases pain (e.g., bending, lifting, sitting, standing, lying, walking, running, coughing, sneezing, straining)

8. Position of greatest comfort
9. Effect of treatment (relieves, does not relieve)
    a. Wet heat
    b. Dry heat
    c. Firm mattress
    d. Position in bed
    e. Supports (e.g., brace, corset, cast, collar)
10. Medication

## Consultation

Most consultations are written up from information readily available because the area of discussion is limited. They usually consist of a summary of findings and a conclusion.

## Orders

To avoid misunderstanding, orders must be specific, or what one physician called "idiot proof." For example, when an order is written for a drug that irritates the stomach, it should specify "TID pc and at bedtime with milk." If the order says only QID, the drug will probably be given at 8, 12, 4, and 8 o'clock, with no regard to food intake.

## Progress notes

Written progress notes are required to provide a chronologic record of the patient's hospitalization. Since some physicians do not see their patients everyday, suspicion is raised when the progress note says "status quo," "no change," or just "seen." Many charts go to the record room lacking a lot, including progress notes. Physicians may then come in and fill in spaces with dates and nonnotes such as those above. Reviewers learn to associate such notes with the fact that most of the orders for the patient are given by telephone.

Good progress notes need not be verbose, but they should say something about the patient. "Color is better," "Not able to swallow; will start IV fluids," or "Hgb 8.9; will order 1 unit of blood" conveys information without rhetoric.

When a physician is called to see a patient, the record should show the problem, the findings, the treatment, the result of treatment, and follow-up. For example:

Patient with fracture C6 and cord compression C5 placed in Vinke tongs 2 hr ago. Called to see patient because BP 80/60 and temperature 96. Will attempt to heat patient up. Appears to be experiencing a sympathetic block.

This patient was next seen by a physician 12 hours later, but there is no mention of the previous problem nor the status of the patient's blood pressure when seen.

If a patient hemorrhages, there should be laboratory studies and progress notes indicating that the physician is aware of the results.

There are many pressures on a physician; having the Utilization Committee upset because a patient has been hospitalized 2 days longer than planned should not be one of them. If consultations have been requested but the consultant has not yet seen the patient or if other studies are delayed, the physician can be freed of responsibility for the delay by writing in the progress notes, "Consultant will be reminded to see the patient today," "Brace has not come; will check with orthotist," and so on.

## THERAPIST DOCUMENTATION

Physical therapists, occupational therapists, inhalation therapists, and speech therapists should chart whatever is necessary to share what they know about the patient. Their record should be a tool for communication with all other health care personnel.

Some therapists write excellent notes; others do not. "Treated as ordered BID" tells nothing except that the patient will be billed for two treatments, and other health care workers may have to look at the physician's orders to learn what the treatments were. Good notes allow another therapist to treat the patient with full knowledge of what he needs and how he reacts and then compare his or her own results. Good notes allow the nurses to keep abreast of the patient's progress or lack of it. For example, a note saying, "After taking two steps, patient became dizzy and faint" not only alerts the next therapist of the difficulty but also prevents nurses who knew that the patient had gone to the physical therapy department for gait training from concluding that he should now be able to ambulate to the bathroom.

Good notes by nurses and therapists allow the physician to adjust the care plan and to estimate how much longer the patient will need to receive treatment or be hospitalized. Changes in reaction, motivation, and so on, should be noted so that the entire health team can look for the cause and try to help solve the problem.

## NURSING DOCUMENTATION

Considerable emphasis is placed here on nursing documentation because, unlike the other disciplines, nursing care is given around the clock. It is in the 24-hour nursing record that the patient's status and progress are most accurately reflected (box, p. 184).

# NURSES' NOTES

| Time | T | P | R | BP | Urine | BM | Medication/ treatment | Fluids/ nourishment | Comments |
|------|---|---|---|----|-------|-----|---------------------|--------------------|----------|
| 1030 | $99^2$ | 100 | 20 | $108/70$ | 300 cc | | MS gr 1/6 rt deltoid — J. Ihll, R.N. | Fruit juice 100cc | Patient c/o severe pain in left leg given for relief of pain (see medica- |
| 1035 | | | | | | | | | tion). Pain relieved, patient dozing. Lab report shows Hgb 9gm; Dr. Nash notified. V. Parks, R.N. |
| 1115 | | | | | | | | | Patient assisted to sit on side of bed; became dizzy and fatigued after 5 min. B. Jones, N.A. |
| 1200 | | | | | | | | Surgical liquid diet | Returned to supine position, c/o mild nausea. B. Jones, N.A. |
| 1230 | | | | | | | Whole blood 500cc | | Started IV in right arm by B. Nair, R.N. |
| 1300 | $101^4$ | 108 | 20 | $100/65$ | | | | | Patient lethargic, less alert than this AM; Dr. Nash notified of elevated temperature, dry skin, nausea. |
| 1400 | | | | | | | | | Patient complains that cast feels very tight and foot feels numb. Toes are cool and pale; poor capillary filling. Dr. Nash notified. A. Kerr, R.N. |
| 1405 | | | | | | | | | Cast saw at bedside. Dr. Nash on his way. |
| 1410 | | | | | | | | | Cast bivalved. Leg elevated. Skin color improved. Pain less. A. Kerr, R.N. |

Currently nursing documentation is in a nationwide flux, with many institutions altering their concepts of the traditional nurses' notes. Many hospitals are using integrated notes wherein nurses and therapists record pertinent information on the progress notes. Thus the information that the physician should know is placed where it is difficult to ignore. It also allows members of each discipline to compare their findings with those of other members of the health team.

Regardless of the form used, the 24-hour record should reflect the patient's status, progress or lack of it, and any signs or symptoms that indicate possible impending complications. It will also show routine care and that specific orders are being carried out.

I feel that as much information as possible should be included on one page so that trends, reactions to treatments or medications, complaints, and signs of progress or deterioration are all together so that cause and effect can be recognized (for example, lethargy, confusion, nervousness, or nausea caused by medication, drop in patient's blood pressure when the head of the bed was raised).

A whole generation of nurses has used separate sheets to record vital signs, medications, fluid balance, and so on. I do not suggest abandoning the use of graphs and such, because they do show trends, and trends are more important than single findings. I would, however, like to see nurse's notes that show medications, treatments, intravenous fluids, and transfusions, on the same page with bedside observations by aides regarding appearance, reaction to position change or activity, and so on. It is unrealistic to expect an aide to correlate dyspnea in a certain position with a possible intrathoracic injury, and if the nurse charts only on the intravenous and medication sheets, the problem will still go unrecognized.

During the acute phase of intensive care or until fluids and electrolytes are balanced after trauma or surgery, an acute care form (box, pp. 186-187) can be very useful as a reminder to check everything and as a format for organizing the information to facilitate evaluation. All the necessary information is recorded on one page, including medication, dose, and route as well as site of intramuscular injections to ensure that they are rotated. Each page covers 8 hours (the form can be adjusted for nurses who work a 10-hour, 4-day week) which prevents nurses from failing to chart information for a full shift, since the empty space will attract attention. If primary nursing is practiced, one nurse signs the sheet for the entire shift; if not, a column can be added for individual nurses' initials.

Without proper monitoring and charting, tragedies can occur, as in the following example.

A mother brought in a happy, healthy little boy but complained that he was sometimes irritable and had fallen a couple of times and that his right eye had a tendency to cross (his mother had the same eye problem). The attending physician, who was not Board certified, decided to do a craniotomy. Postoperatively there was no attempt by the physicians or the nurses to monitor the child's intake and output, weight, or sodium level. He developed intracranial edema and convulsions and was taken back to surgery, where the only finding was cerebral edema. He continued to deteriorate. Finally a pediatrician was called, who rapidly brought the fluid overload under control, but not before the child developed permanent brain damage. When the chart was examined it was found that there were days when two of the three shifts did not chart intake except to note the time when intravenous fluid was started, and there was no output record at all. On one day the output from 7 to 3 o'clock was charted as 20 ml — from a child who had obvious symptoms of fluid overload! The court found in favor of the plaintiff. The hospital's liability was the result of *"a cavalier attitude of the nurses toward proper monitoring and charting."*

## Orthopedic nursing

An orthopedic nurse must be able to recognize and care for any medical or surgical problems the patient may have in addition to the orthopedic injury. Such unrelated systemic problems can be life threatening (for example, diabetes is often out of control following an injury). In addition to basic skills, the orthopedic nurse must be adept at providing good care to patients who are encased in a plaster cast, suspended in traction, or confined in a brace. The nurse must understand the equipment and what it is expected to do, be able to see that it functions as it should, and be able to recognize impending complications caused by the equipment. This means that documentation on the orthopedic nursing service is more complicated than on most other services. In addition, accidental injuries are often followed by lawsuits, and the nurse's documentation comes under more scrutiny. In many cases of bodily injury it is only necessary to establish the type and severity of the injury. However, in some cases there may be end results caused by less than optimum care, resulting in malpractice or negligence suits. These cases involve iatrogenic injuries caused by either a specific action or by failure to take proper action; for example:

1. Dislocation of a hip prosthesis by careless handling, resulting in adduction of the hip
2. Failure to recognize signs and symptoms of ischemia or nerve pressure with resultant

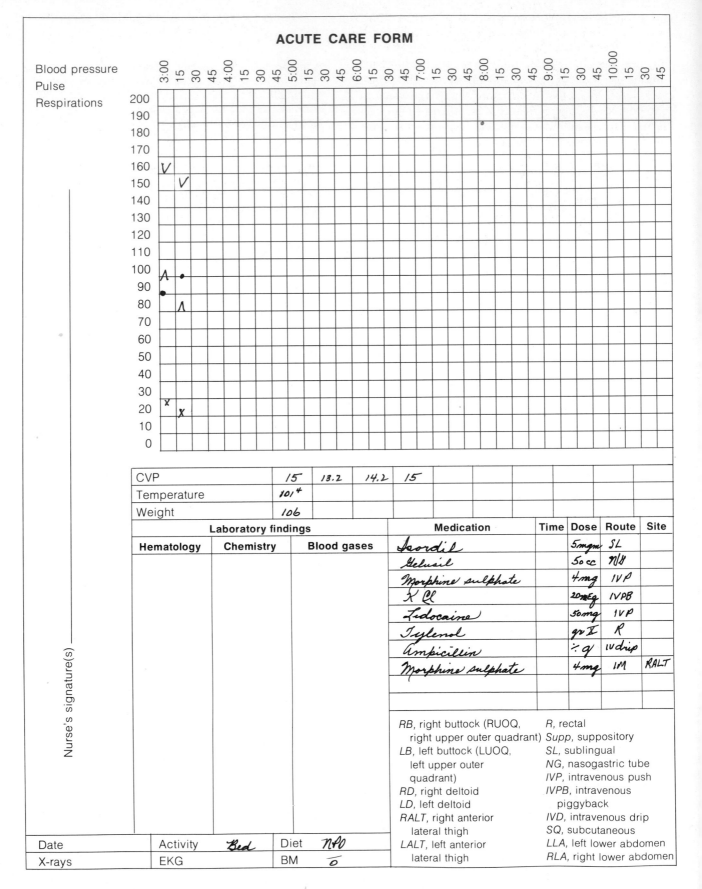

**ACUTE CARE FORM**

Blood pressure
Pulse
Respirations

| | 3:00 | 15 | 30 | 45 | 4:00 | 15 | 30 | 45 | 5:00 | 15 | 30 | 45 | 6:00 | 15 | 30 | 45 | 7:00 | 15 | 30 | 45 | 8:00 | 15 | 30 | 45 | 9:00 | 15 | 30 | 45 | 10:00 | 15 | 30 | 45 |
|---|---|---|---|---|---|---|---|---|---|---|---|---|---|---|---|---|---|---|---|---|---|---|---|---|---|---|---|---|---|---|---|---|

200 / 190 / 180 / 170 / 160 V / 150 V / 140 / 130 / 120 / 110 / 100 A / 90 / 80 A / 70 / 60 / 50 / 40 / 30 / 20 X / 10 / 0

| CVP | | | | 15 | 13.2 | 14.2 | 15 | | | | | | | | |
| Temperature | | | | 101⁺ | | | | | | | | | | | |
| Weight | | | | 106 | | | | | | | | | | | |

| Laboratory findings | | | Medication | Time | Dose | Route | Site |
|---|---|---|---|---|---|---|---|
| **Hematology** | **Chemistry** | **Blood gases** | | | | | |
| | | | Isordil | | 5 mgm | SL | |
| | | | Gelusil | | 50 cc | NG | |
| | | | Morphine sulphate | | 4 mg | IVP | |
| | | | K Cl | | 20 mEq | IVPB | |
| | | | Lidocaine | | 50 mg | IVP | |
| | | | Tylenol | | gr X | R | |
| | | | Ampicillin | | ÷ q / | IV drip | |
| | | | Morphine sulphate | | 4 mg | IM | RALT |

Nurse's signature(s)

RB, right buttock (RUOQ, right upper outer quadrant)
LB, left buttock (LUOQ, left upper outer quadrant)
RD, right deltoid
LD, left deltoid
RALT, right anterior lateral thigh
LALT, left anterior lateral thigh

R, rectal
Supp, suppository
SL, sublingual
NG, nasogastric tube
IVP, intravenous push
IVPB, intravenous piggyback
IVD, intravenous drip
SQ, subcutaneous
LLA, left lower abdomen
RLA, right lower abdomen

| Date | | Activity | Bed | Diet | NPO |
|---|---|---|---|---|---|
| X-rays | | EKG | | BM | 0 |

# ACUTE CARE FORM—cont'd

### Intravenous fluids/transfusions

| Hour | Solution/medication/route/amount/rate |
|------|----------------------------------------|
| 1500 | 800/1000   D5W c̄ 100 mg Nipride LA 50 ml/hr |
|      | 950/1000   R/L   CVP 50cc/hr |
|      | |
|      | |
|      | |
|      | |
|      | |
|      | |
|      | |

### Oral intake

| | |
|------|----------------------------------------|
| 1630 | Gelusil 30cc c̄ NS 20cc N/G |
|      | |
|      | |
|      | |
|      | |
|      | |
|      | |
|      | |
|      | |
|      | |
|      | |
|      | |

### Output

| | GI tube | Drains | Blood loss | Urine (catheter) | Urine (voided) | Vomitus |
|---|---------|--------|------------|------------------|----------------|---------|
| | | | | | | |
| | | | | | | |
| | | | | | | |
| | | | | | | |
| | | | | | | |
| | | | | | | |
| | | | | | | |
| | | | | | | |
| 8-hour total | | | | | | |

See separate neurologic
and vascular sheets

### Comments

permanent disability from ischemic contracture or nerve damage

3. Failure to recognize and correct excessive pressure from a cast or brace or from the part resting on the bed
4. Failure to maintain traction in proper alignment and at a constant force (e.g., too much distraction force can cause joint separation and nonunion, whereas too little force can allow overriding and further soft-tissue damage)
5. Failure to recognize and treat thromboembolic complications
6. Failure to recognize and treat acid-base imbalance or the common problem of fluid overload with dilutional hyponatremia

Nurses' notes should show any positive findings, that the physician has been alerted, and that treatment was initiated. All notations on a medical record should provide needed information regarding the patient, his condition, and his progress or failure to progress. This information can be used by the entire health team on a day-to-day basis to evaluate the patient's needs and improve his care. This same information will be useful if and when the record is ever reviewed for possible legal action.

### Case review

Reviewing a record to determine the extent and severity of an accidental injury should be a simple, straightforward task. However, at times it becomes a frustrating and time-consuming chore because the record lacks necessary information. This may mean that the patient will have to sue to collect from an insurance company even though his claim is legitimate. For example:

A 16-year-old girl had a crush injury to her elbow. She was seen in one emergency room, then sent to another hospital where her family physician was on staff. She was seen in the second emergency room and admitted. Unbelievably, there were no specific descriptions of the area involved, the status of circulation below the injury, or the severity of the crushing effect in either emergency room or on the physical examination. The arm was encased in a massive wet dressing, and the charting was so sketchy that it could not be determined whether that dressing was ever removed or replaced. After 3 months of what appeared to be bumbling care, a plastic surgeon was called in. His was the first recorded description of the appearance of the injured arm! Incidentally, the nurses' notes frequently showed "Arm better," but since the patient went home with a flail arm and the appearance of the arm had not been recorded, one wonders by what criteria the arm was "better." It was interesting that the accident that caused the injury was described in two places, but *the injury was not described!*

Reviewing the record prior to the filing of a malpractice suit is more complex, but the advantage to the reviewer is that he is aware of the consequences and usually has a definite idea of what caused the bad result. It is often possible to pinpoint the act or failure to act from the patient's statement. Therefore the record is reviewed to look for specifics.

Too often nurses' notes offer information about routine care but very little information about the patient. For example, countless charts have notations such as "Complained of pain; medication given as ordered" or "Complained of pain; explained that it was too early for another pain shot." There is no indication where or of what type the pain was, whether the last injection had completely relieved the pain, or any other pertinent information.

The record is expected to give the answers to a number of questions such as:

1. What were the patient's problems when he arrived?
2. What treatment was given?
3. Was the treatment appropriate?
4. What was the reaction to treatment?
5. If there were signs or symptoms of complications, what was done?
6. Does the record show the day-to-day status, or are there notes such as "A little more alert this morning" with no prior notes that the patient had ever been less than alert.
7. Are there notes that the patient is "better" or "worse" without details regarding prior or present condition?
8. Are there physician's orders that say in effect, "Please give oral hygiene," "Please turn the patient," "Please offer oral fluids (or food) and help as needed"? These orders for what should be routine nursing care indicate that the physician is pleading for (or demanding) better nursing care.

In order for the record to answer the reviewer's questions the nurse must understand, among other things:

1. The existing orthopedic problem (injury or disease).
2. The proposed treatment (casts, traction, braces) and how to assist in providing it.
3. What the treatment is expected to accomplish (reduction of fracture, alleviation of pain, relief of muscle spasm).
4. The location, severity, type, and duration of pain to be expected.
   a. Progressively severe, unrelieved, burning pain after a fracture has been immobilized is a sign of impending (or existing) circula-

tory disaster. Immediate release of pressure is mandatory.

b. Pain in an area other than the area of the initial injury may indicate pressure. If the pressure is not recognized and relieved, cessation of pain may indicate that necrosis has already occurred.

5. The types of complications that can be expected and their early warning signs.
   a. Infection secondary to compound fractures.
   b. Decubiti secondary to prolonged immobilization.
   c. Crush syndrome.
   d. Electrolyte imbalance.
6. The problems presented by the patient's age, physical condition, and medical problems.
7. The necessity for *immediate* investigation of untoward signs or symptoms so that remedial action can be taken before the condition is irreversible.

Common errors in orthopedic care include:

1. Failure to investigate the cause of pain before giving medication. Because relief of pain (diminution of sensation) can mask important symptoms, recognition of a problem may be delayed until the condition is irreversible. Questions that should be asked and information that should appear on the record include:
   a. Where is the pain? Is it at the fracture site? Distal to the fracture site? Over a bony prominence?
   b. What kind of pain is it? Burning? Stabbing? Intermittent? Unremitting?
   c. Has medication relieved it completely? Partially?
   d. Does anything make the pain worse?
   e. Does the patient complain of abnormal sensations (paresthesias)? What areas are involved?
   f. Is sensory perception diminished? Check by pinprick or pinch because patients are often unaware of numbness. What areas are involved?
   g. Is there swelling? How severe? Has it increased since the patient was last seen? If the limb is elevated, has elevation decreased the swelling?
2. Failure to care for the whole patient. For example, patients with peripheral vascular disease cannot tolerate routine prolonged elevation of a limb.
3. Failure to recognize and report early signs of complications such as thromboembolic problems, pulmonary problems, acid-base imbalance, infections (soft tissue, bone), and ischemia.
4. Careless handling of patients with spinal injuries or extremity fractures with resultant damage.
5. Failure to recognize injuries not listed on the initial diagnosis. Some of these may be less obvious but more life threatening than the injury being treated.
6. Conclusions based on emotional reactions to the patient rather than on findings. For example, the "bratty" teenager who screams obscenities, lashes out with physical attacks on those who attempt to care for him, and is generally "resistive and combative" may make the staff react negatively. They may think he is a spoiled brat or a drug user or a number of other things and treat him accordingly. He may be restrained, which makes his behavior even more wild. He may be given sedatives or tranquilizers, often without beneficial results and perhaps with detrimental results because the real problem is an undiagnosed head injury.

The record should show (1) that you know what the potential dangers are, (2) that you know what the early warning signs and symptoms are, (3) that you actively assess the patient's condition with specific reference points in mind each time you see him, and (4) that you know what to do in a problem situation. For example, a night nurse makes rounds at midnight and finds a patient in a new leg cast in pain. He states, "The last two pain shots didn't do any good, and the pain keeps getting worse." Charting need not be lengthy but should be specific:

Patient complains of increasing burning pain unrelieved by the last two pain shots. He states the pain is getting worse. His toes are cool and pale. There is no active motion. Pain is increased by passive motion. Dr. Kay notified. Cast bivalved and padding cut to skin full length. Some relief of pain since pressure relieved. Dr. Kay will see the patient in 30 to 45 min to evaluate possible need for fasciotomy.

Such charting indicates that the nurse was alert for signs of compartment syndrome and recognized symptoms that had not been recognized by the nurses who gave the previous medications. The physician was notified and will check the patient, and the pressure was relieved. These few lines of charting will protect that particular nurse legally because they show excellent care.

Sometimes a nurse recognizes and reports signs

of trouble that the physician chooses to ignore. For example, the order for fluids may not be appropriate for the size and condition of the patient. Or the patient may have sacral edema, massive urinary output, massive drainage from a wound or from a Levine tube, copious secretions in the respiratory tract, or symptoms of cerebral edema. The chart may show:

Dr. Blank notified that patient has put out 600 ml/hr for 2 hours, his tracheotomy needs frequent suctioning, his wound has copious drainage, he is restless and confused. Doctor is not concerned; advised to continue with present orders.

At this point the nurse is faced with a real dilemma. A very real danger was recognized and reported, but the danger of the situation was not recognized by the physician. What should the nurse do now? If the physician is an intern, probably the next step is to call the resident. If the physician is the patient's private physician, the nurse should report the problem to the Supervisor or to nursing administration. In these days when hospitals and nurses can be sued for failure to act on behalf of the patient, hospital administrations are much more aware of possible legal responsibilities. If the report to the hospital is made in writing, the nurse should keep a carbon copy for her own protection. It is essential that the nurse chart that such reports were made because the physician may deny being told about the patient's condition. If possible another nurse should also chart that the physician was notified. The chart should also document all findings, both positive and negative, in detail at frequent intervals.

When something goes wrong, chart it. Record all the details while they are fresh in your mind. Legal action may be taken a year or even several years after the incident. Even if you feel that the details are burned into your mind, no jury will accept your description without corroboration by written evidence in the medical record.

Do *not* omit documentation of the incident in an effort to cover up something you have done. For example, if you move a patient in a way that causes injury, chart it. Ordinarily it takes very little effort on the part of an investigator to show that the patient did not have the injury before a specific time and did have the injury after that time. Often the patient knows who caused the injury. If you have failed to chart it, the jury may feel that you knew you were guilty and were trying to avoid responsibility for your act. A jury may be able to understand accidental injury to a patient when you immediately take steps to rectify the problem. They will have little or no sympathy for coverup attempts.

## MULTIDISCIPLINARY DOCUMENTATION

Within the specialty of orthopedics and rehabilitation there is, both by desire and necessity, a need for a multidisciplinary approach to patient care. This approach should be reflected when appropriate in the documentation. If the findings of both the therapists and the nurses are recorded together, any differences will be obvious. It can then be determined whether those differences are actual or if the criteria for evaluation are different. Terms such as "good," "fair," or "moderate amount" have real meaning *only* to the person doing the evaluation and therefore should be avoided in favor of more specific terms.

A multidisciplinary form establishes the patient's initial status (baseline) and shows any changes. These are rarely found in the usual nurses' notes. Obviously this type of form should not be the only charting of patients. There should be notes showing how speech or comprehension or pain level or ability to move has changed.

If activities are being evaluated by physical or occupational therapists as well as by nurses, a double column can be incorporated on the form so that the evaluations can be compared. We all know that the partially paralyzed patient may be able to dress himself in 10 minutes in therapy yet may not be able to do nearly so well in his room, perhaps because he is wakened early after being sedated the night before or because he is tired or upset. Therapists often stay with the patient while he performs, which exerts some pressure. Nurses usually do not have time to stay with the patient, thus there is less pressure and fewer helpful suggestions. Some patients exert great effort during therapy sessions, then have little energy left for performance later. Too often all of these things are not taken into consideration.

The need for 24-hour flow sheets to monitor the specific needs of the patient with an orthopedic injury, disease, or surgery is continuous and multiple in nature. A neurovascular assessment sheet that fulfills these needs is given in Chapter 24. A neurological assessment sheet is shown on p. 191. In many cases it would be advantageous if these forms were combined for the orthopedic patient.

The monitoring of position changes and activity is a necessary part of documentation for the orthopedic patient. This may be accomplished in the nurses' notes, treatment sheet, or all-purpose flow sheet. Bedside flow sheets are useful in circumstances when continuous references or documentation is desired. If these sheets are used for documentation, they should become a part of the permanent record.

## NEUROLOGIC ASSESSMENT SHEET

Patient information

| Time | Right pupil | Left pupil | State of consciousness | Grip L | Grip R | Arm movement L | Arm movement R | Leg movement L | Leg movement R | Remarks |
|------|-------------|------------|------------------------|--------|--------|----------------|----------------|----------------|----------------|---------|
| 1100 | D/NR | N/R | 1+ | ✍ | ✍ | ✍ | ✍ | ✍ | ✍ | |
| | | | | | | | | | | |
| | | | | | | | | | | |
| | | | | | | | | | | |
| | | | | | | | | | | |
| | | | | | | | | | | |
| | | | | | | | | | | |
| | | | | | | | | | | |
| | | | | | | | | | | |
| | | | | | | | | | | |
| | | | | | | | | | | |
| | | | | | | | | | | |
| | | | | | | | | | | |
| | | | | | | | | | | |

### Code

**Pupils**
= equal
N normal
D dilated
C constricted
R reaction
NR no reaction
L light
A accommodation

**State of consciousness**
0 or 0     comatose
1 + (+)     unconscious, responds to painful stimuli
2 + (++)     responds to name
3 + (+++)     groggy, lethargic
4 + (++++)     awake but confused
5 + (+++++)     alert and oriented

**Grip**
R right
L left
S strong
F fair
W weak

**Movement**
R right
L left
V voluntary
I involuntary
A absent
S spastic
H hypotonic

## 192 Anatomy and physiology

Nurses' notes should be set up in a form that presents the information so that it is easy for the medical staff, the nursing staff, and other disciplines to locate significant findings and discover trends so that patient care can be adjusted. If the record is obscure or difficult to read, the information will not be useful.

## LABORATORY DATA DOCUMENTATION

A laboratory summary form (box, below) can be an essential part of care if it is the only way to show trends, but it takes time. Usually a nurse or ward clerk must be assigned to complete this form from the laboratory slips as they arrive on the floor. When mounted, laboratory reports should offer

**LABORATORY SUMMARY SHEET**

**Patient information**

| | 3/1 | 3/2 | 3/3 | 3/4 | 3/5 0800 | 3/5 1600 | 3/5 2400 |
|---|---|---|---|---|---|---|---|
| Hemoglobin/hematocrit | 42 | | 15.2 / 45 | | | | |
| WBC/polys | 16,000 | | 16,800 | | | | |
| Platelets/reticuloendothelium | | | 1.5 | | | | |
| BUN/creatinine | 13 | 19 | 28 | 1.8 | | | |
| Na/K | | | 142 / 50 | 139 / 46 | | | |
| Cl/CO$_2$ | | | 99 / 27 | 98 / 32 | | | |
| Glucose/uric acid | | 85 / 5.9 | 100 / 8.0 | 85 / 6.5 | | | |
| Total protein/albumin | | 6.8 / 4.6 | 6.8 / 4.2 | | | | |
| Ca/PO$_4$/alkyline phosphatase | | 9.5 3.0 64 | 9.0 3.1 90 | 8.9 3.4 90 | | | |
| LDH/SGOT | | 139 / 19 | 130 / 62 | | | | |
| SGPT/T bilirubin | | 1.0 | | | | | |
| D. bilirubin/HAA | | | | | | | |
| FANA/LE prep | | | | | | | |
| Complement | | | | | | | |
| ASO titer | | | | | | | |
| Creatinine clearance | | | | | | | |
| Urine vol/24 hr, urine protein | | | | | | | |
| Sediment, urine | PH 5 RBC | | pH 5 1+ protein | pH 5 | | | |
| Culture, urine | 2+ Bact No casts | | RBC 4+ | | | | |
| Drugs | | | | | | | |

immediate visual comparisons of findings. Medically and economically it is a waste of time to have to make separate summaries, but having all the information where it can be seen readily can be lifesaving. Some laboratories send slips with bright-colored stickers attached to identify abnormal findings. This is extremely helpful, but all reports should be reviewed; someone might fail to use a sticker.

## INTERFACILITY TRANSFER DOCUMENTATION

Interfacility transfer forms (particularly to extended care units) should be filled out carefully and with the knowledge that what you say may do the patient great damage. For example, if it says on the transfer sheet that the patient does not get out of bed or does not feed himself (indicating lack of motivation or effort rather than actual disability), those who care for the patient in the new unit may decide not to bother to help a patient who does not try. In the case of an elderly patient who is left to deteriorate in bed, that interfacility transfer note can be his death warrant. The following scoring system for activities of daily living is recommended to facilitate transfer information:

**dependent** needs complete assistance; unable to perform any part of the task alone.

**assistance** can perform part of the task but must have help.

**supervision** can perform the task but must be instructed, encouraged, and observed during performance.

**difficult** may need mechanical aids, tolerance may be low, may be slow and inefficient, *but* can perform without supervision or assistance.

**independent** may need mechanical aids but can perform at near normal speed with good endurance.

Make comments as positive as possible regarding the patient's cooperation, motivation, and so on. Keep in mind that patients often fear being transferred and having strangers care for them. They feel helpless. Try to give an impression to the new team that here is a person worthy of their best efforts. If the patient feels that the new health care personnel are friendly and concerned, he will work harder to improve.

## DISCHARGE DOCUMENTATION

Discharge documentation involves all health care personnel. Discharge summaries provided by the physician or nurse provide the reader with an overview of the patient's hospitalization. Discharge summary forms vary but should include instructions that were given verbally and should also state that written instructions were given to the patient.

These instructions include:

1. What the patient can and cannot do
2. How to recognize problems that merit the attention of the physician
3. Cast instructions
4. Wound care
5. Ace bandage or elastic stocking instruction
6. Explanation that no weight bearing means placing the involved foot flat on the floor to maintain balance but not supporting the weight of the body on it, not trying to hold the foot 12 inches off the floor and so on.
7. Instructions to look for specific problems, and if they occur to call or come in to be checked

This information is necessary to facilitate follow-up care and to legally protect all health care personnel should postdischarge complications occur.

## SUMMARY

The whole of the record should be greater than the sum of its parts. All information from all sources should be combined to facilitate diagnosis, treatment, and constant reassessment.

The findings should be organized and presented in a manner that makes it easy for all disciplines to find and use the information in order to plan and proceed with the best possible patient care.

Unfortunately some people have advocated that charting should be done with legal accountability and liability in mind. This is neither necessary nor desirable. I firmly believe that we are in the business of *good patient care* and that the best defense in court is evidence of good patient care. If records appear as though written with court action in mind, that fact will be evident and will certainly destroy the credibility of the records. *Only* if something occurs that may well be the basis of future legal action should details be charted for use in court. For example, if a patient is handled in such a manner that a hip prosthesis is dislocated and further surgery is necessary, the record should show how and why this occurred. If patient care is good and that care is reflected in the record, concern for the *patient* will protect the nurse.

### EDITORS' NOTE

The problem-oriented record system (PORS) and similar problem-oriented medical records are not incorporated in this edition. The components of these systems are still in the formulative stages in institutions throughout the United States. Their absence here does not reflect a lack of acceptance or importance but an acknowledgement that these systems are not yet standardized to a degree that permits universal acceptance of methods and principles of implementation.

# PART THREE

# Diagnostic tools

# 9

# Radiography

NANCY E. HILT

Of all the diagnostic tools available to the specialty of orthopedics, none is utilized so frequently as the radiographic examination. The skeletal system, with its connective tissue, lends itself well to this tool because of the normal density of osseous tissue. Radiographic examination, despite its frequent use, should always be an adjunct to the clinical history and physical examination and never a substitute. This assures maximum effectiveness of this tool in providing an accurate diagnosis.

Depending on their responsibilities, various health care personnel are involved to different degrees in the radiographic process. The assumption that the physician is the *only* one involved in the process is erroneous. Generally the physician prescribes the examination, and the radiologist interprets the results. The nurse may be involved in several aspects of the process and, in addition to understanding the general principles of radiography and the musculoskeletal system, should be familiar with the following:

1. Appropriate terminology to accurately transmit or transfer the physician's written order to the form that must ultimately be interpreted by personnel in the radiology department.
2. Required patient history that must be relayed to the radiologist to assist in accurate interpretation. (This is usually accomplished on the appropriate request form and may in some cases be the responsibility of the physician.)
3. Positioning required during the exposure to assure that patient function will permit the accomplishment of the procedure, either independently or dependently, and communication of these judgments to radiology personnel.

In addition radiology technologists are involved in the actual process and procedure of accomplishing the radiographic examination and must therefore be able to accurately position and immobilize the patient to assure that quality films are obtained.

## PRINCIPLES OF RADIOGRAPHIC TECHNIQUES

The principles involved in the production of a radiographic film and the specifics of the equipment involved cannot be outlined within the scope of this chapter. If this information is desired or required, it is suggested that the bibliography provided be consulted as a guide for further exploration. Several principles involving concern for appropriate prescription and implementation of radiographic techniques are discussed in general. Authorities on the topic seem to be in general agreement about most of these principles.

The following principles relate to the potential radiographic hazards and resulting complications of *bone necrosis, cancer, damage to gonads*, and *damage to the hematopoietic system*[2;4,p.34;5,p.11]:

1. Complications of radiographic exposure are related more to high dosages of radiotherapy than to utilization for diagnostic purposes.
2. The greatest concern within the diagnostic range is that of genetic change.
3. The above-outlined principles do not negate the necessity for standard preventive and protective measures during exposure; it is probably because of these measures that hazard incidence is not increased.

**Table 9-1.** Principles of obtaining quality radiographic diagnostic films[6,pp.206-207]

| Quality component | Assurance measures |
| --- | --- |
| Adequate detail | Adequate immobilization of area to avoid blurring |
| | Film positioned as close to area as possible |
| | Focal spot of radiographic tube not too large |
| Adequate contrast | Complete and full development of film |
| | Limitation of beam area |
| | Avoidance of excessive filtration |
| Adequate and standard positioning | Standard positioning requirements and techniques |
| | Immobilization and no movement during exposure |

4. Avoid repetitious exposure in young patients whenever possible.
5. Avoid repetitious exposure in pregnant women.
6. Shield gonads on other than survey films, especially when serial films are anticipated and the patient is young. Survey films, however, are more useful without gonadal shielding to provide a comprehensive comparison baseline for judgment purposes. In all cases care should be taken not to obstruct the diagnostic area with shielding.
7. Discretion in appropriate utilization of radiographic examination can be the greatest factor in control of radiographic hazards and complications. In certain cases where existing statistical value of the radiographic examination is negative or in question, such as in low back pain in the absence of other pathologic factors, it should be utilized as a diagnostic tool *only* after other conservative measures of treatment for a designated period of time have failed to control pain or other symptoms.

For diagnostic purposes it is essential that the radiographic film provide adequate detail and contrast. Standard positioning must be maintained to assure accuracy in interpretation. The acquisition of these factors may be assured by adherence to the principles outlined in Table 9-1. Review of these factors may assist in location of difficulties if continuous problems arise.

## TYPES OF RADIOGRAPHIC PROCEDURES

Many types of radiography may be used in the diagnosis of musculoskeletal diseases, disorders, and injuries. Three basic views are utilized for plain or ordinary radiographic examinations:

**anteroposterior view** accomplished with x-ray tube vertical to body when prone or supine (most often supine).
**lateral view** accomplished with x-ray tube vertical to body when side-lying or standing.
**oblique view** accomplished with x-ray tube tilted at designated angle to body in specified position; utilized for special views.

Despite the effectiveness of these basic views, special radiographic techniques have been designed to assist in the visualization of particular areas of the body and tissues not readily visualized by ordinary films and these basic views. The following are the types most frequently utilized[1-3]:

**arteriography** radiographic visualization of arterial structures by injection of radiopaque dye.
**arthrography** radiographic visualization of joint by injection of radiopaque dye or air.
**cineradiography (videoradiography)** radiographic visualization of joint movement by utilization of movie camera or videotape recorder.
**contrast radiography** radiographic visualization of tissue spaces or cavities by injection of radiopaque dye (e.g., arteriography, arthrography, myelography).
**myelography** radiographic visualization of spinal cord and canal by injection of radiopaque dye into subarachnoid space.
**radiographic magnification** radiographic visualization of small areas through magnification by use of small x-ray tube with small focal spot.
**scanography** accurate measurement of bone lengths.
**stereoscopy** three-dimensional radiographic visualization of superimposed structures.
**tomography (laminography)** radiographic visualization of specific layer of tissue or bone by utilization of technique that blurs those layers above and below focal layer.

Utilization of these radiographic procedures for diagnostic purposes is greatly dependent on relative factors such as the patient's specific history, signs and symptoms (especially severity and duration), degree to which the patient is incapacitated by the disease or deformity, and the patient's response to treatment alternatives. In some cases the specific purpose of and indication for a special radiographic procedure is to attempt to monitor a selected treatment or to establish the status of a complication. Additional information regarding these procedures and their specific application to orthopedics, along with potential complications, is given in Table 9-2. As might be expected, those procedures involving the injection of radiopaque dye or air carry risk of complications.

**Table 9-2.** Special radiographic procedures utilized in orthopedics

| Procedure | Focus | Dye | Air | Orthopedic indications | Potential complications | Comments |
|---|---|---|---|---|---|---|
| Arteriography* | Arterial structures | Yes | No | Bone tumors, soft-tissue tumors: assists in visualization of vessels to and into lesion<br>Traumatic injuries: assists in assessment and management through visualization of disruption of vessels | Reaction to contrast media<br>Infection<br>Hemorrhage<br>Thrombosis of vessels | |
| Arthrography* | Joint structures | Yes | Yes | Hip, shoulder, knee: diagnostic<br>Congenital dislocation of hip: verify positional osseous or soft-tissue damage<br>Soft-tissue injuries surrounding knee | Reaction to contrast media (rare)<br>Infection | Outline of soft-tissue structures of joint not usually visualized on ordinary x-ray film |
| Cineradiography, videoradiography with or without fluoroscopy | Joint motion | No | No | Patterns of joint motion (especially spinal column) | None | May be stored for later comparative purposes<br>Currently many radiologists are using fluoroscopy with video recording for lower doses |
| Myelography* | Spinal cord and column | Yes | No | Questionable pressure on spinal cord or nerve root from lesion or deformity<br>Herniated intervertebral disc | Headache<br>Reaction to contrast media<br>Infection<br>Arachnoiditis | |
| Radiographic magnification | Small area such as bones of feet or hands | No | No | To study trabecular pattern<br>Fine detail of calcification, periosteal new bone, and destruction<br>Subtle fractures<br>Joint diseases | Essentially none | May be combined with tomography |
| Radionuclide imaging (bone scan) | Entire skeleton | No | No | Early detection of infection, ischemia, tumors | Essentially none | Uses radioactive isotopes |
| Scanography | Long bones, usually lower extremities | No | No | Leg length inequality | Essentially none | |
| Stereoscopy | Superimposed structures | No | No | Diagnostic in areas of superimposed structures such as skull, shoulder, spine, and pelvis | Essentially none | Three-dimensional perspective |
| Tomography (laminography) | Predetermined layer of tissue or bone | No | No | Small cavities or areas<br>Possible foreign body or locations of known foreign body<br>Confirmation of union or malunion of bone graft, especially spine<br>Possible lesion or known lesion overshadowed by other structures<br>Abnormalities of joint and spine<br>Lesions within cortex or medullary cavity | Essentially none | |

*Contrast radiography includes these procedures, as well as venography and sinography, and is a collective term used for procedures using a contrast media to clearly define and outline limits of cavities or tissue spaces.

**Table 9-3.** Preparation and postprocedural care

| Procedure | Preparation | Postprocedural care |
|---|---|---|
| Arteriography | Sedation<br>Anesthesia for infants and children<br>NPO 6-8 hours prior to procedure<br>Patient education | Strict bed rest until next morning<br>Check and record:<br>  Groin or axilla for hematoma<br>  Complaints of numbness or tingling<br>  Motion of involved extremity<br>  Arterial pulses (dorsalis pedis or posterior tibial area if femoral; radial or ulnar if axillary) every 15 minutes × 4, every 30 minutes × 2, every hour × 4, every 4 hours × 4<br>  Blood pressures (same schedule as pulses)<br>Call physician if any change |
| Arthrography | Sedation for uncooperative patient<br>Anesthesia for infants and young children<br>Patient education | No strenuous exercise for 3-4 hours<br>Notify physician of any signs of infection |
| Cineradiography-videoradiography with or without fluoroscopy | Patient education | None |
| Myelography | Possible sedation<br>Anesthesia for infants and children<br>NPO 6-8 hours prior to procedure<br>Patient education | Flat in bed for 24 hours<br>Force fluids<br>Check and record:<br>  Temperature<br>  Pulse<br>  Respirations<br>  Blood pressure<br>  Grips upon return to unit, every 30 minutes × 3, every hour × 4, every 4 hours until stable<br>Call physician if any change |
| Radiographic magnification | Patient education | None |
| Scanography | Patient education | None |
| Stereoscopy | Patient education | None |
| Tomography | Patient education | None |

NOTE: Although these general guidelines are provided for review, it is suggested that each individual become familiar with the specific routines of their facility.

## PREPARATION AND POSTPROCEDURAL CARE IN RADIOGRAPHIC PROCEDURES

Some special radiographic procedures are more complicated than others. The degree to which preparation is required or postprocedural care is designated varies slightly from one hospital to another. Typical considerations are outlined in Table 9-3 and are felt to be relatively consistent in principle despite institutional variances. For the most part, only those procedures involving the injection of dye or air require preparation or postprocedural care. All patients should receive an explanation of the procedure.

## REQUESTS FOR RADIOGRAPHIC EXAMINATION

A radiographic examination is ordered for one of the following reasons:

1. To assist in the assessment and evaluation that will ultimately lead to definitive diagnosis of a disease, deformity, infection, or lesion
2. To monitor osseous and related tissue alterations resulting from time or the implementation of therapeutic regimens
3. To identify limitations in function or joint range of motion
4. To assist in the assessment, evaluation, and management of fractures and other traumatic injuries involving the musculoskeletal system

Because the radiographic examination is so important in the diagnosis and management of orthopedic problems, it is essential that it be requested when necessary but always reserved when necessary! The radiographic complications outlined in Table 9-2 reinforce this consideration.

Because of the necessity and frequency of utiliza-

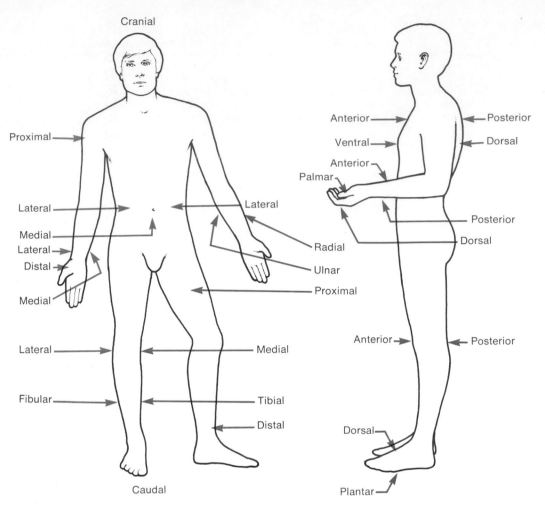

**Fig. 9-1.** Line drawings with standard terminology used in ordering radiographic examinations. Utilization of these terms will assure accuracy and uniformity in interpretation of request. Body planes (Fig. 4-1) may also be used.

tion of this diagnostic tool, maximum benefit and effectiveness should be anticipated. This may only be accomplished, however, if the process of translation and transposition of the physician's order onto the request form, which is sent to the radiology department, is accomplished with accuracy and uniformity of interpretation. It is suggested that the appropriate standard terminology (Fig. 9-1) be utilized by all involved in this process. In addition the following rules or principles are useful in assuring accuracy of interpretation by all levels of personnel as well as the appropriate utilization of this valuable diagnostic tool:

1. The requested radiographic examination should be written completely, utilizing standard terminology, on the physician's order form.
2. Additional instructions should be clear and concise.

3. Transposition from the physician's order form should be exactly as written; it should be assumed that the physician has conveyed in writing the precise and exact films anticipated to assist in diagnosis and management of the orthopedic problem.
4. Nursing personnel, if aware of functional inability that will prevent the patient from assuming or maintaining the position required for the desired view(s), should convey this information to the physician so that alternative views may be considered.
5. If the patient is unable to assume or maintain the required position, a nurse escort should be provided who knows the patient's limitations and who may evaluate and assist with the procedure. It should not be expected that the radiologist or radiology technologist be aware of

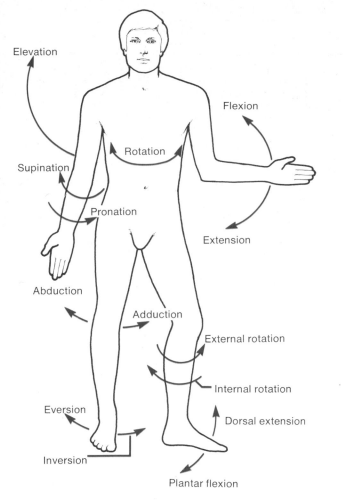

**Fig. 9-1, cont'd.** For legend see opposite page.

all of a patient's possible limitations. Verbal or written communications will sometime suffice, but an escort will assure the least difficulties.

To assure accurate interpretation, all authorities agree on and stress the importance of obtaining a *minimum of two views* (usually anteroposterior and lateral). Errors in judgment may be frequent if this is *not* accomplished. There is controversy, however, regarding the necessity for radiographic examination of the opposite side; some believe it is necessary for comparison, others do not.

## POSITIONING DURING RADIOGRAPHIC EXAMINATION

Proper and standardized positioning for various views during exposure lends credibility to the radiographic examination. Accuracy is necessary to assure both the radiologist and the physician as interpreters that their findings are valid.

All patients should be positioned in the required manner as comfortably as possible. It is recognized that this is not always an easy task, but gentleness in handling the diseased, deformed, or injured part of the body will both ensure the patient's cooperation and reduce the potential complications of mishandling.

To accomplish the x-ray examination, the tube is centered over a predetermined anatomic landmark as standardized by radiographic procedure. The ray direction may be related to the axis of the body or the extremity, depending on the focus of the examination. The central ray is usually directed vertically into the center of the film, but special views may require the tilting of the tube or positioning of the cassette. Special types of views such as stress films or special radiographic procedures may require the presence or assistance of the physician. All films should be labeled appropriately utilizing anatomic nomenclature.

Specific positioning required for the previously outlined radiographic procedures may vary. Specific positioning for plain or ordinary radiographic views may be reviewed in Table 9-4. In addition it is highly recommended that the reader review the referenced source of information for this table. It expands considerably the information provided here and provides radiographic films for each view.

## RADIOGRAPHIC INTERPRETATION

Interpretation of the musculoskeletal radiographic examination is a topic much too broad to cover in depth within this chapter; however, several principles and important factors are reviewed.

The following terminology may be used in reference to radiographic interpretation and is defined to facilitate comprehension:

**decalcification** decreased bone density or undermineralization; may be indicative of bone resorption.
**decreased bone density** radiographic appearance of bone not indicative of specific mechanism or component of bone affected.
**density** radiographic appearance of bone characterized by lightness or darkness of areas of osseous tissue; influenced by age, sex, pathologic determinations, and so on.
**erosion** usually circumscribed area characterized by loss of trabecular pattern of part or full width of the cortex; localized area with loss of bone density.
**osteoporosis** increased translucency of bone indicative of thinning of cortex.
**sclerosis** increased bone density, regardless of cause.
**transradiancy** comparable to radiolucency and is relative to that seen in adjacent bones.

*Text continued on p. 211.*

**Table 9-4.** Positioning for radiographic examination

| Anatomic area of focus | Radiographic view desired | Positioning required |
|---|---|---|
| **Hand and wrist** | | |
| Hand | Dorsopalmar | Palm on cassette |
| | | Wrist joint and fingers extended |
| | | Fingers slightly spread |
| | Lateral | Hand with ulnar side on cassette and strictly lateral |
| | | Wrist and fingers in extension |
| | | Second and fifth fingers overlapping |
| | | Thumb spread toward palm |
| | Oblique | Hand pronated |
| | | Palm against cassette with radial side raised 45° |
| Fingers | Dorsopalmar | Fingers spread |
| | | Palmar surface on cassette |
| | | Fingers extended |
| | Lateral | Fingers separated and/or flexed |
| | | Radial side of designated finger on cassette (second and third) |
| | | Ulnar side of designated finger on cassette (fourth and fifth) |
| Thumb | Dorsopalmar | Hand pronated |
| | | Back of thumb on hand |
| | Lateral | Radial side of thumb on cassette |
| | | Palm toward cassette |
| | | Ulnar side of hand raised sufficiently to make thumb lie exactly lateral |
| Metacarpals | Dorsopalmar | Palm on cassette |
| | Oblique | Hand pronated |
| | | Radial side raised 45° |
| | Fifth metacarpal oblique | Hand supinated |
| | | Ulnar side of fifth metacarpal on cassette |
| | | Back of hand inclined 45° toward cassette |
| Carpus | Dorsopalmar | Hand pronated |
| | | Carpus on cassette |
| | Lateral | Ulnar side of carpus on cassette |
| | | Wrist and fingers extended |
| Scaphoid (navicular) | Dorsopalmar | Hand pronated |
| | | Carpus on cassette |
| | | Fingers slightly flexed (loose fist) |
| | | Thumb gently spread |
| | | Hand held toward palmar side |
| | Lateral | Ulnar side of carpus on cassette |
| | | Hand slightly dorsiflexed |
| | | Loose fist |
| | Oblique radial | Hand pronated |
| | | Hand held toward ulnar side |
| | | Loose fist |
| | | Carpus on cassette |
| | | *Radial* side raised 45° |
| | Oblique ulnar | Hand pronated |
| | | Hand held toward ulnar side |
| | | Loose fist |
| | | Carpus on cassette |
| | | *Ulnar* side raised 45° |
| Pisiform | Pisiform | Hand supinated |
| | | Carpus on cassette |
| | | Radial side raised 60° |
| Triquetrum | Triquetrum | Hand pronated |
| | | Carpus on cassette |
| | | Radial side raised 60° |
| | | Wrist flexed 45° |

Data from Hafner, E., and Meuli, H. C.: Radiographic examination in orthopaedics, Bern, Switzerland, 1976, Hans Huber Medical Publisher; distributed in North and South America by University Park Press, Baltimore.

**Table 9-4.** Positioning for radiographic examination—cont'd

| Anatomic area of focus | Radiographic view desired | Positioning required |
|---|---|---|
| **Hand and wrist—cont'd** | | |
| Carpal tunnel | Carpal tunnel | Hand pronated<br>Wrist on cassette<br>Hand maximally dorsiflexed |
| Wrist | Dorsopalmar | Hand pronated<br>Wrist on cassette<br>Wrist and fingers extended |
| | Lateral | Ulnar side of wrist on cassette<br>Wrist and fingers extended |
| | Oblique | Hand pronated<br>Wrist and fingers extended<br>Radial side raised 45° |
| **Forearm and elbow** | | |
| Forearm | Anteroposterior | Forearm supinated<br>Dorsal side on cassette<br>Wrist and elbow joints extended |
| | Lateral | Patient sitting by edge of table<br>Upper arm abducted 90°<br>Forearm in same plane as upper arm<br>Elbow joint flexed 90°<br>Ulnar side of forearm on cassette<br>Wrist joint extended and strictly lateral |
| Wrist with forearm | Anteroposterior | Forearm supinated<br>Dorsal side with wrist on cassette<br>Wrist joint extended |
| | Lateral | Forearm and wrist with ulnar side on cassette<br>Wrist extended<br>Wrist strictly lateral |
| Forearm with elbow | Anteroposterior | Forearm supinated<br>Dorsal side on cassette<br>Elbow extended |
| | Lateral | Patient sitting by side of table<br>Upper arm abducted 90°<br>Forearm in same plane as upper arm<br>Elbow flexed 90°<br>Forearm and elbow with ulnar side on cassette |
| Elbow | Anteroposterior | Elbow with dorsal side on cassette<br>Elbow extended<br>Hand supinated |
| | Lateral | Elbow flexed 90°<br>Ulnar side on cassette<br>Forearm and upper arm flat on cassette<br>Hand strictly lateral |
| | Groove for ulnar nerve | Patient sitting by side of table<br>Dorsal side of upper arm on cassette<br>Elbow maximally flexed |
| | Coronoid process | Elbow extended<br>Dorsal side against cassette<br>Radial side raised 45° |
| **Upper arm and shoulder** | | |
| Upper arm with elbow and shoulder | Anteroposterior | Patient standing or lying<br>Upper arm with dorsal side on cassette<br>Elbow extended<br>Hand supinated |
| | Lateral | Patient sitting by side of table<br>Upper arm abducted 90°<br>Upper arm with ulnar side on cassette<br>Elbow flexed 90°<br>Hand lateral<br>Head inclined to opposite side |

*Continued.*

**Table 9-4.** Positioning for radiographic examination—cont'd

| Anatomic area of focus | Radiographic view desired | Positioning required |
|---|---|---|
| **Upper arm and shoulder—cont'd** | | |
| Upper arm with elbow | Anteroposterior | Upper arm and elbow with dorsal side on cassette |
| | | Elbow extended |
| | | Hand supinated |
| | Lateral | Patient sitting by side of table |
| | | Upper arm abducted 90° |
| | | Elbow flexed 90° |
| | | Ulnar side of upper arm and elbow on cassette |
| | | Hand strictly lateral |
| Upper arm with shoulder | Anteroposterior | Patient standing or lying |
| | | Dorsal side of upper arm and shoulder on cassette |
| | Lateral | Patient sitting by side of table |
| | | Upper arm abducted 90° |
| | | Medial side of upper arm flat on cassette |
| | | Head inclined toward opposite side |
| Shoulder | Internal rotation | Patient sitting |
| | | Shoulder blade flat on cassette |
| | | Elbow flexed 90° |
| | | Hand supinated |
| | | Upper arm hanging down and internally rotated 45° |
| | External rotation | Patient sitting |
| | | Shoulder blade flat on cassette |
| | | Elbow flexed 90° |
| | | Hand supinated |
| | | Upper arm hanging down and externally rotated 45° |
| | Abduction with external rotation | Patient sitting |
| | | Shoulder blade flat on cassette |
| | | Elbow flexed 90° |
| | | Hand supinated |
| | | Upper arm abducted 90° |
| | | Upper arm maximally externally rotated |
| | Anteroposterior | Patient sitting |
| | | Shoulder blade flat on cassette |
| | | Upper arm hanging down |
| | | Elbow flexed 90° |
| | | Hand supinated |
| | | Forearm vertical to cassette |
| | Transthoracic | Patient sitting lateral to cassette |
| | | Back turned slightly obliquely toward cassette |
| | | Affected shoulder on cassette |
| | | Upper arm hanging down |
| | | Opposite arm overhead |
| | Axillary | Patient recumbent |
| | | Relevant side at edge of table |
| | | Upper arm abducted 90° |
| | | Hand pronated |
| | | Cassette placed on shoulder cranially, vertical on table |
| | Sulcus intertubercularis (bicipital groove) | Patient recumbent |
| | | Relevant side by edge of table |
| | | Arm along body |
| | | Cassette on shoulder cranially, vertical on table and vertical to sagittal plane of body |
| **Scapula, clavicle, and sternum** | | |
| Scapula | Anteroposterior | Shoulder blade flat on cassette |
| | | Opposite side raised 45° |
| | | Arm abducted |
| | | Head turned toward opposite side |
| | Lateral, mediolateral | Arm of affected side over head |
| | | Thorax lateral to cassette |

**Table 9-4.** Positioning for radiographic examination—cont'd

| Anatomic area of focus | Radiographic view desired | Positioning required |
|---|---|---|
| **Scapula, clavicle, and sternum—cont'd** | | |
| | | Ventral side of body slightly oblique to cassette so that dorsal surface of scapula is directed strictly vertical to cassette |
| Acromioclavicular joint | Anteroposterior | Patient standing |
| | | Scapula against cassette |
| | | Arm hanging down |
| | Anteroposterior, bilateral (shoulder girdle) | Patient with back against cassette |
| | | Back fully extended |
| | | Arms hanging down |
| | Anteroposterior, bilateral, with weighting | Patient in hyperlordosis |
| | | Back against cassette |
| | | Arms hanging down |
| | | 3-kg weight in each hand |
| Clavicle | Posteroanterior | Patient standing |
| | | Clavicle on cassette |
| | | Arms hanging down |
| | | Arms internally·rotated |
| | | Head turned to opposite side |
| | Caudocranial | Patient standing or lying |
| | | Clavicle on cassette |
| | | Shoulder raised off cassette sufficiently that clavicle is parallel to cassette |
| Sternoclavicular joint | Oblique | Patient standing |
| | | Sternoclavicular joint on cassette |
| | | Opposite side raised 45° |
| Sternum | Lateral | Patient standing |
| | | Thorax lateral to cassette |
| | | Shoulders pulled dorsally by arms |
| | | Chest in inspiration |
| | Oblique | Patient prone |
| | | Sternum against cassette |
| | | Right (left) arm over head |
| | | Right (left) side of thorax raised 20° |
| **Foot and ankle** | | |
| Foot | Dorsoplantar | Foot plantar flexed |
| | | Sole of foot flat on cassette |
| | Lateral | Lateral edge of foot on cassette |
| | Oblique | Sole of foot against cassette |
| | | Lateral edge of foot raised 45° |
| | Functional exposure, lateral with weighting | Patient standing on pedestal |
| | | Weight on both feet equally |
| | | Cassette in median plane between feet |
| | Functional exposure, lateral in maximal dorsal extension | Medial foot margin on cassette |
| | | Patient lying on side |
| | | Knee flexed 90° |
| | | Foot maximally extended dorsally |
| | Functional exposure, lateral in maximal plantar flexion | Medial foot margin on cassette |
| | | Patient lying on side |
| | | Knee flexed 90° |
| | | Foot maximally plantar flexed |
| Toes | Dorsoplantar | Patient sitting |
| | | Forefoot flat on cassette |
| | Lateral, toes 2 and 3 | Medial side of toe on cassette |
| | | Other toes plantar flexed or dorsally extended by "reins" |
| | Lateral, toes 4 and 5 | Lateral side of toe on cassette |
| | | Other toes plantar flexed or dorsally extended by "reins" |
| Great toe | Dorsoplantar | Plantar side of great toe flat on cassette |
| | Lateral | Medial foot margin on cassette |
| | | Great toe strictly lateral |
| | | Other toes maximally plantar flexed by "reins" |

*Continued.*

**Table 9-4.** Positioning for radiographic examination—cont'd

| Anatomic area of focus | Radiographic view desired | Positioning required |
|---|---|---|
| **Foot and ankle—cont'd** | | |
| Forefoot (metatarsals and toes) | Dorsoplantar | Sole of foot flat on cassette |
| | Lateral | Lateral foot margin on cassette |
| | Oblique | Sole of foot against cassette |
| | | Lateral edge of foot raised 45° |
| | Heads of metatarsals | Patient prone |
| | | Toes maximally dorsally extended |
| | | Plantar side of distal phalanges |
| Tarsus | Dorsoplantar | Sole of foot on cassette |
| | Lateral | Lateral edge of foot on cassette |
| | Oblique | Sole of foot toward cassette |
| | | Lateral edge of foot raised 45° |
| | Held exposure, dorsoplantar (pathologic adduction) | Sole of foot against cassette |
| | | Midfoot forced into adduction in relation to hind part so that gap is produced in line of Chopart's (transverse tarsal) joint |
| Hindfoot (calcaneus and talus) | Dorsoplantar | Foot maximally dorsally extended |
| | | Sole flat on cassette |
| | Lateral | Lateral edge of foot on cassette |
| | Oblique | Sole of foot against cassette |
| | | Lateral edge of foot raised 45° |
| Talocalcanean joint | Internal rotation | Patient recumbent |
| | | Leg extended |
| | | Heel on cassette |
| | | Foot at right angle to lower leg in neutral position |
| | | Lower leg internally rotated 45° |
| | External rotation | Patient recumbent |
| | | Leg extended |
| | | Heel on cassette |
| | | Foot at right angle to lower leg in neutral position |
| | | Lower leg externally rotated 45° |
| Ankle joint | Anteroposterior | Patient recumbent |
| | | Lower leg with heel on cassette |
| | | Foot at right angle to leg in neutral position |
| | | Tip of foot internally rotated 20° |
| | Lateral | Patient lying on side |
| | | Lateral malleolus on cassette |
| | | Foot at right angle to leg in neutral position |
| | | Tip of foot internally rotated so that malleoli are projected on top of each other |
| | Oblique, internal rotation | Patient recumbent |
| | | Lower leg with heel on cassette |
| | | Foot at right angle to leg in neutral position |
| | | Tip of foot internally rotated 45° |
| | Oblique, external rotation | Patient recumbent |
| | | Lower leg with heel on cassette |
| | | Foot at right angle to leg in neutral position |
| | | Tip of foot externally rotated 45° |
| **Lower leg and knee** | | |
| Lower leg | Anteroposterior | Patient recumbent |
| | | Knee extended |
| | | Back of lower leg in neutral position |
| | | Tip of foot internally rotated 20° |
| | Lateral | Patient lying on side |
| | | Lateral side of lower leg on cassette |
| | | Foot at right angle to lower leg in neutral position |
| | | Malleoli must be superimposed on each other |
| Lower leg with ankle joint | Anteroposterior | Patient recumbent |
| | | Lower leg with heel on cassette |
| | | Foot at right angle to lower leg in neutral position |
| | | Tip of foot internally rotated 20° |

**Table 9-4.** Positioning for radiographic examination—cont'd

| Anatomic area of focus | Radiographic view desired | Positioning required |
|---|---|---|
| **Lower leg and knee— cont'd** | Lateral | Patient lying on side<br>Lower leg with lateral malleolus on cassette<br>Foot at right angle to lower leg in neutral position |
| Lower leg with knee joint | Anteroposterior | Patient recumbent<br>Knee extended<br>Lower leg with knee joint on cassette<br>Tip of foot internally rotated 20° |
| | Lateral | Patient lying on side<br>Lateral side of lower leg and knee on cassette<br>Knee extended |
| Knee joint | Anteroposterior | Patient recumbent<br>Hollow of knee on cassette<br>Knee extended<br>Leg internally rotated so that patella is directed forward and lies midway between femoral condyles |
| | Lateral | Patient lying on side<br>Lateral side of knee on cassette<br>Knee flexed 45°<br>Patella strictly lateral<br>Femoral condyles superimposed on each side |
| | Lateral extension | Patient lying on side<br>Lateral side of knee on cassette<br>Knee fully extended<br>Patella strictly lateral |
| | Lateral, 90° flexion | Patient lying on side<br>Lateral side of knee on cassette<br>Knee flexed 90° |
| | Oblique, internal rotation | Patient recumbent<br>Knee extended<br>Hollow of knee against cassette<br>Leg internally rotated 45° |
| | Oblique, external rotation | Patient recumbent<br>Knee extended<br>Hollow of knee against cassette<br>Leg externally rotated 45° |
| | Intercondylar ("tunnel view") | Patient recumbent<br>Knee flexed 45°<br>Hollow of knee against cassette |
| | Lateral soft-tissue exposure | Patient recumbent<br>Leg supported<br>Knee joint slightly flexed<br>Cassette placed on medial side of knee in sagittal plane |
| Patella | Posteroanterior | Patient prone<br>Patella on cassette<br>Knee extended |
| | Lateral | Patient lying on side<br>Lateral side of knee on cassette<br>Knee flexed 45°<br>Patella strictly lateral<br>Femoral condyles superimposed on each other |
| | Distal-proximal | Patient half sitting<br>Knee flexed 45°<br>Cassette held by chest<br>Cassette placed on thigh<br>Cassette vertical to longitudinal axis of patella |
| | Oblique, internal rotation | Patient prone<br>Patella against cassette<br>Leg internally rotated 45° |

*Continued.*

**Table 9-4.** Positioning for radiographic examination—cont'd

| Anatomic area of focus | Radiographic view desired | Positioning required |
|---|---|---|
| **Lower leg and knee—** cont'd | | |
| | Oblique; external rotation | Patient prone<br>Patella against cassette<br>Leg externally rotated 45° |
| **Thigh and hip** | | |
| Thigh with knee and hip joints | Anteroposterior | Patient recumbent<br>Thigh on cassette<br>Leg internally rotated 20° |
| | Lateral | Patient lying on side<br>Lateral side of thigh on cassette<br>Hip and knee joint slightly flexed<br>Leg of opposite side overextended dorsally |
| Thigh with knee joint | Anteroposterior | Patient recumbent<br>Thigh with hollow of knee on cassette<br>Knee extended<br>Leg internally rotated 20° |
| | Lateral | Patient lying on side<br>Knee with lateral side of thigh on cassette<br>Knee flexed 45° |
| Thigh with hip joint | Anteroposterior | Patient recumbent<br>Thigh with hip joint on cassette<br>Leg extended<br>Leg internally rotated 20° |
| | Lateral | Lateral side of thigh and hip on cassette<br>Hip slightly flexed<br>Opposite leg overextended dorsally |
| Leg length measurement (spot scanography, orthoradiography) | | Patient recumbent<br>Leg on cassette<br>Hip and knee joint extended<br>Leg internally rotated 20° |
| Hip joint | Anteroposterior | Patient recumbent<br>Buttocks on cassette<br>Hip extended<br>Leg internally rotated 20° |
| | Lateral, vertical ray direction | Patient recumbent<br>Hip on cassette<br>Opposite side raised 45°<br>Hip slightly flexed |
| | Lateral, horizontal ray direction | Patient recumbent<br>Contralateral hip and knee flexed 90° and propped up<br>Cassette proximal to hip along iliac crest<br>Cassette at 45° angle to median plane of body<br>Cassette vertical on table |
| | Anteroposterior with maximal abduction of thigh | Patient recumbent<br>Buttocks on cassette<br>Legs maximally separated and fixed |
| | Anteroposterior with maximal adduction of thigh | Patient recumbent<br>Buttocks on cassette<br>Legs crossed as far as possible<br>Leg of hip to be examined lying on table with the contralateral leg crossed over it |
| | Anteroposterior, anterior contour | Patient recumbent<br>Hip flexed 45°<br>Hip on cassette |
| | Anteroposterior, posterior contour | Patient recumbent<br>Leg extended<br>Leg internally rotated 20°<br>Hip on cassette |

**Table 9-4.** Positioning for radiographic examination—cont'd

| Anatomic area of focus | Radiographic view desired | Positioning required |
|---|---|---|
| **Pelvis** | | |
| Pelvis | Anteroposterior | Patient recumbent<br>Legs extended and parallel<br>Patellae directed forward<br>Knees touching, if possible |
| Pelvis with both femoral necks | Anteroposterior, normal position | Patient recumbent<br>Both knees flexed 90°<br>Both legs hanging over edge of table<br>Lower legs parallel<br>Patellae directed forward<br>Buttocks on cassette |
| | Lateral, ante-version exposure | Patient recumbent<br>Buttocks on cassette<br>Hips flexed 90°<br>Each thigh abducted 20°<br>Knees flexed 90°<br>Patellae directed forward<br>Lower legs on leg support<br>Buttocks touching support |
| | Anteroposterior, orthograde | Patient recumbent<br>Buttocks on cassette<br>Legs extended<br>Legs internally rotated 20° |
| | Lateral, orthograde | Patient recumbent<br>Buttocks on cassette<br>Hip flexed 90°<br>Each thigh abducted 45°<br>Knee flexed 90°<br>Lower leg supported |
| | Posteroanterior, with abduction and internal rotation | Patient prone<br>Thigh abducted to specified degree<br>Thigh internally rotated to specified degree<br>Knee flexed 90° |
| | Anteroposterior with maximal abduction and internal rotation | Patient recumbent<br>Buttocks on cassette<br>Both legs maximally abducted and internally rotated |
| Apophyses of iliac crests | Anteroposterior | Patient recumbent<br>Both iliac crests on cassette |
| Symphysis | Posteroanterior | Patient prone<br>Symphysis on cassette |
| | Craniocaudal | Patient on table, half sitting with hyperlordosis of back<br>Legs extended<br>Knees flexed over table |
| | Posteroanterior standing (weight bearing) | Patient standing on one leg<br>Symphysis against cassette |
| Sacroiliac joint | Anteroposterior | Patient recumbent<br>Sacrum on cassette<br>Hips and knees slightly flexed |
| | Orthogonal | Patient recumbent<br>Sacrum against cassette<br>Side raised 20° |
| **Vertebral column** | | |
| Cervical spine | Anteroposterior | Patient recumbent or sitting upright and straight<br>Back against cassette<br>Chin raised to level of occiput by tilting head backward |
| | Lateral | Patient sitting upright and straight<br>Neck lateral to cassette |

*Continued.*

**Table 9-4.** Positioning for radiographic examination—cont'd

| Anatomic area of focus | Radiographic view desired | Positioning required |
|---|---|---|
| Vertebral column—cont'd | | |
| | Oblique | Shoulder touching cassette |
| | | Shoulders pulled caudally, chin raised |
| | | Patient sitting with back against cassette |
| | | Side being examined turned 45° from cassette |
| | | Lower jaw raised |
| | Inclination | Patient sitting |
| | | Neck lateral to cassette |
| | | Shoulder by cassette |
| | | Head maximally flexed in median plane with chin pulled down |
| | Reclination (hyperextension) | Patient sitting |
| | | Neck lateral to cassette |
| | | Shoulder by cassette |
| | | Head maximally extended dorsally with chin raised |
| | Lateral inclination (flexion) | Patient recumbent |
| | | Head maximally flexed to right (left) in frontal plane |
| | | Lower jaw held at level of lower margin of occipital bone |
| | Anteroposterior odontoid process of axis | Patient sitting or lying with back against cassette |
| | | Mouth open as wide as possible |
| | | Head tilted backward so that biting edge of upper incisors is at level of lower edge of occipital bone |
| | Lateral inclination of odontoid process of axis (flexion) | Patient recumbent |
| | | Junction occiput-neck on cassette |
| | | Mouth open as wide as possible |
| | | Head maximally flexed to right (left) |
| | | Biting edge of upper incisors at level of lower edge of occipital bone |
| Cervicothoracic junction | Anteroposterior | Patient sitting |
| | | Back against cassette |
| | Lateral | Patient standing lateral to cassette |
| | | Shoulder and upper arm nearest cassette held forward |
| | | Shoulder and upper arm away from cassette held backward, externally rotated and supinated |
| | | Frontal plane of body vertical to cassette |
| Thoracic spine | Anteroposterior | Patient standing |
| | | Back against cassette |
| | | Arms hanging down |
| | | Breath held in expiration |
| | Lateral | Patient standing lateral to cassette |
| | | Arms pulled forward as far as possible |
| | | Elbows as close together as possible |
| | | Hands supinated |
| | | Light respiration with long exposure time |
| Thoracolumbar junction | Anteroposterior | Patient recumbent or standing |
| | | Back against cassette |
| | Lateral in inspiration | Patient standing upright and straight, lateral to cassette |
| | | Breath held in inspiration |
| | Lateral in expiration | Patient standing upright and straight, lateral to cassette |
| | | Breath held in expiration |
| Lumbar spine | Anteroposterior | Patient standing |
| | | Weight on both legs equally |
| | | Back against cassette |
| | Lateral | Patient standing upright and straight, lateral to cassette |
| | | Arms held upward |
| | Oblique | Patient recumbent |
| | | Side to be examined next to cassette |
| | | Contralateral side raised 45° |
| | Inclination (flexion) | Patient standing, lateral to cassette |
| | | Trunk maximally flexed ventrally |

**Table 9-4.** Positioning for radiographic examination — cont'd

| Anatomic area of focus | Radiographic view desired | Positioning required |
|---|---|---|
| **Vertebral column — cont'd** | | |
| | Reclination (hyperextension) | Patient standing, lateral to cassette<br>Trunk maximally extended dorsally |
| Lumbosacral junction | Anteroposterior | Patient recumbent<br>Sacrum on cassette<br>Legs extended |
| | Lateral | Patient standing exactly lateral to cassette |
| Sacrum | Anteroposterior | Patient recumbent<br>Sacrum on cassette<br>Hip and knee slightly flexed |
| | Lateral | Patient lying on side<br>Hips and knees flexed |
| Coccyx | Anteroposterior | Patient recumbent |
| | Lateral | Patient lying on side<br>Hips and knees flexed |
| Whole vertebral column | Anteroposterior standing | Patient standing upright and straight<br>Weight on both legs equally<br>Back against cassette |
| | Lateral standing | Patient standing upright and straight, lateral to cassette<br>Weight on both legs equally<br>Arms held forward |
| | Anteroposterior recumbent | Patient recumbent<br>Middle of back (in scoliosis, maximum of deformity) on center of cassette |

## Principles of radiographic interpretation

The following general principles are applicable to the interpretation of the radiographic examination[14,p.34].

1. General observations of the radiographic examination essential for complete interpretation:
   a. General shape of the bone, including width and curvature.
   b. Relationship of one bone to another in standardized view positioning.
   c. Architecture of the trabecular pattern in the medulla.
   d. Boundary between the cortex and the medulla.
   e. Periosteum, normally not seen unless separated from the cortex.
   f. Uniform density of the bone cortex.
2. Radiographic films should never be interpreted while wet! Judgments may be unreliable under these conditions.
3. Radiographs should always be interpreted on an appropriate viewbox. Holding the film to a light is not sufficient for adequate interpretation.
4. The film should always be placed on the viewbox in anatomic position to facilitate interpretation of relationships.
5. Patient history should be available to the physician and radiologist responsible for interpretation.
6. Because accuracy of interpretation may be dependent on reliability of the positioning or exposure of the view, these must be assured.

### Cardinal radiographic features

Specific radiographic features may be indicative and characteristic of a variety of disease entities (outline, pp. 212-213). It should be noted that these features, despite their specificity, rarely narrow the options to one or a few of the diseases outlined. Serial radiographic examinations may assist in this task, and additional special radiographic procedures in combination with other diagnostic tools may be indicated. Additionally the patient history is extremely important and may frequently assist in the differential diagnosis. Features characteristic of bone growth (skeletal age) and epiphyseal appearance and closure are given in Chapter 3.

# CARDINAL RADIOGRAPHIC FEATURES*

I. Widespread bone density increase
  A. Possible causes
    1. Paget's disease (sclerotic stage)
    2. Osteopetrosis
    3. Pycnodysostosis
    4. Osteopoikilosis
    5. Bone islands
    6. Osteopathia striata
    7. Osteoblastic metastases
    8. Hodgkin's disease
    9. Leukemia
    10. Myelofibrosis
    11. Urticaria pigmentosa
    12. Tuberous sclerosis
    13. Vitamin-D intoxication
    14. Idiopathic hypercalcemia
    15. Fluorosis
    16. Phosphorus intoxication
    17. Heavy-metal intoxication
    18. Renal osteodystrophy
    19. Cretinism
    20. Terminal phalangeal osteosclerosis
    21. Charcot's joint
    22. Healed brown tumors of hyperpara-
        thyroidism
    23. Osteitis condensans illi
  B. Rare causes
    1. Leprosy
    2. Gaucher's disease
    3. Pseudohypoparathyroidism
    4. Multiple myeloma with osteoscle-
       rosis
    5. Craniometaphyseal dysplasia
    6. Sclerosis associated with pheo-
       chromocytoma (infarcts)
    7. Long-standing cyanotic congenital
       heart disease
    8. Hereditary multiple diaphyseal scle-
       rosis
    9. Diffuse familial osteoplastic disease
       (FalchiVallebona disease)
    10. Congenital stenosis of medullary
        spaces with dwarfism
    11. Multiple osteosarcomas
    12. Hypoparathyroidism
    13. Cleidocranial dysostosis
    14. Idiopathic osteosclerosis
II. Widespread areas of bone destruction
  A. Possible causes
    1. Osteolytic metastases (carcinomas,
       sarcomas, lymphomas)
    2. Multiple myelomas
    3. Osteomyelitis of various causes
    4. Leukemia
    5. Burkitt's tumor
    6. Reticuloses
    7. Gout

  B. Rare causes
    1. Massive osteolysis
    2. Intraosseous hemangiomatosis
    3. Cystic lymphangiomatosis of bone
    4. Congenital scattered fibromatosis
    5. Weber-Christian disease
    6. Primary systemic amyloidosis
    7. Electrical injury
III. Bone resorption at specific sites
  A. Distal clavicles
    1. Hyperparathyroidism
    2. Rheumatoid arthritis
    3. Scleroderma
    4. Posttraumatic osteolysis
    5. Progeria
    6. Pycnodysostosis
    7. Reticulohistiocytoma (lipoid der-
       matoarthritis)
    8. Hurler's syndrome
  B. Terminal phalangeal tufts
    1. Scleroderma (may be associated
       with calcification)
    2. Raynaud's disease and allied con-
       ditions
    3. Occlusive vascular disease
    4. Traumatic vascular disease
    5. Thromboangiitis obliterans
    6. Diabetes mellitus
    7. Tabes dorsalis
    8. Syringomyelia
    9. Leprosy
    10. Psoriasis
    11. Epidermolysis bullosa (may be as-
        sociated with calcification)
    12. Pityriasis rubra
    13. Hyperparathyroidism
    14. Osteomalacia
    15. Malabsorption syndrome
    16. Hunger osteopathy
    17. Burns
    18. Frostbite
    19. Electrical injuries
    20. Osteolysis from polyvinyl tank
        cleaners
    21. Acro-osteolysis
    22. Progeria
    23. Pycnodysostosis
    24. Reticulohistiocytoma (lipoid der-
        matoarthritis)
    25. Benign proliferative lesions
    26. Disseminated lipogranulomatosis
    27. Rothmund's syndrome (may be as-
        sociated with calcification)
    28. Sarcoidosis (rare)
    29. Sjögren's syndrome
    30. Gout

*Adapted from Greenfield, G. B.: Radiology of bone diseases, ed. 2, Philadelphia, 1975, J. B. Lippin-
cott Co., pp. 301-401.

C. Superior aspects of ribs
1. Hyperparathyroidism
2. Rheumatoid arthritis
3. Scleroderma
4. Lupus erythematosus
5. Sjögren's syndrome
6. Neurofibromatosis
7. Poliomyelitis
8. Progeria
9. Localized pressure
10. Osteogenesis imperfecta
11. Marfan's syndrome
12. Radiation injury
D. Calcanei
1. Rheumatoid arthritis
2. Hyperparathyroidism
3. Reiter's syndrome
4. Localized osteomyelitis
5. Reticulohistiocytoma
E. Generalized bone resorption
1. Paraplegia
2. Myositis ossificans
IV. Generalized periosteal elevation
A. Characterized by
1. Pulmonary hypertrophic osteoarthropathy
2. Thyroid acropachy
3. Pachydermoperiostosis
4. Infantile cortical hyperostosis
5. Hypervitaminosis A
B. Commonly associated with
1. Prematurity
2. Venous stasis
3. Subacute lupus erythematosus (arteritis)
4. Polyarteritis nodosa
5. Rheumatoid arthritis
6. Reiter's syndrome
7. Psoriatic arthritis
8. Battered child syndrome
9. Thermal injury
10. Widespread osteomyelitis
11. Widespread infarcts of bone (especially hand-foot syndrome in sickle cell anemia)
12. Congenital lves disease
13. Rubella
14. Scurvy
15. Healing rickets
16. Infantile Hurler's syndrome
17. Gaucher's disease
18. Histiocytosis X
19. Myelosclerosis
20. Fluorosis
21. Cornelia de Lange syndrome II (pseudomuscular hypertrophy)
V. Cortical disease
A. Generalized cortical thickening
1. All processes in which periosteal new bone blends with cortex
2. Paget's disease
3. Fibrous dysplasia

4. Progressive diaphyseal dysplasia (Camurati-Engelmann disease)
5. Hereditary multiple diaphyseal sclerosis (Ribbing's disease)
6. Hyperphosphatemia
7. Van Buchem's disease
8. Melorheostosis
B. Splitting of cortex
1. Sickle cell anemia
2. Osteomyelitis
3. Hyperphosphatemia
4. Osteopetrosis
5. Gaucher's disease
6. Battered child syndrome
7. Scurvy
8. Bone graft (local)
C. Scalloping of inner cortical margin
1. Hodgkin's disease
2. Multiple myeloma
3. Leukemia
4. Reticulum cell sarcoma
5. Mastocytosis
6. Histiocytosis X
7. Gaucher's disease
8. Hyperparathyroidism
9. Fibrous dysplasia
10. Osteopetrosis
VI. Bone expansion
A. Primary benign bone tumors
1. Giant cell tumor
2. Enchondroma
3. Benign chondroblastoma
4. Chondromyxoid fibroma
5. Desmoplastic fibroma
6. Lipoma of bone
B. Tumorlike processes
1. Unicameral bone cyst
2. Fibrous dysplasia
3. Aneurysmal bone cyst
4. Eosinophilic granuloma
5. Dermoid inclusion cyst
C. Primary malignant bone tumors
1. Multiple myeloma
2. Malignant giant cell tumor
3. Chondrosarcoma
4. Fibrosarcoma
5. Adamantinoma (long bone)
6. Osteogenic sarcoma (rare)
D. Tumors metastatic to bone
1. Carcinoma of kidney
2. Carcinoma of thyroid gland
3. Treated metastases
E. Differential diagnosis of expansile lesion in rib (most probable lesions)
1. Fibrous dysplasia
2. Multiple myeloma or plasmocytoma
3. Histiocytosis X
4. Chondromyxoid fibroma
5. Aneurysmal bone cyst
6. Chondrosarcoma
7. Gaucher's disease

## SUMMARY

The radiographic examination is one of the most useful diagnostic tools in orthopedics. All health care personnel dealing with this specialty should be familiar, to varying degrees dependent on their involvement, with the principles, positioning, and interpretation of this tool. The chapter reviews those areas felt to be of critical importance and emphasizes the need for increased comprehension of these principles by health care personnel other than those *directly* involved in the procedure and process, although much of the information may be of interest to those directly involved. For a more complete and comprehensive background on the procedures and process, refer to the bibliography.

## REFERENCES

1. Adams, J. C.: Outline of orthopaedics, New York, 1976, Churchill Livingstone.
2. Aegerter, E., and Kirkpatrick, J. A., Jr.: Orthopedic diseases: physiology, pathology, radiology, Philadelphia, 1975, W. B. Saunders Co.
3. Gartland, J. J.: Fundamentals of orthopaedics, Philadelphia, 1974, W. B. Saunders Co.
4. Gillis, L.: Diagnosis in orthopaedics, New York, 1969, Appleton-Century-Crofts.
5. Hafner, E., and Meuli, H. C.: Radiographic examination in orthopaedics, Baltimore, 1976, University Park Press.
6. Simon, G.: Principles of bone x-ray diagnosis, London, 1973, Butterworths.

## BIBLIOGRAPHY

Adams, J. C.: Outline of orthopaedics, New York, 1976, Churchill Livingston.

Aegerter, E., and Kirkpatrick, J. A., Jr.: Orthopedic diseases: physiology, pathology, radiology, Philadelphia, 1975, W. B. Saunders Co.

Brashear, H. R., and Raney, R. B.: Shand's handbook of orthopaedic surgery, ed. 9, St. Louis, 1978, The C. V. Mosby Co.

Cahoon, J. B.: Formulating x-ray techniques, Durham, N.C., 1974, Duke University Press.

Committee on Drugs, Commission on Public Health and Radiation Protection: Prevention and management of adverse reactions to intravascular contrast media, July 1977, American College of Radiology.

Crenshaw, A. H., editor: Campbell's operative orthopedics, ed. 5, St. Louis, 1971, The C. V. Mosby Co.

Edeiken, J., and Hodes, P. J.: Roentgen diagnosis of diseases of bone, Vols. 1 and 2, Baltimore, 1973, The Williams & Wilkins Co.

Gartland, J. J.: Fundamentals of orthopaedics, Philadelphia, 1974, W. B. Saunders Co.

Gillis, L.: Diagnosis in orthopaedics, New York, 1969, Appleton-Century-Crofts.

Greenfield, G. B.: Radiology of bone diseases, Philadelphia, 1975, J. B. Lippincott Co.

Grenlick, W. W., and Pyle, S. I.: Radiographic atlas of skeletal development of the hand and wrist, Palo Alto, Calif., 1959, Stanford University Press.

Hafner, E., and Meuli, H. C.: Radiographic examination in Orthopaedics, Baltimore, 1976, University Park Press.

Jacobs, P.: Atlas of hand radiograph, Baltimore, 1973, University Park Press.

Keats, T. E.: An atlas of normal roentgen variants that may simulate disease, Chicago, 1973, Year Book Medical Publishers, Inc.

Merrill, V.: Atlas of roentgenographic positions and standard radiologic procedure, ed. 4, 3 vols., St. Louis, 1975, The C. V. Mosby Co.

Meschen, I.: Radiographic positioning and related anatomy, Philadelphia, 1968, W. B. Saunders Co.

McInnes, J.: Clark's positioning in radiography, Vols. 1 and 2.

McInnes, J.: Radiographic anatomy, New York, 1975, Appleton-Century-Crofts.

McRae, R.: Clinical orthopaedic examination, New York, 1976, Churchill Livingstone.

Murray, R. O., and Jacobson, H. G.: The radiology of skeletal diseases, Vols. 1 to 4, New York, 1977, Churchill Livingstone.

Ross, P., and DuBonlay, G. H.: An atlas of normal vertebral angiograms, Boston, 1976, Butterworths.

Selman, J.: The fundamentals of x-ray and radium physics, Springfield, Ill., 1977, Charles C Thomas, Publisher.

Sexton, H. M., and Strickland, B.: Practical procedures in diagnostic radiology, New York, 1972, Grune and Stratton.

Siegle, R. L., and Lieberman, P.: A review of untoward reactions to iodinated contrast material, J. Urol. 119: 581-587, 1978.

Simon, G.: X-ray diagnosis for clinical students, London, 1975, Butterworths.

Simon, G.: Principles of bone x-ray, diagnosis, London, 1973, Butterworths.

Snell, R. S., and Wyman, A. C.: An atlas of normal radiographic anatomy, Boston, 1976, Little, Brown and Co.

Squire, L. F., Colaiace, W. M., and Strutynsky, N.: Exercises in diagnostic radiology: bone, Philadelphia, 1972, W. B. Saunders Co.

Tachdjian, M. O.: Pediatric orthopedics, Philadelphia, 1972, W. B. Saunders Co.

Thompson, T. T.: Primer of clinical radiography, Boston, 1973, Little, Brown and Co.

Tzonchev, V., et al.: The radiology of joint diseases, London, 1973, Butterworths.

Witten, D. M., et al.: Acute reactions to urographic contrast medium, Am. J. Roentgenol. Radium Ther. Nucl. Med. **119:**832-840, 1973.

Zimmermann, R. L.: Medical radiographic technology, Indianapolis, 1975, The Bobbs-Merrill Co., Inc.

# 10

# Special procedures

**NANCY E. HILT**

Many diagnostic tools utilized for the orthopedic patient are discussed in Chapters 9, 11, and 12. Each of these chapters provides an overview of what can be considered very broad topics. In this chapter those special diagnostic procedures that are of greatest value when treating musculoskeletal diseases and disorders are considered in greater depth. These include *arthroscopy, bone marrow aspiration, bone scan, electromyography, joint aspiration, knee arthrography, myelography, pulmonary function test,* and *venography of the lower extremity.* Various aspects of each procedure are discussed in relation to specific implications for musculoskeletal diagnoses.

## ARTHROSCOPY

**Definition.** Arthroscopy is a diagnostic tool permitting visualization of internal joint structures through the utilization of an arthroscope. Although arthroscopy may be accomplished in other joints, it is most frequently utilized in the knee. The arthroscope is a telescopic instrument that when inserted in the joint provides flexibility in the field of vision. Photographic capabilities accompany the utilization of this technique. The standard arthroscope (Fig. 10-1) possesses the following abilities, features, and capabilities[4,p.7]:

1. Field of vision: the greatest angle between two light rays going through the lens at which image definition is acceptable

2. Angle of vision: the angle between the axis of the telescope and the centerline of the field of vision
3. Depth of field: the distance over which satisfactory definition is obtained when the lens is in focus for a certain distance
4. Field stop or aperture: an opening, usually circular, in an opaque screen; its diameter determines the field of view of an optical instrument
5. Magnifying power: the ratio of the apparent size of a plane image to the apparent size of the object as the latter would be seen without the magnifying instrument
6. Resolving power: the ability of an optical system to resolve (i.e., separate two entities)
7. Illumination
8. Flexible diameter of instruments
9. Irrigation
10. Photographic capability
11. Ability to be sterilized

**Indications for utilization.** The following are considered to be general indications for utilization of arthroscopy as a diagnostic technique[4,pp.14-15;8,p.170]:

1. Traumatic injuries producing hemarthrosis and no clinical signs of instability
2. Evaluation of visual diagnosis of meniscal tears or injuries
3. Suspected small loose body in the joint
4. Synovial biopsy for suspected processes of the synovial membrane such as synovitis
5. Progression of osteochondritis dissecans
6. Popliteal cyst (when arthrogram does not reveal pathology), postoperative follow-up after knee surgery
7. Determination of severity of pathologic findings, especially with arthritic joint involvement
8. Preoperative confirmation of specific diagnoses to facilitate surgical procedures or to avoid surgery
9. Monitoring of therapeutic modalities and their progression and effect
10. Research

It must be mentioned that arthroscopy is rarely utilized as the initial diagnostic tool. Diagnosis in some cases may already have been established and therapeutic modalities instituted. Considerable effort is most often made in favor of more conservative diagnostic measures, and arthroscopy, due to its complications, is utilized only when lesser tools are insufficient for diagnostic or monitoring purposes.

**Contraindications.** Contraindications for utilization of arthroscopy as a diagnostic tool are (1) any type of injury to the skin (e.g., abscess, laceration, abrasion) surrounding the knee that might render it more susceptible to infection, and (2) fibrous ankylosis of the knee (flexion less than 50°).[4,p.20]

**Preprocedural care.** Arthroscopy may be performed with the patient under local or general anesthesia and prepared according to the specifications of the surgeon. The patient should be provided with a thorough explanation of the procedure, how it is accomplished, and the risks of the procedure. Preoperative medication is prescribed in most circumstances.

**Intraprocedural methodology.** Local or general anesthesia is chosen for the arthroscopic procedure by the orthopedic surgeon. Jackson and Dandy[3,pp.21-22] prefer general anesthesia because (1) if the results of the arthroscopic procedure indicate repair through surgical intervention, it may be accomplished at that time while the patient is under anesthesia, (2) no discomfort is associated with the procedure under general anesthesia if the tourniquet is inflated, and (3) general anesthesia provides total muscular relaxation and permits the surgeon to explore fully all aspects of the knee joint.

Arthroscopy is accomplished as follows*:

1. Patient is placed under local or general anesthesia; this permits a baseline of information regarding his status.
2. Surgical skin preparation is accomplished.
3. Tourniquet is applied but not inflated.
4. Patient is appropriately draped with full exposure of the knee joint.
5. Knee is flexed approximately 40° for insertion of needle.
6. Knee joint capsule is distended and irrigated with sterile normal saline solution.
7. Small incision is made (approximately ¼ inch long) about ½ inch above the lateral tibial plateau and immediately lateral to the patellar tendon while the knee is in approximately 40° flexion.
8. Arthroscope is inserted through the incision, and examination of the knee joint is accomplished from various angles.
9. If indicated the arthroscope may be reinserted at various designated points to promote appropriate visualization of the total knee structures.
10. Joint fluid may be obtained for microscopic examination.
11. Tissue specimens may be obtained for biopsy.

---

*References 3, pp. 22-43; 4, pp. 15-20; 8, pp. 16-30.

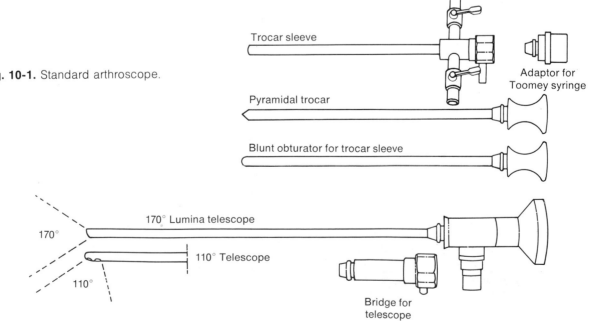

**Fig. 10-1.** Standard arthroscope.

Trocar sleeve

Adaptor for Toomey syringe

Pyramidal trocar

Blunt obturator for trocar sleeve

170°

170° Lumina telescope

110°

110° Telescope

Bridge for telescope

12. Photographic visualization may be obtained through special photographic attachments to the arthroscope.
13. On completion of the arthroscopic procedure, the irrigation system, lighting cable, and arthroscopic telescope are removed from the joint.

14. Joint is irrigated after removal of the instrument.
15. Incision is sutured.
16. Tourniquet is removed.
17. Irrigation of the joint is continued until the fluid is clear. The needle is then removed, and a pressure dressing may be applied to the knee.

**Fig. 10-2.** Arthroscopic views.

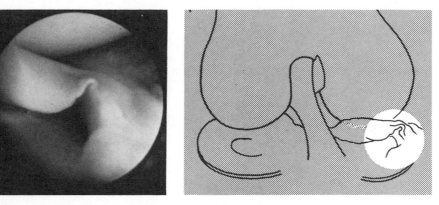

**A,** Anterior portion of longitudinal tear with displacement of inner border toward intercondylar notch (bucket-handle tear).

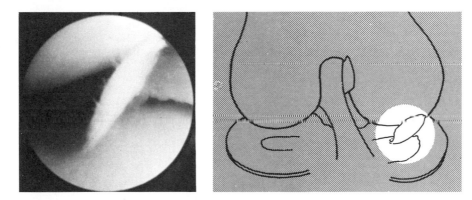

**B,** Small flaplike fragment from inner border of meniscus, combination of longitudinal and radial tearing.

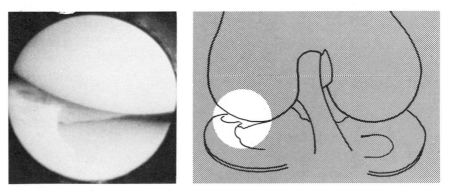

**C,** Radial tear with small longitudinal component in lateral meniscus.

*Continued.*

**Fig. 10-2, cont'd.** Arthroscopic views

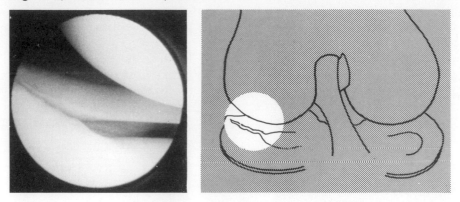

**D,** Pure radial or transverse tear in lateral meniscus.

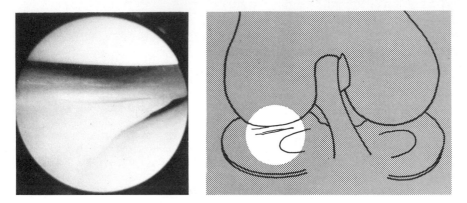

**E,** Undisplaced cleavage tear in posterior horn of lateral meniscus.

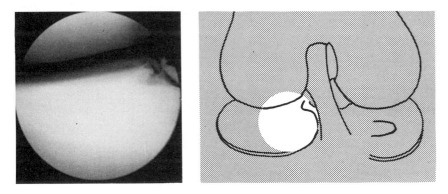

**F,** Intact discoid lateral meniscus with inner border of meniscus close to intercondylar notch.

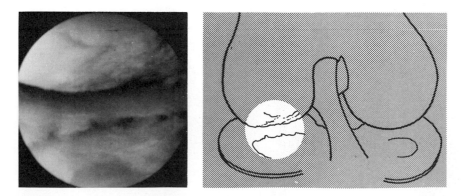

**G,** Degenerative posterior horn of lateral meniscus associated with degenerative changes on articular surface of femoral condyle and tibial plateau.

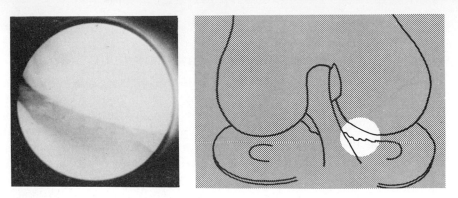

**H,** Degenerative posterior horn of medial meniscus. Note loss of definition of inner border.

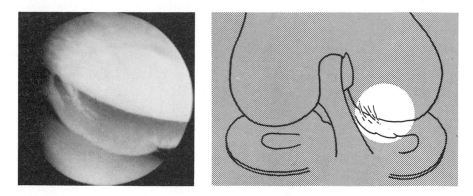

**I,** Disruption of posteromedial corner allows meniscal tissue to bulge in toward center of joint. Presence of tear can be confirmed by insertion of palpating tool into joint or by posteromedial insertion of arthroscope and direct visualization of tear.

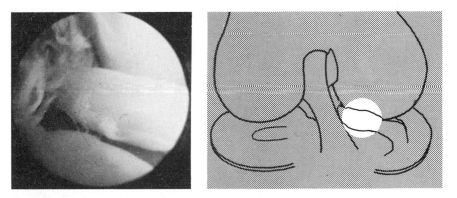

**J,** Displaced fragment of meniscus lying in intercondylar notch obscures visualization of medial compartment of joint and is pathognomonic of bucket-handle tear.

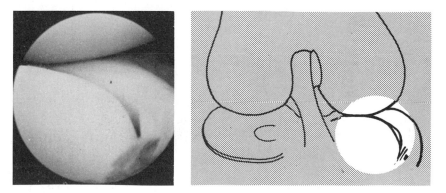

**K,** When meniscotibial attachments are torn anterior horn can extrude from joint, resulting in hypermobile meniscus. (From Jackson, R. W., and Dandy, D. J.: Arthroscopy of the knee, New York, 1976, Grune & Stratton. By permission.)

The entire arthroscopic procedure is performed under strict sterile and aseptic technique. Specific techniques during the actual arthroscopic examination of the joint vary according to the surgeon's preference, the degree of disability, the specific indication for the procedure, and the projected outcome.

**Postprocedural care.** Immediate postprocedural care may be required in the form of monitoring of bleeding from the injection and incisional sites. This is rarely a problem, but additional irrigation of the joint may be required. Ambulation is permitted as soon as the patient is recovered from anesthesia and fully awake. The incisional sutures are usually removed several days after the procedure. Other activities are greatly dependent on the patient's individual response to the procedure and the associated pain. Mild analgesics usually are successful in controlling the associated pain. Some patients complain of numbness surrounding the knee after the procedure, but this usually dissipates within several days. Postprocedural care may be extended considerably if arthrotomy follows the arthroscopic procedure.[4,p.20]

**Diagnostic implications** (Fig. 10-2). Diagnostic implications of arthroscopy, a relatively new procedure in comparison with many outlined in this chapter, must be considered in relation to the established diagnostic findings that are considered indications for the procedure. In addition alternatives, most of which are surgical in nature, may be reviewed in relation to the severity of the diagnostic and treatment projections considered for each preprocedural diagnosis. All indications are that arthroscopy, if utilized when indicated appropriately, provides definitive diagnosis in many of the disease processes, and traumatic injuries of the knee joint especially, without the considerable risk related to exploratory arthrotomy. Despite the fact that arthroscopy may reveal indications for arthrotomy, this surgical procedure may not be necessary for many patients with appropriate utilization of arthroscopy. Microscopic interarticular surgery, arthroscopically accomplished, may be utilized in some cases. At minimum, arthroscopy permits the orthopedic surgeon to relate to further indications for surgical procedures with a more comprehensive view of the problem. The overall usefulness of this tool is yet to be totally explored.

**Complications.** The most frequent complications associated with arthroscopy are infection, injuries to the cartilage and capsule of the joint, hemarthrosis, synovial rupture, thrombophlebitis, and infrapatellar anesthesia.[3,pp.65-71;4,pp.20-22;8,pp.31-34]

## BONE MARROW ASPIRATION

**Definition.** Bone marrow aspiration is a diagnostic procedure that permits microscopic examination of bone marrow obtained through needle aspiration.

**Indications for utilization.** Conditions in which diagnostic bone marrow aspiration is indicated include leukemia, multiple myeloma, Hodgkin's disease, metastatic tumors, infections such as tuberculosis or brucellosis, myelosclerosis, and anemia.[1,p.651;6,pp.159-160;7,p.78]

**Preprocedural care.** The sole preparation required for a bone marrow aspiration is adequate explanation to the patient of the procedure and its purpose.

**Intraprocedural methodology.** The most common sites utilized for bone marrow aspiration are the iliac crest and the upper portion of the sternum, although the vertebral spinous processes and the ribs may also be used. Positioning of the patient varies according to the site to be utilized:

| Site of aspiration | Required position |
| --- | --- |
| Iliac crest | Supine |
| Sternum | Supine |
| Posterior ilium | Lateral recumbent with back at edge of table, knees drawn up to abdomen, head flexed onto chest |
| Ribs | Same as for posterior ilium |

Bone marrow aspiration is accomplished as follows:

1. Patient is appropriately positioned.
2. Site chosen for the aspiration is appropriately cleansed utilizing antiseptic solution.
3. Local anesthetic is utilized to infiltrate the tissues surrounding the site of aspiration.
4. A special type of needle with a stylet is inserted into the bone marrow.
5. Stylet is withdrawn from the needle.
6. A syringe is attached to the hub of the needle.
7. Aspiration of bone marrow is accomplished.
8. Aspirated specimen is appropriately prepared on slides.
9. Additional marrow specimen is placed in appropriate solution.
10. Syringe is removed, and the stylet is replaced.
11. Needle and stylet are removed.
12. Specimens are sent to the laboratory.

**Postprocedural care.** Pressure is applied over the puncture site after the procedure is completed, and the patient is observed for additional bleeding.

**Complications.** Excessive bleeding after the procedure is a complication of bone marrow aspiration from any site. Additional risk accompanies aspiration accomplished from the sternum because of the potential damage to vital structures lying just beneath it. The tibial tubercle is avoided as a site of aspiration because of the proximity to the epiphyseal growth plate.

## BONE SCAN

**Definition.** A bone scan is a diagnostic tool utilizing radioactive isotopes involved in bone metabolism to detect metastatic carcinoma of the bone. Evidence of metastatic tumors of the bone will be reflected on bone scan more readily than may be detectable through normal radiographic examination.

**Indications for utilization.** The major indications for a bone scan are symptomatology reflecting potential metastatic bone disease, usually with a primary site already established, or monitoring of progression of metastatic bone disease. It is also utilized in some cases for detection and monitoring of primary skeletal tumors.

**Preprocedural care.** Explanation of the procedure to the patient is a major preprocedural consideration for a bone scan.

**Intraprocedural methodology.** The radioactive isotopes utilized for a bone scan are those involved in bone metabolism and are injected intravenously approximately 3 hours before the bone scan is scheduled. After this injection the following steps are accomplished:

1. Patient is asked to void immediately prior to the bone scan.
2. Patient is appropriately positioned, dependent on the area to be scanned.
3. Scan is accomplished, with change in positions sometimes being required during the scan.

**Postprocedural care.** No postprocedural care is required.

**Diagnostic implications.** The greatest diagnostic advantage of the bone scan is its ability to detect metastatic and primary bone tumors as early as 3 to 6 months prior to their detection on ordinary radiographic examination. Ordinary radiographic examinations, however, are usually performed after the scan for comparison purposes. Bone scan is not useful in the diagnosis of soft-tissue carcinomas.

## ELECTROMYOGRAPHY

**Definition.** Electromyography (EMG) is a diagnostic tool that provides a graphic readout of the electrical potential generated in an individual muscle. It is usually accomplished with the patient at rest with slight voluntary contraction and followed with maximal contraction. The electrical activity generated through the insertion of a sterile needle electrode into the specific muscle is then amplified and displayed on a cathode ray oscilloscope.

**Indications for utilization.** The electromyogram permits evaluation of muscular activity and assists in the following[5, p.40; 6, p.175]:

1. Diagnosis of neuromuscular abnormalities, especially those involving the lower motor neurons and including disorders of the spinal cord, peripheral nerves, and muscles
2. Determination of management of peripheral nerve injuries
3. Monitoring of progression to assist in the appropriate implementation of rehabilitation programs
4. Differentiation of the apparent paralysis of the malingerer or the patient with hysteria

**Preprocedural care.** It is advantageous to schedule electromyography before utilizing such other diagnostic tools as myelography or muscle biopsy, since the results of this procedure may serve as a better guide to further studies. Electromyography may cause elevation in the muscle serum enzyme levels for up to 10 days following the procedure and for this reason the level should be obtained prior to the procedure if required. Dependent on the pain threshold and the cooperation of the patient, sedation may be required but should be moderate. Adequate preparation in the form of explanation should be provided so that the patient is aware of how the procedure is accomplished and specific expectations related to it.

**Intraprocedural methodology.** Electromyography is accomplished by a physician as follows[5, p.41]:

1. A small needle is inserted into the muscle(s) to be studied. The location of the muscles may vary and will be greatly dependent on the nature of the problems and the symptomatology as well as the preprocedural diagnosis.
2. Electrical activity is observed in each muscle tested on insertion, at rest, during gentle voluntary muscle contraction, and during maximal voluntary effort.
3. Electrical activity is viewed on the oscilloscope screen, and its associated sound equivalents are projected in the amplifier.
4. Permanent recordings may be obtained.

**Postprocedural care.** A slight-pressure dressing is applied over the areas where needles have been inserted.

**Table 10-1.** Electromyographic classification of nerve damage

| Degree of abnormality | Insertional activity | Denervation potentials | Voluntary motor units |
|---|---|---|---|
| 1+ | Increased irritability<br>Prolonged firing of voluntary motor units<br>Scattered denervation potentials | Scattered, not present on all insertions | Present |
| 2+ | Increased irritability<br>Mixed picture of voluntary motor units and denervation potentials | Present in different areas of needle insertion | Decreased, may be poorly formed |
| 3+ | Increased irritability<br>Predominantly denervation potentials | Present on most needle insertions | Rare |
| 4+ | Increased irritability<br>Showers of denervation potentials on all insertions | Profusely present on all needle insertions | Absent |

From Zohn, D. A., and Mennell, J. M.: Musculoskeletal pain: diagnosis and physical treatment, Boston, 1976, Little, Brown & Co.

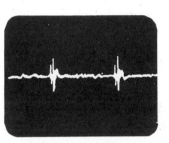

NORMAL VOLUNTARY MOTOR UNIT

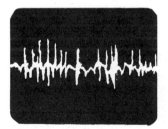

NASCENT MOTOR UNIT

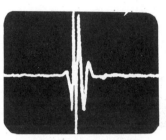

GIANT MOTOR UNIT

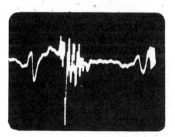

POLYPHASIC MOTOR UNIT

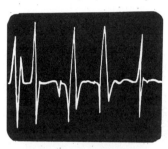

MYOPATHIC MOTOR UNITS

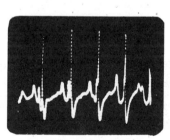

MYOTONIC DISCHARGES

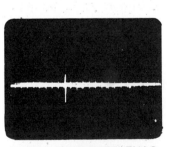

FIBRILLATION POTENTIALS

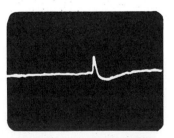

POSITIVE SHARP WAVES

INSERTIONAL (END-PLATE) POTENTIALS

**Fig. 10-3.** Characteristic electromyelographic wave forms. (From Zohn, D. A., and Mennell, J. M.: Musculoskeletal pain: diagnosis and physical treatment, Boston, 1976, Little, Brown & Co.)

**Table 10-2.** Synovial fluid analysis

| Criteria | Normal | Noninflammatory* | Inflammatory† | Purulent‡ |
|---|---|---|---|---|
| Appearance | Straw colored, clear | Straw colored, may be blood tinged | Cloudy | Turbid to opaque |
| Mucin clot | Firm | Firm | Friable | Friable |
| Cell count (% polymorphs) | <200 (<25%) | 200 to 2000 (<25%) | 2000 to 50,000 (50%-75%) | 20,000 to 100,000 (75%) |
| Glucose | 2/3 of blood | 2/3 of blood | Decreased | Markedly decreased |
| Crystals | None | None | May be present§ | None |
| Culture | Negative | Negative | Negative or positive‖ | Positive or negative‖ |

From Zohn, D. A., and Mennell, J. M.: Musculoskeletal pain: diagnosis and physical treatment, Boston, 1976, Little, Brown & Co.
*Osteoarthritis, trauma.
†Rheumatoid arthritis and variants: gout, pseudogout, tuberculosis, acute gonococcal disease, fungal infections.
‡Acute bacterial infections.
§Uric acid, calcium pyrophosphate, cholesterol, steroids.
‖Appropriate culture media necessary.

**Diagnostic implications.** The electromyelogram (Fig. 10-3) is of value in assisting the physician with differential diagnosis of muscle denervation, level or area of nerve injury, presence of dystrophies and myopathies, and recurrence of innervation.

Electromyographic classification of nerve damage is given in Table 10-1.

**Complications.** A hematoma may form around the site of needle insertion, although this is extremely rare.

## JOINT ASPIRATION

**Definition.** Joint aspiration is a diagnostic procedure accomplished by inserting a needle into the synovial capsule of the joint for the purpose of withdrawing fluid for microscopic examination. This may also be accomplished for the relief of pain when effusion and joint swelling are evident. The most common joint to require aspiration is the knee joint.

**Indications for utilization.** The most common indication for joint aspiration for diagnostic purposes is symptomatology (such as pain or joint swelling) indicative of increased joint fluid or joint pathology.

**Preprocedural care.** The only preprocedural care required for most joint aspiration is explanation of the procedure to the patient. Sedation is rarely required, with a possible exception of in young children.

**Intraprocedural methodology.** Joint aspiration (Fig. 10-4) is accomplished by a physician, under aseptic technique, and sometimes with the patient under local anesthesia. The usual steps for aspiration are as follows:

1. Site of aspiration is cleansed with an antiseptic solution.
2. Injection of local anesthetic to infiltrate soft tissues surrounding injection site is accomplished, if desirable.
3. A sterile needle and syringe are prepared with a needle long enough to penetrate the joint capsule and with a gauge large enough to withdraw the synovial fluid.
4. Needle is injected into the joint capsule, and varying amounts of fluid are withdrawn.
5. Fluid is prepared for microscopic examination.
6. Puncture site is again cleansed with antiseptic solution; a small dressing may be applied with some initial pressure.

**Postprocedural care.** Usually no postprocedural care is required with the exception of pressure for approximately 5 minutes. Patients should be cautioned that, if local anesthetic has been utilized, sensation changes may occur for a period of time.

**Diagnostic implications.** Synovial fluid has specific characteristics that are predictable and well defined. Any variation of these normal parameters is an indication of pathologic processes within the joint structure. Table 10-2 shows the normal synovial fluid parameters and variations thereof. It should be noted that some inflammatory or infectious processes may not be evident from joint fluid analysis during the initial stages, and fluid aspiration may have to be repeated.

**Complications.** The major complication of joint aspiration is introduction of infection into the joint capsule due to lack of aseptic technique during the procedure. Slight bleeding may be noted but is usu-

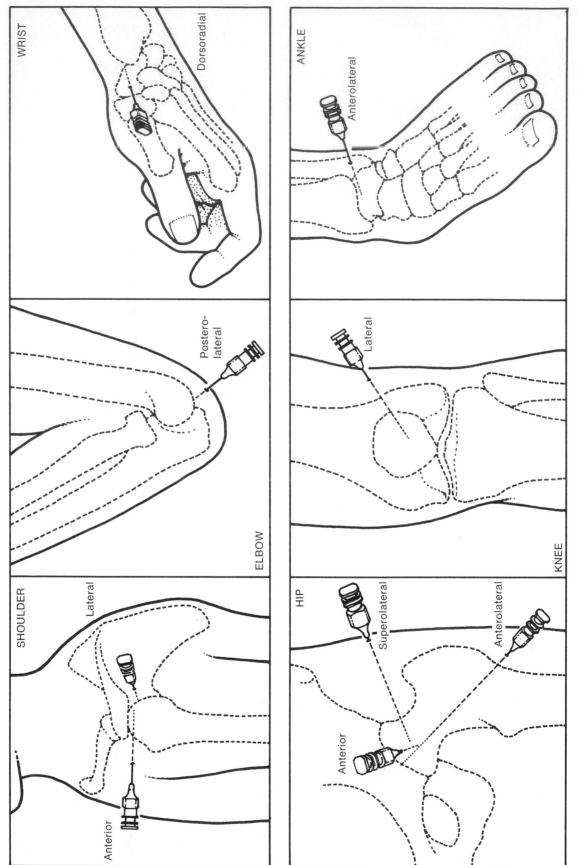

**Fig. 10-4.** Common joint aspiration approaches.

ally alleviated with minimal pressure after the procedure.

## KNEE ARTHROGRAPHY

**Definition.** Arthrography denotes the introduction of air or a radiopaque dye (and sometimes both) into a joint cavity to facilitate visualization of the joint structures. Although arthrography may be accomplished in any joint, it is frequently utilized in the knee.

**Indications for utilization.** The most common indications for the utilization of knee arthrography are (1) suspected meniscus tears or damage, (2) presence of loose bodies, (3) capsular leaks, and (4) other suspected internal derangements.[2,p.13;5,p.237;9,pp.77-78]

**Preprocedural care.** The procedure should be explained to the patient.

**Intraprocedural methodology.** Arthrography is accomplished under aseptic techniques to reduce risk of introduction of infection during the procedure. The procedure is accomplished as follows[5,p.237]:

1. Area is cleansed with antiseptic solution.
2. Area is draped with sterile towels, exposing the site of injection.
3. Soft tissues at the site of injection are infiltrated with a local anesthetic.
4. Joint capsule is entered with a needle.
5. Excess joint fluid is aspirated before injection.
6. Air or a radiopaque dye is injected into the joint capsule.
7. Needle is removed.
8. Motion of the joint is promoted through ambulation or passive exercise.
9. Joint is manipulated with fluoroscopic guidance.
10. Multiple films may be taken throughout the procedure.

**Postprocedural care.** Pain is not always associated with arthrography, but mild analgesics may be prescribed if pain is present. Strenuous exercise is discouraged for approximately 12 hours after the completion of the procedure.

## MYELOGRAPHY

**Definition.** Myelography is a diagnostic tool utilized to increase visualization of lesions or defects of the vertebral column by the introduction of a radiopaque dye into the subarachnoid space.

**Indications for utilization.** The following suspected diagnoses are indications for use of myelography: (1) herniated intervertebral discs, (2) spinal cord compression, (3) tumors, (4) vascular anomalies, and (5) bony structure defects.[2,p.13;9,p.75]

**Preprocedural care.** Because myelography is a lengthy procedure and requires the utilization of a special table, the procedure should be explained to the patient at length. He should also be prepared for the lumbar puncture utilized for introduction of the radiopaque dye. He will be given nothing to eat or drink before the procedure because of the tendency to become nauseated from either the tilting table or the lumbar puncture. Vital signs and neurovascular assessment should be accomplished before the procedure to provide a baseline for postprocedure comparison. Any metal item such as jewelry should be removed before the patient is taken to the radiology department. A preprocedural medication is usually given prior to the procedure.[5,p.29]

**Intraprocedural methodology.** The following steps are followed in the accomplishment of a myelogram:

1. Patient is appropriately positioned for a lumbar puncture (lateral recumbent position with knees flexed toward abdomen and head flexed toward chest).
2. Lumbar puncture is accomplished for injection of the radiopaque dye.
3. A small amount of cerebrospinal fluid is removed.
4. Patient is placed in a prone position.
5. Radiopaque dye is injected.
6. Table is appropriately tilted for proper examination of the suspected lesion in relation to the site of the lumbar puncture.
7. Multiple films are taken; repositioning is sometimes required throughout the procedure.
8. Tilting is accomplished to permit the radiopaque dye to collect near the site of the lumbar puncture.
9. Dye is removed via syringe.
10. Table is leveled.
11. Lumbar puncture needle is removed.
12. Adhesive bandage or very small dressing is placed over the site of the lumbar puncture.

**Postprocedural care.** Postprocedural care is designed to provide frequent monitoring of the patient's status to avoid or detect early signs of complications from the procedure. This care includes (1) neurovascular assessment and vital signs when the patient is returned to his room and frequently thereafter, (2) monitoring of intake and output, (3) the patient remaining flat in bed for 24 hours, and (4) encouragement of increased fluid intake.[5,p.30]

**Complications.** Complications related to myelography are urinary retention, headache, nausea or vomiting, dehydration, chemical meningitis, and radiopaque dye not entirely removed.

## PULMONARY FUNCTION TESTS

**Definition.** Pulmonary function tests (PFT) are diagnostic tools permitting measurement of the flow of air in and out of the lungs as well as lung compliance and diffusing capacity. *Vital capacity* is the total volume of air exhaled with forced expiration after a full inspiration. Under normal circumstances, with absence of pathologic pulmonary involvement or impingement, 80% of the volume is exhaled in 1 second. *Residual volume* is the amount of air that remains in the lung and cannot be removed with forceful expiration. *Total lung capacity* is the volume indicating the greatest capacity for lung inspiration.[6,p.38]

**Indications for utilization.** Pulmonary function tests are indicated under the following circumstances[5,p.161;6,p.99]:

1. Evaluation of preoperative pulmonary status
2. Baseline and follow-up information for patients having thoracic surgery, such as may be seen with anterior spinal fusion
3. Evaluation of thoracic deformities resulting in impingement on the pulmonary cavity
4. Follow-up for specific therapeutic pulmonary regimens

It must be emphasized that these diagnostic tests are not useful in diagnosing specific lesions but for determining the presence or absence of affected pulmonary function by a specific lesion or deformity.

**Preprocedural care.** The most crucial preprocedural preparation required for pulmonary function studies is accurate and extensive explanation provided to the patient. This is extremely important to his ability to cooperate and fully understand the instructions during the actual testing. Restrictive garments should not be worn as they may affect the pulmonary capacity and an inaccurate test result will occur. Preprocedural evaluation of medication should be accomplished, as some medications will affect the total pulmonary capacity and have a tendency to either inflate or deflate the test results.

**Intraprocedural methodology.** Pulmonary function tests provide a massive amount of information regarding not only lung volume but also the flow rates. The following are the specific lung volumes and capacities that are inclusive to this diagnostic tool[5,pp.162-163]:

tidal volume (TV) amount of air inhaled or exhaled during one respiratory cycle.
inspiratory reserve volume (IRV) maximum amount of air

after a normal inspiration that can be inspired from the end of the inspiratory cycle.
expiratory reserve volume (ERV) maximum amount of air during normal expiration that can be expired from the end of the expiratory cycle.
residual volume (RV) amount of air still remaining in the lungs after maximum expiration.
vital capacity (VC) amount of air that can be forcefully inhaled following a maximum expiration or forcefully exhaled following a maximum inspiration (VC = TV + IRV + ERV).
inspiratory capacity (IC) maximum amount of air that can be inspired from the end of the expiratory cycle (IC = TV + IRV).
total lung capacity (TLC) amount of air that remains in the lung following maximum inspiration (TLC = TV + IRV + ERV + RV).
functional residual capacity (FRC) amount of air still remaining in the lungs at the end of the expiratory cycle (FRC = ERV + RV).

Pulmonary function tests are performed as follows[5,pp.163-164]:

1. Patient is seated next to the spirometer, a machine that measures lung capacities and into which the patient breathes for the measurements.
2. Nose clips are applied.
3. Patient is instructed to put the mouthpiece in his mouth and to close his lips tightly around it.
4. For tidal volume he is requested to breathe normally.
5. For inspiratory reserve volume he is requested to take a normal inspiration and then continue with the inspiration until his lungs are completely filled.
6. For expiratory reserve volume he is requested to force all of the air out of his lungs after a normal expiration.
7. Vital capacity and inspiratory capacity are calculated from these determinations.
8. Residual volume, functional residual capacity, and total lung capacity may then be measured through a variety of methods indirectly.
9. Flow rates are then obtained by measurement of inspiratory and expiratory cycles with predetermined measurements of time, such as 1, 2, or 3 seconds.

**Postprocedural care.** No care is required after pulmonary function tests.

**Diagnostic implications.** Pulmonary function studies utilized in orthopedics are of greatest value with thoracic deformities (e.g., scoliosis, kyphoscoliosis), which may impinge on the normal pulmon-

**Table 10-3.** Normal pulmonary function tests

| Test | Age (yr) | | |
|---|---|---|---|
| | 20 to 39 | 40 to 59 | 60+ |
| VC (liters) | | | |
| Men | 3.35-5.90 | 2.72-5.30 | 2.42-4.70 |
| Women | 2.45-4.38 | 2.09-4.02 | 1.91-3.66 |
| FEV L | | | |
| Men | 3.11-4.64 | 2.45-3.98 | 2.09-3.32 |
| Women | 2.16-3.65 | 1.60-3.09 | 1.30-2.53 |
| FEV % (FEV/VC) | | | |
| Men | 77 | 70 | 60 |
| Women | 82 | 77 | 74 |
| Residual volume (liters) | | | |
| Men | 1.13-2.32 | 1.45-2.62 | 1.77-2.77 |
| Women | 1.00-2.00 | 1.16-2.20 | 1.32-2.40 |
| Total lung capacity (liters) | | | |
| Men | 4.80-7.92 | 4.50-7.62 | 4.35-7.32 |
| Women | 3.61-6.18 | 3.41-6.02 | 3.31-5.86 |

From Tilkian, S. M., and Conover, M. H.: Clinical implications of laboratory tests, St. Louis, 1975, The C. V. Mosby Co.

ary capacity. They may be utilized preoperatively or as a means of monitoring continued impingement characterized by progression of these deformities. It must again be emphasized that pulmonary function tests are not diagnostic of specific processes but of the pathologic results of the processes. Normal pulmonary function test results are given in Table 10-3.

## VENOGRAPHY (PHLEBOGRAPHY)

**Definition.** Venography is a radiographic diagnostic tool permitting the visualization of the lower extremity venous system.

**Indications for utilization.** The most frequent utilization of venography is for determination of presence or absence of thrombosis and general venous competence. Upper extremity venography may be accomplished, although it is rarely indicated as compared with the frequency of lower extremity venography.

**Preprocedural care.** The only preprocedural care required for venography is adequate explanation of the procedure to the patient.

**Intraprocedural methodology.** The position of the patient and the site of injection of radiopaque dye vary and are greatly dependent on the locality of symptomatology and the ease with which appropriate viewing may be accomplished. The following steps are associated with venographic procedures[5,pp.140-141]:

1. Venipuncture is accomplished, usually with a scalp vein needle, at the designated site.
2. Utilization of a local anesthetic is dependent on the site and the pain threshold of the client.
3. Radiopaque dye is injected by infusion or manually.
4. Fluoroscopic review is accomplished, and baseline films are obtained.
5. If tourniquets are utilized, they are removed after injection of the radiopaque dye.
6. Various activities are accomplished to promote venous filling.
7. Multiple films are obtained.
8. Patient is returned to the horizontal position.
9. Radiopaque dye is removed by exercise, elevation, massage of the extremity, or injection of normal saline.
10. Venipuncture needle is removed.
11. Pressure dressing is applied over the site of the venipuncture.

**Postprocedural care.** Alternating periods of involved extremity elevation and ambulatory exercise are advocated for total removal of radiopaque dye in an attempt to decrease any possibility of resulting irritation. A designated period of bed rest may be advocated before institution of these measures because of concern related to dislodging of the clot formation at the puncture site. Neurovascular assessments of the involved extremity should be accomplished frequently to assess its general status.

**Diagnostic implications.** The most frequent orthopedic implications of venography are those related to a suspected thrombus or need to further evaluate the general venous status.

## SUMMARY

As may be noted throughout the description of these special diagnostic procedures utilized frequently for the orthopedic patient, great emphasis is placed on the need for adequate explanation to the patient and his comprehension of the procedure to be accomplished, preferably before the procedure begins. This contributes greatly to decreasing anxiety frequently associated with some of these procedures and assists in the assurance of patient cooperation for the most accurate results possible. These diagnostic tools are utilized to varying degrees, but all personnel should be familiar with the procedural information to avoid the communication of erroneous information to the patient.

## REFERENCES

1. Bennington, J., Fouty, R. A., and Hongie, C.: Laboratory diagnosis, New York, 1970, Macmillan Publishing Co.
2. Gartland, J. J.: Fundamentals of orthopaedics, Philadelphia, 1974, W. B. Saunders Co.
3. Jackson, R., and Dandy, D.: Arthroscopy of the knee, New York, 1976, Grune & Stratton.
4. O'Conner, R.: Arthroscopy, Philadelphia, 1977, J. B. Lippincott Co.
5. Skydell, B., and Crowder, A. S.: Diagnostic procedures: a reference for health practitioners and a guide for patient counseling, Boston, 1975, Little, Brown & Co.
6. Tilkian, S. M., and Conover, M. H.: Clinical implications of laboratory tests, St. Louis, 1975, The C. V. Mosby Co.
7. Wallach, J.: Interpretation of diagnostic tests: a handbook synopsis of laboratory medicine, Boston, 1974, Little, Brown & Co.
8. Watanabe, M., Takeda, S., and Ikenchi, H.: Atlas of arthroscopy, New York, 1969, Grune & Stratton.
9. Zohn, D., and Mennell, J.: Musculoskeletal pain: diagnosis and physical treatment, Boston, 1976, Little, Brown & Co.

## BIBLIOGRAPHY

Adams, J. C.: Outline of orthopaedics, Baltimore, 1971, The Williams & Wilkins Co.

Beltham, W., et al.: Physical examination of the joints, Philadelphia, 1965, W. B. Saunders Co.

Bennington, J., Fouty, R. A. and Hongie, C.: Laboratory diagnosis, New York, 1970, Macmillan Publishing Co.

Brashear, H. R., Jr., and Raney, R. B., Sr.: Shands' handbook of orthopaedic surgery, St. Louis, 1971, The C. V. Mosby Co.

Delagi, E., et al.: Anatomic guide for the electromyographer, Springfield, Ill., 1975, Charles C Thomas, Publisher.

Gartland, J. J.: Fundamentals of orthopaedics, Philadelphia, 1974, W. B. Saunders Co.

Goodgold, J., and Dandy, D.: Arthroscopy of the knee, New York, 1976, Grune & Stratton.

Hirshata, K., and Morimoto, K.: Ultrastructure of bone and joint diseases, New York, 1971, Grune & Stratton.

Jackson, R., and Dandy, D.: Arthoscopy of the knee, New York, 1976, Grune & Stratton.

O'Conner, R.: Arthroscopy, Philadelphia, 1977, J. B. Lippincott Co.

Skydell, B., and Crowder, A. S.: Diagnostic procedures: a reference for health practitioners and a guide for patient counseling, Boston, 1975, Little, Brown & Co.

Tachdjian, M. O.: Pediatric orthopaedics, Philadelphia, 1972, W. B. Saunders Co.

Tilkian, S. M., and Conover, M. H.: Clinical implications of laboratory tests, St. Louis, 1975, The C. V. Mosby Co.

Turek, S.: Orthopaedics, Philadelphia, 1977, J. B. Lippincott Co.

Wallach, J.: Interpretation of diagnostic tests: a handbook synopsis of laboratory medicine, Boston, 1974, Little, Brown & Co.

Watanabe, M., Takeda, S., and Ikenchi, H.: Atlas of arthroscopy, New York, 1969, Grune & Stratton.

Zohn, D., and Mennell, J.: Musculoskeletal pain: diagnosis and physical treatment, Boston, 1976, Little, Brown & Co.

# 11

# Laboratory determinations

NANCY E. HILT

Although radiography is the most frequently utilized and most useful diagnostic tool for the orthopedic surgeon, it rarely provides *all* the information required to make an accurate diagnosis and differentially rule out all disease processes that may mimic similar signs and symptoms. In addition many primary musculoskeletal diseases and disorders have systemic manifestations that require assessment and evaluation through other tools, not to mention the multiple systemic manifestations of the many processes with musculoskeletal implications. To assess these manifestations, with their direct and indirect influences, laboratory procedures are critical to the total evaluation of any disease process.

Several aspects of laboratory procedures and determinations are significant within the specialty of orthopedics:

1. Preparation required for specific laboratory procedures
2. Appropriate handling of specimens
3. Normal value range of laboratory procedures
4. Indications for the procedures
5. Abnormal results in relation to our ability to differentially diagnosis pathologic processes

More often than not, it is a combination of results from laboratory procedures and other diagnostic tools that permits differential diagnosis. To facilitate comprehension and in an attempt to provide a more functional outline of these considerations, this information is organized in Tables 11-1 to 11-6.

## PREPARATION FOR LABORATORY PROCEDURES

Table 11-1 gives guidelines for the preparation required for laboratory procedures. Because of the difficulty in determining and categorizing the procedures used only in orthopedics—an impossibility when other implications frequently exist and must be acknowledged for implementation of comprehensive care—most procedures requiring preparation are included. Those not included in the table may be assumed to be those normally not requiring preparation. It must be recognized and emphasized that these are meant to be used as guidelines; some institutional variations may be noted. It is advisable to be familiar with the recommendations specifically required and desired by the laboratory directly handling the specimen.

## HANDLING OF SPECIMENS FOR LABORATORY PROCEDURES

*The reliability of any laboratory procedure is greatly dependent on the handling of the specimen.* Many health care personnel may be directly or indirectly responsible for various aspects of specimen care from the time it is obtained until it reaches the laboratory for processing. All such personnel should be thoroughly familiar with appropriate handling techniques for the particular specimen. Table 11-2 gives guidelines and recommendations for handling of laboratory specimens. It may be assumed that any procedure not listed in the table will not likely require special handling and that there may be some institutional variances from these guidelines.

**229**

*Text continued on p. 240.*

**Table 11-1.** Guidelines for laboratory procedures[1, pp. 8-92]

| Laboratory procedures | Preparation | Laboratory procedures | Preparation |
|---|---|---|---|
| Albumin-globulin ratio, serum | Withhold food<br>May have medications and water | D-xylose absorption | Withhold food and medications<br>May have water |
| Alkaline phosphatase, serum | Withhold food and medications<br>May have water | Electrolytes, serum | May be affected by medications |
| Activated partial thromboplastin time (APTT) | May be affected by medications | Eosinophil count, blood | May be affected by medications |
| Bilirubin, serum | Withhold food<br>May have medications and water | Free fatty acids, (FFA), blood | Withhold food, fluids, and medications for 12 hours<br>May have water |
| Bleeding time | May be affected by medications | Gastric analysis | Withhold food, fluids, medications, and water (NPO) |
| Blood gases | May be affected by medications | Gastrin, serum or plasma | Withhold food and medications |
| Bromsulphalein (BSP) | Withhold food<br>May have medications and water<br>May be affected by medications | Glucose, blood | May have water<br>Withhold food and medications<br>May have water<br>May be affected by medications |
| Calcium, serum | Withhold food<br>May have medications and water | Glucose, blood, postprandial | May be affected by medications |
| Catecholamines, urine | May be affected by medications | Glucose tolerance test | Withhold food and medications |
| Cephalin-cholesterol flocculation, serum | Withhold food<br>May have medications and water<br>*or*<br>Withhold food, fluids, and medications for 12 hours<br>May have water | Glucose, urine, qualitative | May have water<br>May be affected by medications<br>May be affected by medications |
| | | Hemoglobin | May be affected by medications |
| Clotting time, venous (Lee-White) | May be affected by medications | Iodine uptake | May be affected by medications |
| Diagnex blue | Withhold food and medications<br>May have water<br>May be affected by medications | Icterus index, serum | Withhold food<br>May have medications and water |
| | | Insulin, plasma or serum | Withhold food and medications<br>May have water |

**Table 11-1.** Guidelines for laboratory procedures — cont'd

| Laboratory procedures | Preparation | Laboratory procedures | Preparation |
|---|---|---|---|
| Insulin tolerance | Withhold food and medications<br>May have water | Phosphorus, serum | Withhold food<br>May have medications and water |
| Iron, serum | Withhold food<br>May have medications and water | Pregnancy test, urine | May be affected by medications, |
| Lactose tolerance | Withhold food<br>May have medications and water | Protein, total, plasma, or serum | Withhold food<br>May have medications and water |
| Lupus erythematosus (LE) cell test, blood | May be affected by medications | Phenolsulfonphthalein (PSP) test | Withhold food<br>May have medications and water |
| Lipids, total, serum | Withhold food<br>May have medications and water<br>*or*<br>Withhold food, fluids, and medications for 12 hours<br>May have water | Schilling test | Withhold food<br>May have medications and water<br>May be affected by medications |
| Lipoprotein electrophoresis, plasma | Withhold food and medications<br>May have water<br>*or*<br>Withhold food, fluids, and medications for 12 hours<br>May have water | Sugar, urine, qualitative | May be affected by medications |
| | | $T_3$, serum | May be affected by medications |
| | | $T_4$ | May be affected by medications |
| Melanin, urine, qualitative | May be affected by medications | Thorn test | Withhold food and medications<br>May have water |
| Metanephrines, urine | May be affected by medications | Thymol turbidity, serum | Withhold food<br>May have medications and water |
| Protein-bound iodine (PBI), serum | May be affected by medications | Triglycerides, serum | Withhold food, fluid, and medications for 12 hours<br>May have water |
| pH, urine | May be affected by medications | Vitamin $B_{12}$, serum | May be affected by medications |
| Phospholipids, serum | Withhold food<br>May have medications and water<br>*or*<br>Withhold food, fluid, and medications for 12 hours<br>May have water | | |

**Table 11-2.** Recommendations for specimen handling for laboratory procedures[1, pp. 8-92]

| Laboratory procedures | Specimen handling | Laboratory procedures | Specimen handling |
|---|---|---|---|
| Acid phosphatase, serum | Requires immediate attention of laboratory personnel<br>Prevent hemolysis | Carbon monoxide (carboxyhemoglobin), blood | Requires anticoagulant |
| Addis' test, urine | Total collection over a specific period<br>Requires preservative<br>Requires immediate attention of laboratory personnel | Carotene, serum | Requires immediate attention of laboratory personnel |
| | | Catecholamines, urine | Total collection over a specified period<br>Requires preservative<br>Refrigerate or ice during collection |
| Alcohol, ethyl, blood | Requires anticoagulant | Carcinoembryonic antigen (CEA), blood | Collect during laboratory hours<br>Requires immediate attention of laboratory personnel<br>Requires anticoagulant<br>Prevent hemolysis |
| Aldosterone, urine | Total collection over a specified period<br>Requires preservative<br>Refrigerate or ice during collection | | |
| Ammonia, blood | Requires immediate attention of laboratory personnel<br>Refrigerate or ice during collection | Cell count, cerebrospinal fluid | Requires immediate attention of laboratory personnel |
| | | Chloride, serum | Intravenous infusion directly affects results |
| Amylase, urine | Total collection over a specified period<br>Standard specimen container<br>Refrigerate or ice during collection | Cold agglutinins, serum | Collect during regular laboratory hours<br>Requires immediate attention of laboratory personnel |
| Activated partial thromboplastin time (APTT) | Requires immediate attention of laboratory personnel<br>Requires anticoagulant<br>Prevent hemolysis | Colloidal gold curve, cerebrospinal fluid | Requires immediate attention of laboratory personnel |
| | | Coproporphyrins, urine, quantitative | Total collection over a specified period<br>Requires preservative<br>Protect from light<br>Requires immediate attention of laboratory personnel |
| Butanol-extractable iodine (BEI), serum | X-ray contrast media alters results | | |
| Bence Jones protein, urine | Standard specimen container | | |
| Bilirubin, serum | Prevent hemolysis | | |
| Bilirubin, urine | Standard specimen container | Cortisol (hydrocortisone, compound F), plasma | Requires immediate attention of laboratory personnel<br>Requires anticoagulant |
| Blood gases | Requires immediate attention of laboratory personnel<br>Requires anticoagulant<br>Intravenous infusion directly affects results<br>Prevent hemolysis | Creatinine phosphokinase (CPK), serum | Prevent hemolysis |
| | | Creatinine clearance | Total collection over a specified period<br>Standard specimen container |
| Bromsulphalein (BSP) | X-ray contrast media alters results | Creatinine, urine | Total collection over a specified period<br>Standard specimen container |
| Calcium, urine, quantitative | Total collection over a specified period<br>Standard specimen container | | |
| | | Culture | Sterile specimen container |
| Calcium, urine, semi-quantitative | Single voided specimen<br>Standard specimen container | Cystine, urine, qualitative | Single voided specimen<br>Standard specimen container |

**Table 11-2.** Recommendations for specimen handling for laboratory procedures—cont'd

| Laboratory procedure | Specimen handling | Laboratory procedure | Specimen handling |
|---|---|---|---|
| Diagnex blue | Total collection over a specified period | | Refrigerate or ice during collection |
| | Standard specimen container | Hematocrit, blood | Requires anticoagulant |
| | X-ray contrast media alters results. | Hemoglobin, electrophoresis | Requires anticoagulant |
| Electrolyte, serum | Requires immediate attention of laboratory personnel | Hemoglobin, plasma | Requires immediate attention of laboratory personnel |
| | Intravenous infusion directly affects results | | Specimen requires anticoagulant |
| | | | Prevent hemolysis |
| Estriol, urine | Total collection over a specified period | Hemoglobin, urine | Single voided specimen |
| | Requires preservative | | Standard specimen container |
| | Refrigerate or ice during collection | | Collect during regular laboratory hours |
| Estrogens, total, urine | Total collection over a specified period | Hemosiderin, urine | Single voided specimen |
| | Requires preservative | | Standard specimen container |
| | Refrigerate or ice during collection | Homovanillic acid (HVA), urine, quantitative | Total collection over a specified period |
| Fat, feces, quantitative | Total collection over a specified period | | Requires preservative |
| | Refrigerate or ice during collection | 17-Hydroxycorticosteroids, total, urine | Total collection over a specified period |
| Fat, urine, qualitative | Single voided specimen | | Refrigerate or ice during collection |
| Fibrin degradation products (FDP), serum | Requires immediate attention of laboratory personnel | Iodine uptake | X-ray contrast media alters results |
| | Prevent hemolysis | Insulin, plasma or serum | Requires immediate attention of laboratory personnel |
| Fibrinogen, plasma | Requires anticoagulant | | |
| Fibrinolysins | Requires immediate attention of laboratory personnel | Iron, serum | Requires immediate attention of laboratory personnel |
| | Prevent hemolysis | | Prevent hemolysis |
| Folic acid, folate, serum | Requires immediate attention of laboratory personnel | Ketones, urine | Single voided specimen |
| | | | Standard specimen container |
| Follicle-stimulating hormone (FSH), urine | Total collection over a specified period | 17-Ketosteroids | Total collection over a specified period |
| Glucose-6-phosphate dehydrogenase (G6PD), blood | Collect during regular laboratory hours | | Requires preservative |
| | Requires anticoagulant | | Refrigerate or ice during collection |
| Galactose, urine, qualitative | Single voided specimen | Lactic dehydrogenase (LDH), serum | Requires immediate attention of laboratory personnel |
| | Standard specimen container | | |
| Gastrin, serum or plasma | Requires immediate attention of laboratory personnel | | Prevent hemolysis |
| | | Lipoprotein electrophoresis, plasma | Requires anticoagulant |
| Glucose, cerebrospinal fluid | Requires immediate attention of laboratory personnel | Magnesium, serum | Prevent hemolysis |
| | | Melanin, urine, qualitative | Single voided specimen |
| Glucose, urine, quantitative | Total collection over a specified period | | Standard specimen container |
| | Standard specimen container | | Collect during regular laboratory hours |

*Continued.*

**Table 11-2.** Recommendations for specimen handling for laboratory procedures—cont'd

| Laboratory procedure | Specimen handling | Laboratory procedure | Specimen handling |
|---|---|---|---|
| | Requires immediate attention of laboratory personnel | | Requires immediate attention of laboratory personnel |
| Metanephrines, urine | Total collection over a specified period | | Refrigerate or ice during collection |
| | Requires preservative | Porphyrins, urine, qualitative | Single voided specimen |
| Microscopic examination, urine | Single voided specimen | | Standard specimen container |
| | Standard specimen container | | Protect from light |
| | Collect during regular laboratory hours | | Collect during regular laboratory hours |
| Myoglobin, urine, qualitative | Single voided specimen | Potassium, serum | Intravenous infusion directly affects results |
| | Standard specimen container | | Prevent hemolysis |
| | Collect during regular laboratory hours | Potassium, urine | Total collection over a specified period |
| Nitroblue tetrazolium (NBT), blood | Requires immediate attention of laboratory personnel | | Standard specimen container |
| | Requires anticoagulant | Pregnancy test, urine | Single voided specimen |
| Osmolality, serum | Requires immediate attention of laboratory personnel | | Standard specimen container |
| Osmolality, urine | Single voided specimen | Protein, cerebrospinal fluid | Requires immediate attention of laboratory personnel |
| | Standard specimen container | Protein, urine, qualitative | Single voided specimen |
| | Requires immediate attention of laboratory personnel | | Standard specimen container |
| Protein-bound iodine (PBI), serum | X-ray contrast media alters results | Protein, urine, quantitative | Total collection over a specified period |
| pH, urine | Single voided specimen | | Standard specimen container |
| | Standard specimen container | Prothrombin consumption test, blood serum | Requires immediate attention of laboratory personnel |
| | Requires immediate attention of laboratory personnel | | Prevent hemolysis |
| Phenothiazines, urine | Single voided specimen | Prothrombin time, plasma | Requires immediate attention of laboratory personnel |
| | Standard specimen container | | Requires anticoagulant |
| Phosphorus, serum | Requires immediate attention of laboratory personnel | | Prevent hemolysis |
| | | Phenolsulfonphthalein (PSP) test | Standard specimen container |
| | Intravenous infusion directly affects results | Parathyroid hormone (PTH), serum | Requires immediate attention of laboratory personnel |
| | Prevent hemolysis | Red blood cell count, | Requires anticoagulant |
| Pituitary gonadotropins, urine | Total collection over a specified period | Renin, blood | Requires immediate attention of laboratory personnel |
| | Refrigerate or ice during collection | Schilling test | Total collection over a specified period |
| Platelet count, blood | Requires anticoagulant | | Standard specimen container |
| Porphobilinogen, urine, quantitative | Total collection over a specified period | | |
| | Protect from light | Sedimentation rate, blood | Requires anticoagulant |

**Table 11-2.** Recommendations for specimen handling for laboratory procedures—cont'd

| Laboratory procedure | Specimen handling | Laboratory procedure | Specimen handling |
|---|---|---|---|
| Semen analysis | Collect during regular laboratory hours | | Requires immediate attention of laboratory personnel |
| | Requires immediate attention of laboratory personnel | Thrombin time, plasma | Requires immediate attention of laboratory personnel |
| Serum glutamic oxaloacetic transaminase (SGOT) | Prevent hemolysis | | Requires anticoagulant |
| Serum glutamic pyruvic transaminase (SGPT) | Prevent hemolysis | Trypsin, stool | Prevent hemolysis |
| | | | Standard specimen container |
| Sodium, serum | Intravenous infusion directly affects results | | Collect during regular laboratory hours |
| Sodium, urine | Total collection over a specified period | Uric acid, urine, quantitative | Total collection over a specified period |
| | Standard specimen container | | Standard specimen container |
| Specific gravity, urine | Single voided specimen | Urinalysis, routine | Single voided specimen |
| | Standard specimen container | | Standard specimen container |
| | X-ray contrast media alters results | | Collect during regular laboratory hours |
| Sugar, urine, qualitative | Single voided specimen | Watson-Schwartz test | Single voided specimen |
| | Standard specimen container | | Standard specimen container |
| Thromboplastin generation time (TGT), blood | Requires immediate attention of laboratory personnel | | Protect from light |
| | Prevent hemolysis | | Requires immediate attention of laboratory personnel |
| Three-glass test, urine | Standard specimen container | White blood cell count | Requires anticoagulant |

**Table 11-3.** Laboratory procedures and their musculoskeletal implications

| Test | Variance | Clinical implications |
|---|---|---|
| **Blood chemistry** | | |
| Alkaline phosphatase, total serum | ↑ (marked) without liver disease | Paget's disease of bone |
| | ↑ (marked) | Carcinoma with bone metastasis |
| | ↑ (mild) without liver disease and with hypercalcemia | Hyperparathyroidism |
| | ↑ (mild to moderate) with N or ↓ Ca | Osteomalacia |
| Calcium, serum | N with marked ↓ albumin | Hypercalcemia |
| | N with ↑ BUN | Primary or secondary hyperparathyroidism |
| | ↑ with ↓ phosphorus and N BUN | Hyperparathyroidism |
| | ↑ with ↑ gamma globulin | Sarcoidosis, multiple myeloma, malignancies with possible metastasis to bone |
| | ↑ | Severe thyrotoxicosis |
| | ↑ | Malignant tumors with or without bone metastasis |
| | ↑ | Bone fractures |
| | ↑ with ↑ alkaline phosphatase | Paget's disease of bone |
| | ↓ with ↓ albumin fraction of serum protein | Pseudohypocalcemia |
| | ↓ with ↑ phosphorus, N BUN, N creatinine | Hypoparathyroidism |
| | ↓ | Osteomalacia (adults), rickets (children) |
| | ↓ | Respiratory alkalosis |
| Cholesterol, total serum | ↓ (marked) | Diet and malnutrition |
| | ↓ (marked) | Hyperthyroidism |
| Blood glucose | ↑ | Diabetes mellitus |
| | ↑ (mild) with ↑ blood catecholamines | Acute stress |
| | ↑ (mild) with ↑ glucocorticoids | Cushing's syndrome (hyperadrenalism, secondary hyperadrenalism) |
| | ↑ (mild) with ↓ cholesterolemia | Hyperthyroidism |
| | ↑ (moderate) | Diabetes mellitus |
| | ↓ | Pituitary hypofunction |
| Lactic dehydrogenase, serum | ↑ (mild) | Pneumonia, pulmonary emboli |
| | ↑ (mild) | Generalized viral infections |
| | ↑ (mild) | Cerebrovascular accident |
| Phosphorus | ↑ with ↓ Ca, N BUN, N creatinine | Hypoparathyroidism |
| | ↓ with ↑ Ca, N BUN, N creatinine | Hyperparathyroidism |
| | ↓ with N or ↓ Ca and ↑ alkaline phosphatase | Rickets (children), osteomalacia (adults) |
| Potassium, plasma | ↓ with ↑ CO combining power | Cushing's syndrome |
| | ↓ | Anti-inflammatory drugs |
| | ↓ | Poor diet |
| | ↓ | Chronic stress |

Adapted from Tilkian, S. M., and Conover, M. H.: Clinical implications of laboratory tests, St. Louis, 1975, The C. V. Mosby Co.
N, normal; ↑ elevated; ↓ depressed.

**Table 11-3.** Laboratory procedures and their musculoskeletal implications—cont'd

| Test | Variance | Clinical implications |
|---|---|---|
| | ↓ | Chronic diarrhea |
| | ↓ | Diaphoresis |
| | ↓ | Chronic fever |
| Total protein and albumin/ globulin ratio, serum | N with ↓ albumin and ↑ globulin (reversed A/G ratio) | Myeloproliferative diseases, chronic granulomatous infectious diseases |
| Sodium, serum | ↑ with hyperglycemia | Hypothalamic lesion, head trauma, hyperosmolar states |
| | ↓ with ↓ Cl | Vomiting, diarrhea, tube drainage |
| | ↓ | Diaphoresis, burns |
| Serum glutamic oxaloacetic transaminase | ↑ (mild) | Cirrhosis, cholangiolitic jaundice, metastatic liver disease, skeletal muscle disease, posttrauma, generalized infections, dissecting aneurysm, pulmonary infarction, shock, pericarditis |
| Uric acid, serum | ↑ with acute arthritis | Gout |
| | ↑ (mild) | Idiopathic |
| **Hematology** | | |
| White blood cell count | ↑ (mild to moderate) | Infectious disease, mainly bacterial and moderate |
| | ↑ (mild to moderate) | Severe sepsis in elderly persons |
| | ↑ (marked) | Severe sepsis |
| Red blood cell count | ↑ (primary) | Polycythemia vera (leukemia) |
| Differential WBC count Neutrophils | ↑ (mild to moderate) | Bacterial infections, inflammatory disorders, tumors, physical and emotional stress (heat, extreme cold, exercise, electroshock therapy, emotional stimuli), drugs (catecholamines, corticosteroids) |
| Eosinophils | ↑ (90%) | Eosinophilic leukemia |
| | ↓ | Acute and chronic stress (emotional or physical), endocrine causes (excess ACTH, cortisone, epinephrine, intermenstrual period, diurnal variations, acromegaly) |
| Basophils | ↑ | Myeloproliferative disease |
| | ↓ | Anaphylactic reaction |
| | ↓ | Acute hypersensitive reactions, steroids, diurnal changes, hyperthyroidism, pituitary basophilism, radiation therapy, acute and chronic infection, ovulation, pregnancy, aging |
| Lymphocytes | ↑ (80% to 90%) with ↑ (marked) leukocytes | Chronic lymphocytic leukemia |
| | In bacterial infections, ↑ (mild to moderate) with ↑ (mild to moderate) leukocytes | Chronic infectious state |
| **Peripheral smear** | | |
| Platelets | Absolute absence | Aplastic bone marrow, thrombocytopenia (various causes) |
| | ↑ | Polycythemia, splenectomy status, essential thrombocytosis |

*Continued.*

**Table 11-3.** Laboratory procedures and their musculoskeletal implications—cont'd

| Test | Variance | Clinical implications |
|---|---|---|
| **Peripheral smear—cont'd** | | |
| Hemoglobin | ↓ | Anemia |
| Additional findings | Rouleaux formation | Multiple myeloma, macroglobulinemia |
| | ↑Neutrophils, ↑ band forms and toxic granulations | Severe infection |
| | Eosinophilia | Allergy reaction |
| | Blast (primitive) forms | Acute leukemia |
| **Urinalysis** | | |
| Specific gravity | ↓ with ↑ Ca ↓ K | Hypokalemic and hypercalcemic nephropathy |
| Glucose, qualitative | Glycosuria with ↑ blood glucose | Diabetes mellitus |
| Protein, qualitative | Proteinuria (trace) | Follow-up indicated |
| | Proteinuria (more than trace) | Twenty-four hour quantitative urine analysis indicated |
| Microscopic examination | | |
| Crystals | Present with amorphous substances and ↑ uric acid | Possible gouty nephropathy |
| | Calcium oxalate crystals with ↑ serum calcium | Suggest hypercalcemia |
| Color | Dark | Hematuria, bilirubinuria, hemoglobinuria, urobilinuria, porphyria |

**Table 11-4.** Summary of chemical features of diseases with disturbed plasma, calcium, and phosphate

| Disease | Serum | | | Urine | |
|---|---|---|---|---|---|
| | Calcium | Phosphate | Alkaline phosphatase | Calcium | Phosphate |
| Hyperparathyroidism | Increased | Decreased | Normal or increased | Increased | Increased |
| Paget's disease | Normal | Normal | Increased | Normal | Normal |
| Hypoparathyroidism | Decreased | Increased | Normal | Decreased | Decreased |
| Renal insufficiency | Decreased | Increased | Normal or increased | Decreased | Decreased |
| Osteomalacia | Decreased or normal | Decreased | Increased | Decreased | Decreased |
| Senile osteoporosis | Normal | Normal | Normal | Normal | Normal |
| Multiple myeloma | Normal or increased | Normal | Normal | Normal or increased | Normal or decreased |
| Milk-alkali syndrome | Increased | Normal or increased | Normal | Normal or decreased | Normal or decreased |
| Vitamin-D intoxication | Increased | Increased | Normal | Increased | Decreased |
| Metastatic carcinoma | Normal or increased | Normal | Normal or increased | Increased | Normal |
| Sarcoidosis | Increased | Normal or increased | Normal or increased | Increased | Decreased |
| Hyperventilation (alkalosis) | Normal | Normal | Normal | Normal | Normal |

From Bernstein, D. B., and Thorn, G. W. In Wintrobe, M. M., et al., editors: Harrison's principles of internal medicine, ed. 7, New York, 1977, McGraw-Hill Book Co.

**Table 11-5.** Methods of joint fluid examination

| Procedure; amount needed | Container | Test |
|---|---|---|
| Gross and microscopic examination for crystals; approximately 1.5 ml | Any clean, plain test tube | Appearance (e.g., bloody, straw colored, clear, turbid). Does a spontaneous clot appear? Clot size? Crystals (uric acid, calcium pyrophosphate). Pipette a drop, including some clot if present, onto slide and examine microscopically under polarized light for birefringent crystals; visible in plain light too.<br>Mucin: centrifuge to remove clot and cells. To a small volume of supernate add 4 volumes of 1.25% acetic acid. Shake gently. Let stand 1 hour. Observe, shake gently, and read. Report "good mucin" if tight, ropy clump, precipitate, and clear supernate. Report "very poor mucin" if no clot and flecks of precipitate in a cloudy fluid. |
| Cytologic examination; approximately 1 ml | Hematology tubes with buffered oxalate or EDTA anticoagulants | Cell count carried out with counting chamber. Dilute, if needed, with normal saline in a WBC pipette. Acetic acid will cause precipitation. RBC and WBC are distinguished and counted in same chamber. Chamber differential should be attempted.<br>Leukocytes measured if fluid is grossly purulent in Wintrobe hematocrit tube. Smearpack cells by centrifugation; after resuspending in a small volume, smear and stain, one with Wright's and one with Gram's stain. Do differential. |
| Chemical examination; approximately 2 ml | Blood sugar tube with anticoagulant | Send to chemistry laboratory for sugar determination. A simultaneous blood sample is also sent for blood sugar testing. |
| Microbiologic examination; remaining fluid | Culture tube | Send to microbiology laboratory. Orders will depend on nature of disease. Proving neisserian infection is made more likely by early plating. Possible tuberculous fluids should be allowed to clot in sterile vessel. Request anaerobic culture if indicated. |

From Bennington, J., Fouty, R., and Hongie, C.: Laboratory diagnosis, New York, 1970, Macmillan, Inc.

**Table 11-6.** Implications of joint fluid examination

| Diagnosis | Appearance | Mucin clot | WBC/cu mm | PMN (%) | Sugar (100 ml) | Special |
|---|---|---|---|---|---|---|
| Normal | Clear | Good | 60 | 7 | 10 | |
| Trauma | Bloody or clear | Good | 1,250 | 5 | 5 | Cartilage fibers |
| Disseminated joint disease | Clear | Good | 750 | | 0 | Cartilage fibers |
| Gout | Turbid | Poor | 13,000 | 71 | 12 | Uric acid crystal* |
| Rheumatoid arthritis | Turbid | Poor | 14,000-50,000 | 65 | 26 | RA cell |
| Tuberculosis | Turbid | Poor | 19,000 | 60 | 60 | Culture |
| Septic arthritis | Turbid | Very poor | 73,000 | 90 | 71 | Culture |
| Chondrocalcinosis (pseudogout)* | Clear | Poor | 13,000 | Nl | 12 | Calcium pyrophosphorus crystals |
| Reiter's disease | Clear | Poor | 14,000 | Nl | 12 | |

From Bennington, J., Fouty, R., and Hongie, C.: Laboratory diagnosis, New York, 1970, Macmillan, Inc.
*Calcium pyrophosphate crystals are weakly birefringent and are not digested by uricase. These microcrystals produce a disorder simulating gout or septic arthritis.

## MUSCULOSKELETAL IMPLICATIONS OF LABORATORY PROCEDURES

The implications of laboratory procedure results are always relative to the normal range established and accepted by the laboratory accomplishing the procedure. For this reason, variances refer to the ranges for normal values in most cases. The results and their implications are also relative to and used in conjunction with other diagnostic tools, including the history and physical examination, in order that an adequate and accurate diagnosis be concluded. Only the most common musculoskeletal implications are reflected. Normal laboratory values may be reviewed in Appendix I.

## SUMMARY

Results of laboratory procedures reviewed here may generally be considered indicative of specific diagnoses. It cannot be stressed enough, however, that differential diagnostic techniques are important in relation to other clinical findings such as radiographic findings and the physical examination. Laboratory procedures are not only critical to the establishment of definitive diagnoses but also to our ability to monitor progression, regression, and general effects of treatment modalities.

## REFERENCES

1. Strand, M. M., and Elmer, L. A.: Clinical laboratory tests: a manual for nurses, St. Louis, 1976, The C. V. Mosby Co.
2. Tilkian, S., and Conover, M.: Clinical implications of laboratory tests, St. Louis, 1975, The C. V. Mosby Co.

## BIBLIOGRAPHY

Adams, J. C.: Outline of orthopaedics, Baltimore, 1971, The Williams & Wilkins Co.

Bennington, J., Fouty, R., and Hongie, C.: Laboratory diagnosis, New York, 1970, Macmillan, Inc.

Bernstein, D. S., and Thorn, G. W. In Wintrobe, M. M., et al. (editors): Harrison's principles of internal medicine, ed. 6, New York, 1970, McGraw-Hill Book Co.

Eastham, R. D.: A laboratory guide to clinical diagnosis, Chicago, 1976, Year Book Medical Publishers.

Gartland, J. J.: Fundamentals of orthopaedics, Philadelphia, 1972, W. B. Saunders Co.

Holt, S.: Laboratory aids in diagnosis, Baltimore, 1971, The Williams & Wilkins Co.

Ravel, R.: Clinical laboratory medicine: application of laboratory data, Chicago, 1973, Year Book Medical Publishers.

Skydell, B., and Crowder, A.: Diagnostic procedures: a reference for health practitioners and a guide for patient counseling, Boston, 1975, Little, Brown & Co.

Strand, M. M., and Elmer, L. A.: Clinical laboratory tests: a manual for nurses, St. Louis, 1976, The C. V. Mosby Co.

Tachdjian, M. O.: Pediatric orthopedics, Philadelphia, 1972, W. B. Saunders Co.

Tilkian, S., and Conover, M.: Clinical implications of laboratory tests, St. Louis, 1975, The C. V. Mosby Co.

Turek, S.: Orthopaedics, Philadelphia, 1977, J. B. Lippincott Co.

Wallach, J.: Interpretation of diagnostic tests: a handbook synopsis of laboratory medicine, Boston, 1974, Little, Brown & Co.

Widmann, F.: Clinical interpretation of laboratory tests, Philadelphia, 1973, F. A. Davis Co.

# 12

# Pathology

**NANCY E. HILT**

Process: gross pathology
   Inflammatory processes
   Neoplastic process
Procedure: biopsy
Analysis: microscopic pathology
Summary

The term *pathology* refers to several things: a process, a procedure, and the combined results of the process and procedure. As a diagnostic tool, pathology reflects the comparison of normal and pathologic tissue changes that assist in definitive diagnosis. The processes of concern here are those that most frequently produce tissue alterations resulting in defined symptomatology; of particular importance are the *inflammatory* and *neoplastic processes* of the musculoskeletal system. The procedure, of great diagnostic value to the orthopedic diagnostician, is the *biopsy*, permitting microscopic tissue examination that, enhanced by the history, physical examination, laboratory tests, and radiographic examination, considerably increases one's ability to accurately and definitively diagnose specific processes. Pathologic implications of many musculoskeletal processes are reflected in the preceding chapters on other diagnostic tools; reviewed here are those specific to microscopic and to a lesser degree tissue examination.

## PROCESS: GROSS PATHOLOGY

As a diagnostic tool, microscopic tissue examination of the musculoskeletal system is relative to the gross pathology, which establishes an essential "norm" for this system. Many of these features may be reviewed in Chapters 1 and 2. Microscopic tissue examination is used most often in the diagnosis of inflammatory or neoplastic processes. Specific characteristics of both processes are reviewed from a gross pathology view for diagnostic purposes.

### Inflammatory processes

Stages of inflammatory processes of the musculoskeletal system are reflected in the gross appearance of the tissue being examined, for example, *acute, subacute*, or *chronic* stages (Table 12-1). In acute inflammation there is erythema followed by exudation, which may be of a serous, fibrinous, or purulent nature. When tissue destruction occurs an abscess may form. The process of healing may occur through resolution or fibrous tissue replacement. If temporary granulation tissue is identified, the pro-

**Table 12-1.** Gross pathologic characteristics of stages of inflammatory process[1,pp.22-25]

| Stage | Characteristics |
|---|---|
| Acute | Erythema resulting from vascular congestion |
| | Exudation |
| |   Serous |
| |   Fibrinous (pinkish tan) |
| |   Purulent (yellow) |
| Subacute | Erythematous firm tissue |
| | Granulation tissue (capillaries and fibroblastic connective tissue) |
| Necrotic | Destruction of tissue |
| | Formation of grossly observable cystic abscesses |
| | Abscesses contain yellow purulent exudate |
| | May heal completely by fibrous tissue replacement |
| | May progress to chronic stage |
| Chronic | Grayish white firm tissue indicating fibrous scarring |
| | Occasionally, presence of yellow foci indicating presence of cellular breakdown products |
| | Occasionally white chalky deposits indicating calcification |
| Combined | Combination of characteristics of two or more stages |
| | Indicative of persistent inflammatory process |
| Complete resolution | No tissue destruction |
| | Normal gross appearance regained |

cess is in a subacute stage. The chronic inflammatory stage is characterized by erythematous tissue and is always preceded by the acute or subacute stage.

### Neoplastic process

Some neoplastic stages may be difficult to differentiate from inflammatory processes. Table 12-2 gives gross pathologic differentiation characteristics. Additional differentiation, when considering gross pathologic features of the neoplastic process as a separate entity, must encompass the diagnostic characteristics of the benign neoplastic process. The most outstanding characteristic of the benign neoplastic process is the presence of encapsulation or circumscription, while the malignant neoplastic process reveals infiltration into surrounding tissues. Some malignant neoplasms are known to produce pseudoencapsulation, which on microscopic examination reveals tissue infiltration.[1,pp.37-41] Further differentiation is characterized by clinical course, radiographic and microscopic examination.

**Table 12-2.** General gross diagnostic criteria for differentiation of inflammatory and neoplastic processes

| Criteria | Inflammatory process | Neoplastic process |
| --- | --- | --- |
| Weight and size | Organ or tissue may be of normal, increased, or decreased weight and size. Increase in weight and size is explained by inflammatory cellular and fluid accumulation, decrease by atrophy of the organ or tissue. | Organ or tissue is usually of increased weight and size due to presence of new growth. |
| Shape | Organ or tissue usually maintains normal shape unless destruction of tissue occurs with formation of abscesses or scarring. Masses, polyps, and cysts may form. | Organ or tissue usually has altered shape due to presence of new growth. Occasionally when there is diffuse cellular infiltration, as in leukemia, shape of organ is maintained, while size is increased. Masses, polyps, and cysts may form. |
| Color | Inflammatory lesions vary in color depending on chronologic stage of process: Acute: red (due to vascular congestion); pinkish tan (due to fibrinous exudate); yellow (due to purulent exudate). Subacute: red (due to granulation tissue with prominent vascularization). Chronic: yellow (due to accumulation of histiocytes with lipid breakdown products); grayish white (due to fibrosis). | Frequently grayish white. Neoplastic lesions may have various colors due to pigments produced by tumors or due to superimposed inflammatory and ischemic changes. |
| Consistency | Inflammatory lesions may be soft (due to necrosis of parenchymal cells and abscess formation), firm (due to fibrous scarring), or of an in-between consistency. Hardness in an inflammatory lesion may be due to deposition of calcium salts or formation of bone. | Neoplastic lesions may be soft (due to cellularity of lesions with absence of fibrous stroma or necrosis), firm (due to a prominent fibrous stroma), or of an in-between consistency. Hardness in a neoplastic lesion may be due to deposition of calcium salts or formation of bone. |
| Architecture | Organ and tissue cut-surface parenchymal architectural pattern usually preserved unless there is tissue destruction with subsequent abscess formation or fibrous scarring. Ulcer may be present, which on cut surface has a base extending to the normally present underlying architectural structures. | Organ and tissue cut-surface parenchymal architectural pattern is usually replaced by neoplastic process. Occasionally architectural pattern may be preserved, as in leukemic infiltration. Presence or absence or infiltration of lesion into surrounding tissue will usually distinguish benign from malignant neoplasms. Ulcer may be present, which on cut surface has base and walls composed of tumor tissue obliterating normal architectural structures. |
| Location | Usually diffuse involvement of parenchyma or surface and lining membranes of organ or tissue. Focal lesions may also occur. | Usually focal involvement of parenchyma or surface and lining membranes of organ or tissue. Diffuse lesions may also occur. |

From Grossman, I. W.: A primer of gross pathology, Springfield, Ill., 1972, Charles C Thomas, Publisher.

## PROCEDURE: BIOPSY

Gross pathologic features of any musculoskeletal process are determined through exploratory surgery combined with results of radiographic and physical examination. Microscopic tissue examination is accomplished through a *biopsy*, the surgical obtainment of muscular, synovial, or osseous tissue for diagnostic purposes.

Muscular biopsy is most frequently indicated for symptomatology indicative of selected suspected muscle diseases. Many processes, however, do not show definitive diagnostic data on biopsy. Of those that do, the following are some of the most common[3,p.188]:

1. Myasthenia gravis: muscle biopsy reveals lymph.
2. Polymyositis: muscle biopsy reveals neurosis with phagocytosis of fibers and infiltration of inflammatory cells.
3. Muscular dystrophy: muscle biopsy reveals various degenerative changes, late muscle atrophy, and no cellular infiltration.

Synovial biopsy is of most value in the differential diagnosis of inflammatory and arthritic processes. It is as valuable, or more so with the arthritic processes, as a supportive and progressive method of monitoring involvement.

Muscular and synovial biopsy may be accomplished with the patient under local anesthesia, although to facilitate cooperation and additional therapeutic or exploratory procedures general anesthesia is frequently used. With biopsy there is risk of infection, hemorrhage, and minimal to moderate degrees of pain.

The most frequently utilized biopsy of the musculoskeletal system is the *bone biopsy*. The procedure is considered to be more severe in relation to risk involved and is, when utilized diagnostically, accomplished with the patient under general anesthesia. Osseous tissue specimens are necessary for microscopic confirmation of infection and neoplasms. Therapeutic surgical intervention is frequently accomplished immediately after the biopsy procedure.

When accomplished for diagnostic purposes, the site is dependent on the area of the symptomatology. Frozen or demineralized paraffin-imbedded biopsy specimens may be used for the microscopic identification of neoplastic processes identified on radiographic examination.[2,p.62] Success of definitive diagnosis from biopsy is sometimes questionable and must therefore be accompanied by other data that might assist in this effort.

## ANALYSIS: MICROSCOPIC PATHOLOGY

The analysis of biopsy results is reflected in the microscopic pathologic features of the examination and, in many instances, these features are combined with the gross pathologic and other clinical features. Neoplastic microscopic characteristics of individual cells and differential combined benign and malignant neoplastic characteristics are given in Tables 12-3 and 12-4. Selected microscopic characteristics of musculoskeletal pathologic processes are shown in Figs. 12-1 through 12-4.

*Text continued on p. 252.*

**Table 12-3.** Ultrastructure of malignant cells

| Cell structure | Characteristics |
| --- | --- |
| Nucleus | |
| Size | Variable, may be enlarged |
| Shape | Irregular, deep indentations of nuclear membrane |
| Chromatin | Irregularities of heterochromatin; euchromatin may predominate |
| Nucleolus | Enlarged, multiple |
| Mitosis | Often irregular |
| Mitochondria | |
| Number | Often decreased, but may be normal or increased |
| Shape | Irregular |
| Size | Often small |
| Ribosomes | |
| Free | Increased |
| Bound | Decreased |
| Endoplasmic reticulum | Usually decreased |
| Golgi apparatus | Variable |
| Lysosomes | Variable |
| Cytoplasmic inclusions | Often present |
| Oncogenic viruses | Seen in animal tumors |

From Damjanov, I.: General pathology, Flushing, N.Y., 1976, Medical Examination Publishing Co., Inc.

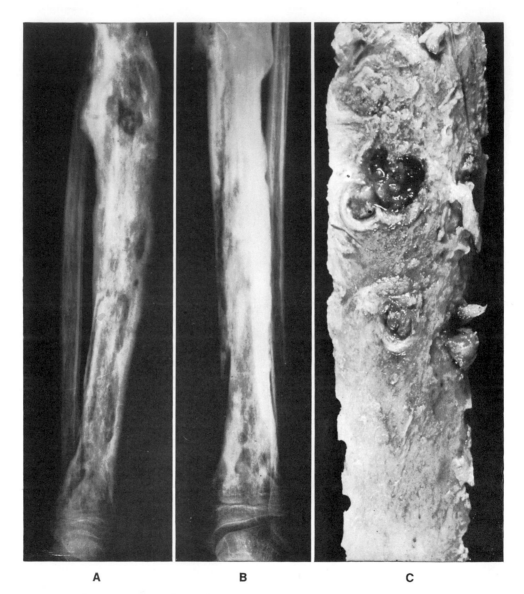

A          B          C

**Fig. 12-1.** Skeletal sepsis. **A** and **B,** Lateral and anteroposterior roentgenograms showing destructive and proliferative changes of long-standing pyogenic osteomyelitis. Sequestrated segments of original tibial shaft visible through shadows cast by ossified granulation tissue (involucrum). **C,** Specimen of bone removed from tibia illustrated in **A** and **B.** Granulation tissue–filled sinus openings clearly evident on external surface of bone. These sinuses formed communications between skin surfaces and sequestrum enclosed in bony cavity. (From Anderson, W. A. D., and Kissane, J. M.: Pathology, ed. 7, St. Louis, 1977, the C. V. Mosby Co.)

**Table 12-4.** Comparison of benign and malignant neoplasms

| Characteristic | Benign | Malignant |
|---|---|---|
| Growth | | |
|   Rate | Slow, may stop or regress, limited | Rapid, progressive |
|   Mode | Expansive | Invasive |
|   Metastasis | None | Frequent |
| Gross appearance | Encapsulated, uniform, regular | Poorly demarcated, mottled, frequent central necrosis |
| Microscopic appearance | | |
|   Architecture | Resembles tissue of origin | Disorganized |
|   Cells | Uniform, normal size and shape | Polymorphous, atypical, enlarged |
|   Nuclei | Normochromic | Hyperchromic, large, irregular |
|   Nucleolus | Inconspicuous | Enlarged or multiple |
|   Nucleocytoplasmic ratio | Normal | Increased |
|   Mitotic figures | Few | Many, often irregular |
| Biologic effects | | |
|   Local | Compression | Compression and destruction |
|   Distant | None | Cachexia, metabolic and mechanical consequences related to metastasis or primary tumor |

From Damjanov, I.: General pathology, Flushing, N.Y., 1976, Medical Examination Publishing Co. Inc.

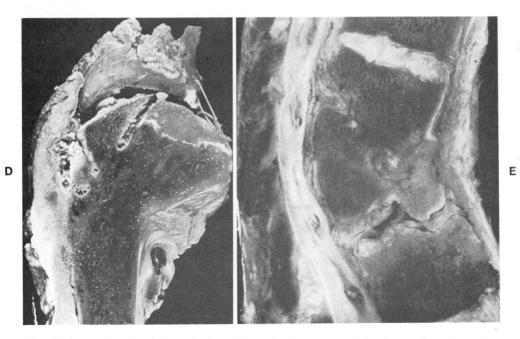

**Fig. 12-1, cont'd. D,** Tuberculosis of hip joint has resulted in destruction of most of femoral caput and acetabular cup. Tuberculous osteomyelitis with extension of sinus tracts into adjacent articular capsule and soft tissues evident on left. **E,** Compression of vertebrae with angulation of spine has resulted from tuberculous osteomyelitis that affected three vertebral bodies and two intervertebral discs.

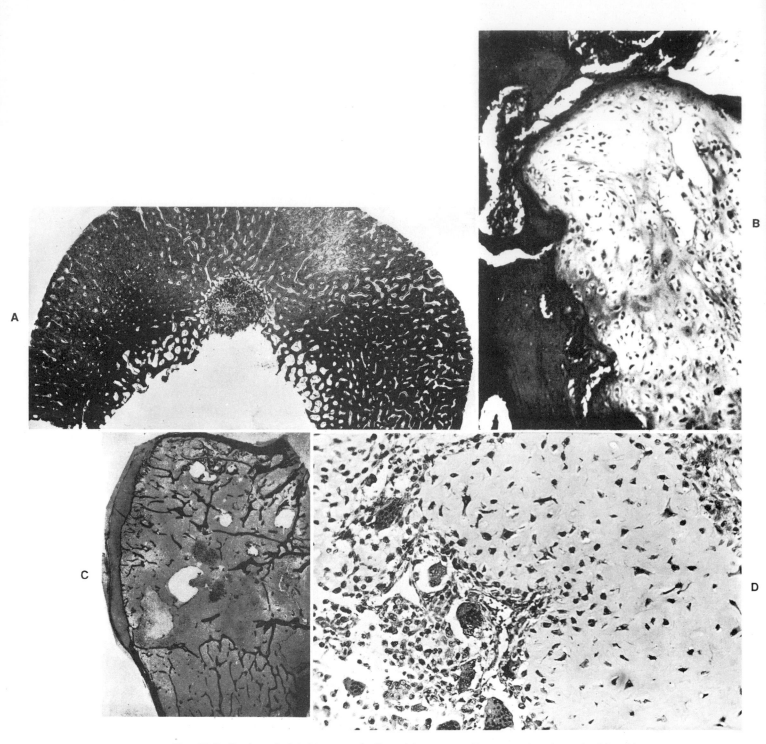

**Fig. 12-2.** Benign skeletal tumors. **A,** Osteoid osteoma. Cross section through nidus. Note thickening and condensation of surrounding cortical bone. **B,** Structural and cytologic features of typical enchondroma. (x130; AFIP 90709.) **C,** Flat osteochondroma of upper end of femur. Note perichondrial layer, growing cartilage, and irregular trabecular bone that has resulted from imperfect endochondral ossification. **D,** Chondromxzoid fibroma showing giant cells, cartilage, and cellular zones. (x200.) (From Anderson, W. A. D., and Kissane, J. M.: Pathology, ed. 7, St. Louis, 1977, The C. V. Mosby Co.)

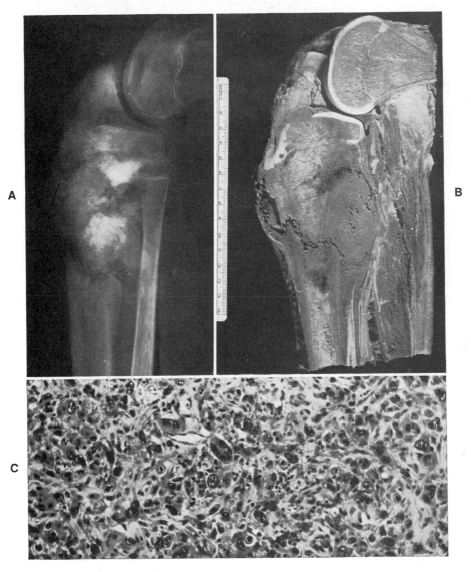

**Fig. 12-3.** Malignant skeletal tumors. **A** and **B,** Destructive and rapidly growing sarcoma of tibia that has resulted in pathologic fracture. **C,** Variation in size and shape of cells, bizarre mitoses, and little or no evidence of bone matrix formation are noteworthy features in this lytic form of osteosarcoma. (x165; AFIP 73613.) (From Anderson, W. A. D., and Kissane, J. M.: Pathology, ed. 7, St. Louis, 1977, The C. V. Mosby Co.)

*Continued.*

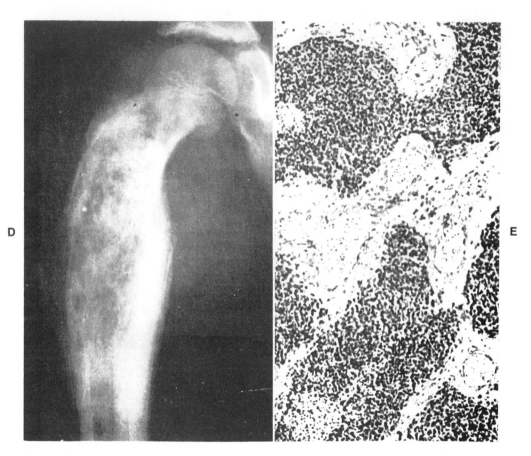

**Fig. 12-3, cont'd. D,** Roentgenographic appearance of Ewing's sarcoma. Note irregular areas of osteoporosis and osteosclerosis, loss of bone architecture, and multilayered periosteal new bone formation. **E,** Closely packed small round cells make up substance of Ewing's sarcoma. Note loosely textured connective tissue containing numerous blood vessels, which forms partitions between masses of tumor cells. (x160; AFIP 73775.)

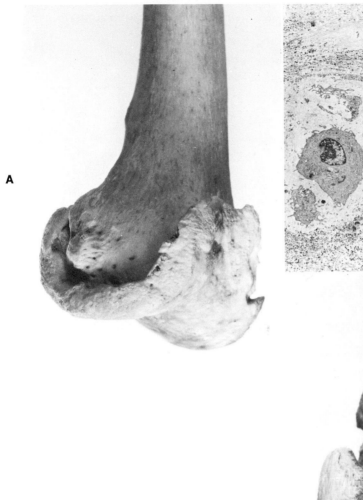

**Fig. 12-4.** Diseases of joint. **A,** Macerated specimen of lower femur. Pronounced osteo-arthrosis of femoral aspect of knee joint with extensive marginal lipping. **B,** Electron micrograph from osteoarthrotic femoral head. Cluster of chondrocytes indicating pro-liferation. Two chondrocytes are shown completely; others are sectioned tangentially and only partly shown. Numerous electrondense granules, some scattered diffusely and others aggregated in crescents, represent lipid derived from disintegrated cells. **C,** Mac-erated specimen of knee joint. Advanced rheumatoid arthritis with bony fusion (ankylosis) at patella, femur, and tibia. (From Anderson, W. A. D., and Kissane, J. M.: Pathology, ed. 7, St. Louis, 1977, The C. V. Mosby Co.; **B** Courtesy Dr. Max Spycher, Zurich.)

*Continued.*

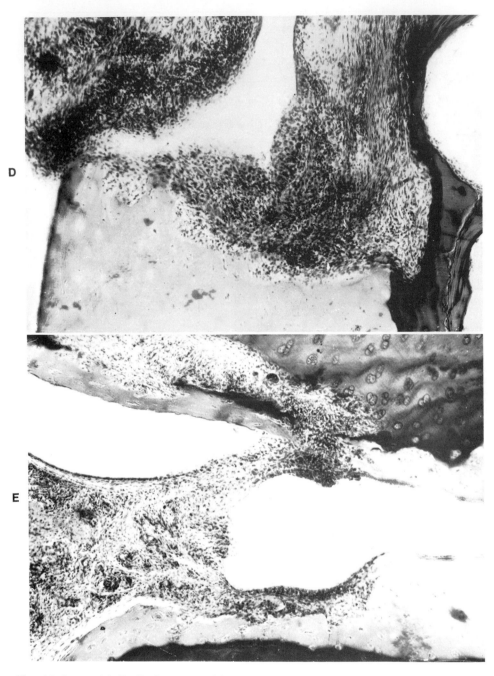

**Fig. 12-4, cont'd. D,** Early stage of fibrous ankylosis. **E,** Granulation tissue projecting inward from margin of interphalangeal joint has formed adhesion across joint space. Nearly all articular cartilage has disappeared beneath pannus, which is clearly shown in lower half.

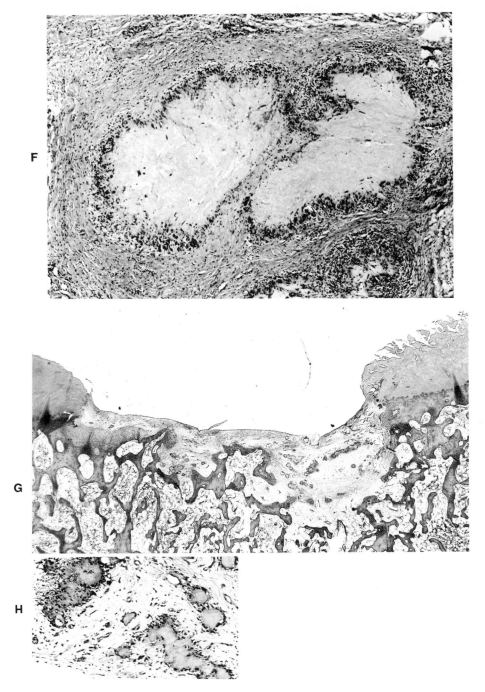

**Fig. 12-4, cont'd. F,** Photomicrograph of portion of gouty tophus in periarticular tissue. Two of several aggregates of which tophus is composed. Urate crystals originally present have been dissolved in processing of tissue and only proteinaceous matrix is preserved in centers. Latter are surrounded by corona of granulation tissue with numerous multinucleated giant cells. (B. H. 69-1754.) **G,** Gouty arthritis. Cartilaginous surface shows large defect, at floor of which urate deposits are seen. Cartilage at left side of ulcer margin is intact, that on right side shows fibrillation of early osteoarthrosis. **H,** Close-up of microtophi at base of ulcer illustrated in **G.**

## SUMMARY

The pathologic examination is an important diagnostic tool when utilized appropriately. It must be emphasized that the reliability of the gross and particularly the microscopic tissue examination is relative to the entire clinical picture obtained from all forms of assessment and evaluation. For this reason it is of utmost importance that the pathologist have all collected data available to assist in the diagnostic task.

## REFERENCES

1. Grossman, I. W.: A primer of gross pathology, Springfield, Ill., 1972, Charles C Thomas, Publisher.
2. Jowsey, J.: The bone biopsy, New York, 1977, Plenum Publishing Corp.
3. Wallach, J.: Interpretation of diagnostic tests: a handbook synopsis of laboratory medicine, Boston, 1974, Little, Brown & Co.

## BIBLIOGRAPHY

Anderson, W. A. D., and Kissane, J. M., editors: Pathology, ed. 7, St. Louis, 1977, The C. V. Mosby Co.

Damjanov, I.: General pathology: medical outline series, Flushing, N.Y., 1976, Medical Examination Publishing Co., Inc.

Gardner, A. F.: Paramedical pathology, Springfield, Ill., 1972, Charles C Thomas, Publisher.

Grossman, I. W.: A primer of gross pathology, Springfield, Ill., 1972, Charles C Thomas, Publisher.

Jowsey, J.: The Bone biopsy, New York, 1977, Plenum Publishing Corp.

Sisson, J. A.: The bare facts of general pathology, Philadelphia, 1974, J. B. Lippincott Co.

Wallach, J.: Interpretation of diagnostic tests: a handbook synopsis of laboratory medicine, Boston, 1974, Little, Brown and Co.

# PART FOUR

# Diagnosis and associated care

# 13

## Upper extremity and shoulder

NANCY E. HILT

SHIRLEY B. COGBURN

Although some diseases and disorders that involve the upper extremity and shoulder are developmental in nature, many are congenital. Tumors, musculoskeletal sepsis, and traumatic injuries of the upper extremity and shoulder are discussed in Chapters 16, 19, and 20. Of greatest concern with all diseases and disorders of this anatomic area is decreased or limited motion, which may considerably impair upper extremity function. This concern increases when the primary arm or hand is involved in a developmental disorder. If the disorder is congenital, however, and of unilateral involvement, the child will frequently develop automatically the utilization of the uninvolved extremity when severe limitations result.

### CARPAL TUNNEL SYNDROME

Carpal tunnel syndrome is a progressive deformity of the wrist and hand caused by narrowing of the carpal tunnel resulting in nerve compression and appropriate accompanying symptomatology.

**Etiology.** Carpal tunnel syndrome may be caused by bony deformity following fracture, osteoarthritis, hypertrophy of the volar ligaments, thickening of flexor tendon sheaths secondary to rheumatoid arthritis or tenosynovitis, and soft tissue masses such as lipomas or ganglia. Occasionally no definite cause is established.[4,p.260]

**Pathology.** Anatomically the structure surrounding the wrist reveals the transverse carpal ligament, a structure with little elasticity, overlying the flexor tendons. The median nerve may be found superficial to the tendons. The structure known as the carpal tunnel is just large enough to house these tendons, the ligament, and the nerve. When the wrist and fingers are held in flexion due to deformity or disease process, the flexor tendons are displaced forward and compress the nerve against the unyielding ligament.[7,p.972]

**Incidence.** Carpal tunnel syndrome is seen more frequently in women, with an approximate 5:1 ratio, between the ages of 40 and 50 years, when wear and tear or degenerative changes may begin. The dominant limb is most often and more severely affected.[7,p.972]

**Signs and symptoms.** The only complaint for several months may be of slight paresthesia. The patient may then describe pain that is spontaneous in nature. This characteristic pain, paresthesia, and numbness along the median nerve distribution, often nocturnal, are the most common symptoms of the syndrome. The patient may complain of attacks of numbness or tingling following manual activities such as writing. During an acute attack the hand may be held in a characteristic position of wrist semiflexion.[7, p. 972]

**Treatment.** Eradication of local causes of nerve compression such as bone deformity following malunion of fractures or neoplasms must be considered first. If this is not the underlying cause of the compression, immobilization and forced rest of the wrist may relieve the symptoms. The aggravation of occupational activity is also stopped in attempts to determine if rest alone will eradicate the symptoms. If this is not successful or if neurologic deficits are progressive, surgical decompression is often necessary.

**Prognosis.** Nonsurgical intervention often relieves the symptoms. When surgical intervention is necessary, permanent disability is not likely to arise.[7, p. 974]

## CONGENITAL ABSENCE OF RADIUS

Congenital absence of the radius (Fig. 13-1) is a common anomaly associated frequently with clubhand.

**Pathology.** Congenital absence of the radius may involve varying degrees of severity, from complete absence to just a portion of the radius. When only a portion is absent, the proximal end usually is present.

**Signs and symptoms.** This congenital anomaly is an obvious deformity. The hand of the affected side deviates radially, and the ulna bows toward the radius. As a result of the deformity the distal upper extremity appears short. A contracture usually exists on the radial side of the forearm.

**Treatment.** Initial treatment consists of release of the contracture. This may be accomplished by splinting in mild cases or surgical release in more severe cases. Arthrodesis of the wrist in a position of function is accomplished as a final procedure.

## CONGENITAL ANKYLOSIS OF ELBOW

Congenital ankylosis of the elbow is a relatively rare congenital anomaly characterized by ankylosis to varying degrees at the elbow joint. It may be seen as a separate entity or in association with additional upper extremity deformities. The type most often seen as a separate entity is frequently characterized by bilateral involvement, while the type commonly associated with other upper extremity deformities may be unilateral or bilateral. Of critical importance is the position in which the elbow becomes ankylosed. Surgical procedures

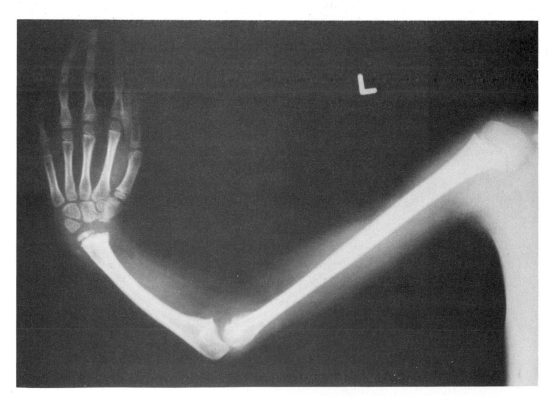

**Fig. 13-1.** Congenital absence of radius. Note hypoplasia of ulna with agenesis of radius.

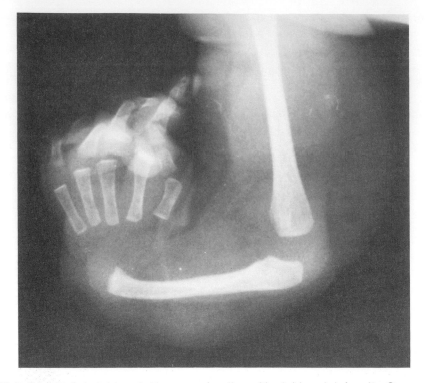

**Fig. 13-2.** Congenital clubhand. Absence of radius with clubhand deformity. Comparison with Fig. 13-1 reveals increased severity of actual deformity.

may be required in attempts to provide a functional degree of flexion at the elbow, which is critical in the ability to maintain and promote maximum degrees of motion.[1,p.172;6,p.102]

## CONGENITAL CLUBHAND

Congenital clubhand (Fig. 13-2) is a rare deformity associated with complete or partial absence of one of the bones of the forearm. It may be bilateral and is sometimes hereditary. Technically, congenital absence of the radius may be classified as congenital clubhand as well.

**Pathology.** Congenital clubhand may be due to defective development of the radial elements of the limbus. With a substantial radial defect, the ulna is shortened and the hand is in a position of radial deviation, as previously described in congenital absence of the radius. If the ulna is the area of primary defect, the hand is carried in a position of ulnar deviation. The thumb may be very small or totally absent.

**Signs and symptoms.** In most cases the forearm is extremely shortened, and although the deformity is obvious and significant, the patient is able to utilize the hand well.

**Treatment.** Congenital clubhand may be treated with a series of corrective cast applications. Surgi-

cal intervention, both soft tissue and bone reconstructive procedures, are directed toward functional rather than cosmetic results.

## CONGENITAL DISLOCATION OF SHOULDER

Congenital dislocation of the shoulder is extremely rare and may be associated with other congenital anomalies. Characteristically the dislocation places the arm in a position of abduction and internal rotation. Radiographically the head of the humerus may be beneath the spine of the scapula. Although it was at one time thought that many congenital dislocations of the shoulder were traumatically induced during the birth process, this is decreasingly thought to be a factor. Some dislocations or subluxations, however, are thought to be secondary to obstetric paralysis. Manipulation of the shoulder to reposition the head of the humerus is indicated only if more than minimal degrees of function limitation are present. Extreme care must be taken during the process not to increase any limited function that already exists. Although arthrodesis of the shoulder joint may be required, this is dependent more on the degree of function limitation resulting from the dislocation than on persistent symptomatology and should be considered on an individual basis.

# CONGENITAL PSEUDARTHROSIS OF CLAVICLE

Congenital pseudarthrosis of the clavicle is a specific type of nonunion or failure of normal ossification of the clavicle and is present at birth.

**Pathology.** Normal ossification and developmental processes of the clavicle stem from ossification centers located at either end of the clavicle. Failure of ossification of the precartilaginous bridge to connect these two masses appears to be the cause of pseudarthrosis.[2,p.1954]

**Signs and symptoms.** Congenital pseudarthrosis of the clavicle produces characteristic features including edema over the clavicular area, drooped shoulder, and little or no limitation of motion. Pain is usually not associated with this deformity. Radiographic examination will frequently reveal slight enlargement at the sight of the pseudarthrosis and a degree of mobility at this site. Differential diagnosis must be made from fractures of the clavicle due to birth trauma and cleidocranial dysostosis. This deformity is rarely associated with other musculoskeletal anomalies.

**Treatment.** Because this deformity rarely causes limitation of motion or function and is rarely associated with pain, no treatment may be required. Surgical intervention, however, may be indicated for cosmetic reasons. Surgical union of the pseudarthrosis requires open reduction by bone grafting. Ideally this is accomplished between the ages of 2 to 4 years. Surgical intervention is recommended for cosmetic reasons more frequently in girls than in boys.[2,p.1954;6,pp.95-96]

# CONGENITAL RADIOULNAR SYNOSTOSIS

Congenital radioulnar synostosis is a rare congenital anomaly involving the fusion of the proximal ends of the radius and ulna, with varying degrees of fixed functional limitation.

**Etiology.** In some cases congenital radioulnar synostosis may be hereditary. Malfunctions, however, in early fetal and embryonic development are often associated with this anomaly, as they are with many congenital anomalies.

**Pathology.** The proximal ulnar and radial fusion associated with this anomaly may occur with or without radial head dislocation.

**Incidence.** Congenital radioulnar synostosis is relatively rare. There is no sex differentiation in regard to incidence.

**Signs and symptoms.** In congenital radioulnar synostosis the forearm most frequently is fixed in a position of pronation or midway between pronation and supination. Extention of the elbow is limited at best, and in the few cases where the synostosis extends to the humerus, absence of the elbow joint may be apparent. Other motions of the wrist and elbow joint are usually within normal limits. The general appearance of the forearm is somewhat twisted, and underdevelopment of the musculature may be seen. Functional limitation to varying degrees depends entirely on the degree of fixed pronation present. Radiographic examination often reveals increased radial bowing relative to the overall severity of the deformity.[1,p.45;6,pp.103-105]

**Treatment.** Many children with congenital radioulnar synostosis learn to compensate for the limited degree of motion through the utilization of increased shoulder motion. If compensation for the functional disabilities is successful, no further treatment may be necessary. Surgical intervention has been utilized in many cases, however, with limited success. Surgical intervention may consist of resection of the upper end of the radius or the osseous tissue that exists between the radius and the ulna, or osteotomy. Surgical intervention may provide an increase in the range of motion, but results are limited.

# CONGENITAL UPPER LIMB DEFICIENCIES

Congenital limb deficiencies (Fig. 13-3) are any congenital anomalies of the upper or lower extremity that result in less than normal development of part or all of the involved extremity. Classification of congenital limb deficiencies, accompanied by universally accepted terminology, was not outlined until 1961. At this time Frantz and O'Rahilly published what is currently considered acceptable terminology and classification. The foundation of this classification is embryologically and teratologically based.[3,p.1202;5,p.135;6,p.108]

"The period of differentiation, known as the embryonic period, takes place during the first 7 postovulatory weeks. At the fourth postovulatory week, limbs begin to develop in the form of small buds on the lateral body wall. During the following 3 weeks, these buds differentiate proximodistally, the hand making its appearance after the arm and forearm. The fetal period is one of embryonic growth."[6,p.108] It is during this development that malfunctions may occur and produce resulting limb deficiencies of varying degrees.

## Terminology

The comprehension of specific terminology utilized in the classification of skeletal limb deficiencies is essential for understanding of the components, concepts, and framework of the clas-

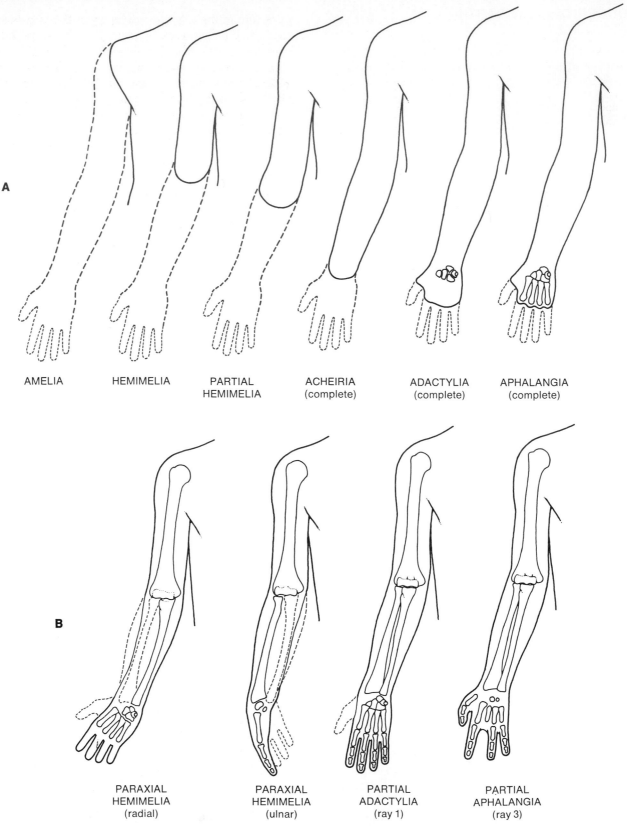

**Fig. 13-3.** Upper extremity deficiencies and classifications. **A,** Terminal transverse. **B,** Terminal longitudinal. (Redrawn from Tachdjian, M. O.: Pediatric orthopedics, Philadelphia, 1972, W. B. Saunders Co.)

sification. The following terms are therefore reviewed[6,p.108]:

**prefix *a*** without; absence.
  **amelia** absence of limb.
  **acheiria** absence of hand.
  **apodia** absence of foot.
  **adactyly** absence of digit.
  **aphalangia** absence of one or more phalanges.
**prefix *hemi*** half.
  **hemimelia** absence or presence of half a limb.
**prefix *phoco*** seallike.
  **phocomelia** limb attached directly to trunk; flipperlike limb.
**paraxial** beside the axis; part of limb absent.
**terminal** all parts distal to and in line with deficient portion affected.
**intercalary** proximal and distal parts present with little part absent.
**transverse** entire width of limb involved.
**longitudinal** only part of limb (preaxial or postaxial) affected.
**ray** digit.
**limb** extremity.

Combinations of the terminology outlined here usually provide an accurate description of the anatomic area of the deficiency as well as its extent.

*Dysmelia* is a general term that represents a group of anomalies, all of which are characterized by hypoplasia or aphasia of the long bones of the extremities. As opposed to distal absence in congenital amputation, dysmelia may involve absence proximally or axially. The deformities in dysmelia range from peripheral hypoplasia of one long bone (as in proximal focal femoral deficiency) to total absence of the extremity (amelia).

**Classification**

The classification of congenital skeletal limb deficiencies, as outlined by Frantz and O'Rahilly in 1961, is shown in the box on p. 260. As may be noted, utilizing the terminology reviewed, the classification is relatively simple and descriptive of the degree of deficiency involved. Visual representation of upper extremity limb deficiency may be seen in Fig. 13-3.

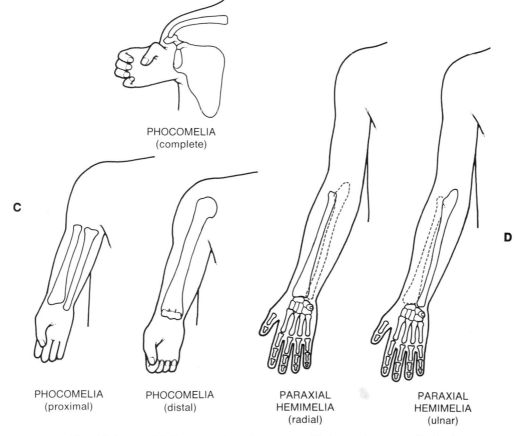

PHOCOMELIA
(complete)

C

PHOCOMELIA
(proximal)

PHOCOMELIA
(distal)

PARAXIAL
HEMIMELIA
(radial)

PARAXIAL
HEMIMELIA
(ulnar)

D

**Fig. 13-3, cont'd. C,** Intercalary, transverse. **D,** Intercalary, longitudinal.

## CLASSIFICATION OF CONGENITAL SKELETAL LIMB DEFICIENCIES

### Terminal (T)

**Transverse (-)**

Amelia: absence of limb

Hemimelia: absence of forearm and hand or leg and foot

Partial hemimelia: part of forearm or leg present

Acheiria or apodia: absence of hand or foot

Complete adactyly: absence of all five digits and their metacarpals or metatarsals

Complete aphalangia: absence of one or more phalanges from all five digits

**Longitudinal (/)**

Complete paraxial hemimelia: complete absence of one of the forearm or leg elements and of the corresponding portion of the hand or foot (R, U, TI, or FI*)

Incomplete paraxial hemimelia: similar to complete paraxial hemimelia, but part of defective element is present (r, u, ti, or fi†)

Partial adactyly: absence of one to four digits and their metacarpals or metatarsals (1, 2, 3, 4, or 5)

Partial aphalangia: absence of one or more phalanges from one to four digits (1, 2, 3, 4, or 5)

### Intercalary (I)

**Transverse (-)**

Complete phocomelia: hand or foot attached directly to trunk

Proximal phocomelia: hand and forearm or foot and leg attached directly to trunk

Distal phocomelia: hand or foot attached directly to arm or thigh

**Longitudinal (/)**

Complete paraxial hemimelia: similar to corresponding terminal defect, but hand or foot is more or less complete (R, U, TI, or FI)

Incomplete paraxial hemimelia: similar to corresponding terminal defect, but hand or foot is more or less complete (r, u, ti, or fi)

Partial adactyly: absence of all or part of a metacarpal or metatarsal (1 or 5)

Partial aphalangia: absence of proximal or middle phalanx or both from one or more digits (1, 2, 3, 4, or 5)

From Frantz, C. H., and O'Rahilly, R.: J. Bone Joint Surg. **43**-A:1204, 1961.

**Code:** FI or fi, fibular; I, intercalary; R or r, radial; T, terminal; TI or ti, tibial; U or u, ulnar. A line below a numeral denotes upper limb involvement; for example, T-2 represents terminal transverse hemimelia of upper limb. A line above a numeral denotes lower limb involvement; for example, I-1 represents intercalary transverse complete phocomelia of lower limb.

*Capital letters, complete paraxial hemimelia.

†Lower case letters, incomplete defect.

**Treatment.** The treatment of congenital upper limb deficiencies is greatly dependent on the degree of deficiency present. When involvement is unilateral, many children learn to utilize the opposite extremity quite well. Minor to moderate degrees of limb deficiencies in the upper extremity may require only education of the patient in regard to utilizing the partial limb in a functional manner. Joint fusions are sometimes advocated to increase stability and function. Prostheses are occasionally utilized but are more commonly associated with limb deficiencies of the lower extremities. Although cosmetic considerations may be of some value, depending on the severity of the deficiency, of greatest importance is the improvement of functional abilities of the child. Treatment and surgical reconstructive procedures are extremely individual and are designed for the specific level of involvement.

## CUBITUS VALGUS OR VARUS

The normal anatomic position of the forearm, as seen from the anterior view, is at an approximately

10° to 15° angle to the upper arm. It depends on the proper relationship between various bones making up the elbow joint. If this angle is abnormally *increased*, the deformity is called *cubitus valgus.* If the angle is decreased it is known as *cubitus varus.*

**Etiology.** Cubitus valgus or varus may result from an improperly reduced fracture, inappropriate healing at a fracture site, or asymmetric epiphyseal growth following a traumatic injury or infection.

**Signs and symptoms.** Obvious deformity exists as outlined, with possible limited elbow motion.

**Treatment.** The treatment of choice for cubitus valgus or varus is surgical intervention if limited motion produces functional disability or pain accompanies the limitation of motion. Wedge osteotomy of the humerus with replacement or removal of the detached lateral condyle is the treatment of choice for cubitus valgus, with a similar type of osteotomy indicated for cubitus varus.

## DUPUYTREN'S CONTRACTURE

Dupuytren's contracture is a contracture of the hand or foot involving flexion at the metacarpophalangeal joint, with occasional distal involvement.

**Etiology.** The cause of Dupuytren's contracture is unknown, but there is a familial tendency. Although trauma is not the cause of the deformity, it may be known to aggravate the already existing condition.

**Pathology.** The major pathologic feature of Dupuytren's contracture is "chronic inflammation of the palmar fascia with progressive fibrosis and contracture, principally of the pretendinous bands of the palmar aponeurosis to the fingers."[1,p.463] Most frequently involved are the ring finger and the little finger. This contracture is often bilateral and symmetric in nature.

**Incidence.** This contracture occurs more frequently in men than in women, with a 7:1 ratio. In men it is seen most frequently after middle age; in women it is usually seen at an earlier age.

**Signs and symptoms.** This condition may take years to reach maximum deformity. The patient infrequently complains of pain; the major complaint is "inability to use the hand due to interference of the flexed fingers."[7,p.959] The deformity frequently starts with the appearance of a small nodule in the palm of the hand near the distal palmar crease and proximal to the ring finger.[7,p.959] A fibrous cord or band forms and gradually thickens. The involved finger then gradually, with the thickening formation, folds into flexion, usually at the metacarpophalangeal joint. The contracture most frequently is seen with no further involvement, but there may be continuous nodule formation distally in the joints of the involved finger. The ultimate result, especially with gradual progression, is a severely flexed finger.

**Treatment.** Surgical intervention is often the treatment of choice. In early cases conservative therapy consisting of stretching exercises of the finger may be utilized, but this has not proved very successful. Resection of the involved palmar fascia may be either conservative or radical in nature depending on the surgeon's preference.

## ERB'S PALSY (OBSTETRIC PALSY, UPPER ARM PARALYSIS)

Symptomatology of Erb's palsy reflects nerve root damage to $C_5$ and $C_6$, resulting in paralysis of the upper arm and shoulder.

**Etiology.** Erb's palsy is most frequently a result of injury to the nerve roots ($C_5$ and $C_6$ specifically) of the brachioplexis during delivery, usually in prolonged or difficult labor and delivery.

**Pathology.** The specific nerve root paralysis referred to involves the adductors and external rotators of the upper arm and shoulder. Varying degrees of paralysis and symptomatology result dependent on the severity of the damage.

**Signs and symptoms.** The typical position of the shoulder and arm in Erb's palsy is internal rotation and adduction with the forearm pronated. The extremity is frequently limp and is held at the side of the body. Little or no muscular activity is reflected over the entire extremity. Passive motion of the involved extremity will frequently produce reactions that indicate pain. Some edema may be apparent. Dependent on the severity of the involvement, varying degrees of returned motion, with decreased swelling and apparent reduction in pain, will be evident several days after birth.[7,p.815]

**Treatment.** The majority of patients with Erb's palsy recover spontaneously with nonsurgical intervention. The utilization of a brace providing a position of abduction and external rotation (of approximately 90°) at the shoulder, flexion at the elbow, supination (full) of the forearm, and slight dorsiflexion of the wrist is often successful. The brace should be removed for skin care and gentle massage to prevent contractures and to assist in maintaining muscular tone. The brace is gradually removed, and active and passive exercises are continued. Frequent observation for contractures is necessary, and the tendency may be counteracted by frequent stretching.[1,p.211;7,p.879]

When nonsurgical intervention has been unsuccessful, surgical procedures may be initiated to restore muscle balance, correct deformities, and alter

# 14

# Lower extremity and hip

**NANCY E. HILT**

**SHIRLEY B. COGBURN**

Many of the musculoskeletal diseases and disorders, both congenital and acquired, are anatomically located in the lower extremity and the hip joint. Not only is the number of diseases and disorders seen in the lower extremity of great concern, but so is the degree to which they can greatly affect, by nature of the disease process or its complications, one's ability to ambulate and become or remain mobile. For this reason early diagnosis and treatment are emphasized for all pathologic processes of the lower extremity and hip in attempts to maximize all mobility potential. Due to the great number of pathologic entities of the lower extremity and hip, only the most commonly seen are reviewed here. To facilitate organization the diseases and disorders are classified anatomically.

## DISEASES AND DISORDERS OF LOWER EXTREMITY
### Foot
#### Accessory bones

Accessory bones of the foot are extra bones anywhere within the structure of the foot.

**Etiology.** Accessory bones are congenital malformations due to errors in embryonic development.

**Pathology.** Accessory bones of the foot may occur anywhere within the structure of the foot and are sometimes also seen within the structure of the ankle. One of the most common sites for an accessory bone is the tarsonavicular joint, usually near the medial end of the navicular bone. In these specific cases the posterior tibial tendon is often attached. Additionally the position of this tendon inappropriately is apt to pose problems with the support of the arch of the foot, resulting in a planovalgus deformity. Other pathologic features of specific accessory bones depend largely on the location of the bone. Common locations are the medial malleolus, talus, os calcis, cuboid, cuneiform, and metatarsals.[8,p.1266]

**Incidence.** Accessory bones are present in approximately 10% of all persons, with locations varying greatly. The accessory bone persists as a separate bone in approximately 2% of the population. It is not at all uncommon for accessory bones to be seen bilaterally.[8,p.1266]

**Signs and symptoms.** Many accessory bones of the foot are asymptomatic. Some, however, are pain producing, especially after long periods of ambulation. Location of this pain will depend primarily on the location of the accessory bone and any compression or pressure that may occur as a result of its position. Bursae may be seen and tenosynovitis may occur as a result of irritation in surrounding structures. It is not uncommon for the diagnosis of an accessory bone to be made accidentally or in connection with associated radiographic examination for traumatic injuries or other reasons.

**Treatment.** Asymptomatic accessory bones require no treatment. Conservative treatment including arch supports, injections of hydrocortisone, and immobilization in a below-the-knee walking cast for several weeks is frequently successful in alleviating mild to moderate symptoms. Symptoms may recur, but surgical intervention is indicated only if symptoms persist over a long time, resulting in con-

tinued pain, signs of resulting deformity due to position of surrounding structures, or compression or pressure caused by the accessory bone. Surgical intervention may include excision of the accessory bone or more conservative procedures and will depend on the location of the bone and the type of symptomatology it has produced. Additional utilization of cast therapy and arch supports may be required after surgery.[8,pp.1267-1269]

#### Claw toe

Claw toe is a deformity characterized by hyperextension of the metatarsophalangeal joint and flexion of the proximal and distal interphalangeal joints.

**Etiology.** Claw toe may be secondary to pes cavus or paralytic in its pathogenesis.

**Signs and symptoms.** Claw toe frequently produces painful callosities, which develop slowly over the dorsum of the interphalangeal joints. Keratosis under the metatarsal heads appears to aggravate the disability. Additional signs and symptoms are frequently not attributable to the claw toe but to its primary origin.[8,p.1411]

**Treatment.** Treatment for claw toe is dependent on the type, the degree of flexibility of the interphalangeal and metatarsophalangeal joints, and the age of the patient. In paralytic claw toe the underlying cause should be corrected. In claw toe secondary to pes cavus the equinus deformity of the forefoot is corrected. Fusion of the interphalangeal joints followed by dorsal capsulotomy of the metatarsophalangeal joint is sometimes indicated.[8,p.1411]

#### Congenital vertical talus (convex pes valgus, congenital rocker-bottom foot)

Congenital vertical talus is a deformity of the foot, present at birth and characterized by apparent dislocation of the talonavicular joint with the talus in a vertical position.

**Etiology.** The cause of congenital vertical talus is unknown, but it is probably due to an error in embryonic development. Other congenital anomalies such as arthrogryposis may be the cause or at least be associated with this deformity. Muscular imbalance may also produce the deformity and may then be associated with certain central nervous system anomalies.[9,p.293]

**Pathology.** A congenital deformity, vertical talus is characterized by dislocation of the talonavicular joint with the talus fixed in a vertical position.

**Signs and symptoms.** In vertical talus the sole of the foot at birth is convex and has the classic "rocker-bottom" appearance. Creases are apparent near

**Table 14-1.** Congenital vertical talus: choice of operative procedures in relation to age of patient

| Procedure | Birth to 2 mo | 3 to 9 mo | 9 mo to 3 yr | 4 to 6 yr | Over 6 yr |
|---|:---:|:---:|:---:|:---:|:---:|
| Soft tissues | | | | | |
|   Stretching cast | + | + | + | + | +* |
|   Elongate contracted musculotendinous units (anterior tibial, toe extensors, peroneals) | − | ± | + | + | +* |
|   Heel cord lengthening | ± | + | + | + | +* |
|   Capsulotomy of posterior part of ankle and subtalar joints | | ± | + | + | +* |
|   Section of calcaneofibular ligament | − | ± | + | + | +* |
| Talonavicular joint | | | | | |
|   Closed reduction | + | − | − | − | − |
|   Open reduction | − | + | + | + | − |
|   Medial incision | − | + | + | + | − |
|   Maintain reduction by plication of capsule inferiorly and medially by tightening calcaneonavicular ligament and posterior tibial tendon | − | + | + | + | − |
|   Internal fixation of talonavicular joint with Kirschner wire | ± | + | + | + | + |
|   May reroute anterior tibial tendon under head of talus | − | + | + | + | − |
|   Both medial and lateral incisions (to release talocalcaneal ligament and calcaneocuboid capsule) | − | − | − | + | − |
| Reconstructive stabilization | | | | | |
|   Triple arthrodesis with partial resection of navicular joint or head and neck of talus or wedge tarsectomy | − | − | − | − | + |

From Tachdjian, M. O.: Pediatric orthopedics, Philadelphia, 1972, W. B. Saunders Co.
Code: +, indicated; −, not necessary; ±, may be required.
*Perform prior to triple arthrodesis when bony growth of foot is complete.

the ankle joint on the dorsolateral aspect of the foot. When the child begins walking the gait is very awkward and clumsy, and almost "pig-like." On physical examination the foot is very rigid, the sole convex, and very tight heel cords are apparent. On weight bearing, the heel fails to touch the floor. Abnormal wearing of the shoes is usually seen, with rapid wearing on the "medial part of the heel and the upper part over the longitudinal arch wearing in just a few weeks."[8,p.1361] Pain is usually not associated with this deformity until adolescence.

**Treatment.** Treatment of congenital vertical talus is directed toward adequate reduction and repositioning of the involved bones with appropriate soft tissue repair. Conservative nonsurgical manipulation often fails but should be utilized with cast therapy, bringing the foot into an equinus position. This stretches the extensor tendons and skin, which is helpful when reduction is achieved through surgical procedures. Many surgical procedures have been developed and utilized in attempts to adequately reduce and maintain reduction of this deformity. Table 14-1 gives some of the options avail-

able to the orthopedic surgeon in relation to the age of the patient.

### Clubfoot (talipes equinovarus)

Clubfoot (Figs. 14-1 and 14-2) is a congenital anomaly characterized by a combination of inversion of the foot, forefoot adduction, and equinus; *all three* components must be present to be classified as true clubfoot.

**Etiology.** The exact cause of clubfoot is unknown and is the source of some controversy. It is theorized that clubfoot may be the result of:
1. Developmental arrest of the fetus in the first trimester of pregnancy, thus explaining the presence of other anomalies often associated with this deformity
2. Intrauterine compression
3. Abnormalities in relative maturity and length of muscles and tendon insertions, often the anterior tibial tendon

**Pathology.** Pathologic features of true clubfoot include (1) *equinus*, (2) *forefoot adduction*, and (3) *inversion*. All degrees of deformity exist, but re-

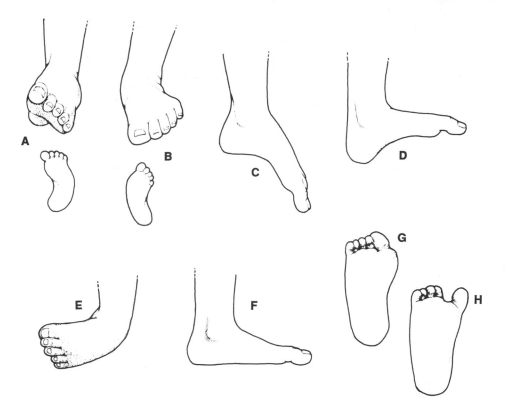

**Fig. 14-1.** Common foot and ankle deformities seen in children. **A,** Talipes varus. **B,** Talipes valgus. **C,** Talipes equinus. **D,** Talipes calcaneus. **E,** Clubfoot. **F,** Flat foot. **G,** Metatarsus adductus. **H,** Metatarsus varus. (From Hilt, N. E., and Schmitt, E. W., Jr.: Pediatric orthopedic nursing, St. Louis, 1975, The C. V. Mosby Co.)

gardless of the severity the Achilles tendon is always shortened. Leg muscles are usually small and may show degenerative changes in some cases. "The joint capsule and ligaments on the medial side are thickened and contracted. The calcaneus is rolled in under the talus, and the navicular is medially displaced on the head of the talus."[9,p.267] It is not uncommon for the talus to be wedge shaped with only its posterior surface opposed to the tibia. The distal portions of the tibia and fibula show slight inward rotation (tibial torsion). As the child grows, changes occur as an adaptive measure for the persistent abnormal position. Radiographic examination usually confirms the pathologic features.

**Incidence.** Clubfoot occurs in 1 in 1,000 live births. There is a 1 in 35 chance of a second child in the family having the same deformity. It is twice as common in boys as in girls.[8,p.1275]

**Signs and symptoms.** Clubfoot is an obvious deformity and is most frequently diagnosed on physical examination. The pathologic features outlined above constitute the signs and symptoms. If diagno-

sis is not made before the infant begins to walk, he is tremendously disabled due to inability of weight-bearing components of the normal gait to function. Pain is usually not associated with clubfoot except during adulthood when arthritic changes have occurred within the bony structures of the foot. If treatment is not begun early, fatigue and marked atrophy of the muscles of the leg may be seen. Bilateral involvement produces the typical "reel" walk with wobbling from side to side. In extreme untreated cases weight is borne on a bursa that has developed over the cuboid and proximal end of the third metatarsal bone. This acts as a shock absorber, like the heel of the normal foot.

**Treatment.** Because clubfoot is one of the oldest recorded deformities, the history of attempts at treatment is too lengthy to review in depth here. Many early attempts to correct clubfoot involved forceful manipulation, which was accompanied by a very high incidence of complications such as fractures and considerable risk. It was not until the 1930s that Kite advocated conservative treatment of clubfoot without the utilization of force.[6,p.39]

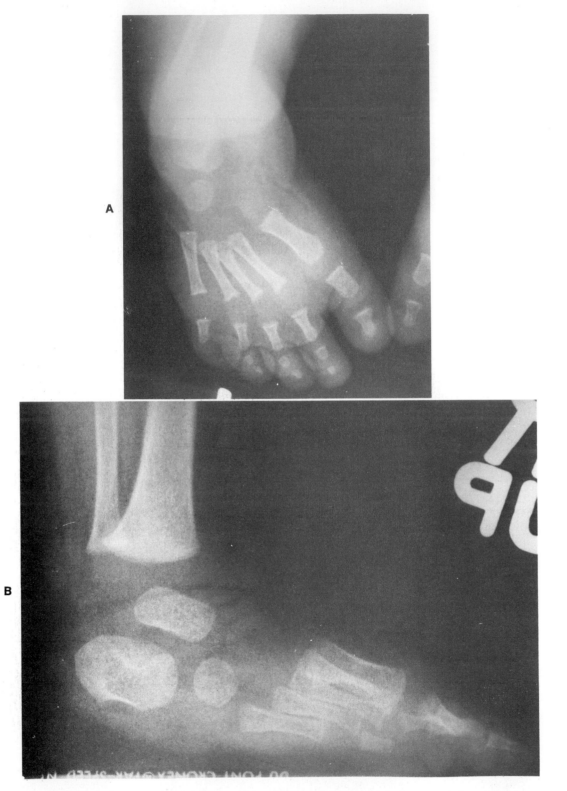

**Fig. 14-2.** Clubfoot, frontal **(A)** and lateral **(B)** projections. Note bony malalignments.

**Table 14-2.** Talipes equinovarus (clubfoot): methods of treatment in various age groups

| Method of treatment | Birth to 2 mo | 3 to 9 mo | 10 to 18 mo | 1½ to 3 yr | 4 to 8 yr | 9 to 11 yr | Over 12 yr |
|---|---|---|---|---|---|---|---|
| **Conservative** | | | | | | | |
| Manipulation, passive stretching | + | + | + | + | + | + | + |
| Adhesive strapping | + | − | − | − | − | − | − |
| Corrective cast | + | + | ± | + | + | ± | ± |
| Dynamic splinting | − | + | − | − | − | − | − |
| Bivalved cast or other night splint to maintain part in corrected position | − | + | + | + | + | − | − |
| Dynamic below-knee orthosis (dorsiflexion assist, valgus strap, tarsal pronator shoe) | − | − | − | + | + | + | − |
| Special shoes | | | | | | | |
|   Prewalker clubfoot | − | + | + | − | − | − | − |
|   Tarsal pronator (reversed Thomas heel, ⅛-inch outer sole and heel wedges) | − | − | − | + | + | + | − |
|   Straight-last shoe (⅛-inch outer sole and heel wedges) | − | − | − | + | + | + | − |
| **Surgical: soft tissue procedures** | | | | | | | |
| Posterior release | | | | | | | |
|   Heel cord lengthening | − | + | + | + | + | + | + |
|   Posterior tibial lengthening | − | + | + | + | + | + | + |
|   Capsulotomy (posterior ankle and subtalar) | − | + | + | + | + | + | + |
|   Section of calcaneofibular, posterior part of deltoid, and talofibular ligaments | − | + | + | + | + | + | + |
| Medial release of hindfoot and midfoot | − | ± | + | + | + | + | ± |
| Mediodorsal release of metatarsotarsal joints (Heyman-Herndon) | − | − | − | + | + | − | − |
| Plantar release | − | ± | + | + | + | + | + |
| Posterior tibial transfer (anterior through interosseous route) | − | − | − | − | ± | ± | ± |
| Anterior tibial transfer laterally | − | − | − | − | − | − | − |
| **Surgical: bony procedures** | | | | | | | |
| Cuboid decancellation | − | − | − | + | + | − | − |
| Evans procedure (resection and fusion of calcaneocuboid joint) | − | − | − | − | + | + | + |
| Dwyer osteotomy of os calcis (open-up) | − | − | − | − | + | + | + |
| Dwyer osteotomy of os calcis (close-up) | − | − | − | − | ± | + | + |
| Metatarsal osteotomy (at their bases) for correction of metatarsus varus | − | − | − | − | − | + | + |
| Triple arthrodesis, tarsal reconstruction by wedge resection, and fusion of midtarsal and subtalar joints | − | − | − | − | − | + | + |
| Astragalectomy | − | − | − | − | ± | + (severe untreated) | + (severe untreated) |
| Dorsal angulation osteotomy of distal tibia and fibula | − | − | − | − | + (rigid equinus) | + (rigid equinus) | + (rigid equinus) |
| Derotation osteotomy of tibia | − | − | − | − | − | + | + |

From Tachdjian, M. O.: Pediatric orthopedics, Philadelphia, 1972, W. B. Saunders Co.
Code: +, indicated; −, not necessary; ±, may be required.

Kite advocated early and persistent nonsurgical intervention in the form of frequent cast application and changes. Manipulation of the deformity was advocated and is still utilized between cast changes, with correction of the three components individually until full correction is obtained.[6,pp.58-63]

Early conservative treatment appears to produce the best results. Preferably the orthopedic surgeon should begin the therapy while the infant is still in the nursery, as soon after birth as possible. This therapy may progress slowly and extend for several years with the gradual manipulation and reduction of the deformity. Overcorrection of the deformity is advocated for best results in maintaining the correction. The technique for cast application and manipulation is critical, but patience must be exhibited throughout the entire process. Kite reviews this special technique very well in his publication. Even with nonsurgical intervention, it is advocated that maintenance of the correction be ensured through appropriate immobilization with various orthotic or other devices for a time.[2,6,pp.77-79]

Despite conservative attempts at correcting clubfoot, surgical intervention is sometimes indicated. This is usually reserved for resistant cases in which conservative measures have failed or the deformity is fixed due to lack of appropriate early intervention. Statistics regarding the success or failure of nonsurgical therapy, resulting in surgical intervention, vary greatly. It is thought by some that this is partially due to the degree of patience exhibited, while others think there are tremendous advantages to early surgical intervention. If surgical intervention is deemed necessary by the orthopedic surgeon, it is frequently limited to soft tissue procedures. These multiple procedures are designed to release soft tissue structures in an effort to increase the pliability of the foot. Tendon transfers and a combination of soft tissue and bony surgical procedures are utilized when the deformity remains severe after the child is 3 to 5 years of age. Various components of treatment for clubfoot at various ages are given in Table 14-2.

### Dupuytren's contracture (of foot)

Dupuytren's contracture is a contracture of the foot (or hand) involving flexion at the metacarpophalangeal joint with occasional distal involvement. (See also Dupuytren's contracture of hand, Chapter 13.)

### Forefoot adduction

Forefoot adduction is a deformity in which the forefoot is deviated toward the midline of the body.

It is one of the major components of clubfoot but may be seen without the other two components. It is treated with serial cast applications with manipulation between cast changes and is much more responsive to this therapy than is true clubfoot. Special shoes or other devices may be utilized to maintain the correction for a time after it has been obtained. Additional information may be found in the section on clubfoot.

### Freiberg's infraction

Freiberg's infraction is characterized by aseptic necrosis of a bone, most commonly the second metatarsal head.

**Etiology.** Vascular insufficiency resulting in aseptic necrosis of the bone is the primary cause of Freiberg's infraction.[8,p.408]

**Pathology.** The major pathologic feature of Freiberg's infraction is aseptic necrosis of the involved bone.

**Incidence.** Freiberg's infraction is most commonly localized in the metatarsal head. It is most frequently seen in adolescents and is more common in females than in males.

**Signs and symptoms.** The most striking sign and symptom of Freiberg's infraction is pain on weight bearing, swelling, and limitation of motion in the metatarsophalangeal joint.

**Treatment.** In the adolescent nonsurgical intervention is advocated. Utilization of a short leg cast may be indicated during the acute painful stages of the process. In the adult with recurrence of symptomatology "resection of the head with a portion of the adjacent shaft are often indicated. To prevent recession of the corresponding toe, it is surgically syndactylized with its adjacent normal toe."[8,p.410]

### Ganglion

A ganglion is a small cyst, seen less frequently on the foot than on the hand. Its very thin wall contains a clear and colorless fluid and frequently extends from or is located near the tendon sheaths or adjacent to the joint lining. If seen on the foot the dorsum, in the midtarsal area, is the most frequent anatomic site. Ganglia may also be seen in the ankle area near the malleoli. Pain may be associated as the most common sign or symptom, and the cyst is frequently palpable on examination. The treatment of choice is complete excision. Rupture of the cyst is usually inadequate and temporary as a form of treatment, and the ganglion often recurs unless surgical intervention is accomplished. (See also ganglion of hand, Chapter 13.)

### Hallux rigidus

Hallux rigidus is a deformity characterized by limited motion, especially dorsiflexion of the great toe, and pain that may ultimately lead to degenerative changes of the involved joints.

**Etiology.** The exact cause of hallux rigidus is unknown, but in adolescence it is often familial.[8,p.1402]

**Pathology.** Pathologic characteristics of hallux rigidus include limited motion accompanied by pain in the great toe with the greatest degree of involvement being dorsiflexion of the metatarsophalangeal joint. Degenerative arthritic joint changes are frequently seen with progression of the deformity.

**Incidence.** Although hallux rigidus may have its onset in early childhood, symptoms may not develop until later, usually after adolescence. The incidence is higher in females during adolescence but the same in both sexes during adulthood.[8,p.1309]

**Signs and symptoms.** Hallux rigidus has a gradual onset, with pain often developing suddenly after trauma. Pain on ambulation is the outstanding symptom. It is often of an aching, throbbing nature and relieved only with rest. Joint stiffness prevents dorsiflexion. Plantar flexion is usually near normal. Some edema and tenderness may be evident over the involved joint, with a fixed position of slight flexion. It is not uncommon for a patient with hallux rigidus to have pronated feet. In the adult progressive stiffness of the great toe may develop with or without pain. Osteoarthritic symptoms of the joint are typical. The characteristic "hopping, short-stepped" gait is observed.[8,p.1405;9,p.1309]

**Treatment.** Treatment of hallux rigidus is greatly dependent on the patient's age at the onset of symptoms and the severity of the deformity and symptoms at the time of diagnosis. With acute symptomatology during the adolescent years, conservative therapy consisting of proper and well-fitted shoes and gait education (heel-to-toe walking) is often successful. During the acute stage additional measures involving rest, heat, and sedation with local injections of corticosteroids to reduce pain and swelling may be initiated. With continued evidence that acute symptomatology is subsiding, manipulation may be considered for restoration of full joint motion. Surgical intervention may be necessary for persistent and recurring symptoms. Surgical intervention is also considered for advanced cases for correction of the deformity and existing disability. Procedure alternatives include arthrodesis, osteotomy, and arthroplasty with depression of the first metatarsal section. Continued pain associated with this deformity may also require continued utilization of appropriate shoe inserts (metatarsal pad or bar).[9,pp.1309-1310]

### Hallux valgus (bunion)

Hallux valgus is a deformity characterized by lateral angulation of the great toe at its metatarsophalangeal joint with enlargement and the development of a bursa or callus over this area.

**Etiology.** There appears to be a familial tendency toward hallux valgus. The following are known to be contributory causes[9,p.1282]:

1. Poorly fitting shoes
2. Osseous wedging of the medial cuneiform, causing the first metatarsal to angle medially
3. Degenerative arthritic changes, especially of the metatarsophalangeal joint
4. Pronated feet (flat feet)

**Pathology.** Hallux valgus causes lateral angulation of the great toe at its metatarsophalangeal joint. The medial side of the head of the first metatarsal bone enlarges, and a bursa or callus forms over this area; this constitutes the *bunion*. The great toe rotates on its long axis medially, and the long toe extensor tendon is displaced laterally. Development of a hammer toe and callus on the dorsum may be seen when the second toe is displaced dorsally.

**Incidence.** Hallux valgus is seen more frequently in females than in males.

**Signs and symptoms.** Varying degrees of the deformity may be seen with symptoms ranging from mild tenderness over the affected area to extreme disability.

**Treatment.** Early diagnosis of hallux valgus is essential for implementation of early therapeutic regimens in attempts to provide comfort and prevent further deformity. Conservative therapy consists of well-fitted shoes allowing for a wide forefoot or "bunion pocket." Bunion pads may be utilized to relieve the pressure of the shoe. "Severely painful bursitis may require incising and hot moist compresses applied for relief. Intra-articular injections of corticosteroids, heat, rest, and salicylate therapy may be necessary for treatment of the osteoarthritic joint involvement."[9,p.1282]

Although severe deformity from hallux valgus may be quite unsightly, surgical intervention is not considered for cosmetic reasons but for the relief of symptomatology. Many surgical procedures have been devised for removal of the deformity and alleviation of the extreme disability that accompanies the severe case.

### Hallux varus

Hallux varus is a deformity characterized by medial angulation of the great toe at the metatarsophalangeal joint.

**Etiology.** Hallux varus may be congenital or the result of trauma, infection, or muscular imbalance.[2]

**Pathology.** The major pathologic feature of hallux varus is the medial angulation of the great toe at the metatarsophalangeal joint.

**Signs and symptoms.** Hallux varus is obvious. Its onset is usually gradual but is greatly dependent on the specific cause of the deformity. The types of hallux varus of congenital origin may be seen as the primary deformity, may be secondary with associated congenital deformities of the forefoot, or may be associated with developmental deformities of the skeletal system.[8,p.1375]

**Treatment.** Depending on the severity of the deformity, no treatment may be required. Surgical intervention, release of the contracted stricture on the medial side of the toe with or without osteotomy, may be required for more severe cases.

### Hammer toe

Hammer toe is a deformity that may involve any toe and is characterized by a flexion contraction of the proximal interphalangeal joint with flexion, neutral extension, or slight hyperextension of the distal interphalangeal joint.

**Etiology.** Hammer toe may be congenital or acquired. If acquired, it is most frequently due to poorly fitted shoes that force the involved toe into flexion. There may be a familial tendency toward this deformity.

**Pathology.** Hammer toe is often bilateral and symmetric. Its most striking pathologic characteristic is that of a flexion contracture of the proximal interphalangeal joint with flexion, neutral extension, or slight hyperextension of the distal interphalangeal joint of the involved toe. The second toe is most frequently involved. Calluses over the proximal interphalangeal joint may result from pressure. This deformity may be associated with hallux valgus.

**Signs and symptoms.** Hammer toe is obvious, and the involved toe(s) tends to point downward. Painful calluses may develop over the tip of the proximal interphalangeal joint.

**Treatment.** Many hammer toe deformities may be treated nonsurgically with appropriate therapeutic implementation of passive stretching exercises. Well-fitted shoes are advocated to decrease pressure over the proximal interphalangeal joint, and appropriate padding and inserts may be prescribed. If the deformity is resistant to improvement with exercises and continued symptomatology is evident, manipulation into extension may be advisable, with positioning maintained by splinting. Arthrodesis of the proximal interphalangeal joint into extension may be indicated if other measures fail.

### Köhler's disease

Köhler's disease is a process attributed to ischemic degeneration of localized bone tissue, most frequently in the navicular bone.

**Etiology.** Köhler's disease may occur simultaneously with Legg-Perthes disease. The cause has not been established, but "the infection seems to fall into a group with localized and self-limited bone diseases of youth that are ascribed to ischemic degenerative changes."[2]

**Pathology.** Pathologic features of Köhler's disease include ischemic degeneration of the affected bone tissue and localized tissue reaction.

**Incidence.** Köhler's disease is relatively uncommon. It occurs more frequently in boys than in girls, with the onset of symptoms at approximately 5 years of age in boys and 4 years of age in girls. Approximately one third of the cases are bilateral.

**Signs and symptoms.** The signs and symptoms of Köhler's disease relate directly to the vascular changes and the resulting surrounding tissue reaction. An antalgic limp is frequently seen, with localized pain and tenderness around the navicular bone. Surrounding tissue edema is not uncommon.[8,pp.406-407]

**Treatment.** Minimal pain produced by this disease process may warrant little treatment other than appropriately fitted shoes with an arch support, which is relatively successful in alleviating the symptomatology. Moderate pain associated with the process usually requires treatment with a short leg walking cast for approximately 6 to 8 weeks. Following the cast removal, appropriately fitted shoes and the avoidance of extreme use of the foot (e.g., running) are indicated. Most of this process resolves itself completely before growth is attained in the foot, and there is no residual deformity or disability.[8,p.408]

### Mallet toe

Mallet toe is a flexion deformity at the distal interphalangeal joint of any of the lesser toes. It is seen less commonly than hammer toe and usually affects a single toe or two adjacent toes. Painful corns may develop on the tip of the toe, but most frequently the deformity is asymptomatic. Symptomatic relief, if necessary, may usually be obtained by padding. If surgery is required, fusion of the distal interphalangeal joint to correct the deformity is the procedure of choice.

### Morton's neuroma (Morton's toe, plantar neuroma)

Morton's neuroma results from impingement on the lateral branch of the medial plantar nerve from the development of a neuroma in the area.

**Etiology.** Morton's neuroma is the result of pressure on the most lateral branch of the medial plantar nerve.

**Pathology.** The lateral branch of the medial plantar nerve lies in the web space between the third and fourth metatarsal heads. It supplies sensation to the third and fourth toes. This third plantar common digital nerve, due to impingement, becomes thickened or forms a neuroma. This is presumably due to traumatization of the nerve trunk. Resulting symptomatology is decreased sensation and pain.

**Incidence.** Morton's neuroma is seen more frequently in females than in males.

**Signs and symptoms.** Morton's neuroma usually affects the fourth toe and is most often unilateral. The patient may complain of a burning sensation in the early stages. This burning may be associated with paresthesia or numbness. The patient later complains of severe pain radiating into the third and fourth toes. The pain is often relieved by removal of the shoe and massage of the ball of the foot.[2]

**Treatment.** Relief of pressure on the neuroma may be accomplished by utilizing a metatarsal arch support. Surgical intervention by excision of the enlarged segment of the nerve is the treatment of choice when conservative measures fail.

### Pes cavus (clawfoot, congenital pes cavus)

Pes cavus (Fig. 14-3) is a deformity characterized by dropping of the forefoot, contracture of the plantar fascia, varus deformity of the heel, and clawing of the toes. The term *clawfoot* is an accurate description of the combination of components that result in this single deformity.

**Etiology.** The cause of pes cavus may be idiopathic or may be secondary to paralytic neurologic diseases or developmental deformities of the spine.[9,p.1289] Specific causes are given in Table 14-3. Due to the vast number of etiologic considerations for this deformity, it is recommended that all possibilities be explored and totally ruled out before the condition is classified as being of idiopathic origin.

**Pathology.** Pathologic features of pes cavus, regardless of cause, include the following:

1. Dropping of the forefoot
2. Contracture of the plantar fascia
3. Varus deformity of the heel
4. Clawing of the toes

**Incidence.** Incidence of idiopathic pes cavus is the same in both sexes. It usually develops after 3 years of age and is often associated with spina bifida occulta.

**Signs and symptoms.** Pes cavus may be seen in varying degrees of severity. The most severe deformities exhibit the following characteristics[9,p.1292]:

1. High arch of foot

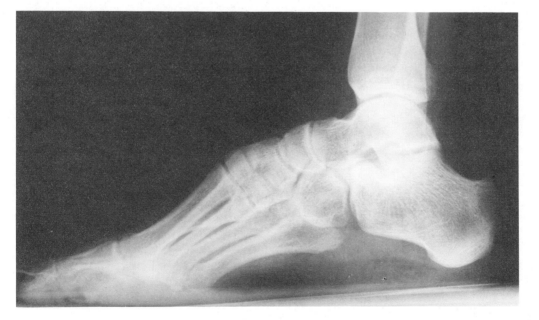

**Fig. 14-3.** Pes cavus (clawfoot). Note severe components of deformity.

**Table 14-3.** Pes cavus: etiologic and pathologic considerations[9,pp.1289-1290]

| | Etiologic classifications | Theories of pathogenesis | Comments |
|---|---|---|---|
| Idiopathic | Often associated with spina bifida occulta | Weakness of intrinsic muscles<br>Overactivity of intrinsic muscles | Most common<br>Develops after 3 years of age<br>Males and females equally affected |
| Secondary | Neurologic disease<br>  Spinocerebellar hereditary degeneration of Mollout<br>  Friedreich's ataxia<br>  Poliomyelitis<br>  Disease of conus medullaris or cauda equina<br>  Spina bifida<br>  Pyramidal or extrapyramidal syndromes<br>  Progressive peroneal palsy (Charcot-Marie-Tooth)<br>Direct trauma to foot<br>Myopathies (muscular dystrophy)<br>Plantar fibromatosis<br>Congenital talipes equinovarus | Associated with paralytic disease:<br>  Acute contracture<br>  Postural contracture<br>  Muscle imbalance<br>    Weak anterior tibial, normal peroneus longus<br>  Weakness of calf muscles | |

**Table 14-4.** Treatment of pes cavus by degree of deformity from least to most severe[9,pp.1292-1302]

| Degree of deformity | Characteristics | Treatment recommendations and considerations |
|---|---|---|
| First | Foot appears relatively normal<br>Minimal cavus deformity | Manipulation daily<br>  Flatten arch by supinating forefoot and everting heel<br>  Dorsiflex first matatarsal forcibly<br>Dorsiflexion exercise; avoid cocking of toes<br>Shoe insert: anterior arch bar<br>Night support: splint; pressure applied behind metatarsal head with dorsiflexion |
| Second | Equinus and pronation of first ray irreducibility<br>Early contracture of plantar fascia<br>Clawing of large toe | Surgical procedure<br>  Jones tenosuspension or similar procedure |
| Third | Involvement of additional metatarsals<br>Increased equinus deformity<br>Increased irreducibility of deformity<br>Calcaneus inversion beginning<br>Resistive passive reduction of calcaneus inversion | Surgical procedures<br>  Extensor shift procedure<br>  Posterior calcaneal osteotomy |
| Fourth | Pronounced deformity, all components<br>Passive correction resisted<br>Some midtarsal motion | Radical surgical intervention<br>Consideration given to preservation of midtarsal motion; not always possible<br>Procedures<br>  Tarsal osteotomy<br>  Anterior tarsal wedge osteotomy<br>  Fusion of first metatarsocuneiform-navicular joints |
| Fifth | Most severe deformities, all components<br>All deformities firmly fixed<br>Toes dislocated distally<br>Plantar fascia, marked contracture<br>Points of pressure evident: proximal interphalangeal joints (dorsally), metatarsal head (volar aspect)<br>Severe disability | Surgical intervention<br>  Correction of midfoot deformities<br>  Correction of hindfoot deformities<br>  Increasing stability<br>Procedures<br>  Bone wedge resection<br>  Triple arthrodesis<br>  Jones procedure<br>  Fusion of proximal interphalangeal joints |

(Degree of deformity column: arrow from "Least severe" to "Most severe")

**Table 14-5.** Classification and causes of pronated feet[9, pp. 1285-1286]

| Classification | Cause |
|---|---|
| **Congenital** | |
| Hypermobile flatfoot | Hereditary |
| | Marked laxity of ligaments |
| | Metatarsal and subtalar joints hypermobile |
| | Archilles tendon short |
| Rigid flatfoot | Common type |
| with tarsal anomalies | Due to bridging between talus and os calcis or navicular and os calis |
| **Acquired** | |
| Osseous | Due to fractures or disease, especially of talus and os calcis |
| Ligamentous | Due to dislocations that may tear and eventually lengthen plantar ligaments |
| Muscle imbalance | Due to weakness of tibials in presence of strong peronei causing a valgus deformity |
| Postural or statis | May be due to internal tibial torsion, excessive weight, muscle fatigue, poorly fitting footwear, bad walking habits, or inherent weakness or laxity of ligaments |
| Arthritis | May be due to arthritis of rheumatoid variety or a development of degenerative arthritis |

2. First metatarsal dropped; pronation present; other metatarsals involved progressively
3. Plantar fascia tight
4. Cock-up deformity of all toes at metatarsophalangeal joints
5. Flexion deformity of all toes at interphalangeal joints
6. Varus deformity of heel
7. Heel not in equinus position

**Treatment.** Of greatest concern in pes cavus are the components of the primary deformity, equinus and pronation of the forefoot, toward which the treatment should be directed. Turek has recommended treatment of this deformity based on the extent of involvement and severity of the combined deformity. The components of this recommended treatment, based on his classification of severity, are given in Table 14-4. As is apparent, all degrees of deformity with the exception of the slightest require surgical intervention, with procedures varying appropriately.

### Pronated foot (flatfoot)

Pronated foot (Fig. 14-4) is a deformity characterized by the absence of the longitudinal arch of the foot.

**Etiology.** Pronated foot may be acquired or congenital (Table 14-5). That of acquired origin may be due to osseous or ligamentous injuries, muscular

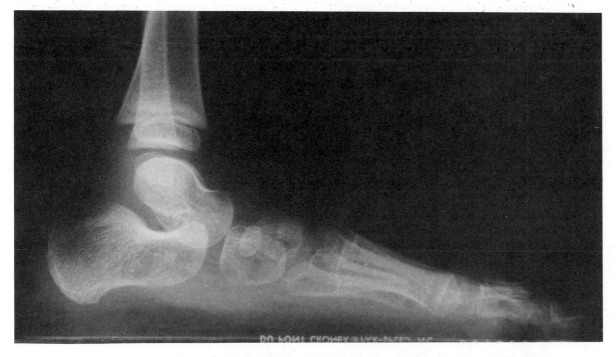

**Fig. 14-4.** Pronated foot (plano valgus). Note that plantar arch is flat, forefoot is adducted, talocalcaneal angle is increased in lateral view, with valgus heel.

imbalance, postural alterations, or arthritic changes. A familial trait is often seen.

**Pathology.** Pronated foot, regardless of cause, reflects a laxity in the ligamentous structures in the longitudinal arch of the foot. There may be a valgus deformity with heel eversion. The term *flatfoot* often is utilized for any deformity of the foot where the longitudinal arch is low. The true pronated foot is characterized by disturbances in the mechanical structure of the ligaments surrounding the arch, which produce medial displacement of body weight resulting in excessive stress and strain on the foot during weight bearing. For this reason it is not "flatness of the longitudinal arch but rather the medial shift in weight bearing that is the important factor in producing foot strain."[8,p.1397]

**Incidence.** Pronated foot is very common in children.

**Signs and symptoms.** The child with pronated feet will frequently "toe-in actively so that the center of gravity of the body is shifted laterally toward the center of the foot."[8,p.1397] On weight bearing the foot is in a valgus position, and the child may complain of pain in the longitudinal arch and extending up the leg. There may be an abnormal degree of fatigue associated with weight bearing and activity. Women may complain of pain in the forefoot from wearing poorly fitting high-heeled shoes.

**Treatment.** Conservative measures in the child are directed toward making the child stand and walk efficiently. The child should not walk barefooted on hard terrain. Shoes should be supportive and provide enough room for the expansion of the foot on weight bearing. Foot strain can be greatly controlled if the weight-bearing pattern can be shifted laterally.[8,p.1399]

In the adult conservative measures are aimed at relieving the symptoms of fatigue, pain, and tenderness. Supportive, well-fitting shoes, and exercises frequently will alleviate some of the symptomatology.

Surgical procedures may be required for persistent symptoms but are not recommended before the age of 10 years. The Grice subtalar extra-articular arthrodesis and triple arthrodesis are procedures that have provided stability and a high degree of alleviation of symptomatology in cases where other measures have failed. They are most frequently accomplished when skeletal maturity has been reached.[9,p.1402]

### Sever's disease of calcaneus

Sever's disease of the calcaneus is a process with onset during puberty and is characterized by fragmentation of areas of the calcaneus surrounding the cartilaginous epiphyseal growth plate resulting in necrosis and eventual resorption.

**Etiology.** Although the specific cause of Sever's disease is unknown, contributing factors may be the stress involved with growth during the preadolescent and early adolescent years.

**Pathology.** The epiphyseal growth plate of the calcaneus is similar in structure and function to all growth plates, with its appearance during preadolescence and its fusion during the midadolescence. Between those years the growth plate in the calcaneus is subjected to a great deal of stress during periods of rapid growth. Pathologic features of Sever's disease may be exhibited through fragmentation of the portion of the calcaneus surrounding this growth plate. With fragmentation necrosis occurs and is identifiable on radiographic examination. Ultimately resorption of the necrotic tissue occurs with evident reconstruction and ossification.[9,p.1314]

**Incidence.** Sever's disease of the calcaneus is seen most frequently between the ages of 11 and 14 years. More boys are seen with this disease than girls.

**Signs and symptoms.** A history of running, hiking, or some type of athletic episode may be taken from the patient with Sever's disease. The patient complains of a gradual onset of pain associated with limp. Low-heeled shoes and standing on tiptoes increase the pain. While walking the patient avoids dorsiflexion of the ankle. The characteristic gait consists of short, halting steps.[9,p.1314]

**Treatment.** Treatment of Sever's disease of the calcaneus is directed toward relief of tension on the epiphysis. In less painful cases the patient is encouraged to decrease activities such as athletics that may aggravate the condition. The foot should be maintained in an equinus position for alleviation of tension on the epiphysis and relief of symptoms; this may be accomplished through heel elevation or adhesive bandage. Only the most severe cases require additional forms of immobilization with cast therapy with the foot in the equinus position.[9,p.1314]

### Tarsal coalition

Tarsal coalition is a deformity characterized by union between two or more tarsal bones.

**Etiology.** The cause of tarsal coalition is unknown, although it is generally thought that it results from an error in embryonic development.

**Pathology.** Tarsal coalition can occur with varying degrees of deformity and involvement. Because of the lack of joint space between the bones involved, the foot is very rigid and motion is extremely limited. The degree of rigidity is dependent on the number of joints involved and the degree of union.

**Signs and symptoms.** When the child with tarsal coalition begins to ambulate, limited motion may be obvious and cause some gait disturbances. Pain is not associated with this deformity in early childhood but may develop later from weight-bearing patterns and the continued stress of ambulation with limited motion. It is not uncommon during adolescence for a severe wrenching injury to occur. Stiffness of the foot is apparent throughout childhood. Spasms of the peroneal muscles may occur but are usually relieved by rest.[8,p.1350;9,p.1303]

**Treatment.** Acute symptoms associated with tarsal coalition are relieved by rest, heat, and immobilization in a cast. Surgical intervention is not accomplished until the preadolescent years, with goals of intervention directed toward creating a stable but more mobile and functional foot for ambulation and alleviation of acute symptoms.[9,p.1305]

### Tarsal tunnel syndrome

Tarsal tunnel syndrome is a disorder caused by compression of the posterior tibial nerve resulting in neurologic symptomatology.

**Etiology.** In most incidences tarsal tunnel syndrome is attributed to "compression neuropathy of the posterior tibial nerve as it passes through the fibro-osseous tunnel beneath the flexor retinaculum on the medial side of the ankle."[9,p.1272]

**Pathology.** Compression of the posterior tibial nerve, as the mechanism responsible for tarsal tunnel syndrome, produces symptomatology (e.g., muscle atrophy, loss of sensation, pain) appropriate to the extent of compression in relation to the length of time the nerve has been compressed.

**Signs and symptoms.** Signs and symptoms of tarsal tunnel syndrome are dependent on the degree of compression and the stage to which the symptoms have progressed at the time of examination. Early signs and symptoms include burning pain, transient ischemia, and paresthesia. In the more advanced stages of compression signs of nerve degeneration are exhibited, and symptoms progress to include numbness, muscle weakness and atrophy, and some reflex alterations. The patient may complain of being awakened by a burning pain and numbness or of burning and tingling after standing and walking.[8,p.735]

**Treatment.** The treatment of tarsal tunnel syndrome and its anticipated success are dependent on the stage of compression at the time of diagnosis. If diagnosed during the early stages, decompression of the nerve is possible and all neurologic functions may return to normal. Hydrocortisone injections have been utilized with some degree of success. Advanced progression of the compression, however, reduces considerably the ability to decompress the nerve without residual symptoms indicative of permanent neurologic damage of varying degrees.

## Lower leg
### Blount's disease (tibia vara, osteochondrosis deformans tibiae)

Blount's disease (Fig. 14-5) is a deformity characterized by disturbances of the epiphyseal growth

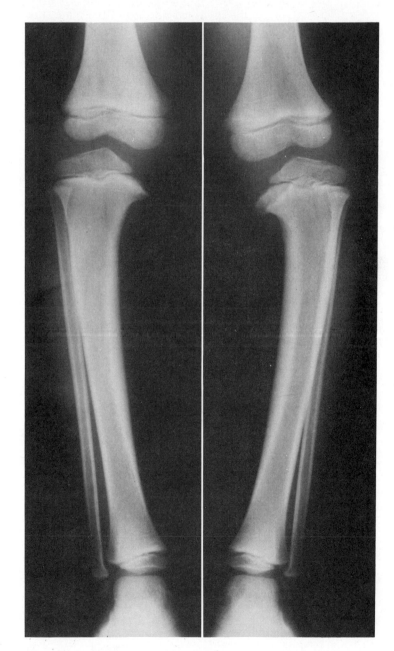

**Fig. 14-5.** Healed Blount's disease with beaking of proximal medial tibial metaphysis and underdevelopment of medial aspect of epiphysis; more marked on left.

plate on the medial aspect of the proximal tibial epiphysis and resulting in tibia vara.

**Etiology.** Blount's disease is the result of either a developmental disturbance of the epiphyseal plate of the proximal tibia or an arrest in the functioning of the epiphyseal growth plate.[2;8,p.341] There may be a history of traumatic injury.

**Pathology.** Two types of Blount's disease characteristically result in the same deformity: the *infantile type* and the *adolescent type*. Regardless of the cause and whether there is an arrest of a portion of the epiphyseal growth plate or disturbance of the growth plate, the involved portion of the plate (the medial aspect of the proximal tibia) ceases to function appropriately and tibia vara results. This deformity results because the remainder of the epiphyseal plate functions, continuing to permit growth on the lateral aspect and creating the angular deformity. It is generally thought that the adolescent type more frequently results from traumatic injuries causing arrest, while the infantile type is created by a developmental disturbance.[8,p.345]

**Signs and symptoms.** Most children with the infantile type of Blount's disease are obese and usually are early walkers (10 to 12 months of age) with increasing bowing of the legs. Approximately one half to three fourths of cases are bilateral. Minimal shortening is exhibited in the involved leg. The adolescent type is of later onset, usually at 8 to 13 years of age. The majority of these cases are unilateral, with bilateral involvement extremely rare. It is not unusual for the involved leg to exhibit significant shortening. There may be a history of trauma and pain, and tenderness may be exhibited on physical examination. On radiographic examination the infantile type reveals medial angulation at the proximal tibia and is a major diagnostic feature of the disease. The adolescent type reveals the center portion of the medial aspect of the epiphyseal growth plate as narrow with increased bone density on the opposite side.[8,p.347] Additional signs and symptoms characteristic of Blount's disease are given in Table 14-6.

**Treatment.** The treatment of Blount's disease depends on the type of deformity and the age of the child. If the angular deformity is between 30° and 45° and the child is between the ages of 2 and 3 years, conservative measures such as support shoes and continued observation for progression of deformity is the recommended treatment. If the de-

**Table 14-6.** Differential findings in Blount's disease

| | Infantile | Adolescent |
|---|---|---|
| Pathogenesis | Dysplasia of growth | Arrest of growth |
| Etiologic factors | Hereditary (recessive) | Trauma |
| | Weight-bearing stresses | |
| | Cartilage necrosis | |
| Age of onset | 1 to 3 years | 8 to 13 years |
| Body habitus | Obese | Normal weight |
| Involvement | Bilateral (50% to 75%) | Unilateral (90%) |
| Pain and tenderness | Absent | Present |
| Internal tibial torsion | Present | Absent |
| Pes planus | Present | Absent |
| Leg shortening | Slight | Significant |
| Deformity | May be excessive | Never excessive |
| Prognosis | Stages I and II: | Depends on progression and time of |
| | complete restoration possible | limitation of treatment |
| | Stages III and IV: | |
| | some restoration possible | |
| | Stages V and VI: | |
| | late sequelae inevitable | |
| Treatment | Less than 30° and under 4 years of age: | Osteotomy |
| | observation and support shoe | |
| | More than 30° and under 4 years: | Epiphyseal closure, osteotomy, and |
| | brace and observation | epiphysiodesis of involved leg |
| | More than 30° and over 4 years: | If of clinical significance, epiphysiodesis of |
| | osteotomy | other leg |
| | Knee laxity and over 9 years: | |
| | elevation of sloping medial condyle of tibia | |
| | followed by osteotomy and lateral | |
| | epiphysiodesis | |

From Tachdjian, M. O.: Pediatric orthopedics, Philadelphia, 1972, W. B. Saunders Co.

formity exceeds 30° and the child is under 4 years of age, lower extremity orthotics along with continued observation to monitor the deformity are recommended. If the child is over 4 years of age and the deformity exceeds 30° surgical intervention in the form of an osteotomy for permanent correction of the deformity is recommended. The adolescent type, due to the stage of growth at the time of diagnosis, requires surgical intervention, usually at the time of diagnosis. Recommended surgical procedures include osteotomy and epiphyseodesis on the involved leg.[8,p.348]

#### Congenital absence of fibula

Congenital absence of the fibula is characterized by absence of the fibula at birth accompanied by varying degrees of associated deformity.

**Etiology.** Congenital absence of the fibula is caused by genetic factors occurring before the eighth embryonic week.[8,p.224]

**Pathology.** Pathologic features of congenital absence of the fibula include varying degrees of the following[9,p.288]:

1. Anterior bowing of the tibia
2. Dimpling of the skin at the distal third of the involved lower extremity
3. Severe talipes equinovalgus
4. Absence of one or more digits of the foot (usually laterally)
5. Absence of one or more tarsal bones, or fusion of two or more tarsal bones
6. Lack of development of the calf and peroneal muscles
7. Shortened involved extremity

**Incidence.** The fibula is the long bone most frequently absent congenitally but rarely occurs despite this fact. It is twice as common in girls as in boys. The right lower extremity is affected more frequently than the left.

**Signs and symptoms.** In congenital absence of the fibula there is a valgus deformity of the foot and ankle. The tibia is often bowed anteriorly (Fig. 14-9, *B*). It may occur with other congenital anomalies. The pathologic features outlined above reflect the additional signs and symptoms that may be seen.

Coventry and Johnson classified deformity of congenital absence of the fibula into three major types, which have specific characteristics[3,p.941]:

*Type I*
1. One extremity affected
2. Affected extremity shortened
3. No bowing of the involved tibia
4. No associated foot deformities

*Type II*
1. One extremity affected
2. More severe shortening of the affected extremity
3. Anterior bowing of the affected tibia
4. Foot deformity: equinovalgus
5. Digits of the foot hypoplastic or absent
6. Tarsal bones hypoplastic or absent

*Type III*
1. Usually bilateral
2. Severe shortening of both extremities
3. Severe tibial bowing anteriorly
4. Severe equinovalgus foot deformities
5. Digits of the foot usually absent
6. Tarsal bones usually absent
7. Frequently in association with other congenital anomalies (e.g., deformities of the femur, spina bifida), especially if unilateral

**Treatment.** The treatment of congenital absence of the fibula is greatly dependent on the type and severity of accompanying deformities and associated involvement. Type I requires the least treatment. An elevated shoe may be appropriate if there is a leg length inequality of more than 1/2 inch accompanied by spinal deformities resulting from the discrepancy. Epiphyseodesis is then recommended at an appropriate age in attempts to equalize the leg lengths. Types II and III present problems that are much more difficult to correct and require more drastic forms of intervention. The prognosis of total correction of these types is poor even with appropriate measures. Contractures of surrounding soft tissue structures are common and frequently require early intervention in the form of excision or release surgically. This should be accomplished as early as possible for best results in the prevention of further deformities of the foot and tibial bowing. Additional procedures may be required if progression of these deformities has not been arrested. Correction of leg length inequality requires intervention, which may vary depending on the severity of the deformities. If the inequality is great, a Syme's amputation may be accomplished to facilitate fitting of a prothesis that will assist in maximally promoting normal function.[8,pp.228-229]

#### Congenital absence of tibia

Congenital absence of the tibia is a deformity characterized by obvious absence of the tibia at birth and frequently is associated with other deformities or multiple lower extremity abnormalities.

**Etiology.** Congenital absence of the tibia is caused by an error in development during the embryonic stages of growth.

**Pathology.** This deformity is characterized by absence of the tibia but very frequently is associated with other congenital anomalies or malformations of the skeletal system, most frequently in the affected extremity. It is not uncommon to have partial or complete absence of the other leg bones of the lower extremity associated with this deformity. The intrauterine development results in a shortened extremity on the affected side and some decrease in total bulk of the lower portion of the leg due to the absence. Bowing of the lower leg is apparent with accompanying deformities. The severity of the associated deformities is dependent on partial or total absence of the tibia.[8,p.224]

**Incidence.** Congenital absence of the tibia is relatively rare, with no difference in incidence noted between boys and girls.

**Signs and symptoms.** Partial or total absence of the tibia may be present and to a great degree affect the severity of the associated deformities (Fig. 14-9). As a result the affected extremity is shortened, decreased bulk is noted by the diameter of the lower leg, fibular bowing is present, and foot deformities exist. The most common foot deformity associated to varying degrees with congenital absence of the tibia is abnormal adduction and inversion. Flexion contractures of the knee joint may be present and again are relative to the degree of absence (partial or total) of the involved bone.[8,p.224]

**Treatment.** Surgical intervention is the treatment of choice for congenital absence of the tibia. The procedure, however, is determined by the severity of the associated deformities. Objectives of reconstructive surgery are to correct the bowing, increase the functional ability of the extremity, and provide appropriate alignment for potential fitting of a prosthesis. The procedures should be considered individually on the basis of the physical examination and the deformities and may vary from fusion of joints to amputation or disarticulation. These procedures are accomplished early to provide the best possible chance for adjustment and increased function. Lesser procedures are accomplished for partial absence of the tibia. Leg length inequalities are evaluated and appropriate measures implemented in relation to the total intervention program for the child.[8,p.224]

### Tibial torsion (internal/external)

Tibial torsion may be defined as the twisting or rotation, either internally or externally, of the tibia on its longitudinal axis.

**Etiology.** Tibial torsion may be congenital or acquired. Intrauterine positioning and stress may be contributing factors in its development.

**Pathology.** A degree of internal and external tibial torsion, within specific limitations, is considered to be a normal physiologic variance; excessive degrees of torsion, however, are considered pathologic. External tibial torsion in excess of 40° is considered pathologic; lesser degrees of internal tibial torsion are considered pathologic. The major pathologic feature of both is the excessive torsion itself.[9,p.289]

**Incidence.** Physiologic variances of tibial torsion are relatively common, with a less common incidence of pathologic internal or external tibial torsion.

**Signs and symptoms.** *Congenital* internal tibial torsion is characterized by the apparent "bowlegs" that develop. This developmental abnormality is only apparent in nature, and on physical examination it may be noted that the deformity is alleviated automatically when the patellae are facing directly forward. The prognosis is poor for those children who receive no treatment. *Acquired* internal tibial torsion is frequently attributed to the child's sleeping on his or her stomach in the knee-chest position with the toes turned in and may be accompanied by similar signs and symptoms.

External tibial torsion reveals excessive degrees of external rotation with the feet pointing lateral to the midline of the medial plane. Apparent valgus deformity of the knees is exhibited when the feet are pointed directly at the midline of the medial plane. There frequently is a history of sleeping patterns (e.g. frogleg position) conducive to the development of this deformity.[9,p.290]

**Treatment.** Congenital internal tibial torsion may be treated with conservative measures such as various types of splints if diagnosed early. After the age of 6 or 7 years, conservative treatment is unlikely to be successful, and surgical intervention in the form of derotational osteotomies may be required. Acquired internal tibial torsion is frequently alleviated through the correction of sleeping habits, through which spontaneous derotation may be anticipated. The utilization of splints or appropriate orthotic devices may assist in the maintenance of the position and alteration of sleeping patterns in the infant and young child. External tibial torsion also responds well to the correction of sleeping patterns and appropriate positional maintenance devices.[9,p.290]

## Knee
### Baker's cyst (popliteal cyst)

Baker's cyst, sometimes known as a popliteal cyst, is a fluid-filled sac located in the posterior portion of the knee structure.

**Pathology.** Baker's cyst is frequently located around or in bursae in or near the knee joint. One of the most common sites is distal to the popliteal crease on the posteromedial aspect of the knee just under the medial head of the gastrocnemius muscle. The developing cyst produces an increasingly distended sac filled with fluid, and swelling may be externally apparent. Additional pathologic features occur only if the growth impinges on the surrounding structures producing pain or other symptomatology.

**Incidence.** Baker's cyst is most frequently unilateral and is twice as common in males as in females. It is not infrequently seen in children.

**Signs and symptoms.** The most frequent sign or symptom of Baker's cyst, which requires diagnostic review, is the presence of a mass in the posterior aspect of the patient's knee. There may also be associated stiffness and local pain.

**Treatment.** Baker's cyst frequently requires no treatment. If the mass is large and causes persistent symptoms, surgical excision may be indicated.

### Chondromalacia of patella

Chondromalacia of the patella is softening of the articular cartilage of the patella resulting in pain, stiffness, and various degrees of instability of the knee joint.

**Etiology.** The cause of chondromalacia is unknown in many patients. Its development may follow traumatic injuries to the patella.

**Pathology.** Chondromalacia of the patella is associated with degeneration of the articular hyaline cartilage lining the undersurface of the patella. When examined grossly the cartilage may appear yellowish white, opaque, and dull, and it lacks resiliency. Edema of the cartilaginous tissue involved may occur and form an elevation on the surface of the area of articulation. This is usually found near the center of the softened area, and pathologic features reveal signs of eruption. Turek has classified pathologic features of this process into the following types: (1) primary idiopathic, (2) secondary adolescent, and (3) adult. Additional specific pathologic features in relation to onset and outcome are given in Table 14-7.

**Incidence.** The incidence of chondromalacia of the patella of the primary idiopathic and secondary types is relatively limited to adolescents and young adults. The adult type may appear at any time throughout adulthood and as early as the second decade of life.

**Signs and symptoms.** The signs and symptoms of chondromalacia are characterized according to the stated classifications and are as follows.

*Primary idiopathic type.* Chronic, aching pain "over the front or anteromedial aspect of the knee, made worse when the knee functions under load in flexion," is characteristic of this type of chondromalacia.[9,p.1191] Stair climbing and descending, as well as sitting with the knees in flexion for prolonged periods, initiates or aggravates the pain.

*Secondary type.* Symptoms seen with secondary type of chondromalacia are similar to those seen in the primary idiopathic type, with additional complaint of instability or "giving way" of the knee accompanied by stiffness and swelling.

*Adult type.* Osteoarthritic alterations are seen with the adult type of chondromalacia, starting as early as the second decade of life. Stiffness, marked limitation in motion, crepitation, and effusion result as the condition progresses.

**Treatment.** The treatment of chondromalacia is also related to the classification as follows.

*Primary idiopathic type.* Conservative treatment modalities include the avoidance of sitting with knees flexed for extended periods, squatting, and stair climbing. Quadriceps strengthening exercises are encouraged. Surgical intervention is indicated when severe symptoms persist and it is apparent

**Table 14-7.** Chondromalacia of patella: categories of syndrome[9,pp.1189-1195]

| Classification | Age group | Onset | Outcome |
| --- | --- | --- | --- |
| Primary idiopathic type | Adolescents and young adults | Chronic, aching pain, worse when knee is functioning under load in flexion (e.g., walking up or down stairs) | Usually subsides with little or no residual symptomatology. Early osteoarthritic changes rare |
| Secondary adolescent type | Adolescents and young adults | Due to direct or repeated trauma. Classic locking or "giving way" of knee are associated symptoms | Osteoarthritis often develops with advancing age |
| Adult type | Adults, as early as second decade | Changes may be asymptomatic until middle age or later | Progressively increasing pain with severe limitation of motion |

that conservative measures have failed. Procedures such as shaving the surface cartilage and excision of the lesion are attempted prior to a patellectomy. This consideration is made because of the tendency of the latter procedure to weaken quadriceps function and thus interfere with activities for some individuals.[9,p.1191]

*Secondary type.* Conservative measures for chondromalacia of the patella are directed toward the avoidance of dislocations and subluxations, which produce the characteristic instability of the knee joint. "Only when pain and patella displacement are intractable and persistently disabling is surgical treatment justified."[9,p.1193]

*Adult type.* Conservative treatment modalities for the adult type of chondromalacia include rest, heat, intra-articular injection of steroids, salicylate therapy, quadriceps strengthening exercises, and avoidance of activities requiring excessive stress on the patellofemoral joint. Surgical intervention in the form of a patellectomy is the treatment of choice when conservative measures have failed. Because osteoarthritic degeneration of the joint is known to result from this type of chondromalacia, it is advantageous for immediate surgical intervention to be accomplished in cases where recurrent subluxations and dislocations are apparent and patellar involvement can be diagnosed in attempts to halt the advancement of this process.[9,p.1198]

### Congenital dislocation of knee

Congenital dislocation of the knee is displacement of the knee joint present at birth.

**Etiology.** Hereditary factors influence the presence of congenital dislocation of the knee, which is often associated with other congenital anomalies, the most frequent of which is congenital dislocation of the hip.[8,p.200]

**Pathology.** Although the degree of displacement may vary, the tibia is usually displaced anteriorly in relation to the femur. Varying degrees of rotational anomaly and lateral subluxation may be evident, producing a noticeable deformity.[8,p.200]

**Incidence.** The incidence of congenital dislocation of the knee as a deformity associated with other anomalies is rare. It is even more rare as a single deformity.

**Signs and symptoms.** The most common form of congenital dislocation of the knee is subluxation rather than dislocation. Involvement is often bilateral, and flexion of the knee is limited to varying degrees. Physical examination will reveal varying degrees of the outlined pathologic features.[8,p.202]

**Treatment.** Treatment of dislocation of the knee should begin in the neonatal period with manipulation of the knee into flexion. The lower extremity is immobilized in a plaster cast, which is replaced at 2-week intervals with gradually increasing degrees of flexion at the knee. The regimen is continued for 6 to 8 weeks or until the knee becomes stable. A bivalved cast may then be utilized to maintain the knee in flexion for 4 to 6 months. The child's leg is exercised by the parents to increase the degree of flexion. Skeletal traction may be utilized when the subluxation cannot be reduced by manipulation. Surgery is indicated when conservative measures have failed. In the adult with arthritis and marked deformity resulting from congenital dislocation of the knee, arthrodesis may be indicated.[8,p.206]

### Discoid meniscus

Discoid meniscus is a developmental anomaly characterized by the cartilaginous meniscus of the knee being discoid rather than similunar in shape.

**Pathology.** The lateral meniscus is most often affected, although the medial meniscus may be. It is characterized by the development of a discoid rather than the usual semilunar meniscus. Increased wear on the affected meniscus apparently contributes to the degeneration that occurs. Tears of the meniscus resulting from the general pathologic degeneration may be seen.[8,pp.721-722]

**Incidence.** Discoid meniscus is often seen bilaterally, with no sex differentiation.

**Signs and symptoms.** Discoid meniscus is asymptomatic in the infant or young child. It occurs most frequently in the child between 6 and 8 years of age. There is frequently a complaint of a "clicking" or "giving way" of the knee joint. The symptoms may follow an injury but may also be seen without traumatic association. Examination demonstrates this "clicking," usually when the knee is moved from flexion to extension, during the last 15° to 20°.[8,p.722]

**Treatment.** Minimal pain and functional disability are not indications for surgery. However, excision of the meniscus may be indicated if symptomatology is recurrent or the "clicking" is of enough concern.

### Recurrent dislocation of patella (slipping patella)

Recurrent dislocation of the patella is displacement of the patella that occurs repeatedly.

**Etiology.** Recurrent dislocation of the patella is relatively uncommon. Its various causes are[8,pp.723,731]:
1. Ligamentous laxity
2. Contracture and abnormal attachments of the iliotibial tract

3. Genu valgum and external torsional deformity of the tibia
4. High-line patella
5. Traumatic injury

**Pathology.** Recurrent dislocation of the patella most frequently occurs with flexion and extension of the knee. The repeated episodes result in degeneration of the patellofemoral joint. Pathologic changes and progressions have been divided by Macrab into five stages[8,pp.731-732]:

*Stage I.* During this initial stage changes are confined to the patella.

*Stage II.* Greater degeneration of the articular surface of the patella occurs.

*Stage III.* Patellofemoral arthritis begins to develop with progressive attrition of the articular cartilage of the patella and opposing femur.

*Stage IV.* Marked patellofemoral arthritis is evident.

*Stage V.* Osteoarthritic changes progress to involve the femorotibial joint.

**Incidence.** There is a very high incidence of recurrent dislocation of the patella in females. It is usually unilateral, with a familial tendency.

**Signs and symptoms.** The patient with recurrent dislocation of the patella usually complains of the knee "giving way," which may be associated with a high degree of edema surrounding the knee. Infrequent attacks are associated with severe pain, which may cause the patient to fall when the dislocation occurs. With frequent episodes of dislocation the pain and disability appear to decrease. Radiographic examination reveals involvement comparable to the stage of progression and positioning of the patella, which is unusually high and lateral. Other bony abnormalities and involvement reflect the wearing of the surrounding structures.

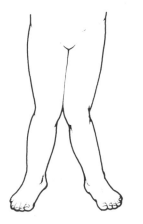

**Fig. 14-6.** Genu valgum. (From Hilt, N. E., and Schmitt, E. W., Jr.: Pediatric orthopedic nursing, St. Louis, 1975, The C. V. Mosby Co.)

**Treatment.** Conservative management of recurrent dislocation of the patella is preferred when the episodes of dislocation are infrequent. Quadriceps strengthening exercises are of some value in conservative management. Passive stretching is advised if a contracture exists. Sports and strenuous exercises are known to initiate or aggravate the condition and should be avoided. The medial side of the heel of the shoe may be raised and toeing-in encouraged in attempts to correct genu valgum deformity if present. Surgical intervention may be necessary if dislocations become extremely frequent. Numerous surgical procedures have been devised. In children only soft tissue procedures should be accomplished.[8,p.732]

### Genu valgum (knock-knee)

Genu valgum (Fig. 14-6) is a deformity characterized by a decreased space between the knees, is physiologic between the ages of 2 and 6 years, and is considered pathologic if it persists after that age.

**Etiology.** When genu valgum is unilateral the most frequent cause is a traumatic injury, usually a fracture to the lateral portion of the epiphyseal growth plates surrounding the knee joint. Due to increased educational emphasis, rickets are rarely a cause of this deformity, although nutritional disorders must be considered if the deformity is bilateral. Severe pronated feet (flatfeet) may be an additional etiologic factor in this deformity.[9,p.1211]

**Pathology.** With traumatic injury to the epiphyseal growth plate, medial growth plate function may continue while lateral function ceases, resulting in genu valgum. When pronated feet are the cause the deformity is developmental in nature and related to the stance and gait associated with the deformity. In all cases outward deviation of the lower leg from the longitudinal axis of the tibia and femur, accompanied by medial angulation of the knee, is the major pathologic feature.[5,pp.377-378]

**Signs and symptoms.** The major sign and symptom of genu valgum is a decreased space between the knees, with lateral angulation below the level of the knee. It may occur unilaterally or bilaterally, and the degree of angulation may be extremely variable. Pain is sometimes associated with this deformity and is most frequently referred to the calf or the anterior aspect of the thigh. It is not unusual for the child with genu valgum to be obese.

**Treatment.** It must be emphasized that genu valgum is physiologic between the ages of 2 and 6 years. Spontaneous correction may be anticipated in this age group. In genu valgum associated with pronated feet, the child may be fitted with a special shoe with appropriate support or inserts in attempts to prevent foot strain and promote toeing-in for correction of the deformity. Surgical intervention is necessary in severe cases, with appropriate procedures varying according to the age of the child and the severity of the deformity as well as its cause. In most cases the surgical procedure of choice includes wedge osteotomies for correction of the deformity.

### Genu varum (bowleg)

Genu varum (Fig. 14-7) is the outward bowing of the knee joints with medial deviation of the femur and tibia.

**Etiology.** With the advent of vitamin D therapy rickets, a once common cause of genu varum, has become rare. Unilateral deformity may be caused by an injury to the medial portion of the upper tibial epiphyseal plate. Infants' sleeping patterns have also been known to contribute to the development of genu varum.[9,p.1214]

**Pathology.** The major pathologic feature of genu varum is the outward bowing or angulation of the knee joint characterized by a wide space between the knees. Deformities resulting from traumatic injuries to the tibial epiphyseal growth plate pathologically reveal continued functioning of the lateral portion of the growth plate, with ceased functioning of the medial portion, resulting in the deformity. The degree of bowing or angulation may involve the tibia or femur or both to varying degrees. Genu varum is physiologic during infancy and up to approximately 2 to 2½ years of age because of the initial stress of weight bearing and the need to provide a wide base during the initial phases of ambulation.

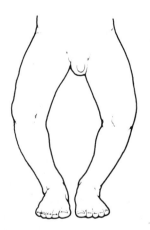

**Fig. 14-7.** Genu varum. (From Hilt, N. E., and Schmitt, E. W., Jr.: Pediatric orthopedic nursing, St. Louis, 1975, The C. V. Mosby Co.)

It is most often seen bilaterally but occasionally affects only one leg and may be associated with genu valgum in the other leg.[8,p.1462]

**Incidence.** Physiologic genu varum is quite common, with tremendously decreased incidence of pathologic genu varum.

**Signs and symptoms.** When the legs are placed together in the extended position during physical examination, the knees do not touch in a patient with genu varum. The child walks with his feet widely separated and toes turned in. This causes the characteristic waddling or rolling gait as the child shifts his body weight with each step. Radiographic examination reveals medial tilting of the transverse plane of the knee and ankle joints and the obvious angulation with normal epiphyseal appearance and development. When involvement is bilateral, radiographic features are usually symmetric.[8,p.1464]

**Treatment.** Because genu varum is physiologic during the first 2 to 2½ years of life, the greatest contribution to treatment in this age group is reassurance directed to the parents that the bowing appearance of the leg is normal and will probably spontaneously correct itself. Severe and persistent deformity associated with older children usually requires surgical intervention in the form of an osteotomy.

### Osgood-Schlatter disease (osteochondritis of tibial tubercle)

Osgood-Schlatter disease (Fig. 14-8) is characterized by pain and swelling of the patellar tendon and enlargement of the tibial tubercle.

**Etiology.** The most frequent contributing factor to Osgood-Schlatter disease is a traumatic injury, frequently during adolescence. An additional consideration may be forced flexion of the knee with the presence of a tight quadriceps muscle.[9,p.204]

**Pathology.** The major pathologic feature of Osgood-Schlatter disease is necrotic fragmentation associated with swelling of the patellar tendon and enlargement of the tibial tubercle. It is unclear as to whether this disease is truly one of the group known as *osteochondrosis*, characterized by primary disturbances of the circulation to a specific bony structure resulting in vascular necrosis to the area, or whether the necrosis occurs after the fragmentation.

**Incidence.** Osgood-Schlatter disease occurs most frequently during puberty, is seen more frequently in boys than in girls, and is often bilateral.

**Signs and symptoms.** Tenderness and soft tissue swelling associated with Osgood-Schlatter disease are usually localized over the tibial tubercle. Pain is associated with this process and appears to increase with localized pressure created by specific activities such as kneeling, running, bicycle riding, and stair climbing. The symptomatology is chronic and may persist for several years but is known to cease at approximately 18 years of age. Occasionally minor symptoms associated with this disease persist into the adult years.[5,p.90;9,p.1205]

**Treatment.** Nonsurgical intervention in the form of cast application with the knee in full extension for several months is frequently successful. This extension releases the tension on the quadriceps, permitting "revascularization and reossification of the tibial tubercle."[9,p.1205] If surgical intervention is necessary, either because of persistent symptoms or indication of failure of nonsurgical treatment modalities, the most common and useful procedure recommended permits revascularization by means of holes drilled through the tubercle into the main shaft or portion of the bone. Because tubercle enlargement commonly associated with this disease may be progressive and may pose some cosmetic difficulties, removal may be indicated.

### Rupture of collateral ligaments of knee

Rupture of collateral ligaments of the knee is a painful and often disabling condition resulting from forceful abduction of the knee.

**Etiology.** Stress on the collateral ligaments with

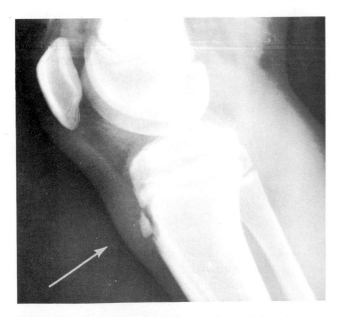

**Fig. 14-8.** Osgood-Schlatter disease showing irregularity of epiphysis, tibial tuberosity, and swelling of overlying soft tissues. (From Brashear, H. R., and Raney, R. B.: Shand's handbook of orthopaedic surgery, ed. 9, St. Louis, 1978, The C. V. Mosby Co.)

the knee slightly flexed and forceful abduction of the knee, such as may occur in a football "clip" or skiing accident, is frequently the cause of rupture of these ligaments.

**Pathology.** The collateral ligaments may be torn from their attachments or ruptured completely. Damage to the cruciate ligament often accompanies rupture of the collateral ligaments. The "terrible triad" exists when, following severe trauma, tearing of the collateral ligaments, the cruciate ligament, and the medial meniscus occurs simultaneously.

**Incidence.** Rupture of the collateral ligaments of the knee occurs most often in young or athletic individuals.

**Signs and symptoms.** The patient with a rupture of the collateral ligaments of the knee complains of tenderness over the area of the injury. With rupture there is swelling and increase of joint fluid, and the patient may complain of instability or "catching" in the knee joint. Stress x-ray films of the partially flexed affected knee while adduction force is applied to the joint confirms the diagnosis. "Opening of the medial side of the joint indicates rupture of the medial collateral ligament; opening of the lateral side indicates rupture of the lateral collateral ligaments."[5,p.373]

**Treatment.** Decreased activities and only partial weight bearing for 3 to 4 weeks is the therapy of choice for the mild injury. Quadriceps setting exercises for strengthening are prescribed. In moderate injuries, especially with knee instability, immobilization in a long leg cast with the knee joint in slight flexion is advocated. When there is complete ligamentous rupture, surgical intervention as soon after the injury as possible is indicated, followed by a period of 5 to 6 weeks of immobilization in a long leg cast.

### Rupture of cruciate ligaments of knee

Rupture of the cruciate ligaments of the knee is caused by severe trauma and involves great degrees of swelling and instability of the knee joint.

**Etiology.** Severe trauma to the knee is the most frequent contributing factor to rupture of the cruciate ligaments of the knee.

**Pathology.** The anterior cruciate ligament may rupture in association with tears of the medial meniscus and rupture of the medial collateral ligament. Rupture of the anterior cruciate ligament may be caused by forced hyperextension of the knee and internal rotation of the tibia on the femur. Forced displacement of the tibia backward on the femur with the knee flexed may cause rupture of the posterior cruciate ligament.

**Incidence.** Rupture of the cruciate ligaments of the knee most frequently occurs in the young or athletic individual.

**Signs and symptoms.** Instability of the knee joint and swelling follow rupture of the cruciate ligaments. The pain and spasms encountered in an acute cruciate ligament injury make examination very difficult and may obscure the degree of instability.

**Treatment.** Surgical intervention is the treatment of choice, especially if the "terrible triad" (rupture of the collateral ligament and the cruciate ligament and tear of the medial meniscus) exists. Conservative therapy consisting of immobilization in a cast for 2 months followed by utilization of a leg brace may be chosen for the older patient.

## Upper leg
### Femoral torsion (anteversion)

Femoral torsion, or anteversion, is an extreme twisting or torsion of the femur anteriorly on its longitudinal axis.

**Etiology.** Femoral torsion is a developmental deformity frequently resulting from reverse tailor's sitting position.

**Pathology.** Femoral torsion reveals pathologic features of anterior or forward twisting of the axis of the femoral neck. Other pathologic indications reveal features secondary to this singular primary feature.

**Incidence.** Femoral torsion is relatively common and is seen twice as often in girls as in boys.

**Signs and symptoms.** The patient with femoral torsion usually walks with a clumsy, awkward gait and toeing-in. On examination with the feet aligned, the legs appear bowed and the patellae face inward. When the hips are laterally rotated and the patellae face forward, the legs and feet point outward and the bowleg appearance is corrected. Limited lateral hip rotation with increased internal rotation is often seen when the hip is examined in extension. With the hip in flexion, however, lateral rotation is usually increased. Adaptive alterations in response to the abnormal and extreme femoral anteversion include valgus deformity of the hindfoot, lateral torsion of the tibia, and toeing-in. A history of the reverse tailor's sitting position is frequently obtained.[8, p. 1448]

**Treatment.** The parents of the young child with femoral torsion are instructed to strongly encourage the tailor's sitting position rather than the reverse tailor's position if, as in most cases, this latter pattern has been established. Corrective shoes are utilized for the valgus deformity. The child should be examined at regular intervals and the parents en-

couraged that the condition will in all probability correct itself spontaneously by the age of 7 to 8 years. If spontaneous correction is not obtained, immobilization of the hip and forced external rotation may be advocated for those children under 7 to 8 years of age. If spontaneous correction does not occur in children over this age, osteotomy of the femur is indicated. Surgical intervention in these cases should be accomplished during preadolescence to avoid further developmental deformities.[8, p. 1452]

### Dysgenesis of proximal femur

Dysgenesis of the proximal femur is a skeletal growth disorder presumably congenital in origin. There is a familial tendency. It is characterized by shortening of the femur and decrease of the neck-shaft angle, occurring with varying degrees of severity. The localized forms of dysgenesis are sub-classified as (1) congenital coxa vara, (2) congenital short femur with coxa vara, and (3) congenital bowed femur with coxa vara. Dysgenesis may be due to a localized disturbance or a manifestation of generalized growth dysfunction.[8, p. 180] (See also coxa vara.)

## General lower extremity diseases and disorders
### Congenital hemihypertrophy

Congenital hemihypertrophy is a condition of asymmetric overgrowth of one side of the body.

**Etiology.** The specific cause of congenital hemihypertrophy is unknown, but factors to be considered are[8, p. 1514]:

1. Endocrine and lymphatic abnormalities
2. Vascular anomalies
3. Lesions of the brain
4. Embryonic defects of the autonomic system
5. Hereditary influences
6. Embryogenic variants

**Pathology.** With true hemihypertrophy the entire side of the body is affected, although the lower extremity alone may be involved or more pronounced. The classic pathologic feature is asymmetric overgrowth of the involved side, with inclusion of blood vessels, muscles, and bones.[8, p. 1514]

**Signs and symptoms.** The signs and symptoms associated with hemihypertrophy are greatly dependent on the degree of involvement. Segmental involvement is associated with the extremities only, with the left side more frequently involved than the right. Crossed hypertrophy may occur, with one extremity involved on one side and one extremity involved on the opposite side. The most extensive involvement is seen with true hemihypertrophy, where an entire side of the body is involved. Other associated anomalies may be seen in conjunction with hemihypertrophy, the most frequent of which are syndactylism, polydactylism, congenital heart disease, synostosis, and mental deficiencies (in approximately 15% to 20% of the cases). At the end of the growth period the overgrowth appears to cease; however, the disproportionate size is often cosmetically and functionally unacceptable.[8,p.1514]

**Treatment.** The treatment of hemihypertrophy varies according to the extensiveness of the involvement and is directed toward cosmetic and functional restoration. Surgical intervention in the form of epiphyseodesis is almost always required to equalize the leg lengths.[8,p.1515]

### Dyschondroplasia (Ollier's disease, enchondromatosis)

Dyschondroplasia is a "rare developmental condition characterized by disorderly and excessive proliferation of cartilage cells at many of the epiphyseal plates."[2]

**Pathology.** Excessive proliferation of irregularly shaped cartilaginous cells are found in the metaphyses of the bones, characterizing this disease process and reducing longitudinal growth. Microscopically the cells are of varying sizes in maturation. Differential diagnosis between dyschondroplasia and multiple exostosis is often confusing. One distinguishing pathologic feature is that dyschondroplasia is characterized by involvement within the metaphysis, while multiple exostosis is characterized by involvement projecting outward from the surface of the metaphysis.

**Incidence.** Dyschondroplasia manifests itself during the growth period, with the main sites of involvement in the long bones at the actively growing ends.[9,p.320]

**Signs and symptoms.** The major sign and symptom of dyschondroplasia is reduced longitudinal growth of the long bones. The lesions appear to affect the bones on one side of the body. The pathologic feature, therefore, is a shortened limb with valgus or varus deformities when growth is retarded unequally at the epiphyseal line.

Radiographic examination reveals the metaphysis filled with clear spaces of cartilage in varying sizes and shapes. The metaphysis is expanded and the diaphysis is short and occasionally curves. As the growth period of adolescence is approached, the areas of cartilage become less defined and the suggestion of ossification with appearance of dense spots within the bone is observed.[9,p.320]

**Treatment.** The resulting deformities of mild to moderate severity may be treated conservatively. In severe deformity osteotomy may be necessary. Epiphyseodesis may be indicated to combat limb length inequality.[9,p.320]

### Leg length discrepancy (leg length inequality, anisomelia)

Leg length discrepancy is a very common orthopedic problem caused by a variety of conditions and resulting in inequality of the leg lengths.

**Etiology.** A number of causes of leg length discrepancy are given in Table 14-8.

**Pathology.** The pathologic features of leg length discrepancies are dependent on the cause. The one obvious feature common to all etiologic origins is that of the inequality in the leg lengths. The actual inequality may occur in the upper or the lower leg or both.

**Table 14-8.** Summary of etiologic origins of leg length discrepancy[8,p.1469]

| General classification | Specific etiologic origin |
|---|---|
| I Congenital anomalies of skeletal system | Congenital short femur |
| | Dysgenesis of proximal femur |
| | Congenital dislocation of hip |
| | Congenital absence or hypoplasia of long bones of lower extremity |
| | Congenital hemihypertrophy |
| II Tumorous conditions of skeleton | Fibrous dysplasia |
| | Enchondromatosis |
| | Multiple hereditary exostosis |
| | Unicameral bone cyst |
| III Infections of bones and joints | Osteomyelitis |
| | Tuberculosis |
| IV Trauma | Epiphyseal growth plate injuries |
| | Metaphyseal injuries |
| | Fractures of shaft of femur or tibia |
| V Miscellaneous skeletal diseases and disorders | Rheumatoid arthritis |
| | Legg-Perthes disease |
| | Slipped capital femoral epiphysis |
| VI Neuromuscular diseases with asymetric paralysis | Cerebral palsy |
| | Poliomyelitis |
| | Myelomeningocele |
| | Peripheral joints |
| VII Soft tissue abnormalities | Arteriovenous fistula |
| | Hemangiomatosis |
| | Neurofibromatosis |

**Incidence.** The incidence of leg length discrepancy is widely varied due to the multiple causes. It is generally thought that many discrepancies of a minor degree exist that are not symptomatic and therefore are not diagnosed and treated.

**Signs and symptoms.** The signs and symptoms associated with leg length discrepancy vary considerably with the severity of the inequality and the cause. Moderate to severe discrepancies cause a moderate to significant limp. Posture is usually asymmetric and relative to the degree of discrepancy. While standing the patient usually tilts the pelvis downward on the side that is short. Secondary scoliosis convex to the short side is usually apparent. Radiographic examination in the form of scanography (growth study films) confirms the specific location of the discrepancy and localizes the malfunction in either the lower or upper leg or both. Pain is rarely associated with leg length discrepancy unless secondary to resulting deformities and is comparable to the severity of the associated deformities.[2,8,p.1469]

**Treatment.** Many factors are taken into consideration in the determination of treatment of leg length discrepancy. Of utmost importance is the definitive diagnosis of cause whenever possible. The chronologic and skeletal age of the child is crucial in determination of the preferred treatment modality. The predictory process involves the collection of data to determine the exact status of discrepancy at this time compared to related future status; techniques have been perfected to assist in this process and are relatively accurate. Tachdjian has compiled multiple normal growth patterns and predictory information to assist in this process. After collection of the data is accomplished, Tachdjian recommends the following tabulations for a composite view of current and future status of the discrepancy[8,p.1485]:

1. Actual and apparent anthropometric measurements of height and leg length
2. True lengths of both tibia and femurs measured by scanography (growth study films)
3. Clinical and radiographic measurement of the total femoral and tibial leg length discrepancy
4. Establishment of the relative maturity reflected by the skeletal age and determined on review of radiographic examination of the hands and wrists
5. Examination for appearance of secondary sexual characteristics
6. Establishment of pelvic and trunk balance as reflected by specific lifts under the short leg adequate to sufficiently balance both
7. Miscellaneous information such as wearing of an above-the-knee orthosis or previous and future contemplated surgery on the lower extremities or vertebral column
8. Serial standing photographs of the child with and without a lift under the short leg

The tabulation of this information provides the orthopedic surgeon with the required information to make adequate judgments in relation to the treatment of choice.

Minor discrepancies in leg length may frequently be treated successfully with a lift in the shoe on the short leg. Extreme and severe discrepancies accompanied by massive deformity of the lower extremity may require appropriate amputation and fitting for a prosthesis as the treatment of choice. Those cases between the minimal and severe may be corrected with selective surgical procedures.

Multiple surgical procedures are available for eventual maximal equalization of the leg lengths. *Epiphyseodesis* provides permanent arrest of growth of the long leg, and specifically the bone that is shortened. This procedure is accomplished at a specific time calculated to permit equalization when full growth is attained. *Epiphyseal stapling* does not totally arrest the growth of the extremity but provides for some retardation or partial arrest of growth. This procedure is also calculated so that it is accomplished at a specific time in skeletal growth to obtain maximum benefit from the procedure. When full skeletal growth is already achieved at the time of diagnosis, procedures involving the epiphyseal growth plate are no longer valid and reliable. In these cases *shortening* of the specific bone may be accomplished through recession techniques to equalize the leg lengths. In some cases it is advantageous not to accomplish procedures that will ultimately shorten the long leg for equalization; this decision is made on the basis of the previously outlined tabulations and calculations of predicted growth. The surgical alternative is *lengthening* of the short extremity by osteotomy and distraction utilizing pins and an external apparatus to gradually distract the short bone over a period of time or by stimulation of the epiphyseal growth. Considerable risk and an increased number of complications, both in relation to incidence and severity, are related to the lengthening procedures. For this reason these procedures are reserved only for those cases when lesser procedures will not provide adequate equalization and functioning.[8,pp.1489-1514]

### Congenital lower limb deficiencies

Congenital limb deficiencies refer to any congenital anomaly of the upper or lower extremity that result in less than normal development of part or all of the involved extremity. Classifications of congenital limb deficiencies, accompanied by universally accepted terminology, were not outlined until 1961. At that time Franz and O'Rahilly published what is currently acceptable terminology and classification. The foundation of this classification is embryologically and teratologically based.[4;7;8,p.108]

"The period of differentiation, known as the embryonic period, takes place during the first 7 postovulatory weeks. At the fourth postovulatory week, limbs begin to develop in the form of small buds on the lateral wall. During the following 3 weeks, these buds differentiate proximodistally, the hand making the appearance after the arm and forearm. The fetal period is one of embryonic growth."[8,p.108] It is during this development that malfunctions may develop and produce resulting limb deficiencies of varying degrees.

**Terminology.** The comprehension of specific terminology utilized within the classification of skeletal limb deficiencies is essential for understanding of components, concepts and framework of the classification. The following terms are therefore reviewed:

**prefix a** without, absence.
    **amelia** absence of a limb.
    **achieria** absence of a hand.
    **apodia** absence of a foot.
    **adactyly** absence of a digit.
    **aphalangia** absence of one or more phalanges.
**prefix hemi** half.
    **hemimelia** absence or presence of half a limb.
**prefix phoco** seallike.
    **phocomelia** limb attached directly to the trunk, flipper-like limb.
**paraxial** beside the axis; part of the limb absent.
**terminal** all parts distal to and in line with the deficient portion affected.
**intercalary** proximal and distal parts present with middle part absent.
**transverse** involving entire width of limb.

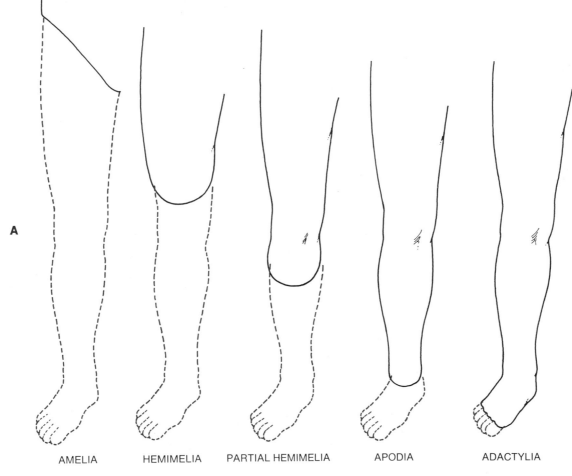

| | | | | |
|---|---|---|---|---|
| AMELIA | HEMIMELIA | PARTIAL HEMIMELIA | APODIA | ADACTYLIA |

**Fig. 14-9.** Lower limb deficiencies and classifications. **A,** Terminal transverse.

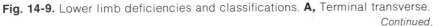

*Continued.*

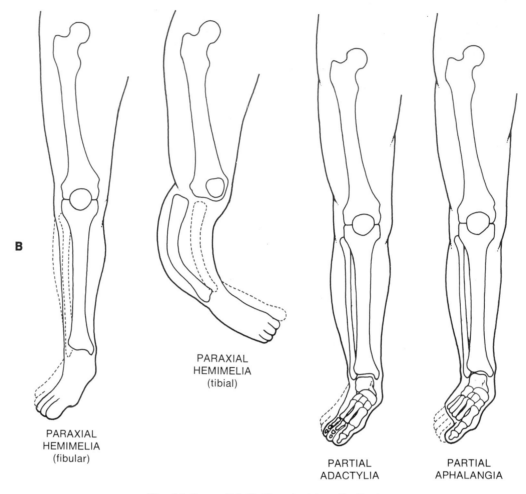

B

PARAXIAL
HEMIMELIA
(fibular)

PARAXIAL
HEMIMELIA
(tibial)

PARTIAL
ADACTYLIA

PARTIAL
APHALANGIA

**Fig. 14-9, cont'd. B,** Terminal longitudinal.

**longitudinal** only part of the limb (preaxial or postaxial) affected.

**ray** digit.

**limb** extremity.

Combinations of the terminology outlined here usually provide an accurate description of the anatomic area as well as the extent of the deficiency.

*Dysmelia* is a general term that represents a group of anomalies, all of which are characterized by hypoplasia or aplasia of the long bones of the extremities. As opposed to distal absence in congenital amputation, dysmelia may involve absence proximally or axially. The deformities in dysmelia range from peripheral hypoplasia of one long bone (as in proximal phocofemoral deficiencies) to total absence of the extremity (amelia).

Specific types of lower extremity deficiencies are reviewed in brief elsewhere in this chapter (e.g., congenital absence of tibia).

**Classification.** The classifications of congenital and skeletal limb deficiencies, as outlined by Frantz and O'Rahilly in 1961 may be reviewed in Table 13-1. As may be noted the classification is relatively simple and descriptive of the degree of deficiency involved. Visual representation of lower extremity limb deficiencies is given in Fig. 14-9.

**Treatment.** Treatment of congenital limb deficiencies is greatly dependent on the degree of deficiency present. Lower extremity limb deficiencies are of greater concern than upper limb deficiencies because of their interference with ambulation and lower extremity functioning. The objective of treat-

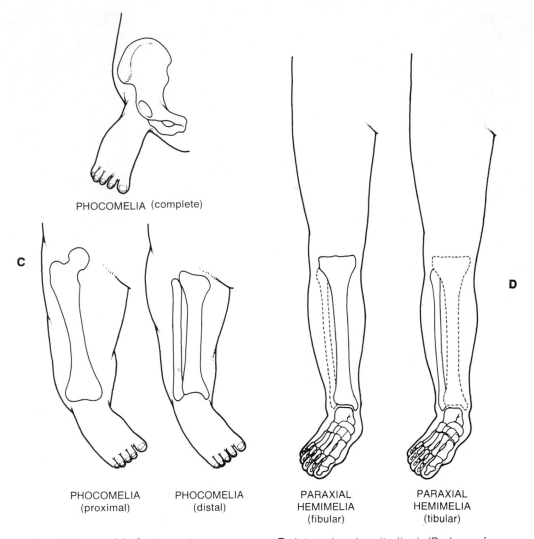

PHOCOMELIA (complete)

**C**

| PHOCOMELIA (proximal) | PHOCOMELIA (distal) | PARAXIAL HEMIMELIA (fibular) | PARAXIAL HEMIMELIA (tibular) |

**D**

**Fig. 14-9, cont'd. C,** Intercalary transverse. **D,** Intercalary longitudinal. (Redrawn from Tachdjian, M. O.: Pediatric orthopedics, Philadelphia, 1972, W. B. Saunders Co.)

ment of lower extremity limb deficiencies is to maximize functioning for promotion of appropriate ambulation, resulting in as normal an activity level as possible, with additional focus on prevention of resulting deformities associated with these deficiencies during growth. Minor to moderate degrees of limb deficiencies in the lower extremity may require only utilization of a shoe lift or appropriate conservative measure to equalize leg lengths to permit ambulation. Joint fusion is sometimes advocated to increase stability and function. Depending on the severity of the deficiency, amputation may be the treatment of choice, with appropriate fitting of a prosthesis. Treatment and surgical reconstructive procedures are individual and are designed for the level of involvement.

## DISEASES AND DISORDERS OF HIP
### Congenital dislocation of hip

Congenital dislocation of the hip (Fig. 14-10) is the displacement of the femoral head from the acetabular socket and is present at birth or shortly thereafter.

**Etiology.** The specific cause of congenital dislocation of the hip is unknown, but contributing factors are thought to be ligamentous laxity, breech presentation, and intrauterine positioning. Hereditary factors are influential, and it is not unusual to see several members of one family with this deformity.[8,pp.130-131;9,p.244]

**Pathology.** The femoral head, the acetabulum, and the hip joint capsule are well developed and proportioned at approximately 10 weeks of em-

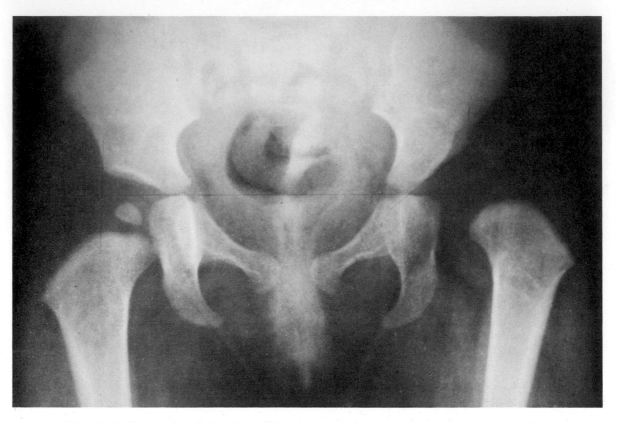

**Fig. 14-10.** Congenital dislocation of hip. Untreated at 1 year of age; lateral and superior dislocation of left hip and dysplastic left acetabulum; hypoplastic capital femoral epiphyseal ossification center.

bryonic development. The correct relationship between the femoral head and the acetabulum must exist for continued growth and development without deformity. The displacement seen in congenital dislocation of the hip causes a structural alteration in the entire upper portion of the femur. The femoral head is found posterior and superior to the acetabulum, thus causing the hip joint capsule to become stretched and elongated. The angle of anteversion is increased and becomes increasingly greater. If the dislocation is not diagnosed and treated early, continued activity and stress on the hip joint through ambulation and weight bearing continue to cause pathologic features of the entire joint structure. The wear and tear on the acetabulum with ambulation decreases the bony structures surrounding the head of the femur and results in decreased ability for the head of the femur to anatomically reduce itself. A secondary acetabulum on the wing of the ilium may develop. Postural vertebral compensation in the lumbar area may result. The pelvis, due to the posterior positioning of the head of the femur, tilts forward, resulting in increased lumbar lordosis. Partial dislocation or *subluxation* may occur with patho-

logic features decreased to the extent of dislocation.[8,pp.131-135;9,p.244]

**Incidence.** Dislocation of the hip may be present at birth or occur shortly thereafter. Girls are more commonly affected, at a ratio of 9:1. A geographic and cultural differential incidence may be noted, with a strikingly high incidence in those geographic areas where culture dictates carrying the infants with their hips bound in extension; in contrast a strikingly low incidence of this deformity occurs in geographic regions where cultures dictate the carrying of infants with hips in abduction, flexion, and external rotation. Barlow found, after examining 9,289 infants over a period of 5 years, that one in 60 were born with instability in one or both hips. Of these, 60% recovered in the first week and 88% in the first 2 months; dislocation in the remaining 12% persisted, with an overall incidence of 1.55 per thousand.[1,8,p.130]

**Signs and symptoms.** The signs and symptoms of congenital dislocation of the hip (Fig. 14-11; Table 14-9) are evident on physical examination. The most common initial signs of congenital dislocation of the hip are listed on p. 298.

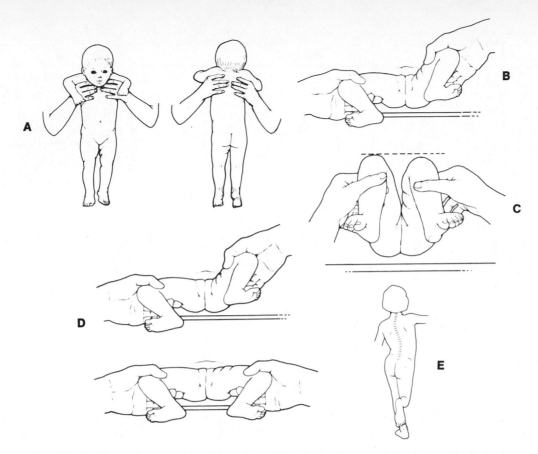

**Fig. 14-11.** Signs of congenital dislocation of hip. **A,** Asymmetry of gluteal and thigh folds. **B,** Limited hip abduction as seen in flexion. **C,** Apparent shortening of femur as indicated by knees in flexion. **D,** Ortolani's sign if infant is under 4 weeks of age. **E,** Trendelenburg's gait on weight bearing. (From Hilt, N. E., and Schmitt, E. W., Jr.: Pediatric orthopedic nursing, St. Louis, 1975, The C. V. Mosby Co.)

**Table 14-9.** Signs and symptoms of congenital dislocation of hip[8, pp. 135-138]

| Signs and symptoms | Technique of examination | Results indicative of congenital dislocation of hip |
|---|---|---|
| Thigh or gluteal folds | Usually apparent in any position | Asymmetry |
| Leg length | Upright or recumbent | Apparent shortening on side of dislocation |
| Hip abduction | Recumbent with hip and knees flexed Abduct hips bilaterally | Limited abduction on side of dislocation |
| Femoral length | Recumbent with hips and knees flexed Examine level of knees | Apparent shortening on side of dislocation (Galeazzi's sign) |
| Ortolani's sign | Recumbent with hip and knees flexed Abduct, then adduct hips | Palpable click with reduction in abduction and dislocation in adduction; sign present |
| Barlow's test | Recumbent with hips flexed 90% and knees fully flexed | Thumbpressure applied over the lower trochanter posteriorly can dislocate hip joint |
| | Long finger of each hand over greater trochanter | Release of thumb pressure relocates hip |
| | Thumb opposite lesser trochanter on medial aspect of proximal thigh | Indicative of hip *instability*, not dislocation |
| | Hips brought into midabduction | |
| Piston mobility | Recumbent with hip adducted | Abnormal mobility or feeling of telescoping |
| | Alternate hip flexion and extension | |
| | With each, hip pushed in piston fashion with finger over greater trochanter | |
| Hip and knee flexion contractures | Recumbent | Normal during first few months of life |
| | Thomas test | Absent contractures indicative of dislocation |
| | Check hyperextension of knee | |
| Nélaton's line | Line drawn between anterosuperior iliac spine and ischial tuberosity | Tip of greater trochanter proximal to this line |
| Trendelenburg's sign | Standing on one leg with other leg lifted off floor. | Normally able to maintain pelvis level |
| | | With dislocation, when standing on dislocated side unable to elevate pelvis opposite side |
| | | May be apparent with gait |
| | | Bilateral dislocation produces waddling gait |

**Table 14-10.** Radiographic features of congenital dislocation of hip*[8, pp. 137-141]

| Radiographic feature | Explanation |
|---|---|
| Hilgenreiner's line or Y line | Draw horizontal line through the top of clear areas in depth of acetabulum<br>Represents triradiate or Y cartilage. |
| Ombredanne's vertical line or perkin's line | Draw line from most lateral ossified margin of roof of acetabulum, perpendicularly downward through Y line to form quandrants<br>Normal hip shows nucleus of ossific femoral head below Y line and within lower medial quadrant |
| Acetabular index | Draw line passing through depth of acetabulum at Y line to most lateral ossified margin of roof of acetabulum<br>Measure angle between this line and Y line.<br>Measurement should be 27° to 30° at birth and decrease to approximately 20° at 2 years of age<br>Dislocation of hip will produce measurement over 30° |

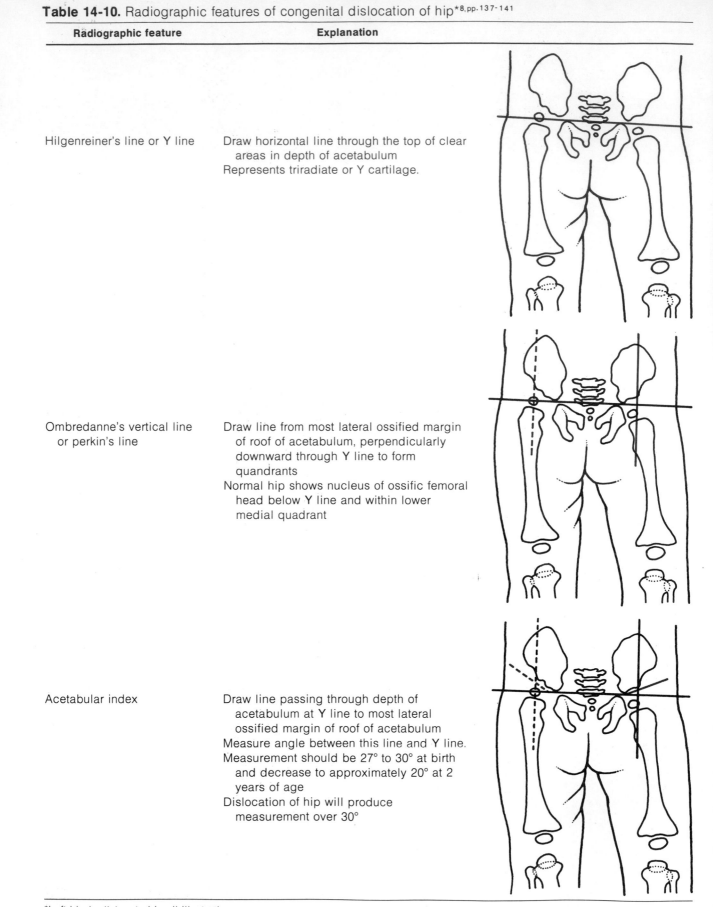

*Left hip is dislocated in all illustrations.

**Table 14-10.** Radiographic features of congenital dislocation of hip—cont'd

| Radiographic feature | Explanation | |
|---|---|---|
| Y coordinate (Ponseti) | Measure distance from center of gravity to midsacrum to center of ossified nucleus of femoral head, or measure distance from medial aspect of protruding tip of ossified femoral neck to sacrum<br>Dislocation of hip reveals discrepancies in this measurement<br>Determines lateral displacement of hip | |
| CE angle of Wiberg | Draw line from most lateral ossified margin of acetabular roof to ossified nucleus center of femoral head<br>Measure angle between this line and Ombredanne's vertical line<br>Determines lateral displacement of hip | |
| Shenton's line or Menard's line | Draw line between medial border of femoral neck and superior border of opturator foramen<br>Normal hip reveals continuous line<br>Dislocated hip reveals broken line<br>Measures superior displacement of hip | |

*Continued.*

**Table 14-10.** Radiographic features of congenital dislocation of hip—cont'd

| Radiographic feature | Explanation |
|---|---|
| Von Rosen's superior displacement measurement | Draw Y line<br>Draw a line parallel to Y line through upper margin of symphysis<br>Measures superior displacement of hip<br>Dislocation of hip with superior displacement reveals encroachment of ossified shadow of proximal femoral shaft on space between these lines |
| Von Rosen's abduction measurement | Radiographic film with hips in 45° of abduction and internally rotated<br>Draw lines through center of femoral shaft to extend through pelvis<br>Normal hip reveals this line bisecting lateral corner of acetabulum<br>Dislocation of hip reveals this line bisecting anterosuperior iliac spine |

1. Asymmetry of gluteal or thigh folds
2. Limited hip abduction
3. Apparent shortening of femur (Galeazzi's sign)
4. Positive Ortolani's sign
5. Positive Trendelenburg's sign or gait

Other signs and symptoms may be seen but are less frequently diagnostic.

Greater difficulty is encountered in diagnosing a subluxation or partial dislocation. A part of the difficulty is due to the stage of the ossification process in existence during infancy and early childhood, making it extremely difficult to determine radiographically the exact position of the head of the femur and the acetabulum. Arthrography assists in this effort when ordinary radiographic films are not sufficient.

Even under the best circumstances and with full dislocation, the ossification process makes the diagnosis difficult to establish without the utilization of specific established lines (Table 14-10) that may be drawn to determine the exact position of the femoral head within the acetabulum. These constitute radiographic features that assist in the determination of treatment. It should be emphasized that radiographic examination is necessary, in addition to the clinical features or signs and symptoms, to establish definitive diagnosis and implement a therapeutic regimen.

The ability to provide optimum correction of this deformity is greatly dependent on the age of the infant or child at the time of diagnosis. The severity of treatment as well as the prognosis are directly proportionate to the child's age at the time of diagnosis and implementation of treatment. Many dislocations of the hip are still not diagnosed until the child reaches the weight-bearing age. It is obvious that considerable destruction can be produced by the stress of the weight-bearing process. The importance of diagnosing this deformity at an early stage cannot be emphasized enough. It is highly recommended that *screening programs* be instituted in all newborn nurseries, well-baby clinics, pediatricians' offices, and hospital units with children under 3 to 4 years of age. Adequate screening techniques may be easily taught as a necessary part of the nursing assessment. Increased emphasis on screening programs can contribute tremendously to the early diagnosis and implementation of treatment and the prevention of resulting deformities. It should be noted that this screening process should be limited to assessment and evaluation of the gluteal or thigh folds, hip abduction, extremity length, and femoral length because of the special techniques required to assess some of the more complicated signs and symptoms. Screening for these few but relatively reliable signs and symptoms requires very little time, and any suspect results may then be followed by appropriate consultation.

**Treatment.** Although various opinions exist relative to the specific treatment modalities advocated for the child with congenital dislocation of the hip, several principles are acknowledged by all:

1. Regardless of the choice of treatment modality, early diagnosed dislocated hips require positioning placing the hip in abduction, flexion, and some external rotation.
2. The earlier the age at the time of diagnosis, the less severe and intense the treatment need be.
3. The earlier the age at the time of diagnosis and implementation of treatment, the better the prognosis for correction of the deformity with the least risk of complications.
4. The best response to treatment is encountered

if the dislocation is diagnosed before the weight-bearing age.
5. Treatment modalities are chosen according to the child's age at the time of diagnosis.

Treatment for congenital dislocation of the hip is begun as soon after the condition is detected as possible. The treatment of congenital dislocation of the hip is discussed by all authorities in relation to different age groups; however, on reviewing the literature there is obvious variance of opinion regarding ideal treatment within these age spans. The treatment modalities offered at various ages are somewhat different according to Brashear and Raney, Tachdjian, and Turek, as is their age differentiation for determination of treatment (Table 14-11). These authors recommend the following.

*Birth to 2 months.* If congenital dislocation of the hip is diagnosed during the first few months of life, gentle manipulation of the hip will usually be sufficient for reduction. The reduced position (abduction and flexion) is maintained for a period of 2 to 3 months with a short leg hip spica cast, Frejka pillow, or other commercial abduction device. Diagnosis and implementation of treatment at this age is extremely successful with few complications.

*Two to 12 months.* Because the soft tissue structures surrounding the hip joint have already begun to accommodate to the dislocated position, additional effort is often required for gradual reduction. Skin traction (bilateral split Russell traction or Bryant traction) is utilized for a period of several weeks to extend the hip, placing the head of the femur in a better position under the acetabulum, with gradual abduction to "seat" the head of the femur in relation to the acetabular socket. A closed reduction with the patient under anesthesia is usually required after traction therapy to assure adequate positioning before the application of a hip spica cast or other positioning device. The maintenance of this position is required for up to 6 months to assure the appropriate development of the acetabular socket to assist in maintenance of the position and to decrease the risk of redislocation. There is a relatively high success rate, but some dislocations do not respond to the closed reduction and may require an open reduction. Complications in this age group are slightly increased.

*Twelve to 18 months.* For most infants in this age group weight bearing has already begun. For this reason a degree of acetabular damage has already been encountered, making reduction with skin traction only more difficult. Infants in this age group usually require a combination of skin and skeletal traction with a wire or pin in the distal femur to pro-

**Table 14-11.** Comparison of treatment modalities for congenital dislocation of hip

| Brasshear and Raney* | | Tachdjian† | | Turek‡ | |
|---|---|---|---|---|---|
| **Age** | **Treatment** | **Age** | **Treatment** | **Age** | **Treatment** |
| Birth to 1 year | Reduction with gentle abduction<br>Skin traction for 1 to 3 weeks with gradual abduction<br>Maintenance of position with splint or cast | Birth to 2 months | Gentle manipulation of hip into flexion and abduction<br>Maintenance of position Frejka pillow or hip spica cast for 2 to 3 months | Birth to 1 year | Both hips maintained in abduction<br>Pillow or abduction mattress between thighs<br>Continued for several months until radiographic examination confirms relocation with adequate formation of acetabular roof |
| One to 3 years | Skeletal traction<br>Gradual increasing abduction<br>Manipulation under general anesthesia if hip not reduced with traction<br>After reduction, bilateral hip spica cast (moderate abduction, 90° external rotation, 90° flexion, knees in 90° flexion, ankles in neutral position)<br>If hip unstable, internal rotation used<br>Six months' immobilization advised in this position<br>New cast, bilateral hip spica (45° abduction, external rotation and flexion) applied after 2 to 3 months<br>Ambulation after closed reduction and immobilization<br>If closed reduction not successful, open reduction with osteotomy<br>Hip spica cast immobilization<br>Deep pool therapy<br>Maintenance of position with long leg brace<br>Night splints | Two to 18 months | Skin traction (younger age group)<br>Bilateral split Russell traction<br>Gradual abduction<br>Skeletal traction (older age group)<br>Split Russell with distal femoral Kirschner wire<br>Gradual abduction<br>After reduction with traction<br>Closed reduction under anesthesia<br>Hip spica cast for 6 months<br>Open reduction may be indicated if closed reduction not successful | | Complete dislocation<br>Closed reduction with nontraumatizing manipulation under anesthesia<br>If reduction stable, wide hip abduction maintained for several months in cast with gradual decrease of abduction and flexion after initial few months |
| | | Eighteen months to 3 years | Percutaneous or open adduction myotomy to release tight soft tissues<br>Skeletal traction<br>Two weeks<br>Gradual abduction and extension<br>Open reduction with osteotomy<br>Hip spica cast<br>Derotation osteotomy may be required | One to 3 years | Traction<br>Slow reduction<br>Abduction (gradual) until femoral head is opposite acetabulum<br>Continued for 2 months<br>Effective in two thirds of cases<br>Surgical intervention<br>To provide stability<br>Rotation osteotomy for excessive anteversion<br>Innominate osteotomy |
| | | Four to 7 years | Skeletal traction<br>Soft tissue releases<br>Open reduction with osteotomy<br>Derotation osteotomy after 8 to 10 weeks<br>Capsular arthroplasty may be required | Over 3 years | Surgical intervention<br>Open reduction<br>Salter innominate osteotomy<br>Chiari shelf operation<br>Other |
| Three to 6 years | Skeletal traction for at least 3 weeks<br>Closed reduction under anesthesia<br>Possible adductor tenotomy<br>If closed reduction unsuccessful, open | Over 8 years | Treatment postponed until degenerative changes and pain develop<br>Then arthrodesis or arthroplasty | | |

*Data from Brashear, H. R., Jr., and Raney, R. B., Sr.: Shand's handbook of orthopaedic surgery, ed. 9, St. Louis, 1978, The C. V. Mosby Co.
†Data from Tachdjian, M. O.: Pediatric orthopedics, Philadelphia, 1972, W. B. Saunders Co., pp. 141-176.
‡Data from Turek, S.: Orthopaedics, Philadelphia, 1977, J. B. Lippincott Co., pp. 249-266.

Lower extremity and hip 301

**Table 14-11.** Comparison of treatment modalities for congenital dislocation of hip—cont'd

| Brashear and Raney* | | Tachdjian† | | Turek‡ | |
|---|---|---|---|---|---|
| Age | Treatment | Age | Treatment | Age | Treatment |
| Over 6 years | reduction with osteotomy<br>Arthroplasty may be indicated, followed by derotational osteotomy<br>Reduction usually impossible and inadvisable<br>Surgical procedures to improve disability and increase support<br>Chiari shelf<br>Abduction osteotomy of femur<br>Arthroplasty<br>Arthrodesis<br>Corrective shoes or corset for relief of strain | | Total hip replacement arthroplasty may be indicated | | |

vide an increased degree of traction. Gradual abduction will again be obtained during traction therapy to assist in the appropriate positioning of the reduction. Closed reduction with the child under anesthesia is accomplished, followed by the application of a hip spica cast for approximately 6 months. There is increased risk of redislocation in this age group, and many of these patients later require open reduction with an innominate osteotomy.

*Eighteen months to 3 years.* Of increased concern for the child in this age group with congenital dislocation of the hip is further destruction to the acetabular socket and its general inability to maintain reduction. Skeletal traction for several weeks to several months is always required as the initial therapeutic prescription. Gradual abduction and extension is maintained throughout the traction therapy. Soft tissue releases may be required either before or after the application of skeletal traction to increase the flexibility of the hip joint and increase the possibility of reduction with traction. Surgical intervention in the form of an open reduction with an osteotomy is required to provide stability to the reduced hip and to assist in maintaining or creating an acetabular shelf to assure the reduction. A hip spica cast is applied postoperatively. A rotational osteotomy may be required to correct excessive anteversion.

*Three to 7 years.* As the age of the child at the time of diagnosis increases, assumptions may be made of comparable damage to the bony joint structures. Skeletal traction with associated soft tissue releases is usually required, followed by an open reduction and osteotomy or a surgical acetabular shelf procedure. Excessive anteversion is more common in this age group and may be corrected with a rotational osteotomy 8 to 10 weeks after the major procedure. Capsular arthroplasty may be required. Complications and risk of redislocation are extremely high in this age group, and reduction is rarely accomplished without use of all indicated procedures and therapy. It is not uncommon that some of these procedures be repeated to assure a successful outcome.

*Over 7 years.* Reduction of a dislocated hip in the child over 7 years of age is often impossible and not advisable. Treatment is usually not advocated unless signs of degenerative changes or pain are present. The ages at which these develop vary considerably. At the time that these clinical signs are evident, arthrodesis, arthroplasty, acetabular shelf procedures, or osteotomies may be required. It is not unlikely that more than one procedure will have to be accomplished. Total hip replacement arthroplasty may be indicated if it is apparent that destruction of the joint structures is of such severity that lesser alternatives are not feasible. Shoe lifts may be utilized to relieve the pain associated with strain or limp.

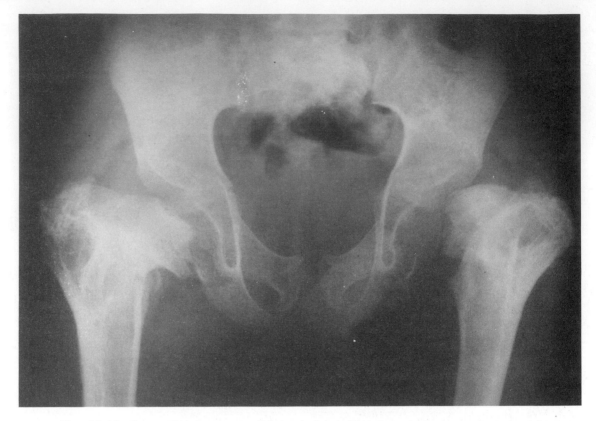

**Fig. 14-12.** Congenital coxa vara. Bilateral dysplastic changes in femoral neck and acetabulum.

It is obvious that the later the age of diagnosis of congenital dislocation of the hip, the more severe the treatment involved. For this reason the necessity to implement thorough and adequate screening programs to detect this deformity cannot be stressed enough. Because many of these deformities are diagnosed in the older child, we know that not enough screening programs have been adequately implemented to determine their impact on the incidence of congenital hip dislocation.

**Complications.** Complications of congenital dislocation of the hip include (1) redislocation, (2) avascular necrosis of the femoral head, (3) fractures, and (4) nerve paralysis.

The degree of risk involved with these complications is directly proportional to the age at the time of diagnosis and implementation of treatment.

### Congenital coxa vara (infantile coxa vara, developmental coxa vara)

Congenital coxa vara (Fig. 14-12) is the reduction or decrease of the normal 120° to 140° angle of the femoral neck and is present at birth or shortly thereafter.

**Etiology.** The cause of congenital coxa vara is probably an embryonic developmental error. This deformity is found or diagnosed usually at birth or shortly thereafter.

**Pathology.** The normal angle of the infant femoral neck in relation to the longitudinal axis of the femur is 120° to 140°. Congenital coxa vara is characterized by (1) progressive decrease of the neck-shaft angle, (2) shortness of the neck of the femur, (3) an extension upward of the greater trochanter, (4) shortening of the femur, and (5) malposition of the proximal femur causing secondary degenerative changes in the acetabulum. The head of the femur is normal in configuration.[9,pp.284-285]

**Signs and symptoms.** If congenital coxa vara is diagnosed prior to weight bearing, the major sign or symptom is that of a deformity or asymmetry of the configuration of the hip and upper thigh as compared with the normal hip. After weight bearing the initial complaint is that of a painless limp. On physical examination the involved extremity is found to be shorter, and there is a positive Trendelenburg's sign. With bilateral involvement the characteristic waddling gait may be observed. Radiographic examination reveals a shortened femoral neck with beaking of the greater trochanter. The femoral head may be larger than anticipated and translucent. Distal slipping of the femoral head, epiphyseal cartilage, and triangular fragment may be apparent.[9,p.285]

**Treatment.** The treatment of congenital coxa vara is "aimed at obliterating the neck defect and thereby halting progression of the deformity."[9,p.285] Subtrochanteric osteotomy is the surgical procedure of choice.

**Prognosis.** The prognosis of congenital coxa vara is guarded. Recurrence is often possible, especially during rapid growth periods.

### Legg-Perthes disease (coxa plana)

Legg-Perthes disease is one of a group of diseases called *osteochondroses*. It is a self-limiting disease characterized by avascular necrosis of the femoral head in which the necrotic tissue is absorbed and then replaced by reparative osseous tissue. The process is relatively predictable in regard to pathologic phases and results in varying degrees of deformity and limited hip motion.

**Etiology.** The cause of Legg-Perthes disease is unknown. What is known is that avascular necrosis of the epiphyseal ossification center of the femoral head is the cause of the deformity. Theories about the primary cause of the avascular necrosis, however, differ, and it is attributed variously to hereditary, metabolic, chemical, and mechanical dysfunctions.

**Pathology.** The primary pathologic feature of Legg-Perthes disease is avascular necrosis of the epiphyseal ossification center as a result of loss of blood supply. Resorption of the dead bone and replacement with newly formed immature bone cells takes place in various stages and are predictable in their characteristics.

*Incipient or synovitis stage.* The first stage of Legg-Perthes disease is characterized by pathologic features of the soft tissue structures of the hip joint. The synovium is hyperemic and edematous. Joint fluid is increased. This stage lasts 1 to 3 weeks.

*Aseptic necrotic or avascular stage.* The entire or anterior half of the nucleus of the femoral head ossification center is necrotic in this stage. The necrosis remains relatively unchanged throughout the entire stage, and no regeneration is evident. The normal progression of this stage is from several months to a year.

*Regenerative or fragmentation stage.* The primary characteristic of this stage is the resorption of necrotic bone with initial replacement. The replacement is accomplished by immature new bone cells. The contour of the newly formed soft bone develops in response to the external forces. This stage lasts from 1 to 3 years.

*Healed or residual stage.* This stage is characterized by formation and replacement of the resorbing bone cells by normal bone cells. Any residual pathologic features are greatly influenced by the promptness of treatment.

Each of these stages, in addition to pathologic characteristics, also has radiographic characteristics from which the pathologic features may be determined in relation to the specific stage of progression. These features are given in Table 14-12.

**Incidence.** Statistics related to Legg-Perthes disease vary in regard to the affected age group. Tachdjian outlines the age group usually affected as that between 4 and 8 years of age, while Turek relates a predominance in 3- to 12-year-olds, with a peak at 6 years. The incidence in the general population is approximately 1 in 1,200. Predominance of incidence in boys is evident in the literature, ranging from 4:1 (Turek) to 5:1 (Tachdjian). Hereditary influence may be considered but is not always established.

**Signs and symptoms.** Legg-Perthes disease has an insidious onset with a prolonged course of symptoms characteristic of the disease process. An antalgic gait is typical and usually of several months' duration. The patient usually complains of pain in the groin or in the medial aspect of the thigh or knee. Motion of the hip in certain types of activities appears to aggravate the pain; rest relieves the discomfort. In the synovitis stage the child may hold the extremity in slight flexion and abduction. Physical examination may reveal limited hip motion, especially of rotation. A hip contracture may be noted. A traumatic injury may be seen in approximately 25% of the cases.

Radiographic features of Legg-Perthes disease are classified according to the specific stage of the disease process (Table 14-12) and are characteristic of those seen with necrosis and associated rapair and epiphyseal thinning (i.e., flattening and ultimate fragmentation, shortened femoral neck, and acetabular alterations that accommodate to the shape of the femoral head).

**Treatment.** Because the pathologic features of Legg-Perthes disease are predictable, the aim of therapy is directed toward reduction of the deformity during the healing of the avascular necrosis, the preservation of a normal femoral head with normal relationship with the acetabulum, and preservation of normal range of motion whenever possible. If these objectives are not achieved or diagnosis and treatment implemented during the early stages, increased risk of residual damage to the hip joint may be reflected during adulthood. Although a variety of treatment alternatives are available to accomplish these objectives, consideration must be given to the patient's ability to remain immobilized or in bed for

*Text continued on p. 308.*

**Table 14-12.** Pathologic and radiographic features of stages of Legg-Perthes disease[8,pp.1097-1098;9,pp.387-396]

| Stage | Pathologic characteristics | Radiographic characteristics |
|---|---|---|
| Incipient or synovitis stage (1 to 3 weeks) | Soft tissue alterations<br>Synovium edematous<br>Synovium hyperemic<br>Increased joint fluid | Swelling of capsular shadows<br>Soft tissue thickening<br>Widening of articular cartilage<br>Possible decalcification of inferior osseous tissue of metaphysis (adjacent to epiphyseal plate) |
| Aseptic necrotic or avascular stage (several months to a year) | Necrosis of entire or anterior femoral head ossification nucleus<br>Necrosis includes bone and bone marrow<br>Bone softer than normal<br>No evidence of bone regeneration | Increased opacity of femoral head (homogenous) and no areas of rarefaction<br>Flattening of ossification nucleus to varying degrees<br>Possible subchondrial thinning<br>Possible lateral displacement of femoral head<br>Possible increased joint space |

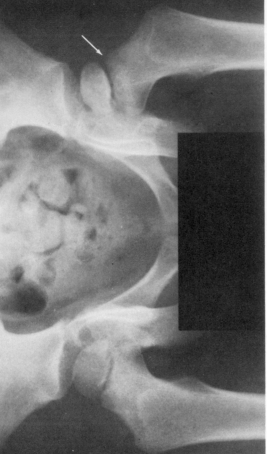

Increased joint space with increasing density of femoral head.

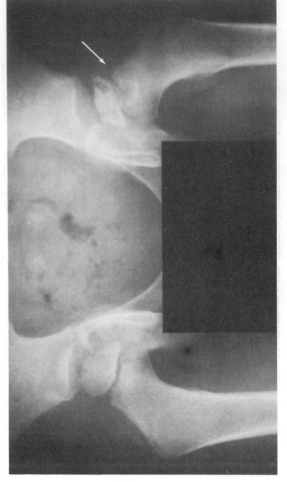

Marked collapse of femoral neck with sclerosis and beginning fragmentation. Radiolucent metaphyseal defect can be seen.

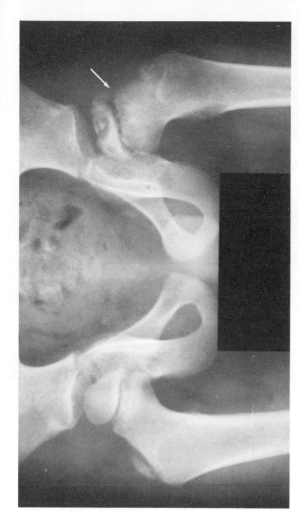

Regenerative or
fragmentation
stage (1 to
3 years)

Resorption of necrotic
bone
Replacement of
necrotic bone by
immature, newly
formed bone
Cartilage change
similar to necrotic
stage

Compression and
fragmentation of
femoral head
Rarefied areas
Widened femoral
neck
Normal cartilage
shape of femoral
head on
arthrography

Beginning regeneration phase. Sclerosis and flattening of femoral head with fragmentation still noted.

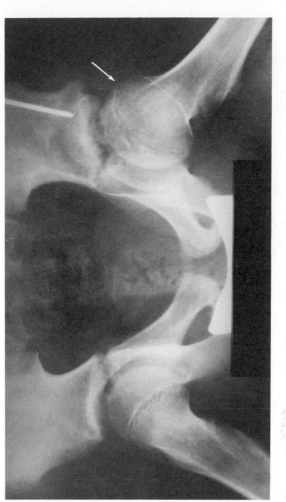

Healed or
residual stage

Normal bone replaces
resorbing necrotic
bone

Rarefied areas
disappearing grad-
ually
Normal bone
trabeculae
appearing
Femoral head normal
or flattened
Femoral neck
widening
Enlargement of
acetabulum
(adaptive)
Possible residual
coxa magna

Regeneration almost complete with coxa magna deformity (overgrowth effect). Healed postosteotomy changes in left ileum.

**Table 14-13.** Classifications of slipped capital femoral epiphysis[8, p.463]

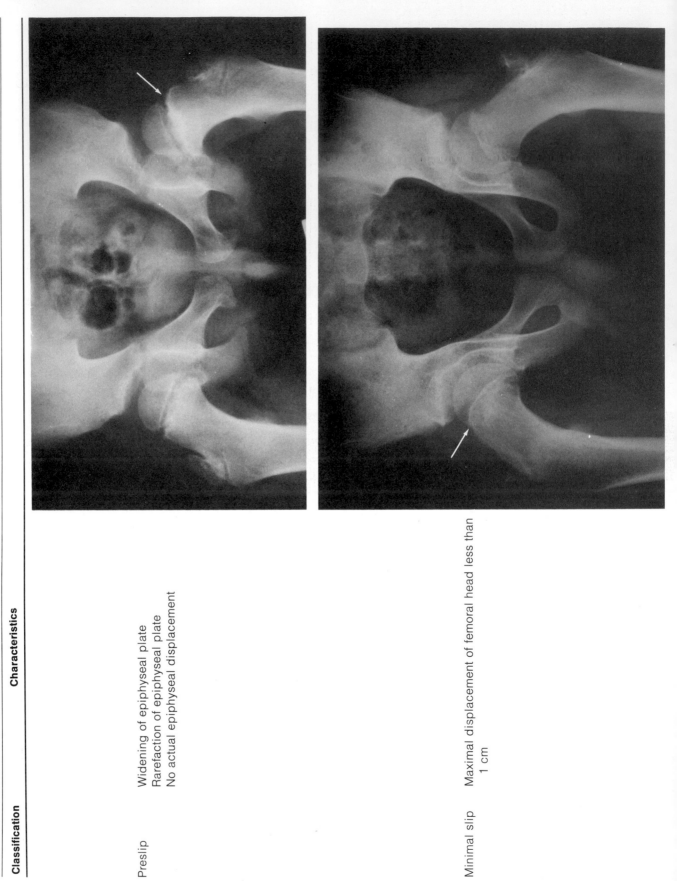

| Classification | Characteristics |
|---|---|
| Preslip | Widening of epiphyseal plate<br>Rarefaction of epiphyseal plate<br>No actual epiphyseal displacement |
| Minimal slip | Maximal displacement of femoral head less than 1 cm |

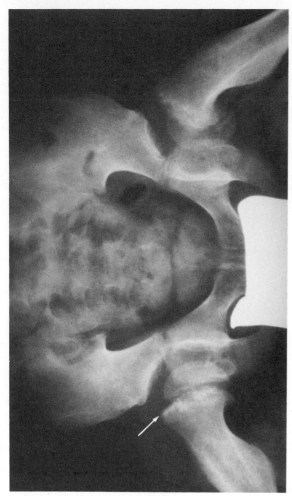

Moderate slip    Displacement of femoral head more than 1 cm but less than two thirds of diameter of femoral neck

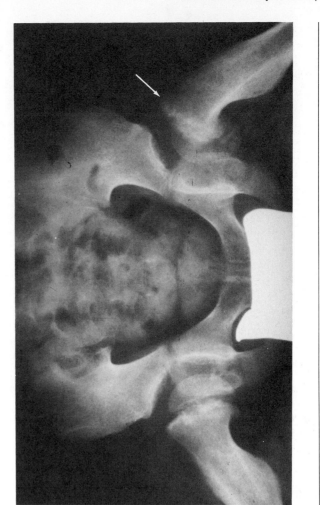

Severe slip    Displacement of femoral head is greater than two thirds of diameter of femoral neck

the long periods required for the normal healing process. It is generally accepted that no direct femoral head weight bearing on the affected extremity is advocated. The methods by which this may be accomplished vary and are classified by Tachdjian as follows[8,p.399]:

1. Conservative therapy
2. Recumbent therapy
   a. Bed rest with or without traction or rolling platform
   b. Hip spica traction
   c. Broomstick plaster method
   d. Hip abduction brace to prevent hip flexion
3. Ambulatory therapy
   a. Bilateral long leg cylinder spica walking cast
   b. Bent knee brace with crutches
   c. Sam Browne belt with crutches
   d. Schneider sling with crutches
   e. Patten bottom brace with ischial ring
   f. Containment splint
4. Operative therapy
   a. Innominate osteotomy
   b. Intrapelvic opturator neurectomy
   c. Varization osteotomy of proximal femur
   d. Bone grafting, drilling, or both
   e. Osteoplasty of extruded lateral portion of femoral head if limiting abduction

The specific treatment alternative to be utilized is determined by the physician's preference and the stage of progression at the time of diagnosis. Additional consideration is given to the radiographic features evident, the age of the child at the time of diagnosis, and the length of time since onset of symptoms. It is agreed that direct femoral head weight bearing on the affected extremity is not desirable and if permitted will deter the normal healing process. Even if another form of treatment is chosen by the physician, rest and traction or a cast application may be utilized initially to relieve pain and muscle spasms. All braces are designed to alleviate femoral head weight bearing. Treatment is continued until radiographic determination of the progression of healing is completed, which usually takes 2 to 3 years.[5,p.88;8,pp.399-406]

**Prognosis.** The prognosis of Legg-Perthes disease is dependent on the stage of progression at the time of diagnosis and implementation of treatment. Many patients show signs of degenerative changes of the hip joint in adulthood.

### Slipped capital femoral epiphysis (adolescent coxa vara, epiphyseal coxa vara)

Slipped capital femoral epiphysis is displacement downward and backward of the capital femoral epiphysis. It occurs during the rapid growth period of adolescence with resulting disabling external rotation deformity of the lower extremity.

**Etiology.** The cause of slipped capital femoral epiphysis is unknown; however, some authorities think an underlying endocrine or metabolic imbalance may be a contributing factor. Specific body types, if not contributing to the potential stress on the epiphyseal plate, appear with a high degree of frequency with this deformity. These are the obese type and, less frequently, the tall, thin type (frequently associated with a growth spurt).

**Pathology.** The basic pathologic changes of slipped capital femoral epiphysis occur in the cartilage of the growth plate. Displacement of the epiphysis inferiorly and posteriorly occurs through the layer of hypertrophied cartilage cells adjacent to the calcified cartilage layer. Separation causes the interval, which fills with fibrous tissue, embryonic cartilage, and callus. This weakens the attachment of the epiphysis to the femoral neck, resulting in displacement. Persistent displacement produces degenerative alterations within the joint structure. The pathologic features in relation to the severity of the slippage are determined radiographically. The specific characteristics (preslip, minimal slip, moderate slip, and severe slip) are given in Table 14-13.

**Incidence.** Slipped capital femoral epiphysis occurs during adolescence with a male-female differentiation due to difference in the skeletal growth in the sexes. It is seen most frequently between the ages of 13 and 16 years in boys and between the ages of 11 and 14 years in girls. This deformity occurs two to five times more frequently in boys. It is seen most frequently in the obese or overweight adolescent, with less frequency in the tall, thin adolescent after a rapid growth spurt. There is a higher incidence in the left hip than in the right hip, and one of four cases show bilateral involvement.[8,p.463;9,pp.1081-1082]

**Signs and symptoms.** Slipped capital femoral epiphysis has an insidious onset and is usually progressive in nature. The clinical picture associated with this deformity varies according to severity and stage of progression at the time of diagnosis. During the preslip or minimal slip stages the patient usually complains of discomfort in the groin, which subsides with rest. The patient may walk with a slight limp. Symptoms remain rather vague, often with no objective findings. As the slip progresses to the chronic stage the patient complains of increasingly intense pain. A persistent antalgic limp develops. The objective findings include limitation of motion and tenderness about the hip. A deformity gradually develops with adduction and external rotation apparent. Bilateral slipping causes the characteristic waddling gait. Fixed deformity associated with the most severe slips is accompanied by limp, external rotation, adduction, and shortening of the femur; pain and muscle spasms, however, are no longer present.

Radiographic features are also diagnostic and significant in the various stages of progression of this deformity. In the *preslip stage* the growth plate is abnormally widened and irregular. There is no actual displacement of the epiphysis. The first slipping may be revealed on a lateral rather than anterior radiographic view. *Minimal* degrees of slippage reveal the epiphyseal edge flush with the upper border of the femoral neck. In addition the continuity of Shenton's line is broken. With progression of the deformity and slippage, the epiphysis is exposed at the upper medial border of the femoral neck. Eventually callus fills this space between the femoral head and neck. Recalcification of the metaphysis is evident when healing is complete, and the epiphyseal line again becomes normal in width. *Moderate* to *severe* slips are apparent radiographically, while the minimal slip poses the greatest problem to the diagnostician.[8,pp.465-467;9,pp.1083-1084]

**Treatment.** "Slipped capital femoral epiphysis is an emergency, and it is imperative that it be treated immediately, since minor trauma may cause further or complete displacement of the femoral head."[8,p.468] Non-weight bearing and bed rest are advocated as soon as the diagnosis is made. Traction is useful in assisting with this task and decreasing the muscle spasms commonly associated with this deformity. An internal rotation strap may be utilized if an external rotation contracture exists. A short period of this nonsurgical therapy permits the diagnostician to collect data preparatory to surgical intervention. The primary objectives of surgical intervention are correction of the deformity resulting from the slippage and creation of premature epiphyseal closure to prevent continued or recurrent slippage. In the preslip stage no significant deformity between the head and neck of the femur exists; thus the surgeon may concentrate efforts on accomplishing operative closure of the growth plate through epiphysiodesis. With moderate and severe slips it is necessary to correct the alignment of femoral neck and head through osteotomy and the insertion of a pin or pins to assure the correction.

## SUMMARY

It must be emphasized that the diseases and disorders of the lower extremity and joints are of great significance to the orthopedic surgeon. The bones and joints of the lower extremity are subjected to more weight and stress due to the weight-bearing process and ambulation than any other bones or joints in the body. For this reason any disruption that might hinder ambulatory goals is of great concern. These are of greatest concern when they are of a congenital or developmental nature and ultimately capable of producing devastating effects on ambulation and mobility. All diseases and disorders in this category are, for this reason, treated as early as possible, with early diagnosis of critical value and importance, and as a result have received the greatest emphasis within this chapter.

## REFERENCES

1. Barton, T. G.: Early diagnosis and treatment of congenital dislocation of the hip, J. Bone Joint Surg. **44:** 292, 1962.
2. Brashear, H. R., Jr., and Raney, R. B., Sr.: Shand's handbook of orthopaedic surgery, ed. 9, St. Louis, 1978, The C. V. Mosby Co.
3. Coventry, M. B., and Johnson, E. W.: Congenital absence of the fibula, J. Bone Joint Surg. **34-A:**941, 1952.
4. Frantz, C. H., and O'Rahilly, R.: Congenital skeletal limb deficiencies, J. Bone Joint Surg. **43:**1202, 1961.
5. Gartland, J. J.: Fundamentals of orthopaedics, Philadelphia, 1974, W. B. Saunders Co.
6. Kite, J. H.: The clubfoot, New York, 1964, Grune & Stratton, Inc.
7. O'Rahilly, R.: Morphological patterns in limb deficiencies and duplications, Am. J. Anat. **89:**135, 1951.
8. Tachdjian, M. O.: Pediatric orthopaedics, Philadelphia, 1972, W. B. Saunders Co.
9. Turek, S.: Orthopaedics, Philadelphia, 1977, J. B. Lippincott Co.

## BIBLIOGRAPHY

Adams, J. C.: Outline of orthopaedics, Baltimore, 1971, The Williams and Wilkins Co.
Aegertu, E., and Kirkpatrick, J.: Orthopaedic diseases, Philadelphia, 1975, W. B. Saunders Co.
Brashear, H. R., Jr., and Raney, R. B., Sr.: Shand's handbook of orthopaedic surgery, ed. 9, St. Louis, 1978, The C. V. Mosby Co.
Crenshaw, A. H., editor: Campbell's operative orthopaedics, ed. 5, St. Louis, 1971, The C. V. Mosby Co.
Gartland, J. J.: Fundamentals of orthopaedics, Philadelphia, 1974, W. B. Saunders Co.
Goldstein, L. A., and Dickerson, R. C.: Atlas of orthopaedic surgery, St. Louis, 1974, The C. V. Mosby Co.
Tachdjian, M. O.: Pediatric orthopaedics, Philadelphia, 1972, W. B. Saunders Co.
Turek, S.: Orthopaedics, Philadelphia, 1977, J. B. Lippincott, Co.

# 15

# Cervical and spinal diseases and disorders

NANCY E. HILT

SHIRLEY B. COGBURN

Diseases and disorders of the cervical and spinal vertebrae vary in cause, clinical features, and severity of symptoms. The implications of these processes vary as well. In this chapter are discussed those diseases and disorders commonly seen by orthopedic surgeons. It is suggested that the anatomy and physiology of the musculoskeletal components of the vertebral column and the spinal cord be reviewed in Chapters 1 and 2. Tumor processes that may involve the vertebral column are discussed in Chapter 19.

## CERVICAL DISEASES AND DISORDERS
### Cervical disc syndrome (cervical root syndrome)

The terms *cervical disc syndrome* or *cervical root syndrome* are used to describe the symptoms and signs produced by compression or irritation of cervical nerve roots in or about intervertebral foramina before they divide into anterior and posterior rami.[1]

**Etiology.** Cervical disc syndrome may be caused by ruptured cervical intervertebral discs, degenerative cervical disc disease, or cervical injuries of varying types and degrees.

**Pathology.** Cervical disc syndrome caused by ruptured cervical intervertebral discs or degenerative disease may produce varying degrees of malalignment causing nerve root compression. Most cervical disc syndromes from injuries involve hyperextension, which because of the anatomic structures causes compression. Flexion injuries in the cervical area do not result in nerve compression. In all cases cervical root irritation including some edema usually occurs.

**Signs and symptoms.** The most common symptom of cervical disc syndrome is pain, usually in the cervical area but may radiate down the arm to the fingers. The pain may be increased with cervical motion and, as with any intervertebral disc problem, may also be sharply increased with coughing, sneezing, or radical movement. Some paresthesia may be noted. Decreased skeletal function and hand grip may be associated with or without pain on the affected side. It is not uncommon for headache, blurred vision, or other generalized symptoms to accompany the pain. As a protective measure the patient may avoid cervical motion in an attempt to control the pain and other symptoms associated with cervical disc syndrome. Physical examination may reveal varying degrees of muscular atrophy, some sensory disturbances, muscular weakness, and decreased reflexes. Radiographic examination may reveal a loss of the normal lordosis seen in the cervical vertebrae, and occasionally some minor malalignment of the vertebrae may be noted. Differential diagnosis is recommended to distinguish cervical disc syndrome from other disease entities such as tumor processes, vertebral fractures, or dislocations.

**Treatment.** Nonsurgical intervention is usually successful in the treatment of cervical disc syndrome and may include immobilization of the cervical vertebrae in an attempt to decrease the irritation and provide rest for the area. Methods may include intermittent traction, Thomas collar, and heat therapy. Mobilization in any form of cervical hyperextension is contraindicated. Exercises may be utilized in some cases. Mild analgesics are usually successful in control of pain when utilized in conjunction with immobilization. Surgical intervention is only recommended when the signs and symptoms persist despite nonsurgical treatment.

**Prognosis.** The prognosis for cervical disc syndrome is good; however, recurrence of symptoms is not uncommon.

## Congenital short neck (Klippel-Feil syndrome)

Congenital short neck, or Klippel-Feil syndrome, is a rare congenital malformation of the cervical spine in which the vertebrae are fused into one mass of bone with resulting decrease of neck motion and cervical length and sometimes with neurologic involvement.

**Pathology.** Klippel-Feil syndrome involves fusion of the cervical vertebrae, usually in pairs. The posterior portions of the laminar arches in the cervical area, either totally or in part, are not fully developed. This results in spina bifida in the cervical region, usually involving the lower cervical vertebrae and sometimes one or two of the upper thoracic vertebrae.[1] It is not unusual to find a cervical rib or hemivertebrae associated with this deformity. Neurologic manifestations such as nerve root compression and peripheral nerve symptoms are secondary to deformities of the vertebral bodies.

**Signs and symptoms.** The most common sign of congenital short neck is the obvious deformity, that is, extreme shortness of the neck, which allows only limited motion, lateral bending, and rotation. Neurologic manifestations vary depending on the pathologic findings. With nerve root compression symptoms of peripheral nerve involvement may be apparent, such as pain or burning sensation; with nerve root compression symptoms of weakness, paralysis, hyperesthesia, or paresthesia may be seen. Spinal cord involvement may present signs of

lower extremity involvement with associated signs of an upper motor lesion.[6,p.302] Differential diagnosis between Klippel-Feil syndrome and Pott's disease or congenital torticollis should be established.

**Treatment.** Klippel-Feil syndrome may require no treatment. Mild associated symptoms may be alleviated with traction, cast application, or cervical collars. Surgical intervention may be necessary to relieve neurologic manifestations.

## Torticollis (congenital wryneck)

Torticollis, or congenital wryneck (Fig. 15-1), is a deformity in which the sternocleidomastoid muscle is shortened, resulting in flexion of the neck toward the affected side with the chin toward the unaffected side.

**Etiology.** The cause of torticollis has not been established. It is frequently seen following difficult delivery or breech presentation and in infants of primiparas.

**Pathology.** The first sign of torticollis frequently is a firm, nontender lump or enlargement, which may be palpated within the sternocleidomastoid muscle. This lump may regress and even disappear in 3 to 6 months. When it does not regress and results in fibrous contracture and shortening of the sternocleidomastoid muscle, a secondary contracture may develop in the soft tissue of the neck. It is not uncommon for torticollis to be associated with hemivertebrae in the cervical area or Klippel-Feil syndrome. Associated congenital dislocation or subluxation of the hip may also be observed.

**Incidence.** Torticollis is seen more frequently in girls than in boys.

**Signs and symptoms.** There is limited cervical motion, and the mass may be palpated by the observant parent or health care professional shortly after birth. In the severe case the head is tilted toward the side of the shortened muscle and the chin points toward the opposite side, or away from the shortened muscle. After 2 to 3 months the characteristic facial asymmetry develops, possibly resulting from impaired blood supply to the depressed side of the head.

Secondary to the deformity the patient may develop eye strain as a result of ocular imbalance. If the deformity persists untreated, compensatory curvature of the cervical and upper thoracic spine, along with elevation of the shoulder on the affected side, may be observed.

**Treatment.** If the deformity is slight and detected shortly after birth, some correction may be achieved through gentle stretching exercises accomplished routinely several times daily by the par-

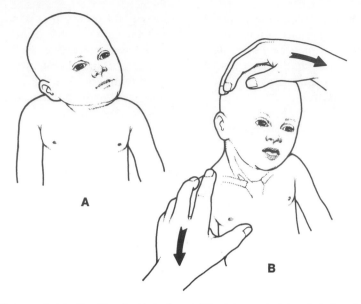

**Fig. 15-1.** Congenital torticollis. **A,** Note head tilted toward side of deformity with chin pointed in opposite direction. **B,** Note prominence of sternocleidomastoid muscle when head is flexed laterally. (Redrawn from Tachdjian, M. O.: Pediatric orthopaedics, Philadelphia, 1972, W. B. Saunders Co.)

ents. Surgical intervention is necessary when the contracture is not corrected through exercise. Maintenance of correction is accomplished with a cervical collar or brace or by traction accompanied by the continuation of the exercise program. Recurrence of the deformity is possible, necessitating another surgical procedure.

**Prognosis.** Proper and timely treatment often results in complete cure. The facial asymmetry in cases treated early may completely disappear.

### Acquired torticollis

Acquired torticollis occurs within the first decade of life. The patient complains of pain, which may be due to infection, injury, or trauma of the throat, neck, or cervical spine. Psychogenic factors may also be the cause of acquired torticollis.

Treatment is directed toward the cause. With severe contracture, surgical intervention may be the treatment of choice. Often in acute or inflammatory cases nonsurgical intervention such as exercise and heat application may resolve the condition.

### Spasmodic torticollis

Spasmodic torticollis is most frequently seen in the adult and is of gradual onset. The patient may complain of a drawing sensation and twitching, which pulls the head toward the affected side. The symptoms gradually develop into convulsive spasms, with or without regular patterns of rhythm,

with forcible pulling of the head to one side. Excitement appears to accelerate the symptoms. It is interesting to note that often the convulsive spasms can be inhibited by the light pressure of a finger against the head.

Conservative measures for the treatment of spasmodic torticollis are often successful. Such measures may include an exercise program, support and immobilization of the neck with a cervical collar, or the utilization of an appropriate brace. Although such therapy often results in resolution of the condition, psychotherapy or surgical intervention may be indicated.

## SPINAL DISEASES AND DISORDERS
### Ankylosing spondylitis (Marie-Strumpell disease)

Ankylosing spondylitis (Marie-Strumpell disease) (Fig. 15-2) is sometimes classified as a form of arthritis, although it has characteristics that indicate that it is a specific disease process. It was first clinically described in the late 1800s by the physicians for whom it was named. The specific characteristics include ossification of the ligaments surrounding the sacroiliac joint, ultimately progressing to other portions of the spine. In some cases ligaments of the hip and shoulder joints are involved.

**Etiology.** The cause of ankylosing spondylitis is not known.

**Pathology.** The pathologic alterations in ankylosing spondylitis are very similar to those seen in

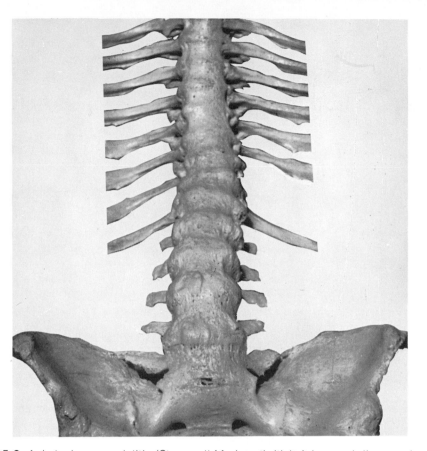

**Fig. 15-2.** Ankylosing spondylitis (Strumpell-Marie arthritis). Advanced disease showing bony ankylosis of vertebrae and sacroiliac joint. (From Brashear, H. R., and Raney, R. B.: Shand's handbook of orthopaedic surgery, ed. 9, St. Louis, 1978, The C. V. Mosby Co.)

rheumatoid arthritis. The ligamental ossification is progressive in nature and begins with general synovial inflammation surrounding the joints. Later stages of the disease process reveal progressive ankylosis of the fibrous and bony structures of the spine. Characteristically with progression of the disease the entire spinal column becomes ankylosed into a single bony mass.

**Incidence.** Ankylosing spondylitis is much more common in men than in women. It is seen most frequently in the third decade of life, with a smaller degree of incidence in the fourth decade.

**Signs and symptoms.** The most characteristic symptoms of ankylosing spondylitis are pain and spinal stiffness. The pain may be in the lower back or may radiate into the hip, buttocks, or lumbosacral region. The pain may occur before actual stiffness is noted, and in some cases there may be stiffness without pain. Varying degrees of both pain and stiffness may be seen depending on the stage of progression at the time of examination. Radiographic examination may not reveal the disease process during its early stages. Later stages may show varying degrees of joint erosion and narrowing with apparent ossification and ankylosis. A radiographic feature of this disease process is sacroiliac involvement. The blood sedimentation rate is elevated in the majority of the cases. Differential diagnosis between ankylosing spondylitis and rheumatoid arthritis may be made in the absence of the rheumatoid blood factor.

**Treatment.** If ankylosing spondylitis is diagnosed during the early stages, the major goal of treatment is to maintain the spine straight and erect throughout the progression of the disease, thus preventing the deformities related to later stages. If diagnosed during the later stages, nonsurgical measures may not be sufficient and spinal osteotomy or other appropriate surgical intervention may be required. Exercises and heat therapy are of some value in both the relief of pain and prevention of deformity. Additional pain control may be achieved with salicylate therapy. Occasionally additional anti-inflammatory drugs are of some value.

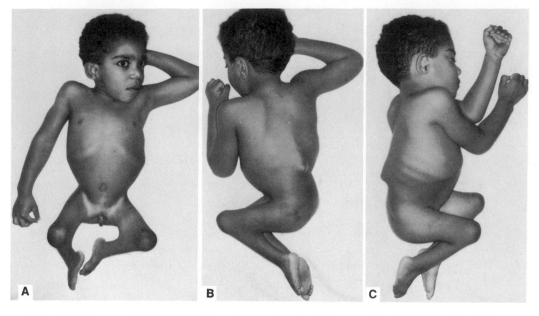

**Fig. 15-3.** Congenital absence of lumbosacral spine in 6-year-old child. (From Tachdjian, M.: Pediatric Orthopaedics, Philadelphia, 1972, W. B. Saunders Co.)

## Congenital absence of sacrum and lumbar vertebrae

Congenital absence of the sacrum and lumbar vertebrae (Fig. 15-3) is an anomaly present at birth to varying degrees. Obvious deformities are apparent at birth and vary according to the severity of the anomaly.

**Etiology.** This deformity is most likely the result of dysfunction in early embryonic development of the specified areas.

**Incidence.** Congenital absence of the sacrum and lumbar vertebrae is relatively rare.

**Pathology.** Various degrees of this deformity may be present at birth, from absence of the lower segment of the coccyx to absence of the entire sacrum and all lumbar vertebrae.

**Signs and symptoms.** Lesser degrees of this congenital anomaly may involve so few signs that marked deformities are not present, and the condition may therefore not be diagnosed unless found accidently on radiographic examination. More severe forms of the anomaly evince not only gross deformities but associated neurologic deficits. Signs and symptoms of the more severe types of this deformity may include short stature, flattened buttocks, muscle paralysis to varying degrees, muscle atrophy in the lower extremities, cross-legged appearance in position of lower extremities, foot deformities, contractures of the hips and knees, and varying degrees of sensation loss, particularly distal to the knees. Definitive diagnosis as to the extent of the absence may be made by radiographic examination.[5,p.1180]

**Treatment.** The treatment of congenital absence of the sacrum and lumbar vertebrae varies greatly and is dependent on the severity of the anomaly. Surgical intervention is usually required for maximum mobility with the greatest degree of spinopelvic stability. Surgical intervention may be reconstructive or may involve disarticulation procedures at various levels. Fusion of the remaining vertebrae may be accomplished. With a combination of appropriate procedures many patients, again dependent on the severity of the deformity, can be provided with enough stability to sit and to ambulate with some assistance.

**Prognosis.** With appropriate surgical intervention, patients with slight to moderate degrees of this deformity can attain some stability and mobility. The most severe forms of this deformity, however, are incompatible with life.

## Hemivertebra

Hemivertebra (Fig. 15-4) is a congenital failure of a vertebra to develop completely. Usually half of the vertebra involved is completely or partially developed, with obvious absence of the other half. Involvement may be seen with one or more vertebrae and produces varying degrees of balanced or unbalanced congenital scoliosis.

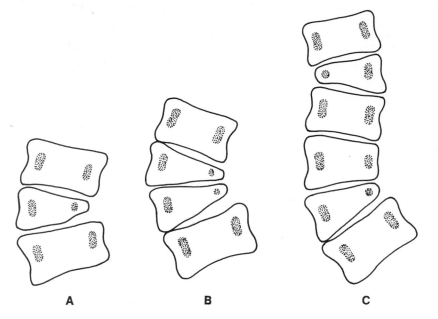

**Fig. 15-4.** Hemivertebra. **A,** Complete unilateral failure of formation of one vertebra. **B,** Double hemivertebra, unbalanced with complete unilateral failure of formation of more than one vertebra. **C,** Double vertebra, unbalanced with complete unilateral failure of formation of one vertebra with involvement on opposite sides.

**Etiology.** Hemivertebra is a developmental error of the spine due to lack of formation of a vertebral body growth center.

**Pathology.** The failure of the growth center on one side of the vertebral body to appropriately develop produces a wedge-shaped vertebra. As a result the adjacent vertebral bodies are expanded or tilt to fit the deformity. The intervertebral spaces are usually well preserved. Varying degrees of balanced or unbalanced congenital scoliosis result from the deformity, and other developmental abnormalities may be present. Hemivertebra may be classified in one of three categories[5,p.1147]:

1. Hemivertebra due to the complete failure of the growth center of one vertebral body, creating slight to moderate unbalanced congenital scoliosis.
2. Hemivertebra involving two vertebral bodies with failure of development of one growth center of each vertebral body on the same side, resulting in moderate to severe unbalanced congenital scoliosis.
3. Hemivertebra involving failure of development of two vertebral bodies (with involved growth centers on opposite sides), creating balanced congenital scoliosis.

**Signs and symptoms.** Singular hemivertebra may pose few if any signs and symptoms. Dependent on the degree of congenital scoliosis present, obvious deformity may be noted with progression of growth. Hemivertebra of the other types, especially those that involve unbalanced congenital scoliosis, are known to progress considerably and have a relatively poor prognosis unless an early spinal fusion to prevent progression of curvature is accomplished.[6,p.1461]

**Treatment.** No treatment may be necessary for hemivertebra that results in balanced curvature. Unbalanced types, which are known to result in progression of curvature, require early intervention in the form of spinal fusion. If surgical intervention is accomplished at an early stage, the prognosis is relatively good.

Additional information regarding hemivertebra may be found in the section on congenital scoliosis.

### Kyphosis (round back)

Kyphosis is the posterior convexity of the thoracic portion of the vertebral column. This is a normal curvature but becomes pathologic if excessive.

**Etiology.** Excessive kyphosis may be the result of poor posture. It may also be secondary to tuberculosis, chronic arthritis, osteoporosis in the elderly, and compression fractures of the thoracic vertebrae. Kyphosis in children may be caused by Scheuermann's disease, the most common type of pathologic kyphosis. (See also the section on Scheuermann's disease.)

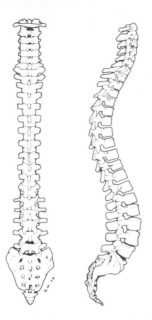

**Fig. 15-5.** Normal spine. Note normal physiologic curves on lateral view. (From Hilt, N. E., and Schmitt, E. W., Jr.: Pediatric orthopedic nursing, St. Louis, 1975, The C. V. Mosby Co.)

**Pathology.** The normal physiology of the spine (Fig. 15-5) reveals a degree of normal curvature when viewed laterally. Normal posterior convexity, varying from one individual to another, is seen in the thoracic region. Normal concavity in the cervical and lumbar areas usually balances the degree of kyphosis of the thoracic area. Excessive degrees of curvature may result in decreased pulmonary capacities and various fixed or irreversible deformities.

**Incidence.** Pathologic kyphosis is seen most frequently in children and young adults. If seen in middle-aged or elderly persons it is referred to as *adult round back.*

**Signs and symptoms.** The most common sign of kyphosis is the obvious round-back deformity that results from the excessive curvature. Depending on the cause, other signs and symptoms may be absent. Depending on the degree of kyphosis, decreased pulmonary function and general poor posture may be noted.

**Treatment.** Kyphosis caused by poor posture, if treated early, may be successfully corrected with exercises and adequate patient instruction on appropriate posture. Other types of kyphosis, however, of pathologic cause, may require additional exercises, which may still be relatively unsuccessful. Braces and surgical intervention may be indicated in some cases.

## Lordosis (hollow back)

Lordosis is an accentuation of the cervical or lumbar curvature beyond physiologic levels.

**Etiology.** Lordosis may be idiopathic, secondary to disease processes of the vertebral bodies in the cervical or lumbar area, or the result of traumatic injury.

**Pathology.** The normal physiologic structure of the spine, as viewed laterally, reveals concavity directed posteriorly in the cervical or lumbar areas (Fig. 15-5). As with kyphosis, this degree may vary normally from one individual to another. Of concern is curvature excessive enough to create deformities, impinge on surrounding tissues, or produce symptoms sufficient to require relief. Excessive lordosis in the lumbar area is often seen with flexion contractures of the hip, obesity, congenital dislocation of the hip, and coxa vara.[1]

**Signs and symptoms.** Contrary to what may be seen with kyphosis, excessive lordosis may be accompanied by pain. Fatigue may also be a complaint, and low back pain may be associated with fatigue. The pain may be persistent and vary in severity. Protrusion of the abdomen may be noted. Lordosis in children is commonly asymptomatic.

**Treatment.** Postural exercises or support garments may be relatively successful in the relief of pain and other symptoms in some patients. It should be noted, however, that relief from these measures is frequently not permanent. The cause of the lordosis should be determined, and appropriate treatment prescribed.

## Pott's disease

Pott's disease (Fig. 15-6) is tuberculosis of the spinal column, the most common site of tuberculosis of bone or joints.

**Etiology.** Pott's disease is caused by a tuberculous infection with vertebral involvement.

**Pathology.** Tuberculous infection in Pott's disease may be found anywhere within the vertebral column or the vertebral body or arches. Usually the vertebral body is affected with minimal destruction of bone and surrounding tissue. The infection invades not only the bone tissue of the specific vertebrae but may involve surrounding tissue at varying points of progression. Total destruction of bone and surrounding tissue with invasion into adjoining vertebrae is not uncommon with progression of the process. Deformity may result from the destruction and collapse of the vertebral structure. Healing of the infectious process is accomplished through gradual fibrosis and eventual new bone forma-

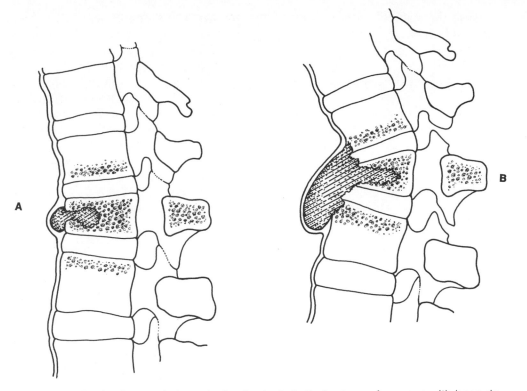

**Fig. 15-6.** Pott's disease (tuberculosis of spine). **A,** Early stage of process with bone destruction and minimal abscess formation. **B,** Late stages of process with extensive bone destruction and abscess formation. (Redrawn from Brashear, H. R., Jr., and Raney, R. B., Sr.: Shand's handbook of orthopaedic surgery, ed. 9, St. Louis, 1978, The C. V. Mosby Co.)

tion, which results in ankylosis of the affected area.[1,5,p.687]

**Incidence.** The spinal column is the most common site of tuberculosis of bone tissue, representing half or more of diagnosed cases. The most commonly involved area of the vertebral column is the lower thoracic vertebrae, although any portion of the spine may be affected. Pott's disease is most frequently seen in adults, since improved public health measures over the past few decades have alleviated the incidence in children.[5,pp.686-687]

**Signs and symptoms.** Because the evolution of this disease process is usually somewhat slow, the onset of associated signs and symptoms may be insidious. The early symptoms are more likely to be of a general nature and may include weight loss, general malaise, easy fatigability, and loss of appetite. Pain may not be associated with the early signs and if present is usually minimal and intermittent. Low-grade fever may be noted especially during the late afternoon and evening. Progression of the disease process may reveal increased pain, muscle

spasms, and limited motion. Radiographic examination usually reveals features compatible with the degree of progression; extremely early stages of the disease may not be seen on x-ray films. Differential diagnosis should be established between various types of benign and malignant tumors and other infectious processes. Extremely advanced forms of Pott's disease may result in varying degrees of paralysis of the lower extremities with associated disturbances of gait, hyperactive reflexes, and sensory and sphincter alterations.[1,5,pp.687-689]

**Treatment.** The treatment of Pott's disease includes recumbency during the preoperative phase, followed by surgical intervention and postoperative immobilization. Preoperative recumbency may be achieved through the utilization of a Bradford frame, various types of special beds, or cast therapy. Traction or orthotic devices may be used if the cervical area of the vertebral column is involved. Local infectious abscesses require the initiation of a chemotherapeutic regimen. Surgical intervention is accomplished to eradicate the focus of tuberculous infection and increase the stability of the involved vertebrae with the additional objective of prevention of further deformity. Postoperative immobilization may be accomplished with various types of cast therapy to support the healing process of the fusion and promote appropriate alignment conducive to the healing process. Other forms of immobilization may be advocated in some cases. Recumbency throughout the postoperative process is advised for a period of several months.

### Ruptured intervertebral disc

Ruptured intervertebral disc (Fig. 15-7) is the complete or partial herniation of the nuclear material of the intervertebral disc. This herniation or rupture into the spinal canal may cause compression of the spinal nerve roots in the area, resulting in characteristic symptoms.

**Etiology.** The cause of a ruptured intervertebral disc is somewhat obscure. Although trauma or poor body mechanics may be precipitating factors, small tears in surrounding tissues may be responsible for the rupture.

**Pathology.** Throughout life the intervertebral discs are subjected to almost continuous wear and tear. Degenerative changes begin to occur within the nucleus. It becomes softened through cellular changes and loses its firm, glistening appearance. The annulus becomes progressively weaker and

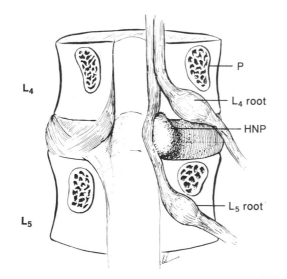

**Fig. 15-7.** Diagram of herniated nucleus pulposus *(HNP)* as seen from back with spinous processes and laminae removed from pedicles *(P)*. Note that disc protrusion between fourth and fifth lumbar vertebrae impinges on fifth lumbar nerve root. (From Brashear, H. R., and Raney, R. B.: Shand's handbook of orthopaedic surgery, ed. 9, St. Louis, 1978, The C. V. Mosby Co.)

thinner. The turgor of the nucleus causes stretching of the posterior fibers, resulting in the bulging of the disc into the floor of the spinal canal.[6,p.1325] With the bulging, compression of the spinal nerve roots in the area, as they exit from the spinal canal, results in specific pathologic signs and symptoms.[3,p.330]

**Incidence.** A ruptured (herniated) intervertebral disc is seen most commonly between the ages of 20 and 45 years. It is more commonly seen in men than in women, which may be indicative of their level of activity and the associated degree of wear and tear on these tissues.

**Signs and symptoms.** The characteristic clinical picture does not appear until some of the nuclear material actually herniates or ruptures causing compression of or pressure on the nerve root, although the degenerative process may have been occurring for years. Its onset may be sudden with severe low back pain following a traumatic injury of some type. The episodes of pain subside in a few days but recur with progressive intensity and at shorter intervals. Sciatic pain follows, beginning as a dull pain in the buttocks. This pain is followed by the characteristic leg pain, which may extend to the ankle, heel, and foot. The pain is usually unilateral and radiating and is exaggerated by sneezing, coughing, or straining.

On examination limited forward bending is frequently seen. During acute stages of the process additional limited mobility may be observed. A characteristic list or lean away from the affected side is often noted during standing or ambulating. Tenderness may be elicited with deep pressure over the affected area. Straight leg raising may produce sciatic nerve pain.[6,pp.1328-1330]

Although degrees of lower extremity muscle atrophy and weakness may be noted in most lumbar disc involvement, additional symptoms may be related to the level of involvement (Table 15-1). If the *third lumbar disc* is involved, sensory deficits may be noted on the medial aspects of the ankle and foot, with additional sensory deficits noted on the anterior and medial aspects of the leg. *Fourth lumbar disc* involvement, where the majority of these lesions occur, may produce difficulty or total inability to walk on the heel and varying degrees of decreased strength in dorsiflexion of the great toe. At this level sensory deficits are most frequently noted over the medial aspect of the dorsum of the foot, the dorsum of the great toe, and the anterolateral aspect of the leg. Occasionally sensory deficits may also be seen over the dorsum of the second toe. With involvement of the *fifth lumbar disc* there is often difficulty or inability to walk on the toes. Sensory

**Table 15-1.** Characteristic common and differential symptoms of ruptured intervertebral disc

| Symptom | Most lesions | Third lumbar disc | Fourth lumbar disc | Fifth lumbar disc |
|---|---|---|---|---|
| Pain | Sudden onset; severe; subsides in few days | | | |
| | Recurrent episodes, increasing in intensity and severity, at close intervals | | | |
| | May radiate to foot, heel, and ankle | | | |
| | Unilateral | | | |
| | Exaggerated by sneezing, coughing, straining, lifting | | | |
| | Often relieved by rest | | | |
| Motion | Limited forward bending | | | |
| | Acute stages, all motion decreased | | | |
| Posture or gait | List or lean away from affected side | | Difficulty or inability to walk on heels | Difficulty or inability to walk on toes |
| Tenderness | Elicited by deep pressure over affected vertebral interspace | | | |
| Tests | Sciatic nerve pain reproduced by straight leg raising | | | |
| Motor | Lower extremity muscle atrophy | | Decreased strength of dorsiflexion of great toe | |
| | Lower extremity muscle weakness | | | |
| Sensory deficit | To varying degrees | Medial aspect of ankle | Dorsum of great toe (sometimes second toe) | Last two or three toes |
| | | Medial aspect of foot | Medial aspect of dorsum of foot | Lateral aspect of foot |
| | | Anteromedial aspect of leg | Anterolateral aspect of leg | Posterior and lateral aspects of lower leg |

deficits at this level are usually seen on the lateral and possibly the posterior aspect of the lower leg, the foot, and the last two or three toes.[6,pp.1328-1330]

Ruptured intervertebral discs may reveal some definite or suspected pathology on radiographic examination. Most frequently seen is a decrease in the intervertebral disc space. Myelography is often utilized to confirm the diagnosis. Additionally epidural venography may be utilized in cases where myelographic accuracy is limited. Differential diagnosis should be made between other diseases that have similar exhibitions, such as spondylolisthesis, Marie-Strumpell disease, osteoporosis, infections, tumors, hip and pelvic conditions, malformation of lumbar spinal nerve roots, varicosities, and vascular insufficiency.[6,pp.1332-1333]

**Treatment.** The treatment of a confirmed ruptured intervertebral disc involves a relatively massive and comprehensive program. Success or failure of the treatment is dependent on the patient's adherence to all portions of the program. The comprehensive plan includes the following components.

*Bed rest* is recommended to remove weight bearing pressure from the affected intervertebral disc. Placing the patient in a recumbent position allows the disc bulge, which is producing the symptoms, to move away from the nerve root. There is the possibility of resolution through conservative therapy with formation of scar tissue over the tear in the annulus.

*Exercise programs* are utilized to strengthen back

extensor, abdominal, and quadriceps muscles. Although the specific exercise program may vary, the goal of strengthening these specific muscles is generally agreed upon. In addition proper posture is reviewed with the patient and encouraged.

*Traction and heat* are often utilized to assist in the decrease of muscle spasms and the relief of symptoms. The type of traction utilized may vary from leg or pelvic sling traction to 90-90 traction (see p. 522). The traction is applied to distract the disc interval and allow replacement of the bulging tissue. A firm mattress and bed board are advocated. Heat may be applied at intervals to the lower back.

*Support* may be provided through the utilization of an appropriately fitted garment. Ambulation is not advocated without the garment.

*Education* of the patient about the overall program is extremely important in gaining cooperation and adherence. The patient should be advised to follow the exercise program carefully, and with recurrence of symptoms bed rest should be resumed. The patient should be advised not to participate in any sports or activities that might initiate or aggravate the condition. The patient is encouraged to maintain proper weight through dieting or close observation of proper diet. Compliance with the recommendations is dependent on the education of the patient by health care professionals when treatment is initiated.

This program may be sufficient to maintain the patient relatively free of symptoms. However, with repeated attacks of increasing intensity and duration, failure of conservative (nonsurgical) therapy, and positive and progressive neurologic signs, surgical removal or fusion of the disc may be necessary. The need for surgical intervention frequently does not negate the need for some of the components of the nonsurgical therapy program. Certain portions of this program may be continued postoperatively.

**Prognosis.** Even when conservative therapy has been successful, surgical intervention in the form of a spinal fusion may be necessary with aging because of degenerative arthritis or instability of the spinal column. Recurrence of symptoms following disc removal and spinal fusion may require another fusion.

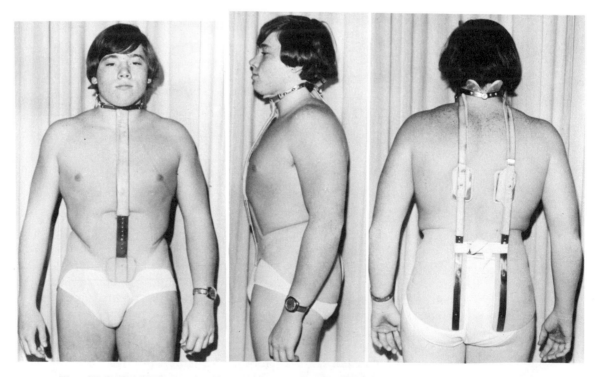

**Fig. 15-8.** Scheuermann's disease (excessive kyphosis). Patient shown in Milwaukee brace, commonly utilized for treatment. (From Hilt, N. E., and Schmitt, E. W., Jr.: Pediatric orthopedic nursing, St. Louis, 1975, The C. V. Mosby Co.)

## Scheuermann's disease (juvenile kyphosis, adolescent kyphosis, adolescent vertebral epiphysitis)

Scheuermann's disease (Fig. 15-8) is a fixed kyphosis that develops at puberty and is caused by wedge-shaped deformities of one or multiple vertebrae.[5,p.1240]

**Etiology.** The cause of Scheuermann's disease is unknown. It has been speculated that this disease may result from infection, inflammatory processes, aseptic necrosis, disc deterioration, mechanical influences, inadequate circulation during rapid growth, and disturbances of epiphyseal growth resulting from protrusion of the intervertebral disc through deficient or defective cartilaginous plates.[1,5,p.1241]

**Pathology.** The most striking pathologic feature of Scheuermann's disease is the presence of wedge-shaped vertebral bodies seen on radiographic examination. These wedge-shaped vertebrae create a curvature in excess of the normal curvature.

**Incidence.** Scheuermann's disease is seen most frequently in children between the ages of 12 and 16 years with onset shortly after puberty. It occurs more frequently in girls than in boys.

**Signs and symptoms.** Scheuermann's disease has an insidious onset. Often there is a history of unusual strenous physical activity or participation in sports. The most frequent sign is poor posture with accompanying symptoms of fatigue and pain in the involved area. Tenderness or stiffness may be seen in the involved area and sometimes along the entire spinal column. In most cases the kyphosis is within the thoracic vertebrae; however, in some cases the vertebrae below this level may be involved. If the patient is seen shortly after the onset of the dis-

**Table 15-2.** Classification of scoliosis

| Brashear and Raney[1] | Tachdjian[5] | Cobb[2] |
|---|---|---|
| I. Postural or nonfunctional scoliosis | I. Functional or postural scoliosis | |
| II. Structural scoliosis | II. Structural scoliosis | II. Structural scoliosis |
|   Congenital |   Congenital |   Osteopathic |
|     Hemivertebrae |   Acquired |     Congenital |
|     Congenital anomalies |     Idiopathic (unknown origin) |     Thoracogenic |
|   Paralytic |       Lumbar |     Other |
|     Poliomyelitis |       Dorsolumbar |   Neuropathic |
|     Infantile muscular atrophy |       Dorsal (infantile, juvenile, adolescent) |     Congenital |
|     Progressive muscular |       Combined dorsal and lumbar |     Postpoliomyelitis |
|       dystrophy |       Cervicodorsal |     Other |
|     Freidrich's ataxia |     Neuromuscular |   Myopathic |
|     Syringomyelia |       Poliomyelitis |     Congenital |
|     Spastic paralysis |       Neurofibromatosis |     Muscular dystrophy |
|   Idiopathic |       Intraspinal tumors |     Other |
| |       Friedreich's ataxia |   Idiopathic |
| |       Syringomyelia | |
| |       Spastic paralysis, cerebral palsy | |
| |       Muscular dystrophies and other | |
| |         myopathies | |
| |       Arthrogryposis multiplex congenita | |
| |     Postirradiation scoliosis | |
| |     Thoracogenic (postempyema, | |
| |       postthoracoplasty) | |
| |     Scoliosis in children with congenital | |
| |       heart disease | |
| |     Scoliosis due to affections of the | |
| |       vertebral column | |
| |       Osteochondrodystrophy | |
| |       Osteogenesis imperfecta | |
| |       Fracture, dislocation | |
| |       Tumors such as osteoid osteoma | |
| |       Inflammatory conditions such as | |
| |         rheumatoid, pyogenic, or | |
| |         tuberculous spondylitis | |

ease process the associated posture may be corrected actively and passively. It does, however, become fixed within a period of 6 to 9 months. Radiographic examination reveals the wedge-shaped vertebrae along with possible disturbances of ossification around the epiphysis.[5, p. 1244] Differential diagnosis should be made between Scheuermann's disease, tuberculosis of the spine, and osteochondritis. Such differentiation is not difficult, because tuberculosis shows marked rigidity of the spine usually not seen with Scheuermann's disease and osteochondritis is known to develop at an earlier age and rarely is seen in more than one vertebral body.

**Treatment.** The most effective treatment for Scheuermann's disease is immobilization with a plaster cast or Milwaukee brace. It is recommended that the immobilization be continuous for 10 to 12 months, with additional immobilization at night for approximately the same length of time. An exercise program is accomplished throughout and after the immobilization period. In adulthood persistent pain in the thoracic area may indicate a degenerative alteration secondary to this disease process, and spinal arthrodesis may be necessary for relief of symptoms.

### Scoliosis

Scoliosis is lateral curvature of the spine. In the normal spinal column (Fig. 15-5) no curvature is present; *any* lateral curvature, therefore, is abnormal. Scoliosis may occur from specific pathologic processes or may be idiopathic. It may result from a deformity in one or many vertebral bodies. The extent to which the vertebrae are involved may vary from several to the entire spinal column. The degree of curvature may be mild, moderate, or severe. It is not uncommon as the spine begins to curve for the involved vertebrae to rotate, which may produce rib cage deformities and decrease pulmonary capacity. Because the classification of scoliosis (Table 15-2)

has changed over recent years, the following terminology is provided for clarification:

**functional, postural, or nonstructural scoliosis** (Table 15-3) lateral curvatures resulting from temporary postural influences; spinal structures not abnormal; easily correctable.
**structural scoliosis** lateral curvature characterized by spinal structural changes of various causes; more difficult to correct, with success highly dependent on the severity of curvature.
**congenital scoliosis** lateral curvature of the spine present at birth, most frequently resulting from specific congenital spinal anomalies.
**acquired scoliosis** lateral curvature resulting from some cause not present at birth.
**paralytic scoliosis** lateral curvature resulting after specific neurologic diseases such as poliomyelitis or progressive muscular dystrophy.
**idiopathic scoliosis** lateral curvature resulting from an unknown cause; manifests itself during the preadolescent or adolescent years; most common type of scoliosis.

Scoliosis may also be classified by the characteristic of the curvature itself, as follows:

**functional curvature** lateral curvature with no structural alterations within the vertebral column; posturally induced curvature; curvature can be corrected by postural alterations.
**structural curvature** lateral curvature resulting from structural alterations within the vertebral column.
**S-shaped curvature** double curvature comprised of a major curve (usually primary) and a compensatory curve above or below the major curve.
**C-shaped curvature** lateral curvature involving all or most of the lumbar and thoracic areas; most frequently associated with paralytic disease.
**double major curve** lateral curvature comprising two primary curves of equal or almost equal degree; almost always a balanced curvature.
**primary curvature** major curvature; the most prominent curvature; the curvature involving greatest deformity.

**Table 15-3.** Characteristics of functional versus nonfunctional scoliosis[1, p. 123; 6, p. 1325]

|  | Functional | Nonfunctional |
|---|---|---|
| Most common area | Thoracolumbar | Thoracic or thoracolumbar but may vary |
| Single/multiple | Single | Usually multiple |
| Compensatory curvature | No | Frequently |
| Convexity | Left | Right most common |
| Rotation | Rarely, toward concavity | Frequent, toward convexity |
| Flexibility | Disappears with recumbency | No voluntary correction |
|  | Disappears with suspension | Part of curvature fixed |
|  | Voluntary correction | Flexibility variable |
| Radiographic examination | No structural change | Structural changes |
|  |  | Variable flexibility with some fixed curvature |

**compensatory curve** lateral curvature that results after the development of a primary curvature, in the opposite direction and immediately above or below the primary curvature; develops in an attempt to maintain balance; secondary curvature.

**tertiary curvature** curvature that results above or below a secondary or compensatory curvature; usually of minimal severity.

Scoliosis may develop in a localized area of the spinal column (e.g., cervical, cervicothoracic, thoracic, thoracolumbar, lumbar) or may involve the entire spinal column (as is seen with the C-shaped curvature). The characteristics of the curvature are important in the determination of appropriate treatment. Of significance are the degree of *rotation* and the degree of *balance*. Rotation is of greatest significance because of its ability to impinge on the rib cage, resulting in decreased pulmonary and cardiac capacity. Rotation of even mild to moderate degrees can result in obvious rib cage deformity. The degree of balance is significant in its overall effect on spinal stability and trunk mobility. The resulting deformity can drastically affect gait patterns.

Although all types of scoliosis are of concern, emphasis here is on congenital and idiopathic scoliosis, both structural in nature, because of their high incidence in relation to total scoliosis cases. The general incidence of types of scoliosis reveals no significant difference relative to race. Because of decreased incidence of poliomyelitis and tuberculosis, scoliosis from these diseases is seen less frequently.

### Congenital scoliosis

Congenital scoliosis is a lateral curvature of the spine, present at birth, and resulting from specific congenital rib and vertebral anomalies.

**Etiology and pathology.** The etiologic and pathologic characteristics of congenital scoliosis are classified into six categories[4,7]:

   I. Partial unilateral failure of formation of a vertebra
  II. Complete unilateral failure of formation of a vertebra
 III. Bilateral failure of segmentation with absence of disc space
 IV. Unilateral failure of segmentation with unsegmented bar
  V. Fusion of ribs
 VI. Unclassifiable

Characteristics of each category are given in Table 15-4 and corresponding Fig. 15-9.

Class IV scoliosis (unsegmented unilateral bar) appears to progress more rapidly and has the highest degree of deformity. Other congenital deformities not associated with the vertebral column have been noted with a relatively high degree of frequency in these patients (e.g., congenital heart disease).

**Signs and symptoms.** Depending on the cause of congenital scoliosis, there will be a varying degree of obvious deformity. This deformity increases with growth and age, usually progressing slowly during periods of slow trunk growth. Diagnosis of the specific congenital anomaly may be confirmed with radiographic examination. Specific rate of progression of many congenital curvatures cannot be predicted, and sometimes there is little correlation in relation to the severity of the curvature at the time of diagnosis.

**Treatment.** Treatment of congenital scoliosis may be nonsurgical or surgical. Nonsurgical intervention includes exercise programs, utilization of orthotic devices such as a scoliosis splint, Milwaukee brace, Risser localizer, or turnbuckle cast for prevention

**Table 15-4.** Classification of etiologic and pathologic characteristics of congenital scoliosis[4,7]

| Classification | Major characteristic | Features |
|---|---|---|
| I | Partial unilateral failure of formation of vertebra | Wedge-shaped vertebra<br>Small vestigial pedicle may be seen on x-ray film |
| II | Complete unilateral failure of formation of vertebra | Hemivertebra produced<br>May be unbalanced or balanced |
| III | Bilateral failure of segmentation | Absence of disc space |
| IV | Unilateral failure of segmentation | Unsegmented bar<br>Two or more vertebrae may be involved<br>Vertebral body, posterior elements, or both may be involved |
| V | Fusion of ribs | May fuse close to or with vertebrae<br>May fuse anteriorly |
| VI | Unclassifiable | Those anomalies not fitting into other classifications |

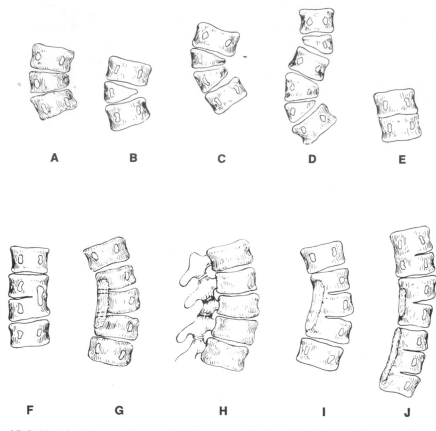

**Fig. 15-9.** Vertebral anomalies producing congenital scoliosis. **A,** Wedge vertebra due to partial unilateral failure of formation of vertebra. **B,** Hemivertebra due to complete unilateral failure of formation of vertebra. **C,** Double hemivertebra, unbalanced. **D,** Double hemivertebra, balanced. **E,** Bilateral symmetric failure of segmentation; note absence of disc interspace and fusion of adjacent vertebral bodies. **F,** Asymmetric failure of segmentation, unsegmented bar. **G,** Asymmetric failure of segmentation, unsegmented bar involving posterior elements only, anteroposterior view. **H,** Asymmetric failure of segmentation, oblique view; note intact disc space and confinement of lack of segmentation to posterior elements only. **I,** Unsegmented bar involving both disc area and posterior elements. **J,** Multiple unsegmented bars, unbalanced. (From Winter, R. B., Moe, J. H., and Eilers, V. E.: Congenital scoliosis: a study of two hundred thirty four patients treated and untreated, J. Bone Joint Surg. **50**-A:3, 1968.)

of progression of the curvature. Surgical intervention is in the form of an anterior or posterior spinal fusion. Careful evaluation for curvature progression must be accomplished. In rare circumstances additional surgical procedures such as spinal osteotomy or halo traction may be required.

### Idiopathic scoliosis

Idiopathic scoliosis is the type most frequently seen and is characterized by lateral curvature of unknown cause.

**Pathology.** Idiopathic scoliosis may occur at any age, although the three types are commonly associated with certain age groups:

1. *Infantile type:* 1- to 3-year-olds
2. *Juvenile type:* 3- to 10-year-olds
3. *Adolescent type:* preadolescents and adolescents

Specific characteristics are seen with each type, as shown in Table 15-5.

As previously stated, the degree of deformity that may occur with scoliosis varies considerably. Of critical concern to the diagnostician are the *degree* of curvature, the *balance* of the curvature(s), and the *rotational component* of the curvature. All three pathologic features must be taken into consideration for a total view of the process and to predict progression. The rotational component is instrumental in causing rib cage deformities and impingement on pulmonary and cardiac status.

**Table 15-5.** Characteristics of types of structural idiopathic scoliosis[5,pp.1191-1194; 6,p.1416]

| Type | Age group | Most common curvature | Sex | Comments |
|------|-----------|----------------------|-----|----------|
| Infantile | 1 to 3 years | Left thoracic curvature | Males predominately | May resolve itself spontaneously |
| Juvenile | 3 to 10 years | Right thoracic curvature | Both sexes | |
| Adolescent | 10 years to skeletal growth completed | Right thoracic curvature<br>Right thoracolumbar curvature | Females predominately | High familial tendency |

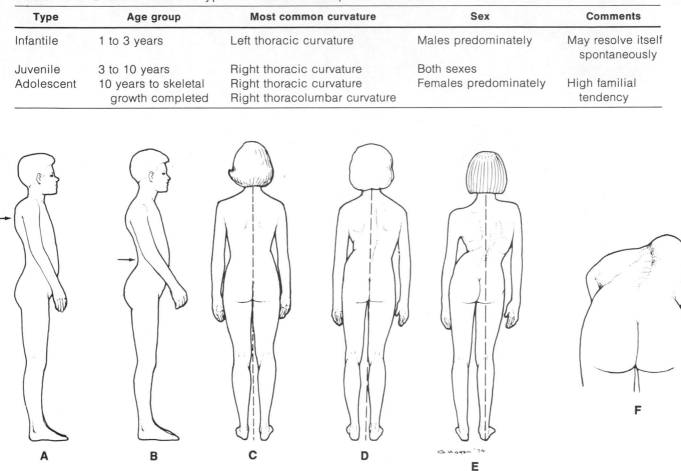

**Fig. 15-10.** Scoliosis. **A,** Kyphosis. **B,** Lordosis. **C,** Normal spine and balance. **D,** Mild scoliosis and balance **E,** Severe scoliosis, uncompensated, not in balance. **F,** Rib hump and flank asymmetry seen in flexion due to rotary component. (From Hilt, N. E., and Schmitt, E. W., Jr.: Pediatric orthopedic nursing, St. Louis, 1975, The C. V. Mosby Co.)

**Incidence.** Idiopathic scoliosis is seen in approximately 70% of all patients with scoliosis and in up to 80% of those with structural scoliosis. Further incidence patterns are given in Table 15-5 according to the specific type of idiopathic scoliosis.

**Signs and symptoms.** The signs and symptoms of idiopathic scoliosis are relatively clear cut. It must be emphasized, however, that especially in the adolescent type (the one most frequently seen) early diagnosis is difficult. Many of the obvious signs of idiopathic scoliosis may be somewhat hidden with clothing, and therefore diagnosis and treatment are delayed. Many states have now begun to implement *scoliosis screening programs* in the school system to improve ability to detect this process at an early stage. Most of these programs have been quite successful and are highly recommended for continued implementation.

The signs commonly associated with scoliosis are (1) unlevel shoulders, (2) prominent scapula, (3) prominent breast, (4) prominent flank area (flattening of flank area), (5) unlevel or prominent hip, (6) poor posture, and (7) obvious curvature. Throughout the examination and screening process it is critical that the adolescent be examined for *all* of these signs. Some may be subtle. It is necessary to view the patient from the front, from the back, and while bending. If a rotational component is associated with the curvature, the rib hump will become obvious in flexion (Fig. 15-10, *F*). In addition to the signs noted, the patient may complain of difficulty with uneven hemlines, occasional transient pain, and fatigue. Sometimes the deformity is accidentally discovered on routine chest radiographic examination.

Decreased pulmonary function may be noted,

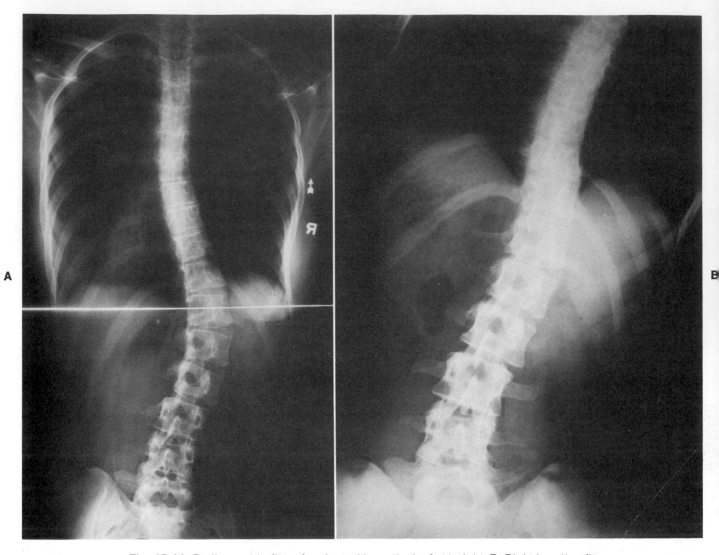

A

B

**Fig. 15-11.** Radiographic film of patient with scoliosis. **A,** Upright. **B,** Right bending film; note the degree of correction.

dependent on the degree of deformity and rotational component creating rib cage alterations. Confirmation of the diagnosis is accomplished through extensive radiographic examination. Bending films (Fig. 15-11, *B*) are extremely important in ascertaining the flexibility of the curvature and the degree of spontaneous correction potential.

It is not uncommon with severe curvature for neurologic deficits to occur. These deficits will vary according to the extent to which the curvature has impinged on the integrity of the spinal cord. Reflex, sensation, and motor alterations of the lower extremity may be noted.

**Treatment.** Treatment of idiopathic scoliosis is dependent on the clinical picture obtained through physical and radiographic examination. All compo-

nents of the deformity are taken into consideration before prescribing an intervention program. Additional consideration is given to the present stage of the growth cycle, since we know that progression of the deformity ceases at or shortly after completion of bone growth. Thus there is more concern if a moderate degree of curvature exists in a 12-year-old girl than in a 17-year-old.

Three specific measures are utilized for nonsurgical intervention: *observation*, an *exercise program*, and the *Milwaukee brace*. Observation and an exercise program are frequently the only treatment required. Observation is carried out through frequent physical examination and monitoring of the progression of the curvature through radiographic examination. Exercise programs are designed to

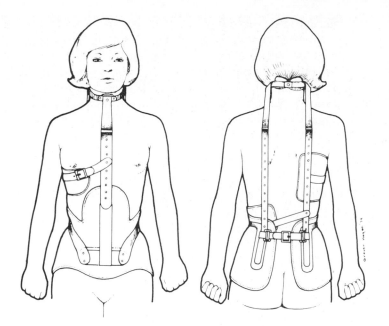

**Fig. 15-12.** Milwaukee brace utilized for nonsurgical treatment of scoliosis, kyphosis, and lordosis. (From Hilt, N. E., and Schmitt, E. W., Jr.: Pediatric orthopedic nursing, St. Louis, 1975, The C. V. Mosby Co.)

promote the maximum degree of correction possible as indicated by the degree of flexibility shown on the initial x-ray studies. In some cases compliance with the exercise program can increase the flexibility of the curvature. Observation and an exercise program are utilized with patients who have a curvature under 15° to 20°. Degrees of curvature over 15° to 20° usually require utilization of a Milwaukee brace (Fig. 15-12) in addition to observation and an exercise program. The major objective of the Milwaukee brace is to control progression of the curvature, although some degree of correction may be obtained. The Milwaukee brace is worn 23 hours a day. Lateral pads are applied to specific areas for application of pressure over the apex of the curvature. Careful attention is given to the skin to maintain appropriate integrity. The major part of the exercise program is carried out during the time that the adolescent is out of the brace, and additional exercises are accomplished while in the brace. It is of the utmost importance that the health care professionals relate the need for compliance with the program to the adolescent. Because the adolescent years are normally traumatic, compliance may not be achieved without support from family and health care professionals. Utilization of the Milwaukee brace has been extremely successful in the management of scoliosis with a curvature between 15° to 20° and 40°, and in some cases has been successful

in higher degrees of curvature. If successful in halting the progression of the curvature, it can be anticipated that the brace will be utilized until full bone growth is achieved, and there is some indication that it may be advantageous to extend the utilization of the brace for a short time thereafter.

If the curvature has progressed to 40° or beyond at the time of diagnosis or if a slightly lesser degree of curvature exists with a high degree of rotational component or imbalance, surgical intervention may be required. Surgical intervention is required for approximately 5% to 10% of patients with idiopathic scoliosis.[5,p.1208] All forms of surgical intervention involve fusing the involved vertebrae to prevent the progression of the deformity. Preoperative traction such as *Cotrel traction* (see p. 528) or *halo-femoral traction* may be utilized. Cotrel traction is a form of skin traction, utilized not so much to obtain additional correction and increased flexibility of the curvature as it is to permit gradual tissue alterations and decrease postoperative complications. It is quite successful in accomplishment of these objectives and permits frequent exercise with a special attachment. The patient is placed in traction for a period of 5 to 10 days preoperatively.

Halo-femoral traction is utilized to provide for gradual tissue adjustment and to increase the flexibility of the curvature in more severe cases. Because it is skeletal traction (see p. 529), there is risk of osteomyelitis. The time required to accomplish specific goals varies, but most patients require 1 to 3 weeks of traction preoperatively. Some physicians choose to obtain a degree of immobilization and preadjustment to the postoperative cast by applying a cast for 1 to several weeks preoperatively. A preoperative cast may also be utilized in cases when a relatively severe degree of curvature exists and extensive time elapses before surgery can be scheduled.

At one time spinal fusion was the only form of surgical intervention accomplished. Advances in the past few decades, however, have considerably improved our ability to provide surgical correction of the curvature as well as the prevention of progression of the deformity. It must be noted, how-

ever, that even with surgical intervention it is impossible to totally correct the curvature or to totally alleviate the deformity.

The two surgical methods currently utilized are *Harrington rod instrumentation* and *Dwyer cable instrumentation* (Fig. 15-13). The Harrington rod is a mechanical device that assists in obtaining curvature correction through a posterior approach. The Dwyer cable is a device that permits surgical correction through an anterior approach. In both cases fusion accompanies insertion of the device, and the major purpose of the device is to assist in holding the corrected curvature while the fusion heals. The devices are usually not removed unless there is a postoperative indication of displacement or associated symptoms. Harrington rod instrumentation is utilized much more commonly because of

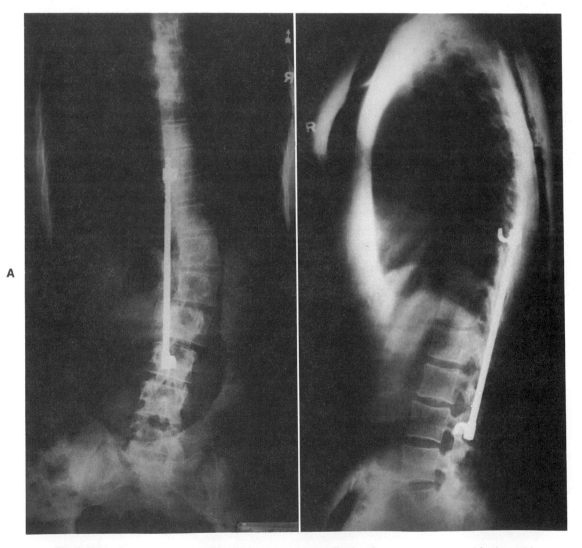

**Fig. 15-13. A,** Radiographic film of patient with scoliosis after posterior spinal fusion with Harrington rod instrumentation, anteroposterior and lateral views.

the decreased risk with the posterior approach, which requires no surgical intervention through the pulmonary cavity and rib cage. When an anterior approach is required, a posterior spinal fusion is also frequently required several weeks later.

Initial postoperative immobilization is obtained through utilization of a posterior plaster shell, Milwaukee brace, windowed cast, or log-rolling on a regular bed. A Stryker frame, Foster frame, or CircOlectric bed also may be utilized. Blood replacement may be required postoperatively, and appropriate intravenous therapy is recommended for several days.

Additional immobilization in the form of cast therapy is required after the initial acute postoperative phase. This may be required for 8 to 12 months or until there is absolute evidence of bony union of the fused area. The type of cast utilized frequently is the Risser localizer cast (see p. 481), which is applied with a degree of traction. The Risser turnbuckle cast (see p. 481) is utilized occasionally

when instrumentation has not been used. If and when lesser immobilization is desired, the Milwaukee brace or a plaster body jacket may be used.

### Spina bifida

Spina bifida is a congenital deformity involving a developmental anomaly in the posterior vertebral arch.

**Incidence.** Spina bifida is a relatively common congenital anomaly, seen in approximately 10 to 20 per 1,000 births.

**Pathology.** Spina bifida is characterized by a developmental gap in one or more of the posterior vertebral arches. It may occur with only a small deformed lamina separated by a midline gap or complete absence of laminae encompassing a large area. If this separation is large enough, the contents of the spinal canal protrude posteriorly, and a larger deformity known as myelomeningocele (see Chapter 18) is seen. This more serious deformity carries with it gross deficits not normally associated with

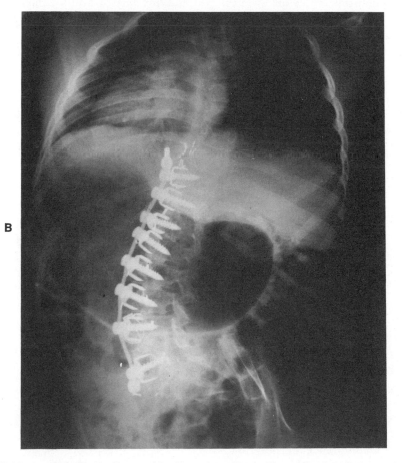

**Fig. 15-13, cont'd. B,** Radiographic film of patient with scoliosis after anterior spinal fusion with Dwyer instrumentation.

spina bifida. Referred to here are only those deformities that reflect a bony abnormality with no herniation of spinal canal contents or meninges.

**Signs and symptoms.** Neurologic deficits are not usually associated with the anomalies involving only bony deformity. Direct signs and symptoms are rarely associated and are frequently accidentally diagnosed when radiographic examination is required for other reasons.

**Treatment.** Spina bifida involving only bone deformity, with no herniation of meninges or spinal canal contents, rarely requires treatment.

### Spinal cord injuries

Spinal cord injuries of various types have associated musculoskeletal involvement. Trauma such as fractures, dislocations, and gunshot wounds may cause damage to the spinal column and the spinal cord with resulting degrees of paraplegia or quadraplegia. Injuries below the first thoracic vertebra produce paraplegia; above this level they are associated with quadraplegia. Complete transection of the cord results in permanent loss of motor and sensory abilities supplied by neurons below the level of the lesion.

Spinal cord injuries place the body in a state of spinal shock, which is characterized by placid paralysis and complete loss of skin sensation occurring initially after the injury. Within a few weeks the affected muscles become spastic, and the loss of skin sensation may become markedly decreased. These motor and sensory losses are permanent. Musculoskeletal complications are associated with the neurologic involvement. In addition prevention of decubitus ulcers and treatment of loss of bladder and bowel control are continuing concerns.

Orthopedic involvement varies considerably, depending on severity of the injury and availability of health care facilities. At minimum the orthopedic specialist is involved with the prevention of decubitus ulcers and the prescription of appropriate orthotics and ambulatory techniques to increase the patient's ability to become mobile. An exercise program, of an active nature for the uninvolved muscles to promote ambulatory skills and of a passive nature for the involved muscles, is prescribed. An interdisciplinary approach to rehabilitation is necessary and requires extensive and comprehensive program planning. Specific musculoskeletal implications beyond this scope are greatly dependent on the degree of initial attention provided to prevent deformities and on the maintenance of muscular performance to promote alternate goals and maximum rehabilitation. Individual psychological and physical program planning is essential.

### Spondylolisthesis

Spondylolisthesis is the forward slipping or gliding of a vertebra on the vertebral body below. When the vertebral body is not displaced the condition is known as *spondylolysis.*

**Etiology.** The cause of spondylolisthesis is not known.

**Pathology.** Spondylolisthesis has a characteristic defect, that is, an "interruption and continuity of the isthmus of the neural arch, usually of the fifth lumbar vertebrae."[6,p.1364]

**Incidence.** Spondylolisthesis is seen most often in women. It occurs most frequently at the L-4 to L-5 level. It is commonly seen in individuals past middle age and is associated with some degree of frequency with severe osteoarthritis of the spine.[6,p.1364]

**Signs and symptoms.** Patients with spondylolisthesis frequently have a history of weakness and possibly of fatigue associated with the lower back. These complaints may be recurrent. They may be localized in the lumbosacral region but may radiate down one or both legs like sciatic pain. In cases of extensive slipping the torso is actually shortened, the ribs may rest on the iliac crest, and the abdomen may protrude. An awkward, waddling gait may be noted.[1]

Radiographic examination demonstrates the isthmus defects on oblique views with apparent forward slipping of the body of the vertebra onto another. The anomaly is found at the L-4 to L-5 level, most commonly with the fourth vertebra displaced on the fifth. Differential diagnosis should be made between other deformities or disease processes such as tuberculosis and rickets.

**Treatment.** Conservative treatment of spondylolisthesis including posture exercises and immobilization or support with a cast or brace may be utilized when symptoms are mild. Surgical intervention in the form of spinal fusion and decompression is necessary with progression and recurring episodes of pain. Occasionally a laminectomy may be required.

**Prognosis.** Mild spondylolisthesis is usually resolved through rest and immobilization and an adequate exercise program. Surgical intervention, when required, is relatively successful.

### REFERENCES

1. Brashear, H. R., Jr., and Raney, R. B., Sr.: Shand's handbook of orthopaedic surgery, ed. 9, St. Louis, 1978, The C. V. Mosby Co.
2. Cobb, J. R.: Outline for the study of scoliosis, AAOS Instructional Course Lectures **5:**261, 1948.
3. Gartland, J. J.: Fundamentals of orthopaedics, Philadelphia, 1974, W. B. Saunders Co.
4. MacEwen, G. D.: Congenital scoliosis with a unilateral bar, Radiology **90:**711, 1968.

5. Tachdjian, M. O.: Pediatric orthopaedics, Philadelphia, 1972, W. B. Saunders Co.
6. Turek, S.: Orthopaedics, Philadelphia, 1977, J. B. Lippincott Co.
7. Winter, R. B., Moe, J. H., and Eilers, V. E.: Congenital scoliosis: a study of 234 patients treated and untreated, J. Bone Joint Surg. **50:**1, 1968.

## BIBLIOGRAPHY

Adams, J. C.: Outline of orthopaedics, Baltimore, 1971, The Williams & Wilkins Co.

Aegertu, E., and Kirkpatrick, J.: Orthopedic diseases, Philadelphia, 1975, W. B. Saunders Co.

American Orthopaedic Association: Manual of orthopaedic surgery, Chicago, 1972, The Association.

Aston, J. N.: A short textbook of orthopaedics and traumatology, London, 1972, The English Universities Press Ltd.

Blount, W. P., and Moe, J. H.: The Milwaukee brace, Baltimore, 1973, The Williams & Wilkins Co.

Brashear, H. R., Jr., and Raney, R. B., Sr.: Shand's handbook of orthopaedic surgery, ed. 9, St. Louis, 1978, The C. V. Mosby Co.

Cobb, J. R.: Outline for the study of scoliosis, AAOS Instructional Course Lectures **5:**261, 1948.

Crenshaw, A. H., editor: Campbell's operative orthopaedics, St. Louis, 1971, The C. V. Mosby Co.

Enneking, W. G., and Sherrard, M. G.: Physical diagnosis of the musculoskeletal system. Gainesville, Fla., 1969, Storter Printing Co.

Farfan, H. F., editor: Symposium on the lumbar spine, Orthop. Clin. North Am. **6**(1), January 1975.

Gartland, J. J.: Fundamentals of orthopaedics, Philadelphia, 1974, W. B. Saunders Co.

Goldstein, L. A., and Dickerson, R. C.: Atlas of orthopaedic surgery, St. Louis, 1974, The C. V. Mosby Co.

Hoppenfeld, S.: Scoliosis: a manual of concept and treatment, Philadelphia, 1967, J. B. Lippincott Co.

Iversen, L. D., and Clawson, D. K.: Manual of acute orthopaedic therapeutics, Boston, 1977, Little, Brown & Co.

MacEwen, G. D.: Congenital scoliosis with a unilateral bar, Radiology **90:**711, 1968.

Rubin, A.: Handbook of congenital malformations, Philadelphia, 1969, W. B. Saunders Co.

Tachdjian, M. O.: Pediatric orthopaedics, vols. 1 and 2, Philadelphia, 1972, W. B. Saunders Co.

Turek, S.: Orthopaedics, Philadelphia, 1977, J. B. Lippincott Co.

Winter, R. B., Moe, J. H., and Eilers, V. E.: Congenital scoliosis: a study of 234 patients treated and untreated, J. Bone Joint Surg. **50:**1, 1968.

# 16

## Trauma

NANCY E. HILT

A broad range of traumatic injuries to the musculoskeletal system may occur, varying tremendously in severity, intensity, ease of correction and treatment, and anticipatory results. A number of the most common injuries of varying severities are presented here with little emphasis on the initial management or emergency treatment of these injuries; these aspects of care are covered in some depth in Chapter 22.

Musculoskeletal traumatic injuries may occur as a single entity or, as is frequently seen in automobile accidents, for example, in combination with other injuries. Those outlined within this chapter are viewed as single entities with no complications other than those directly related to the injury to the musculoskeletal system.

### TERMINOLOGY

Knowledge of specific terminology related to traumatic injuries of the musculoskeletal system is essential to the comprehension of their consequences and management. The major categories of injuries are defined here, with more detailed definitions provided for subcategories in the individual sections on specific traumatic entities. Major categories of musculoskeletel traumatic injuries may be classified and defined as follows:

**contusion** minimal traumatic injury, usually involving soft tissue hemorrhage into subcutaneous, adipose, or muscular tissue, resulting in a bruised area.

**sprain** acute musculoskeletal injury involving the incomplete tearing of the capsule or ligaments surrounding the joint structure, including potential disruption of the continuity of the synovial membrane but not involving instability of the involved joint.

**strain** traumatic musculoskeletal injury of an acute or chronic nature resulting from utilization of a specific structure beyond its intended or functional ability; is not always associated with a one-time injury but with cumulative effects of overutilization over time.

**subluxation** traumatic injury to the joint structure resulting in partial or incomplete dislocation or separation of the surfaces of the joint.

**dislocation** musculoskeletal traumatic injury resulting in the disruption of continuity of joint configuration and articulation to the extent that the articulating surfaces are no longer in contact.

**fracture** traumatic injury resulting in partial to complete disruption in the continuity of osseous tissue of a bone.

### CONTUSION

A contusion is a minimal traumatic injury, usually involving soft tissue hemorrhage into subcutaneous, adipose, or muscular tissue, resulting in the appearance of a bruised area. A contusion may occur anywhere in the body and may vary as to the extent of involvement. It rarely requires medical attention or treatment and, even in its most severe form, usually resolves spontaneously through absorption. The length of time for this resolution to occur is dependent on the severity of the injury.

### SPRAIN

A sprain (Fig. 16-1) is an acute musculoskeletal injury involving the incomplete tearing of the capsule or ligaments surrounding a joint structure, including potential disruption of the continuity of the synovial membrane but not involving instability of

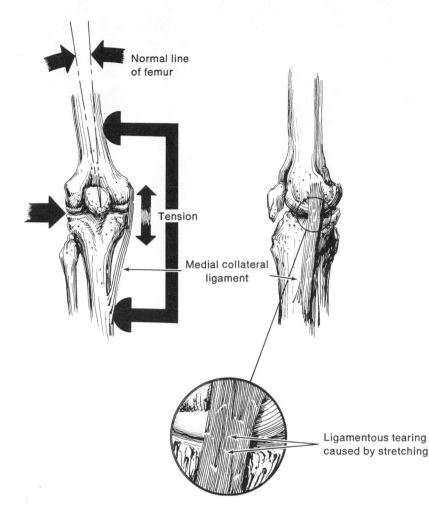

Normal line
of femur

Tension

Medial collateral
ligament

Ligamentous tearing
caused by stretching

**Fig. 16-1.** Sprains, mechanism and pathology. (From Schneider, F. R.: Handbook for the orthopaedic assistant, ed. 2, St. Louis, 1976, The C. V. Mosby Co.)

the involved joint. It is a much more significant injury than a contusion and usually requires medical attention.

**Etiology.** The most common cause of a sprain is a twisting injury, usually of a sudden nature.

**Pathology.** The twisting injury resulting in a sprain produces incomplete tearing of the ligaments and capsule surrounding the joint. There may be minor hemorrhage surrounding the involved tissue. The injury usually does not result in disabling pathologic features, although soft tissue swelling may be seen, which may produce limited function to varying degrees.

**Incidence.** Sprains are relatively common, especially in the ankle or the knee. A relatively high incidence of cervical sprains, known as whiplash, are associated with automobile accidents when the individual has been hit from the rear by another vehicle.

**Signs and symptoms.** The cause of a sprain frequently is a sudden, twisting injury to the involved

joint. Varying degrees of pain are usually associated with the injury. Limitation of joint motion is common, and edema surrounding the joint is usually apparent. A superficial bruise may be present indicating soft tissue hemorrhage. On physical examination the joint appears to be stable. Tenderness over the involved joint is present. No evidence of sprain is seen on radiographic examination, with a possible exception of soft tissue swelling.[9,pp.80-82]

A sprain of the cervical spine, or whiplash, usually reveals similar signs and symptoms of pain and limitation of cervical motion. Slight swelling may be apparent. Other associated symptoms such as headache, dizziness, visual disturbances, and nausea may develop and are related to the location of the injury. There is usually localized tenderness to varying degrees. Results of radiographic examination are negative.[9,p.83]

**Treatment.** The treatment of a sprain includes minimizing the soft tissue swelling associated with the injury and maximizing comfort to decrease pain and promote healing. Application of ice to the involved joint may be somewhat successful in the control of edema if the injury has been diagnosed at an early stage. If diagnosed later the most effective means of control of edema is elevation of the extremity and possible use of a compression bandage. Comfort may be promoted through immobilization of the joint, utilizing a splint or a cast for several weeks. Isometric exercises of the involved joint and active exercise of other exposed joints assist in

promotion of healing. A cervical collar may be utilized for immobilization of the neck after whiplash injury.[9,pp.83-84]

**Prognosis.** Most sprains completely heal with appropriate immobilization in approximately 4 to 6 weeks.

## STRAIN

A strain is a traumatic musculoskeletal injury resulting from utilization of a specific structure beyond its intended or functional ability. It is not

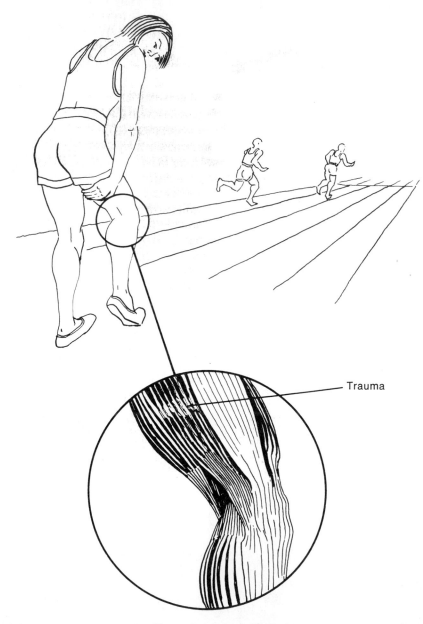

Trauma

**Fig. 16-2.** Acute muscle strain. (From Schneider, F. R.: Handbook for the orthopaedic assistant, ed. 2, St. Louis, 1976, The C. V. Mosby Co.)

always associated with a one-time injury but with the cumulative effects of overutilization over time. Strains may be acute (Fig. 16-2) or chronic.

**Etiology.** An acute muscular strain is usually the result of a sudden, forced motion that causes a specific muscle to become stretched beyond its normal capacity. Chronic muscular strain is caused by the repetitious utilization of a muscle beyond its normal capacity.

**Pathology.** An acute strain frequently produces disruption of tissue surrounding the involved muscle. Hemorrhage into the localized tissue is not uncommon, and surrounding tissue reaction indicative of inflammation may be present. Chronic strain usually produces similar pathologic features, but its onset is gradual rather than sudden.

**Signs and symptoms.** Pain is associated with both acute and chronic muscle strain. The pain associated with acute strain is more severe and is usually accompanied by a specific injury from excessive or improper motion. In contrast chronic strain has a more insidious onset, with less severe, aching pain. Limitation of motion may be apparent with both types of strain. Symptomatology of acute strain is aggravated by activity, and the associated disability is more severe.[9,pp.85-86]

**Treatment.** The treatment of strain encompasses the relief of associated symptoms. Immobilization in a splint or cast is not indicated. If the injury is acute and the patient is seen immediately after the injury, ice may be applied to control edema. After the first few days the application of heat may be

helpful in controlling pain. In both acute and chronic strain, rest with minimal activity of the involved area is usually recommended initially. After the first healing stages gradual exercise is advocated. Mild analgesics may be required.[9,p.86]

**Prognosis.** Acute or chronic strain usually responds to rest and symptomatic treatment within 4 to 6 weeks.

## LIGAMENTAL TEARS

Ligamental tears are injuries involving the partial or complete tearing of ligamentous structures connecting the bones and surrounding the joints. Although ligamental tears may occur at any site, the knee is the most vulnerable structure; therefore discussion of this injury is limited to ligamental tears of the knee.

**Etiology.** Ligamental tears are caused by injuries to the involved joint; in the case of the knee the injury is usually a forceful blow or twisting, which places stress or stretching forces on the ligamentous structures surrounding the knee joint.

**Pathology.** The pathologic features of ligamental tears of the knee are dependent on the location and severity of the injury. The most common ligaments involved in knee injuries are the medial, lateral, and posterior ligaments and the anterior and posterior cruciate ligaments.

More often than not, ligamentous injuries involve more than one structure because of the manner in which they connect and support each other. Definite patterns are attributable to specific combina-

**Table 16-1.** Etiologic and pathologic features of ligamental injuries of knee[4]

| | Structures commonly involved | Common etiology | Common pathologic features |
|---|---|---|---|
| Medial injuries | Medial collateral ligament<br>Anterior cruciate ligament<br>Medial meniscus<br>Posterior capsule | Flexed leg is forced into external rotation while force is applied to lateral knee; knee may be in extension | Tearing of involved structures<br>Posterior structures may be spared if injury occurs with knee in flexion<br>Patellar retinaculum may tear<br>Patellar tendon may avulse or tear<br>Lateral meniscus may be involved |
| Lateral injuries | Fibular collateral ligament<br>Iliotibial band<br>Lateral meniscus<br>Posterior cruciate ligament | Force applied laterally with knee in extension | Tearing of involved structures<br>Biceps tendon may be damaged<br>Peroneal nerve may be involved<br>Popliteus tendon may be involved<br>Medial meniscus may be damaged |
| Posterior injuries | Posterior capsule<br>Posterior cruciate ligament<br>Medial collateral ligament<br>Medial meniscus | Hyperextension<br>Force applied to anterior tibia with knee flexed | Tearing of involved structures<br>Fibular collateral ligament may be torn<br>Peroneal nerve may be damaged |

tions of injuries and reflect certain etiologic and pathologic features of the ligamental injuries and tears (Table 16-1).

Mild injuries are likely to produce little damage, with no functional loss such as weakness of the ligament or instability of the joint. Only a few fibers may be torn, around which a small hematoma may develop. Moderate injuries produce a very definite tear of the ligament with varying degrees of surrounding tissue involvement. Varying degrees of instability may be noted. With severe injury complete tear of the involved ligament(s) is apparent and is accompanied by functional instability of the knee joint.[4, pp.621-622]

**Incidence.** Ligamental tears of the knee joint are extremely common in athletic individuals and usually are associated with sports injuries.

**Signs and symptoms.** Ligamental tears of the knee may produce a variety of signs and symptoms. The most common are:

1. Effusion surrounding the knee joint
2. Varying degrees of edema
3. Differences in the configuration of the knee joint as viewed from various angles
4. Tenderness on palpation
5. Crepitation
6. Instability of the knee joint to varying degrees
7. Possible ecchymosis

Radiographic examination may reveal varying degrees of displacement resulting from the ligamental tears, but the primary ligamentous injuries are not visible on x-ray films.[4, pp.622-623]

**Treatment.** The treatment of ligamental tears of the knee, which may be termed a form of sprain, is greatly dependent on the severity of the injury (Table 16-2). Mild injuries involving tears of only a few fibers usually do not require any treatment and resolve spontaneously with time. If treatment is advocated, it is usually of a symptomatic nature and includes rest and compression but rarely requires immobilization. Moderate ligamental tears require protective treatment. Rest is essential to the healing process. Aspiration of the excessive joint fluid may be required. Compression may be of value in controlling swelling and further effusion. Support of the joint by means of a splint or other device may be required. A special method of taping may be utilized to provide this support and is commonly used in sports injuries. The severe ligamentous injury of the knee requires restorative treatment. Although the nonsurgical intervention recommended for the moderate injury may be effective, surgical intervention may be advocated for the most severe injuries with multiple ligamentous tears and gross instability

**Table 16-2.** Characteristic signs, symptoms, and treatment of knee ligament tears

| Injury | Signs and symptoms | Treatment |
|---|---|---|
| Mild (little damage) | Positive Tenderness Swelling Stress pain Negative No effusion No hematoma No pain on motion No instability | Minimal Rest Injection Compression Cold or heat No immobilization Early use |
| Moderate (definite tear) | Positive Pain Tenderness Swelling Effusion Disability Negative No instability | Protective Rest Aspiration Injection Compression Cold or heat Support Rehabilitation |
| Severe (complete tear) | Severe disability Knee gives way Severe pain Blood in joint Blood in tissues Swelling Abnormal motion Positive stress x-ray | Restorative Nonsurgical (frequently ineffective) Same as for moderate injury Surgical (effective and more certain) Early intervention Complete repair of all tears |

associated with severe disability. Surgical procedures are designed to repair the complete tears and vary according to the location of the injury and the damage found during the surgical procedure. Exercises are of value postoperatively to strengthen the knee structures.[4, pp.633-634]

## MENISCAL TEARS

The most common injury to the menisci of the knee is a tear, an injury associated with sports activities and a variety of motions resulting in instability of the knee joint. Injuries to the menisci are frequently seen in combination with injuries to ligamentous components.

**Etiology.** The causes of a torn meniscus include the following[8, pp.649-650]:

1. A sharp, sudden, violent pivot
2. A direct blow to the knee
3. Restraining motions on the posterior capsule medially by the semimembranous or antero-lateral capsule laterally as the tibia is fixed and the thigh moves forward
4. Forced internal rotation of the tensed biceps tendon laterally
5. Attrition of the surrounding structures, such as from wear or repetitive squatting and climbing activities

The individual with ligamentous laxity of the knee joints is extremely vulnerable to meniscal tears.

**Pathology.** The menisci serve specific functions in relation to the ability of the knee joint to maintain stability with the stress of weight bearing. The most important of these functions are (1) acting as a shock absorber, (2) assisting, with other structures, in stabilization of the knee joint, and (3) controlling rotary stability. A torn meniscus decreases these functions and over time can contribute to additional wear and tear on various other components of the knee joint. It is not unusual to see meniscal injuries in combination with ligamentous damage because of the interlocking nature of the surrounding structures.

**Incidence.** Torn menisci are frequently associated with sports injuries and are very common in the athletic individual.

**Signs and symptoms.** Dependent on the degree of the tear involved, a torn meniscus may be asymptomatic. More severe tears or continued stress and injury to the meniscus may produce edema, limited motion, especially of flexion or extension, pain to varying degrees, and a limp that may be aggravated by running, climbing, stopping suddenly, squatting, walking, or jumping.[8,pp.649-650] The symptoms may occur with varying severity, but if persistent or extremely severe are usually brought to the attention of medical personnel for diagnosis and treatment. When symptoms occur the patient may also complain of "locking" or "slipping" of the knee. Arthrography or arthroscopy are useful in the diagnosis of meniscal tears. Both procedures provide additional information in relation to the specific location and the type of tear, which may assist the diagnostician in determination of the treatment modality to be chosen. (For examples of arthroscopic evaluation of this injury see Chapter 11.)

**Treatment.** The treatment chosen is dependent on the severity and persistence of the specific symptoms associated with the injury. Nonsurgical treatment modalities include exercises designed to strengthen the stability of the knee such as quadri-

ceps strengthening, straight leg raising, and progressive resistance exercises. If surgical intervention is required, it may be necessary to protect the knee joint from further injury until the procedure is accomplished. The surgical procedure of choice is a meniscectomy.[8,pp.652-653]

## DISLOCATION

A dislocation (Fig. 16-3, *A*) is a musculoskeletal injury resulting in the disruption of continuity of joint configuration and articulation to the extent that the articulating surfaces are no longer in contact. A dislocation may occur in any joint and is usually due to a traumatic injury.

**Etiology.** A dislocation of any joint is the result of an injury that places excessive stress in an abnormal direction on one or more bones near the joint.

**Pathology.** The traumatic injury resulting in dislocation of a joint reveals a lack of contact between the articulating surfaces of the bones of that joint. The direction of the dislocation is dependent on the physiologic structure of the specific joint involved and the nature of the force or injury. The displacement of the bone alters the normal contour and configuration of the involved joint. Disruption of the joint capsule occurs to accommodate for the displacement. The surrounding ligamentous structures may be torn. Damage to the surrounding soft tissue structures occurs to varying degrees.

**Signs and symptoms.** The dislocated joint reveals obvious deformity with loss of normal configuration and motion. The degree of deformity may be somewhat obscured by soft tissue edema surrounding the joint. Pain is associated with the injury and is usually localized around the involved joint. Neurovascular status may be impaired to varying degrees dependent on the ability of these structures to accommodate to the injury. Some dislocations are known to reduce themselves. Radiographic examination reveals the distinct displacement of the involved bones. Because the direction of the dislocation may be difficult to determine because of soft tissue swelling, it is advantageous to obtain radiographic films in at least two planes to assure adequate diagnosis.

**Treatment.** The most effective treatment of a dislocated joint is early anatomic reduction (Fig. 16-4). If this is accomplished, either through manual or surgical manipulation involving open or closed procedures, adequate joint functioning frequently returns. Radiographic examination is utilized to confirm appropriate reduction. Immobilization following reduction is required to promote rest, which is necessary to permit soft tissue healing. Active mo-

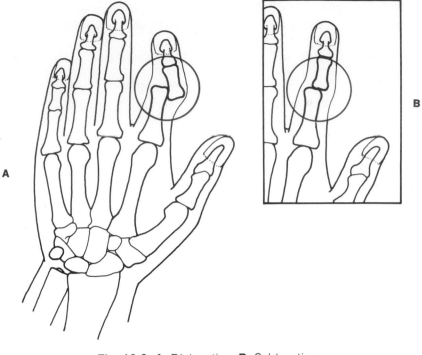

**Fig. 16-3. A,** Dislocation. **B,** Subluxation.

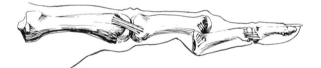

Dislocation of proximal interphalangeal
joint (PIP)

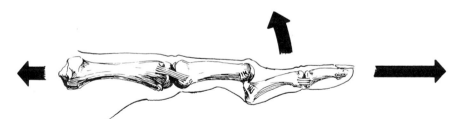

Gradual application of traction and countertraction forces
fatigues the muscles about the joint

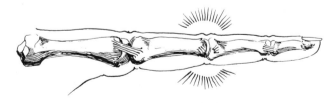

Joint surfaces realigned

**Fig. 16-4.** Anatomic reduction of dislocation. (From Schneider, F. R.: Handbook for the orthopaedic assistant, ed. 2, St. Louis, 1976, The C. V. Mosby Co.)

tion may be restricted for a period of time after immobilization until indications of complete healing are exhibited. Gradual exercises are then promoted with increased active motion.

## SUBLUXATION

A subluxation (Fig. 16-3, *B*) is a traumatic injury to the joint structure resulting in incomplete dislocation of the surfaces of the joint. It may occur in any joint. Subluxations are caused by traumatic injuries of the same nature as are responsible for dislocations but are usually less severe. The pathologic features are similar, but there is less tissue damage because the displacement is only partial.

Diagnostic signs and symptoms are also similar but usually not as obvious and severe. The treatment of subluxation is the same or similar as that of dislocation but usually requires less healing time.

## FRACTURE

A fracture (Fig. 16-5) is a traumatic injury resulting in partial or complete disruption in the continuity of osseous tissue of a bone. Fractures may occur in any bone and are the result of a variety of types of traumatic injuries. Pathologic fractures may occur if, because of immobilization or normal physiologic processes, increased porosity of the bones exists. The specific type of fracture is frequently

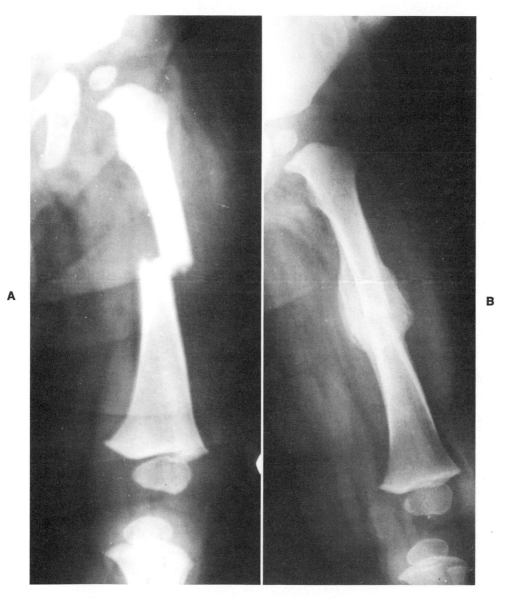

**Fig. 16-5. A,** Fractured femur. **B,** Six-month postfracture film showing callus formation. (From Hilt, N. E., and Schmitt, E. W., Jr.: Pediatric orthopedic nursing, St. Louis, 1975, The C. V. Mosby Co.)

indicative of the anatomic area involved, the structure of the specific bone involved, and the type of injury.

Fractures are described anatomically according to the bone involved and the area of the bone in which the fracture occurs (e.g., distal, medial, proximal). The types of fractures are as follows:

**incomplete fracture** fracture that does not disrupt continuity of entire thickness of bone involved.

**complete fracture** fracture that disrupts continuity of tissue of entire thickness of bone involved.

**undisplaced fracture** fracture in which fragments or ends of fracture sites are not separated.

**displaced fracture** fracture in which fragments or ends of fracture sites are separated.

**comminuted fracture** fracture in which there are several definite disruptions in continuity of tissue of involved bone, creating two or more fragments.

**segmental fracture** fracture in which proximal and distal segments of shaft of long bone are fractured, with free central segment or fragment.

**butterfly fracture** fracture in which center fragment of two disruptions in continuity of tissue creates a triangular effect.

**spiral fracture** fracture in which disruption of bone tissue is spiral, oblique, or transverse to long axis of involved bone.

**impacted fracture** fracture in which fragmented ends (disruption of tissue) are locked together or driven into each other.

**compression fracture** fracture, usually in a short bone, in which disruption of tissue causes collapse of involved bone.

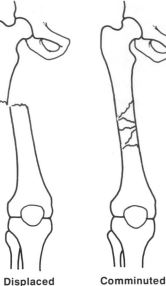

Displaced     Comminuted     Segmental

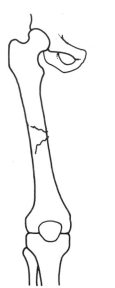
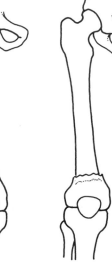

Butterfly     Spiral     Impacted

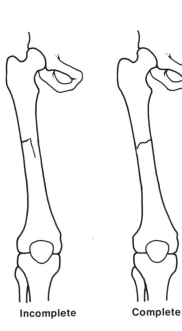

Incomplete     Complete     Undisplaced

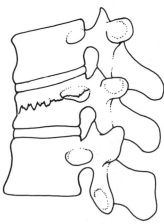

Compression

Although these general types of fractures may occur singly, it is not unusual to have a combination of types of fractures.

Fractures may be *open* or *closed*. The closed fracture is one in which the bone has not disrupted soft tissue and projected through the skin. An open fracture is one in which the disruption of osseous tissue has projected through soft tissue and the skin. A closed fracture is also known as a *simple* fracture, while an open fracture is *compound*.

In addition to these general types of fractures there are specific types, which are indicative of anatomic areas or pathologic features of the fracture. The following are some of the most common of these specific types of fractures:

**agenetic fracture** spontaneous fracture due to imperfect osteogenesis.

**angulated fracture** fracture in which fragments are angulated.

**angulation fracture** fracture caused by angulation of spine or shaft of long bone.

**apophyseal fracture** fracture separating apophysis from bone where there is strong tendinous attachment.

**articular fracture** fracture involving articular surfaces of a joint; also called intra-articular fracture, joint fracture.

**atrophic fracture** spontaneous fracture due to atrophy.

**avulsion fracture** fracture caused by tearing away of bone fragment where pull of strong ligamentous tendinous attachment forcibly pulls fragment away from rest of bone.

**Barton's fracture** fracture of distal articular surface of radius; may be accompanied by dorsal dislocation of carpus on radius.

**Bennett's fracture** fracture of first metacarpal bone that runs obliquely through base of bone and into carpometacarpal joint, detaching greater part of articular facet; may be associated with dorsal subluxation or dislocation of thumb metacarpal.

**bending fracture** fracture resulting from bending of the extremity.

**bent fracture** incomplete greenstick fracture.

**blow-out fracture** fracture of floor of orbit produced by blow causing sudden increase in intraocular pressure.

**boxer's fracture** fracture of one or more metacarpal bones (usually fourth or fifth); often distal, angulated, and impacted; produced by striking hard object with closed fist.

**bucket-handle fracture** fracture involving tear in semilunar cartilage along medial side, through loop of cartilage and into intercondyler notch.

**bursting fracture** fracture resulting in multiple fragments, usually at or near end of bone.

**buttonhole fracture** fracture caused by perforation of bone by bullet.

**capillary fracture** hairlike fracture.

**central fracture (of pelvis)** acetabular fracture in which there is central displacement.

**chauffer's fracture** fracture of radial styloid process produced by twisting or snapping injury.

**chip fracture** fracture, usually involving a bony process and near a joint, in which there is small fragmental fracture.

**chisel fracture** fracture in which there is oblique detachment of fragment from head of radius.

**cleavage fracture** fracture involving shelling off of cartilage with avulsion of small fragment of bone from distal portion of lateral condyle of humerus.

**Colles' fracture** fracture of and through epiphysis of distal radius within $\frac{1}{2}$ to 1 inch of articular surface, and characterized by dorsal displacement and angulation of distal fragment, producing characteristic "silver-fork" deformity.

**complex fracture** closed fracture resulting in severe soft tissue damage.

**condylar fracture** fracture of round end of hinge joint, usually occurring at distal humerus or femur and frequently resulting in small fragment that includes condyle, which has separated from bone.

**cortical fracture** fracture which involves cortex of bone.

**Cotton's fracture** *see* trimalleolar fracture.

**cough fracture** fracture of rib, usually fifth or seventh, caused by violent coughing.

**dentate fracture** fracture resulting in fragmented ends being serrated and opposing each other, fitting together like teeth on a gear.

**depressed fracture** fracture, usually within skull, in which fragment(s) is depressed below surface of skull.

**diacondylar fracture** transcondylar fracture; occurring across the line of condyle.

**direct fracture** fracture resulting at specific point of injury and due to injury itself.

**displaced fracture** fracture in which fragmented ends are separated from each other.

**dishpan fracture** depressed skull fracture; otherwise known as derby hat fracture.

**double fracture** fracture of bone resulting in more than two segments, with fractures in two places.

**dome fracture (of pelvis)** fracture of acetabulum, specifically the weight-bearing surface.

**Dupuytren's fracture** *see* Galeazzi's fracture; Pott's fracture.

**Duverney's fracture** fracture of ilium just below anterior superior spine.

**dyscrasic fracture** fracture caused by weakening of specific bone from debilitating disease.

**endocrine fracture** fracture resulting from weakness due to endocrine disorder (e.g., hyperparathyroidism).

**epicondylar fracture** fracture involving medial or lateral epicondyle of long bone.

**epiphyseal fracture** fracture involving epiphyseal growth plate of long bone, resulting in separation or fragmentation; also called epiphyseal slip fracture, Salter's fracture, or Salter-Harris fracture.

**extracapsular fracture** fracture occurring near joint but not directly involving or entering joint capsule; extremely common in hip.

**fatigue fracture** fracture resulting from excessive physical activity, often associated with metatarsal bones and not due to a single injury.

**fissure fracture** fracture resulting in crack (fissure) extending in one cortex of bone but does not extend through entire bone.

**fracture-dislocation** fracture involving bony structures of joint with associated dislocation of same joint.

**fragmented fracture** fracture resulting in multiple fragments.

**Galeazzi's fracture** fracture of distal radius accompanied by dislocation of distal ulna; also known as Dupuytren's fracture.

**Gosselin's fracture** V-shaped fracture of distal tibia that extends into ankle.

**greenstick fracture** fracture in which periosteum on one side of bone is disrupted, creating incomplete fracture with angulation, occurs in growing bones of children where some degree of flexibility is still present; also known as infraperiosteal fracture, hickory-stick fracture, or willow fracture.

**grenade thrower's fracture** fracture of humerus resulting from tremendous muscular contraction.

**Guerin's fracture** fracture of maxilla.

**gunshot fracture** fracture resulting from bullet or other missile.

**hangman's fracture** fracture of posterior elements of cervical vertebrae with dislocation anteriorly of C-2 on C-3.

**hickory-stick fracture** *see* greenstick fracture.

**indirect fracture** fracture resulting from specific injury or blow but occurring at a site other than direct area of injury.

**inflammatory fracture** fracture of bone weakened from inflammation.

**infraction fracture** fracture of pathologic origin resulting in small radiolucent line and most commonly associated with metabolic dysfunction.

**intercondylar fracture** fracture between condyles of bone.

**intertrochanteric fracture** fracture of proximal femur between greater and lesser trochanters.

**interperiosteal fracture** incomplete fracture in which periosteum is not disrupted.

**intra-articular fracture** *see* articular fracture.

**intracapsular fracture** fracture within joint capsule.

**intraperiosteal fracture** fracture that does not involve rupture of periosteum.

**intrauterine fracture** fracture occurring during fetal life.

**Jefferson fracture** bursting type of fracture of ring of atlas (first cervical vertebra).

**joint fracture** *see* articular fracture.

**lead pipe fracture** fracture involving compression at point of impact and linear fracture on opposite side.

**Le Fort's fracture** fracture of maxilla.

**linear fracture** fracture that extends parallel to long axis of bone with no displacement.

**lip fracture (of hip)** fracture of posterior lip of acetabulum; may be associated with hip dislocation.

**Lisfranc's fracture** fracture-dislocation of foot with displacement of proximal metatarsals.

**mallet fracture** avulsion fracture of dorsal base of distal phalanx that involves extensor apparatus insertion, creating dropped flexion of distal segment.

**Malgaigne fracture (of pelvis)** multiple fractures of pelvis, which include wing of ilium or sacrum and ipsilateral pubic rami with associated upper displacement of hemipelvis.

**march fracture** stress fracture of one or more metatarsals; usually attributed to excessive marching.

**missile fracture** penetration fracture caused by missile such as bullet or shrapnel.

**Monteggia's fracture** fracture of proximal third or half of ulna, associated with radial dislocation or disruption of annular ligament, resulting in angulation or overriding of ulnar fragments.

**Montercaux's fracture** fracture of neck of fibula associated with diastasis of ankle mortise.

**Moore's fracture** fracture of distal radius with associated dislocation of ulnar head resulting in securing of styloid process under annular ligaments.

**multiple fracture** several fracture lines in one bone or fracture of several bones from one injury.

**neoplastic fracture** fracture in bone weakened by neoplasm or malignancy.

**neurogenic fracture** fracture resulting from destruction of nerve supply to specific bone.

**oblique fracture** fracture that occurs at slanted or oblique angle to longitudinal axis of bone.

**occult fracture** fracture that cannot be detected on radiographic examination initially but may be evident radiographically weeks later; accompanied by usual clinical signs of pain, history of trauma, and occasionally soft tissue edema.

**paratrooper fracture** fracture of distal tibia and malleolus as result of extreme force on ankles.

**parry fracture** *see* Monteggia's fracture.

**pathologic fracture** spontaneous fracture resulting in tissue weakened from disease or neoplastic processes rather than traumatic injury.

**Pauwels' fracture** fracture of proximal femoral neck with varying degrees of angulation.

**perforating fracture** open fracture created by a missile creating small surface wound.

**periarticular fracture** fracture located near joint but not directly involving joint.

**piedmont fracture** oblique fracture of distal radius with fragments pulled into ulna.

**pillion fracture** T-shaped fracture of distal femur with displacement of condyles posterior to femoral shaft; caused by severe blow to knee.

**plafon fracture** fracture that involves buttress part of malleolus.

**Pott's fracture** fracture of distal fibula, usually of spiral oblique type, with associated ligamentous damage or medial malleolus injury with lateral displacement of the foot; also called Dupuytren's fracture.

**pressure fracture** fracture created by pressure resulting from tumor.

**puncture fracture** fracture created by projectile creating loss of bone tissue without disruption of continuity of involved bone.

**Quervain's fracture** fracture of navicular bone accompanied by dislocation of lunar bone.

**reverse Barton's fracture** fracture of volar articular surface of radius with associated displacement of carpus on radius.

**Rolando's fracture** fracture of base of first metacarpal.

**Salter's fracture** *see* epiphyseal fracture.

**secondary fracture** *see* pathologic fracture.

**segmental fracture** fracture resulting in several large fragments of shaft of single bone.

**silver-fork fracture** *see* Colles' fracture.

**Skillern's fracture** open fracture of distal radius associated with greenstick fracture of distal ulna.

**Smith's fracture** fracture involving volar displacement and angulation of distal fragment; also called reverse Colles' fracture.

**splinter fracture** fracture comminuted with thin, sharp fragments.

**spontaneous fracture** *see* pathologic fracture.

**sprain fracture** fracture resulting from separation of tendon or ligament at its insertion site, with portion of bone being separated with it.

**sprinter's fracture** fracture of anterior superior or anterior inferior spine of ilium created by fragment of bone being forcibly pulled by violent muscle spasm.

**stellate fracture** fracture involving central point of impact or injury, from which numerous fissures radiate.

**Steida's fracture** fracture of internal condyle of femur.

**stress fracture** fracture, often of metatarsals, resulting from repeated, abnormal, or prolonged stress; occurs gradually

**subcapital fracture** fracture occurring distal to head of bone (ball-and-socket joint).

**subperiosteal fracture** fracture of bone that has not disrupted periosteal covering and essentially occurs beneath periosteum.

**subtrochanteric fracture (of hip)** fracture of femur occurring transversally just below lesser trochanter.

**supracondylar fracture** fracture involving area between condyles of humerus or femur.

**T-fracture** intercondylar fracture in which fracture lines are shaped like a "T."

**teardrop fracture** fracture, usually located in short bone such as vertebra, in which fracture is of avulsion type and is in general shape of teardrop.

**torsion fracture** fracture of spiral type, usually caused by torsion-type injury.

**torus fracture** *see* lead pipe fracture.

**transcondylar fracture** fracture occurring transversally and distal to epicondyles.

**transverse fracture** fracture occurring at right angles to longitudinal axis of involved bone.

**trimalleolar fracture** fracture involving medial malleolus, lateral malleolus, and posterior lip of tibia; also called Cotton's fracture.

**trophic fracture** fracture in bone weakened by nutritional disturbance.

**tuft fracture** fracture of distal phalanx.

**Wagstaffe's fracture** fracture involving separation of internal malleolus.

**wedge fracture** fracture of vertebral structures with anterior compression.

**willow fracture** *see* greenstick fracture.

**Y fracture** intercondylar fracture shaped like a "Y."

Although these specific fractures usually occur singly, multiple fractures may be seen. In most cases each fracture is viewed as a separate entity and treated accordingly. The exception would be when multiple fractures occur within a relatively limited area such as to the same bone or to the same extremity.

**Etiology.** The most common cause of fracture is traumatic injury. The site of the injury is not necessarily the site of the resulting fracture; for example, severe blows to a joint may produce a fracture above or below that joint. A fracture that occurs at the specific site of injury is known as a *direct* fracture, while a fracture resulting from injury to an area above or below the specific site is known as an *indirect* fracture.

Some fractures are the result of rotation or torsion in excess of the capacity of the bone and surrounding structures. When this is the case the specific fracture is frequently of an oblique or spiral type.

Still other types of fractures are the result of processes other than direct injury or blows to the area. Such is the case with the *stress* or *fatigue* fracture, resulting from prolonged or excessive stress or strain on a specific area such as the metatarsals, or the *pathologic* fracture, which occurs in bony structures weakened from disease, inflammation, or a neoplastic process.

**Signs and symptoms.** The most common signs and symptoms of a fracture are pain, soft tissue edema, and excessive motion at the site. The pain varies in severity and is greatly dependent on the type of fracture and injury accompanying the fracture. Soft tissue edema in surrounding structures is a reaction to the trauma of the fracture and may or may not be indicative of the severity of the underlying damage. The area surrounding the fracture site may feel warm to the touch. Excessive motion frequently exists at the site of the fracture, especially if the site is not near a joint or is not splintered by surrounding soft tissue structures.

Obvious deformity may be present, dependent on the type of fracture and the degree of displacement. Muscle spasms surrounding the fracture site may alter the notable deformity between the time of the injury and when the patient is seen and appropriately treated. Certain types of fractures are accompanied by open wounds, which sometimes mask the degree of damage. Neurovascular impairment may result from fragmentation of bone and soft tissue alterations. Radiographic examination gives a relatively accurate picture of the fracture but does not always reveal the severity of soft tissue damage associated with it; this is more specifically and accurately reflected from the clinical picture.

**Stages of tissue reaction and healing.** The process of tissue reaction surrounding a fracture and the healing of the bone and surrounding tissues that follows are characteristic and with few exceptions predictable. The stages in this process of tissue reaction and healing (Fig. 16-6) are as follows.[5,pp.24-25;9,pp.44-46]

STAGE I. *The injury causing the fracture disrupts the blood vessels supplying nutrition to the bone tissue, creating a hematoma at the fracture site.*

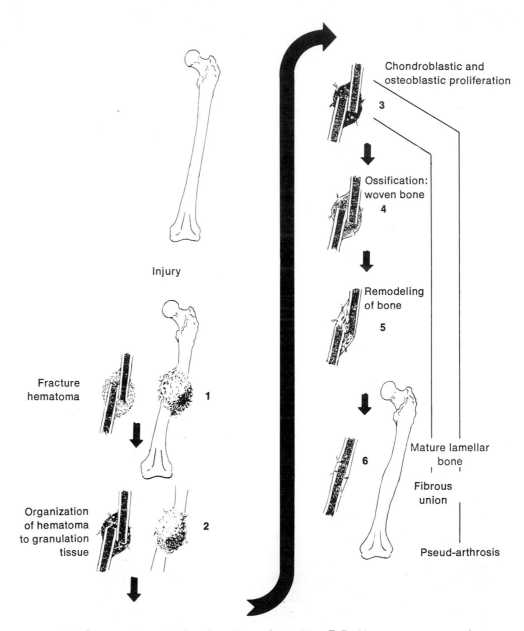

**Fig. 16-6.** Stages in fracture healing. (From Schneider, F. R.: Handbook for the orthopaedic assistant, ed. 2, St. Louis, 1976, The C. V. Mosby Co.)

This hematoma or blood clot, alters chemical compositions and consistency of the blood during the first 48 to 72 hours after the injury, forming a network that attacks the fragments. The accompanying loss of blood supply resulting from the vascular damage and initial trauma ultimately leads to necrosis of the osseous and periosteal cells.

STAGE II. *The characteristic physiologic process of Stage II is the development of external granulation or callus formation of the fibrous or cartilaginous type.* This formation is the result of the combined processes of fibroblastic activity, the presence of a rich capillary blood supply, and phagocytosis.

STAGE III. *The healing process is continued by the infiltration of the hematoma by chondroblasts and osteoblasts, creating a nonosseous union.* It is generally thought that this stage is greatly influenced by the degree of immobilization achieved at the fracture site, affecting not only the process but the length of time required for accomplishment of this stage.

STAGE IV. *Firm union of the fragments is characteristic of stage IV as evidenced by external callus formation.* This callus formation is the result of new bone formation and is the first stage in which an actual bony union occurs.

STAGE V. *After callus formation, remodeling occurs with the resorption of necrotic cells.* Remodeling serves to restore the traumatized bone to a more normal shape and contour with maximum posttraumatic strength. Normal density is usually apparent in this stage on radiographic examination.

The stages of healing are segmental in nature; inappropriate or incomplete staging results in a variety of complications. The length of each stage is somewhat predictable but dependent on (1) type and severity of injury, (2) type of fracture, (3) degree of displacement, (4) appropriate immobilization of the fragment(s), and (5) health and age of the patient.

**Treatment.** Treatment modalities available to the diagnostician for fractures are dependent on the type of injury and fracture, the age and general health of the patient, and severity of displacement and associated tissue damage. With these considerations in mind, alternatives of treatment are generally adopted to promote, restore, and maintain maximum function of the involved area. Additional considerations are given to cosmetic results, but these are of secondary importance. Only the principles of management of the single fracture are considered here; emergency treatment of musculoskeletal trauma including multiple injuries is discussed in Chapter 22.

A major consideration in the choice of treatment of any fracture is optimal *reduction.* The ability to reduce a fracture is dependent on the degree of displacement and whether the fracture is closed. The ability to replace bone fragments in an appropriate anatomic position is dependent on the degree of displacement and complicated when an open fracture is involved because of the massive tissue destruction often associated with this type of fracture. Reduction of the fracture may be accomplished through one of the following methods.[3]

*Manipulation.* Manipulation of a closed fracture is often successful in realignment of the bone fragments and total reduction. Manual manipulation, with distraction and pressure over the appropriate displaced fragment, may be accomplished with no anesthesia (for minor displacements), local anesthesia, or in some cases general anesthesia; this is usually dictated by the degree of displacement involved and the ability of the client to cooperate throughout the procedure.

*Traction.* Dependent on the location of the fracture, the degree of displacement, and the physician's preference, a sling or other traction device may be utilized to provide distraction and appropriate pressure to promote or restore anatomic alignment. Traction may be applied as an emergency measure but also may be utilized as a reduction device. It may also serve to immobilize and maintain reduction.

*Open reduction.* Reduction of open fractures and comminuted fractures is especially difficult to achieve through manipulation or traction techniques; these and other severe types of fractures may require open surgical reduction. Internal fixation devices, when open reduction procedures are necessary, are often utilized to maintain and immobilize the reduction. The greatest advantage of the open reduction, as well as its greatest indication for utilization, is the opportunity it offers to examine and correct soft tissue damage, which may both impair reduction by other methods and be the source of delayed healing, neurovascular impairment, or other complications. Open reduction is most frequently utilized for fractures in older adolescents and adults but rarely is required for the treatment of fractures in children.

It should be mentioned that some fractures of minimal or no displacement will not require reduction if satisfactory anatomic position is assured. This may be confirmed through radiographic examination. When satisfactory reduction is assured, maintenance of the reduction is required through *immobilization* of the fracture site to decrease friction at the site and maintain anatomic position until healing is complete. Inability to maintain appropriate immobilization during the healing process will delay healing and increase the risk of deformity at the fracture site. Immobilization can be maintained throughout the healing process by one or a combination of the following methods.[3]

*External fixation (cast or splint).* Splints or casts may be utilized to maintain reduction of a fracture obtained through manipulation, traction, or in some cases open reduction. It is one of the most common forms of immobilization utilized throughout the healing process. Splints are utilized for minimally displaced fractures and other fractures that do not require reduction. The splint utilized is dependent on the area to be immobilized, such as aluminum padded splints for fingers, commercial splinting devices for various anatomic areas, or plaster or fiberglass custom-molded splints usually utilized for larger areas such as the lower arm. Splints are utilized more commonly in the upper extremity than in the lower extremity because of the stress and wear and tear involved with weight-bearing. A cast may be utilized as an immobilization device following any of the common methods of reduction. The cast may be constructed of plaster of paris or fiberglass and most frequently extends above and below the fracture site to assure total immobilization of the involved area. Specific molding techniques during the cast application procedure may serve to assist in the appropriate positioning of the fracture. Certain risks are involved with cast therapy, such as pressure areas under the cast, but these may be decreased considerably with adequate padding and good application techniques. Specific types of casts are discussed in Chapter 23.

*Traction.* Traction may be utilized as a method of immobilization and maintenance of reduction as well as a method of obtaining and accomplishing the reduction. Traction utilized for this purpose is usually necessary for several days to several weeks or until there is appropriate indication on radiographic examination of callus formation. Additional immobilization with a cast is often required after traction therapy. The types of traction utilized most frequently are adhesive skin traction and skeletal traction. Lower extremity fractures are most frequently managed by the utilization of Buck's extension, Russell traction, Bryant traction, or balanced suspension. Lower extremity traction as a mechanism of maintenance of reduction is utilized more frequently for femoral fractures than for tibial or fibular fractures. Steinmann pins or Kirschner wires may be utilized through the distal femur or proxi-

mal tibia to assist in obtaining or maintaining reductions of femoral fractures with moderate to severe displacement. Upper extremity fractures, especially supercondylar fractures of the elbow, may be effectively immobilized with Dunlop traction with or without a pin or wire. Cervical tongs, such as Crutchfield or Vinke, are utilized as methods of skeletal traction for cervical vertebral fractures. Specific types of traction are discussed in Chapter 24.

*Internal fixation.* Methods of immobilization and maintenance of reduction classified as internal fixation are accomplished in conjunction with open surgical reduction of the fracture. Many internal fixation devices, offering a high degree of success, are available, including plates and nails, transfixion screws, and intramedullary rods. The device utilized is dependent on the type of fracture, effective open reduction obtained, and the anatomic area involved. Risks from these devices include infection, migration of the device, and tissue reaction. With current improvement in the metal composition of these devices, tissue reaction has been tremendously decreased. Whether the device should be removed after the healing process is complete is determined by the physician's preference and the patient's response to the device.

When the osseous healing process is complete, treatment is still required to promote maximum functioning of the area involved. The immobilization required during the healing phase almost always results in a degree of joint stiffness and muscle atrophy. Restoration of adequate function of the involved area is dependent on the ability to restore normal muscle tone and full joint range of motion. This process must be accomplished gradually; rapid increase of motion should be discouraged immediately after the period of immobilization. Exercises that promote gradual increase in the level of functioning are prescribed. Heat and massage may contribute to comfort throughout this process.

Open fractures are most commonly reduced through open reduction and internal fixation. Additional treatment regimens are required for damage that results from bone fragments impinging on the surrounding soft tissue. The degree of vascular and nerve damage resulting from the injury may require more severe methods of treatment. Occasionally amputation of the limb is necessary because of neurovascular loss. The risk of infection is extremely high and can further complicate success of the chosen treatment modality. The initial care of the open wound is extremely important to provide optimal success of treatment.

**Complications.** Specific complications are associated with fractures or their treatment (Table 16-3). All individuals caring for a patient with a fracture should be thoroughly familiar with the signs and symptoms of these complications and their implications. Specific complications of fractures seen with relative frequency include *delayed union, malunion, or nonunion of the fracture, fat embolism, nerve compression syndromes,* and *compartmental syndromes.*

*Delayed union of fracture.* Delayed union is failure of the fracture to consolidate within the time usually required for union. This complication is indicative of retardation of the healing process but does not mean resulting deformity or failure of union. The healing process in these cases requires additional time, but solidarity of the bone eventually occurs. The following may be contributory factors to delayed union of a fracture[3]:

1. Inaccurate reduction of the fracture
2. Immobilization that is inadequate or interrupted during the healing process
3. Severe tissue trauma surrounding the fracture site
4. Circulatory disturbances to or around the fracture site following surgical intervention
5. Infection of bone or surrounding tissues in open fractures
6. Loss of bone tissue such as might be encountered in the excision of necrotic fragments
7. Excessive distraction from traction or an internal fixation device causing separation of the fragments

Any of these factors may cause delayed union; two or more factors increase the risk of delayed union considerably. Prevention of delayed union is best accomplished by appropriate implementation of sound principles of fracture management. When delayed union is encountered the cause should be identified and corrected if possible. Additional immobilization is required to promote proper alignment throughout the extended healing process. Evidence indicates that when delayed union exists in a fracture of the tibia or femur, weight bearing with appropriate immobilization tends to accelerate the healing process.

*Malunion.* Malunion is indicative of union of the fracture but with an increased degree of angulation or deformity at the fracture site. Malunion of a fracture may be detected at any stage throughout the healing process or after it is complete. Before completion of the healing process, excessive deformity at the fracture site may be corrected to varying degrees through realignment and reimmobilization.

Some degrees of malunion are not worth the risk of repeated attempts to correct the alignment because of increased incidence of delayed union or nonunion that accompanies these attempts. If the healing process is near completion, correction of the alignment must be accomplished by surgical intervention. A degree of spontaneous alignment is obtained, especially in children, with growth and continuation of the healing process.

*Nonunion.* Nonunion is the failure of a fracture site to consolidate and produce a complete, firm, and stable union. Nonunion is characterized by excessive mobility at the fracture site, creating a false joint or *pseudarthrosis.* Common contributory factors to nonunion of a fracture are[3]:

1. Varying degrees of separation of the bone fragments at the fracture site
2. Loss of bone tissue, especially from necrosis or excision of fragments
3. Inappropriate and inadequate external or internal fixation of the fracture, which permits excessive motion at the fracture site
4. Repeated attempts to manipulate the fracture to obtain correction of alignment, thereby disrupting the normal healing process and development of callus formation, possible production of circulatory damage
5. Fragmentation of bone resulting in soft tissue placement between the bone fragments, which serves as a deterrent to the normal healing process
6. Infection resulting from an open fracture or surgical intervention
7. Circulatory impairment resulting from the initial injury or reduction of the fracture associated with severe soft tissue trauma

The mobility characteristic of nonunion or pseudarthrosis exists in all directions. Pain is rarely associated with nonunion, with the possible exception of lower extremity involvement, in which case the pain may be elicited by weight bearing. Atrophy of the surrounding muscles is gradual but may become severe. The joints above and below the nonunion may reveal decreased motion. The treatment of nonunion is accomplished through the utilization of appropriate orthotic devices or by surgical intervention. Braces promote stability and prevent deformities. The most common surgical procedure accomplished is that of a bone graft. The type of graft is greatly dependent on the general condition of the bone and its anticipated ability to accept a graft. Common grafts include (1) *cortical graft* (often obtained from the tibia), (2) *cancellous graft* (usually obtained from the ilium), (3) *subperiosteal*

Osteoperiosteal graft

Inadequate internal or external fixation permitting mobility at fracture site
Disruption of healing process through repeated manipulations
Placement of soft tissue between bone fragments causing disruption of healing process
Infection, usually associated with open

**Table 16-3.** Complications of fractures[3. pp.275-293; 6. pp.34-39]

| Complication | Contributory factors | Signs and symptoms | Treatment | Prevention | Comments |
|---|---|---|---|---|---|
| Delayed union | Inappropriate or inaccurate reduction<br>Immobilization that is inadequate or interrupted during healing process<br>Severe traumatization to | Healing phase beyond predicted time as evidenced through radiographic examination | Determine cause of delayed union and correct if possible<br>Longer immobilization period | Appropriate implementation of principles of fracture management<br>Early, accurate, gentle reduction<br>Appropriate | Union accomplished but over longer time<br>May be encountered with any fracture |

**Table 16-3.** Complications of fractures—cont'd

| Complication | Contributory factors | Signs and symptoms | Treatment | Prevention | Comments |
|---|---|---|---|---|---|
| | | Possible patchy pulmonary infiltrates on chest x-ray examination<br>Possible presence of fat in urine | | Appropriate splinting and emergency treatment of fracture | |
| Nerve compression syndromes<br>Carpal tunnel syndrome (median nerve entrapment at wrist)<br>Ulnar nerve syndrome (at wrist)<br>Ulnar nerve syndrome (at elbow)<br>Radial nerve compression (at elbow)<br>Tarsal tunnel syndrome (posterior tibial nerve compression)<br>Common peroneal nerve compression<br>Sciatic nerve compression | Impingement on nerve structures in specific anatomic area due to:<br>Displacement of bone fragment<br>Soft tissue alteration (such as stretching of nerve) due to injury<br>Fracture management | Pain or discomfort<br>Burning sensation<br>Generalized or specific muscular weakness or paralysis<br>Muscle atrophy<br>Limitation of motion<br>Altered reflexes<br>Altered sensory status | Relief of source of compression<br>Surgical intervention may be required to relieve compression or correct resulting deformity | Accurate initial and frequent assessment of neurovascular status to detect early alterations | |
| Compartmental syndrome | Decrease in size of specific compartment due to constrictive force such as cast or dressing<br>Increase in contents of compartment due to hemorrhage, increased pressure, and so on | Sensory alterations indicative of structures involved<br>Motor alterations<br>Pain on passive motion<br>Tenseness on palpation over area | Decompression within 12 hours after onset of symptoms | Early detection | |
| Infection (see Chapter 20) | Open fracture<br>Open reduction | Pain<br>Fever<br>Erythema<br>Drainage | Antibiotic therapy intravenously<br>Surgical irradication of infected tissue<br>Immobilization | Appropriate initial wound care of open fractures<br>Strict aseptic techniques during surgical open reduction | |

*graft,* and *osteoperiosteal graft* (obtained from the tibia or rib). Many grafts require internal fixation devices.[3]

*Fat embolism.* Fat embolism is a syndrome exhibited by "self-limited pulmonary disease that usually occurs within 3 days after a fracture."[6,p.34] Signs and symptoms indicative of fat embolism are[6,pp.34-35;11]:

1. Altered level or disturbances of consciousness
2. Tachycardia
3. Dyspnea
4. Hypovolemic shock
5. Petechial skin hemorrhages, especially over the chest and shoulders and petechia in the conjunctiva
6. Fever
7. Platelet count below 150,000/cu mm
8. $Pao_2$ less than 60 mm Hg
9. Increased serum lipase
10. Possible patchy pulmonary infiltrates seen on chest radiographic examination
11. Possible presence of fat in the urine

In addition certain electrocardiographic alterations may be suggestive of a fat embolism (Table 16-3). Treatment of fat embolism includes (1) treatment for shock, (2) respiratory support including oxygen and intubation if necessary, and (3) administration of corticosteroids.[6,p.35] The most important preventive measure for fat embolism is immediate and appropriate management of the fracture area with splinting.

*Nerve compression syndromes.* Nerve compression syndromes are a collective indication of compression of specific nerve roots resulting in temporary or permanent impairment of nerve function and status. The syndromes are classified according to the anatomic area affected. The most common are the following[6,pp.35-38]:

1. Carpal tunnel syndrome, median nerve entrapment at the wrist
2. Ulnar nerve syndrome at the wrist
3. Ulnar nerve syndrome at the elbow (tardy ulnar nerve palsy, cubital tunnel syndrome)
4. Radial nerve syndrome at the elbow
5. Tarsal tunnel syndrome, posterior tibial nerve compression
6. Compression of the common peroneal nerve over the fibular head
7. Sciatic nerve compression

Nerve compression syndromes may be the direct result of impingement on the specific nerve involved by bone fragments, alterations in tissue structures (such as stretching) due to the injury and bone displacement, or complication of the treatment. Regardless of the specific area, certain signs and symptoms are indicative of nerve compression:

1. Pain or discomfort
2. Generalized or specific muscular weakness or paralysis
3. Burning sensation
4. Muscular atrophy
5. Limitation of motion
6. Altered reflexes of the specific area
7. Altered sensory status of the area

The initial treatment of nerve compression syndromes is directed toward the relief of the source of compression if possible. If conservative measures fail to accomplish this goal, surgical intervention may be required. Permanent destruction resulting from nerve compression requires attention to the specific deformities that may result. Appropriate splinting and emergency treatment of fractures may assist in the avoidance of this complication. Accurate initial and frequent assessments of neurovascular status are essential to detect alterations and thus provide the best potential for relief of the compression.

*Compartmental syndrome.* Compartmental syndrome is "a condition in which increased pressure within a space compromises the circulation of the contents of that space."[6,p.38] Compartmental syndrome may occur in the upper or the lower extremity and is caused by decreased size of the specific anatomic compartment due to constrictive forces, such as a dressing or cast, or increased contents within the compartment due to hemorrhage or increased pressure. The signs and symptoms of specific compartment syndromes are reflective of the anatomic area and the surrounding structures. Disturbances of sensory status are indicative of the distribution of the contents of the compartment involved. Motor disturbances are reflected by weakness in specific surrounding muscular tissues. Pain is often elicited on passive motion. Tenseness may be noted on palpation of the area. The signs and symptoms of compartment syndrome are progressive. Decompression must be accomplished within a short time after the onset of symptoms to prevent permanent damage. Early detection, therefore, is essential.

*Infection.* Infection associated with a fracture is most frequently seen in open fracture or open reduction of a fracture. Signs and symptoms of infection are pain, fever, erythema, or drainage. The treatment of infections of the musculoskeletal system includes antibiotic therapy intravenously, surgical eradication of the infected tissue, and appropriate support through immobilization. Initial wound care of open fractures is critical in the prevention of infection, as is strict aseptic techniques during open surgical reductions.

## Epiphyseal fractures

During childhood and adolescence growth of the skeletal system and individual bones is controlled by the epiphyseal growth plate. This growth plate appears at both ends of long bones between the epiphysis and diaphysis and controls overall growth, limb length equality, and specific function of anatomic areas and joints. Disturbances of the growth plate during the growth period may retard or stop growth. After full growth is attained, function of the growth plate ceases, and therefore the risk of growth disturbance from fractures is lessened. Until growth is complete, however, there is great concern when a fracture occurs near or involves the epiphyseal growth plate. If an epiphyseal fracture occurs, monitoring of the growth pattern in the extremity is necessary even after healing of the fracture is completed. Evidence of deformity or limb length inequality is then dealt with appropriately. This may involve surgical intervention in the form of rotation osteotomies (to correct angular deformity) or epiphysiodesis (for leg length equality).

## Childhood fractures

In addition to concern regarding injury to the epiphyseal growth plate, the following are of importance in the diagnosis and treatment of fractures in children[10,p.1533]:

1. Exact and accurate anatomic reduction of a fracture is not quite so critical in children as in adults because the normal remodeling process during the growth years appears to realign fragments more efficiently. Spontaneous correction of angular deformities, with the possible exception of rotation, is almost always complete as a result of the remodeling process.
2. The increase in circulation from fractures stimulates growth in the involved bone. For this reason it is not only acceptable but desirable to have some overriding of the fragments to accommodate for this overgrowth. This is especially significant and important in the long bones of the lower extremity.
3. Several physiologic features of young, immature bones, such as the abundant blood supply and thickened periosteum, contribute greatly to rapid bone healing. Union of the fracture site is accomplished much more readily in

younger patients, and solid and stable union of the fragments is more readily assured. Nonunion is almost nonexistent in childhood fractures, and open reduction is rarely required.

## Battered child syndrome

Exploration of battered child syndrome is not possible within the context of this chapter. It is important to consider, however, that any child who has multiple soft tissue injuries in association with a fracture or multiple fractures at various stages of healing *may* be a battered child. Although specific laws vary, most states require further exploration of such physical findings and require reporting of suspicions. The bibliography at the end of this chapter gives several sources relative to diagnosis of battered child syndrome, legal obligations of health care personnel, and intervention with the family when child abuse or neglect are suspected or confirmed.

## SUMMARY

Traumatic injuries to the musculoskeletal system constitute a high percentage of the orthopedic cases seen on an inpatient and outpatient basis. All personnel should be thoroughly familiar with the implications of such injuries and the appropriate emergency intervention as well as the biophysiologic considerations. For review of emergency intervention, see Chapter 22.

## REFERENCES

1. Aston, J. N.: A short textbook of orthopaedics and traumatology, London, 1972, The English Universities Press, Ltd.
2. Blauvelt, C. T., and Nelson, F. R. T.: A manual of orthopaedic terminology, St. Louis, 1977, The C. V. Mosby Co.
3. Brashear, H. R., Jr., and Raney, R. B., Sr.: Shand's handbook of orthopaedic surgery, ed. 9, St. Louis, 1978, The C. V. Mosby Co.
4. Donoghue, D. H.: Treatment of acute ligamentous injuries of the knee, Orth. Clin. North Am. 4(3): 617-645, 1973.
5. Gartland, J. J.: Fundamentals of orthopaedics, Philadelphia, 1974, W. B. Saunders Co.
6. Iverson, L. D., and Clawson, D. K.: Manual of acute orthopaedic therapeutics, Boston, 1977, Little, Brown & Co.
7. Kerr, A.: Orthopedic nursing procedures, Baltimore, 1969, The Williams & Wilkins Co.
8. Nicholas, J. A.: Injuries to the menisci of the knee, Orthop. Clin. North Am. 4(3):647-664, 1973.
9. Schneider, F. R.: Handbook for the orthopaedic assistant, ed. 2, St. Louis, 1976, The C. V. Mosby Co.

10. Tachdjian, M. O.: Pediatric orthopaedics, Philadelphia, 1972, W. B. Saunders Co.
11. Turek, S.: Orthopaedics, Philadelphia, 1977, J. B. Lippincott Co.

## BIBLIOGRAPHY

Adams, J. C.: Outline of orthopaedics, Baltimore, 1971, The Williams & Wilkins Co.

Aegertu, E., and Kirkpatrick, J.: Orthopedic diseases, Philadelphia, 1975, W. B. Saunders Co.

Astor, J. N.: A short textbook of orthopaedics and traumatology, London, 1972, The English Universities Press, Ltd.

Ballinger, W. F., et al.: The management of trauma, ed. 2, Philadelphia, 1973, W. B. Saunders Co.

Blauvelt, C. T., and Nelson, F. R. T.: A manual of orthopaedic terminology, St. Louis, 1977, The C. V. Mosby Co.

Blount, W. P.: Fractures in children, Baltimore, 1955, The Williams & Wilkins Co.

Brashear, H. R., Jr., and Raney, R. B., Sr.: Shand's handbook of orthopaedic surgery, ed. 9, St. Louis, 1978, The C. V. Mosby Co.

Collins H. R., editor: Symposium on sports injuries, Orthop. Clin. North Am. 4:3, 1973.

Crenshaw, A. H., editor: Campbell's operative orthopaedics, ed. 5, St. Louis, 1971, The C. V. Mosby Co.

Donoghue, D. H.: Treatment of acute ligamentous injuries of the knee, Orth. Clin. North Am. 4(3):617-645, 1973.

Ebeling, N. B., and Hill, D. A.: Child abuse: intervention and treatment. Publishing Sciences Group Inc., Acton, Mass., 1975.

Gartland, J. J.: Fundamentals of orthopaedics, Philadelphia, 1974, W. B. Saunders Co.

Goldstein, L. A., and Dickerson, R. C.: Atlas of orthopaedic surgery, St. Louis, 1974, The C. V. Mosby Co.

Kempe, C. H., and Helfer, R. E., editors: Helping the battered child and his family Philadelphia 1972, J. B. Lippincott Co.

Kerr, A.: Orthopedic nursing procedures, Baltimore, 1969, The Williams & Wilkins Co.

Nicholas, J. A.: Injuries to the menisci of the knee, Orthop. Clin. North Am. 4(3):647-664, 1973.

Rang, M.: The growth plate and its disorders, Baltimore, 1969, The Williams & Wilkins Co.

Schneider, F. R.: Handbook for the orthopaedic assistant, ed. 2, St. Louis, 1976, The C. V. Mosby Co.

Tachdjian, M. O.: Pediatric orthopaedics, Philadelphia, 1972, W. B. Saunders Co.

Turek, S.: Orthopaedics, Philadelphia, 1977, J. B. Lippincott Co.

# 17

# Joint diseases and disorders

NANCY E. HILT

SHIRLEY B. COGBURN

The major function of any joint is motion. Any permanent damage to the structure of the joint considerably threatens that function and as a result may also threaten one's ability to remain mobile.

A major portion of this chapter is devoted to the various types of arthritis. Arthritis poses the ultimate threat to the joint structures and their functions. Degenerative arthritis is a complication of all joint disorders and diseases discussed. The various forms of arthritis are the most common of all joint diseases.

## ANKYLOSIS

Ankylosis is the limitation or restriction of normal range of motion due to tissue alterations in or out of the joint cavity. It may be seen in the absence of another disease, or it may be the result of another disease process or disorder of the joint structures.

**Etiology.** Ankylosis is often the result of either incomplete healing or restoration of joint structures damaged by chronic arthritis, infection, or in some cases traumatic injuries.[1]

**Pathology.** Tissue alterations resulting in ankylosis may occur with the joint in a functional position or in one of deformity. It may be *fibrous* or *bony*. Fibrous ankylosis occurs when connective tissue adhesions are not accompanied by bony union. Bony ankylosis occurs when solid bone is formed between the articular surfaces.

**Signs and symptoms.** With fibrous ankylosis some motion of the joint is possible. Pain may accompany movement of the joint. With bony ankylosis no motion is possible. Radiographic examination may show the presence of bony trabeculae across the area of the former joint space.

**Treatment.** When a known disease process or joint injury is diagnosed, immediate and appropriate treatment is the best assurance of preventing ankylosis. When it has occurred, however, fibrous ankylosis may be treated with physical therapy to increase or maintain joint range of motion. Manipulation may be necessary with the patient under anesthesia. Joint function is improved if adhesions and contractures can be overcome with a minimum of effort. Extreme care must be given to the adjoining bones because they fracture easily. Arthroplasty may be the treatment of choice if the ankylosis has resulted in a functional position of the joint. With undesirable joint positioning, surgical intervention to restore joint motion or to correct deformity may be indicated.

**Prognosis.** Success of treatment of ankylosis is variable.

## ARTHRITIS

Arthritis may be defined, as strictly translated from the Greek, as inflammation of a joint. Structur-

354

al changes within the joint often arise from the inflammation and resulting damage. Arthritis may be *acute* or *chronic, monoarticular* or *polyarticular.* Various types of arthritis are discussed on the following pages, without classification.

The most promising modality of treatment for all types of arthritis, as the result of advanced technology in recent years, is total joint replacement. Most joints may now be replaced, decreasing the pain and limited motion associated with arthritis. This form of surgical intervention is discussed briefly throughout this chapter, although it has not been available to all patients with arthritis.

### Gouty arthritis

Gouty arthritis (Fig. 17-1) is a hereditary metabolic disorder characterized by sodium urate crystals within the joint spaces. It may be acute or chronic.

**Etiology.** Although the cause of gouty arthritis is unknown, the following predisposing factors have been established: (1) heredity, (2) sex, (3) age, (4) adrenal cortex activity, (5) vascular changes, (6)

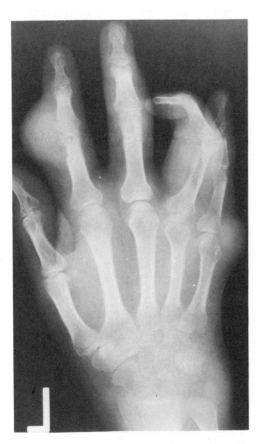

**Fig. 17-1.** Gouty arthritis. Note the large soft tissue tophi with "punched-out" periarticular bone lesions.

altered electrolyte balance, and (7) decreased urinary 17-ketosteroids.[3,p.195]

**Pathology.** *Acute* gouty arthritis is characterized by sodium urate crystals within the joint space and may be differentiated from the *chronic* form characterized by disposition of these crystals in cartilage, bone, subcutaneous tissue, and the kidneys. These deposits are known as *tophi.*

**Incidence.** Gouty arthritis occurs in families, is not sex linked, although it is seen predominately in men, and is common at age 40 years or older.

**Signs and symptoms.** Gouty arthritis has an abrupt onset with periods of remission. It may involve one or more joints, usually the peripheral joints. Gout should be suspected in the patient with symptoms of swelling, tenderness, or pain in the peripheral joints or "hot" peripheral joints. The fingers, toes, ankles, and wrists are most often involved, although the knees, elbows, or other joints may be. Results of radiographic examination may be negative unless tophi are present. Laboratory findings show presence of sodium urate crystals in the synovial fluid. An elevated blood uric acid level may also be noted.

**Treatment.** The acute stage of gouty arthritis is often controlled by anti-inflammatory drugs such as calchicine or corticosteroids. The chronic stage of the process requires control through the use of uricosuric agents such as probenecid (Benemid) or allopurinol to lower the serum uric acid level. Surgical intervention is only necessary to excise tophi in rare cases.

### Hemophilic arthritis

*Hemophilia* is a hereditary disease of the blood occurring in males and transmitted by females. It is characterized by repeated and excessive hemorrhage into tissues. Of concern here is hemorrhage into the joint space.

**Etiology.** Repeated joint hemorrhage causes articular cartilage degeneration.

**Pathology.** As a result of hemorrhage and degeneration, the bone becomes atrophic, and subchondral bone cysts may occur.

**Incidence.** Hemophilic arthritis occurs only in males and is transmitted by females. Although any joint may be subject to damage from repeated hemorrhage, the knee is the most common joint affected.

**Signs and symptoms.** The first episode of hemophilic arthritis may occur during early or middle childhood. With hemorrhage the joint shows distention, tenderness, and extreme pain on motion. Fever may accompany excessive hemorrhage. Repeated hemorrhage results in edema, muscle atrophy, and contractures.

**Treatment.** With acute hemarthrosis immobilization of the extremity is necessary. Protection from trauma is essential. Orthotics designed to limit knee motion may be utilized. Physical therapy and traction, bracing, or casting (e.g., Quengle's cast) for gradual correction of contractures may be used to minimize trauma. Injections of hyaluronidase for absorption of the blood may be used.

**Prognosis.** Initially the hemorrhage is usually absorbed. Avoidance of trauma is advocated, but joint damage is inevitable with repeated episodes of hemorrhage, resulting in increasing disability.

### Juvenile rheumatoid arthritis

Juvenile rheumatoid arthritis (Figs. 17-2 and 17-3) is chronic, with onset during childhood. It is more severe than the adult form but exhibits similar deterioration of joint structures. The fulminating systemic form is known as *Still's disease*.

**Etiology.** The cause of juvenile rheumatoid arthritis is undetermined.

**Pathology.** Juvenile rheumatoid arthritis may be *monoarticular, polyarticular, or acute febrile.* The monoarticular type involves only one joint; the polyarticular type exhibits multiple joint involvement; and the acute febrile type includes multiple systemic and acute clinical symptoms. The joint inflamma-

tory process often destroys the growth cartilage, thus arresting long bone growth in the child. *Persistent joint involvement in one or more joints is the most valid criterion for diagnosis.* The usual laboratory findings in the adult type of rheumatoid arthritis (RA factor) are not always seen in the juvenile type. Typical laboratory findings include increased white blood cell count (rarely above 20,000/cu mm), elevated erythrocyte sedimentation rate (ESR), and possible positive C-reactive protein test results. One half of all cases of juvenile rheumatoid arthritis are polyarticular, with similar joint pathologic processes as in the adult form except for the thickened cartilage and effect on adjacent epiphyseal growth plates.

**Incidence.** Juvenile rheumatoid arthritis is diagnosed in approximately six to eight per 100,000 children annually. It is more common in girls than in boys, with a 7:3 ratio. Onset occurs most often between the ages of 1 to 4 years and 9 to 14 years.[3,p.360]

**Signs and symptoms.** The signs and symptoms associated with juvenile rheumatoid arthritis vary

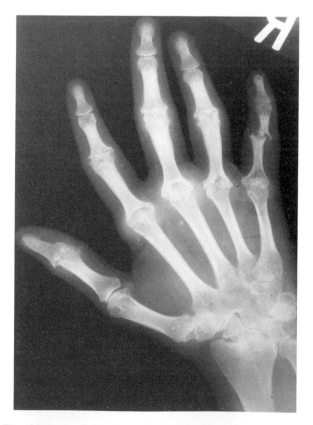

**Fig. 17-3.** Juvenile rheumatoid arthritis. Deformities are similar to those of adult rheumatoid arthritis, although there is greater tendency to fusion later in life. Note almost total fusion of carpals.

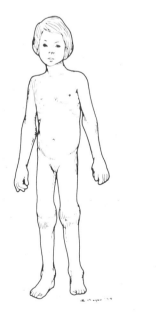

**Fig. 17-2.** Typical appearance of severe juvenile rheumatoid arthritis. Note the thickening of the joint areas, apparent deformities, and characteristic facial expression. (From Hilt, N. E., and Schmitt, E. W., Jr.: Pediatric orthopedic nursing, St. Louis, 1975, The C. V. Mosby Co.)

**Table 17-1.** Comparison of types of juvenile rheumatoid arthritis[3, pp. 360-366]

| | Monoarticular | Polyarticular | Acute febrile |
|---|---|---|---|
| Clinical picture | Comprises 30% of all cases<br>Involvement of one joint only, frequently knee<br>Often accelerates epiphyseal growth, causing temporary limb length discrepancy<br>Onset insidious with mild joint symptoms<br>Joint symptoms may be more severe if hip is involved<br>Highest incidence of all types of iridocyclitis | Comprises 50% of all cases<br>Onset characterized by simultaneous symmetric involvement of usually four or more joints, usually hands, feet, wrists, ankles, knees<br>If cervical involvement:<br>  Apophyseal joint limits motion<br>  Stiffly held head<br>  Vertebral growth retardation results in shortened trunk<br>Premature epiphyseal closure may produce limb length discrepancy<br>Weight loss due to anorexia may be present<br>Child may appear ill with low-grade fever, rash, lymphadenopathy<br>Splenomegaly, subcutaneous nodules rare | Comprises 20% of all cases<br>Child generally appears ill<br>Listlessness and irritability<br>Anorexia with weight loss<br>Fever<br>Rash<br>Splenomegaly<br>Lymphadenopathy<br>Pericarditis or myocarditis may be present<br>Pneumonia or pleuritis may be present<br>All symptoms need not be present for definitive diagnosis |
| Laboratory findings | ESR often normal<br>White blood cell count often normal | Elevated ESR<br>Elevated white blood cell count<br>Positive C-reactive protein test results<br>RA factor positive in 10% of children under 12 years of age | Elevated ESR<br>Neutrophilic leukocytosis<br>Normocytic hypochromic anemia<br>Normal serum electrophoresis with possible high alpha and gamma globulins |
| Differential diagnosis | Infection arthritis<br>Osteochondritis dissicans<br>Meniscal injury | Rheumatic fever<br>Systemic lupus erythematosus<br>Septic arthritis<br>Leukemia<br>Reiter's syndrome<br>Congenital agammaglobulinemia<br>Acquired hypogammaglobulinemia<br>Allergic reactions<br>Viral diseases | Systemic lupus erythematosus<br>Leukemia<br>Polyarticular arthritis |
| Course | Becomes polyarticular in 25% of cases<br>Marked with periods of remission and exacerbation<br>Chronic iridocyclitis with resulting blindness a threat | Intermittent periods of remission and exacerbation for years<br>Episodes may be severe, resulting in marked deformities | Periods of remission and exacerbation each year in 50% of cases, with adulthood attacks subsiding; leaves no deformities<br>Becomes polyarticular in 50% of cases, continuing into adulthood with periods of remission and exacerbation; deformities likely |

with the type. The following are the most commonly associated signs and symptoms seen with each form.

*Monoarticular*

1. Involvement of one joint, often the knee
2. Accelerated epiphyseal growth resulting in temporary leg length discrepancy
3. Onset insidious with mild joint pain and stiffness
4. White blood cell count and ESR often normal
5. High incidence of iridocyclitis

*Polyarticular*

1. Simultaneous symmetric joint involvement, usually four or more joints (e.g., hands, feet, wrists, ankles, knees)
2. Joints involved may be tender, painful, stiff, or warm to the touch
3. Premature epiphyseal closure common
4. Leg length discrepancy may result from premature epiphyseal closure
5. Weight loss due to anorexia may be seen
6. Child frequently appears ill, with low-grade fever, rash, generalized lymphadenopathy, splenomegaly (subcutaneous nodules rare)
7. Elevated white blood cell count
8. Elevated ESR
9. Positive C-reactive protein test
10. RA factor positive in 10% of children under 12 years of age

*Acute febrile*

1. Child appears generally ill, listless, and irritable
2. Anorexia with weight loss
3. Fever
4. Rash
5. Splenomegaly
6. Lymphadenopathy
7. Pericarditis or myocarditis may be present
8. Pneumonia or pleuritis may be present

(*Note:* The above clinical findings may be present in any combination; all need not be present for definitive diagnosis.)

9. Elevated ESR
10. Neutrophilic leukocytosis
11. Normocytic hypochromic anemia
12. Normal serum electrophoresis with possible high alpha and gamma globulins

Considerations for differential diagnosis as well as comments regarding the general clinical course of each type are given in Table 17-1.

**Treatment.** Early diagnosis and appropriate treatment are essential to prevent the possible severe sequelae such as crippling joint deformities, heart disease, or blindness. Nonsurgical treatment modalities are designed to control, prevent, and correct deformities, preserve joint motion, and prevent serious sequelae.[3,p.366] These modalities include rest, exercise, heat, immobilization, or physical therapy and may be used in a variety of combinations tailored to the child's specific needs as well as the severity of joint involvement. Immobilization may be accomplished through bed rest, splints, casts, traction, orthotics, or any combination thereof.

Pharmacologic therapeutic regimens are designed to decrease the inflammatory process and other systemic reactions to the disease. *Aspirin,* plain or buffered, is usually prescribed at dosage levels compatible with the child's body weight. Doses are given four to six times daily to maintain an adequate level in the blood. The blood salicylate level is frequently monitored to assure adequate dosage and to avoid toxicity. It is recommended that the level be maintained at 20 to 25 mg/100 ml. In addition to monitoring blood salicylate levels, observation for gastrointestinal tract irritation, bleeding, and other signs of toxicity should be accomplished. *Intra-articular corticosteroids, systemic corticosteroids, gold injections,* and *indomethacin* (Indocin) may also be used, depending on the severity of the process and response to other therapeutic regimens.

Surgical intervention may be indicated at varying stages of the disease process. This, too, is dependent on the severity of joint involvement and resulting structure destruction as well as response to nonsurgical intervention. Of the procedures that may be indicated, synovectomy, osteotomy, arthrodesis, contracture release, and total joint replacement are the most commonly required. The purpose of surgical intervention is to improve function and to alleviate pain.

## Osteoarthritis (degenerative joint disease)

Osteoarthritis (Fig. 17-4), or degenerative joint disease, is a progressive joint disorder found commonly in middle-aged and elderly individuals. It is characterized by degenerative changes of the articular cartilage and overgrowth at joint margins and thus by joint deformities.

**Etiology.** Although the precise cause of osteoarthritis is unknown, age, sex, heredity, and obesity are known to be predisposing factors.

**Pathology.** Osteoarthritis attacks primarily the weight-bearing joints. Early alterations appear in the articular cartilage, with thinning and widespread degeneration. Osteophytes form early around the cartilaginous edges and are viewed on radiographic films as spurs. These may in turn form loose bodies within the joint. As degeneration progresses, bony

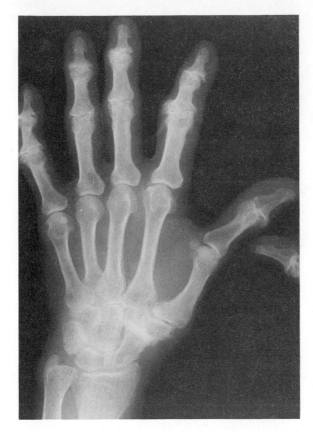

**Fig. 17-4.** Osteoarthritis. Typical location involving distal interphalangeal and proximal joints and base of thumb with cartilaginous thinning and hypertrophic osteophytes.

deformities become apparent and functional limitations may be noted.

Osteoarthritis appears to begin in the second decade of life, but degenerative changes are not evident until middle age. By 55 to 65 years of age, approximately 85% of patients have x-ray evidence of the disease.

**Incidence.** Osteoarthritis affects men and women equally until about age 54 years, after which it is more severe in women.

**Signs and symptoms.** Early stages of osteoarthritis are characterized by stiffness, pain, and swelling of one or more joints. The pain is characteristically "achy." The stiffness is relieved with moderate motion; continued motion produces discomfort, which is usually relieved by heat and rest with support. These symptoms of osteoarthritis increase in cold, wet weather.

Some noticeable alteration of affected joints may be observed as slight enlargement (e.g., Heberden's nodes). There may be mild tenderness on examination.

The later stages of osteoarthritis reveal marked joint limitation with considerable disability. Pain may be present when the joint is at rest as well as in motion. Malalignment is frequently noted with crepitation. Fatigue may be a complaint, especially if the patient is obese.

Definitive diagnosis is accomplished through careful analysis of the history and observation of joint alterations by x-ray and physical examination. Osteoarthritis is difficult to distinguish from rheumatoid arthritis, and they sometimes coexist.[1]

**Treatment.** Nonsurgical treatment may include but is not limited to combinations of the following:

1. *Rest* of the involved joint to decrease aggravation of symptoms
2. *Exercise* including full range of motion of the joint
3. Use of *ambulatory aids* (walker, crutches) to avoid full weight bearing on the involved joint
4. *Immobilization* of the joint with traction in the acute inflammatory phase of the process
5. Carefully planned *physical therapy*
6. Utilization of appropriate *splints* and *braces*
7. Warm, dry climate if possible
8. Drug therapy including corticosteroids, salicylates, or indomethacin (Indocin).

Surgical intervention may be indicated to improve or maintain joint motion, relieve pain, or correct deformity. In advanced cases artificial implants create a new joint through partial or total joint replacement surgical procedures. Arthrodesis may be considered when other measures are not possible or have failed.

### Rheumatoid arthritis

Rheumatoid arthritis (Figs. 17-5 and 17-6) is a chronic inflammatory systemic disease of unknown cause characterized by destruction and proliferation of the synovial membrane, resulting in joint destruction, ankylosis, and deformity.

**Etiology.** The cause of rheumatoid arthritis is unknown, but infection, allergic reaction, endocrine or metabolic imbalance, or stress may be contributory factors.

**Pathology.** The synovial membrane is the major target organ of rheumatoid arthritis. Immunologic mechanisms appear to play an important role in the initiation and perpetuation of the disease.[2, p. 94] The presumption is that once the articular changes begin, the antigen-antibody reaction occurs within the synovial cavity. Marked proliferation of the synovium in turn damages the articular cartilage and surrounding tissue through the release of proteolytic enzymes. The disease process is then perpetuated by the injurious enzymes.

Synovial inflammation with effusion of the joint, along with alterations within the capsule and periarticular soft tissue, cause swelling, decreased joint motion, and tenderness. Bone and muscle in the region may atrophy. In the chronic stage joint effusion is not present, as this is when the disease is active. With no definitive treatment available, the antigen causes a constant state of inflammation. With continued inflammation the synovium forms a granulomatous mass called *pannus*. The pannus spreads and leaves behind still further destruction of cartilage, tendons, and ligaments adjacent to the joint. The result is progressive, crippling joint deformity and loss of motion.

**Incidence.** The insidious onset of rheumatoid arthritis usually begins before 40 years of age. It is seen predominately in women, with a 3:1 ratio. There is a slight familial tendency.[2, pp.94-95;4,pp.348-349]

**Signs and symptoms.** The onset of rheumatoid arthritis is insidious. The patient often complains of fatigue, weakness, and sweating with no fever. Inflammation is symmetric when the interphalangeal joints of the hand are involved. Knees, feet, and wrists are next in frequency of occurrence of inflammation. The overlying skin is characteristically stretched and shiny. Swelling limits motion, and the joints assume a semiflexed position. The extremities may be clammy and cold. Subcutaneous nodules are seen over bony prominences; 20% of these are seen at the elbow. Lymphadenopathy, splenomegaly, and weight loss with malnutrition are general manifestations of the disease as it progresses.

According to the American Rheumatism Association, the following have been established as *criteria for diagnosis of rheumatoid arthritis:*

*Symptoms:*
1. Morning stiffness
2. Pain on motion or tenderness in at least one joint
3. Swelling (soft tissue thickening or fluid, not bony outgrowth alone) in at least one joint continuously for not less than 6 weeks
4. Swelling of at least one other joint
5. Symmetric joint swelling
6. Subcutaneous nodules
7. X-ray changes typical of rheumatoid arthritis
8. Positive latex fixation test results
9. Poor mucin clot
10. Characteristic histologic changes in synovial membrane
11. Characteristic histologic changes in nodules

*Probable diagnosis:* Any *three* of the above for at least 4 weeks

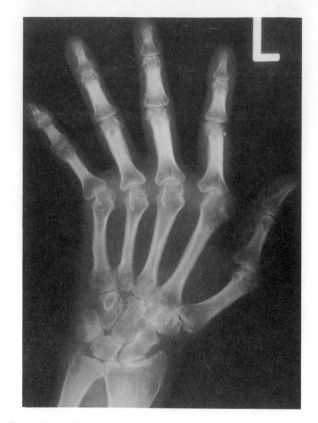

**Fig. 17-5.** Rheumatoid arthritis. Note extensive periarticular demineralization and erosions with subluxation and ulnar deviation.

*Definite diagnosis:* Any *five* of the above for at least 6 weeks

*Classic diagnosis:* Any *seven* of the above for at least 6 weeks

**Treatment.** Treatment for rheumatoid arthritis is directed toward the general care of the whole patient and the affected joints. The multidisciplinary team approach is utilized in the rehabilitation of these patients with participation of the orthopedic surgeon, rheumatologist, and physiatrist.

Nonsurgical intervention includes rest and physical therapy, with maintenance of joint function as the primary goal through the use of exercise, heat, and splints. Increased caloric and vitamin intake is often prescribed. It is advantageous to encourage an atmosphere of decreased anxiety if possible.

There is currently no specific curative drug available to the patient with rheumatoid arthritis. Salicylate, steroid, gold injection, and other pharmacologic therapies are used for their anti-inflammatory effects. These are prescribed in regular daily doses (four to eight) to provide adequate levels in the blood.

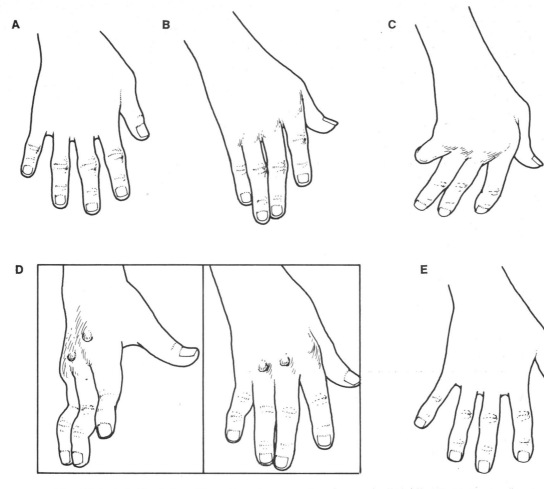

**Fig. 17-6.** Arthritic deformities of hand apparent on gross examination. **A,** Early stages of rheumatoid arthritis with fusiform swelling of proximal interphalangeal joints. **B,** Moderate involvement of rheumatoid arthritis with edema of metacarpophalangeal joints and early ulnar deviation. **C,** Advanced stages of rheumatoid arthritis with marked ulnar deviation, subluxation of metacarpophalangeal joints, extension of proximal interphalangeal joints, flexion of distal joints, and deformed thumb. **D,** Swan-neck deformities of fingers in rheumatoid arthritis with flexion of proximal joints, hyperextension of middle joints, and flexion of distal joints associated with contractures of intrinsic muscles; subcutaneous nodules may be evident. **E,** Osteoarthritis of hand with enlargement of distal joints.

Aspiration of joint fluid may be indicated for relief of pain from recurrent effusion. Intra-articular injections of steroids may also be useful in reducing inflammation and decreasing associated pain.

Surgical intervention may be indicated for relief of pain, correction of associated deformities, and improvement of motion and function. The surgical procedures vary according to the joint involved and include the following[3,pp.357-359]:

*Knee*
1. Synovectomy
2. Total knee arthroplasty
3. Osteotomy
4. Arthrodesis

*Hip*
1. Arthrodesis
2. Cup arthroplasty
3. Total hip arthroplasty

*Elbow*
1. Total elbow arthroplasty
2. Arthrodesis
3. Excision of radial head

*Shoulder*
1. Excision of acromion

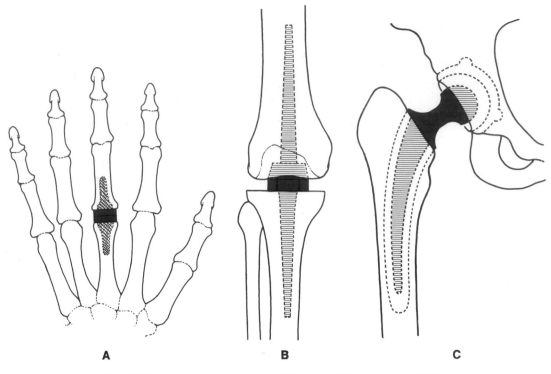

A                                B                                C

**Fig. 17-7.** Joint replacement for **(A)** finger, **(B)** knee, and **(C)** hip.

2. Rotational osteotomy of humerus
3. Arthrodesis
4. Total shoulder arthroplasty
*Wrist*
1. Radiocarpal fusion (grasp position)
2. Resection of distal ulna
*Hand*
1. Synovectomy
2. Total phalangeal arthroplasty
3. Capsulotomy
4. Arthrodesis
5. Tendon transfers
*Spine*
1. Osteotomy
2. Fusion

As mentioned, total joint arthroplasties (Fig. 17-7) developed in recent years provide hope that did not previously exist for the patient with rheumatoid arthritis. These procedures, however, are still utilized in many cases only when lesser measures have not fulfilled optimal function and relief of pain. They should not and are not used as the first option, because of the irreversibility of the procedures and the risk of infection.

Rheumatoid arthritis is characterized by periods of remission during which slight joint alterations may disappear. With the team approach and proper care and cooperation instituted as early as possible, good results can be obtained.

**Differentiation between osteoarthritis and rheumatoid arthritis.** Osteoarthritis and rheumatoid arthritis not only have similar manifestations but it is possible for them to coexist. Table 17-2 gives differential characteristics of these two processes.

### Traumatic arthritis

Arthritis may develop in any joint that has been previously damaged. The term *traumatic arthritis* implies that arthritis of the joint is a result of recent trauma. This, however, is not always the case. Osteoarthritis may occur in a joint whose articular cartilage has been damaged or joint surface altered by previous trauma.

**Etiology.** Traumatic arthritis is usually the result of trauma to the joint.

**Pathology.** Pathologically and roentgenographically, traumatic arthritis is indistinguishable from osteoarthritis except that the involvement is limited to the injured joint.

**Signs and symptoms.** Occupational stress may affect the wrist, elbow, or aeromyoclavicular joints. A history of previous major trauma such as dislocation or displaced fracture is usually noted (Fig. 17-8). Especially prone to the development of

**Table 17-2.** Differentiation between rheumatoid arthritis and osteoarthritis

| | Rheumatoid arthritis | Osteoarthritis |
|---|---|---|
| **Clinical** | | |
| Geographic distribution | Most common in temperate climates<br>Rare in tropical climates | Climate not a factor |
| Family history | Often history of rheumatic fever or rheumatoid arthritis in a member of immediate family | Frequently history of similar form of arthritis in one or both parents |
| Past history | Occasionally history of rheumatic fever<br>Frequently tonsillitis or sinusitis | Rheumatic fever, tonsillitis, sinusitis not characteristics<br>Sometimes history of trauma or faulty body mechanics |
| Age at onset | Any age<br>Over 80% between 20 and 50 years | Rare before 40 years |
| Mode of onset | Rarely acute<br>Usually subacute or insidious<br>Often accompanied by migratory pains | Insidious<br>Not accompanied by migratory pains |
| General condition | Usually undernourished, anemic, and "chronically" ill<br>Frequently slight fever (+37.2 C [+99 F]) and slight leukocytosis | Well nourished<br>Frequently obese, not anemic<br>No fever, no leukocytosis |
| Involvement of joints | Symmetric and generalized<br>Proximal interphalangeal joints especially involved | Usually weight-bearing joints (spine, hips, knee)<br>Distal joints of fingers (Heberden's nodes) |
| Appearance of joints | Early: periarticular swelling, fusiform fingers<br>Late: ankylosis, extreme deformity, ulnar deflection | Early: slight articular enlargement<br>Late: more pronounced articular enlargement; limitation of motion usually slight; ankylosis, Heberden's nodes |
| Muscular atrophy | Often pronounced, particularly in later stages | Not characteristic |
| Cutaneous changes | Extremities frequently cold, clammy; skin atrophic and glossy; redness of thenar and hypothenar eminences<br>Psoriasis occasionally present | No characteristic features |
| Subcutaneous nodules | Present in 15% to 20% of cases | Not present |
| **Laboratory** | | |
| Agglutination reactions | Positive in over 50% of typical cases | Never definitely positive |
| Sedimentation rate | Usually greatly increased<br>Tends to return to normal as arthritis improves | Normal or only slightly increased |
| Roentgenologic appearances | Early: osteoporosis, periarticular swelling, joint effusion<br>Late: narrowing of joint space, bone destructs, ankylosis, and deformities | Early: No osteoporosis; slight lipping at joint margins<br>Late: Marked lipping, osteophytes, narrowing of joint space, deformation of articular bone ends |

Data from Turek, S.: Orthopaedics, Philadelphia, 1977, J. B. Lippincott Co., p. 374.

traumatic arthritis are the weight-bearing joints (ankles, knees, hips).

The classic symptoms are those of most types of arthritis and include pain, stiffness, and swelling. X-ray examination shows osteoarthritis with previous traumatic deformity.

**Treatment.** The treatment for traumatic arthritis is the same as for osteoarthritis.

## BURSITIS

A bursa is a closed sac that exists in some 52 anatomic areas for the purpose of lubrication to diminish friction on movement. Bursae are located beneath the skin and tendons and overlying joints. Bursitis is inflammation of a bursa.

**Etiology.** Bursitis may be the result of trauma, excessive utilization of the area, infection, gout,

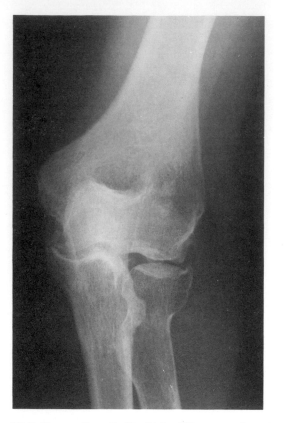

**Fig. 17-8.** Traumatic arthritis: Note difference of contour indicating previous fracture with secondary hypertrophic and degenerative alterations.

rheumatoid arthritis, metabolic diseases, neoplasms, or occupational stress.

**Pathology.** The synovial membrane, as a result of overstimulation from inflammation, produces excess fluid and thus distention of the bursa. Trauma produces bloody fluid, while gout produces urate crystals in the fluid.

**Incidence.** Bursitis may occur at any age.

**Signs and symptoms.** Symptoms vary according to the location of the bursitis.

### Prepatellar bursitis

Prepatellar bursitis is the result of excessive and repeated utilization of the knee joint such as in kneeling (e.g., "housemaid's knee" or "nun's knee"). It may also be produced from traumatic injury. A well-circumscribed localized mass is usually observed on the anterior aspect of the knee. The knee joint itself is not necessarily involved.

**Treatment.** Spontaneous subsidence may occur if the pressure against the front of the knee is relieved or eliminated by padding. Aspiration of the fluid, injections of corticosteroids, and a pressure dressing may be necessary if symptoms persist. If there

is infection, incision and drainage with antibiotic therapy may be necessary. Surgical excision may be necessary for chronic recurrence.

### Olecranon bursitis

Olecranon bursitis is usually the result of a single localized injury or continued trauma of varying degrees. It may also be seen with gout and rheumatoid arthritis. Chronic enlargement is known as "bartender's elbow."

**Treatment.** Treatment is usually the same as that for prepatellar bursitis.

### Radiohumeral bursitis (tennis elbow, epicondylitis)

The cause of radiohumeral bursitis is unknown, but in some cases irritation of tissue overlying the radiohumeral joint capsule appears responsible. Continual or excessive utilization of the joint such as is required in tennis is a common cause. Pain on the lateral aspect of the elbow with spreading of pain into the forearm is common. Hand grip may be weak. Passive movement does not produce pain and is unaffected. Extension against resistance results in discomfort. Results of radiographic examination are usually negative.

**Treatment.** Immobilization for a time with a sling or a cast is frequently indicated. Additional utilization of heat or injections of procaine or steroids may be indicated. Manipulation of the elbow with the patient under anesthesia or surgical intervention and excision may be indicated if conservative measures are unsuccessful.

### Deep trochanteric bursitis

The deep trochanteric bursa is located behind the greater tronchanter and in front of the insertion of the gluteus maximus muscle. The chief complaint when this bursa is inflamed is marked tenderness with pain radiating down the posterior aspect of the thigh. The patient may tend to hold the leg in abduction and external rotation for comfort. Motion of the hip joint frequently produces pain. Differential diagnosis must be made between hip joint infection and osteomyelitis of the femur.

**Treatment.** Rest and heat are usually sufficient to relieve symptoms of deep trochanteric bursitis. With pyogenic infection, appropriate antibiotic therapy should be initiated.

### Superficial trochanteric bursitis

The superficial trochanteric bursa is located between the greater trochanter and the skin. Inflammation of this bursa may produce localized tenderness and edema. No pain is elicited on movement of the leg and affected hip.

**Treatment.** Conservative measures such as rest of the extremity and heat are quite successful.

### Iliopectineal or iliopsoas bursitis

The iliopectineal or iliopsoas bursa is located between the iliopsoas muscle and the iliopectineal eminence on the anterior surface of the hip joint capsule and frequently communicates with the joint cavity. Pain over the anterior aspect of the hip with femoral nerve involvement causing radiating pain down the anterior aspect of the leg is frequent. For comfort the hip may be held in flexion, abduction, and external rotation.

**Treatment.** Heat and rest of the hip joint through immobilization with traction to the lower extremity is usually successful. Antibiotic therapy should be utilized if infection is present.

### Bursitis of heel

Several bursae are found in the region of the heel. These may give rise to symptoms of pain from inflammation. Causative factors appear to be ill-fitting shoes and irritation from excessive walking or running.

**Treatment.** Heat, sponge rubber pads, or local injections with corticosteroids are often successful in treating bursitis of the heel.

### Subacromial or subdeltoid bursitis

Subacromial or subdeltoid bursitis results when the large flat bursa that covers the upper end of the humerus laterally and the shoulder joint becomes inflamed. It is often seen in persons between 40 and 50 years of age and is more common in women and in sedentary individuals. The associated pain may be extremely severe in the shoulder and may radiate into the entire upper extremity.

**Treatment.** Rest and support with application of heat are often successful. Surgery is inadvisable unless conservative measures fail.

### NEUROPATHIC JOINT DISEASE (CHARCOT JOINTS)

Neuropathic joint disease (Charcot joints) (Fig. 17-9) is a chronic progressive degenerative arthropathy affecting one or more peripheral or supinal joints.[2,p.118]

**Etiology.** Underlying neurologic disorders that may give rise to Charcot joints are tabes dorsalis of syphilitic origin, diabetic neuropathy, syringomyelia, myelomeningocele, spinal cord compression, peripheral nerve section, leprosy, and con-

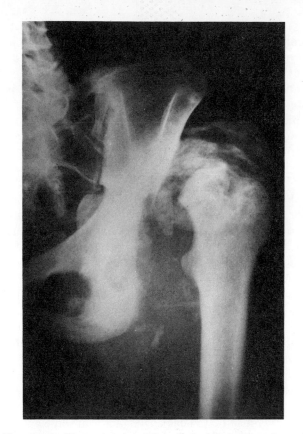

**Fig. 17-9.** Charcot joint (hip). Note total disruption of joint with extensive reactive soft tissue ossification.

genital absence of pain sensation.[2,p.118] Persons with absence or depression of pain sensation lose the protective reaction in the joint, and thus the joint is subjected to repeated strains and fractures, resulting in chronic instability of the joint.

**Pathology.** The constant destruction outstrips the process of repair of a joint with marked swelling, hemorrhage, and localized heat with both atrophic and hypertrophic bone changes.

**Incidence.** Neuropathic joint disease is seen more frequently in men than in women. It is most commonly seen in persons over the age of 40 years.

**Signs and symptoms.** The most common sign of neuropathic joint disease is notable absence of pain accompanied by swelling in the unstable joint. The involvement may be multiple in tabes-related conditions and is seen in the knee, hip, ankle, shoulder, elbow, and spine. Some patients complain of pain associated with the swelling, but not to the degree expected from the clinical and radiographic appearance of the joint. X-ray examination reveals marked osteoarthritis. Joint effusion often occurs. Compression fractures and loose bodies in the joint cavity may also occur.

**Treatment.** Early recognition is the best treatment for neuropathic joint disease to alert medical personnel and the patient to appropriate protection of the joint. Often, however, the patient is not seen until damage has already occurred and the joint is abnormal and clinically unstable. Surgical intervention is often unsuccessful because of poor healing and nonunion. In some cases amputation is necessarily the treatment of choice.

## SYNOVITIS

Synovitis is a process involving inflammation of the synovial membrane of a joint. Two forms are common: the toxic type, often seen in toddlers, and the traumatic type, which is the result of a traumatic injury.

**Etiology.** Toxic synovitis is of unknown cause. A history of streptococcal infection is occasionally seen, but it is thought that this type is most often the result of excessive utilization of the joint or undetected traumatic injury. Traumatic synovitis usually follows a twisting or jarring injury to a weight-bearing joint such as the knee or hip, which causes irritation of the membrane and formation of synovial effusion within the joint. Viral inflammation may also be the causative factor in some cases.

**Pathology.** Little pathologic change is noted in synovitis other than synovial membrane inflammation and effusion.

**Incidence.** Toxic synovitis is most frequently seen in toddlers. Traumatic synovitis may be seen at any age.

**Signs and symptoms.** The most frequent sign of synovitis is limited joint motion. Pain often accompanies the limited motion. A painful limp may result with accompanying muscle spasms. A low-grade fever may be seen with toxic synovitis. An afebrile clinical course and negative results of radiographic examination and joint aspiration differentiate synovitis from pyogenic septic joint, possible Legg-Perthes disease, or tuberculosis of the joint or bone. Results of radiographic examination are almost always negative except for possible evidence of capsule distention resulting from increased fluid accumulation within the joint.

**Treatment.** Rest of the joint with utilization of traction for immobilization is quite successful in reducing the symptoms of synovitis. Occasionally with toxic synovitis it is possible that rest without traction will accomplish the objectives, provided the rest provides for no weight bearing. Local application of heat may assist in alleviation of pain. Joint distention may be relieved by aspiration of excess joint fluid. Synovitis, in contrast to other joint disease processes, usually runs a relatively benign course and responds well to rest and immobilization.

## SUMMARY

Diseases and disorders of the joint and joint structures may be seen at any age. Multiple joint involvement may produce more significant damage, depending on the specific disease process. The multiplicity of the involvement, however, is of great concern to the diagnostician. The purpose of any joint is to permit motion. Any disease or disorder of these structures, by nature of the process or its complications (and sometimes even the treatment), endangers this function considerably. Decreased or ceased motion of major joints can cause considerable impairment of one's ability to function, and multiple joint involvement may be devastating. Early diagnosis and treatment are advocated whenever possible to avoid or minimize possible permanent joint damage and ultimate joint destruction.

## REFERENCES

1. Brashear, H. R., Jr., and Raney, R. B., Sr.: Shand's handbook of orthopaedic surgery, ed. 9, St. Louis, 1978, The C. V. Mosby Co.
2. Gartland, J. J.: Fundamentals of orthopaedics, Philadelphia, 1974, W. B. Saunders Co.
3. Turek, S.: Orthopaedics, Philadelphia, 1977, J. B. Lippincott Co.

## BIBLIOGRAPHY

Adams, J. C.: Outline of orthopaedics, Baltimore, 1971, The Williams & Wilkins Co.

Aegertu, E., and Kirkpatrick, J.: Orthopedic diseases, Philadelphia, 1975, W. B. Saunders Co.

American Orthopaedic Association: Manual of orthopaedic surgery, Chicago, 1972, The Association.

Arthritis Foundation: Arthritis manual for allied health professionals, Atlanta, 1973, The Foundation.

Aston, J. N.: A short textbook of orthopaedics and traumatology, London, 1972, English Universities Press, Ltd.

Brashear, H. R., Jr., and Raney, R. B., Sr.: Shand's handbook of orthopaedic surgery, ed. 9, St. Louis, 1978, The C. V. Mosby Co.

Brewer, E. J.: Juvenile rheumatoid arthritis, Philadelphia, 1970, W. B. Saunders Co.

Crenshaw, A. H., editor: Campbell's operative orthopaedics, ed. 5, St. Louis, 1971, The C. V. Mosby Co.

Enneking, W. F., and Sherrard, M. G.: Physical diagnosis of the musculoskeletal system, Gainesville, Fla., 1969, Storter Printing Co., Inc.

Gartland, J. J.: Fundamentals of orthopaedics, Philadelphia, 1974, W. B. Saunders Co.

Goldstein, L. A., and Dickerson, R. C.: Atlas of orthopaedic surgery, St. Louis, 1974, The C. V. Mosby Co.

Iversen, L. D., and Clawson, D. K.: Manual of acute orthopaedic therapeutics, Boston, 1977, Little, Brown & Co.

Millender, L., and Sledge, C., editors: Symposium on rheumatoid arthritis, Orthop. Clin. North Am. 6(3): 601-602, 1975.

Rosenbaum, M. G.: Understanding arthritis, St. Louis, 1975, Warren H. Green, Inc.

Rubin, A.: Handbook of congenital malformations, Philadelphia, 1969, W. B. Saunders Co.

Tachdjian, M. O.: Pediatric orthopaedics, Philadelphia, 1972, W. B. Saunders Co.

Turek, S.: Orthopaedics, Philadelphia, 1977, J. B. Lippincott Co.

# 18

# General skeletal, muscular, and associated neurologic and metabolic diseases and disorders

NANCY E. HILT

SHIRLEY B. COGBURN

Accessory muscle
Achondroplasia
Apert's syndrome (acrocephalosyndactylism)
Arthrogryposis multiplex congenita
Cerebral palsy
  Classification and terminology
Congenital absence of muscles
Diaphyseal aclasis (hereditary deforming chondroplasia, multiple cartilaginous exostosis)
Diastrophic dwarfism
Ehlers-Danlos syndrome
Fibrous dysplasia
Freidreich's ataxia
Gaucher's disease
Hyperparathyroidism (generalized osteitis fibrosa cystica, von Recklinghausen's disease of bone)
Hyperpituitarism
  Acromegaly
  Gigantism
Hypothyroidism (cretinism)
Infantile muscular atrophy (Werdnig-Hoffmann disease, amyotonia congenita, Oppenheim's disease, infantile spinal muscular atrophy)
Marfan's syndrome (arachnodactyly)
Metaphyseal dysostosis
Metaphyseal dysplasia
Mucopolysaccharidoses
  Hurler's syndrome
  Hunter's syndrome
  Sanfilippo's syndrome
  Morquio's syndrome
  Scheie's syndrome
  Maroteaux-Lamy syndrome

Muscular dystrophy (progressive muscular dystrophy, pseudohypertrophic muscular dystrophy, Duchenne muscular dystrophy)
Myasthenia gravis (Erb-Goldflam disease)
Myelomeningocele (spina bifida occulta)
  Terminology
Neurofibromatosis (von Recklinghausen's disease)
Osteogenesis imperfecta
Osteomalacia (adult rickets)
Osteopetrosis (Albers-Schonburg disease, marble bone disease)
Paget's disease (osteitis deformans)
Peroneal muscular atrophy (Charcot-Marie-Tooth disease)
Poliomyelitis
Progressive diaphyseal dysplasia (Engelmann's disease)
Rickets
Scurvy

Many of the diseases and disorders discussed thus far are relative to a specific anatomic area of the musculoskeletal system. These diseases, however, comprise only a portion of the total number that may affect the musculoskeletal system. Some muscular and skeletal processes are more general and have effects on the entire system. In addition many neurologic and metabolic processes have musculoskeletal implications. These diseases and disorders are presented in this chapter. They are not categorized specifically or classified as to cause or origin because of their multiple effects. It is suggested that the anatomy and physiology of the musculoskeletal and neurologic systems be reviewed for total comprehension of the implications of these processes (see Chapters 1 and 2). In most cases the pathophysiologic implications of these diseases and disorders are not discussed in depth; rather, those disease processes that have significant musculoskeletal implications are presented.

## ACCESSORY MUSCLE

An accessory muscle is the anatomic duplication of a muscle. It may appear anywhere in the muscular system but is relatively rare. The most common sign associated with an accessory muscle is the appearance of a soft tissue mass. Differential diagnosis without surgical intervention and exploration is difficult because of the similar appearance of some tumors or soft tissue masses such as ganglia. The appearance of the soft tissue mass may be transient or constant, depending on the location of the accessory muscle in relation to motion. In many cases specific treatment is not indicated unless the accessory muscle interferes with normal function.

## ACHONDROPLASIA

Achondroplasia is the most common type of dwarfism, resulting from a developmental abnormality of endochondral ossification in which there is failure of normal ossification of the long bones but not of the flat bones.

**Etiology.** The primary cause of achondroplasia is a germ plasm defect that results in failure of endochondral ossification. This is usually apparent at approximately the end of the second month of fetal development. It is transmitted by an autosomal dominant gene, with transmission occurring from a male achondroplastic by mendelian dominance, resulting in a 50% chance that the disease will appear in the offspring. There is some consideration currently being given to maternal age as a possible contributing factor.[5,pp.278-279]

**Pathology.** In achondroplasia the endochondral ossification process at the epiphyseal growth plate of the long bones is disturbed. Normal calcification of the cartilage is replaced by a process producing vascularization and degeneration. The longitudinal growth of the bone is retarded, while periosteal ossification continues at a normal rate and assures the appropriate diameter of the bones.[5,p.279;6,p.323]

**Incidence.** Achondroplasia is seen more frequently in females than in males.

**Signs and symptoms.** Characteristic skeletal features of achondroplasia are obvious at birth. The trunk length is normal while the limbs are short and the head enlarged. The hands present the typical trident appearance: the overall appearance of the hand is short and broad, with the second and third fingers spread, forming a V-shaped space. The musculature of the body is often overdeveloped. Intelligence and sexual development are usually normal. Differential diagnosis must be established between achondroplasia and a number of disorders that simulate this process, such as osteogenesis imperfecta, rickets, cretinism, and Morquio's and Hurler's syndromes.[5,p.287;6,p.323]

Radiographic features of achondroplasia are relatively characteristic. All of the long bones are short, although the clavicles and fibulae are less affected; therefore the fibulae may be longer than the tibiae. Diaphyses of the long bones are normal in diameter. The sacrum is narrowed, and the spine is of normal length, but ossification centers in the vertebrae may be small. The skull is large with marked shortness in the base because of the retarded growth. The foramen magnum is small and funnel shaped. Except for the characteristic flattened appearance of the face, with the root of the nose depressed, the facial bones are not involved.[5,pp.281,286]

**Treatment.** Premature births are frequent with achondroplasia, most being stillbirths or failing to survive beyond the first year of life. Those who do survive are usually healthy and have normal life spans. Achondroplasia does not usually require specific treatment, although ruptured intravertebral discs in the adult may necessitate laminectomy and excision. Gait and appearance may be improved by correction of the varus deformity of the tibia or femur.[6,p.323]

## APERT'S SYNDROME (ACROCEPHALOSYNDACTYLISM)

Apert's syndrome is a rare condition of unknown cause with characteristic craniofacial appearance in combination with partial or complete syndactyly of the hands and feet.

**Etiology.** The specific cause of Apert's syndrome is unknown, but it appears to be the result of a primary germplasm defect.

**Pathology.** Characteristic pathologic features of Apert's syndrome include premature synostosis of the cranial bones and syndactyly of the hands and feet, with resultant growth disturbances.

**Incidence.** Apert's syndrome is relatively rare.

**Signs and symptoms.** The following are characteristic signs of Apert's syndrome[5,p.252]:

1. Head characteristically peaked and vertically elongated
2. Eyes widespread and bulging
3. Increased intracranial pressure with associated signs and symptoms

4. High, arched posterior palate often present with bony defects of the maxilla and mandible
5. Mental retardation may be present
6. Partial or complete syndactyly of metatarsals, metacarpals, or digits

The degree of syndactyly present varies greatly; it may be complete with apparent fusion of all digits externally.

**Treatment.** Osteotomy of the cranial bones is performed to prevent increased intracranial pressure. If the infant survives the syndactyly is surgically corrected, with the specific procedure depending on the severity of the deformity.

## ARTHROGRYPOSIS MULTIPLEX CONGENITA

Arthrogryposis multiplex congenita (Figs. 18-1 and 18-2) is an extremely disabling condition of unknown origin characterized by multiple congenital contractures of joints, particularly the hips, knees, elbows, and wrists, as a result of incomplete fibrous ankylosis of the involved joints.

**Etiology.** The cause of arthrogryposis multiplex congenita is unknown. It has been suggested that it is the result of a congenital defect of the anterior horn cells of the spinal cord in association with the maintenance of a fixed position in utero.[6,p.630]

**Pathology.** The pathologic features of arthrogryposis multiplex congenita are suggestive of several disease entities (Table 18-1); therefore, the condition is considered a syndrome. Tachdjian subdivides this syndrome into the following forms, which are reflective of their pathologic features[5,p.235]:

1. *Neuropathic:* shows reduction in number and size of anterior horn cells and in size of spinal cord; brain may be underdeveloped

**Fig. 18-1.** Arthrogryposis. **A,** Dysplastic hips with bilateral dislocation, severe muscle atrophy. **B,** Forearm flexion contracture at wrist, extension contracture at elbow, severe muscle atrophy.

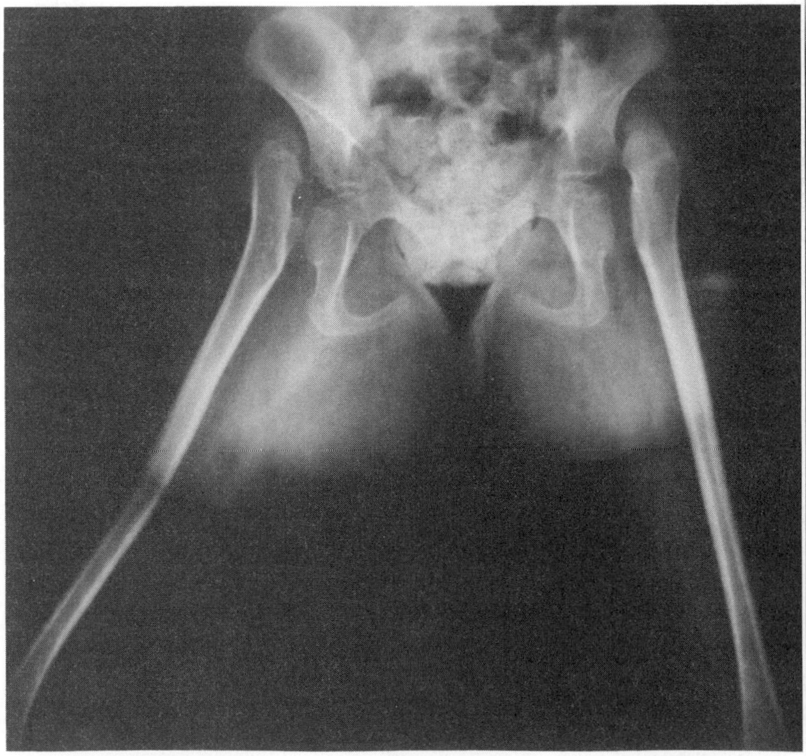

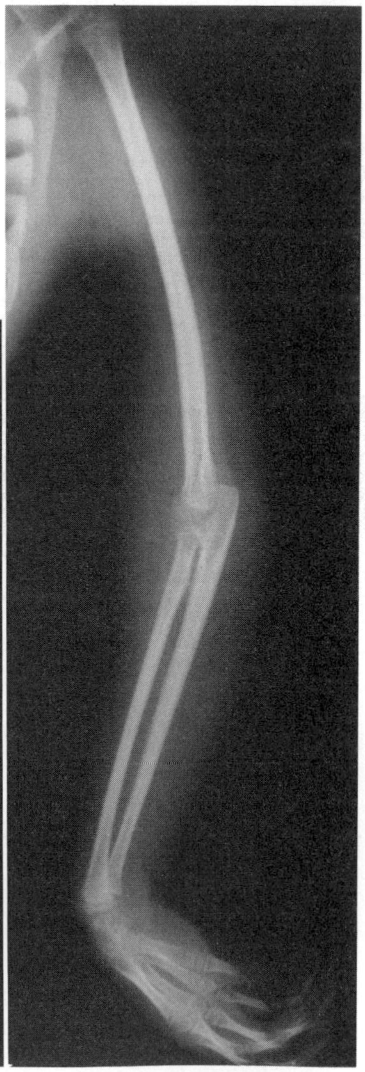

2. *Myopathic:* demonstrates fibrous fatty muscular alterations
3. *Mixed:* demonstrates findings of both neuropathic and myopathic forms

In the *neuropathic form* the outstanding feature is reduction, degeneration, or absence of the anterior horn cells. The spinal cord is decreased in size, usually in the lumbar and cervical regions. In the affected limb the muscles may be normal or they may be small or even absent and replaced by fat and fibrous tissue. In the *myopathic form* alterations of the central nervous system are not present. On microscop-

ic examination the affected muscles reveal fibrous and fatty degeneration. There is an increase in the endomysial connective tissue. Alterations in the joints are similar to those found in the neuropathic form. The *mixed form* may reveal varying degrees of pathologic findings of the other two forms.[5, p. 242]

The pathologic features associated with the joint structures are similar in all types of arthrogryposis multiplex congenita. The gross pathologic feature is contracture of the involved joints attributed to the apparent lack of musculature surrounding the joint. The joints most frequently involved are the ankles,

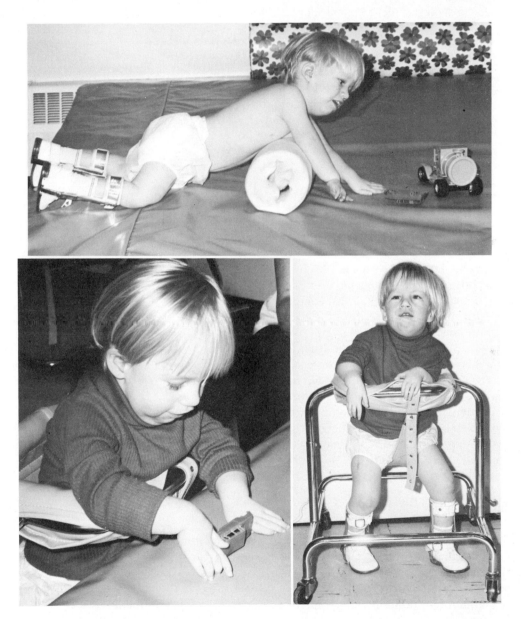

**Fig. 18-2.** Arthrogryposis multiplex congenita. Typical joint deformities acquired from this process as well as limitation of motion may be noted in this child. (From Hilt, N. E., and Schmitt, E. W., Jr.: Pediatric orthopedic nursing, St. Louis, 1975, The C. V. Mosby Co.)

**Table 18-1.** Pathologic features of classifications of arthrogryposis multiplex congenita[5, pp.235,242]

| Classification | Pathologic features |
|---|---|
| Neuropathic | Reduction, degeneration, or absence of anterior horn cells |
| | Spinal cord decreased in size, usually in the lumbar and cervical regions |
| | Muscles normal, small, or absent and replaced by fat and fibrous tissue |
| | Muscle biopsy shows denervation atrophy |
| | Possible cerebral defects and corticospinal tract atrophy |
| | Joints show destruction of articular surfaces; degenerative changes and capsular thickening occur later |
| Myopathic | No central nervous system alterations |
| | Muscles show fibrous and fatty degeneration |
| | Increase in endomysial connective tissue |
| | Joints show findings similar to neuropathic form with late degenerative changes |
| Mixed | Varying degrees of features of neuropathic and myopathic forms |

**Table 18-2.** Surgical procedures utilized for common deformities of arthrogryposis multiplex congenita[5,p.243; 6,p.631]

| Deformity | Surgical procedure(s) |
|---|---|
| Equinovarus of foot | Heel cord lengthening |
| | Soft tissue release and Achilles tenotomy |
| | Posterior tibial tendon transfer |
| | Capsulotomy of ankle, subtalar and tarsometatarsal joints |
| | Metatarsal osteotomy |
| | Cuboid decancellation |
| | Dwyer osteotomy of os calcis |
| | Triple arthrodesis |
| Knee flexion contracture | Supracondylar osteotomy |
| | Posterior capsulotomy |
| | Hamstring tenotomy |
| Hip flexion deformity | Adductor tenotomy |
| | Osteotomy at skeletal maturity |
| Dislocation of hip | Open reduction if closed reduction fails |
| | Salter's innominate osteotomy |
| Thumb contracture | Adductor myotomy |
| Wrist contracture | Arthrodesis at skeletal maturity |
| | Osteotomy to improve functional position |
| Elbow contracture | Capsulotomy |
| | Pectoralis major transfer |
| Shoulder contracture | Derotational osteotomy of upper third of humerus |
| Spinal deformities | Fusion for severe scoliotic curvature with possible intraoperative instrumentation |

knees, hips, elbows, and wrists. Microscopic or radiographic pathologic features in the joint structures are not apparent early in the process. Many of the later alterations, including degeneration and destruction of the articular surfaces, are secondary to the primary deformities.

**Signs and symptoms.** Arthrogryposis multiplex congenita involves a variety of deformities that are present at birth. The symptoms are not progressive but may be quite severe initially. One or all four extremities may be involved, although the latter is most frequently seen. The axial skeleton is rarely involved, although in rare instances associated spinal deformities may be seen. The syndrome is clinically characterized by the following signs and symptoms present to varying degrees in the affected extremities[5,p.242]:

1. Muscular wasting
2. Decreased active and passive motion of the joints
3. Absence of normal skin creases
4. No sensory deficit
5. Diminished or absent deep tendon reflexes
6. Possible mental retardation in the neuropathic form
7. Dislocated hips, clubfeet, subluxed or dislocated knees, and subluxed or dislocated shoulders, elbows, and wrists

The overall appearance of the infant is that of a wooden doll. The joints are fixed in flexion and external rotation at the hips, flexion and internal rotation at the shoulders, and severe flexion at the elbows and knees. Limited mobility is characteristic. Scoliosis is sometimes present with trunk involvement.

**Treatment.** Although the deformities associated with arthrogryposis multiplex congenita are not progressive, lack of treatment can lead to worsening of the condition. In addition the deformities tend to recur after treatment. Treatment is begun early and continued throughout the growth period because of the strong tendency toward recurrence of the deformities. Initially deformities are corrected by cast therapy, and correction is maintained through the

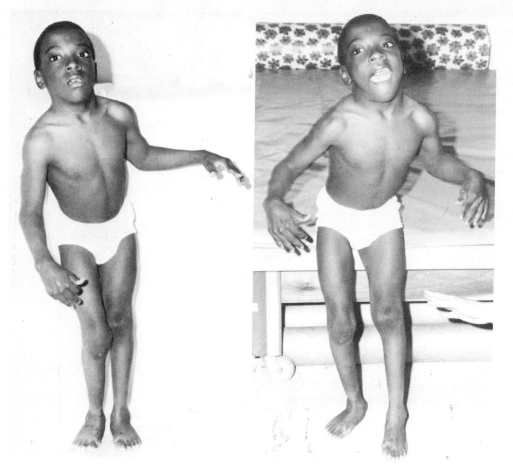

**Fig. 18-3.** Cerebral palsy. Note spasticity characteristic of this disease. (From Hilt, N. E., and Schmitt, E. W., Jr.: Pediatric orthopedic nursing, St. Louis, 1975, The C. V. Mosby Co.)

utilization of bivalved casts and braces. Surgical intervention is required when conservative measures fail. Even with use of both casts and braces, full range of motion and function are not possible, but considerable improvement may be obtained. Weight bearing and ambulation are the primary objectives of treatment of the lower extremity deformities, while maximum function is the therapeutic goal for the upper extremities. If surgical intervention is required, the procedure of choice is dependent on the anatomic area of the deformity, the degree of correction already obtained through nonsurgical methods, and the desired result. Some of the most common procedures chosen for the correction of arthrogryposis multiplex congenita are given in Table 18-2. Early diagnosis and implementation of treatment are of utmost importance to maximize the result potentials.[1;5,p.243]

## CEREBRAL PALSY

Cerebral palsy (Fig. 18-3) includes muscular dysfunction and other associated symptomatology re-

sulting from a fixed, nonprogressive brain lesion that develops during the prenatal period, at birth, or during the early postnatal period.[5,p.769] The signs and symptoms of cerebral palsy are quite broad and sometimes rather obscure. In some cases musculoskeletal involvement is quite incapacitating, while in others it may produce only minimal muscular dysfunction and related dysfunctions of speech and hearing. Convulsions or mental retardation may be the primary handicap associated with cerebral palsy. More often than not a combination of symptoms of varying degrees exists.

**Classification and terminology.** Multiple classifications for cerebral palsy and its associated symptomatology have been suggested, and no single classification is utilized uniformly. These classifications are based on state of muscle tone, alterations in muscle tone, clinical manifestations, neurologic involvement, and etiologic factors. Tachdjian has extensively reviewed many of the classifications proposed and utilized over the last 30 years. He suggests that the most commonly utilized are modifications of the Phelps classification, generally based on the state of muscular tone present or absent, as follows[3;5,p.772]:

| | |
|---|---|
| Spastic | Tremor |
|   Aspastic |   Unclassified |
|   Spastic |     Paraplegia |
|     Monoplegia |     Quadriplegia |
|     Hemiplegia |     Monoplegia |
|     Paraplegia |     Recovered |
|     Triplegia | Rigidity |
|     Quadriplegia |   Intermittent |
|   Basilar |   Continuous |
| Athetosis |   Miscellaneous |
|   Tension |     Hemiplegia |
|   Nontension |     Paraplegia |
|   Dystonic |     Triplegia |
|   Flail |     Quadriplegia |
|   Arm, neck | Tremor |
|   Deaf |   Intention |
|   Shudder |   Constant |
|   Hemiathetoid | Ataxia |
|   Cerebellar release |   Cerebellar |
|   Rotary |   Eighth nerve |
|   Emotional release | |

The classifications of cerebral palsy are not only useful in defining the area of involvement but also may be descriptive of this involvement. It is suggested that all classifications as outlined by Tachdjian be reviewed to further familiarize the reader with the process of cerebral palsy.

Common to all of the classifications proposed for the diagnosis of cerebral palsy are terms reflective of the area of involvement. Familiarization with this terminology is helpful in the comprehension of the total process:

**monoplegia** involvement of single extremity.
**diplegia** involvement of both upper extremities.
**hemiplegia** involvement of upper extremity and lower extremity on same side of body.
**paraplegia** involvement of both lower extremities.
**triplegia** involvement of three extremities.
**quadriplegia** involvement of all four extremities.
**tetraplegia** utilized interchangeably with quadraplegia.

**Etiology.** The etiologic factors of cerebral palsy are multiple and may occur *prenatally, during birth,* or *postnatally* (Table 18-3).

Prenatal considerations include the following:
1. Family history of cerebral palsy, neurologic disease, mental retardation
2. Maternal disease during the first trimester of pregnancy
3. Inborn errors of metabolism

Etiologic factors occurring during the birth process include the following:

1. Premature birth
2. Mechanical trauma
3. Prolonged labor
4. Fetal hypoxia
5. Prolonged anoxia as a result of excessive sedation, umbilical cord around the infant's neck, and so on
6. Aspiration of mucus or amniotic fluid

Postnatal causes of cerebral palsy include:
1. Infection
2. Convulsions
3. Head trauma
4. Vascular lesions
5. Rh incompatability

A higher incidence of postnatal factors is apparent in premature infants.

**Pathology.** The pathologic features of cerebral palsy are greatly dependent on the clinical type.

**Table 18-3.** Etiologic factors in cerebral palsy[1,5,6]

| | Possible cause |
|---|---|
| Prenatal | Maternal disease during first trimester of pregnancy (e.g., rubella, toxoplasmosis, syphylis) |
| | Toxemia of pregnancy |
| | Inherited metabolic defects |
| | Excessive irradiation |
| | Known family history of cerebral palsy, congenital malformation, or neurologic disease |
| | Congenital anomalies |
| During birth process | Traumatic injury |
| |   Improperly applied forceps |
| |   Excessive uterine contractures |
| |   Precipitous delivery causing sudden pressure alterations |
| | Prematurity |
| | Excessive maternal sedation |
| | Infant aspiration of mucus or amniotic fluid |
| | Anoxia-hypoxia |
| |   Umbilical cord around infant's neck |
| |   Tracheal obstruction |
| | Cerebral hemorrhage |
| Postnatal | Convulsions |
| | Head injury |
| | Encephalitis, meningitis, other infectious diseases |
| | Vascular lesions |
| | Rh incompatability |

Pathologic alterations within the central nervous system are reflected through varying degrees of spasticity, hyperkinesia, athetosis, and ataxia. Each of these pathologic features, regardless of severity, is considered abnormal and reflective of the process. Intracranial hemorrhage and resultant tissue destruction appear to be the major pathologic features. The specific features are also reflective of the area of the brain to which damage and destruction have resulted. Specific pathologic features relative to the clinical type of the disease and the area to which the damage has occurred are given in Table 18-4. The severity of the characteristics in most cases reflects the extent to which destruction or damage has occurred.

**Incidence.** Incidence of cerebral palsy is relatively high, being seen in approximately seven of 100,000 births. Of these seven, approximately one child does not survive infancy, two are severely mentally retarded, one is severely handicapped to the extent that treatment is often ineffective, and one is affected to such a mild degree that treatment is often not required. A relatively high number of patients with cerebral palsy were born prematurely. There is also a high incidence of cerebral palsy in children of mothers who had complications during the pregnancy or previous abortions. Approximately 50% to 60% of patients with cerebral palsy have the spastic type, approximately 20% to 25% have the athetoid type, 1% to 5% have the ataxic type, 5% to 7% have the rigid type, and the remainder have a mixed variety of symptoms.[1,2,p.149;5,p.780]

**Signs and symptoms.** The clinical picture associated with cerebral palsy varies depending on the location and extent of the lesion. The infant with cerebral palsy is late in the normal developmental

**Table 18-4.** Pathophysiologic features of central nervous system involvement in cerebral palsy[5,pp.778-780]

| Clinical type | Causative factor | Incidence | Characteristics |
|---|---|---|---|
| Spastic: increased muscular tension with passive lengthening | Lesion in cerebral cortex (tends to eliminate motor control system) permits reception of excessive impulses from lower motor neurons | 70% | Hyperreflexia<br>Spasticity pulls limbs into flexion<br>Elbow flexed, forearm pronated, wrist flexed, fingers flexed with thumb adducted in palm<br>Lower extremity adducted, hip joint flexed and internally rotated, knees flexed, equinus deformity of foot, dorsiflexed great toe<br>Scissor gait characteristic if both extremities affected |
| Athetoid: fluctuation of posture superimposed on persistent attitude | Subcortical lesion in basal ganglia | 20% | Purposeless, involuntary muscular movements<br>  Excitement exaggerates movements<br>  Attempts to accomplish purposeful movements tend to exaggerate purposeless movements<br>Reflexes normal<br>Absent stretch reflex<br>Rh incompatability<br>  Hearing loss<br>  Limited vertical eye movement<br>Possible muscular tremor<br>Possible muscular rigidity |
| Ataxic: destruction of all kinesthetic sense producing lack of control and coordination | Cerebellum | 10% | Disruption of balance<br>Asynergy or dysynergy<br>  Loss of muscular control<br>  Loss of muscular coordination<br>Dysdiadochokinesia or adiadochokinesia<br>  Alternate movements carried out slowly, irregularly, or clumsily<br>Dysmetria<br>  Inability to judge distance, speed, or power of movement<br>Intention tremor<br>Hyporeflexia<br>Muscular rigidity<br>Nystagmus |

milestones requiring muscular control, such as sitting, standing, and walking. The face may be expressionless, and the child may drool or grimace. Motion is usually uncoordinated and jerky.

The characteristic deformities of the upper extremity are shoulder adduction with internal rotation, elbow flexion with forearm pronation, wrist and finger flexion, and thumb adduction into the palm. The child, when supported under the arms in a standing position, holds the lower extremities tightly together in a scissors fashion. The heels frequently cannot be placed flat on the floor when standing or walking. Attempts of the child to move one part of the extremity precipitate other muscular spasms; clonus is often seen. Athetosis gradually appears within the first 2 years. On physical examination the deep reflexes are usually hyperactive. The child may have convulsions to varying degrees of frequency and severity. Speech disturbances may be present or speech development may be retarded. Other sensory disturbances, including difficulties with perception and hearing, are frequent. Some degree of mental retardation is common.[5,pp.780-786;6,pp.497-498]

Other signs and symptoms reflective of the specific area involved are given in Table 18-5. It must be emphasized that the symptomatology exhibited may vary tremendously from very mild to very severe and does not have to be all-inclusive. The severity of the lesion determines not only the severity of the symptoms but also the combination of symptoms seen.

**Treatment.** A multidisciplinary approach is necessary in the planning and implementation of a total therapeutic regimen for the patient with cerebral palsy. Health care professionals most frequently involved include the nurse, occupational and physical therapists, pediatrician, orthopedic surgeon, neurologist, psychologist, speech therapist, audiologist, and social worker. The treatment plan must be individualized because of the multiple implications of the disease process. Treatment considerations are long term and planned around the developmental changes that occur with growth. The overall goal of treatment is to make the child as independent as possible, with function and mobility of primary importance. The degree of mental retardation present is a great consideration in the determination of a treatment modality and, if incapacitating, may be a deterrent to functional goals otherwise obtainable. Many of the decisions involved in the treatment of children with cerebral palsy must be made as a team effort for achievement of maximum goals and objectives. Decisions made regarding treatment during childhood are crucial in relation to ability to function independently as an adult.

Although the specific therapeutic modalities included in an individualized treatment plan are greatly dependent on the severity and type of cerebral palsy, nonsurgical intervention is always utilized to varying degrees in an attempt to rehabilitate the child through reeducation. Training in techniques of balance and posture, mobility or locomotion, muscular relaxation, rhythmic exercises, and speech is started as soon after the diagnosis is made as possible. Bracing may be required to assist in stability for ambulation and to provide general muscular control. Coordination exercises are also of great value in improving and maintaining control of various muscle groups. Diversion exercises and repetitious unaided individual efforts are also somewhat effective and contribute to improvement of muscular control. Continued stress on the growing skeleton from muscle imbalance results in structural bony deformity, especially of the hip joint.[6,p.498]

With progressive development of deformity, the

**Table 18-5.** Location of lesion and manifestations of cerebral palsy[6,p.498]

| Location of lesion | Manifestations |
| --- | --- |
| Cerebral cortex | |
| Premotor area | Increased muscular tone |
| | Exaggerated deep tendon reflexes |
| | Clonus |
| | Pathologic reflexes |
| | Stretch reflex |
| Motor area | Decreased muscular tone |
| | Decreased deep tendon reflexes |
| | Abnormal elongation of muscle |
| Cerebellum | Ataxia |
| | Loss of sense of balance |
| | Lack of muscular coordination |
| | Dysdiadochokinesia |
| | Nystagmus |
| | Dizziness |
| Basal ganglia | Athetosis (irregular, arrhythmic, involuntary movements) |
| | Expressionless face, uncontrolled facial twitching, grimacing |
| | Increased muscular tension during attempts to control involuntary movements |
| Diffuse | General muscular rigidity |
| | Loss of muscular elasticity |
| | No stretch reflex |
| | Mental deficiency (usually) to varying degrees |

treatment of choice is surgical intervention, even when conservative measures are being implemented. Patients with spastic cerebral palsy benefit most from surgical procedures. Surgery is contraindicated in the athetoid form of cerebral palsy and in those who are severely mentally retarded. If possible surgery should be postponed until the child is 5 to 7 years of age.[2,p.152;6,p.500] Goals of surgical intervention include the following:

1. Diminishment of muscle spasm through surgical procedures on motor nerves (e.g., neurectomy)
2. Correction of joint contractures and deformities
3. Restoration of muscle balance by equalizing the power of opposing muscles (e.g., tendon transplants)
4. Stabilization of poorly controlled joints (e.g., fusion)

The most common deformities associated with cerebral palsy and seen in the foot and ankle are equinovarus and valgus deformities. Although these deformities may pose problems in ambulation, the equinus deformity is of the greatest concern. A heel cord lengthening procedure is often required to alleviate this deformity and permit weight bearing with the foot flat on the floor. Deformities of the hip including adduction, flexion, and external rotation are also extremely common in patients with spastic cerebral palsy. These deformities produce the commonly associated scissors gait and frequently require release of the tight musculature through an adductor tenotomy, adductor myotomy, or other procedures. Other flexion deformities, especially of the knee and elbow, may require surgical release for ambulatory and functional considerations. Of all deformities of the upper extremity, those that act as a deterrent to actualization of functional utilization of the hands and arms are those that most frequently require surgical release or transfer procedures in attempts to promote maximum potential. Numerous surgical procedures may be accomplished for the patient with cerebral palsy but must be individualized to the specific needs of the patient.[5,pp.786-787]

Specific postoperative considerations are important. Muscle spasms are frequent with the types of immobilization utilized and are of special concern when a cast is required; continued friction over joints from the spasms may be the source of pressure areas under the cast and requires accurate and continued observation for early detection of problems. After the acute phase of immobilization following a surgical procedure, exercises are accomplished to maintain improved motion; difficulties may be encountered in accomplishing these exercises, dependent on the age of the child and the degree of mental retardation present. Continuation of the total therapeutic regimen postoperatively is important to maximize the results of the surgical procedure and to ensure that there is no loss of function in other areas.

## CONGENITAL ABSENCE OF MUSCLES

Congenital absence of muscles is relatively uncommon. A skeletal muscle may be partially or entirely absent and, although a singular muscle is usually affected, a group may be absent. Any muscle may be affected, with the pectoralis the most frequently involved. The condition is most often unilateral, although bilateral involvement may be seen. The signs and symptoms associated with this anomaly are dependent on the area and function of the muscle involved. Congenital absence of a muscle is nonprogressive and produces functional disabilities to varying degrees.

## DIAPHYSEAL ACLASIS (HEREDITARY DEFORMING CHONDROPLASIA, MULTIPLE CARTILAGINOUS EXOSTOSIS)

Diaphyseal aclasis is a relatively uncommon disease of the skeletal system. It is hereditary and characterized by multiple exostoses or bony protrusions.

**Etiology.** Diaphyseal aclasis is hereditary and transmitted as a dominant trait. Approximately half of the children of an individual with diaphyseal aclasis exhibit varying degrees of manifestations of the disease.

**Pathology.** The exostoses or bony protrusions that are characteristic of diaphyseal aclasis are radiographically and microscopically similar to osteochondroma. Diffuse involvement is seen, with the long bones usually affected more severely and more frequently than the short bones. Dependent on the specific area involved, various angular or rotational deformities may result.[5,p.498]

**Incidence.** Diaphyseal aclasis is usually bilateral and is seen more frequently in boys than in girls.

**Signs and symptoms.** Although diaphyseal aclasis is hereditary, manifestations are usually not evident until 2 years of age or older. It is not uncommon for children to be examined solely because a parent has the condition. Pain is not usually associated with the exostoses and if present is usually minimal. The major sign of the process is the noticeable protrusions in the areas of the exostoses. Deformities of the extremities may be noted depending on the severity and location of the exostoses. Radiographic examination reveals a broadened metaphyseal area, and the specific lesion is exhibited by abnormal continuity and decreased density.[5,pp.498,501]

**Treatment.** Asymptomatic lesions characteristic of diaphyseal aclasis generally require little or no treatment other than continued observation. Those lesions located near the joint that interfere with joint motion or produce neurovascular impairment from pressure may be surgically excised. Angular or rotational deformities resulting from the lesions may require surgical correction to facilitate improved function. Lower extremity length inequalities resulting from unilateral involvement may require epiphysiodesis. A small percentage of these lesions may undergo malignant transformation.[5,pp.501-502]

## DIASTROPHIC DWARFISM

Diastrophic dwarfism is an extremely rare type of micromelic dwarfism associated with and accompanied by clubfeet, scoliosis, and hitchhiker's deformity of the hand.

**Etiology.** Diastrophic dwarfism is transmitted as an autosomal-recessive trait.

**Pathology.** The major pathologic feature of diastrophic dwarfism appears to be a "lack of normal columnation and calcification within the growth plate, indicating a disorder of cartilage cells and a deficit of motor neurons."[5,p.335]

**Incidence.** Diastrophic dwarfism is extremely rare.

**Signs and symptoms.** Signs and symptoms of diastrophic dwarfism are apparent at birth and include the following[5,p.339]:

1. Severely dwarfed body with extremely short extremities
2. Bilateral clubfoot
3. Deformities of ear
4. Possible cleft palate
5. Short, broad hands
6. Thumb fixed in a position perpendicular to the other digits ("hitchhiker's thumb"), the most distinguishable feature of this type of dwarfism

Scoliosis associated with this type of dwarfism is not present at birth but develops as the child begins to sit and walk. Lower extremity dislocations at the knee and the hip are also common as these developmental milestones are reached. Ambulation and functional abilities are tremendously hindered by the multiple deformities. Radiographic examination reveals the deformities appropriate for the age of the child, with appearance of the ossification centers of the epiphyses of long bones delayed. The long bones are short and thick with flared metaphyses.[5,p.339]

**Treatment.** Conservative and supportive measures are the treatment of choice for diastrophic dwarfism. The deformities that exist or result are frequently nonresponsive to usual treatment modalities, and even when some success is encountered, the deformities often recur. Orthoses are sometimes useful in the prevention of deformity progression. Surgical intervention may be required to correct components of clubfeet sufficiently to promote ambulation or correct resulting dislocations.[5,p.341]

## EHLERS-DANLOS SYNDROME

Ehlers-Danlos syndrome is a hereditary disorder characterized by hypermobility of the joints, increased elasticity of the skin, and fragility of the walls of the blood vessels.

**Etiology.** Ehlers-Danlos syndrome is a rare inherited autosomal-dominant trait "caused by faulty organization of collagen bundles into an intermeshing network."[5,p.250]

**Signs and symptoms.** Ehlers-Danlos syndrome is characterized by hypermobility or hyperextensibility of the joints, creating what is commonly known as an increased degree of "loose-jointedness." The joints may be longitudinally extended or pulled apart to a greater degree than usually seen. Associated with these joint features are increase in the elasticity of the skin as well as increased fragility of the walls of the blood vessels, creating easy bruising of the tissues. Recurrent joint dislocations, especially of the knee, hip, and shoulder, are often seen, and genu recurvatum may also be present. Scoliosis may develop but is not a striking clinical feature.

**Treatment.** Specific treatment of Ehlers-Danlos syndrome is not usually indicated. Management is directed toward symptomatic relief.

## FIBROUS DYSPLASIA

Fibrous dysplasia is a generalized skeletal condition characterized by the fibrous displacement of osseous tissue within the affected bones.

**Etiology.** The specific cause of fibrous dysplasia is unknown; indications are that it is of developmental or congenital origin.

**Pathology.** Pathologic features of fibrous dysplasia reveal three distinct classifications[1;5,p.515]:

**monostotic** only one bone involved.
**polyostotic** more than one bone involved.

**polyostotic with associated endocrine disturbances** more than one bone involved and associated with a variety of endocrine abnormalities including precocious puberty and hyperthyroidism (Albright's syndrome).

Any bone may be affected with the monostotic type; with the polyostotic type a segmental distribution of the involved bones is usually seen. All of the bones involved have varying degrees of the characteristic fibrous replacement of the osseous tissue. Irregular continuity of bone involvement is usually present, and angular deformities may be seen. Bulging of the involved tissue may be noted with a thin cortex.[6,p.637]

**Incidence.** The onset of fibrous dysplasia is usually during childhood, progressing beyond puberty and through adulthood. There is discrepancy in the relationship of incidence among the sexes, varying from being equal to females being affected two to three times as frequently.[1,5,p.515,6,p.637]

**Signs and symptoms.** The onset of symptoms associated with fibrous dysplasia is usually during early childhood, although diagnosis may be delayed until adolescence or even early adulthood if symptoms are minimal. The initial complaints are a limp, pain, or fracture at the affected site. The female may have early onset of menses and breast development and early epiphyseal closure. Albright's syndrome usually is diagnosed on the basis of a triad of symptoms including the polyostotic type of fibrous dysplasia, café au lait patches on the skin, and precocious puberty. Pathologic fractures are frequently associated with this process, and angulation deformities may follow. The involved extremity may be shortened, with the classic "shepherd's crook" deformity of the femur common. Radiographic examination reveals a well-circumscribed lesion occupying all or a portion of the shaft of the long bone, with appearance very similar to a unicameral bone cyst. Differential diagnosis must be established.[1,5,p.515,6,pp.638-639]

**Treatment.** When symptoms are mild and limited, fibrous dysplasia usually progresses slowly. Fractures heal with conservative treatment; however, often there are residual deformities. Weight-bearing bones that fracture should be treated by open reduction, bone graft, and internal fixation. Radiation therapy may provoke malignant degeneration and is therefore not advocated. If there is increased pain or alterations seen on radiographic examination, biopsy should be performed. Epiphyseal arrest may be utilized for leg length discrepancies resulting from the primary process or its resultant deformities.[5,p.525,6,639-642]

## FRIEDREICH'S ATAXIA

Friedreich's ataxia is a hereditary or familial disorder involving primarily the posterior columns of the spinal cord. It is progressive and is characterized by ataxia, weakness of the lower extremities, and a characteristic gait.

**Etiology.** Friedreich's ataxia may be hereditary or familial and is a disorder exhibiting both dominant and recessive inheritance patterns.[2,p.155]

**Pathology.** The primary pathologic feature of Friedreich's ataxia is "an extensive degeneration or sclerosis of the posterior columns of the spinal cord" with possible "involvement of the spinocerebellar tracts and later of the corticospinal tracts."[1]

**Incidence.** Males and females are affected equally, with manifestations usually occurring between 5 and 20 years of age. The highest incidence of onset is at puberty.

**Signs and symptoms.** The onset of Friedreich's ataxia is insidious. The characteristically ataxic gait may progress to severe disability. Over a period of years the child may also develop ataxia of the upper extremities. He may have difficulty with writing or simple maneuvers such as handling silverware while eating. Cavus deformity, or clawfoot, characterized by a high, curved longitudinal arch, prominence of the metatarsal heads, and clawing of the toes, is present. The gait is very unsteady with a wide base. The stance is also unsteady. There may be a positive Romberg's sign. Babinski's sign is present with decreased or absent deep reflexes. The speech is slurred and staccato, and there is tremor of the head. Tachycardia and cardiac failure may be seen as complications of the disease process. Thoracic scoliosis is present in approximately 80% to 90% of the patients. All of the signs and symptoms are progressive, with severity relative to the time span of progression.[1,5,p.877]

**Treatment.** Curative treatment is not available to the patient with Friedreich's ataxia. Orthoses may be useful to varying degrees in the prevention of associated deformities and maintenance of an ambulatory status. Correction of the foot deformity allows the patient to remain ambulatory for as long as possible and is preferred when lack of progression of the disease process is demonstrated, thereby decreasing potential recurrence. Spinal fusion may correct the scoliosis and is especially useful when there is a question of cardiopulmonary compromise. Death usually is due to myocardial failure.[5,p.877]

## GAUCHER'S DISEASE

Gaucher's disease is a relatively rare metabolic disorder in which there is an accumulation of

Gaucher's cells in the spleen, liver, bone marrow, and other sites.

**Etiology.** Gaucher's disease is hereditary, transmitted as an autosomal-recessive trait and occasionally as autosomal-dominant. The pathologic alterations are the result of an accumulation of large numbers of Gaucher's cells in the spleen, liver, bone marrow, and other sites.

**Pathology.** Although pathologic features of Gaucher's disease include the accumulation of Gaucher's cells, histiocytes laden with a cerebroside known as *kerasin* may involve the spleen, liver, bone marrow, and other sites. Of primary importance here are the accumulation in the bone and bone marrow. The major pathologic feature of accumulation within the skeletal system is the infiltration of these cells to tumorlike proportions, which erode the involved tissue and cause expansion of the cortex. The process may be acute or chronic.[5,p.427;6,p.669]

**Incidence.** A high incidence of Gaucher's disease is seen in Jewish persons. Both sexes are affected equally, with the acute form most often seen in infants and the chronic form associated with children and adults.

**Signs and symptoms.** Gaucher's disease may be *acute* or *chronic*. The acute form is seen in infants and primarily involves the central nervous system, resulting in death at approximately 18 months of age. The chronic form has an insidious onset. The course varies from patient to patient in relation to the severity and manifestations. The patient may have symptoms of pain in the hip, knee, shoulder, or spine. Avascular necrosis and pathologic fracture, frequently in the femur, are common. Necrosis of any bone may occur, however. Avascular necrosis of the femoral head is usually bilateral. Classic radiographic signs associated with Gaucher's disease with bone involvement include modeled translucencies, which may be localized or diffuse, along with thinning and erosion of the cortex with some noticeable expansion. Diagnosis is made by identifying Gaucher's cells in a bone marrow smear.[6,p.671]

**Treatment.** Avascular necrosis of the femoral head resulting from Gaucher's disease in children is treated by bed rest with no weight bearing. If bed rest is not possible, an ischial weight-bearing brace may be utilized. In the adult a total hip replacement is the surgical treatment of choice. Pathologic fractures of the long bones should be treated conservatively whenever possible. Patients with Gaucher's disease are highly susceptible to infection and hemorrhage. When open reduction and internal fixation are necessary, such as in femoral neck fractures, they should be accomplished with great care. In the older patient local curettage, intermedullary nailing, additional fixation with acrylic cement, and supplemental bank bone are utilized and may assist in earlier ambulation. Utilization of steroids may be indicated for their antiinflammatory effect. Splenectomy may be required in some cases.[5,pp.429-430;6,p.672]

## HYPERPARATHYROIDISM (GENERALIZED OSTEITIS FIBROSA CYSTICA, VON RECKLINGHAUSEN'S DISEASE OF BONE)

Hyperparathyroidism is a disease process characterized by the secretion of increased amounts of the parathyroid hormone resulting in decreased bone density and osteoporosis.

**Etiology.** Hyperparathyroidism is caused by a variety of factors, the most frequent of which is the occurrence of tumors of the parathyroid gland in adults.

**Pathology.** Excessive amounts of parathormone are secreted by the parathyroid gland, causing gradual resorption of bone trabeculae and replacement by fibrous tissue. This excessive osteoclastic resorption results in calcium and phosphorus metabolic disturbances, ultimately resulting in a decrease in bone density and osteoporosis. Microscopic manifestations of the bone involvement may simulate the giant cell tumor or reflect the new bone formation with excessive osteoids and osteoblasts. The ultimate result of the process is reflected by a general loss of strength, leading to compression, pathologic fractures, or curvature.[1;2,p.179]

**Incidence.** Hyperparathyroidism may occur at any age but is seen most often during middle age.

**Signs and symptoms.** The patient with hyperparathyroidism may complain of general lassitude or muscle hypertonia, which are the direct result of hypercalcemia. There may be severe skeletal pain and pathologic fractures. Renal complications are also frequently associated with hyperparathyroidism. Radiographic examination of the involved area reveals decreased density as a result of loss of bone. Radiographic films of the spine may show cupping, wedging, or crushing of the vertebral bodies. Kyphosis and "pigeon breast" deformity of the chest may also be observed.[1]

**Treatment.** The treatment of hyperparathyroidism, especially if due to a tumor, is a parathyroidectomy. Marked improvement usually follows the procedure. Orthopedic intervention consisting of supportive measures, orthoses, and splints to prevent deformities is required. Osteotomy or other corrective surgical procedures may be indicated after bone strength has been restored.

## HYPERPITUITARISM
### Acromegaly

Acromegaly is caused by hypersecretion of growth hormones produced by the anterior lobe of the pituitary gland, resulting in gradual bony thickening. Seen in adults, it corresponds to gigantism in children.

**Etiology.** The most common cause of acromegaly is an eosinophilic or acidophilic adenoma located on the anterior lobe of the pituitary gland.

**Pathology.** Excessive secretion of the growth hormone produced by the anterior lobe of the pituitary gland stimulates growth just under the periosteum. Particularly vulnerable to this overgrowth are areas of extreme stress such as those to which ligaments and muscles are attached and areas of compression such as near the ends of long bones.[1,6,p.114]

**Signs and symptoms.** Circumferential bone growth is greatly affected in acromegaly, resulting in thickened bones. Characteristically the patient with acromegaly has a large skull and jaw with excessively enlarged ears, nose, lower lip, and tongue. The hands and feet are huge, with thick fingers and toes. Kyphosis is common. Other signs and symptoms such as disturbances of vision may be the direct result of intracranial tumor.

**Treatment.** The treatment of acromegaly is directed to the cause, usually a tumor. It may be treated by radiation or by surgical intervention and sometimes by both. Orthopedic intervention is supportive and designed for symptomatic relief and prevention of deformity.

### Gigantism

Gigantism is caused by hypersecretion of the growth hormone during childhood and is characterized by excessive longitudinal growth of long bones. Gigantism is the equivalent of acromegaly in adults.

**Etiology.** Gigantism is most frequently the result of an eosinophilic or acidophilic adenoma of the anterior lobe of the pituitary gland.

**Pathology.** Pathologic features of gigantism are manifested before epiphyseal closure. Excessive production of the growth hormone results in thickening of the long bones near both ends and increased length. Premature or delayed epiphyseal closure is usually not a manifestation of this process.

**Signs and symptoms.** Children with gigantism often show subnormal sexual development and mentality. Characteristically the bones show thickening and increased length. The excessive growth is generally limited to the subperiosteal area and the epiphyseal growth plate. Other signs and symptoms associated with the process are rare.[6,p.114]

**Treatment.** The treatment of gigantism is usually implemented by the endocrinologist or the neurologist. The orthopedist may become involved or be the first medical specialist consulted for definitive diagnosis. Although orthopedic follow-up after diagnosis is not required, the process is of "orthopaedic interest in demonstrating clearly a close relationship between skeletal development and endocrine function."[1]

## HYPOTHYROIDISM (CRETINISM)

Hypothyroidism, or cretinism, results from severe deficiency in the production or secretion of the thyroid hormone. It is characterized by dwarfism and often accompanied by mental deficiency.

**Etiology.** The decreased secretion of thyroid hormone causing hypothyroidism is congenital. It is reflective of either inadequate thyroid tissue to produce sufficient quantities of the hormone or a defect in the production or secretion mechanism within the thyroid gland.

**Pathology.** Sufficient quantities of the thyroid hormone are required for skeletal growth. Insufficient quantities, characteristic of hypothyroidism, delay to varying degrees the overall skeletal ossification process, producing retardation of longitudinal growth and ultimate dwarfism.[2,p.179]

**Incidence.** Hypothyroidism is three times as common in girls as it is in boys.

**Signs and symptoms.** Typical features of hypothyroidism include overweight, general sluggishness, considerable dwarfism, and mental retardation. These features are usually not evident diagnostically until the child is 6 to 12 months of age. The skin is dry, and the hair is coarse and scanty. The face is expressionless, and developmental milestones such as sitting and standing may be somewhat delayed. Endochondral bone formation is greatly disturbed, with the skeleton considerably immature for the chronologic age. The head is large in relation to the body. The spine at the level of the second lumbar vertebra is wedge shaped. Lumbar kyphosis develops when the child begins to sit. Radiographic examination reveals late appearance of the ossification centers with modeling, and their size is smaller than normal when they do appear.[5,p.461]

**Treatment.** Early diagnosis and treatment of hypothyroidism, with the administration of thyroid hormone, provide a good prognosis for normal mental development and skeleton maturation.

## INFANTILE MUSCULAR ATROPHY (WERDNIG-HOFFMANN DISEASE, AMYOTONIA CONGENITA, OPPENHEIM'S DISEASE, INFANTILE SPINAL MUSCULAR ATROPHY)

Infantile muscular atrophy, or Werdnig-Hoffmann disease, is a disease of the anterior horn cells and the motor neurons of the fifth to twelfth cranial nerves, characterized by progressive degeneration resulting in paralysis. Onset is during infancy, and the disease is usually fatal by 4 or 5 years of age.

**Etiology.** The specific cause of infantile muscular atrophy is unknown; it is transmitted as an autosomal-recessive trait.[5,p.879]

**Pathology.** Infantile muscular atrophy is characterized by degenerative changes of the anterior horn cells of the spinal cord and the motor neurons of the fifth through twelfth cranial nerves. Generalized muscular weakness and hypotonia are secondary to these changes, with gradual and progressive denervation atrophy of skeletal muscle. Involuntary muscular alterations do not occur.[5,p.879;6,p.420]

**Incidence.** Infantile muscular atrophy affects both sexes.

**Signs and symptoms.** Some differentiation of signs and symptoms may be noted when onset is between birth and the end of the first month of life as compared with onset between the second and twelfth months of life. Both types show generalized muscular weakness with signs of progressive degeneration. The differentiation is seen in the severity and extent of the signs and symptoms. Infrequently onset may begin during the second year of life or thereafter.

If the disease is fully developed at birth or shortly thereafter, it is called *amyotonia congenita* or *Oppenheim's disease*. The infant is extremely flaccid and assumes a position with the hips in flexion, abduction, and external rotation; the shoulders in abduction and external rotation; the forearms pronated, and the hands elevated above the head. The chest and lower ribs flare into a bell shape. Deep tendon reflexes are absent. The infant eventually loses the sucking and gag reflexes. The facial expression is bland due to paralysis of the facial muscles. The predisposition to pneumonia and atelectasis, resulting from bulbar muscle weakness and respiratory insufficiency, greatly accelerates the rapid progression of the disease, and the infant often dies of respiratory infection before he is 1 year of age.[1,p.195;5,p.879]

The type of infantile muscular atrophy with onset between the second and twelfth month of life is usually referred to as *Werdnig-Hoffman disease*. The onset is usually more insidious, with signs and symptoms somewhat less severe than in amyotonia congenita. Muscular weakness is generally more localized, with the lower extremities affected to a greater degree than the upper extremities. The onset of active motion in the infant usually reveals a fine tremor of the upper extremities. Developmental milestones may be delayed, but sitting and crawling, and less frequently standing, are achieved. Most children who have onset of the disease between 2 and 12 months survive up to approximately 4 years.[5,pp.879-880]

A third type of infantile muscular atrophy, also known as Werdnig-Hoffman disease, has its onset during the second year of life or thereafter. More localized muscular weakness is characteristic, with less overall effect on the achievement of developmental milestones. The major muscles involved are the thigh muscles and the gluteus maximus. Sitting is usually accomplished at the normal time, with slight delay seen in standing and walking. Although some children may survive into the third decade of life, the average survival rate is approximately 7 years of age.[5,pp.879-880]

**Treatment.** Each child with infantile muscular atrophy must be individually assessed as to potential ability. No specific therapy is applicable to all of these patients. No orthopedic measure is specifically offered if onset of disease occurs between birth and the first month of life. If onset is between the second and twelfth month of life, assistive devices may be required for support in locomotion. Scoliosis, if present, may be treated conservatively with a body jacket or occasionally with stabilization by spinal fusion and Harrington rod fixation. If onset is after 2 years of age, treatment other than supportive devices is rarely required. Continued monitoring of progress of the disease is essential.[5,p.880]

## MARFAN'S SYNDROME (ARACHNODACTYLY)

Marfan's syndrome (Fig. 18-4) is a relatively rare disorder characterized by elongation of the bones, often with associated abnormalities of the eyes and the cardiovascular system.

**Etiology.** Marfan's syndrome is inherited as an autosomal-dominant trait.

**Pathology.** Marfan's syndrome produces a "disturbance of mesenchymal tissue affecting the musculoskeletal, cardiovascular, and ocular systems."[6,p.243] Musculoskeletally the major pathologic changes are underdevelopment of the muscles, ligamentous laxity, joint hypermobility, and elongation of the bones. Pathologic alterations associated with the cardiovascular system appear to produce fragmentation of the elastic fibers in the media of the

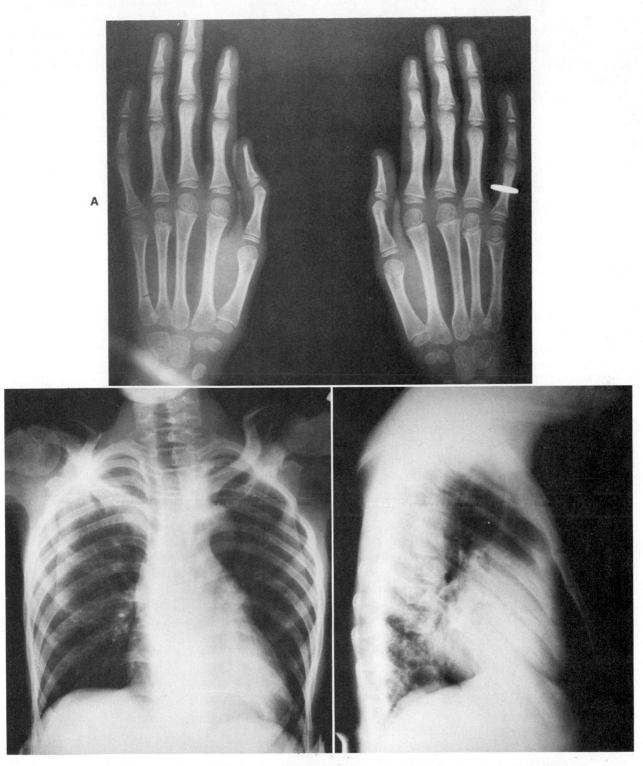

**Fig. 18-4.** Marfan's syndrome. **A,** Arachnoidactyly of right hand. **B,** Anterior and lateral views of bowing deformity of sternum, large aortic shadow.

aorta, which may lead to aneurysm. Ocular changes may include a variety of eye abnormalities with dislocation of the lens. Cardiac and ocular involvement occurs in approximately half of the patients with Marfan's syndrome.

**Incidence.** Marfan's syndrome is uncommon but not rare and affects both sexes equally.

**Signs and symptoms.** The patient with Marfan's syndrome is tall, frequently over 6 feet as an adult. The extremities are extremely long and slender with elongated metacarpals, metatarsals, and phalanges, which creates spiderlike fingers and toes. The skull is asymmetric in most of the patients. Pectus excavatum is common, and lateral curvature of the spine may develop and increase during years of rapid vertebral growth with kyphoscoliosis developing to varying degrees. Eye deformities with dislocation of the lens and cardiovascular complications are present in a high percentage of patients. Severe ligamental laxity and joint hypermobility may be seen on physical examination and often results in pes valgus and genu recurvatum.[1;5,p.243]

**Treatment.** No specific treatment is advocated for Marfan's syndrome, and management is often symptomatic. Resulting deformities including kyphoscoliosis may be treated with orthoses or surgical procedures as indicated.

## METAPHYSEAL DYSOSTOSIS

Metaphyseal dysostosis is a generalized skeletal disorder caused by a disturbance of the mineralization of the metaphyseal area of the bones and resulting in dwarfism. This disease has been classified as follows[5,p.329]:

1. *Gansen type:* characterized by metaphyseal alterations similar to those of achondroplasia but not involving the skull or the epiphysis of long bones
2. *Schmidt type:* characterized by developmental changes from the weight-bearing age to approximately 5 years, again similar to achondroplasia and resulting in moderate dwarfism
3. *Spahr-Hartmann type:* characterized by skeletal changes and severe genu varum
4. *Cartilage-hair hypoplasia:* characterized by severe dwarfism and the presence of hair that is sparse, short, and brittle

Mental retardation is not usually associated with this disease process. Radiographic examination in all types reveals characteristic widening of the metaphyses of tubular bones with normal diaphyseal and epiphyseal ossification centers. Treatment is supportive and symptomatic with no specific modality advocated.[5,p.335]

## METAPHYSEAL DYSPLASIA

Metaphyseal dysplasia (Fig. 18-5) is a "familial and perhaps hereditary disease of the endochondral bone growth resulting in a failure of normal cylindrical bone modeling."[5,p.335] It may involve any bone(s), with the distal femur or proximal tibia most often affected. The most characteristic radiographic feature is "Erlenmeyer flask" deformity. The metaphyseal circumference is enlarged with a decreased medullary area. The involvement is limited to long bones.[5,p.335]

## MUCOPOLYSACCHARIDOSES

Mucopolysaccharidoses is the term utilized to describe metabolic disturbances in mucopolysaccharide metabolism. These disturbances have been classified by McKusick into various categories that reflect their clinical and radiographic features as follows[4]:

Type I: Hurler's syndrome
Type II: Hunter's syndrome
Type III: Sanfilippo's syndrome
Type IV: Morquio's syndrome
Type V: Scheie's syndrome
Type VI: Maroteaux-Lamy syndrome

Clinical features of these syndromes are compared in Table 18-6, which reviews the differential diagnosis of mucopolysaccharidoses including the biochemical defect associated with each type.

### Hurler's syndrome

Hurler's syndrome is a type of mucopolysaccharidosis transmitted as an autosomal-recessive trait and resulting in severe mental retardation. The onset of symptoms is within the first few months of life. Enlargement of the liver and spleen are characteristic, and cardiovascular involvement is often seen. Facial characteristics include a low forehead and enlargement sometimes resulting from hydrocephalus. Corneal clouding is common, and the neck is short. Marked kyphosis is apparent at the dorsolumbar level. The hands and fingers are short and broad. Flexion contractures are common. Radiographic features are consistent with the characteristics outlined with multiple skeletal alterations. Death usually results during childhood from cardiac or pulmonary complications.[4;5,pp.287-295]

### Hunter's syndrome

Hunter's syndrome is seen less frequently than Hurler's syndrome and is transmitted as a sex-linked recessive trait. Liver and spleen involvement are not associated with this type of mucopolysaccharidosis, nor are corneal clouding and kypho-

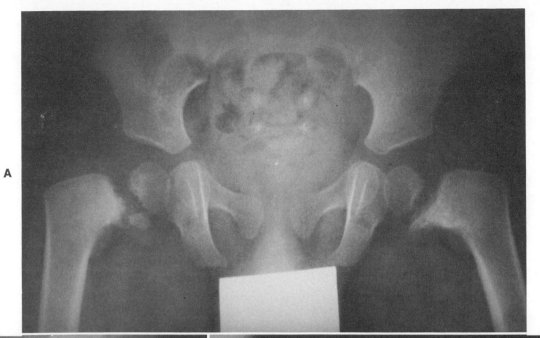

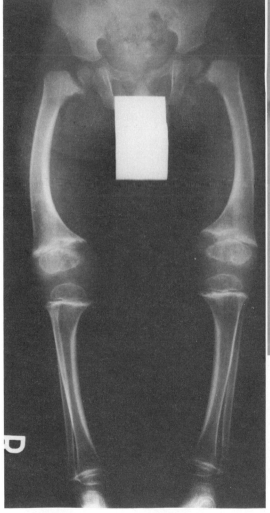

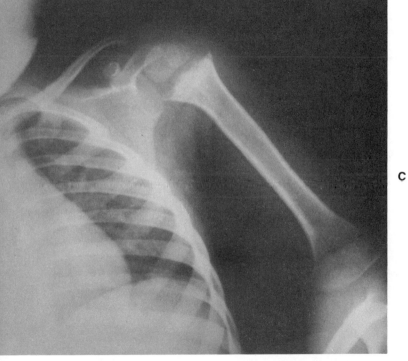

**Fig. 18-5.** Metaphyseal chondrodysplasia (metaphyseal dysplasia; metaphyseal dysostosis, Schmidt type). **A,** Varus deformities of pelvis with irregular metaphyseal margins. **B,** Bowing of femurs. **C,** Irregular metaphysis of proximal humerus.

**Table 18-6.** Genetic mucopolysaccharidoses (as classified in 1972)

| | Designation | Clinical features | Genetics | Excessive urinary MPS | Substance deficient |
|---|---|---|---|---|---|
| MPS I H | Hurler's syndrome | Early clouding of cornea, grave manifestations, death usually before age 10 | Homozygous for MPS IH gene | Dermatan sulfate Heparan sulfate | α-L-iduronidase (formerly called Hurler's corrective factor) |
| MPS I S | Scheie's syndrome | Stiff joints, cloudy cornea, aortic regurgitation, normal intelligence, ?normal life-span | Homozygosity for MPS IS gene | Dermatan sulfate Heparan sulfate | α-L-iduronidase |
| MPS I H/S | Hurler-Scheie compound | Phenotype intermediate between Hurler's and Scheie's | Genetic compound of MPS I H and I S genes | Dermatan sulfate Heparan sulfate | α-L-iduronidase |
| MPS II A | Hunter's syndrome, severe | No clouding of cornea, milder course than in MPS IH but death usually before age 15 years | Hemizygous for X-linked gene | Dermatan sulfate Heparan sulfate | Hunter's corrective factor |
| MPS II B | Hunter's syndrome, mild | Survival to 30s to 50s, fair intelligence | Hemizygous for X-linked allele for mild form | Dermatan sulfate Heparan sulfate | Hunter's corrective factor |
| MPS III A | Sanfilippo's syndrome A | Identical phenotype | Homozygous for Sanfilippo's A gene | Heparan sulfate | Heparan sulfate sulfatase |
| MPS III B | Sanfilippo's syndrome B | Mild somatic, severe central nervous system effects | Homozygous for Sanfilippo's B (at different locus) | Heparan sulfate | N-acetyl-α-D-glucosaminidase |
| MPS IV | Morquio's syndrome (probably more than one allelic form) | Severe bone changes of distinctive type, cloudy cornea, aortic regurgitation | Homozygous for Morquio's gene | Keratan sulfate | Unknown |
| MPS V | Vacant | | | | |
| MPS VI A | Maroteaux-Lamy syndrome, classic form | Severe osseous and corneal change, normal intellect | Homozygous for M-L gene | Dermatan sulfate | Maroteaux-Lamy corrective factor |
| MPS VI B | Maroteaux-Lamy syndrome, mild form | Severe osseous and corneal change, normal intellect | Homozygous for allele at M-L locus | Dermatan sulfate | Maroteaux-Lamy corrective factor |
| MPS VII | β-glucuronidase deficiency (more than one allelic form?) | Hepatosplenomegaly, dysostosis multiplex, white cell inclusions, mental retardation | Homozygous for mutant gene at β-glucuronidase locus | Dermatan sulfate | β-glucuronidase |

From McKusick, V. A.: Heritable disorders of connective tissue, ed. 4, St. Louis, 1972, The C. V. Mosby Co.

sis. Although mental retardation is also associated with this form, it is much later in onset and usually progresses more slowly. Deafness is often characteristic. Although cardiac complications are frequently a contributing factor in the death of patients with Hunter's syndrome, survival is often into the third decade of life.[4;5,p.295]

## Sanfilippo's syndrome

Sanfilippo's syndrome is transmitted as an autosomal-recessive trait and results in severe mental retardation. Corneal clouding and cardiovascular abnormalities are usually not seen, and liver and spleen involvement if present is usually minimal to moderate. Skeletal involvement is usually less than is seen in the other mucopolysaccharidoses. Most patients survive into the third or fourth decade of life.[4;5,p.296]

## Morquio's syndrome

Morquio's syndrome (Fig. 18-6) is a form of mucopolysaccharidosis transmitted as an autosomal-recessive trait and characterized by "dwarfism, flattening of the vertebral bodies, marked

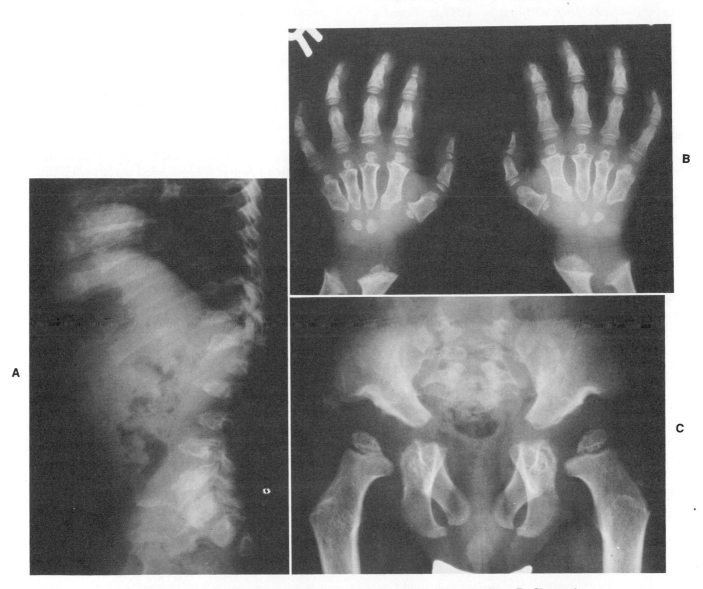

**Fig. 18-6.** Morquio's syndrome. **A,** Diffuse flattening of vertebral bodies. **B,** Shortening of metacarpal bones with constriction of proximal ends of metacarpals, distal ends of radius and ulna directed toward each other. **C,** Dysplastic changes in hip joints, flaring of illiac bones anteriorly, straightening of femoral neck angle, broadening of ischial and pubic bones.

kyphosis, widespread affection of the epiphyses, and normal intelligence."[5,p.296] The child with Morquio's syndrome progresses normally, or appears to, until he begins to walk. With growth the development of the characteristic features of the syndrome become evident. The kyphotic deformity, shortened neck, and valgus angulation of the knees are extremely apparent by the fourth year of life. Dwarfing is general; however, the arms may be relatively long. The epiphyses are enlarged. The child stands in the characteristic crouched position with hips and knees in flexion, the hands placed on the thighs, and the head thrust forward and tucked between the shoulders. The gait is waddling. There is valgus deformity of the feet and ankles. Intelligence is normal. The facies is normal, although the head may appear large in contrast to the diminished size of the trunk. The chest is narrowed in the transverse diameter and elongated in the anteroposterior diameter (pectus carinatum). There may be ligamentous laxity with hypermobility of the hands and feet. The digits are short and broad. Characteristic radiographic features are observed in the spine and hips. Flattened vertebrae are specifically pronounced in the lumbar and thoracic areas. There is wedging of the anterior portion of the vertebrae at the cervicolumbar and dorsolumbar junctions. Flattening of the femoral head with fragmentation is present. Treatment of Morquio's syndrome is directed toward correction of deformities. Implementation of therapy to control progression of deformities through supportive or surgical means is important in the minimization of degenerative joint disease that may result with age. Most patients have a normal life span.[4;5,pp.296-297;6,pp.313-315]

### Scheie's syndrome

Scheie's syndrome is transmitted as an autosomal-recessive trait and is characterized by corneal clouding and cardiovascular disease. Carpal tunnel syndrome is frequent. Neither liver and spleen involvement nor mental retardation are associated. Most patients with Scheie's syndrome survive into adulthood.[4;5,p.302]

### Maroteaux-Lamy syndrome

Maroteaux-Lamy syndrome is transmitted as an autosomal-recessive trait and is characterized by severe skeletal involvement including dwarfism, genu valgum, kyphosis of the lumbar area, and protrusion of the sternum anteriorly. Corneal clouding is present and liver and spleen enlargement is common, but there is no cardiovascular involvement. Mental retardation is not associated. Longevity of patients with Maroteaux-Lamy syndrome cannot be determined from currently available data.[4;5,p.302]

## MUSCULAR DYSTROPHY (PROGRESSIVE MUSCULAR DYSTROPHY, PSEUDOHYPERTROPHIC MUSCULAR DYSTROPHY, DUCHENNE MUSCULAR DYSTROPHY)

Muscular dystrophy is a general term inclusive of genetically determined primary degenerative diseases resulting in progressive muscular atrophy. Differential diagnosis of the principal types of muscular dystrophy is given in Table 18-7. The most common form encountered and described here is pseudohypertrophic muscular dystrophy, or Duchenne muscular dystrophy.

**Etiology.** The specific cause of muscular dystrophy is unknown. It is transmitted as a sex-linked recessive trait.[1;2,p.161]

**Pathology.** Pathologic features of muscular dystrophy include hypertrophy of extremity muscles with atrophy of the muscles, especially surrounding the shoulder girdle. Eventual fragmentation of muscular fibers results, accompanied by fatty deposits. Muscles formed first in embryo are the first to be involved in the dystrophic process.[1;5,p.1082]

**Incidence.** Symptoms of muscular dystrophy appear within the first 3 to 5 years of life. This disease is seen almost exclusively in males.

**Signs and symptoms.** The first symptoms associated with muscular dystrophy are severe fatigue and weakness of the lower extremities. The calf muscles appear enlarged. The child stands with an obvious lumbar lordosis, walks with a waddling gait, and falls frequently. He has difficulty climbing stairs or arising from the floor as a result of increased weakness of the extensor muscles of the lower extremity. *Gowers' sign* is a positive sign of this weakness. Pseudohypertrophy is characteristic in 80% of the patients and is the result of accumulation of fatty deposits in the muscles. Weakness around the shoulder girdle is also characteristic. Facial muscle weakness causes inability to close the eyes, and the characteristic facial expression is "mask-like." Intelligence is approximately 15% to 20% lower than that of the child's normal peers.[1;5,pp.1084-1087]

Electromyography is sometimes useful as a diagnostic tool, usually reflecting "a decrease in the amplitude of motor unit potentials on voluntary muscle contraction as well as an increase in polyphasic potentials and absent fibrillations."[1] The serum creatine phosphokinase level is elevated during the early stages of the disease process; signifi-

**Table 18-7.** Differential diagnosis of principal types of muscular dystrophy

| Clinical features | Duchenne muscular dystrophy | Limb girdle muscular dystrophy | Facioscapulohumeral muscular dystrophy | Distal muscular dystrophy | Progressive dystrophia ophthalmoplegia | Congenital or infantile muscular dystrophy |
|---|---|---|---|---|---|---|
| Incidence | Most common | Less common, but not infrequent | Not common | Rare | Rare | Rare |
| Age at onset | Usually before 3 yr; sometimes between 3 and 6 yr | Variable (usually by second decade, occasionally later) | Variable (usually in second decade) | 20 to 77 yr (mean 47 yr) | Any age | At or soon after birth |
| Sex preponderance | Male | Either sex | Male and female equally affected | Either sex | Either sex | Not yet determined |
| Inheritance | Sex-linked autosomal-recessive less than 10% | Autosomal-recessive; on rare occasions autosomal-dominant | Autosomal-dominant usually; autosomal-recessive rarely | Autosomal-dominant | Simple dominant or simple recessive | Unknown |
| Pattern of muscle involvement | Proximal: pelvic and shoulder girdle muscles affected early, spreads to periphery of limbs late in course | Proximal: shoulder and pelvic girdle early, spreads to periphery late | Face and shoulder girdle, later spreads to pelvic girdle | Distal: hand first, anterior tibial and calf of leg | Usually limited to external ocular muscles | Generalized |
| Muscles spared until late | Gastrocnemius, toe flexors, posterior tibial, hamstrings, hand muscles, upper trapezius, biceps, triceps, face, jaw, pharyngeal, laryngeal, ocular | In upper extremity brachioradials and hand; calf muscles | Back extensors, iliopsoas, hip abductors, quadriceps | Proximal | Ocular | |
| Pseudohypertrophy | 80% of cases (calf muscles) | Less than 33% of cases | Rare | Not seen | Not seen | Not seen |
| Myotonia | Absent | Absent | Absent | Absent | Absent | Absent |
| Contractural deformities | Common | Develop late in course less severe than in Duchenne | Mild, late | Mild, late | | Severe |
| Scoliosis and kyphoscoliosis | Common in late stage | Mild, late stage | Mild, late | | | |
| Heart involvement | Hypertrophy and tachycardia common; in late stages widespread degeneration, fibrosis, fatty infiltration | Very rare | Very rare | Very rare | Not seen | Not seen |
| Endocrine changes | Not seen | Not seen | Not seen | Not seen | Not seen | ? |
| Intellectual level | Commonly decreased | Normal | Normal | Normal | Normal | ? |
| Course | Steady rapid progression | Slow progression, considerable variation in pace of disease | Progresses insidiously | Comparatively benign | Slow progression | Steady progression |

From Tachdjian, M. O.: Pediatric orthopedics, Philadelphia, 1972, W. B. Saunders Co., p. 1093.

cant elevation may also be present in female carriers of this disease. Muscle biopsy also serves as a useful diagnostic tool in muscular dystrophy.[1]

Because of the progressive nature of this disease the child is usually confined to a wheelchair by the age of 10 to 15 years. Skeletal deformities (e.g., flexion contractures) then become a severe problem. Scoliosis results from weakness of the trunk and abdominal muscles. Most patients die of respiratory or pulmonary problems or cardiac failure. Few survive the age of 20 years.[1;5,p.1087]

**Treatment.** No specific treatment modality is available for muscular dystrophy. Conservative and supportive measures including psychological support are of great value. Maintenance of mobility for as long as possible is extremely important in the care of these children. Orthotic support is determined carefully as it may be cumbersome and serve as a deterrent to mobility; utilization for support and ambulation is useful, however. With progression of the disease, scoliosis may require support by means of a plastic body jacket. Surgical measures such as soft tissue release of contractures may be useful in the correction of deformities that hinder mobility and ambulation.

## MYASTHENIA GRAVIS (ERB-GOLDFLAM DISEASE)

Myasthenia gravis is a disease characterized by extreme weakness of voluntary muscles. It may occur at any age, is usually not progressive, and is characterized by periods of remission.

**Etiology.** The specific cause of myasthenia gravis is unknown.

**Pathology.** The major pathologic feature of myasthenia gravis is disuse muscular atrophy with the muscles otherwise appearing normal.

**Incidence.** Females are twice as predisposed to myasthenia gravis as are males. Although it may occur at any age, it is most prevalent in the fourth decade.

**Signs and symptoms.** The patient with myasthenia gravis may consult the orthopedic surgeon because of pain in the back and lower limbs. There is fatigue, which is exaggerated by exertion, is usually worse at the end of the day, and often is relieved by rest. The characteristic "sad" expression is due to facial muscle weakness. The patient often has difficulty chewing, and complains that his tongue feels thick. He complains of heaviness in the chest, and respiratory compromise may cause serious problems. There are characteristic periods of remission, and in most cases the disease process is not progressive. The disease usually remains benign if it has been present more than 10 years. Differential diagnosis must be established between myasthenia gravis and muscular dystrophy or poliomyelitis.[6,p.633]

**Treatment.** It is of critical importance that the orthopedic surgeon, when the diagnosis of myasthenia gravis is either considered or confirmed, refer the patient immediately to permit adequate and appropriate medical management of the process. Pharmacologic therapeutics prescribed include neostigmine (Prostigmin), pyridostigmine (Mestinon), and ambenonium (Mytelase) in variable doses depending on the age of the patient, severity of the disease, and response to the medication. A respirator may be required if pulmonary compromise is encountered. Tracheostomy may be needed if excessive pooling of secretions results from pharyngeal muscular weakness. Orthopedic management is rarely required after referral.[5,p.1112;6,p.633]

## MYELOMENINGOCELE, SPINA BIFIDA OCCULTA

Myelomeningocele (Fig. 18-7) and spina bifida occulta reflect a group of defects or disorders involving the spinal column, spinal cord, or both. The classifications and terminology associated with these defects vary slightly depending on the source. The general classifications of these defects, according to Tachdjian and Brashear and Raney are given in Table 18-8. The following terminology associated with these defects is provided to facilitate comprehension of the information to follow[1;5,p.886]:

**spina bifida** congenital developmental defect of spinal column characterized by failure of fusion between one or more vertebral arches, occurring with or without protrusion of intraspinal contents, and associated with varying degrees of neurologic deficits; broad term utilized for all types of such defects.

**myelodysplasia** general term used to denote developmental defect of spinal cord with associated peripheral neurologic deficits.

**anterior spina bifida** form of spina bifida denoting anterior rather than usual posterior protrusion of meninges and its contents; relatively rare.

**spina bifida occulta** failure of fusion of one or more laminae with no protrusion of meninges or intraspinal contents; frequently diagnosed accidentally and is in most cases of little clinical significance.

**meningocele or spina bifida with meningocele** failure of fusion of one or more vertebral arches with protrusion of meninges containing cerebrospinal fluid but no nerve tissue involvement.

**myelomeningocele or spina bifida with myelomeningocele** failure of fusion of one or more vertebral arches with

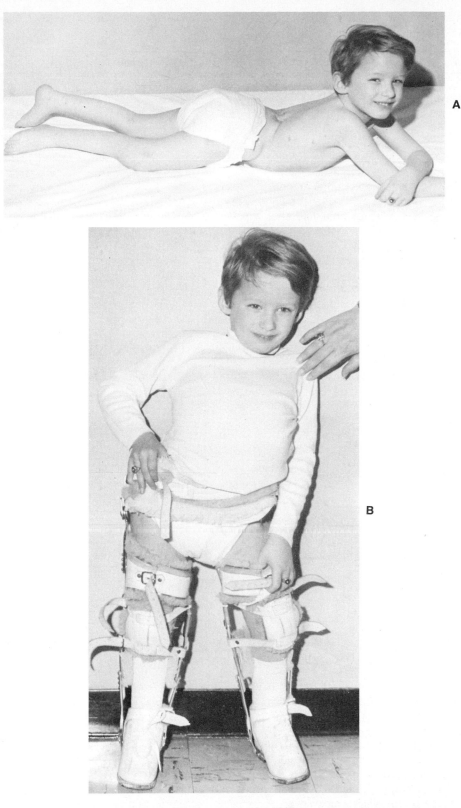

**Fig. 18-7.** Myelomeningocele. **A,** Surgical correction of defect accomplished. **B,** Utilization of orthotic devices is common to provide stability for ambulation and gait training. (From Hilt, N. E., and Schmitt, E. W., Jr.: Pediatric orthopedic nursing, St. Louis, 1975, The C. V. Mosby Co.)

**Table 18-8.** Major classifications of spina bifida according to Tachdjian and Brashear and Raney[1; 5, p. 886]

| Tachdjian | | Brashear and Raney | |
|---|---|---|---|
| **Classification** | **Characteristics** | **Classification** | **Characteristics** |
| I. Spina bifida occulta | Incomplete closure of laminae, one or more vertebrae<br>Absence of protrusion of intraspinal contents to surface<br>Possible overlying cutaneous defect, neurologic deficit, spinal cord dysplastic changes | I. Spina bifida occulta | Bony defect of spinous process and laminae, one or more vertebrae<br>No protrusion<br>Possible skin alterations (indentations, pigmentations, telangiectasis, hypertrichosis [hairy patches])<br>Possible associated tumors inside or outside vertebral canal (lipoma, angioma, dermoid cyst)<br>Possible alterations with growth, gradual incomplete paralysis |
| II. Meningocele | Unfused vertebral arches<br>Visible meningeal sac filled with cerebrospinal fluid and composed of dura mater or arachnoid, no nerve tissue<br>Myelodysplasia of spinal cord absent<br>Sensory, motor, reflex status intact<br>No sphincter disturbance | II. Spina bifida with meningo-cele | Unfused vertebral arches<br>Herniation of meninges contains cerebrospinal fluid; no involvement of nerve tissue |
| III. Myelomeningocele | Unfused vertebral arches<br>Cystic distention of meninges, nerve tissue within or adherent to sac<br>Spinal cord myelodysplasia<br>Neurologic deficits (sensory, motor, reflex, sphincter) caudal to level of lesion | III. Spina bifida with myelo-meningocele | Unfused vertebral arches<br>Herniation of meninges<br>Neurologic deficit (sensory, motor, reflex, spincter) caudal to level of lesion |
| | | IV. Spina bifida with syringo-myelocele | Same as spina bifida with myelomeningocele but more severe<br>Herniated spinal cord contains greatly dilated central canal and distended with cerebrospinal fluid |
| | | V. Spina bifida with myelocele | Most severe form<br>Wide bony deficit<br>Open groove with imperfectly or inadequately formed spinal cord tissue, draining cerebrospinal fluid<br>Infection common |

protrusion of meninges containing cerebrospinal fluid, the spinal cord or nerve roots, with resultant neurologic (sensory, motor, reflex, sphincter) deficits of varying degrees caudal to level of lesion.

**syringomyelocele or spina bifida with syringomyelocele** more severe form of myelomeningocele in which herniated spinal cord contains central canal greatly dilated and extended with cerebrospinal fluid.

**myelocele or spina bifida with myelocele** most severe form of spina bifida resulting in wide bony defect that forms open groove partially lined by inadequately formed or developed spinal cord tissue and characterized by draining cerebrospinal fluid.

**rachischisis** spina bifida or spina bifida with myelocele.

**spina bifida manifesta** general term utilized to denote presence of soft tissue tumor due to herniation of meninges, characterized and inclusive of spina bifida occulta, meningocele, myelomeningocele, and syringomyelocele.

**spina bifida cystica** general term utilized to describe meningocele and myelomeningocele and inclusive of those classifications descriptive of external cystic protrusion of nerve tissue components.

**Etiology.** Although the various forms of spina bifida reflect early embryonic developmental defects, the specific cause is unknown. However, the incidence in more than one child in a family is great enough that genetic counseling for the parents should be encouraged, especially when any of the more severe forms exist.

**Pathology.** The pathologic features associated with spina bifida reflect the severity of the form encountered. With all types there is failure of bony fusion between the vertebral arches of one or more vertebrae of the spinal column. The extent of this bony defect reflects specific vulnerability in relation to protrusion of the meninges and the intraspinal contents, which is associated with the more severe forms. A protrusion in one form or another is present in all types except spina bifida occulta. The protrusion of the meninges creates a visible herniated sac filled with cerebrospinal fluid. A meningocele is characterized by lack of nerve tissue involvement. In myelomeningocele and syringomyelocele there is nerve tissue involvement with the herniated sac, resulting in varying degrees of sensory, motor, reflex, and sphincter deficits. The myelocele is characterized by an incomplete lined protrusion which drains cerebrospinal fluid through to the surface. [5,pp.889-891]

The herniated sac associated with the more severe types of spina bifida may be covered by normal skin or by a very thin membrane. In many cases this covering is incomplete, with the meninges above and below the lesion appearing normal. The extent of nerve tissue involvement ranges from absent in spina bifida occulta and meningocele to severe involvement ranging from an absent, split, or dysplastic spinal cord. Peripheral nerve development appears to be normal in myelomeningocele. [5,p.890]

The lesions associated with spina bifida are predominantly seen in the lumbosacral region. They may, however, occur higher in the thoracolumbar or thoracic region. Hydrocephalus to varying degrees is almost always present but may be controlled clinically in many cases with a ventricular shunt. [5,p.891]

**Incidence.** The incidence of spina bifida in its various forms differs throughout the world. The approximate incidence in the United States is 1.22 per 1,000 births with approximately 1 in 1,000 being sufficiently severe to produce clinical deformity. Approximately 50% of the latter survive infancy. [1,] [5,pp.887-888] Incidence of the least severe form, spina bifida occulta, is higher, with authorities reporting that "approximately 25% of all infants and young children show some minor defect of the vertebral arches on radiographic examination." [5,pp.887-888]

**Signs and symptoms.** Frequently the diagnosis of spina bifida occulta is made accidentally on radio-

graphic examination for other purposes. Most cases have no clinical significance and require no therapy. When the neural axis is involved the patient may require surgical intervention. The skin over the lesion may show (1) an abnormal patch of hair, (2) dimpling of the overlying skin, (3) subcutaneous lipoma, or (4) hemangioma. Complaints or objective findings such as disturbances in bowel and bladder control, motor or sensory deficits, or musculoskeletal deformity of the lower extremities should be investigated through myelography but are rarely associated with this form of spina bifida. [5,p.887]

The more severe forms of spina bifida produce clinical manifestations to varying degrees within three major categories: (1) herniated sac or soft tissue protrusion, (2) neurologic deficits reflecting the degree of nerve tissue involvement, and (3) other associated deformities. The herniated protrusion varies mainly in relation to the size permitted by the severity of the bony defect and its contents. Transillumination usually reveals a translucent sac. The bony defect is best evaluated through radiographic examination. Neurologic deficits may range from slight to extremely severe impairment or loss of sensory, motor, reflex, and sphincter control distal to the lesion. Total paraplegia may be seen. The highest percentage of deformities associated with this defect involve the musculoskeletal system and include clawfoot, clubfoot, scoliosis, kyphosis, lordosis, unilateral or bilateral dislocation of the hips, and contractures. Hydrocephalus may be present. [5,pp.887-888]

Although many of the signs and symptoms associated with the more severe forms of spina bifida and myelomeningocele are present at birth, alterations may be noted only with the normal growth and developmental sequence. Sphincter control, for example, may not be totally evaluated until late infancy. During the earlier stages of evaluation shortly after birth, continuous observation for leakage of cerebrospinal fluid must be accomplished. These infants are extremely vulnerable to infection, and meningitis is responsible for most of the deaths that occur during infancy.

**Treatment.** The least severe form, spina bifida occulta, usually requires no specific therapeutic intervention; however, increasing neurologic deficits should be investigated and surgical intervention utilized when indicated. Cosmetic procedures may be indicated for removal of large hairy patches or skin nevi. It is generally accepted that with the more severe types neurosurgical exploration and excision of the meningocele is an emergency measure. The overall approach to the implementation of treatment is multidisciplinary. All aspects of the care of these children are extremely important if they are to receive adequate and proper care.

The orthopedist should begin evaluation of the infant from the day of birth if possible. Paralysis and deformities of the lower extremities require extensive treatment with surgery, cast therapy, or orthoses. Each deformity should be considered both as a separate entity and in combination with the other deformities that exist. Clubfeet and dislocated hips are of significant concern as deterrents to ambulation. Nonsurgical intervention for both should be attempted, but resistance to permanent correction is sometimes encountered.[5,p.896]

Of critical importance in the decisions to be made early in relation to the surgical intervention for these deformities is the overall goal of orthopedic intervention: "to have these children walking with appropriate orthotic support by the age of 18 months."[5,p.896] This ambulatory goal is crucial to the ability of these children to achieve and maintain an independent status as early as possible. Other considerations that should, of course, be appropriately weighed and that may require alterations of this goal include (1) the level of the lesion, especially if it is extremely high, (2) the degree of mental capacity existing, and (3) parental compliance. In most cases, however, all treatment instituted at an early age should be directed toward achieving ambulation.

An additional consideration throughout the course of early and late intervention is the avoidance of pressure areas. Casts and traction therapy, as well as immobilization, considerably increase the risk of skin problems, even in the patient with normal skin integrity. These patients, however, are known to have sensitive skin and are at increased risk because of sensory deficits. Constant attention must be given to avoid pressure areas, especially if the time required to achieve the above goals is lengthy.

It is important to mention here that to some degree the total approach and intervention pattern for the patient with myelomeningocele is still not totally agreed upon. Until several decades ago the health care professions had little or nothing to offer these children, and those who survived infancy often needed a tremendous amount of care because of hydrocephalus. With the advent of the ventricular shunt all infants with any level of severity of lesion were aggressively treated. Many are now questioning the wisdom of this philosophy, particularly in children with high thoracic lesions. Regardless of the trend of philosophical and moral considerations

associated with the treatment of myelomeningocele, it must be stressed that parental education and support requires utmost commitment from health care personnel working with these children. At minimum the problems associated with this defect are very complex, and multidisciplinary treatment modalities are no less complex. The need for coordination of treatment and continued communication with the parents to both educate them regarding the associated problems, potential problems, and progress of their child in relation to ultimate goals are critical to their compliance with therapeutic regimens and are no less than what these parents should obtain from the health care system. Without this commitment from health care personnel, the child is likely to be functionally independent but unable to cope within the family unit, which functions as a model for his societal interactions.

## NEUROFIBROMATOSIS (VON RECKLINGHAUSEN'S DISEASE)

Neurofibromatosis is a disease characterized by multiple neurofibromas of spinal nerves, cranial nerves, or peripheral nerves; multiple fibrous pedunculated soft tissue tumors; and multiple spots of light brown pigmentation on the skin (café au lait spots).

**Etiology.** Neurofibromatosis is a congenital abnormality transmitted as a dominant trait but not sex linked.

**Pathology.** The major pathologic features of neurofibromatosis involve the supportive tissue of the central and peripheral nervous systems, resulting in (1) multiple neurofibromas of the spinal, cranial, or peripheral nerves; (2) multiple fibrous pedunculated soft tissue tumors; and (3) multiple pigmentations of the skin resulting in light brown spots known as *café au lait spots.* The resulting pathologic features include a variety of abnormalities of the skeletal system, skin, and soft tissue.[1, 2,p.168;5,p.539]

**Incidence.** Neurofibromatosis may appear at any age and affects males more frequently than females.

**Signs and symptoms.** Nonskeletal manifestations of neurofibromatosis include café au lait spots ranging in size from a few millimeters to several centimeters, subcutaneous tumors, growth along the course of the peripheral nerves, and localized neurofibromas in nerve trunks. The orthopedic interest in this process lies in the skeletal complications seen in approximately 50% of patients with neurofibromatosis. Scoliosis is frequently an associated complication. Gigantism of all or part of an extremity may be seen. The fibromatous lesions may cause local erosion, and cysts may occur within the medullary cavity. Pseudarthrosis of the tibia or fibula may exist. Tumors associated with neurofibromatosis possess the ability to undergo malignant alteration.[1;2,p.168;5,p.541]

**Treatment.** The patient with skeletal complications as a result of neurofibromatosis may require surgical intervention of various forms. Scoliosis if present may be treated with spinal fusion if the curve progresses rapidly. Gigantic digits may be amputated for cosmetic purposes. Hypertrophied soft tissue and nodular masses may be excised. Local recurrence is common; therefore more radical excision is indicated in the initial surgical treatment of these masses. Neurofibromatosis is often fatal, especially if malignant transformation occurs.[1;5,p.541]

## OSTEOGENESIS IMPERFECTA

Osteogenesis imperfecta (Fig. 18-8) is a hereditary but uncommon disorder of the general connective tissue and is characterized by severe fragility of the bones, ligamentous laxity surrounding the joints, blue sclerae, and potential deafness. It is often referred to as "brittle bone" disease.

**Etiology.** The specific cause of osteogenesis imperfecta is unknown, but some cases are of congenital origin and the hereditary factor is demonstrable in many, with the disease usually transmitted as an autosomal-dominant trait.[6,p.309]

**Pathology.** The primary pathologic features of osteogenesis imperfecta result from a defect in the formation of osteoblasts. Endochondral ossification at the epiphyseal plate appears to proceed normally "as far as the stage of provisional calcification of cartilage."[6,p.309] Metaphyseal areas are composed of calcified cartilage rather than osseous tissue. Gross pathologic features of osteogenesis imperfecta reveal bones that are shorter and thinner than usual. The bone density is varied and uneven on radiographic examination. Multiple fractures result, creating a variety of deformities of a rotational and angular nature. Abundant callus formation

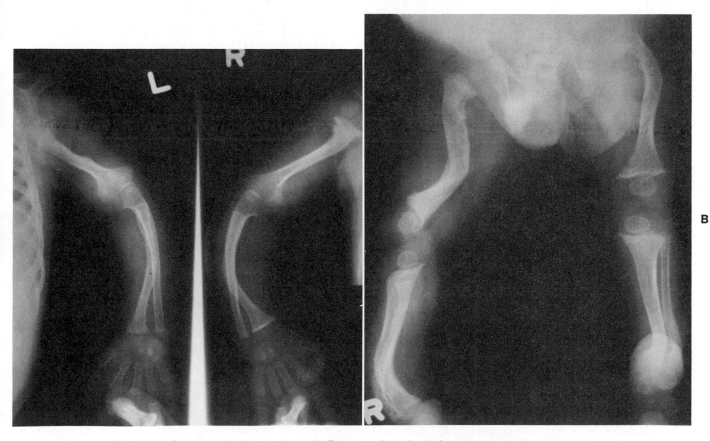

**Fig. 18-8.** Osteogenesis imperfecta. **A,** Fracture of shaft of left humerus; marked demineralization in both views. **B,** Severe bowing deformities evident in lower extremities.

is usually apparent, with fracture healing resulting from hyperplastic and tumorlike bone formation.[1;5,p.303;6,p.309]

**Incidence.** Osteogenesis imperfecta is relatively rare, with the congenital type occurring in approximately 1 of every 40,000 births. It is somewhat more frequent in females than in males.[5,p.303]

**Signs and symptoms.** The clinical characteristics of osteogenesis imperfecta vary according to the type encountered (Table 18-9).

*Type I. Fetal or prenatal form: osteogenesis imperfecta congenita.* This is the most severe form of osteogenesis imperfecta, with multiple fractures present at birth, often the result of the trauma of the birth process. The skull is soft and membraneous. The infant may be stillborn or may die at birth or within the first few weeks. If he survives, continued multiple fractures exist with minimal trauma, and a loss of stature is the eventual result.

*Type II. Infantile form: osteogenesis imperfecta tarda, gravis form.* This form is less severe, with multiple fractures occurring during infancy. The skull is thin and globular and may resemble that seen in hydrocephaly. Multiple fractures frequently continue. Survival past the first few years increases the chance of lessening of this tendency and continued survival. The loss of stature is also noted with this type as a result of deformities resulting from fractures.

*Type III. Adolescent form: osteogenesis imperfecta tarda, levis form.* With this, the least severe of all types of osteogenesis imperfecta, the child is normal at birth. Fractures from minimal trauma occur later in childhood and are sometimes not seen until adolescence. With increasing age the tendency to fracture is lost. Delayed ambulation may be noted.

Blue sclerae are usually associated with all types or classifications of osteogenesis imperfecta.

When considering osteogenesis imperfecta as a total entity, the following are common characteristics[5,p.310;6,pp.309-310]:

1. Multiple fractures accompanied by slight or no pain, which heal well but with deformity; tendency decreases with growth
2. Blue sclerae as a result of abnormal thinness of the sclerae
3. High incidence of otosclerosis often resulting in deafness
4. Ligamentous laxity surrounding the joints
5. Feeble musculature
6. Dwarfism as an eventual result
7. Broad skull
8. Poorly calcified deciduous teeth

In addition scoliosis, kyphosis, or both result from compression fractures of the vertebral bodies as a result of laxity of the ligaments.

**Treatment.** Of primary concern to the physician and parents, especially in the prenatal or infantile forms of osteogenesis imperfecta, is to afford as much protection from fracture as possible. A tremendous degree of support is required to teach the parents how to appropriately accomplish this task without instilling such fear that it results in the parents' lack of handling the infant and fulfilling appropriate contact needs necessary for healthy growth and development. Continued counseling and support are required to accomplish this necessary balance and to alleviate parents' guilt feelings about fractures occurring after the birth process.

A balance must also be achieved when fractures do occur between enforced immobilization, which results in disuse atrophy, and a period of immobilization for normal healing. Alignment of the fractures is vital to avoid deformities. Adequate vitamin intake is essential. Estrogen administration may be of value; however, prolonged administration may cause osteoporosis with resultant compression fractures of the vertebrae.[5,p.310;6,p.312]

**Table 18-9.** Classification of osteogenesis imperfecta[5,p.303;6,p.309]

| Classification | Characteristics* |
| --- | --- |
| I. Fetal or prenatal form: osteogenesis imperfecta congenita | Severe with multiple fractures throughout body at birth<br>Skull soft and membranous<br>Infant may be stillborn or die at birth or within a few weeks<br>Loss of stature |
| II. Infantile form: osteogenesis imperfecta tarda, gravis form | Less severe<br>Multiple fracture during infancy<br>Skull thin and globular, may resemble that seen in hydrocephaly<br>Loss of stature<br>Survival after first few years increases chance of lessening frequency of fractures and continued survival |
| III. Adolescent form: osteogenesis imperfecta tarda, levis form | Normal at birth<br>Fracture due to minimal trauma later in childhood<br>Delayed ambulation<br>With increasing age, tendency to fracture is lost |

*Blue sclerae are usually associated with all types.

Surgical intervention may be the treatment of choice to correct severe deformities or fractures of long bones. Rotational osteotomies with intermedullary instrumentation is the procedure of greatest value in the realignment of the long bones. When a long bone is extremely fragile, homogeneous bone, either from the parent of the child or bone bank, may be utilized. Union occurs rapidly, generally with no disturbance of epiphyseal growth.[5,p.310; 6,p.312]

## OSTEOMALACIA (ADULT RICKETS)

Osteomalacia, in its strictest interpretation, refers to the softening of bone as a result of undermineralization of the bone matrix, but the term is more commonly utilized to refer to the adult type of rickets resulting from a nutritional deficit and corresponding to infantile rickets and its pathologic features.

**Etiology.** The most common cause of osteomalacia is deficiency of vitamin D as a result of inadequate absorption of calcium and phorphorus from the intestines.

**Pathology.** Lack of sufficient vitamin D causes the bones to become soft and the cortex to become thin. "Heart-shaped" pelvis is characteristic of this disease. The spine is often shortened, and the tibia and femur are usually bowed.

**Incidence.** The incidence of osteomalacia in the United States is rare in comparison with those countries that by culture have diets consistently deficient in vitamin D and that promote activities that are less likely to subsidize vitamin D intake through exposure to sunlight.

**Signs and symptoms.** The patient with osteomalacia complains of extreme tenderness in the areas of the pelvis, back, or hips. Progressive muscular weakness is present. Pathologic fractures are common. The spine, pelvis, and long bones may develop deformities resulting from undermineralization. Radiographic examination reveals the characteristic "heart-shaped" pelvis, tibial and femoral bowing, and a shortened spine, all of which may be present to varying degrees. Radiographically the long bones usually appear elongated and thin with bulbous ends, while vertebral bodies are frequently shallow, biconcave, and translucent.[1]

**Treatment.** The cause of osteomalacia must be accurately determined for appropriate treatment prescription. If due to malabsorption, this underlying process must be treated. If, however, as existent in the majority of cases, dietary deficiencies are the cause, appropriate alteration of dietary habits with sufficient quantities of vitamin D supplements pro-

vided in large doses is necessary. Supplements of calcium and phosphorus may also be useful in the overall therapeutic regimen. Exercises are of some value in the prevention of resulting deformities, with surgical intervention the treatment of choice if severe deformities exist. Rotational osteotomies are especially useful in the correction of angulation deformities in the lower extremities.[1]

## OSTEOPETROSIS (ALBERS-SCHÖNBERG DISEASE, MARBLE BONE DISEASE)

Osteopetrosis (Fig. 18-9) is a general skeletal disease characterized by widespread areas of increased bone density, creating a marbled effect, usually including the long bones of the extremity as well as the pelvis, vertebral column, and skull.

**Etiology.** The cause of osteopetrosis is unknown, but there is a familial or hereditary tendency transmitted as an autosomal-recessive or autosomal-dominant trait.

**Pathology.** The major factor affecting the pathogenesis of osteopetrosis is the "failure of osteoclastic resorption of the primary spongiosa."[1]

**Incidence.** Osteopetrosis is relatively rare. The most severe form is usually seen in the newborn, with less severe forms not apparent until later in life.

**Signs and symptoms.** The most severe form of osteopetrosis, the type transmitted as an autosomal-recessive trait, exhibits generalized bone alterations in the newborn, which often result in early death from osteosclerotic anemia. The less severe form, transmitted as an autosomal-dominant trait, is characterized by the same type of bone involvement with increased density but is present to a lesser degree. Although multiple problems may eventually be present, such as hepatosplenomegaly, blindness, malnutrition, and hydrocephalus, longevity is usually relatively normal. Pathologic fractures may occur with both types but usually heal with little difficulty. Radiographic examination reveals the extent to which the bone density is altered, with widespread areas of increase usually noted.[1]

**Treatment.** No curative treatment is available for osteopetrosis. Treatment is designed to relieve symptoms when present and to be supportive. No specific treatment modality is advocated.

## PAGET'S DISEASE (OSTEITIS DEFORMANS)

Paget's disease is a chronic skeletal disease with an insidious onset and is characterized by progressive development of skeletal deformities resulting from increased resorption accompanied by increased and abnormal regeneration.

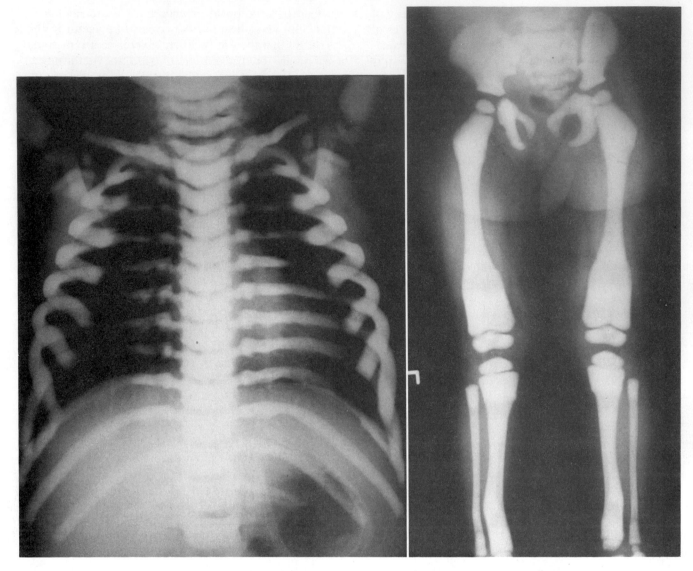

**Fig. 18-9.** Osteopetrosis (marble bones). Severe generalized osteosclerosis; severe mottling error with broadening of metaphyseal segments; marked sclerosis of hips and spine.

**Etiology.** The cause of Paget's disease is unknown.

**Pathology.** The major pathologic features of Paget's disease are the characteristic structural changes that result from disorganized acceleration of resorption and excessive, abnormal regeneration of osseous tissue. The lone bones become thickened, with apparent bowing. The cortex has an irregular surface creating a characteristic mosaic pattern. The cranium also usually shows signs of generalized thickening. Singular or multiple bone involvement may be seen.[1;2,p.185]

**Incidence.** Onset of Paget's disease is primarily during middle age and late adulthood. Approximately 3% to 4% of the population over 45 years of age are affected. Men are affected more frequently than women.[2,p.184]

**Signs and symptoms.** Paget's disease is often found accidentally on radiographic examination. The bones most frequently involved are the pelvis, femur, skull, tibia, and spine. The onset is insidious, with the initial complaint being pain in the lower back or lower extremities. The tibiae and vertebrae are most frequently involved in the early stages. The pain varies in type and intensity, ranging from an ache to a severe intractable pain. The tibiae may bow anteriorly, and the femurs may bow anteriorly and laterally. The head enlarges, and with vertebral involvement kyphosis and scoliosis result. The characteristic picture is that of the "patient standing in a crouched position with the head thrust forward, the trunk bent, and the lower extremities widely bowed outward."[6,p.653] The major complications associated with Paget's disease are pathologic fractures and malignant degeneration, with approximately 5% of cases undergoing malignant degeneration with resultant osteogenic sarcoma, fibrous sarcoma, or round cell sarcoma.[6,p.653] Progressive neurologic deficits due to vertebral compression may also result. Radiographic examination reveals characteristics relative to the area involved. Long bone involvement reveals bowing, enlarged and thickened cortex, and a loss of the usual definitive line between the cortex and the medulla. Pelvic involvement reveals an extremely prominent and coarse trabecular pattern, with the skull examination showing thickening and obliteration of sutures.[1]

**Treatment.** The treatment for Paget's disease is symptomatic and supportive. Salicylate therapy, sex hormones, vitamins, and x-ray therapy may be a part of the treatment regimen. Suppressive agents such as thyrocalcitonin and mithramycin have been used with some success. The patient must be kept active, but if fracture occurs he should be observed for signs and symptoms of hypercalcemia (nausea and vomiting, difficulty swallowing, dryness of the nose or throat). Hypercalcemia may be controlled by a low-calcium diet, magnesium salts, and fluids. Cardiovascular complications, pathologic fractures, and malignant regeneration are treated accordingly.[1,6,p.655]

## PERONEAL MUSCULAR ATROPHY (CHARCOT-MARIE-TOOTH DISEASE)

Peroneal muscular atrophy, or Charcot-Marie-Tooth disease, is a hereditary disease of a progressive nature resulting in atrophy and paralysis, beginning with the peroneal muscles and eventually involving the rest of the lower extremities and the upper extremities.

**Etiology.** The specific cause of peroneal muscular atrophy is unknown; it is transmitted as a dominant-recessive sex-linked trait.

**Pathology.** Peroneal muscular atrophy is a degenerative process that affects the anterior horn cells and the peripheral nerves. The resulting pathologic feature is muscular atrophy and paralysis of a progressive nature. The peroneal muscles are involved initially, with progression to the rest of the lower extremities, and eventually to the upper extremities.[6,p.420]

**Incidence.** Boys are more frequently affected than girls, with the onset of symptoms most frequently occurring between the ages of 5 and 10 years.

**Signs and symptoms.** Initial complaints of the patient with peroneal muscular atrophy are pain and paresthesia of the lower extremities. Tightening of the heel cords may also occur to varying degrees during the early stages. The gait may be a clumsy, steppage gait resulting from the equinovarus deformity. Progression results in stumbling and gait unsteadiness. Atrophy of the leg muscles and the intrinsic muscles of the feet occurs gradually. Eventually the patient walks with a toe-heel gait with progression of the equinovarus deformity and claw-toes. The upper extremities are comparably involved as the disease progresses, causing mild clawing of the hands. Reflexes are usually hypoactive or absent.[1,6,421]

**Treatment.** Nonsurgical intervention during the earliest stages of peroneal muscular atrophy is often successful in decreasing or at least delaying the progression of some of the deformities. Passive stretching exercises and night splinting are of some value. Surgical intervention may be required depending on the progression of heel cord tightening. These initial considerations are extremely important in the delay or prevention of the deformities, which considerably impair gait. Active exercises for maintenance of strength of weakened muscles are necessary on an ongoing basis. Additional surgical procedures and orthoses are prescribed to correct and prevent deformities.[1,5,p.1062]

## POLIOMYELITIS

Poliomyelitis is an acute viral infectious disease that results in temporary or permanent damage to the central nervous system with associated deformities and paralysis (Table 18-10).

**Etiology.** Poliomyelitis is caused by a "filterable virus with a special affinity for the anterior horn cells of the spinal cord and for certain motor nuclei of the brainstem."[5,p.944] The chief pathway for entrance of the virus is thought to be the gastrointestinal and respiratory tracts with subsequent invasion to the central nervous system.

**Pathology.** The virus responsible for poliomyelitis damages or destroys the anterior horn cells of the spinal cord and brainstem. "Anterior horn cell changes early show swelling of the cell, enlargement of the nucleus, and disappearance of the Nissl bodies. Next the nucleus undergoes chromatolytic degeneration, and basophilic granules fill the cytoplasm. Then changes may cease at this stage with reversibility and restoration of the cell, or the destruction of the cell may progress to comple-

**Table 18-10.** Stages, symptoms, and treatment of poliomyelitis[1, pp. 190-193; 6, pp. 448-449]

| Stage | Duration | Characteristic symptoms | Treatment | Prognosis |
|---|---|---|---|---|
| Acute | 1 to 4 weeks | Fever<br>Malaise<br>Cervical lymphadenopathy<br>Spinal fluid normal | Objective: symptomatic relief<br>  Moist heat<br>  Massage<br>  Exercises | Variable |
| Prepar-<br>alytic | | Stiff neck<br>Headache<br>Severe prostration<br>High temperature<br>Hypersensitivity to touch<br>Irritability<br>Possible positive Kernig's sign<br>Absent superficial reflexes |   Muscle relaxant drugs<br>Objective: prevention of<br>  deformity<br>  Maintenance of body<br>    alignment<br>  Splinting to avoid<br>    contractures | Recovery may occur<br>  with no paralysis |
| Paralytic | | Resistance to muscle-<br>  stretching movement<br>Onset on second or third day | | Recovery usually<br>  with varying de-<br>  grees of paralysis |
| Spinal | | Constitutional signs continue<br>Meningeal signs continue<br>Flaccid muscle weakness<br>Paralysis<br>Decreased deep reflexes<br>  Sporadic<br>  Asymmetric<br>Spasms, opposing muscles<br>Contractures | | |
| Bulbar | | Constitutional symptoms<br>  extreme<br>Meningeal symptoms extreme<br>Possible encephalitis<br>Somnolence, stupor<br>Emesis<br>Absent gag reflex<br>Possible involvement of<br>  medullary respiratory center | | High mortality |
| Conva-<br>lescent | Up to 2 years | Decrease in muscular<br>  tenderness<br>Increase in muscular power | Objective: attainment of<br>  maximum muscle power,<br>  restoration of loss of joint<br>  motion, prevention of<br>  deformities<br>  Gentle active exercises<br>    begun slowly and<br>    gradually increased to<br>    increase function and<br>    strength<br>  Passive exercises to<br>    prevent joint contrac-<br>    tures, avoiding muscle<br>    fatigue<br>  Exercise program<br>    directed by orthopedist<br>  Braces and crutches for<br>    support and ambulation | Varying degrees of<br>  recovery |
| Residual | Remainder<br>  of life | Remaining paralysis<br>  permanent<br>Residual deformities of<br>  varying severity | Objective: correction of<br>  deformities and improvement<br>  of function<br>  Physical therapy<br>  Orthoses<br>  Surgery | No further sponta-<br>  neous recovery |

tion."[6,p.448] Destroyed cells that innervate a particular muscle will never be repaired or replaced; therefore that muscle will exhibit complete and permanent flaccid paralysis.[2,p.153]

**Incidence.** With the advent of the polio vaccine only sporadic cases of poliomyelitis are seen today. However, because of decreased emphasis on the necessity for receiving immunization, concern relative to potential revitalization of this disease is now being exhibited by health care personnel.

**Signs and symptoms.** Two forms of poliomyelitis clinically exist. The *spinal type* is characterized by flaccid muscle weakness and paralysis of the extremities, back, abdomen, and respiratory muscles. The *bulbar type* is characterized by extreme constitutional and meningeal symptoms and is often associated with encephalitis. The gag reflex is absent. Somnolence, stupor, and emesis are common.[1,6,p.449]

The *acute stage* of poliomyelitis lasts from 1 to 4 weeks. The characteristic symptoms of this stage are fever, malaise, cervical lymphadenopathy, headache, and some muscle stiffness. The spinal fluid is normal during this stage. Progression from the preparalytic to the paralytic phase of the acute stage is characterized by increased signs of paralysis and resistance to muscle-stretching motions, with onset usually on the second or third day. The *convalescent* stage may last up to 2 years. Its major characteristics are a decrease in the muscular tenderness and increase in muscular power to varying degrees. *The residual stage* follows the convalescent stage. No further spontaneous recovery is seen during this stage. Any remaining paralysis is permanent. Residual deformities exist at varying locations and to varying degrees.[1,6,pp.448-449]

**Treatment.** The treatment of poliomyelitis in the acute stage is primarily directed by the pediatrician or internist; however, the orthopedic surgeon should be consulted early regarding the management of the musculoskeletal system. When the patient becomes afebrile, total care is accomplished by the orthopedist. The specific management or prescriptions are dependent on the stage of the disease process. During the acute stage symptomatic relief and prevention of deformity are of primary importance. Moist heat, muscle-relaxant drugs, massage, and exercises may be utilized for the former, while the maintenance of appropriate body alignment and splinting to avoid contractures is helpful in assisting with the latter. The focus of musculoskeletal management during the convalescent stage shifts to the attainment of maximum muscle power recovery, restoration of loss of joint motion, and prevention of deformities. Gentle active exercises may gradually be increased during this stage to maximize function and strength; passive exercises assist in the prevention of joint contractures and maximum joint motion. Orthotics and crutches may be utilized for support in the achievement of ambulatory goals. Treatment goals during the residual stage are directed toward the correction of any existing deformities, the prevention of further deformities, and the improvement of function. The physical therapy program, orthotic devices, and surgical intervention are individually prescribed and greatly dependent on the residual paralysis and deformities.[1,5,pp.945-946,6,p.448-449]

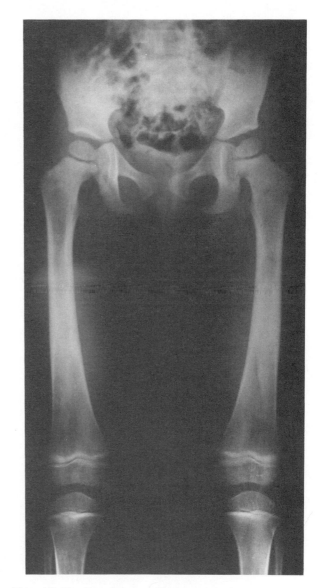

**Fig. 18-10.** Progressive diaphyseal dysplasia. Note marked sclerosis of diaphysis with minimal mottling error.

## PROGRESSIVE DIAPHYSEAL DYSPLASIA (ENGELMANN'S DISEASE)

Progressive diaphyseal dysplasia (Fig. 18-10) is a "rare developmental syndrome of the skeleton characterized by widened fusiform diaphyses with excessive periosteal and subcortical new bone formation and sclerosis, but with no involvement of the epiphyses or physes."[5,p.316]

**Etiology.** The cause of progressive diaphyseal dysplasia is unknown, but a familial tendency is often seen.

**Pathology.** The major pathologic features of progressive diaphyseal dysplasia include periosteal and subcortical new bone formation incorporated into the cortex of the long bones. The cortex as a result becomes markedly thickened with evidence of narrowing of the medullary cavity.[1,5,p.316]

**Incidence.** Progressive diaphyseal dysplasia is seen slightly more frequently in males than in females.

**Signs and symptoms.** Pain in the lower extremities is frequently associated with progressive diaphyseal dysplasia. Generalized muscular weakness may be seen with increased fatigability. A waddling gait is often seen. Increased lumbar lordosis may be present. Although upper extremities may be involved, most initial symptoms are seen in the lower extremities. Other associated signs and symptoms

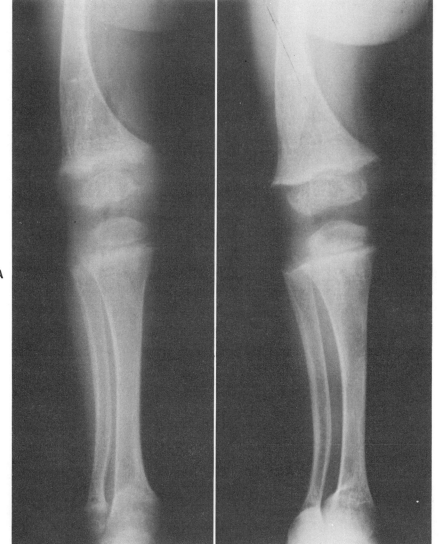

**Fig. 18-11.** Rickets. **A,** Pretreatment. Severe changes resulting in demineralization of bone with "B" wing of diaphysis, irregular metaphyseal margins. **B,** Healing stage after treatment shows regeneration of bone and metaphysis.

include delayed puberty, hypogonadism, skull changes (when involved), and potential neurologic alterations. Radiographic examination reveals increased bone density and widening of the cortex of the diaphyses but no epiphyseal alterations. The diaphyses are widened, and the medullary cavity is narrowed.[1,5,pp.316-319]

**Treatment.** No specific treatment modality is advocated for progressive diaphyseal dysplasia. Management is usually symptomatic in nature.

## RICKETS

Rickets (Fig. 18-11) is a disease of children and infants in which there is vitamin D deficiency or dietary lack of calcium and phosphorus causing softening of the bones and resulting deformities.

**Etiology.** The primary cause of rickets is deficiency of vitamin D or dietary lack of calcium and phosphorus. The four principle causes of this deficiency that may result in rickets are primary vitamin D deficiency, renal tubular insufficiency, chronic renal insufficiency, and hypophosphotasia.[5,p.434]

**Pathology.** The major pathologic feature of rickets is widespread increase of osteoid tissue resulting in epiphyseal thickening, enlargement of the cartilage at the costochondral junctions (rachitic rosary), and craniotabes.

**Signs and symptoms.** Early signs and symptoms of rickets include general lethargy and muscular weakness. The rachitic infant or child has a protruding abdomen, and developmental milestones such as standing, walking, and sitting are delayed. Craniotabes results from softening and thinning of the skull. Beading of the ribs (rachitic rosary) results from enlargement at the costochondral junction. Thickening of the knees, ankles, and wrists are classic manifestations of rickets as a result of epiphyseal widening. As growth progresses and body weight is exerted on the lower extremities, the softened long bones bow resulting in genu varum or valgum. There may also be deformities of the spine, and greenstick fractures are not uncommon.[5,p.434]

Radiographic examination of the infant or child with rickets reveals generalized osteoporosis and thinning of the cortices and bone trabeculae. Widening of the growth plate is noted. Areas of the most rapid bone growth show the most involvement (e.g., distal femur, proximal tibia). The affected epiphyses appear irregular and fuzzy. Varying degrees of bowing of the lower extremities may be noted.[2,p.172]

**Treatment.** A high calcium diet and large doses of vitamin D are components of the most useful treatment modality for rickets. Many of the skeletal deformities regress spontaneously with correction of the deficiency. The residual orthopedic deformities may be corrected by orthoses or surgical intervention (rotational osteotomy).[2,p.172]

## SCURVY

Scurvy is a nutritional disease resulting from dietary deficiency of vitamin C and resulting in subperiosteal hemorrhage and fractures with minimal trauma.

**Etiology.** Scurvy is caused by a dietary deficiency of vitamin C.

**Pathology.** Deficiency of vitamin C results in pathologic alterations throughout intracellular components of tissues, producing hemorrhage of the subperiosteal and submucosal tissues.

**Incidence.** Scurvy is rarely seen in the United States.

**Signs and symptoms.** The initial signs and symptoms of scurvy include loss of appetite, hemorrhage of the gums, irritability, and evidence of subperiosteal hemorrhage of the distal portion of the femur, tibia, or humerus. The lower extremities are often swollen. Beading of the ribs at the costochondral junction may develop. Delayed wound healing is common. Hemorrhage and fractures result from minimal trauma.[1,5,p.453]

**Treatment.** Treatment of scurvy includes daily oral and parenteral administration of vitamin C. With this therapy symptoms usually disappear and body growth resumes.

## REFERENCES

1. Brashear, H. R., Jr., and Raney, R. B., Sr.: Shand's handbook of orthopaedic surgery, ed. 9, St. Louis, 1978, The C. V. Mosby Co.
2. Gartland, J. J.: Fundamentals of orthopaedics, Philadelphia, 1974, W. B. Saunders Co.
3. Hellebrant, F. A.: Trends in the management of cerebral palsy (based on Phelps classification), Lectures at Medical College of Virginia, 1950-1951. Unpublished manuscript.
4. McKusick, V. A.: Heritable disorders of connective tissue, ed. 4, St. Louis, 1972, The C. V. Mosby Co.
5. Tachdjian, M. O.: Pediatric orthopaedics, Philadelphia, 1972, W. B. Saunders Co.
6. Turek, S.: Orthopaedics, Philadelphia, 1977, J. B. Lippincott Co.

## BIBLIOGRAPHY

Adams, J. C.: Outline of orthopaedics, Baltimore, 1971, The Williams & Wilkins Co.
Aegertu, E., and Kirkpatrick, J.: Orthopedic diseases, Philadelphia, 1975, W. B. Saunders Co.
American Orthopaedic Association: Manual of orthopaedic surgery, Chicago, 1972, The Association.

Arthritis Foundation: Arthritis manual for allied health professionals, Atlanta, 1973, The Foundation.

Aston, J. N.: A short textbook of orthopaedics and traumatology, London, 1972, English Universities Press, Ltd.

Brashear, H. R., Jr., and Raney, R. B., Sr.: Shand's handbook of othopaedic surgery, ed. 9, St. Louis, 1978, The C. V. Mosby Co.

Brewer, E. J.: Juvenile rheumatoid arthritis, Philadelphia, 1970, W. B. Saunders Co.

Crenshaw, A. H., editor: Campbell's operative orthopaedics, ed. 5, St. Louis, 1971, The C. V. Mosby Co.

Enneking, W. F., and Sherrard, M. G.: Physical diagnosis of the musculoskeletal system, Gainesville, Fla., 1969, Storter Printing Co., Inc.

Gartland, J. J.: Fundamentals of orthopaedics, Philadelphia, 1974, W. B. Saunders Co.

Goldstein, L. A., and Dickerson, R. C.: Atlas of orthopaedic surgery, St. Louis, 1974, The C. V. Mosby Co.

Iverson, L. D., and Clawson, D. K.: Manual of acute orthopaedic therapeutics, Boston, 1977, Little, Brown & Co.

Millender, L., and Sledge, C., editors: Symposium on rheumatoid arthritis, Orthop. Clin. North Am. **6**(3): 601-602, 1975.

Rosenbaum, M. G.: Understanding arthritis, St. Louis, 1975, Warren H. Green, Inc.

Rubin, A.: Handbook of congenital malformations, Philadelphia, 1969, W. B. Saunders Co.

Tachdjian, M. O.: Pediatric orthopaedics, Philadelphia, 1972, W. B. Saunders Co.

Turek, S.: Orthopaedics, Philadelphia, 1977, J. B. Lippincott Co.

# 19
# Tumors

**NANCY E. HILT**

**SHIRLEY B. COGBURN**

Many types of tumors are associated with the musculoskeletal system. The tumors discussed in this chapter are found in *all* tissues within this system. Because the musculoskeletal system comprises various types of tissue, it is helpful to understand the terminology utilized within the classification of these tumors:

**benign** abnormal growth but not malignant.
**malignant** abnormal growth; cancerous; usually associated with poor prognosis; frequently of recurrent nature.
**osteogenic** arising from osseous tissue.
**chondrogenic** arising from cartilaginous tissue.
**collagenic** arising from connective tissue such as tendon.
**myelogenic** arising from bone marrow.
**blastoma** granular tumor formed by single type of tissue (includes fibromas and chondromas)
**chondroma** cartilaginous tumor of slow growth.
**fibroma** fibrous, encapsulated, connective tissue tumor.
**sarcoma** malignant tumor.

With this terminologic foundation, classification of tumors of the musculoskeletal system can be easily comprehended.

Tumors may be *benign* or *malignant*. Benign tumors may be *osteogenic, chondrogenic*, or *collagenic*. Malignant tumors may be *osteogenic, chondrogenic, collagenic*, or *myelogenic*. *Primary* malignant tumors arise directly from musculoskeletal tissue or at least have the potential to do so. *Secondary* tumors arise from tissues other than musculoskeletal and have the potential of metastasizing to musculoskeletal tissue. Specific tumor classifications are given in Table 19-1. The focus of this chapter is on benign and primary malignant tumors. It should be emphasized, however, that some of the primary malignant tumors outlined only have the *potential* for arising directly from musculoskeletal tissue but are included to provide a comprehensive scope of the topic. In addition collagenic tumors, also because of their potential, are included.

**Table 19-1.** Classification of tumors arising from musculoskeletal tissue

| Tissue origin | Benign | Malignant (primary) |
|---|---|---|
| Osteogenic | Benign osteoblastoma<br>Giant cell tumor (osteoclastoma)*<br>Multiple chondromatosis (hereditary multiple exostosis)<br>Osteoid osteoma<br>Osteoma<br>Osteochondroma<br>Unicameral bone cyst | Osteosarcoma (osteogenic sarcoma)<br>Parosteal sarcoma |
| Chondrogenic | Benign chondroblastoma<br>Chondromyxoid fibroma<br>Enchondroma | Chondrosarcoma |
| Collagenic | Aneurysmal bone cyst<br>Angioma<br>Nonosteogenic fibroma (nonossifying fibroma)<br>Subperiosteal cortical defect | Angiosarcoma<br>Fibrosarcoma |
| Myelogenic | None | Ewing's sarcoma<br>Hodgkin's disease<br>Plasma cell myeloma<br>Reticulum cell sarcoma |

*Has potential to become malignant.

## BENIGN TUMORS

The benign musculoskeletal tumors are compared in Table 19-2. Radiographic findings are shown in Table 19-5.

### Osteogenic
#### Benign osteoblastoma

The benign osteoblastoma is a lesion of the bone. It is most frequently found in the spine but may be seen elsewhere.

**Etiology.** The cause of benign osteoblastoma is unknown.

**Pathology.** Benign osteoblastoma is similar to osteoid osteoma except for the presence of large numbers of osteoblasts; differential diagnosis is required.

**Incidence.** Benign osteoblastoma is relatively uncommon. It occurs more frequently in males, children, and young adults.

**Signs and symptoms.** The most common symptom is pain in the area of the lesion, sometimes indistinguishable from the pain associated with osteoid osteoma. The pain may be relieved dramatically with salicylate therapy. Vertebral location of the lesion may produce generalized back pain, paresthesia, and paraplegia.

**Treatment.** Benign osteoblastoma may be self-healing; because the duration is long and painful, however, this is contraindicated. Treatment by conservative measures, curettage or excision, is the choice dependent on the location of the lesion.

**Prognosis.** Recurrence of benign osteoblastoma is unlikely, and progression to malignancy is considered rare.

### Giant cell tumor (osteoclastoma)

Giant cell tumor (Fig. 19-1) is a very aggressive and destructive lesion with malignant potential. It occurs in young adults.

**Etiology.** The cause of giant cell tumor is unknown.

**Pathology.** The giant cell tumor is an eccentric lesion that invades the overlying cortex from within the bone. It exhibits characteristically multiple irregular chambers producing a "soap bubbles" effect. It has a high potentiality for malignant change and is sometimes considered to be a malignant tumor.

**Incidence.** The giant cell tumor occurs most frequently in young adults. It is infrequently seen in persons over 40 years of age. Its incidence is slightly higher in women than in men. The most common sites of giant cell tumor are the distal femur, proximal tibia, and distal radius, occurring in the region of the former epiphyseal plate of long bones after closure of the growth plates. It is infrequently seen in the vertebrae.

**Signs and symptoms.** The most common and frequently the only symptom is pain. Dependent on location, joint motion limitation and weakness may be seen.

**Treatment.** Treatment for giant cell tumor de-

*Text continued on p. 414.*

**Table 19-2.** Comparison of benign musculoskeletal tumors

| Tumor | Origin | Incidence | Site | Signs & symptoms | Preferred treatment | Prognosis | Comments |
|---|---|---|---|---|---|---|---|
| Benign osteo-blastoma | Osteogenic | ↑ Males<br>↑ Children and young adults | 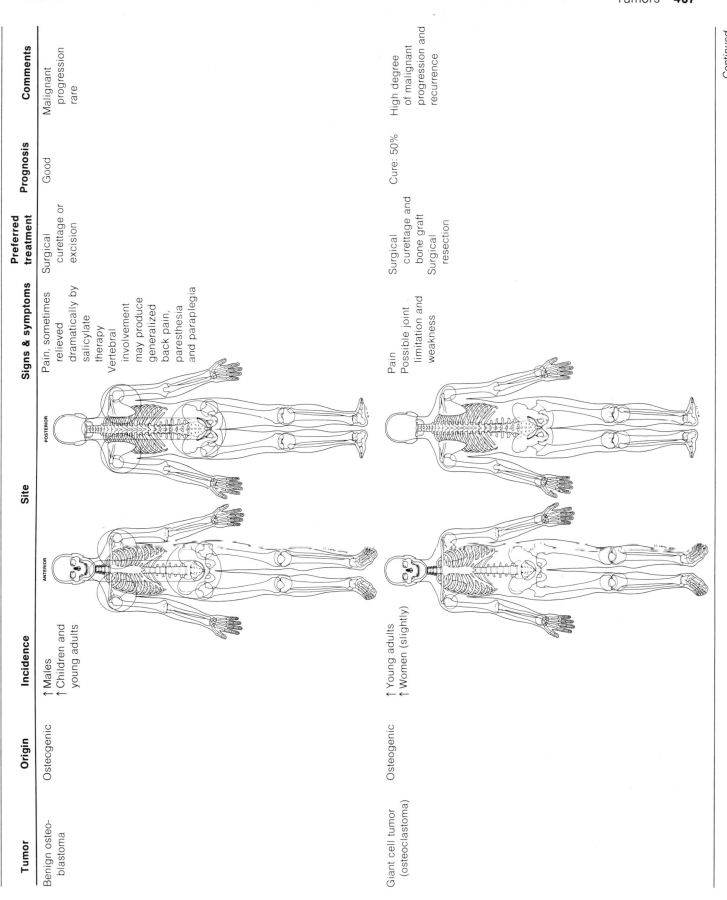 | Pain, sometimes relieved dramatically by salicylate therapy<br>Vertebral involvement may produce generalized back pain, paresthesia and paraplegia | Surgical curettage or excision | Good | Malignant progression rare |
| Giant cell tumor (osteoclastoma) | Osteogenic | ↑ Young adults<br>↑ Women (slightly) | | Pain<br>Possible joint limitation and weakness | Surgical curettage and bone graft<br>Surgical resection | Cure: 50% | High degree of malignant progression and recurrence |

*Continued.*

**Table 19-2.** Comparison of benign musculoskeletal tumors—cont'd

| Tumor | Origin | Incidence | Site | Signs & symptoms | Preferred treatment | Prognosis | Comments |
|---|---|---|---|---|---|---|---|
| Multiple osteo-chondromatosis (hereditary multiple exostosis) | Osteogenic | ↑ Males (3:1) Familial | | Asymptomatic If irritating to surrounding tissues, possible pain or neurovascular impairment | Surgical intervention only for alleviation of pain or correction of deformity | Good | Chondrosarcoma *may* occur but is rare |
| Osteoid osteoma | Osteogenic | ↑ Males ↑ Second and third decades of life | | Pain ↑ in time from intermittent to intense and sharply defined Pain may be localized or referred; may be relieved by salicylate therapy | Surgical resection | Good | Recurrence rare with complete resection |

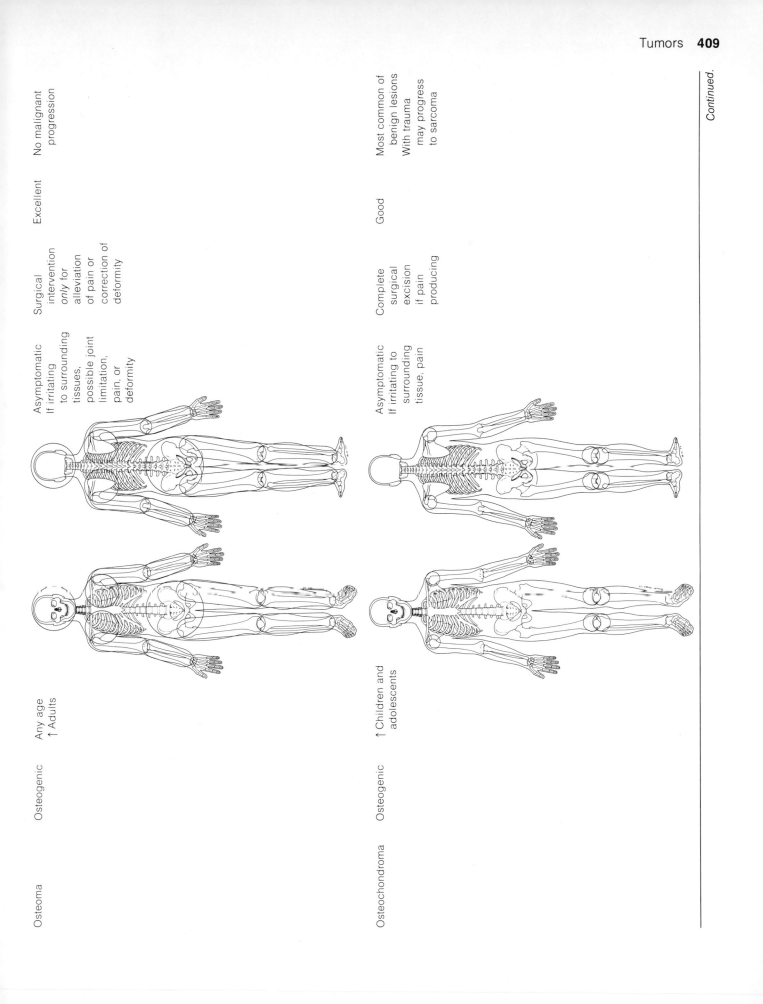

| Osteoma | Osteogenic | Any age<br>↑ Adults | Asymptomatic<br>If irritating to surrounding tissues, possible joint limitation, pain, or deformity | Surgical intervention *only* for alleviation of pain or correction of deformity | Excellent | No malignant progression |
| Osteochondroma | Osteogenic | ↑ Children and adolescents | Asymptomatic<br>If irritating to surrounding tissue, pain | Complete surgical excision if pain producing | Good | Most common of benign lesions<br>With trauma may progress to sarcoma |

*Continued.*

**Table 19-2.** Comparison of benign musculoskeletal tumors—cont'd

| Tumor | Origin | Incidence | Site | Signs & symptoms | Preferred treatment | Prognosis | Comments |
|---|---|---|---|---|---|---|---|
| Unicameral bone cyst | Osteogenic | ↑ First and second decades | | Asymptomatic Vague symptoms or mild discomfort Possible pathologic fracture | Spontaneous healing If fracture, surgical curettage with bone graft or resection | Good | Malignant changes rare |
| Benign chondro-blastoma | Chondrogenic | ↑ Adolescents ↑ Males | | Pain referred to joint Muscle atrophy Joint stiffness | Surgical curettage with bone graft | Good | No malignant progression Occasional recurrence |

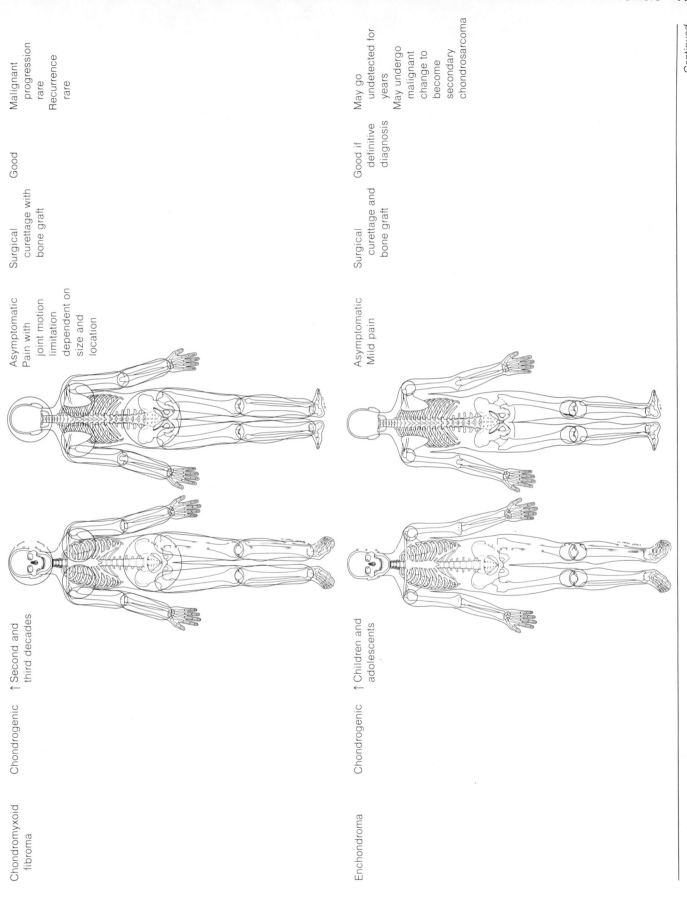

| | | | | | | | |
|---|---|---|---|---|---|---|---|
| Chondromyxoid fibroma | Chondrogenic | ↑ Second and third decades | | Asymptomatic Pain with joint motion limitation dependent on size and location | Surgical curettage with bone graft | Good | Malignant progression rare Recurrence rare |
| Enchondroma | Chondrogenic | ↑ Children and adolescents | | Asymptomatic Mild pain | Surgical curettage and bone graft | Good if definitive diagnosis | May go undetected for years May undergo malignant change to become secondary chondrosarcoma |

*Continued*

**Table 19-2.** Comparison of benign musculoskeletal tumors—cont'd

| Tumor | Origin | Incidence | Site | Signs & symptoms | Preferred treatment | Prognosis | Comments |
|---|---|---|---|---|---|---|---|
| Aneurysmal bone cyst | Collagenic | ↑ Adolescents and young adults | 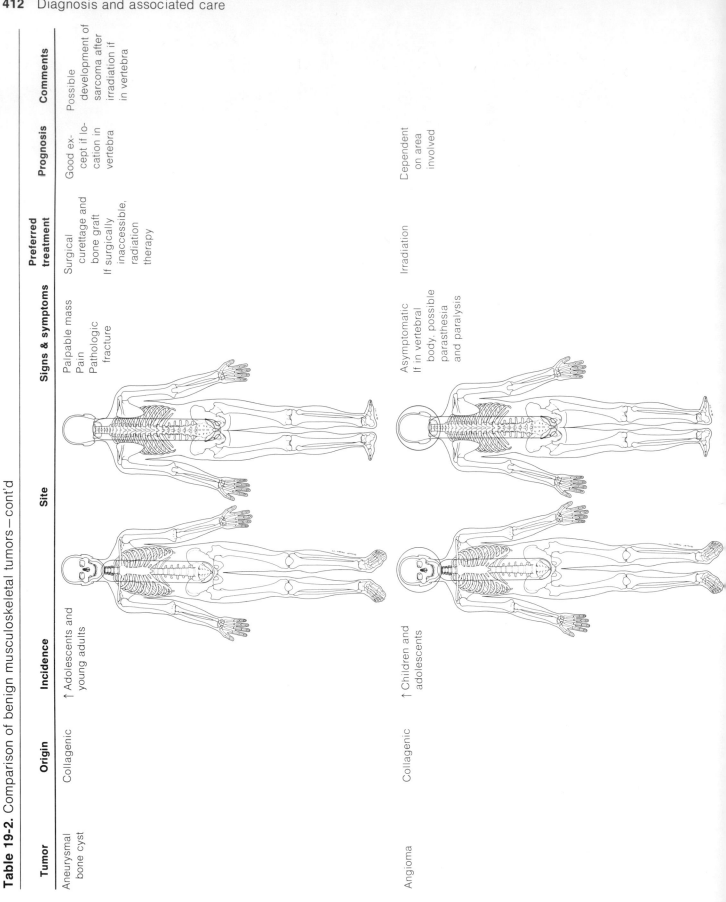 | Palpable mass Pain Pathologic fracture | Surgical curettage and bone graft If surgically inaccessible, radiation therapy | Good except if location in vertebra | Possible development of sarcoma after irradiation if in vertebra |
| Angioma | Collagenic | ↑ Children and adolescents | | Asymptomatic If in vertebral body, possible parasthesia and paralysis | Irradiation | Dependent on area involved | |

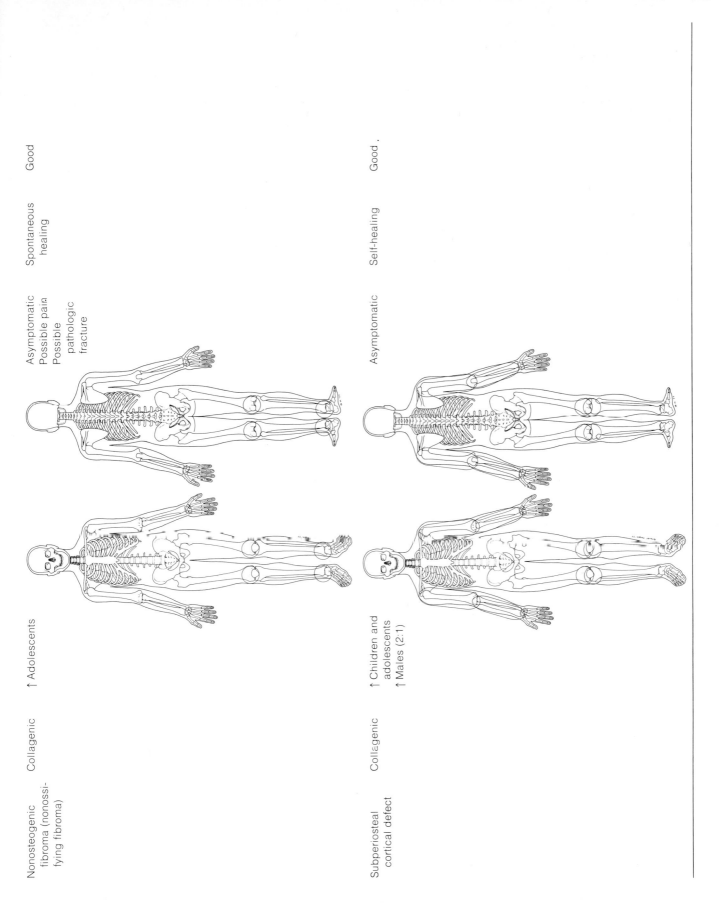

Nonosteogenic fibroma (nonossifying fibroma)

Collagenic

↑ Adolescents

Asymptomatic
Possible pain
Possible pathologic fracture

Spontaneous healing

Good

Subperiosteal cortical defect

Collagenic

↑ Children and adolescents
↑ Males (2:1)

Asymptomatic

Self-healing

Good

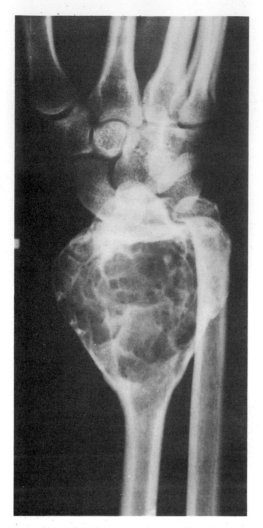

**Fig. 19-1.** Giant cell tumor of right radius. Note characteristic multiple irregular chambers, producing "soap bubbles" effect.

pends on the location. If accessible, curettage and bone grafting may be attempted. With this type of treatment, however, the tumor tends to recur, so more aggressive resection is the treatment of choice. Radiation therapy is contraindicated except in inaccessible lesions. In some cases amputation may be indicated.

**Prognosis.** Probable recurrence of this tumor with its malignant tendencies reduces the ultimate cure to approximately 50%.

### Multiple osteochondromatosis (hereditary multiple exostoses)

Multiple osteochondromatosis is a familial disease in which multiple bony overgrowths are present with growth disturbances. It is differentiated from the solitary osteochondroma by its number and familial trait.

**Etiology.** The cause of multiple osteochondromatosis is unknown.

**Pathology.** This anomaly of skeletal development produces multiple exostoses. In over 50% of patients, this lesion may be traced to an affected parent, usually the father. It may be similar in appearance to the solitary osteochondroma.

**Incidence.** Multiple osteochondromatosis is familial and is three times more common in males than females. Several children in one family may be affected. It appears most often in the long bones of the extremities.

**Signs and symptoms.** These lesions are usually asymptomatic unless irritation of surrounding tissues causes inflammation. They may cause pain from pressure on nerves or interference with vascular supply by compressing the blood vessels. Incomplete longitudinal growth of the ulna and fibula results in a characteristic curvature at the elbow and knee.

**Treatment.** Surgical intervention is not indicated for multiple osteochondromatosis except for alleviation of pain or for correction of a resulting deformity. Chondrosarcoma may occur but is rare in the young patient. If there is unusually rapid growth of the lesion, it should be excised.

**Prognosis.** With or without surgical intervention, the prognosis is most often good.

#### Osteoid osteoma

Osteoid osteoma (Fig. 19-2) is a relatively infrequent and benign osteoblastic lesion with limited growth potential.

**Etiology.** The cause of osteoid osteoma is unknown.

**Pathology.** Osteoid osteoma occurs within bone and less frequently may be seen between periosteum and cortex. It consists of a nidus or core of osteoid and bone surrounded by an area of sclerosis.

**Incidence.** Osteoid osteoma is more common in males than females. It develops most frequently in the second and third decades of life.

**Signs and symptoms.** The symptoms of osteoid osteoma are relatively distinct. The pain associated with this lesion increases in time from intermittent discomfort to intense and sharply defined pain. The pain, as with many other bone lesions, is usually worse at night but is often relieved by salicylate therapy. The pain may be localized or referred. If the lesion is located in the proximal femur the pain may mimic that of a herniated intervertebral disc, or it may be referred to the hip joint and produce a limp. The radiographic features are distinctive and diagnostic.

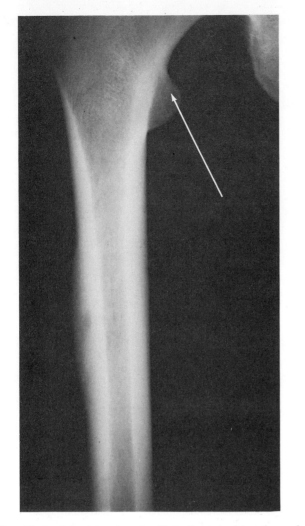

**Fig. 19-2.** Osteoid osteoma. Note lucent nidus *(arrow)* in center of area of thickened cortex.

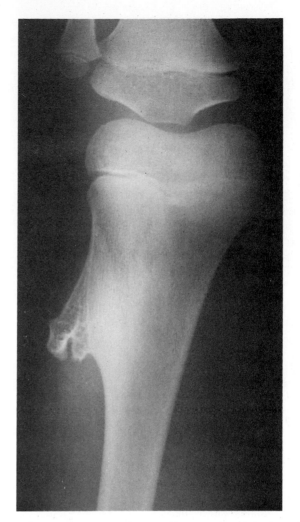

**Fig. 19-3.** Osteochondroma. Note cortex intact and trabecular structure within lesion.

**Treatment.** The preferred treatment of osteoid osteoma is resection of the involved area to relieve pain. Spontaneous healing without surgical intervention has been known to occur; however, this may be a long and painful process and thus is not the preferred treatment.

**Prognosis.** Osteoid osteoma has been known to recur, but with complete removal of the nidus patients may expect complete recovery.

### Osteoma

Although classified as an osteogenic tumor, the osteoma is no more than an exaggerated example of fibro-osseous tissue found in the skull and facial bones, especially in the paranasal sinuses.

**Etiology.** The cause of osteoma is unknown.

**Pathology.** Osteoma is found only in areas where bones are produced directly by cartilage.

**Incidence.** Osteoma usually occurs singly. Although it may occur at any age, it is most frequently seen in adults.

**Signs and symptoms.** Osteoma remains asymptomatic unless it intrudes on surrounding tissues and structures.

**Treatment.** Surgical intervention is indicated only if the lesion intrudes on surrounding tissues to the extent of unrelievable pain, limited function, or deformity; this is a rare occurrence.

**Prognosis.** The prognosis for osteoma is excellent with no evidence of neoplastic growth.

### Osteochondroma

An osteochondroma (Fig. 19-3) is a benign lesion that consists of a large spur or projection of bone covered by a cartilage cap.

**Etiology.** The cause of osteochondroma is unknown.

**Pathology.** Osteochondroma is thought to originate within the periosteum as a cartilaginous nodule. It is usually seen on the metaphysis of a long bone near the epiphyseal plate. The most frequent sites are the proximal humerus, distal femur, and proximal tibia.

**Incidence.** Osteochondroma is the most common of the benign bone tumors. It usually begins to develop during the growth period and may cease with skeletal maturation.

**Signs and symptoms.** Osteochondroma may be asymptomatic and thus may be found only by accident when the patient discovers a lump near a joint. Pain may exist due to irritation of surrounding structures. This lesion rarely causes a fracture but may, with trauma to the area, undergo change and become a sarcoma.

**Treatment.** The treatment of choice for osteochondroma is complete surgical excision if the lesion is large enough to have produced pain. It rarely recurs, but when it does it is usually the result of incomplete excision and therefore requires additional surgical excision.

**Prognosis.** The prognosis of a completely excised osteochondroma is good. Recurrence is usually in the form of chondrosarcoma.

### Unicameral bone cyst

A unicameral or solitary bone cyst (Fig. 19-4) is a benign cystic lesion of osteogenic origin, most frequently seen in the proximal humerus or femur.

**Etiology.** The cause of unicameral bone cyst is unknown.

**Pathology.** Unicameral bone cyst is thought to arise during childhood and adolescence. The single chamber is lined with a thin layer of soft tissue and characteristically contains a bloody, amber, or clear fluid, depending on age. Radiographic examination usually discloses an oval defect in the bone.

**Incidence.** Unicameral bone cyst occurs relatively frequently during the first two decades of life.

**Signs and symptoms.** A unicameral bone cyst may be present without symptoms. Frequently only vague symptoms of mild discomfort exist and are overlooked. The lesion may only become apparent after pathologic fracture has occurred.

**Treatment.** Unicameral bone cyst has been known to heal spontaneously. Reduction of the fracture, if it occurs, is not always dependable because of the tendency to refracture. The treatment of choice is either surgical curettage with bone graft or resection of the lesion.

**Prognosis.** Malignant changes in unicameral bone cyst have been reported but are rare.

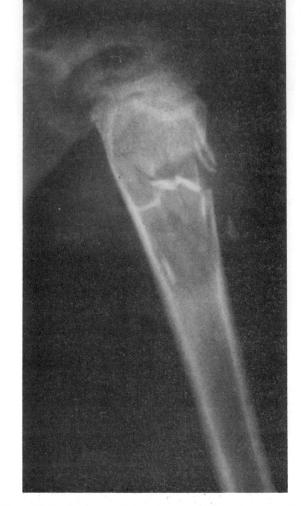

**Fig. 19-4.** Unicameral bone cyst. Fallen fragment indicates cystic rather than solid tumor.

## Chondrogenic
### Benign chondroblastoma

Benign chondroblastoma is a rare lesion arising from cartilaginous tissue.

**Etiology.** The cause of benign chondroblastoma is unknown.

**Pathology.** Benign chondroblastoma arises from young chondroblasts in the growth plate.

**Incidence.** Chondroblastoma is seen most frequently in the epiphyses of adolescents. It is seen in males more frequently than in females. The site affected most frequently is the humerus.

**Signs and symptoms.** Because of the epiphyseal involvement of this lesion, the pain it produces is usually referred to the joint. The lesion apparently grows slowly and with enlargement muscle wasting and joint stiffness may occur.

**Treatment.** The treatment of choice for benign chondroblastoma is surgical curettage and bone graft (usually from the iliac crest).

**Prognosis.** Benign chondroblastoma occasionally recurs but exhibits no tendency toward malignancy.

### Chondromyxoid fibroma

Chondromyxoid fibroma is a relatively rare benign lesion arising from cartilaginous tissue. It is not thought to be a true fibroma.

**Etiology.** The cause of chondromyxoid fibroma is unknown.

**Pathology.** Chondromyxoid fibroma may resemble hyaline cartilage, which is characteristically lobular. It is usually located in the metaphyseal region and may involve the epiphysis.

**Incidence.** Chondromyxoid fibroma is most frequently seen during the second and third decades of life. Although it may be seen in the flat bones, it is most often found in the long tubular bones near the knee.

**Signs and symptoms.** Chondromyxoid fibroma may be asymptomatic. Pain may occur with limitation of joint motion, depending on location and size of the lesion.

**Treatment.** The treatment of choice for chondromyxoid fibroma is curettage and bone grafting. Radiation therapy is contraindicated.

**Prognosis.** Recurrence of chondromyxoid fibroma has been documented, but wide resection is usually successful. Malignant changes are rare.

### Enchondroma

An enchondroma (Fig. 19-5) is a circumscribed, oval lesion containing cartilage cells and found in the metaphysis.

**Etiology.** The cause of enchondroma is unknown.

**Pathology.** This spheroid mass is comprised of a resilient substance and is pale and bluish. It never invades bone but may push it aside or cause lysis by pressure. Radiographic differentiation between some giant cell tumors, unicameral bone cysts, and enchondromas is sometimes difficult and complicates diagnosis of this lesion.

**Incidence.** Enchondroma is thought to begin to develop during the growth period in childhood or adolescence. It may go undetected for years and may undergo malignant change to become a secondary chondrosarcoma.

**Signs and symptoms.** Mild pain associated with this lesion is infrequent, and as a result the enchondroma may go undetected until a pathologic fracture occurs.

**Treatment.** Differential diagnosis between an

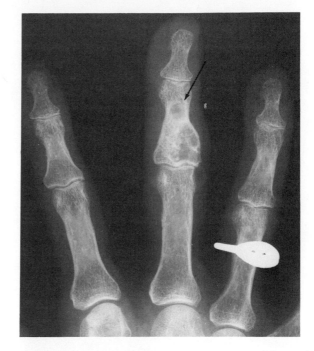

**Fig. 19-5.** Enchondroma of middle phalanx with small amount of cartilaginous calcification typical of this tumor.

enchondroma and a neoplasm is difficult but necessary for prescription of appropriate treatment. If the lesion occurs in the small bones of the hands or feet it is most often diagnosed as an enchondroma; chondrosarcoma is more frequently diagnosed if the lesion occurs in the flat bones or the metaphyses of large cylindrical bones. Confirmation of invasion or rapid growth may also assist in differential diagnosis. A problematic or questionable lesion is more likely to be treated radically. A confirmed enchondroma is treated by surgical curettage and bone grafting.

**Prognosis.** The prognosis for enchondroma is dependent on definitive diagnosis.

## Collagenic
### Aneurysmal bone cyst

An aneurysmal bone cyst (Fig. 19-6) is a benign lesion that is thought to arise from vascular tissue in bone. Characteristically it produces a "bubble" appearance on x-ray examination.

**Etiology.** The cause of aneurysmal bone cyst is unknown.

**Pathology.** Aneurysmal bone cyst, thought to arise from vascular tissue in bone, is classified as a neoplasm because of its tendency to destroy bone and its tumorlike characteristics. The lesion consists of large spaces filled with blood.

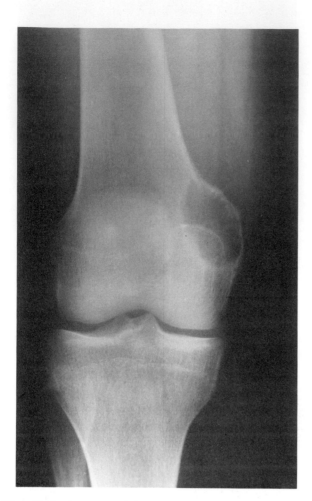

**Fig. 19-6.** Aneurysmal bone cyst. Note characteristic "bubble" appearance.

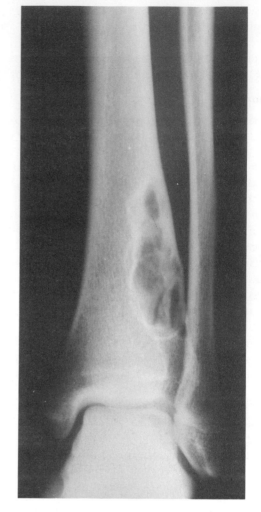

**Fig. 19-7.** Nonossifying fibroma (fibrous cortical defect). Note characteristic irregular circular area with scalloped border of sclerotic bone.

**Incidence.** Aneurysmal bone cyst develops with frequency in the adolescent and young adult. It may occur in any bone but is seen with some frequency in the vertebra.

**Signs and symptoms.** A palpable mass may be the first sign of aneurysmal bone cyst. Pain, depending on the size and location of the lesion, may occur. Pathologic fractures are occasionally seen.

**Treatment.** The treatment of choice is surgical curettage and bone grafting. Radiation therapy may be required for those lesions not easily accessible to surgical intervention such as the vertebral body. Differential diagnosis is important to avoid overtreatment.

**Prognosis.** The prognosis for aneurysmal bone cyst is usually considered to be good with curettage or irradiation. The exception is in vertebral involve-

ment in which development of sarcomas has been reported after radiation therapy.

### Angioma

An angioma is a highly vascular lesion that may occur singly but frequently is multiple.

**Etiology.** The cause of angioma is unknown.

**Pathology.** The angioma is a cavernous lesion filled with red blood cells. It may involve any part of the bone. Multiple lesions are known as angiomatosis of the bone.

**Incidence.** Angioma is found most frequently in children and adolescents.

**Signs and symptoms.** The majority of angiomas are asymptomatic. If the lesion involves the vertebral body, collapse with pressure on the spinal cord and nerves and subsequent paresthesia and paralysis may be the outcome.

**Treatment.** Surgical excision of angioma is risky due to its highly vascular nature. It may be treated with irradiation with good results.

**Prognosis.** The prognosis of angioma is highly dependent on the area involved.

### Nonosteogenic fibroma (nonossifying fibroma)

Nonosteogenic fibroma (Fig. 19-7) is a very common bone defect questionably classified as a true tumor. It occurs with frequency in children 10 to 15 years of age, in the long bones of the lower extremity.

**Etiology.** The cause of nonosteogenic fibroma is unknown.

**Pathology.** Nonosteogenic fibroma exhibits an irregular circular area with a scalloped border of sclerotic bone.

**Incidence.** Nonosteogenic fibroma occurs most frequently in adolescents and is most commonly seen in the large bones of the lower extremity. The highest incidence is in the femur.

**Signs and symptoms.** Nonosteogenic fibroma is frequently asymptomatic, and as a result the diagnosis is usually made on incidental x-ray examination. In some cases, however, pain or pathologic fracture may be seen.

**Treatment.** Spontaneous healing may occur with nonosteogenic fibroma. Differential diagnosis must be made between this lesion and bone cyst, fibrous dysplasia, giant cell tumor, bone infarct, and chronic osteomyelitis.

**Prognosis.** The prognosis for nonosteogenic fibroma is good, especially in view of the fact that many such lesions undergo spontaneous healing.

### Subperiosteal cortical defect

A benign lesion, subperiosteal cortical defect is questionably categorized as a tumor. It frequently occurs in children and adolescents, is usually asymptomatic, and may be referred to as a "bone island."

**Etiology.** The cause of subperiosteal cortical defect is unknown.

**Pathology.** Sometimes referred to as a "bone island," this lesion involves cortical bone craters filled with fibrous tissue. Although not a true tumor, its inclusion is significant because of the necessity for differential diagnosis.

**Incidence.** Subperiosteal cortical defect is seen most frequently in children and adolescents and is most commonly found in the long cylindrical bones of the lower extremity. It is twice as common in males as in females.

**Signs and symptoms.** Subperiosteal cortical defect may remain asymptomatic and therefore untreated.

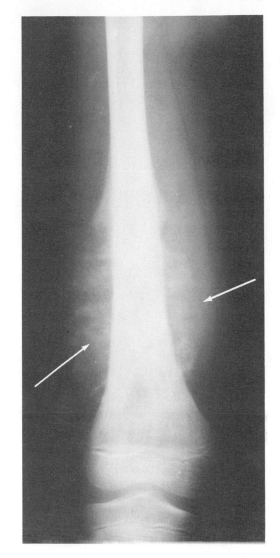

**Fig. 19-8.** Osteosarcoma of femur.

**Treatment.** The need for differential diagnosis is of utmost importance; overtreatment due to faulty diagnosis can be tragic. Frequently no treatment is necessary other than definitive diagnosis to rule out other types of lesions.

**Prognosis.** Subperiosteal cortical defect may be self-limiting and self-healing over a period of several years.

## PRIMARY MALIGNANT TUMORS

The primary malignant musculoskeletal tumors are compared in Table 19-3. Radiographic findings are shown in Table 19-4.

### Osteogenic
#### Osteosarcoma (osteogenic sarcoma)

Osteosarcoma (Fig. 19-8) is one of the most frequently seen primary malignant tumors of bone as well as the most fatal.

*Text continued on p. 425.*

**Table 19-3.** Comparison of primary malignant musculoskeletal tumors

| Tumor | Origin | Incidence | Site | Signs & symptoms | Preferred treatment | Prognosis | Comments |
|-------|--------|-----------|------|------------------|---------------------|-----------|----------|
| Osteosarcoma (osteogenic sarcoma) | Osteogenic | ↑ Males<br>↑ Second and third decades | 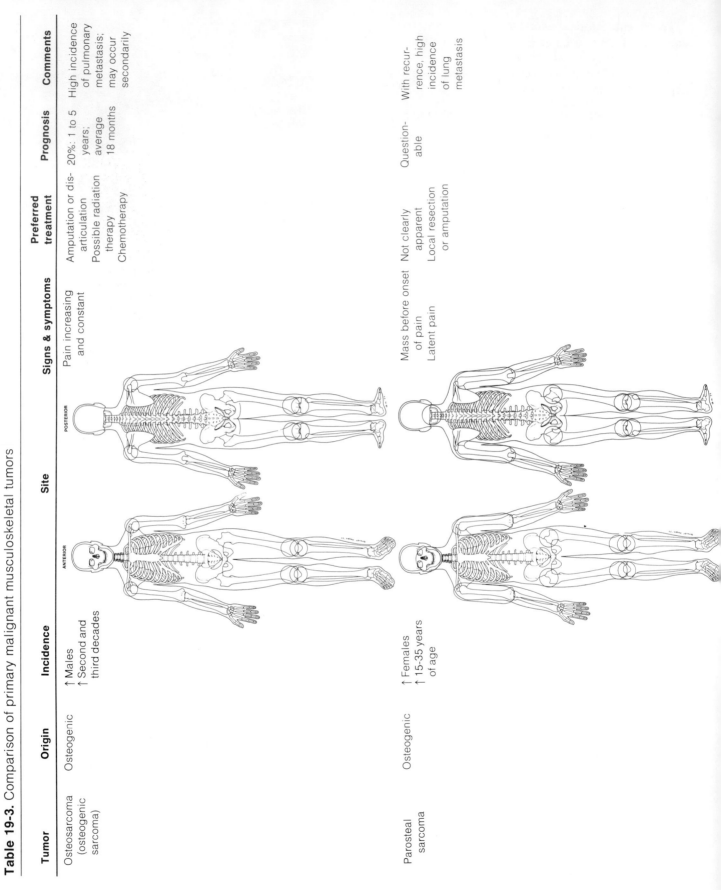 | Pain increasing and constant | Amputation or dis-articulation<br>Possible radiation therapy<br>Chemotherapy | 20%: 1 to 5 years; average 18 months | High incidence of pulmonary metastasis; may occur secondarily |
| Parosteal sarcoma | Osteogenic | ↑ Females<br>↑ 15-35 years of age | | Mass before onset of pain<br>Latent pain | Not clearly apparent<br>Local resection or amputation | Question-able | With recur-rence, high incidence of lung metastasis |

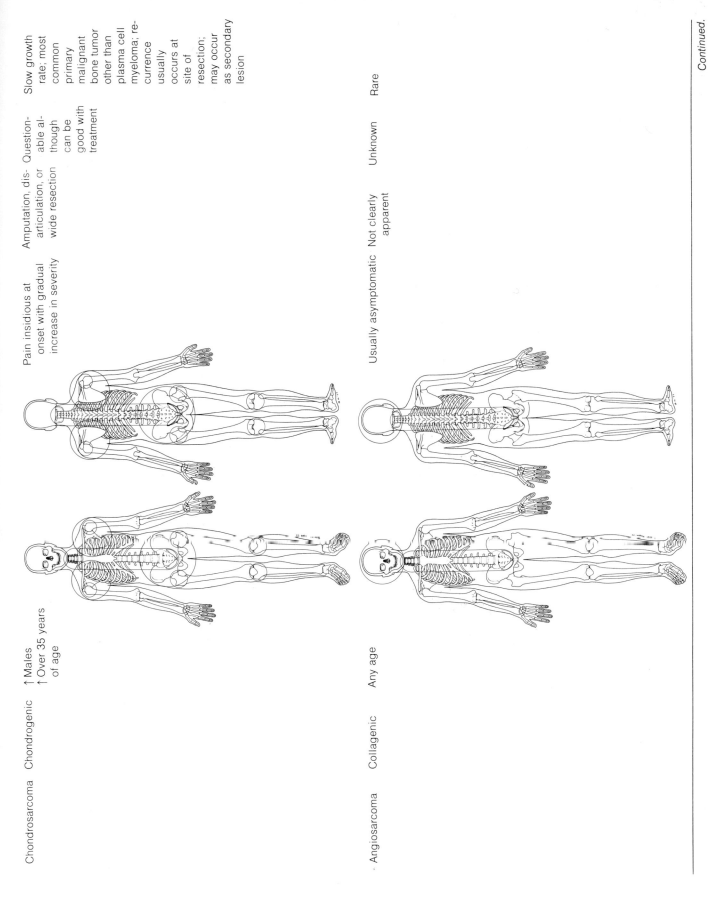

| | | | | | | |
|---|---|---|---|---|---|---|
| Chondrosarcoma | Chondrogenic | ↑ Males<br>↑ Over 35 years of age | Pain insidious at onset with gradual increase in severity | Amputation, disarticulation, or wide resection | Questionable although can be good with treatment | Slow growth rate; most common primary malignant bone tumor other than plasma cell myeloma; recurrence usually occurs at site of resection; may occur as secondary lesion |
| Angiosarcoma | Collagenic | Any age | Usually asymptomatic | Not clearly apparent | Unknown | Rare |

*Continued.*

**Table 19-3.** Comparison of primary malignant musculoskeletal tumors—cont'd

| Tumor | Origin | Incidence | Site | Signs & symptoms | Preferred treatment | Prognosis | Comments |
|---|---|---|---|---|---|---|---|
| Fibrosarcoma | Collagenic | ↑Middle age | | Pain at site<br>Swelling at site | Amputation<br>Chemotherapy | Better than osteosarcoma or chondrosarcoma | Slow growing |
| Ewing's sarcoma | Myelogenic | ↑Second decade of life | | Systemic manifestations: fever, leukocytosis<br>Pathologic fractures | Radiation therapy<br>Chemotherapy | Mortality high; life expectancy averages 2 years | Metastasizes to other bone rather than other tissue |

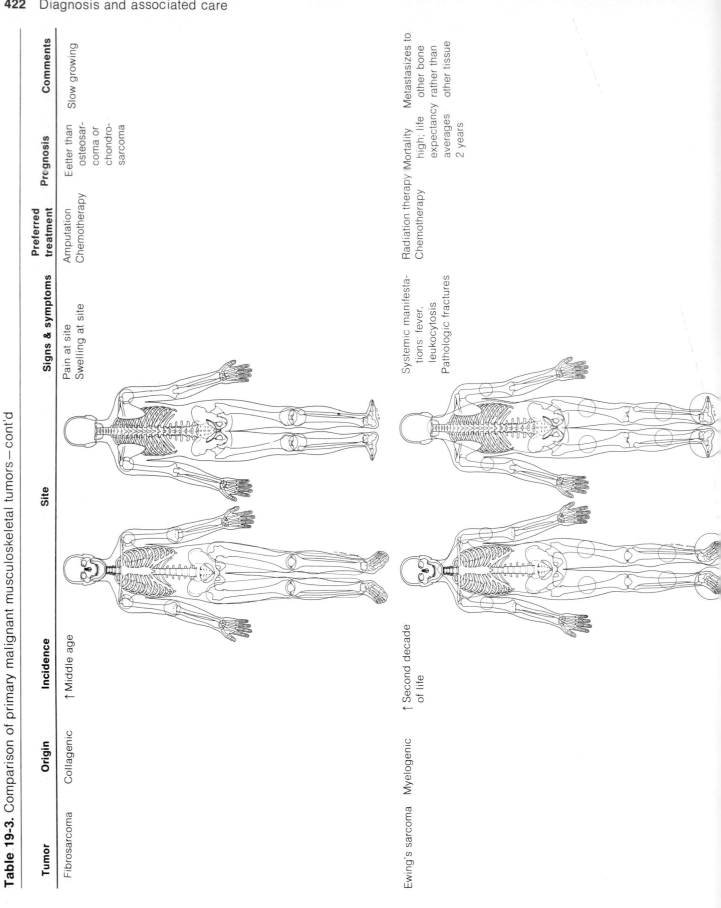

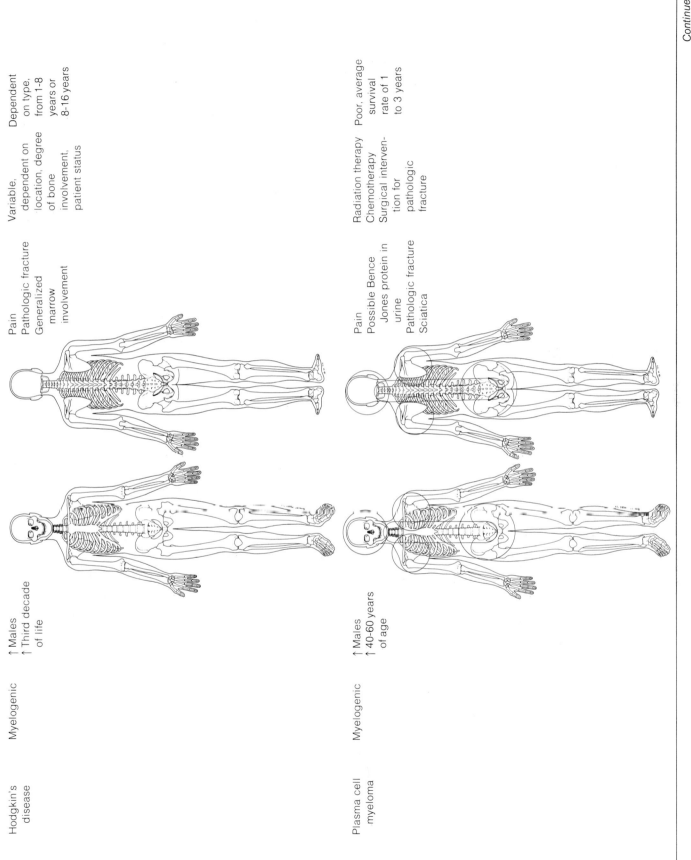

Hodgkin's
disease

Myelogenic

↑ Males
↑ Third decade
  of life

Pain
Pathologic fracture
Generalized
  marrow
  involvement

Variable,
dependent on
location, degree
of bone
involvement,
patient status

Dependent
on type,
from 1-8
years or
8-16 years

Plasma cell
myeloma

Myelogenic

↑ Males
↑ 40-60 years
  of age

Pain
Possible Bence
  Jones protein in
  urine
Pathologic fracture
Sciatica

Radiation therapy
Chemotherapy
Surgical interven-
  tion for
  pathologic
  fracture

Poor, average
survival
rate of 1
to 3 years

*Continued.*

**Table 19-3.** Comparison of primary malignant musculoskeletal tumors—cont'd

| Tumor | Origin | Incidence | Site | Signs & symptoms | Preferred treatment | Prognosis | Comments |
|-------|--------|-----------|------|------------------|--------------------|-----------|----------|
| Reticulum cell sarcoma | Myelogenic | ↑ Adults | | Pain Pathologic fracture | Differential diagnosis from Ewing's sarcoma Radiation therapy Chemotherapy | Good with radiation therapy and early diagnosis | |

**Table 19-4.** Radiographic findings of musculoskeletal tumors

| Radiographic finding | Benign | Malignant |
| --- | --- | --- |
| Margin of lesion | Clear-cut and well defined; may have sclerosed margin | No clear-cut margin; invasive and abnormal bone fades into normal bone |
| Periosteal reaction | Rarely occurs except in the following:<br>Osteoid osteoma: reaction is well formed and consolidated as opposed to irregular reaction of malignant tumor<br>Aneurysmal bone cyst: periosteal (blowout) or part of bone contour<br><br>Chondroblastoma: may produce slight periosteal reaction | Common and occurs in all malignant forms of bone tumor except:<br>Reticulum cell sarcoma (entirely destructive)<br><br>Endosteal type of fibrosarcoma; may be absent in osteogenic sarcoma or Paget's disease |
| Expansion | Not uncommon in benign tumors | Malignant tumor grows too rapidly to expand bone; it perforates and destroys cortex *except* in central chondrosarcoma (relatively benign) |
| Soft tissue swelling (high-quality films required, at least two views) | Absent | Usually present except in endosteal fibrosarcoma (unless late and eroding cortex) |

From Gillis, L.: Diagnosis in orthopaedics, New York, 1969, Appleton-Century-Crofts.

**Etiology.** The cause of osteosarcoma is unknown.

**Pathology.** Osteosarcoma arises from osteoblasts and primitive cells. Except for marrow tumors, it is the most common and most fatal of the primary malignant bone tumors.

**Incidence.** Osteosarcoma is seen most frequently in men during the second and third decades of life. The most common sites are near the epiphyseal growth plates of long bones.

Osteosarcoma has been known to occur secondarily in Paget's disease, irradiated bone, and rarely in osteochondroma.

**Signs and symptoms.** The common symptom seen with osteosarcoma is increasing and constant pain due to bone destruction and erosion. Radiographic diagnosis is relatively significant, but confirmation must be made by biopsy.

**Treatment.** The treatment of choice for osteosarcoma is amputation or disarticulation if an extremity is involved. This may be accomplished for relief of pain. Radiation may be utilized for control of local symptoms but has little effect on the lesion, since it is radiosensitive. Cytotoxic drugs or other chemotherapeutic regimens are utilized in conjunction with surgical or radiographic intervention.

**Prognosis.** Only 20% of patients with osteosarcoma survive for 5 years, with an average survival of 18 months. The patient frequently succumbs to pulmonary metastasis.

**Parosteal sarcoma**

Parosteal sarcoma is a less common malignant lesion arising from periosteal tissue.

**Etiology.** The cause of parosteal sarcoma is unknown.

**Pathology.** Parosteal sarcoma arises from the periosteum and frequently involves the metaphyseal region.

**Incidence.** Parosteal sarcoma is considerably less common than osteosarcoma, chondrosarcoma, or fibrosarcoma. It affects more females than males and is most often seen between the ages of 15 and 35 years. The most common site of involvement is the proximal femur.

**Signs and symptoms.** The patient is frequently aware of a mass before the onset of pain, which may be considerably latent compared with many malignant lesions. Pathologic fracture is usually not seen, since actual bone destruction does not occur with the severity seen with other tumors.

**Treatment.** The treatment of parosteal sarcoma is not clearly defined. Diagnosis by biopsy may lead to conservative measures; however, there is incidence of recurrence after only local resection. More radical treatment, therefore, with amputation is often necessary.

**Prognosis.** The prognosis for parosteal sarcoma is questionable and often dependent on the aggressiveness of the initial treatment. With recurrence there is a high incidence of lung metastasis.

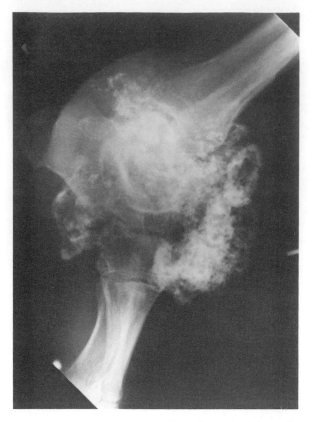

**Fig. 19-9.** Chondrosarcoma. Note flocculent formation of tumor.

## Chondrogenic
### Chondrosarcoma

Chondrosarcoma (Fig. 19-9) is a malignant musculoskeletal tumor arising from cartilaginous tissue and ultimately grows into a large cartilaginous growth. It is the only chondrogenic lesion with anticipated malignant behavior.

Chondrosarcoma may be classified as either *primary* (arising without a known preexisting lesion) or *secondary* (arising from or in association with a preexisting lesion). This becomes apparent with review of the potentialities of the benign lesions.

**Etiology.** The cause of chondrosarcoma is unknown.

**Pathology.** Chondrosarcoma exhibits characteristic multichambered areas of bone destruction containing scattered areas of calcification. It arises from chondroblasts and collagenoblasts.

**Incidence.** Chondrosarcoma is the most common primary malignant bone tumor other than plasma cell myeloma. It occurs about half as frequently as osteosarcoma. It is seen more frequently in men than in women. It is infrequently seen in patients under 30 years of age, but the incidence rises considerably after 35 years of age. The most common sites are the bones of the trunk, shoulder, and hip.

**Signs and symptoms.** The signs and symptoms exhibited are dependent on the area involved. Pain, however, is a consistent symptom and usually is insidious at the onset with a gradual increase in severity. The symptoms may not be recognized for years because of the slow growth rate of this lesion.

**Treatment.** Amputation, disarticulation, or extremely wide resection is the treatment of choice for chondrosarcoma. The specific choice is greatly dependent on the location and size of the lesion. Radiation therapy is contraindicated because this lesion is radioresistant. Cytotoxic drugs are of questionable value.

**Prognosis.** The prognosis for chondrosarcoma is questionable, although it is felt to be good if there is no recurrence. The fact that this lesion grows slowly and usually metastasizes late is favorable. If there is recurrence it is usually at the site of resection.

## Collagenic
### Angiosarcoma of bone

Angiosarcoma is a malignant lesion of vascular origin that infiltrates the healthy areas surrounding the primary site and metastasizes very early.

**Etiology.** The cause of angiosarcoma is unknown.

**Pathology.** Angiosarcoma may be composed of one or a combination of the following cell types: hemangioendothelioma, hemangiosarcoma, hemangiopericytoma, or hemangioblastoma.

**Incidence.** Angiosarcoma found in the bone as a primary lesion is rare. It may occur at any age and occurs with greater frequency in the skull and vertebrae.

**Signs and symptoms.** Most angiosarcomas remain asymptomatic. If within the vertebral body, weakening due to lysis and collapse with spinal cord pressure, resulting nerve infringement, and subsequent symptoms of the involved area may occur.

**Treatment.** The treatment of choice for angiosarcoma of bone is not clearly defined and depends on the size and location of the lesion.

**Prognosis.** The prognosis for angiosarcoma is not known.

### Fibrosarcoma

Fibrosarcoma is a relatively slow growing primary malignant lesion occurring less frequently than osteosarcoma.

**Etiology.** The cause of fibrosarcoma is unknown.

**Pathology.** Fibrosarcoma arises from fibrous connective tissue of bone. It tends to recur but not to metastasize.

# Myelogenic
## Ewing's sarcoma

Ewing's sarcoma (Fig. 19-10) is a highly malignant primary sarcoma of bone. It is the third most common primary tumor.

**Etiology.** The cause of Ewing's sarcoma is unknown.

**Pathology.** Ewing's tumor arises from cells within the marrow reticulum. It begins in the medullary region and causes bone destruction from within.

**Incidence.** Ewing's sarcoma is seen in patients under 30 years of age, with the highest incidence in the second decade of life. Although it may be seen in any bone, the highest incidence is associated with the flat bones.

**Signs and symptoms.** Manifestations of Ewing's tumor are often systemic. Fever is likely to be present at the onset (38 C to 40 C [100 F to 105 F]), and leukocyte count ranges from levels of 20,000 to 40,000/cu mm. Pathologic fractures may be seen due to bone necrosis. This lesion has a tendency to metastasize to other bone rather than to other tissue.

**Treatment.** Irradiation and cytotoxic drugs are the treatment of choice because of their local and systemic effects. A combination of both is likely to be prescribed.

**Prognosis.** The prognosis for Ewing's sarcoma has improved in the past few years. Although 3- to 5-year survival is not always expected, it is not uncommon.

## Hodgkin's disease

Hodgkin's disease involving bone is similar to that in soft tissue or viscera.

**Etiology.** The cause of Hodgkin's disease is unknown.

**Pathology.** Hodgkin's disease involves the lymphoid reticulum arising from tissues in the lymph nodes, spleen, liver, skin, thymus gland, and intestinal follicles. Its characteristic lymphatic leukemia usually infiltrates the bone marrow and may produce bone changes.

**Incidence.** Hodgkin's disease is predominant in males and is seen most frequently in the third decade of life.

**Signs and symptoms.** The specific symptoms related to the musculoskeletal involvement of Hodgkin's disease depend on the location and degree of involvement. Pain and pathologic fractures may be seen.

**Treatment.** Surgical intervention and irradiation are the treatments of choice but greatly vary according to the location, degree of involvement, and patient status.

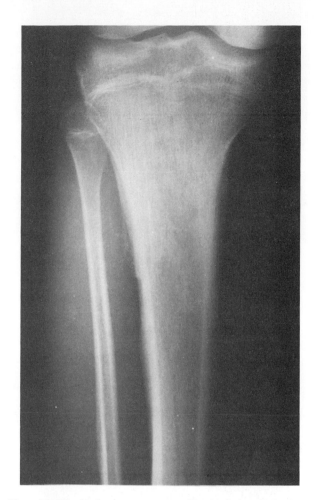

**Fig. 19-10.** Ewing's sarcoma. Typical laminated or "onionskin" periosteal reaction with some vertical spiculation. "Hair on end" periosteal reaction. Subtle finding soft periosteal reaction and blurring of trabecular pattern.

**Incidence.** Fibrosarcoma is seen approximately one third as often as osteosarcoma. It occurs in the long bones of the lower extremity, most frequently the femur or tibia. Although it may be seen at any age, the most common incidence is during middle age.

**Signs and symptoms.** Pain and swelling at the site of the lesion are the most common symptoms. Pathologic fractures are not often seen in association with fibrosarcoma.

**Treatment.** Because fibrosarcoma is radioresistant, amputation of the involved part is the treatment of choice. Cytotoxic drugs or other chemotherapeutic regimens are also utilized.

**Prognosis.** The prognosis for fibrosarcoma with treatment is better than for osteosarcoma or chondrosarcoma.

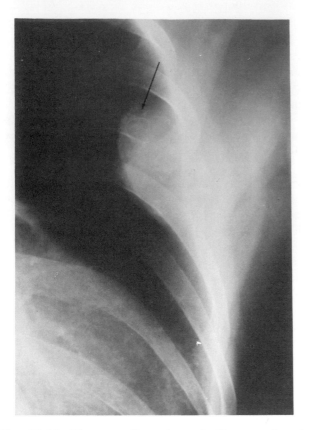

**Fig. 19-11.** Plasma cell myeloma (solitary myeloma) with expanded and destroyed cortex.

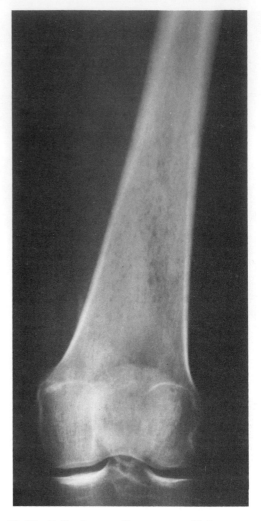

**Fig. 19-12.** Reticulum cell sarcoma. Note permeated pattern within shaft of bone.

**Prognosis.** Hodgkin's disease and its characteristic involvement has recently been divided into six types. The prognosis is dependent on the type and survival rates may range from 8 to 16 years or 1 to 8 years. The degree of musculoskeletal involvement is not necessarily indicative of overall prognosis.

### Plasma cell myeloma (multiple myeloma, myelomatosis)

Plasma cell myeloma (Fig. 19-11) is the most common of the primary malignant bone lesions.

**Etiology.** The cause of plasma cell myeloma is unknown.

**Pathology.** Plasma cell myeloma arises from plasma cells in bone marrow.

**Incidence.** Plasma cell myeloma is seen more frequently in men than in women. The highest incidence is found between 40 and 60 years of age.

**Signs and symptoms.** The most common symptom of plasma cell myeloma is pain, which may vary considerably. Bence-Jones protein is found in the urine of more than 50% of the patients. Pathologic fracture may occur. Involved nerve root compression of the vertebrae elicits symptoms correspond-

ing with the involved area. Sciatica may be the chief complaint.

**Treatment.** Irradiation and chemotherapeutic drugs are the treatment of choice. Biopsy is accomplished for the purpose of diagnosis. Additional surgical intervention may be required if a pathologic fracture occurs.

**Prognosis.** The prognosis for plasma cell myeloma is poor, with average survival rates of 1 to 3 years.

### Reticulum cell sarcoma

Reticulum cell sarcoma (Fig. 19-12) is a relatively uncommon malignant lesion and is the slowest growing and least malignant of all marrow tumors.

**Etiology.** The cause of reticulum cell sarcoma is unknown.

**Table 19-5.** Metastatic musculoskeletal tumor classification

| Classification | |
|---|---|
| **Predominantly osteolytic** | **Predominantly osteoblastic** |
| Source of metastasis | Source of metastasis |
| Carcinoma of breast | Carcinoma of breast |
| Carcinoma of kidney | Carcinoma of intestinal |
| Carcinoma of thyroid | tract |
| gland | Bronchogenic carcinoma |
| Neuroblastoma | Carcinoma of prostate |
| | gland |

**Pathology.** Reticulum cell sarcoma arises from cells of the marrow reticulum.

**Incidence.** Reticulum cell sarcoma may be found in the long or flat bones. The highest incidence is in adults.

**Signs and symptoms.** Pain is the most outstanding symptom of reticulum cell sarcoma. The fever and leukocytosis associated with Ewing's sarcoma is not usually seen. Pathologic fracture may occur.

**Treatment.** Cellular differential diagnosis from Ewing's sarcoma may be difficult; however, reticulum cell sarcoma affects older patients and is slower growing and less malignant. Treatment of choice involves irradiation and cytotoxic drug therapy. Surgical intervention for diagnostic purposes or treatment of pathologic fracture is indicated.

**Prognosis.** Good prognosis is possible with irradiation and early diagnosis.

## SECONDARY MALIGNANT TUMORS

Secondary musculoskeletal tumors are those associated with, arising from, or metastasizing from a primary tumor of another origin. The most common sites from which primary tumors metastasize to bone are (1) the breast (adenocarcinoma of the breast is the most frequent source of metastasis to bone), (2) the kidney, (3) the lung, (4) the prostate gland, and (5) the thyroid gland. Musculoskeletal involvement may invade the bone or associated tissues by direct extension or by way of the blood or lymphatic transport systems.

**Table 19-6.** Chemotherapeutic agents commonly utilized with malignant musculoskeletal lesions

| Drug | Dosage route of administration | Side effects | Toxicity | Precautions | Major indications |
|---|---|---|---|---|---|
| Cyclophosphamide (Cytoxan) | 500-1500 mg/sq m as single dose IV; or 60-120 mg/m/ day PO; dosage decreased if severe leukopenia develops | Nausea and vomiting | Bone marrow depression, alopecia, cystitis | Maintain adequate fluid intake to avoid cystitis | Hodgkin's disease and other lymphomas, multiple myeloma, neuroblastoma, carcinomas of the breast, ovary, lung |
| Dacarbazine (DTIC-Dome) | 150-120 mg/sq m/day IV x 5 or 950-1,200 mg/m IV once | Nausea and vomiting diminishing with continued dose; occasional flu-like syndrome | Bone marrow depression | Use lower dose in patients with impaired marrow or renal function | Melanoma, Hodgkin's disease |
| Dactinomycin (actinomycin D, Cosmegen | 15-40 μg/kg/ week IV for 3-5 weeks in adults; 15 μg/kg/day IV x 5 in children | Pain on local infiltration with skin necrosis; nausea and vomiting in many patients 2 hr after dose; occasional cramps and diarrhea | Bone marrow depression, stomatitis, diarrhea, erythema, hyperpigmentation with occasional desquamation in areas of previous irradiation | Administer through running IV infusion; use with care in liver disease and in presence of inadequate marrow function; prophylactic antiemetics are helpful | Wilms' tumor, neuroblastoma, embryonal rhabdomyosarcoma, Ewing's sarcoma, choriocarcinoma, testicular and carcinoid tumors |

Adapted from Marsh, J. C., and Mitchell, M. S.: Chemotherapy of cancer: overview of clinical pharmacology; drugs in current use, Drug Therapy (hospital edition), September 1976, pp. 8-15; October 1976, pp. 43-47; November 1976.

*Continued.*

**Table 19-6.** Chemotherapeutic agents commonly utilized with malignant musculoskeletal lesions—cont'd

| Drug | Dosage route of administration | Side effects | Toxicity | Precautions | Major indications |
|---|---|---|---|---|---|
| Doxorubicin (Adriamycin) | 60-100 mg/sq m IV q 3 wk | Nausea, vomiting, fever, local phlebitis, necrosis if extravasated, red urine (not blood) | Bone marrow depression, alopecia, cardiac toxicity related to cumulative dose, stomatitis | Administer through running IV infusion; avoid giving to patients with significant heart disease, follow-up for ECG abnormalities and signs of heart failure | Acute lympho-blastic leuke-mia, sarcomas, neuroblastoma, lymphoma, Ewing's sarcoma, carcinoma of the bladder, breast, thyroid gland, lung |
| Methotrexate (MTX, amethopterin) | Choriocarcinoma: 10-30 mg/day PO or IM x 5 Acute leukemia, maintenance: 1.25-5 mg/day PO in children; 5-10 mg/day PO in adults; 30 mg/sq m IM or PO twice weekly in both Meningeal leukemia: 0.2-0.4 mg/kg intrathecally Head and neck tumor: 50 mg/day intra-arterially with concomitant or sequential systemic anti-dote, leucovorin | None | Bone marrow depression, megalo-blastic anemia, diarrhea, stomatitis, vomiting, alopecia less common, occasional hepatic fibrosis, vasculitis, pulmonary fibrosis | Adequate renal function must be present, and urine output must be maintained | Choriocarcinoma, acute leukemia, carcinoma of head and neck, breast and testicular tumors, adjuvant for osteosarcoma |
| Vincristine (Oncovin) | 0.4-1.4 mg/m IV weekly in adults; 2 mg/sq m weekly in children | Local inflam-mation if extra-vasated | Paresthesia, weakness, loss of reflexes, constipation; abdominal, chest, and jaw pain; hoarseness, footdrop, mental de-pression; marrow toxicity generally mild, anemia and reticulo-cytopenia most prominent; alopecia | Administer through running IV in-fusion or inject with great care to prevent extra-vasation; de-crease dosage in liver disease; patients with underlying neurologic problems may be more susceptible to neurotoxicity; alopecia may be prevented by use of scalp tourniquet for 5 minutes during and after administration | Acute lympho-blastic leuke-mia, lymphomas, Wilms' tumor, neuroblastoma, testicular tumors, carcinoma of breast |

Metastatic tumors may be classified as *osteolytic* (bone destroying) or *osteoblastic* (bone forming). The areas of metastasis and their appropriate potential in relation to these classifications are given in Table 19-5.

The most common symptom of metastatic bone disease is bone pain, which is highly suggestive of a positive diagnosis if a prior diagnosis of primary carcinoma in other tissues has been confirmed. Pathologic fractures are quite common as a result of bone destruction and disruption associated with metastasis.

Aspiration or surgical biopsy is used to establish diagnosis and identify the primary site. The metastatic bone deposits usually produce cellular patterns similar to those of the original (primary site) tumor. The treatment of choice, which may include irradiation, chemotherapy, hormone therapy, or surgical intervention, is dependent on the site of metastasis, the type of origin of the primary tumor, and the patient's status. Intervention for pathologic fractures may be required, usually accomplished in the form of internal fixation when possible to reduce pain or impending pathologic fracture.

## CHEMOTHERAPEUTIC REGIMENS

Because of the nature of both primary and secondary musculoskeletal tumors, chemotherapeutic regimens may be utilized in combination with radiation therapy or surgical intervention as the treatment of choice. These regimens may vary considerably as new combinations of drugs are continually being explored in attempts to improve the prognosis associated with many of these lesions. In addition new drugs are continually being discovered and placed on experimental status. For these reasons no attempt is made here to outline all of the chemotherapeutic drug combinations to which a patient or health care personnel might be exposed; rather, the basic types of drugs currently being utilized within a variety of known combinations, their usual dosages, and side effects are shown in Table 19-6. It is recommended that all personnel be thoroughly familiar with this information in anticipation of their possible use under the outlined prescriptive circumstances.

## SUMMARY

This brief review of musculoskeletal tissue lesions, both benign and malignant, exposes the reader to several commonalities that are apparent in view of the total scope of the topic. The following are important when considering the limitations of as well as exposure to information available on the subject:

1. In review of incidence of musculoskeletal lesions by age it is apparent that the majority of the tumors have the highest incidence in children, adolescents, and young adults. This is a significant factor and should be weighed heavily during the evaluation and diagnostic process when applied to these specific age groups.

2. The cause of all the lesions is essentially unknown. We are able to identify to a high degree the characteristic manners in which these tumors act, their radiographic appearance, and their characteristics under the microscope, but, as with most of the malignancies, the actual cause is not known. This certainly is justification for the continuation of research in the field.

3. The most common symptom of all of the tumors is pain. The pain is not necessarily characteristic of one lesion or another and therefore in most cases is not diagnostically reliable. It should, however, be the source of a high index of suspicion until a lesion is otherwise ruled out.

4. The treatment of choice for most musculoskeletal lesions, at least in part, involves the surgical excision, curettage, grafting, or resection of the tumor. In the case of malignant tumors, more radical surgical intervention such as amputation or disarticulation may be required. The prognosis is often directly related to the success of treatment. An additional consideration in view of the nature of the more radical components of surgical intervention is the necessity for adequate and accurate diagnosis.

5. The last and probably most important of the commonalities between lesions is the need for accurate differential diagnosis. Some lesions appear similar pathologically as well as radiographically. It is necessary to assure that the radiologist and pathologist have adequate historical information to assist in the differential diagnosis of lesions that tend to act or appear similarly. Errors in diagnostic judgment can prove to be tragic. Avoiding such errors is rarely easy.

With both the specific and common areas of exploration of tumors of the bone and related tissues, it is believed that the reader can become familiar with the foundation that may permit prescription and implementation of an appropriate plan of care. Specific care has not been outlined because of the variety of measures that may be required and is dependent on the size, site, method of treatment, and prognosis. It is suggested that care plans based on individual diagnosis and treatment be reviewed in other chapters (e.g., cast or traction therapy). The bibliography may provide further information.

## BIBLIOGRAPHY

Ackerman, L. V., and Rosai, J.: Surgical pathology, ed. 5, St. Louis, 1974, The C. V. Mosby Co.

Adams, J. C.: Outline of orthopaedics, Baltimore, 1971, The Williams & Wilkins Co.

Aegertu, E., and Kirkpatrick, J.: Orthopedic diseases, Philadelphia, 1975, W. B. Saunders Co.

American Orthopaedic Association: Manual of orthopaedic surgery, 1972, The Association.

Aston, J. N.: A short textbook of orthopaedics and traumatology, London, 1972, English Universities Press, Ltd.

Brashear, H. R., Jr., and Raney, R. B., Sr.: Shand's handbook of orthopaedic surgery, ed. 9, St. Louis, 1978, The C. V. Mosby Co.

Crenshaw, A. H., editor: Campbell's operative orthopaedics, ed. 5, St. Louis, 1971, The C. V. Mosby Co.

del Regato, J., and Spjut, H. J.: Ackerman and del Regato's cancer: diagnosis, treatment, and prognosis, ed. 5, St. Louis, 1977, The C. V. Mosby Co.

Enneking, W. F., and Sherrard, M. G.: Physical diagnosis of the musculoskeletal system, Gainesville, Fla., 1969, Storter Printing Co., Inc.

Gartland, J. J.: Fundamentals of orthopaedics, Philadelphia, 1974, W. B. Saunders Co.

Iversen, L. D., and Clawson, D. K.: Manual of acute orthopaedic therapeutics, Boston, 1977, Little, Brown & Co.

Lichtenstein, L.: Bone tumors, ed. 5, St. Louis, 2977, The C. V. Mosby Co.

Rubin, A.: Handbook of congenital malformations, Philadelphia, 1969, W. B. Saunders Co.

Sutow, W. W., Vietti, T. J., and Fernbach, D. J.: Clinical pediatric oncology, ed. 2, St. Louis, 1977, The C. V. Mosby Co.

Tachdjian, M. O.: Pediatric orthopedics, Philadelphia, 1972, W. B. Saunders Co.

# 20

# Sepsis

NANCY E. HILT

SHIRLEY B. COGBURN

Brodie's abscess
Osteomyelitis
    Acute osteomyelitis
    Chronic osteomyelitis
    Pin tract infections
Pyogenic arthritis (infectious arthritis, septic
    arthritis, septic joint, suppurative arthritis)
Tuberculosis of bones and joints
Wound infections
Antimicrobial agents
Summary

Orthopedic sepsis can be one of the most devastating diseases. It has been known to deform, to cripple, and to add tremendous burden in the form of cost to the patient and the health care system. The results of orthopedic sepsis may be quite destructive and damaging to musculoskeletal tissues. With persistent and continued symptomatology, some bone infections may drain for years and develop direct sinus tracts to external structures. For these reasons preventive aspects (see Chapter 26) cannot be emphasized enough.

*Osteomyelitis* indicates infection of the bone (despite its suffix *itis*, which literally means inflammation). The term is utilized to encompass pyogenic infection of solid bone tissue. Other terminology is used for joint infection (e.g., arthritis), indicating that the joint is involved rather than solid bone substance. Although other types of musculoskeletal infections are discussed here, osteomyelitis encompasses a major portion of all orthopedic sepsis.

Radiographic features of musculoskeletal sepsis are shown in Table 20-1.

## BRODIE'S ABSCESS

Brodie's abscess is a chronic, localized abscess, usually the result of a staphylococcal organism of

**Table 20-1.** Differential radiographic features of musculoskeletal sepsis

| Septic process | Radiographic features |
| --- | --- |
| Brodie's abscess | Decreased density<br>Well-defined lytic lesion surrounded by denser sclerotic bone |
| Acute osteomyelitis | No evidence may be present until 7 to 10 days after onset of symptoms<br>Early<br>  Hazy or mottled metaphysis<br>  Irregular areas of decalcification<br>Late<br>  New bone formation under periosteum<br>  Evidence of shaft destruction (localized) |
| Chronic osteomyelitis | Irregularly shaped islands, denser than surrounding bone tissue<br>Cavities may be seen |
| Pyogenic arthritis | May be negative<br>Evidence of joint capsule expansion or swelling<br>Widening of joint space |
| Tuberculosis of bone and joints | Early<br>  Negative or only slight alterations<br>Late<br>  Decalcification<br>  Faint joint outlines<br>  Irregularities of joint surfaces<br>  Area of decreased density surrounded by sclerosis<br>  No new bone formation<br>Spine<br>  Decreased disc space<br>  Vertebral erosion<br>  Collapse of vertebral bodies |

low virulence. Although it is characteristic in its manifestations, it is a form of osteomyelitis.

**Etiology.** Brodie's abcsess is usually caused by a staphylococcus organism of low virulence.

**Pathology.** Radiographic examination reveals a well-defined lytic lesion surrounded by an area of dense sclerotic bone.

**Incidence.** Brodie's abscess occurs more frequently in older children and young adults than in any other age group.

**Signs and symptoms.** Brodie's abscess is manifested by gradual onset of bone pain. The pain is usually worse at night, and there may be tenderness over the site of the lesion. Brodie's abscess is most commonly seen at the distal end of the tibia. Differential diagnosis must be made between this infection and neoplasms that frequently exhibit the same symptoms and radiographic manifestations, such as osteoid osteoma, osteogenic sarcoma, and unicameral bone cysts.

**Treatment.** Surgical intervention with draining of the abscess and excision is usually indicated. Utilization of bone graft usually assists in the healing process. Local and systemic antibiotics are administered, and immobilization is recommended with cast application after surgery.

## OSTEOMYELITIS

Osteomyelitis, infection of bone tissue, may be *acute* or *chronic*. The acute form usually indicates a more rapid onset with a febrile course and systemic as well as local manifestations. In contrast chronic osteomyelitis may have a more insidious onset but more often indicates the continuation of persistent symptoms or clinical findings after an acute episode. Chronic osteomyelitis may exist for years after an initial acute episode and may encompass a series of acute courses with periods of decreased symptoms between acute phases.

### Acute osteomyelitis

**Etiology.** Acute osteomyelitis (Fig. 20-1) may be caused by a number of bacteria, most commonly *Staphylococcus aureus, Streptococcus, Haemophilus influenzae, and Escherichia coli.* Predisposing factors include traumatic injuries and infections and

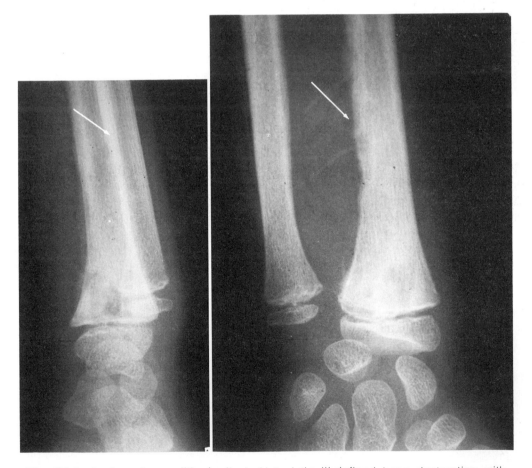

**Fig. 20-1.** Acute osteomyelitis (radius). Note lytic ill-defined bone destruction with morphous periosteal reaction.

infections at other sites such as a boil or tonsillitis. Hematogenous spread frequently occurs from a preexisting focus.

**Incidence.** Acute pyogenic osteomyelitis occurs most frequently in infants and children. It most commonly originates in the metaphysis of growing long bones. It is seen twice as often in boys.

**Signs and symptoms.** Systemic signs and symptoms of acute osteomyelitis include headache, elevated temperature, elevated white blood cell count (as high as 30,000/cu mm), and elevated pulse rate. Muscle spasms of the extremity may be noted, and the patient may semiflex the extremity for comfort. Movement of the extremity frequently initiates pain. The soft tissue surrounding the infected bone becomes edematous and red with the formation of a subperiosteal abscess. If untreated, further and more severe systemic manifestations follow, including unconsciousness and possibly death. Radiographic examinations are frequently negative until a week to 10 days after the initial symptoms when the bone destruction may be absorbed. Definitive diagnosis can only be accomplished with aspiration of the suspect bone tissue. Differential diagnosis must be accomplished to rule out rheumatoid arthritis, Ewing's sarcoma (acute febrile form), and acute suppurative arthritis.

**Treatment.** Surgical aspiration of the infected tissue is advocated as early as possible to confirm diagnosis. Excision and drainage of the area surgically may be accomplished at the same time. Immobilization of the area with a splint, cast, or traction is usually indicated. Irrigation tubes may be inserted at the focal point of the infected tissue at the time of surgical aspiration, excision, and drainage. These tubes may be utilized to irrigate the area with antibiotic solutions at frequent intervals during the first week to 10 days after surgery. Massive intravenous antibiotic therapy is begun postoperatively and is sometimes initiated prior to definitive diagnosis. The intravenous antibiotic therapy may continue for 1 to 2 weeks dependent on the course of the disease. The patient is then given antibiotics orally for 6 to 8 weeks to maintain adequate blood levels. With appropriate and early excision, drainage, and antibiotic therapy the initial acute course subsides and many patients do well. There is, however, a small percentage of patients in whom chronic osteomyelitis persists as a result of the initial acute episode.

## Chronic osteomyelitis

Chronic osteomyelitis (Fig. 20-2) usually indicates recurrence of an acute pyogenic febrile course

related to one or more sites of infected bone tissue. It also is an indication diagnostically of resistance to response to treatment for acute episodes of osteomyelitis. In some cases there is apparent response to treatment with exacerbation of the symptomatology at a later time at the original site of infection. Continued symptomatology is frequently an indication for long-term antibiotic therapy, immobilization, and continued observation through examination and radiographic monitoring of the area. It is not uncommon with continued infection for considerable bone tissue destruction to occur, jeopardizing the stability of the bone. It is also not uncommon for a sinus tract to develop through bone and soft tissue to the surface of the skin as a result of continual drainage. Although the percentage of cases of acute osteomyelitis that become

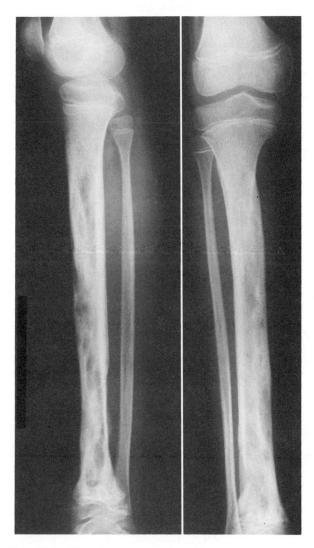

**Fig. 20-2.** Chronic osteomyelitis (tibia). Note lytic destruction with reactive new bone and distortion of contour.

chronic is relatively small, persistent resistance to the usual therapy emphasizes the need for early diagnosis and comprehensive treatment of acute cases. Extensive bone tissue damage from chronic osteomyelitis may require multiple surgical interventions to debride the infected bone tissue or to graft bone in an attempt to improve stability. Response to grafting procedures is frequently dependent on the ability to rid the surrounding tissue of the infected tissue cells.

## PIN TRACT INFECTIONS

Pin tract infections are a complication of skeletal traction. They may manifest themselves in the form of minor superficial infections, deeper soft tissue infections, or osteomyelitis. The major concern with skeletal traction is that there is a direct tract to the bone, and therefore a superficial infection may very rapidly become osteomyelitis. For this reason most physicians choose to remove the skeletal pin or wire at the early signs of superficial infection. In some cases the pin or wire may be reinserted at a different site, and sometimes alternative methods of traction are utilized.

Early signs of pin tract infections include erythema at the pin site, drainage, and fever. Deeper infections may develop if attention is not given to these early signs of superficial infection. There may be increased severity of earlier signs and pain. Continued observation of pin sites is crucial so that early signs may be detected and reported to the physician.

In addition to general observation of the pin sites for early signs of infection, various procedures and routines may be adopted for routine care of pin sites (e.g., utilization of antibiotic or antiseptic solutions or sprays at the pin site) and can considerably decrease potential of infection at these sites. A crust usually develops superficially around the pin sites externally and is the body's normal response to the inflicted trauma. Continual removal of this crust is likely to produce increased vulnerability to infection. Some physicians incorporate plaster around the pin sites to assure that the area is not disturbed or the crust removed and to decrease the possibility of pin migration. We do not advocate this despite some of the apparent advantages because it does not permit continued observation of the area and may therefore considerably delay recognition of early signs and symptoms of superficial infection. Other routines and utilization of antibiotic or antiseptic materials around the area do not seem as important as nonremoval of the crust. (For information relative to pin care, see Chapter 24.)

In addition to possible pin removal and reinsertion, treatment of a pin tract infection is greatly dependent on the depth of infection and the individual's ability to respond to usual treatment protocol. Superficial infections may require nothing more than local antibiotic therapeutics in addition to pin removal. Deeper infections may require the oral or intravenous administration of antibiotics or extensive treatment as outlined for acute osteomyelitis. It cannot be emphasized enough that the comprehensive care required for osteomyelitis resulting from pin tract infections can be alleviated in many cases if early attention is provided when the initial signs and symptoms of superficial infection appear. Additionally considerable emphasis should be placed on aseptic technique during the pin insertion procedure.

## PYOGENIC ARTHRITIS (INFECTIOUS ARTHRITIS, SEPTIC ARTHRITIS, SEPTIC JOINT, SUPPURATIVE ARTHRITIS)

Pyogenic arthritis (Fig. 20-3) is inflammation of the synovial lining of a joint and is caused by a pus-forming organism.

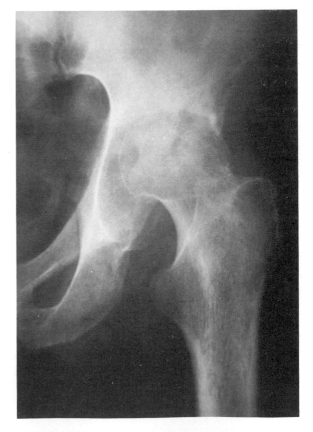

**Fig. 20-3.** Septic joint (hip). Note extensive destruction of cartilage with loss of acetabular cortex.

**Etiology.** The most common etiologic organism of pyogenic arthritis is *Staphylococcus aureus*. *Streptococcus hemolyticus* is the next most common organism seen, but with much less frequency. Even less frequently seen are a variety of microorganisms including salmonellae, brucellae, bacilli, pneumococci, and gonococci. The organisms are introduced through a variety of routes:

1. Vascular transfer (through the bloodstream) from a focus of infection such as upper respiratory infection or an infected wound
2. Direct extension of a musculoskeletal infection of adjacent bone tissue
3. Direct introduction into a joint through failure to utilize strictly aseptic technique for injection or aspiration of a joint

**Pathology.** Initial pathologic alterations indicative of pyogenic arthritis are limited edema of the synovial membrane with moderate increase of the synovial fluid. On examination the fluid may be cloudy with an increased cell count. More advanced stages of infection may reveal fibrous layers forming over the synovial membrane and infiltration of polymorphonuclear leukocytes. Even more advanced stages of the process reveal purulent effusion with involvement of all of the articular structures of the joint. The cartilage, especially at points of pressure, erodes through chondrolysis. Fibrous or bony ankylosis of the joint or spread of the infection through the development of osteomyelitis of adjacent bony structures may occur.

**Incidence.** Pyogenic arthritis is seen more commonly in males than in females. It is seen most frequently in children, with the highest incidence in 1- to 2-year-olds. It occurs most often in the hip and the knee.

**Signs and symptoms.** The symptoms of pyogenic arthritis may vary considerably with the degree of joint inflammation and the stage to which the infection has progressed. Mild pain is usually present with a moderate degree of edema surrounding the joint structures. There may be fever and mild leukocytosis. The patient will frequently flex the joint to promote expansion of the capsule for comfort. Motion of the joint usually initiates mild to severe pain. With progression of the process there may be increased pain and indications of joint inflammation. The purulent stage of the process produces temperature elevations to 40 C to 41 C (104 F to 105 F) and increased leukocytosis. On palpation, if possible, the joint shows marked tenderness, is warm to the touch, and may show varying degrees of edema. Radiographic examination is frequently negative or reveals only capsule expansion with soft tissue in-

flammation unless bony destruction or extension of the infection in the form of osteomyelitis has occurred.

**Treatment.** Differential diagnosis between pyogenic arthritis and acute rheumatoid arthritis, tuberculosis, or other disease processes that may cause joint pain, as well as confirmation of diagnosis, may only be accomplished with aspiration of the joint fluid for microscopic smear and culture. On definitive diagnosis prompt and vigorous therapy must be initiated. Hip involvement may require surgical intervention with the insertion of irrigation tubes to the joint involved. Postoperative irrigation may be accomplished with antibiotic solution. Antibiotic therapy intravenously for 2 to 3 weeks followed by antibiotic therapy orally is indicated. Immobilization of the joint is required to obtain maximum rest and decreased irritation from motion by placing the joint and adjacent areas in a splint, cast, or traction.

**Prognosis.** Early diagnosis and prompt therapy give a good prognosis. With the advanced or purulent stage of the disease there is risk of limited motion, possible ankylosing of the bone, extension of the infection to adjacent bone structures, and later degenerative joint changes. If septicemia occurs with pyogenic arthritis or results from the process, death may ensue.

## TUBERCULOSIS OF BONES AND JOINTS

Tuberculosis of bone or joint structures (Fig. 20-4), an infection caused by the tubercle bacillus, has decreased considerably in the past few decades.

**Etiology.** Tuberculosis of bones and joints, caused by the tubercle bacillus, is always secondary to tuberculosis elsewhere in the body; the primary source of infection is usually the lungs.

**Pathology.** Tuberculosis may invade any bone or joint structure through direct hematogenous routes or indirectly from infected adjacent bone or joint tissues. Specific pathologic features of tuberculosis of the spine, known as *Pott's disease*, are given in Chapter 15. Characteristically this infectious process destroys bone tissue with little evidence of new bone formation in the areas of tissue destruction. For this reason its progressive nature lends itself easily to multiple resulting deformities and extension into surrounding tissues. If near a joint, joint structures are easily involved.

**Incidence.** Tuberculosis of bones or joints is seen most frequently in the spinal column and the bone and joint structures surrounding the hip and the knee. The incidence of tuberculosis has decreased considerably in the United States but is still some-

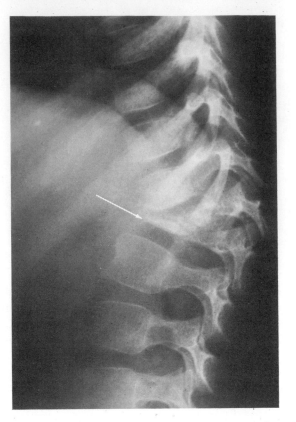

**Fig. 20-4.** Tuberculosis (of spine). Note destruction of vertebral body and disc with localized kyphosis (gibbus deformity).

what common in some of the underdeveloped countries. There is a degree of concern about the possibility of increased incidence of tuberculosis with increased virulence and resistance to the present antibiotic therapy. The majority of cases that do exist and have musculoskeletal involvement are seen in children; there appears to be a degree of immunity in the adult population.

**Signs and symptoms.** The signs and symptoms of a tuberculous infection invading bone or joint structures are usually insidious. Dependent on the location of the infection, mild to moderate pain with some tenderness may be present. When involving the joint or extending into the joint structures, stiffness with some limitation of motion may be seen. Muscle atrophy may be apparent to varying degrees, and there may be increased joint fluid. Progression of the infection may reveal muscle spasms and, if located in the lower extremity, may produce some gait variations. Low-grade fever, especially in the afternoon, is also characteristic of this infection. Generalized symptomatology such as decreased weight, anemia, night sweats, and tachycardia may be identified. Radiographic examination reveals

deterioration and invasion of bone and joint structures compatible with the stage of progression at the time of diagnosis. Tuberculin skin test results are often positive. An elevated sedimentation rate may be seen. Radiographic examination and intravenous pyelogram may confirm the involvement of the lungs, kidneys, and lymph nodes.

**Treatment.** Treatment of tuberculosis of the bone and joint structures may be classified into those measures provided for the specific treatment of the local lesion and those prescribed for generalized tuberculosis infection. Treatment of the local lesion requires immobilization of the joint or extremity involved and possible surgical intervention to eradicate abscess formation at the site of infection. In addition various surgical procedures may be required depending on the extensiveness of the tissue destruction resulting from the infection. General methods of treatment include appropriate pharmacologic therapy in the form of drugs that specifically attack the tubercle bacillus. The most effective drug utilized currently is isoniazid, although other drugs may also be prescribed. Bed rest and adequate nutrition are maintained for relatively long periods until the infection is adequately controlled.

**Prognosis.** The prognosis for tuberculosis of bone or joint structures is variable and dependent on the stage of progression or resulting deformities at the time of diagnosis. Early and appropriate intervention is advocated.

## WOUND INFECTIONS

Wound infections may be a complication of orthopedic surgical procedures. Preventive aspects of wound infection are emphasized in rigid aseptic technique before, during, and after surgical procedures, specifically in preoperative skin preparation, operating room techniques conducive to decreased risk of introduction of infection during surgical procedures, and postoperative wound care and dressing changes. Preoperative skin preparation should include, at minimum, antiseptic and antibacterial soap scrubs several times prior to surgery, appropriate nail care of extremities prior to surgery, and a clean shave immediately before surgery or in the operating room. Any violations of skin integrity prior to admission or existing immediately prior to surgery should be well documented and examined carefully in relation to their potential for introduction of infection if the surgical procedure is carried out. Extreme care and caution must be exhibited in relation to nail care and the preoperative shave so as not to pose additional threats to skin integrity. The general atmosphere in the operating

**Table 20-2.** Antimicrobial agents commonly used initially in acute bone and joint infections

| Antibiotic | Usual susceptible organisms | Daily dosage (intravenous route) | Comments |
|---|---|---|---|
| Methicillin | Penicillinase-producing *Staphylococcus aureus;* will also treat streptococci, pneumococci, non-penicillinase-producing staphylococci, but is not agent of choice for these | Birth to 2 weeks: 75-100 mg/kg<br>2 weeks to 1 month: 100-200 mg/kg<br>1 month to 12 years: 200-300 mg/kg<br>12 years to adult: 8-12 g | Agent of choice for penicillinase-producing staphylococci |
| Nafcillin | Same as methicillin | Birth to 2 weeks: 50-75 mg/kg<br>2 weeks to 1 month: 100 mg/kg<br>1 month to 12 years: 150-200 mg/kg<br>12 years to adult: 8-12 g | Reasonable alternative to methicillin |
| Cephalothin | Same as methicillin and nafcillin; also effective against some gram-negative organisms such as *Klebsiella pneumoniae* | Birth to 2 weeks: 100 mg/kg<br>2 weeks to 1 month: 100-200 mg/kg<br>1 month to 12 years: 200 mg/kg<br>12 years to adult: 8-12 g | Alternative drug to methicillin; primary use is in patients suspected of being allergic to penicillin |
| Penicillin G (aqueous) | Streptococci (not enterococci, pneumococci, gonococci, penicillin-susceptible staphylococci | Birth to 2 weeks: 50,000-100,000 units/kg<br>2 weeks to 1 month: 150,000-250,000 units/kg<br>1 month to 12 years: 250,000-400,000 units/kg<br>12 years to adult: 12 million to 20 million units | Agent of choice for listed susceptible organisms |
| Ampicillin | Same as penicillin G; also *Haemophilus influenzae,* some strains of *E. coli, Proteus,* and *Salmonella* | Birth to 2 weeks: 75-150 mg/kg<br>2 weeks to 1 month: 150-250 mg/kg<br>1 month to 12 years: 250-300 mg/kg<br>12 years to adult: 8-12 g | Agent of choice for *Haemophilus influenzae* infections |
| Carbenicillin | Same as ampicillin; also some strains of *Pseudomonas* | Birth to 2 weeks: 400-500 mg/kg<br>2 weeks to 1 month: 500-600 mg/kg<br>1 month to 12 years: 600 mg/kg<br>12 years to adult 20-30 g | Usually reserved only for proved or suspected *Pseudomonas* or resistant *Proteus* infections; combination with gentamicin often synergistic against *Pseudomonas* strains |

From Hansen, S. T., Jr., Ray, C. G., and Clawson, D. K.: Antibiotics in orthopaedics. In Kagan, B. M., editor: Antimicrobial therapy, ed. 2, Philadelphia, 1974, W. B. Saunders Co.

*Continued.*

**Table 20-2.** Antimicrobial agents commonly used initially in acute bone and joint infections—cont'd

| Antibiotic | Usual susceptible organisms | Daily dosage (intravenous route) | Comments |
|---|---|---|---|
| Clindamycin | Staphylococci, pneumococci, streptococci (not enterococci); many *Bacteroides* strains | Dosage for infants and children not yet clearly established<br>Adult dosage: 600 mg q6-8h | Considered an excellent agent for *Bacteroides fragilis* infections |
| Gentamicin | Gram-negative bacteria (e.g., *E. coli*, *Proteus*, *Klebsiella*, *Serratia*, *Pseudomonas*) | Birth to 1 week: 5 mg/kg<br>1 week to 2 years: 7.5 mg/kg<br>2 to 12 years: 5-6 mg/kg<br>12 years to adult: 4.5-5.0 mg/kg | May be given either IV or IM<br>Renal function must be carefully checked, and therapy beyond 10 days must be administered cautiously because of potential toxicity<br>May be synergistic with carbenicillin against some strains of *Pseudomonas;* also usually synergistic with penicillin against enterococci |
| Kanamycin | Gram-negative bacteria, as with gentamicin; not effective against *Pseudomonas* | Birth to adult: 12.5-15.0 mg/kg | May be given IV or IM<br>Renal function and duration of therapy must be watched closely, as with gentamicin |

**Table 20-3.** Tentative selection of therapy when organism not immediately identified

| | Organism suspected | Suggested antibiotic |
|---|---|---|
| **Birth to 1 month:**<br>Osteomyelitis<br>Septic arthritis | Staphylococcus<br>Streptococcus<br>Gram-negative bacteria including *E. coli*, *Klebsiella*, *Proteus*, *Pseudomonas* | Methicillin plus gentamicin |
| **1 month to 4 years:**<br>Osteomyelitis<br>Septic arthritis | Staphylococcus<br>*Haemophilus*<br>Staphylococcus<br>Streptococcus | Methicillin, nafcillin, or cephalothin<br>Methicillin plus ampicillin |
| **4 to 12 years:**<br>Osteomyelitis<br>Septic arthritis | Staphylococcus | Methicillin, nafcillin, or cephalothin |
| **12 years to adult:**<br>Osteomyelitis<br>Septic arthritis | Staphylococcus<br>Staphylococcus | Methicillin, nafcillin, or cephalothin<br>Methicillin or nafcillin (penicillin or ampicillin if gonococcus strongly suspected) |
| **Chronic hemolytic disorders**<br>Osteomyelitis<br>Septic arthritis | Staphylococcus<br>Pneumococcus<br>Salmonella | Methicillin, nafcillin,* or cephalothin |
| **Infections following puncture wounds of foot** | *Pseudomonas* | Carbenicillin plus gentamicin |
| **Infections following trauma or surgery** | Staphylococcus<br>Streptococcus<br>Gram-negative organisms | Methicillin, nafcillin, or cephalothin plus gentamicin |

From Hansen, S. T., Jr., Ray, C. G., and Clawson, D. K.: Antibiotics in orthopaedics. In Kagan, B. M., editor: Antimicrobial therapy, ed. 2, Philadelphia, 1974, W. B. Saunders Co.
*Infections due to Salmonella should be documented by culture and sensitivity testing before initiating empirical treatment with agents such as ampicillin or chloramphenicol.

room is crucial, and recent emphasis has been placed on the attire and grooming of operating room personnel, techniques, and "clean air" systems that reduce potential infection. Postoperative wound care including dressing changes and suture removal must be accomplished with strictest emphasis on aseptic technique and handwashing. Treatment for wound infections varies according to the depth of the infection and may include antibiotic therapy (local, oral, or intravenous), debridement, or promotion of open drainage.

## ANTIMICROBIAL AGENTS

Selection of antimicrobial agents to combat bone and joint infections vary depending on pharmacologic breakthroughs and recommendations for sensitivity to specific organisms. Those currently in common use with definitely identified organisms are presented in Table 20-2; those recommended when the organisms are not immediately known are given in Table 20-3.

## SUMMARY

Because of the devastating and long-lasting effects that may result from musculoskeletal sepsis, prompt diagnosis and treatment with definitive diag-

nosis is advocated whenever possible. Appropriate preventive techniques in the operating room and aseptic emphasis on pin and wire care, dressing changes, and joint aspiration and injections cannot be stressed enough.

## BIBLIOGRAPHY

Adams, J. C.: Outline of orthopaedics, Baltimore, 2971, The Williams & Wilkins Co.

Aegertu, E., and Kirkpatrick, J.: Orthopaedic diseases, Philadelphia, 1975, W. B. Saunders Co.

Brashear, H. R., Jr., and Raney, R. B., Sr.: Shand's handbook of orthopaedic surgery, ed. 9, St. Louis, 1978, The C. V. Mosby Co.

Crenshaw, A. H., editor: Campbell's operative orthopaedics, ed. 5, St. Louis, 1971, The C. V. Mosby Co.

Gartland, J. J.: Fundamentals of orthopaedics, Philadelphia, 1974, W. B. Saunders Co.

Goldstein, L. A., and Dickerson, R. C.: Atlas of orthopaedic surgery, St. Louis, 1974, The C. V. Mosby Co.

Kelly, P. J., and Fitzgerald, R., editors: Symposium on infections in orthopaedics, Orthop. Clin. North Am. **6**(4), 1975.

Tachdjian, M. O.: Pediatric orthopaedics, Philadelphia, 1972, W. B. Saunders Co.

Turek, S.: Orthopaedics, Philadelphia, 1977, J. B. Lippincott Co.

# PART FIVE

# Rehabilitation

# 21

# Rehabilitation: philosophy, concepts, and principles

**BARBARA H. DUNN**

The history of rehabilitation is bound to the development of the specialty of physical medicine and the growth of social awareness and responsibility among the public. Concepts of rehabilitation have not been well incorporated into the educational programs of health care professionals, causing a lag in knowledge, education, and particularly practice. Because of this lag and the social stigma attached to the disabled by professionals and the public, few professionals have concentrated in the rehabilitation field, believing it to be uninteresting, depressing, or unproductive. This chapter will acquaint the reader with current philosophy, concepts, and principles of rehabilitation and will attempt to dispel the myths and misinformation that are so apparent in the current practice of health care professionals and in the mind of the public.

## REHABILITATION DEFINED
## Terminology

Rehabilitation has been defined in various ways. The National Council on Rehabilitation has stated that rehabilitation involves "restoration of the handicapped to the fullest physical, mental, vocational and economic usefullness of which they are capable."[6,p.74] More recently there have been attempts to integrate concepts of rehabilitation into all aspects of health care delivery and to redefine rehabilitation to stress the habilitative aspects of care. This habilitation assists individuals to maximize their capabilities and to cope with current and anticipated situations in order to provide a meaningful life within the boundaries established by an altered level of health.[1,p.7]

The use of such terms as *handicapped* and *disabled* are socially stigmatizing and suffer from unclear definition and misinterpretation. An individual with a physical or mental disability is not necessarily handicapped although he or she is automatically classified as such by most persons. Stryker understands the essence of this when she states that disability is the degree of impairment that can be objectively described, while a handicap refers to a person's total adjustment to a disability.[5,p.21] Likewise her concept of rehabilitation is in concert with current interpretation. "Rehabilitation is a creative process that begins with immediate preventative care in the first stage of an accident or illness. It is continued through the restorative phase of care and involves adaptation of the whole being to a new life."[5,p.13]

It should be emphasized that thinking of rehabilitation as a process that begins only after the acute phase of illness further fragments the delivery of health care and makes restoration to a condition of health or useful and constructive activity much more difficult. Rehabilitation must be perceived as a process that begins when the person first suffers an acute illness or injury, for preventive and maintenance measures are necessarily part of acute care.[5,p.35] Rehabilitation is both a treatment and socialization process,[6,p.74] the objectives of which are (1) to prevent further impairment, (2) to maintain existing abilities, and (3) to restore maximal functioning.[5,p.35]

Rehabilitation: philosophy, concepts, and principles  **445**

## Population

The population of persons requiring rehabilitative services spans the continuum from birth to death. Rehabilitation will be needed by most persons at some time during their lifetime. With the increase in specialized medical knowledge and treatment there has been a relative decrease in the number of children born with congenital anomalies, more effective treatment of chronic medical illness, and almost complete disappearance of certain diseases such as polio. However, a greater number of children with chronic conditions are living into adulthood, and a greater number of adults are being successfully treated for conditions that previously would have shortened their life span. Because of the increased life expectancy of all persons there is also an increased incidence of chronic disease and disability. In addition there is a tremendously increased incidence of accidental injury and trauma in all age groups.

Although disabling conditions are traditionally thought of in terms of visibly apparent disorders, such as cerebral palsy, spinal cord injury, spina bifida, and other congenital musculoskeletal anomalies, they include conditions of virtually every major organ system. Those conditions most frequently seen in rehabilitation settings for children also include cardiovascular, pulmonary (asthma, cystic fibrosis), kidney, and neurologic disease; hearing, vision, and speech disorders; and juvenile rheumatoid arthritis, acute rheumatic fever, diabetes mellitus, mental retardation, cerebral vascular accidents, and childhood cancer. In adult rehabilitation the scope is essentially the same, with a preponderance of cardiovascular and pulmonary disorders or their sequelae and adult-onset neuromuscular disorders or cancer.

Many of these disorders and illnesses, regardless of origin, have musculoskeletal implications as a result of limited activity and immobility, and large numbers continue to involve the system directly. Patients with these disorders generally require continuous services or at least an intensive period of rehabilitation followed by occasional services.

In comparing chronic disease in the adult and child populations, obviously it is of greater significance and complexity in children because of their potential longevity.[3,p.1] The care and treatment provided the child will ultimately determine those services required by the adult population and will reflect the priorities of the health care industry and the general public.

## PHILOSOPHY OF REHABILITATION

"All in all, it is in the carefree audacity to try it, to put a straw in a wine goblet, and smile."[2,p.244]

### Access and quality of health care

When rehabilitation is separated from acute and convalescent care, there is an implication that it follows after everything else has been done. This situation deprives the individual of preventive care and maximal efforts to maintain existing abilities; it prevents the individual from visualizing a realistic future, and does not assist the family to prepare themselves and their environment for the return of the disabled family member.[5,p.10] A major liability of the health care industry is its organization to provide episodic care, which is not usually effective in such areas as health maintenance and anticipatory guidance; parent, child, or adult education; and psychologic/behavioral counseling.[3,p.542]

### Individual self-actualization

In reality, the whole and the disabled live together in a state of more intellectual than emotional acceptance,[3,p.552] and attitudes tend to define persons in terms of their deviance from the norm, their conformity or lack thereof, and their limitations. These attitudes that attempt to define, limit, or compare are handicapping in themselves.[2,p.235] An existential approach to rehabilitation, in which there is a reciprocal appreciation of one person for another,[6,p.158] will help the disabled person and family make their unique physical, mental, and emotional adjustment, as well as assist them in acquiring the necessary hope, insight, and strength to take up the challenge of self-actualization.[2,p.5] It is the tendency to classify and categorize that focuses our energy on limitations rather than on the limitless potential of every human being.[2,p.63]

Certain knowledge, skills, and attitudes regarding rehabilitation must be basic to all phases of health care; without this, the professional deprives the individual recipient of care of realistic expectations. The ultimate goal of rehabilitation is to promote ego integrity and feelings of self-worth in the individual.[5,pp.11,20] In order to develop self-esteem, the disabled individual and the family must be active participants in the rehabilitation process. Only through development of ego integrity and self-worth will a person be able to recognize that, above all else, he must be himself, that it is not what was lost that is important, but what remains; and if the person is being who he is, people will accept and even help him.[2,p.245]

### Elements of philosophy

Boroch has delineated five elements that are essential to an understanding of the philosophy of rehabilitation. Rehabilitation (1) is patient/family oriented; (2) requires cooperation of the patient and family; (3) is a continuous process with varying degrees of emphasis in all phases of altered levels of health; (4) is goal-directed; and (5) requires the collaboration of health team professionals.[1,p.7]

### Rights of the disabled and their families

What are disabled persons and their families entitled to in their dealings with the health care system and society? The disabled person is entitled to[2,pp.199-204]:

1. Accurate and adequate knowledge regarding the disability
2. Equal status in society and within the family
3. A voice in family decisions and plans
4. Self-determination
5. Education
6. Act and react with "normal" individuals

The families have the right to expect[2,pp.108-109]:

1. Sound medical knowledge
2. Continual reevaluation of the disabled family member
3. Helpful, relevant, and specific information about their role in the rehabilitation process
4. Knowledge of educational opportunities, community resources, and rehabilitative services
5. Some hope, reassurance, and human consideration
6. Help in seeing the disabled person's potentialities
7. Good reading material
8. Interaction with other families of disabled persons
9. To actualize their personal rights as individuals

## CONCEPTS AND PRINCIPLES OF REHABILITATION
### The rehabilitation process

Whether a disability is congenital, occurs during early childhood, is acquired in adult life, is progressive or stable, or is the result of an accident or trauma, certain processes and problems will be similar and will differ primarily in kind and value judgment.

A child with a congenital or acquired disability is more *like* other children than different from them. Much of the child's growth and development will be determined by the feelings, attitudes, and values of parents and family.[2,pp.34-35] The individual with a congenital disability has no other standard to go by and only gradually learns that he or she is different from others; by contrast, an acquired disability in later life is usually of sudden onset and may require a change of mental set and self-image. Both the affected individual and the family go through the stages of mourning their loss: grief, acknowledgement and handling of anger, dealing with their anxieties, and making adjustments in their way of life.[3,p.548] Buscaglia has called these stages disintegration (shock, disorganization), beginning acceptance (denial, partial acceptance), and reintegration.[2,p.209]

The degree of loss and ultimate adjustment will depend on a number of variables. Internal factors include age, onset, prognosis, personality, intelligence, aptitude and interest, and physical dependency. In relation to age, with congenital conditions there are problems with growth and development, play and school adjustment, but not in adapting to an altered body image. The adolescent is primarily concerned with body image (physical strength, beauty), activity, and identity; while the adult experiences a sense of loss of both function and a way of life. Disability may be more expected in the elderly, but it is no less distressing. The onset, whether acute or slowly progressive, will cause differing responses because the acute disability usually stabilizes while the progressive disorder causes anxiety and uncertainty and adjustment must be related to the stage of the disease. The psychological impact may be more intense in accidental injury because of the factors contributing to the accident and feelings of guilt, although parents and families usually experience feelings of chronic guilt nonetheless. Obviously, the prognosis will affect individual and family adjustment, but even with a fatal prognosis, there can be effective use of time, enabling the individual to live as full a life as possible. The individual's premorbid or previous personality as well as intelligence will affect the ability to adjust to disability, although motivation may compensate to some degree. Aptitude and interests will affect adjustment insofar as educational and vocational modifications must be made; and finally, the more dependent the person is on others to have physical needs met, the more difficult will be the adjustment.[5,pp.15-17]

External factors that will affect individual response and adjustment may include the psychological environment (family, friends, professionals), the physical environment, economic conditions, social expectations, and community resources.[5,p.18]

An individual's perceptions of himself and his world, whether accurate or inaccurate, will be the primary facilitators of behavior.[6,p.103] The degree or extent of the sense of loss will depend on (1) the desirability of the part or function; (2) the visibility of the altered function; and (3) the social and cultural values attached to performance of the affected skill or activity.[1,p.118]

The degree of discomfort associated with the interference caused by disability, according to Boroch, is related to[1,p.142]:

1. The point in life at which it occurs
2. The perceived meaning attached to the interference as it relates to the future
3. The degree of past success in goal achievement
4. The area of disability and need for it to accomplish a goal
5. The amount of time, energy, and money already invested
6. The desired primary and secondary gains associated with goal achievement
7. The amount of guilt associated with the occurrence[1,p.142]

All disabled persons share similar areas of concern regarding self-development, interpersonal relations, frustration, rejection and acceptance, limitation of experience, suffering, and inferiority and lowered status.[2,183-191] The individual's world—environment, interpersonal, and self-consciousness—must be in a state of balance for healthy outcome and adjustment.[6,p.159] The disabled person and the family must realize that there can be no return to the prior or previous state or stage of experience, regardless of other circumstances. Ultimately, the success of any rehabilitation program will depend on certain psychologic adaptations by the individual and family[5,p.15]; at the least, it requires cooperation or lack of resistance to the program. Any rehabilitation program, whether for child or adult, must be based on the belief that the individual with a disability is an individual first and foremost.[4,p.39]

### The rehabilitation setting

The traditional setting in which rehabilitation takes place is in the country, in a bucolic setting. The trend in modern rehabilitation toward integration of rehabilitation principles into all phases of health care, however, defies description of a single setting. For persons who require long-term or intensive rehabilitation over an extended period of time, the unit or institution needs to convey a generally positive, hopeful outlook. The atmosphere should be more relaxed than the usual hospital acute care unit, with emphasis on tasteful, bright decoration,

ample space for mobility, rooms that allow for privacy and a limited number of inhabitants, and the wearing of street clothes.

The personnel involved in a rehabilitation setting will necessarily be multidisciplinary, usually including medicine, nursing, social work, physical therapy, occupational therapy, recreational therapy, speech and hearing, education and/or vocational rehabilitation, psychology, dietary, housekeeping, and administration. The key professional or discipline in any instance will vary according to the specific needs of the individual. The main function of the rehabilitation team will be to communicate knowledge in order to execute a plan of care for each disabled individual that all will share in.[2,p.271] The problem-solving and goal-setting process must involve the individual and the family as active participants in the care. The environment must be conducive to open communication, staff motivation, actualization of the growth potential of each individual, and fulfillment of mutual performance expectations that directly relate to meaningful staff-patient relationships.[1,p.9] Regardless of the philosophy espoused by the institution or agency, the quality of care delivered will reflect the true beliefs or philosophy of the care providers.[1,p.13]

Because of the number of hours of service and the variety of services performed by nursing personnel, they are perhaps the most crucial persons in the rehabilitation setting. Their attitude and approach can do more toward rehabilitating or discouraging rehabilitation than any other single factor; they may actively contribute to or retard the growth of individual patients during the rehabilitation process.[4,p.455;3,p.562] Primary nursing as a system of nursing care delivery is particularly appropriate and feasible in this setting and facilitates both coordination and continuity of care to the disabled individual and the family.

### SUMMARY

Rehabilitation is a creative process that begins during the acute phase of any illness or injury. It is a treatment and socialization process requiring multidisciplinary care planning, implementation, and evaluation in conjunction with the disabled individual and the family. Rehabilitation is an integral part of all quality health care provided and seeks to bring the individual to maximal functioning ability and to realize his or her potential for self-actualization. Although all rehabilitation is not necessarily concerned with orthopedics, it may be said that all orthopedics is concerned with rehabilitation.

## REFERENCES

1. Boroch, R. M.: Elements of rehabilitation in nursing: an introduction, St. Louis, 1976, The C. V. Mosby Co.
2. Buscaglia, L.: The disabled and their parents: a counseling challenge, Thorofare, N.J., 1975, Charles B. Slack, Inc.
3. Downey, J., and Low, N., editors: The child with disabling illness: principles of rehabilitation, Philadelphia, 1974, W. B. Saunders Co.
4. Ince, L. P.: The rehabilitation medicine services, Springfield, Ill., 1974, Charles C Thomas, publisher.
5. Stryker, R. P.: Rehabilitative aspects of acute and chronic nursing care, Philadelphia, 1972, W. B. Saunders Co.
6. Zamir, L. J.: Expanding dimensions in rehabilitation, Springfield, Ill., 1969, Charles C Thomas, Publisher.

## BIBLIOGRAPHY

Boroch, R. M.: Elements of rehabilitation in nursing: an introduction, St. Louis, 1976, The C. V. Mosby Co.

Buscaglia, L.: The disabled and their parents: A counseling challenge, Thorofare, N.J., 1975, Charles B. Slack, Inc.

Downey, J., and Low, N. editors: The child with disabling illness: Principles of rehabilitation, Philadelphia, 1974, W. B. Saunders Co.

Ince, L. P.: The rehabilitation medicine services, Springfield, Ill., 1974, Charles C Thomas, Publisher.

Jones, S. L.: Orthopedic injuries: illness as deviance— Am. J. Nurs., 75(11):2030-2033, 1975.

Stryker, R. P.: Rehabilitative aspects of acute and chronic nursing care, Philadelphia, 1972, W. B. Saunders Co.

Zamir, L. J.: Expanding dimensions in rehabilitation, Springfield, Ill., 1969, Charles C Thomas, Publisher.

# PART SIX

# Treatment alternatives

# 22

# Emergency care

NANCY E. HILT

Emergency care of the musculoskeletal injury is extremely important to the outcome of the injury. Appropriate and accurate assessment of the injury, accompanied by the initial treatment, is essential to the continued management of the specific injury. Although a high percentage of musculoskeletal injuries occur as a singular entity, multiple injuries are often associated with automobile accidents and the like. Emphasis in this chapter has been placed on the single musculoskeletal injury, but principles have been outlined that also relate to patients with multiple injuries. In these cases, priorities are frequently such that the musculoskeletal injuries are secondary to life-saving measures. Initial treatment of the musculoskeletal injury may be delayed, but the principles involved in the treatment of that injury are not necessarily altered.

## GENERAL EMERGENCY CARE PRINCIPLES

General emergency care principles of traumatic injuries revolve around two major factors: *treatment of life-threatening conditions* and *assessment or review of total injuries with appropriate implementation of necessary emergency measures.* The former, obviously, takes priority over the latter. Those components of a traumatic injury that are generally considered to be life-threatening are: (1) cardiac and/or respiratory arrest, (2) shock, and (3) hemorrhage. Only when these life-threatening considerations have been reviewed and appropriate treatment implemented should there be an additional systematic survey to assess the need for other emergency measures. Additional consideration should also be given at this time to the patient's state of consciousness, which can alter considerably the recommended handling of the patient throughout continued treatment and assessment. Appropriate emergency measures acceptable for life-threatening situations are reviewed in Fig. 22-1 and Table 22-1.

Multiple traumatic injuries require additional assessment after the life-threatening measures have been successfully implemented. Injuries that are not life-threatening but require emergency care before mobilization are: (1) brain and spinal cord injury, (2) fractures, and (3) wounds. Each of these

**Table 22-1.** Priorities for treating components of multiple injuries—emergency measures and/or triage[1, p.45]

| Priorities | | |
|---|---|---|
| **First** | **Second** | **Third** |
| Airway and breathing difficulties | Burns | Fractures or other minor injuries |
| Cardiac arrest | Major multiple fractures | Obviously mortal wounds where |
| Uncontrolled or suspected severe bleeding | Back injuries with or without spinal cord damage |    death appears reasonably certain |
| Severe head injuries | | |
| Severe medical problems (e.g., poisonings, diabetic complications) | | |

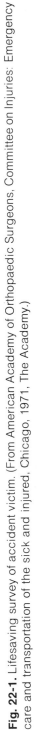

**LIFESAVING SURVEY OF ACCIDENT VICTIM**
(The following should be done simultaneously)

**OBSERVE**

For breathing
- Clear airway
- Mouth-to-mouth resuscitation
- Seal chest wound
- Stabilize flail chest

For bleeding
- Use hand pressure, then large dressing with bandages
- Use tourniquet only if necessary

**TALK**

Reassure
Inquire for painful areas

Determine state of consciousness
If in coma:
- Handle carefully as if spine injured
- Check pupils

Multiple casualties:
Survey systematically, stopping to treat only those with life-threatening problems

**FEEL**

Pulse

None
Cardiac arrest:
- Give cardiac compression
- Give mouth-to-mouth resuscitation

Weak
Shock:
- Elevate legs
- Cover
- Eliminate cause

**Fig. 22-1.** Lifesaving survey of accident victim. (From American Academy of Orthopaedic Surgeons, Committee on Injuries: Emergency care and transportation of the sick and injured, Chicago, 1971, The Academy.)

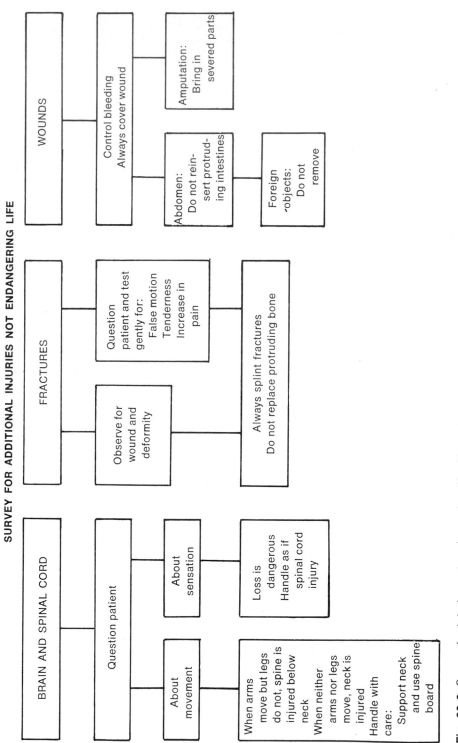

**SURVEY FOR ADDITIONAL INJURIES NOT ENDANGERING LIFE**

**Fig. 22-2.** Survey for injuries not endangering life. (From American Academy of Orthopaedic Surgeons, Committee on Injuries: Emergency care and transportation of the sick and injured, Chicago, 1971, The Academy.)

major areas should be systematically evaluated and appropriate measures implemented as indicated in Fig. 22-2. Further elaboration of emergency measures of the musculoskeletal injuries is reviewed separately.

## CONTROL OF HEMORRHAGE

Traumatic hemorrhage may be *internal* or *external* in origin. Internal hemorrhage results from injury to internal organs that are not protruded through the surface; abdominal hemorrhage or hemorrhage from a closed fracture are common examples. The most common signs of internal hemorrhage are[1,p.83]:

1. Pulse—weak or rapid
2. Skin—cold or clammy
3. Eyes—dull
4. Pupils—dilated and slow to respond to light
5. Blood pressure—low and irratic
6. Nausea and vomiting—may be present
7. Anxiety—may be evident

Evidence of internal bleeding through exhibition of these signs requires initial treatment and emergency measures[1,p.83]:

1. Treat the patient for shock.
2. Maintain recumbent position; loosen collar and belt.
3. Give the patient nothing by mouth.
4. Treat hemorrhage into an extremity, as evidenced by rapid increase in swelling, by the application of pressure and a splint.
5. Give the patient oxygen, if available.
6. Transport the patient gently and efficiently.

External hemorrhage results from an injury that breaks the surface of the skin. The most common and efficient method of controlling external hemorrhage is to apply pressure, which decreases or stops the flow of blood, permitting normal mechanisms to control the hemorrhage through the development of a blood clot. Several options are available to control external hemorrhage. They are: (1) direct pressure of the apparent wound, (2) pressure-point control, and (3) tourniquet.

*Direct pressure* over the wound is easily accomplished by using a pressure dressing. When available, a sterile dressing is preferred, however, a clean cloth or handkerchief may be used if necessary. Manual pressure can be used in the absence of other mechanisms of applying a pressure dressing. *Pressure-point control* should be used if pressure dressings are not available or have not been successful in controlling the hemorrhage. Pressure points must be proximal to the wound for effective application. This method of control is accomplished by pressing the artery against the bone; the most common areas are major arteries of both extremities. The last alternative available for control of external hemorrhage is the use of a *tourniquet*. A tourniquet should *not* be used unless other methods of control are unsuccessful or not possible, because of the risk of damage and complications. Hemorrhage can most often be controlled by the other measures outlined and will rarely require a tourniquet. If it is determined that a tourniquet is the only way to control the hemorrhage, the following precautions must be noted[1,p.81]:

1. If a rubber tube or a blood pressure cuff is not available, use a wide bandage and tighten securely.
2. Do not use wire or any type of material that will cut the skin.
3. Do not cover a tourniquet and be sure to indicate to other emergency staff members that a tourniquet has been applied.

The patient should receive the attention of a physician as soon as possible when a tourniquet has been applied, and the tourniquet should be released periodically when utilized over an extended time. If not applied properly and accurately, tourniquets may result in nerve and circulatory damage, which can ultimately be more destructive than the original injury.

## EMERGENCY CARE OF DISLOCATIONS

Dislocations may occur with traumatic injury at any joint. Some dislocations are very difficult to distinguish from a fracture or a fracture-dislocation. For this reason, emergency treatment and care are similar to that for a suspected or confirmed fracture. Dislocations will most often result in deformity surrounding the involved joint, with pain, swelling, and tenderness. Dislocation of the hip joint frequently causes internal rotation not common with fractures. Shoulder and finger dislocations are the most common dislocations.

With any apparent or suspected dislocation, appropriate immobilization and splinting are required to decrease further tissue disruption. Immobilization should be accomplished in the *position of deformity* until medical attention is received in a physician's office or emergency room. Various types of splinting available for dislocations and fractures are reviewed later. Again, it must be stressed that the emergency treatment of many dislocations is similar to that of a potential fracture in the same area and that definitive diagnosis at the time of injury is frequently difficult to determine.

## EMERGENCY CARE OF FRACTURES
### Closed fractures

Closed fractures are usually accompanied by a specific history of trauma, pain, tenderness, and varying degrees of swelling over the area. The most effective emergency measure for any closed fracture is appropriate splinting, which should include the joint below and above the suspected area of fracture whenever possible. Adequate immobilization with the splinting must be accomplished to prevent further and additional tissue damage. Patients with closed fractures accompanied by signs of internal hemorrhage should be treated for shock. Lower extremity, pelvic, and spinal fractures require recumbency with no weight-bearing from the time of injury until medical treatment is obtained. Spinal cord injury is of particular concern when there is a spinal fracture. Initial assessment of neurovascular status will assist in the determination of these factors, but appropriate handling using log rolling techniques and a spinal board are indicated with *all* spinal injuries.

### Open fractures

Emergency measures for the treatment of open fractures involve several additional considerations. With closed fractures, we are primarily concerned with the immobilization of the fracture site until reduction can be accomplished to prevent further tissue damage. With open fractures, we are concerned about the fracture itself, the protrusion through tissues and skin causing massive tissue destruction, potential neurovascular damage, and the open wound that accompanies the fracture. The fracture itself may be immobilized through appropriate splinting. The massive tissue destruction caused by the fracture fragments and neurovascular alterations may be considered together because of their associated interaction. With open fractures, there is usually a force or injury that has been sufficient enough to drive the fragment ends through to the surface of the skin. Although soft tissue destruction is of great concern in relation to potential infection and loss of muscular function, of greater concern is tissue destruction and damage involving

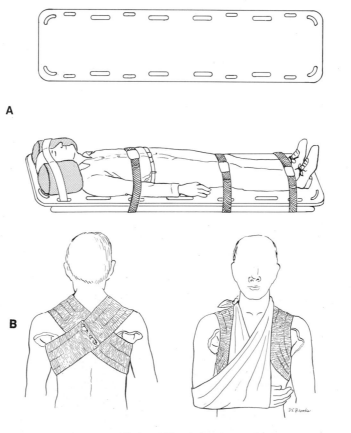

**Fig. 22-3.** Common emergency splints utilized for musculoskeletal injuries. **A,** Back board for cervical and spinal injuries. **B,** Figure-of-eight splint for clavicle fractures.

neurovascular structures, which may ultimately result in the loss of an extremity. Control of hemorrhage when major blood vessels are involved must be accomplished immediately, with additional vascular repair being required later. Nerve damage should be adequately assessed initially, and in many cases may be appropriately stabilized with splinting until transportation is accomplished. Specific care of any wounds involved with open fractures is mandatory to the restoration of function, efficient reduction of the fracture, and prevention of infection. Although wounds may vary in size considerably, the principles involved with the emergency care of the wound remain the same. Considerations

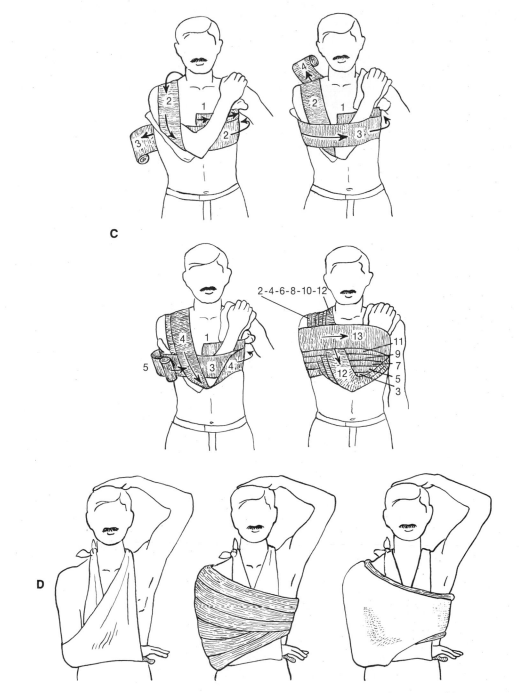

**Fig. 22-3, cont'd. C,** Velpeau bandage for shoulder dislocations, fractures of humerus, and some elbow fractures. **D,** Sling-and-swathe bandage for shoulder dislocations, fracture of humerus, and some elbow fractures.

*Continued.*

and principles involved with this care are as follows[7,p.11]:

1. Cover the wound immediately with a sterile dressing. If available, it is advisable for the dressing to be moistened with a balanced electrolyte solution.
2. Do *not,* under any circumstances, probe the wound.
3. Do *not* soak the wound.
4. Do *not* replace protruding soft tissue or bone back into the wound in an attempt to realign the fragments or close the wound. All protruding material is considered contaminated and, if replaced, considerably increases the risk of infection. In addition, there is considerable risk of damaging adjacent tissue structures if realignment is attempted.
5. Splinting of the open fracture should be accomplished without replacing tissue or bone in the wound.

Tetanus prophylaxis and antibiotic therapy may be required. Further debridement of the wound, repair of the soft tissue including neurovascular structures, and reduction of the fracture are usually accomplished in the operating room under sterile technique. Delayed primary closure is often the treatment of choice with open fractures and is accomplished over a period of 3 to 5 days.[2,p.13]

## METHODS OF EMERGENCY SPLINTING

Splints for musculoskeletal injuries may generally be classified as those utilized for *spinal injuries,* *upper extremity injuries*, and *lower extremity injuries*. Splints range from those made of very simple and common items to elaborate and sophisticated commercial splints. The type of splint used is not always as important as the manner in which it is applied and the degree to which the splinting provides adequate immobilization.

Appropriate splinting should be used for any suspected *cervical* or *spinal injury.* The most common form of splinting for a spinal injury is a *back board* (see Fig. 22-3, *A*). Sandbags should be used to immobilize the head and neck in the neutral position. The patient should be secured to the back board when being transported.

*Upper extremity splints* are used for suspected fractures, fracture-dislocations, and dislocations. Commercial *air splints* can be used for distal portions of the upper extremity, but they are not useful with shoulder girdle involvement. Air splints should not be maintained on the extremity for extended

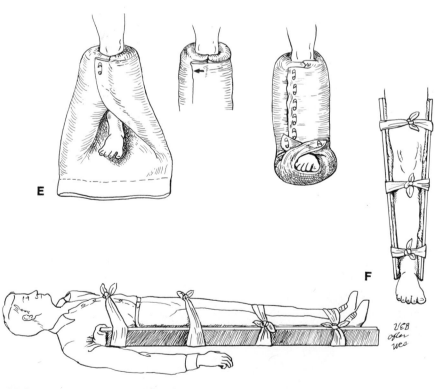

**Fig. 22-3, cont'd. E,** Pillow splint for distal lower extremity injuries. **F,** Board splint for extremity fractures.

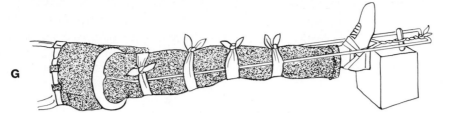

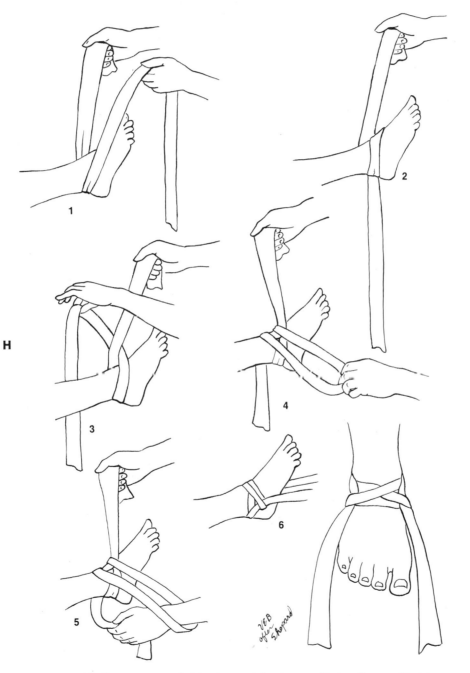

**Fig. 22-3, cont'd. G,** Thomas splint for femoral fractures with traction applied by means of Collins hitch. **H,** Method of application of Collins hitch for Thomas splint. (From Iverson, L. D., and Clawson, D. K.: Manual of acute orthopaedic therapeutics, Boston, 1977, Little, Brown & Co.)

periods of time because of the risk of skin maceration. The inflatable splint permits continued observation of the extremity through a clear plastic. Care should be taken during inflation to assure that vascular compromise is not resulting from overinflation.

Other splints commonly used for fractures of the humerus and shoulder girdle involvement are the *figure-of-eight splint*, the *Velpeau bandage*, and the *sling-and-swathe bandage* (Fig. 22-3, *B, C,* and *D*). The figure-of-eight splint is most common for clavicular fractures, while the Velpeau and sling-and-swathe bandages are used for shoulder dislocations, fractures of the humerus, and some elbow fractures.[2,pp.45-47] It should be noted that before the application of any splint to the upper extremity, *all rings or bracelets should be removed* to prevent circulatory compromise with continued edema.

The type of splint used for *lower extremity* fractures, dislocations, or fracture-dislocations is often dictated by the material available. The most common splints for these injuries are the *board splint* and the *pillow splint* (Fig. 22-3, *E* and *F*). For the board splint a board is put on either side of the extremity, which is tied on with cloth ties at intervals. For distal lower extremity injuries, the other extremity can be used as a splint. A board is placed on the side of the injury and cloth ties are wrapped around the patient's body to secure the board. A *Thomas splint* may be used, if available, to provide both immobilization and, in conjunction with a Collins hitch, a degree of traction to the extremity. If utilized, the traction must be applied very carefully and slowly, to avoid excessive traction. This splint is most useful with femoral fractures (Fig. 22-3, *G* and *H*).[2,pp.48-50]

Several general guidelines are useful in the application of all splints to avoid complications. Among the guidelines are:[2,p.51]

1. *Take measures to avoid circulatory compromise.* Splints or bandages must be wrapped with a sufficient degree of securement to provide the necessary immobilization, but extreme caution must be exhibited to avoid too much pressure, which may function as a tourniquet. Splints should be checked periodically to assure that movement has not produced such an effect to the extremity.

2. *Open fractures should be splinted in the position of deformity,* with no attempt to reduce the fracture or correct any malalignment.

3. Closed fractures should be splinted after a skilled attempt to reduce any gross angulation through the utilization of gentle traction in the direction of the angulation, followed by additional gentle traction in the direction of the long axis of the extremity or bone. If one is not skilled in this area, it is better to splint the fracture as is.

4. Open wounds should be cared for and treated before splinting, utilizing the techniques indicated under open fracture management.

## SUMMARY

Emergency care of the musculoskeletal injury is critical to the anticipated outcome of the injury. The patient with multiple injuries must be appropriately evaluated so that life-threatening conditions receive the highest priority. Fractures, fracture-dislocations, and dislocations should be appropriately splinted to provide for optimal immobilization during transportation until primary care is received.

## REFERENCES

1. American Academy of Orthopaedic Surgeons: Manual of orthopaedic surgery: emergency care and transportation, Chicago, 1972, The Academy.
2. Iverson, L. D., and Clawson, D. K.: Manual of acute orthopaedic therapeutics, Boston, 1977, Little, Brown & Co.

## BIBLIOGRAPHY

American Academy of Orthopaedic Surgeons: Manual of orthopaedic surgery, Chicago, 1972, The Academy.

Aston, J. N.: A short textbook of orthopaedics and traumatology, London, 1972, The English Universities Press Ltd.

Committee on Injuries, American Academy of Orthopaedic Surgeons: Emergency care and transportation of the sick and injured, Chicago, 1971, The Academy.

Iverson, L. D., and Clawson, D. K.: Manual of acute orthopaedic therapeutics, Boston, 1977, Little, Brown & Co.

Kerr, A.: Orthopedic nursing procedures, New York, 1961, Springer Publishing Co., Inc.

# 23

# Cast and splint therapy

NANCY E. HILT

SHIRLEY B. COGBURN

Of all the tools associated with orthopedics, casts and splints are more readily identified with this "specialty" than any other. Plaster methods of immobilization have been utilized for centuries and, despite modern technology, have not lost their usefulness.

This chapter deals with the broad spectrum of plaster techniques in reference to the most common types of cast and splint applications. It does not explore specific types of casts currently being used for specific conditions, such as the cast-brace in the treatment of fractures or the postoperative application of the cast-prosthesis. Rather, this chapter deals with the general principles associated with cast and splint therapy, with emphasis on application, removal, types, and nursing care.

## DEFINITIONS AND TERMINOLOGY

A *cast* may be defined as a method of temporary immobilization that circumferentially incorporates a part or parts of the body. Most casts are constructed of plaster of Paris incorporated into gauze material, which permits flexibility in application. Other materials have been substituted to provide the same degree of immobilization and yet alleviate some of the disadvantages of plaster, such as its inability to become damp after drying without becoming soft and losing its effective rigidity. Many of these materials are still experimental; however, fiberglass is becoming increasingly popular for specific types of cast applications and is therefore reviewed briefly.

The major categories of casts are (1) upper extremity, (2) lower extremity, (3) spinal and cervical, and (4) spica casts. *Extremity* casts incorporate all or a portion of the designated extremity. *Spinal* and *cervical* casts incorporate all or a portion of the trunk of the body or the cervical area. The term *spica* refers to a cast that incorporates part or all of the trunk of the body and a part or all of one or more extremity.

459

The term *cast* implies that the plaster or fiberglass encases the entire part of the body, in contrast to a *splint*, which supports rather than encases the trunk or extremity. A splint provides less immobility, is frequently used on a part-time rather than full-time basis, and is removable.

## PRINCIPLES OF APPLICATION

Adherence to specific principles of cast and splint application will provide for maximal comfort and alleviation of complications of cast and splint therapy. Although a brief portion of this section outlines use of the fiberglass cast, major emphasis is on the more common plaster casts and splints.

### Equipment and supplies

The following are the materials and supplies necessary for the application of a plaster cast:

1. Stockinette
    a. Commercially available in various sizes; most common sizes are 2 through 12 inches.
    b. Stretches easily.
    c. Size must be carefully chosen to avoid wrinkles.
    d. Layers of thickness will vary from application to application.
    e. One thickness usually used for extremity casts; two thicknesses may be used for casts incorporating the trunk of the body.
    f. Certain circumstances and physician preferences may reflect choice of no stockinette lining.
    g. May be applied to extremity or trunk easily if rolled.
    h. Applied against skin; first layer of cast application.

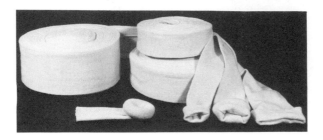

2. Cotton padding
    a. Available in many commercial types and sizes; most common sizes are 2, 3, and 4 inches.
    b. Is flexible and conforms to the contour of the body.
    c. Size should be chosen appropriately for size of extremity or trunk.
    d. Should be applied wrinkle free to avoid potential pressure areas.
    e. Is the first layer of cast application against the skin if stockinette is not used; is the second layer if stockinette is used.
    f. Thickness will vary, but two to three layers are usually sufficient for protection of skin integrity.
    g. Additional padding may be provided over bony prominences.

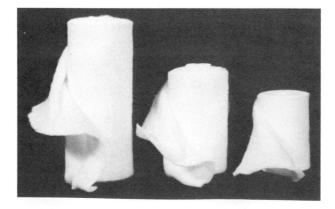

3. Felt padding
    a. Available by the yard in several thick-nesses; ¼- or ½-inch thickness most fre-quently desired.
    b. Is flexible when cut to fit specific area.
    c. Used over bony prominences or joints as extra padding for those areas that are par-ticularly vulnerable to skin breakdown.
    d. Is incorporated within the cotton padding.
    e. Felt padding may be omitted at the dis-cretion of the physician.

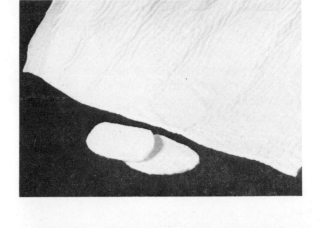

4. Plaster rolls
    a. Available in various commercial types and sizes; most frequently utilized sizes are 2, 3, 4, 5, 6, and 8 inches.
    b. Is flexible when wet and conforms to con-tour of body part.
    c. Size is chosen according to the size of the extremity or body part; several sizes may be used for one cast application.
    d. Layers desired will be dependent on the thickness desired.
    e. Layers must be continually smoothed dur-ing application to provide for necessary meshing of layers into one solid cast.
    f. Is applied over the cotton padding.

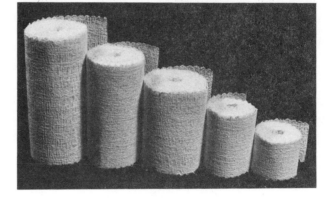

5. Plaster splints
    a. Available commercially in various types and sizes; most frequently used sizes are 3 × 15, 4 × 15, and 4 × 30 inches; com-mercial preparation provides for splints already cut in desired length.
    b. Flexible when wet and conforms to contour of body part.
    c. Size chosen will be dependent on size of extremity or body part.
    d. Layers desired will be dependent on desired thickness; most frequently used in four to eight layers.
    e. Incorporated between plaster rolls.
    f. Used to add strength over specific areas where the cast is vulnerable to breakage (e.g., over a joint such as the knee in a long leg cast).
    g. Layers must be smoothed well after appli-cation to provide for necessary meshing of layers.

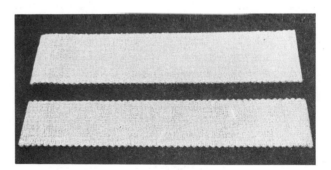

6. Bucket of water
   a. Water should be fresh and changed at the beginning of each application.
   b. More than one bucket may be required for large cast applications, or water may be changed midway through the application.
   c. Lukewarm water most frequently desired.
   d. Cold water may be used if physician desires slower "setting" or hardening of the plaster.
   e. *Never* use hot water.

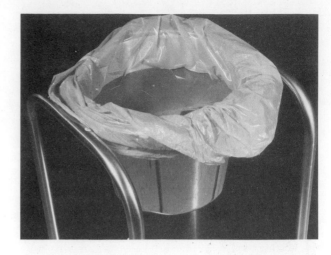

7. Knives
   a. Knives are available commercially in various types and models.
   b. Type used will frequently be designated by physician preference.
   c. Used for trimming the edges of the cast immediately after application.

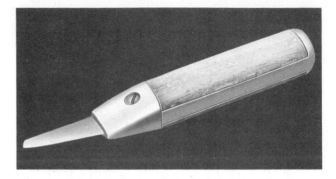

8. Scissors
   a. May be required for cutting felt, throughout application, for trimming after application, and so on.
   b. Large 7-inch plaster scissors are most efficient except with small children.

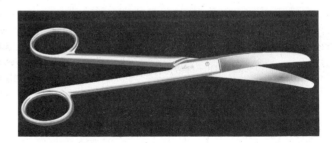

9. Plaster cart (optional)
   a. May be used as a method of organizing the above supplies.
   b. Provides for mobility of supplies when required in areas other than Plaster Room.

**Application procedure**

The actual cast application procedure has been alluded to in the previous section, in which the supplies and equipment are outlined. Essentially, the following steps apply, in varying degrees, to the application of all types of plaster casts:

1. Stockinette, if utilized, is rolled onto the extremity or torso under the area where the plaster will be applied. This stockinette will usually extend several inches above and below the anticipated area where the plaster will end. The stockinette should be taut but not constrictive. It may be cut over joints where wrinkles occur to alleviate potential pressure areas.

2. Cotton padding is applied over the stockinette but does not extend above or below it. If the stockinette is not utilized, application of the cotton padding will be the first step in the procedure. Several layers are applied in the appropriate size.

3. Felt padding, if desired, is incorporated within the layers of cotton padding.

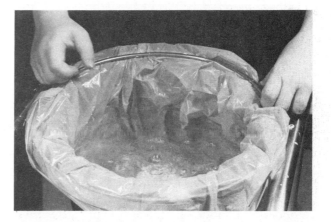

4. A plaster roll is submerged in water until the bubbles disappear, indicating that saturation has occurred.

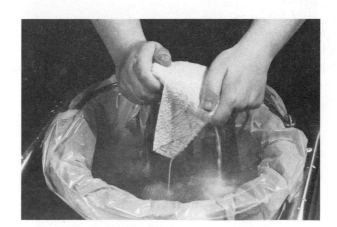

5. The plaster roll is removed from the water, gently squeezed at either end to remove excess water, and applied. One to many rolls may be applied, depending on the size of the area.

6. Splints are then applied. They are submerged in the water in thicknesses of four to eight layers.

7. The splints are removed from the water and fanfolded to remove the excess water. They are then applied to the designated area requiring additional strength. Under some circumstances splints are not utilized at all.

8. Additional rolls of plaster are applied as desired to establish required thickness.
9. If stockinette has been used to line the cast, it may be pulled over the edges and incorporated into the last few layers of plaster roll.

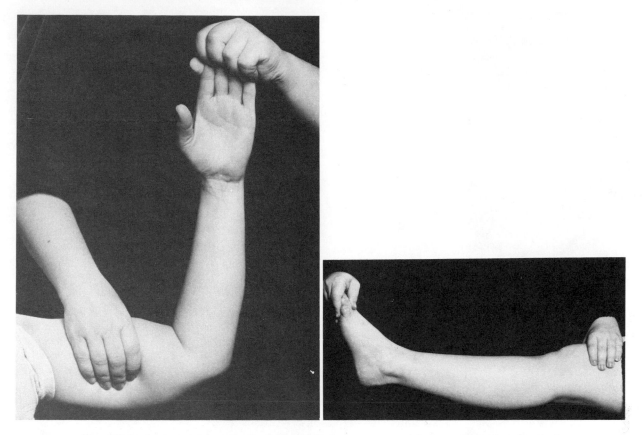

**Fig. 23-1.** Appropriate method of immobilizing upper and lower extremities for cast application to ensure maintenance of desired position and adequate exposure of area to which cast is being applied.

Despite the fact that these steps are general enough to apply to all cast applications, alterations in this process may be applicable to specific types of casts. The amount of plaster, padding, and so on applied will obviously also vary greatly depending on the size of the area to which the cast is being applied. Application of this process and procedure for specific types of casts is discussed on the following pages.

An additional factor that is applicable to all cast applications is immobilization during the procedure itself. If immobilization is not maintained throughout cast application, undesirable positioning may result and pressure areas are likely to develop. All health care personnel should know the proper methods of immobilization during cast application.

Extremity casts require manual immobilization. This is not an easy task even with a cooperative patient because of the amount of weight involved in manually holding an extremity and the length of time required to apply the cast. If the patient is uncooperative, such as an infant or toddler, the task becomes even more difficult and requires tremendous strength. The best methods for manual immobilization of an extremity during cast application are shown in Fig. 23-1. Spinal, cervical, and spica cast applications do not usually require this degree of manual immobilization, since the tables used provide immobilization and exposure of the body area to which the cast is being applied.

**Specific cast applications.** The procedure for applying extremity, spinal, and spica casts is given below.

*Extremity casts.* Extremity cast applications are the simplest in reference to the amount of time and materials required. They become more complicated, however, if molding is necessary to correct a deformity or align a fracture. The specific steps in the application of a short arm and short leg cast follows.

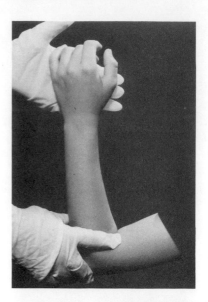

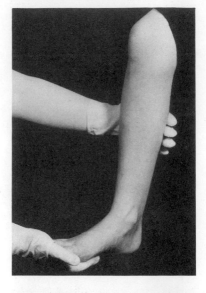

The extremity should be as clean as possible *before* the cast application.

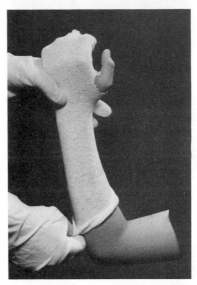

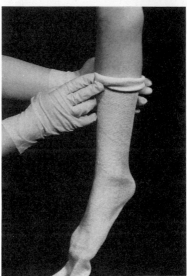

Stockinette is carefully rolled on extremity to avoid any wrinkles over joints.

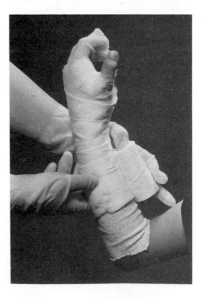

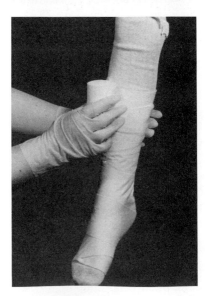

Cotton padding is applied smoothly and wrinkle-free.

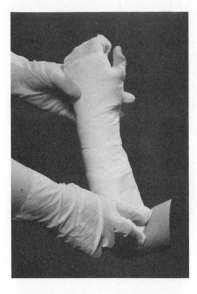

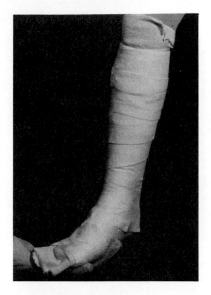

Several layers of cotton padding are applied without covering edges of the stockinette.

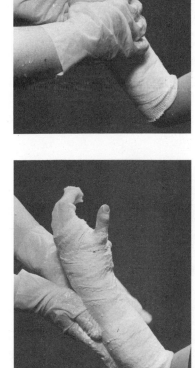

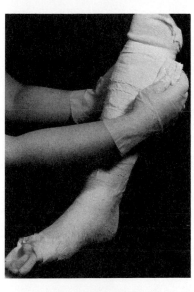

A plaster roll is applied over the cotton padding.

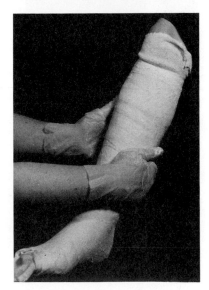

Additional plaster rolls are applied as required. Plaster is smoothed as applied to permit meshing of layers.

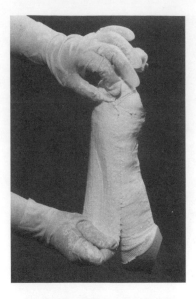

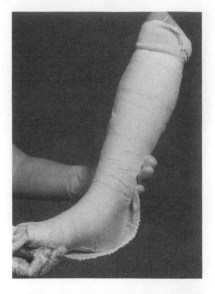

Splints are applied over areas requiring additional strength and smoothed to permit meshing of layers.

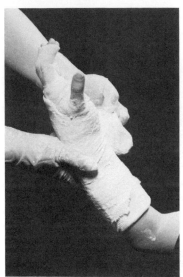

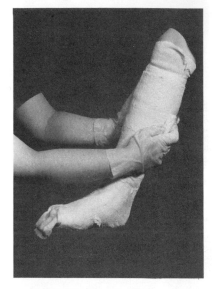

Additional rolls are applied as desired to the designated thickness.

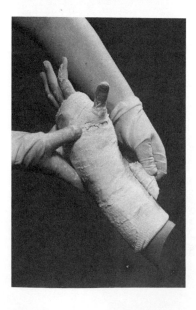

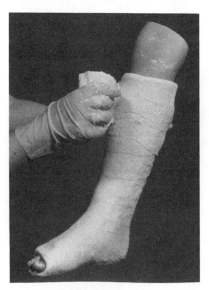

The stockinette at the edges is pulled over the edge of the plaster and incorporated into the last layers of plaster.

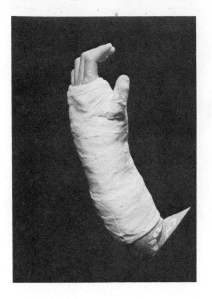

The cast is now complete. If stockinette had not been used, trimming around the edges with the cast knife may have been required.

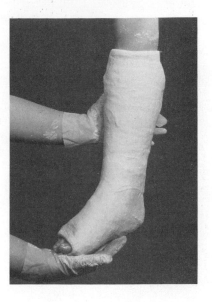

A long arm or leg cast merely requires extending all material to the upper arm or leg. The major alteration required for the application of the leg cylinder cast is in the preparation of the skin and initial layers of padding to avoid the common problem of the cast slipping during ambulation, which would create potential pressure areas over the maleoli. Although this may be a source of controversy, we believe the following is the most satisfactory method:

1. Spray the leg with tincture of benzoin.
2. Do not use stockinette.
3. Apply the cotton padding to the skin while it is still "tacky" or "sticky."
4. Apply the remainder of the cast as usual.

It might be advantageous to confirm the specific procedure alteration desired by the physician for this cast.

Lower extremity casts may be used for ambulation with the addition of a "walker." There are two forms of walkers available commercially: those made of hard rubber and incorporated into the cast, and those applied over the cast like a shoe or "boot" (Fig. 23-2). Both forms are currently in wide use. The rubber walker may be added either at the initial cast application or later. It should be properly mounted to permit neutral foot alignment.

Ambulation should not be permitted on a walking cast until the plaster is totally dry. Ambulation is facilitated in a cast that incorporates the foot if the plantar aspect of the foot is totally supported; that is, the plaster should be extended beyond the toes for support and protection.

*Spinal and cervical casts.* Spinal and cervical casts are applied on a cast table, which permits maximal flexibility in positioning, immobilization and security during the application, and exposure of large portions of the trunk and extremities. Many of the tables available commercially may be used in the operating room as well as the plaster room. It would not be advantageous here to outline all of the positioning methods for spinal and cervical casts, for physician preference may dictate many varied procedures. In addition, individual alterations frequently depend on the specific needs of the patient. Two of the common methods of scoliosis cast application using such tables are shown in Fig. 23-3.

Recommended alterations in the outlined cast application procedure for spinal and cervical casts are as follows:

1. Two layers of stockinette are usually used under these casts, especially for patients who will be in cast therapy during the summer, since perspiration and body odor may become a tremendous problem. This permits removal of inside layer (with great care and skill) about midway through cast therapy schedule.
2. Many long splints are used to reinforce the thickness of the cast around the trunk.
3. Felt pads are used in several areas.

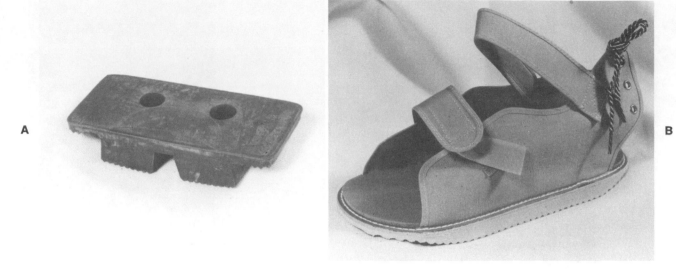

**Fig. 23-2.** Walkers for conversion of short or long leg cast to ambulatory cast. **A,** Rubber walker is applied and secured to cast with additional plaster. **B,** Boot or shoe type of walker, which is utilized over cast and secured by lacing or straps.

*Spica casts. Shoulder* spica casts can be applied with the patient in a sitting position or on a cast table. No special alterations in application are required.

*Hip* spica casts are applied on either an infant spica table or a cast table. The infant spica table, the length of which can be adjusted, is used for infants, toddlers, and preschoolers. Older children, adolescents, and adults are placed on the cast table for immobilization and positioning. The only alteration in application procedure is the use of felt pads in various areas.

### Fiberglass cast application

Although plaster casts have been used for centuries, there are several disadvantages. One is the weight of the plaster. Under ordinary circumstances and with small casts, the weight does not pose a major problem; with large casts, however, especially for a patient who does not have good muscular control, the weight of the plaster cast may inhibit ambulatory potential. An additional disadvantage of the plaster cast is its inability to maintain immobility when it becomes wet.

These disadvantages have prompted research over the years to develop a material that will offer the same degree of immobilization as plaster but will alleviate the disadvantages. Within the past decade, fiberglass immobilization has been introduced. This form of cast alleviates some of the dis-

advantages of plaster but it is quite expensive. It is currently used by some orthopedic surgeons and institutions, but on a selective rather than general basis. Its degree of popularity, however, at least warrants familiarity with the equipment and materials used in its construction.

A fiberglass cast is applied with special supplies, materials and equipment (Fig. 23-4). The lining or padding of the casts is a specially designed stockinette that is much heavier than the type used with a plaster cast. A coarsely woven padding is rolled over the stockinette. The fiberglass material is supplied in rolls and splints of various sizes. It is open-meshed and the application is similar to that of plaster. The fiberglass material has a rather strong odor until it is "cured" and should be applied in a well-ventilated room. Rubber gloves and a special cream facilitate handling of the fiberglass material. Because the edges tend to be extremely sharp, a special compound is used to smooth the edges. In addition, a finishing tape, made of a finer mesh, secures the stockinette and padding over the edges of the cast.

A special ultraviolet light is used to "cure" or harden the fiberglass. The time required depends on the size of the cast and the number of layers of fiberglass applied. Because the cast is porous it dries fairly quickly. Of course, the larger the cast the longer the drying period necessary. The weight of this cast is considerably less than a plaster cast.

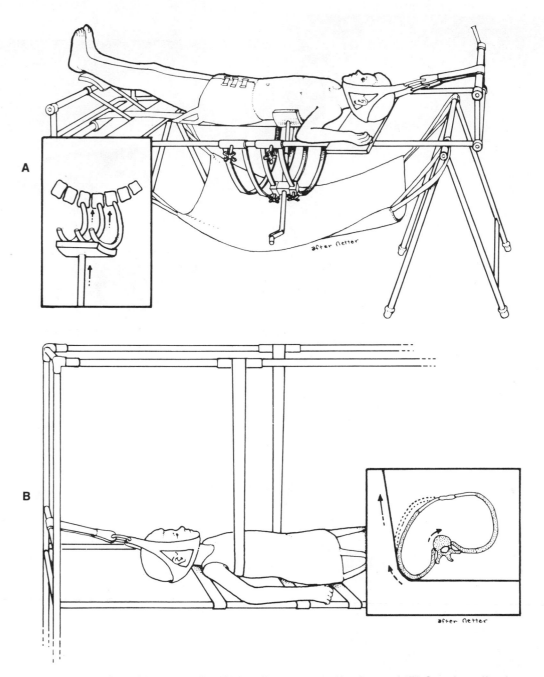

**Fig. 23-3.** Cast table setups for **(A)** localizer cast application and **(B)** Cotrel application of scoliosis casts. (From Hilt, N. E., and Schmitt, E. W., Jr.: Pediatric orthopedic nursing, St. Louis, 1975, The C. V. Mosby Co.)

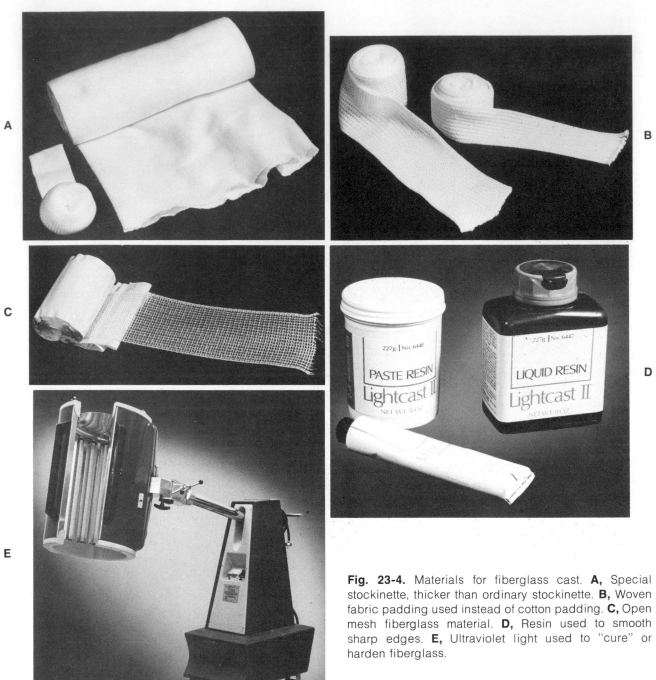

**Fig. 23-4.** Materials for fiberglass cast. **A,** Special stockinette, thicker than ordinary stockinette. **B,** Woven fabric padding used instead of cotton padding. **C,** Open mesh fiberglass material. **D,** Resin used to smooth sharp edges. **E,** Ultraviolet light used to "cure" or harden fiberglass.

**Plaster splint application**

Splints, as previously mentioned, are used for lesser degrees of immobilization and frequently are viewed as an intermittent form of immobilization because they may be easily removed. Although many types of splints may be used for the same purpose, the most common, and probably the easiest type to construct, is outlined here. The following are the steps of construction for a short arm splint.

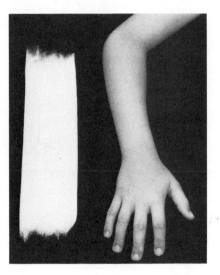

1. Cotton padding is arranged in several thicknesses of the desired length and width.

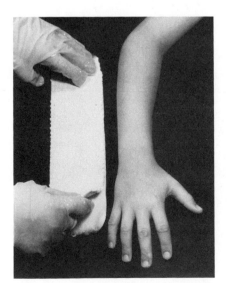

2. Approximately 10 to 15 layers of plaster splints are submerged in water, excess water removed, and placed over the cotton padding and smoothed.

3. Several layers of cotton padding are placed over the plaster splints.

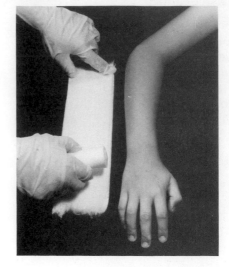

4. Stockinette is carefully rolled over the padding and plaster splints.

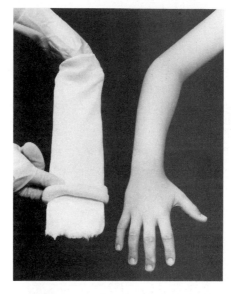

5. The ends of the stockinette are tucked in.

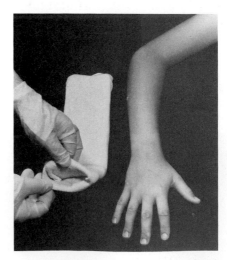

6. The splint is appropriately placed on the extremity.

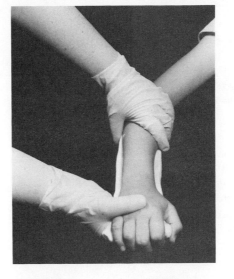

7. The splint is secured with an elastic bandage.

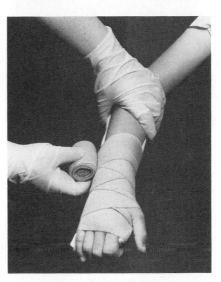

8. The splint should remain on the extremity, with proper support, at least until it has set or hardened. If desired, it may then be removed until dry.

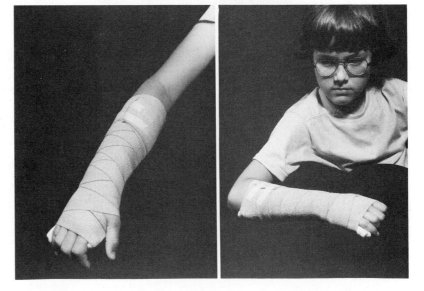

## Additional principles

Certain principles apply to *all* cast and splint applications and should be maintained for maximal effectiveness. These are as follows:

1. *Maintain desired position throughout cast application.* Alterations in positioning during the application will create wrinkles on the inside of the cast. These wrinkles become potential pressure areas, as well as sources of potential neurovascular impairment.

2. *Use caution in handling of the cast until it has set or become hardened.* The palms rather than the fingertips should be used to support the cast. Until the cast has hardened, which usually takes from 10 to 20 minutes, it is extremely impressionable. Fingerprints can cause indentations, which may become potential pressure areas or the source of neurovascular impairment.

3. *Prepare the patient for the cast application by providing appropriate education.* Some cast applications are more traumatic than others. All, however, require realistic patient education. The procedure for the specific type of cast to be applied should be explained. If a cast table is to be used, it may be beneficial for the patient to see it (or photographs of it) and to be shown how he will be secured on the table. Patients should be told that they will feel heat during the application and hardening process, followed by the feeling of coldness and dampness. Patients who will have a cast applied to the chest should be prepared for a feeling of shortness of breath that may occur; they should be instructed to breath normally to permit appropriate chest expansion. Relief should occur after the patient is removed from the table.

All instructions should be age appropriate. Young children respond well to instruction through play therapy; they may assist in the application of a cast on a doll. Photographs are also appropriate. Adolescents respond well if they are able to speak with another adolescent who has or has had the same cast application. Adults usually will respond best to explanation.

4. *Provide the patient with privacy before and during the cast application.* Extremity cast applications do not, for the most part, violate a patient's privacy to the degree that body and spica cast applications do. It is possible, however, to provide privacy for these applications as well, if all health care personnel are educated in methods to facilitate this assurance. Stockinette should be placed on the patient in the privacy of his or her room. It should be extended below and above the area to which the cast is being applied; this assures nonexposure of the perineal and chest area. After placing the patient on the cast table, a towel may be tucked over the perineal area to assure further privacy. Many patients fear violations of their privacy during the cast application procedure and health care personnel should function as patient advocates in this respect. It is recommended that all female patients be provided with a female health care chaperone who can function in this manner. Maintenance of privacy, however, is just as important for the male patient.

## GENERAL USE

Cast and splint therapy is generally used for temporary immobilization of a part or parts of the body. The most frequent justifications for this therapy are to:

1. Obtain correction of a deformity
2. Maintain correction of a deformity
3. Promote appropriate and/or desired alignment
4. Provide for the treatment of a dislocation, sprain, damaged soft tissue, or fracture
5. Provide for postoperative immobilization and/ or positioning
6. Promote rest for disease processes

## SPECIFIC TYPES OF CASTS AND THEIR USE

Many adaptations and alterations of basic types of casts may be encountered to conform to individual patient needs. More frequently than not, however, even these adaptations and alterations will begin with the construction of a basic cast. We will not outline all of the possible alterations, but rather the specific types of casts and how they are most frequently used.

### Upper extremity casts

**Type:** Short arm cast*
**Placement:** Hand to below the elbow
**Use:** 1. Fractures of the hand or wrist
    2. Postoperative positioning or immobilization of the hand or wrist
    3. Correction or maintenance of correction of deformities of the hand or wrist

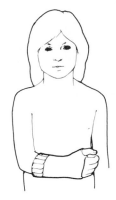

**Type:** Long arm cast*
**Placement:** Hand to upper arm
**Use:** 1. Fractures of the forearm or elbow
    2. Fractures of the humerus
    3. Postoperative positioning of the distal arm, elbow or upper arm
    4. Correction or maintenance of correction of deformities of the distal arm, wrist, or elbow

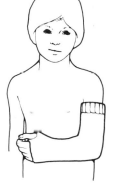

**Type:** Arm cylinder cast*
**Placement:** Wrist to upper arm
**Use:** 1. Dislocation of the elbow
    2. Postoperative immobilization or positioning of the elbow
    3. Correction or maintenance of correction of deformity of the elbow
**Comment:** The long arm cast may serve the same purpose as the cylinder arm cast because its extension over the wrist and hand control supination and pronation to a greater extent.

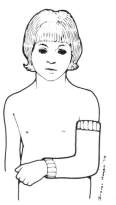

*Illustration from Hilt, N. E., and Schmitt, E. W., Jr.: Pediatric orthopedic nursing, St. Louis, 1975, The C. V. Mosby Co.

### Lower extremity casts

**Type:** Short leg cast*
**Placement:** Toes to knee
**Use:** 1. Fractures of the foot, ankle, and distal leg
    2. Severe sprains and torn soft tissue of the ankle
    3. Postoperative positioning and immobilization of the foot and ankle
    4. Correction or maintenance of correction of deformity of the foot or ankle

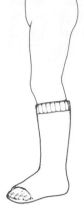

**Type:** Short leg cast with walker*
**Placement:** Toes to knee; addition of rubber walker
**Use:** 1. Same indications as short leg cast
    2. Weight-bearing ambulation desired
**Comments:** The same weight-bearing ambulation may be achieved with the use of a "boot" walker with a short leg cast.

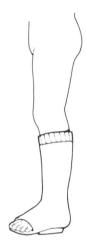

**Type:** Long leg cast*
**Placement:** Toes to upper thigh
**Use:** 1. Fractures of the distal leg, knee, and distal femur
    2. Dislocation of the knee
    3. Torn soft tissue surrounding the knee
    4. Postoperative positioning and immobilization of the knee, distal leg, and ankle
    5. Correction or maintenance of correction of the foot, distal leg, and knee

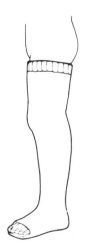

---

*Illustration from Hilt, N. E., and Schmitt, E. W., Jr.: Pediatric orthopedic nursing, St. Louis, 1975, The C. V. Mosby Co.

**Type:** Long leg cast with walker*
**Placement:** Toes to upper thigh; addition of rubber walker
**Use:** 1. Same indications as long leg cast
2. Weight-bearing ambulation desired
**Comments:** The same weight-bearing ambulation may be achieved with the use of a "boot" walker with a long leg cast.

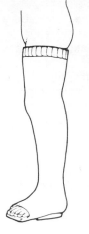

**Type:** Leg cylinder cast*
**Placement:** Ankle to upper thigh
**Use:** 1. Fractures of the knee
2. Dislocation of the knee
3. Torn soft tissue surrounding the knee
4. Postoperative positioning and immobilization of the knee
5. Correction or maintenance of correction of deformities of the knee
**Comment:** The long leg cast may be used rather than the leg cylinder cast because its enclosure of the foot may assure a greater degree of immobilization.

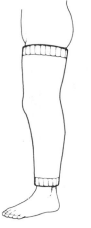

**Type:** Abduction boots
**Placement:** 1. Short leg—foot to knee, bilateral, bar incorporated at ankle level to provide for hip abduction
2. Long leg*—foot to upper thigh, bilateral, bar incorporated at ankle level to provide for hip abduction
**Use:** 1. Postoperative positioning and immobilization after hip adductor releases
2. Promotes proper positioning during the healing phases after surgery

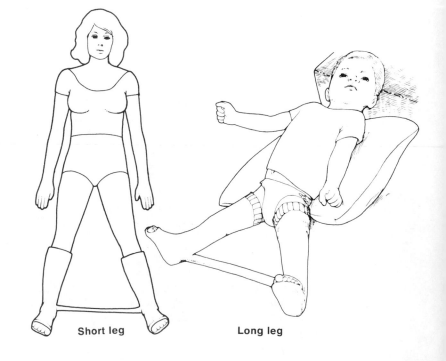

Short leg          Long leg

**Type:** Quengle cast
**Placement:** Foot or ankle to below knee and above knee to upper thigh, special hinges incorporated medially and laterally at the knee level
**Use:** 1. Knee contractures; provides for the gradual correction
**Comment:** Other types of knee-hinge casts may be used to achieve the same purpose.

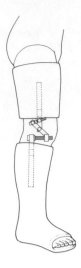

## Spinal and cervical casts

**Type:** Body jacket*
**Placement:** Incorporates the trunk only; does not extend over cervical area, may or may not have shoulder "straps"
**Use:** 1. Spinal injuries
2. Scoliosis
3. Postoperative positioning and immobilization after spinal surgery

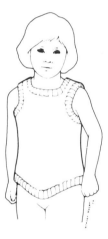

**Type:** Minerva cast
**Placement:** Upper trunk (to the sternum and distal rib border anteriorly and across distal rib border posteriorly); incorporates the head with facial area and area over the ears cut out
**Use:** 1. Torticollis
2. Cervical injuries
3. Cervical spinal infections
**Comment:** This cast is not utilized so frequently as it once was because of advancement in the field of orthotics.

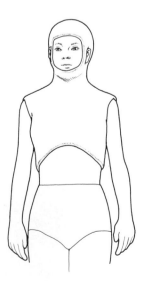

---

*Illustration from Hilt, N. E., and Schmitt, E. W., Jr.: Pediatric orthopedic nursing, St. Louis, 1975, The C. V. Mosby Co.

**Type:** Risser cast*

**Placement:** Over the entire trunk of the body, extends over the cervical area to the chin, may extend over the hips to the knees in rare circumstances

**Use:** 1. Scoliosis (cast will extend to knees if curvature is low)
2. Preoperative or postoperative correction or maintenance of correction of scoliosis

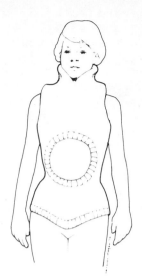

**Type:** Turnbuckle cast*

**Placement:** Over entire trunk, one arm to elbow and opposite leg to knee, cut after application and hinges incorporated

**Use:** 1. Scoliosis
2. Hinges are placed at the level of the apex of the curvature
3. Preoperative and postoperative positioning

**Comment:** The Risser cast is used more frequently than the turnbuckle cast since the availability and improvement of surgical instrumentation for scoliosis. An adaptation of this cast is used occasionally as a hyperextension cast for kyphosis or kyphoscoliosis.

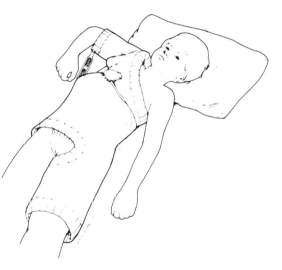

**Type:** Halo cast*
**Placement:** Over the trunk of the body, usually with shoulder "straps," halo apparatus and outrigger incorporated
**Use:** 1. Cervical injury
2. Cervical dislocation
3. Postoperative positioning and immobilization for cervical surgery

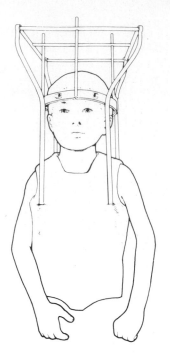

## Spica casts

**Type:** Shoulder spica cast*
**Placement:** Over the trunk, usually to the hips; incorporates the shoulder involved (may have shoulder "strap" over opposite shoulder), involved arm to the wrist or hand; bar may be incorporated to maintain desired position (which may vary)
**Use:** 1. Shoulder dislocation
2. Injury of the shoulder
3. Postoperative positioning and immobilization for shoulder surgery

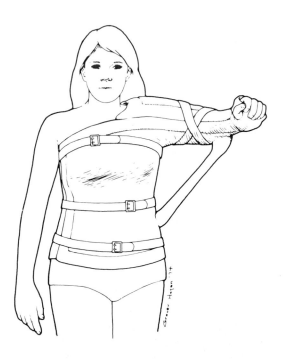

---

*Illustration from Hilt, N. E., and Schmitt, E. W., Jr.: Pediatric orthopedic nursing, St. Louis, 1975, The C. V. Mosby Co.

**Type:** Hip spica casts*
**Placement:** 1. Short leg—trunk of the body to waist or nipple line; both legs to knee
 2. Unilateral long leg—trunk of the body to waist or nipple line, one leg to toes
 3. One-and-a-half—trunk of the body to waist or nipple line, one leg to toes and opposite leg to knee
 4. Bilateral long leg—trunk of the body to waist or nipple line, both legs to toes
**Use:** All types of hip spica casts are used for correction or maintenance of correction of hip deformity.
 1. Short leg—congenital dislocation of hip
 2. Unilateral long leg—rest for hip disease process; fractured femur
 3. One-and-a-half—postoperative positioning or immobilization after hip surgery; fractured femur
 4. Bilateral long leg—fractures of the femur, acetabulum, or pelvis; postoperative positioning or immobilization after hip surgery
**Comment:** The determination of the type of hip spica cast used will depend on specific purpose of the cast and physician preference.

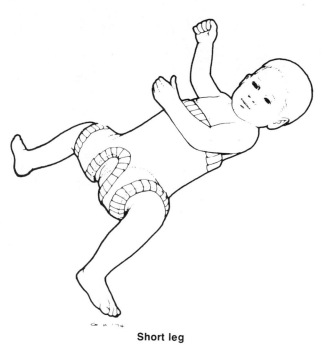

**Short leg**

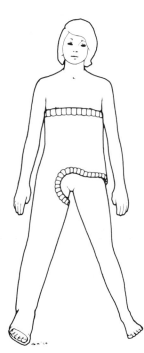

**Unilateral long leg**

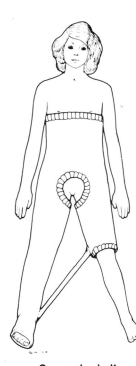

**One-and-a-half**

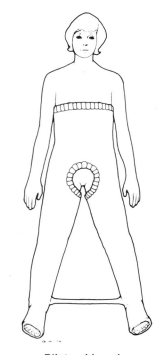

**Bilateral long leg**

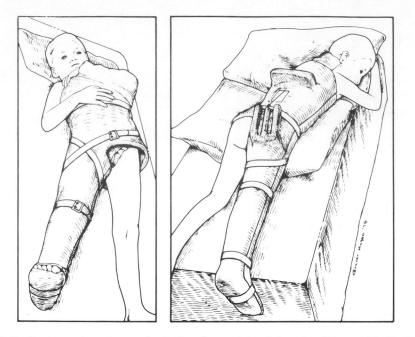

**Fig. 23-5.** Cast used postoperatively for Sprengle's deformity. (From Hilt, N. E., and Schmitt, E. W., Jr.: Pediatric orthopedic nursing, St. Louis, 1975, The C. V. Mosby Co.)

As previously mentioned, most alterations and adaptation of casts are from these basic types and designs. Such an example may be viewed in Fig. 23-5. This cast appears somewhat more complicated than those outlined above. It is used postoperatively after surgery for Sprengle's deformity (congenital elevation of the scapula or failure of descent of the scapula). The specific adaptations permit traction to be applied directly to the scapula by means of a wire that exits through the incision and is attached to a scale device designed for this purpose. Despite the fact that this cast appears more complicated, its basic design is that of the long leg hip spica cast, and the alterations have been constructed after this basic design.

### NURSING CARE

The care of the patient in a cast will vary depending on the type of cast and the degree of independence the patient can maintain (Table 23-1). For example, a patient who has rheumatoid arthritis and accompanying severe deformities has a short arm cast. The care involved with this cast, as compared with some of the other larger casts, is ordinarily less complex but will be complicated by the existence of the patient's other deformities. Therefore, care plans should be altered to accommodate the specific needs of each patient.

### Drying of the cast

Any plaster cast or splint that has been applied will require time to become completely dry, which will vary according to the size and thickness of the cast. As a general rule, extremity casts and splints require 24 to 48 hours, while body and spica casts require 48 to 72 hours.

Measures to assist and facilitate the drying process, such as using of a dryer or fan, are *not* recommended. These measures merely facilitate the drying of the outer portion of the cast. To assure that the cast is solid and stable, drying should occur naturally, from the inside out. The most acceptable measures that will facilitate drying of the cast are: (1) exposure of the cast to the air, and (2) frequent change of positioning (every 1 to 2 hours) to aid in the total exposure of the cast.

To accomplish these measures, sheets and blankets should be placed only over areas of the body that do not have the cast. Many patients experience chilling and feel cold and damp under the areas where the cast has been applied; covering the cast, however, will not relieve this feeling and will only delay the drying process. Splints, of course, will require less time to dry, and the above measures may not be as critical in facilitation of the process.

Frequent change of position is sometimes not

**Table 23-1.** Summary of care of patient in cast

| Care | Type of cast | Specifications | Frequency | Rationale |
|------|-------------|----------------|-----------|-----------|
| Application of cast | All types | Precast education and preparation | Before cast application | To prepare patient for application process |
| | | Role of patient advocate; provide privacy | During cast application | To protect patient's privacy |
| Skin care | All types | Use alcohol; no lotions, oils, or powders | Every 4 hours | To toughen skin |
| | | Around edges and over exposed bony prominences and joints | Every 2 hours: Myelomeningocele Paraplegia Quadraplegia History of sensitive skin Reddened areas. | To maintain skin integrity |
| | If on bedrest | To back, buttocks, coccyx | | |
| | All types | Petal all edges of cast with adhesive tape or moleskin | After cast has dried completely | To decrease skin irritation at edges of cast |
| | | Stockinette, if used to line cast | Replace as necessary | |
| Neurovascular assessments | All types | Precast assessment | Before cast application | To establish "normal" |
| | | Assess all components and document: Color Temperature Capillary filling Edema Pulse Sensation Numbness/tingling Motion | Every hour for first 24 hours after application Then, if "normal" for that patient, every four hours | To facilitate early detection of neurovascular impairment so that treatment may be initiated |
| Postoperative and post-traumatic control of edema | All types applied after surgery or injury | Elevate extremity by bed gatch, pillows, or suspension | Immediately after cast application | To alleviate possibility of neurovascular impairment caused by edema |
| | | Maintain extremity above level of heart | | |
| | | Initiate elevation immediately after cast application | | |
| Postoperative and post traumatic drainage | All types applied after surgery or injury | Monitor drainage (circle) | At change of shifts | To monitor amount of drainage and identify excess |
| | | Document intensity of drainage | At minimum, every shift | |
| | | Add roll of fresh plaster over stains | Before discharge, if drainage has ceased and no further drainage anticipated by physician | |
| Positioning and turning | All types— nonweight bearing | Reposition—rotate: Prone Supine Right side Left side | Every 1-2 hours until cast is totally dry Every 4 hours Every 2 hours: Myelomeningocele Paraplegia Quadriplegia History of sensitive skin | To promote drying of the cast To maintain skin integrity and decrease complications associated with bedrest and immobilization |
| | | Avoid pressure on toes, etc., during repositioning process | | |

*Continued.*

**Table 23-1.** Summary of care of patient in cast—cont'd

| Care | Type of cast | Specifications | Frequency | Rationale |
|---|---|---|---|---|
| Observation for pressure areas under cast | All types | Observe for signs of pressure: Irritability Restlessness Fussiness Drainage Odor Elevated temperature Complaints of burning or pain | Every shift | To detect early signs and symptoms |
| Maintaining cast clean and dry | Leg casts Spinal casts Hip spica casts Shoulder spica casts | See Table 23-2 | See Table 23-2 | To maintain cast clean and dry |
| Joints not in cast | All types | Range of motion exercises: Active Active assisted Passive Provide activities | Depends on condition and status of patient | To discourage joint stiffness and muscle atrophy |
| Nutritional requirements | All types | Monitor diet Encourage balanced diet Encourage juices and roughage | Every shift | To promote healing and decrease constipation |
| Bladder and kidney function | All types— nonweight bearing | Monitor intake and output Limit milk and milk products to meals only Force fluids to twice usually accepted amount | Every shift | To decrease infection and renal calculi |
| Bowel function | All types— nonweight bearing | Monitor bowel movements Juices and roughage in diet Monitor diet Laxatives and enemas as necessary to prevent impaction | Every shift | To decrease constipation |

accomplished because the health care personnel caring for the patient are under the impression that handling of the cast may dent it. Any cast that has been applied with the proper thickness and is handled properly (that is, with the palm of the hand rather than by the fingertips) should not be in danger of cracking or denting during the repositioning process.

**Skin care**

A very important consideration in the care of the patient in a cast or splint is appropriate and frequent skin care. Preventive measures are required to as-

sure the maintenance of skin integrity and to alleviate potential skin breakdown. Skin care for the patient in a cast or splint incorporates the following components:

1. Application of an agent designed to toughen the skin in areas particularly vulnerable to pressure and breakdown
2. Observation of the areas of skin particularly vulnerable to pressure and breakdown
3. Relief of any pressure and potential pressure areas during the repositioning process

We recommend using alcohol as a skin toughener since oils and lotions tend to soften the skin, thereby rendering it more vulnerable to skin breakdown. Powders tend to "cake" and, in combination with skin secretions, may be an additional source of skin irritation.

Skin care should be given to *all* areas vulnerable to pressure and breakdown. These include (1) all areas of skin around the edges of the cast, (2) any exposed joints and bony prominences, such as elbows, knees, etc., and (3) the back and buttocks (if the patient is on bedrest).

The frequency of skin care depends on the patient's history and diagnosis. If the patient has a history of sensitive skin, previous skin breakdown, or a primary or secondary diagnosis indicating potential skin problems (e.g., myelomeningocele, paraplegia), skin care should be provided every 2 hours during the day and every 3 hours during the night. For other patients, skin care every 4 hours is usually sufficient.

An essential component of skin care is observation. Reddened areas may be the first sign of pressure. If reddened areas are noted, the frequency of skin care should be increased—from every 4 hours to every 2 hours, for example. The reddened area should also be relieved of all pressure. This may involve bending the cast edge slightly away from the skin or maintenance of proper positioning.

**Petaling edges.** The edges of a plaster cast can be the source of extreme irritation to the skin if they are not as smooth as possible. The process of making the edge of the cast smooth is called *petaling*. Two types of petaling are explained below.

If *stockinette* has been used to line the cast and has been incorporated into the last few layers of plaster (as shown in the beginning of this chapter), this is an acceptable method of petaling—provided that the plaster has not been applied above the level of cotton padding. If the plaster has been stopped at a level before the edge of the cotton padding, the process of pulling the stockinette over the edge for incorporation into the cast provides for a smooth and padded edge. If, however, the plaster has been applied above the level of cotton padding, the edge may be rough and irritating. It is best, therefore, not to assume that just because stockinette is covering the edge, that it is smooth. If the edge is rough, the stockinette may be cut, several layers of padding applied over the edge of the cast, and the stockinette then secured on the exterior portion of the cast with tape. This, of course, should be accomplished only *after* the cast is totally dried.

If stockinette has not been used to line the cast, the edges may be petaled with *tape*. The procedure for petaling in this manner is shown in Fig. 23-6, *A*.

The process itself becomes relatively clear after reviewing this illustration, but some helpful hints follow.

1. Petaling may be accomplished with adhesive tape or moleskin. However, adhesive tape does not roll at the edges as easily as moleskin and is, therefore, more desirable, although either will serve the purpose. *Non*waterproof tape seems to be more adherent.
2. The cast should never be petaled until it is totally dry.
3. Rolling of the edges of the tape may be alleviated if they are rounded as shown in Fig. 23-6, *A*.
4. *All* edges of the cast should be petaled. The patient or a family member should be taught how to replace the tape if it becomes necessary after discharge.
5. A tongue blade or other utensil should never be used in the process of petaling.
6. Edges of the tape on the interior portion of the cast must be secure to prevent rolling and discomfort.

### Neurovascular assessment

Neurovascular assessment is one of the most important aspects of care required for the patient in a cast. Neurovascular impairment may occur as a direct result of the application itself or weeks or months later. Impairment resulting from the cast application may be caused by improper handling of the extremity or cast during and shortly after application. Normal wear-and-tear of the cast after weeks or months may cause softening or indentations that are the source of difficulty. In addition, postoperative or posttraumatic edema may pose additional threats to neurovascular structures. For these reasons, neurovascular status should be assessed carefully, accurately, and frequently.

Considerable focus and attention must be placed on the education of staff members responsible for the implementation of such assessments. Emphasis must be placed on the consequences of neurovascular impairment, as well as the necessity for early recognition of signs and symptoms of impairment. It is possible for a patient's neurovascular status to be adequate at the beginning of a shift, yet change so rapidly that the use or life of the extremity is in jeopardy by the end of the shift! A very fine margin exists between reversible and irreversible damage to neurovascular structures. If early signs are not recognized and appropriate measures are not taken to assure the integrity of these structures, irreversible damage will result with loss of the extremity or,

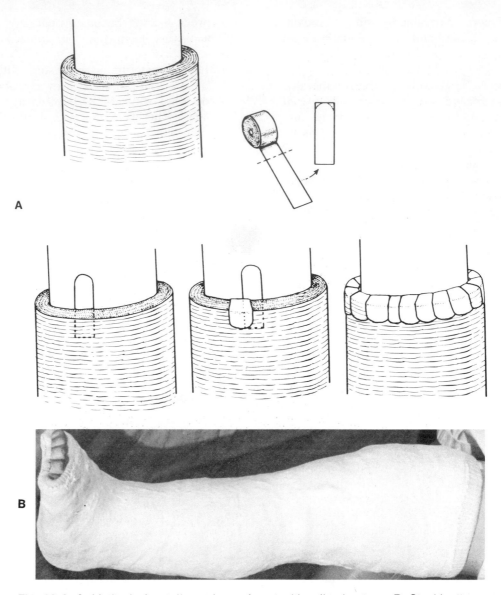

**Fig. 23-6. A,** Method of petaling edges of cast with adhesive tape. **B,** Stockinette over edges of cast. (From Hilt, N. E., and Schmitt, E. W., Jr.: Pediatric orthopedic nursing, St. Louis, 1975, The C. V. Mosby Co.)

at minimum, loss of function. Responsibility for the detection of neurovascular impairment is that of the nursing personnel who assume the 24-hour care of the patient. This does not, however, relieve the medical staff of the responsibility, accountability, or liability of actions taken, or failed to be taken, when such signs of impairment are documented or reported to them.

A precast neurovascular assessment should be the basis for comparison with post-application status. It is not acceptable to merely compare the status of the extremity with a cast to the extremity without a cast. Many patients have "normal" dif-

ferences in neurovascular status from one extremity to the other. In addition, assumptions as to a patient's status should not be made on the basis of the diagnosis. Each patient's "normal" should be established and can be the only valid basis for accurate judgment of status after the cast application.

Frequency of assessment depends on the status of the patient and the length of time after the application. The following are general guidelines that may be adopted as reasonable and valid:

1. Neurovascular assessments should be made every *hour* on all patients for the first 24 hours after cast or splint application.

2. If the status has returned to normal for that particular patient 24 hours after application, the assessments may be done every 4 hours.
3. If the status has *not* returned to normal for that patient, hourly assessments are continued until it has; then assessments are done every 4 hours.
4. If the patient's status is altered or is questionable, hourly assessments are resumed.
5. Neurovascular assessments should be accomplished for the entire duration of cast or splint therapy; this means that neurovascular assessment must be a part of discharge instructions.

To assure both accuracy of judgment and interpretation of status, all components of the neurovascular assessment must be accomplished for *each* assessment. Components of a complete neurovascular assessment may be reviewed in Table 24-2. Documentation of each component must be accurate and complete; the neurovascular assessment sheet shown in Fig. 24-4 will facilitate this process. The areas of assessment for specific cast applications are shown in the boxed material below. Guidelines and cautions about neurovascular assessment, which are outlined in Chapter 24, are applicable to all patients in a cast as well as traction. These should be reviewed in detail and all personnel responsible for this care should be totally familiar with them, since they incorporate many of the common errors encountered in assessing a patient's neurovascular status.

### Postoperative and posttraumatic control of edema

Edema is always likely following surgery or trauma. Because a cast does not allow for expansion, there is considerable threat to the neurovascular status if edema is not controlled.

The most effective measure to control edema is *elevation of the extremity*. This may be accomplished by appropriate elevation of the bed, use of pillows, or suspension of the extremity (Fig. 23-7). The latter is particularly effective for infants and young children, retarded individuals, and elderly or senile patients.

Two principles involved in maximizing effectiveness of elevation in the control of edema are:
1. Elevation should be established as a preventive measure for effective control of edema. It should begin *immediately* after application of the cast, rather than several hours later when some edema is already present.
2. Effective elevation requires the extremity to be placed *above* the level of the heart. Elevation of the lower extremity, for example, is not effective if the head of the bed is elevated as well.

If these principles are maintained, the less desirable measure of treating edema (bivalving of the cast) may frequently be avoided and thus position of the surgical area or traumatized extremity not jeopardized.

Unfortunately, perineal edema is not always as easily controlled as extremity edema. Frequently, surgical procedures involving perineal edema also involve the application of abduction "boots" or a hip spica cast. Because elevation of the area is obviously not as logical or possible, less effective methods of control, such as ice packs, are used. Perineal edema, therefore, takes longer to subside. Observation must be frequent to determine whether or not the edema is posing a problem with pressure or neurovascular status around the edges of the perineal cutout.

### Postoperative and posttraumatic drainage

Surgical procedures and traumatic injuries, depending on their extent, may produce drainage through the cast. Because the plaster is wet when applied, any drainage will be absorbed and may rapidly spread. The area and intensity of the drainage

---

**AREAS OF NEUROVASCULAR ASSESSMENT FOR SPECIFIC CASTS AND SPLINTS**

| Cast or splint | Area of neurovascular assessment |
|---|---|
| Lower extremity cast or splint | Involved lower extremity |
| Upper extremity cast or splint | Involved upper extremity |
| *All* spica casts | All four extremities |
| *All* cervical and spinal casts | All four extremities |
| Halo cast | All four extremities *and* assessment for cranial nerve impairment including: Diplopia Blurred vision Lateral eye movement Equality and reaction of pupils Difficulty swallowing Difficulty with speech Difficulty with tongue control |

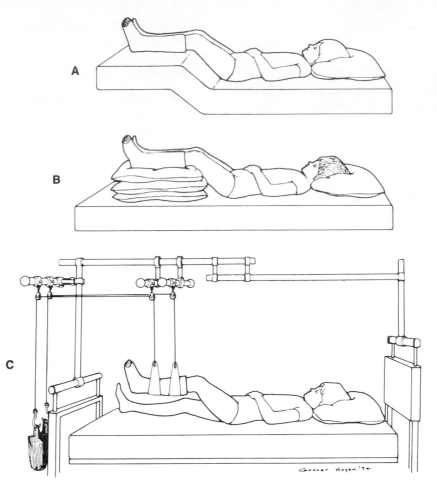

**Fig. 23-7.** Elevation of lower extremity cast to control edema with **(A)** bed gatching, **(B)** pillows, and **(C)** suspension. (From Hilt, N. E., and Schmitt, E. W., Jr.: Pediatric orthopedic nursing, St. Louis, 1975, The C. V. Mosby Co.)

visible on the exterior portion, therefore, do not necessarily indicate the degree and amount of actual drainage. Some types of surgical procedures, such as triple arthrodesis, are expected to produce drainage through the cast.

Monitoring of this drainage is critical for the first 24 to 72 hours after surgery or injury. Monitoring of the drainage should be accomplished by circling the diameter *at the change of shifts only.* This should be labeled with the time and date. Alterations in intensity of drainage should be recorded and documented on the chart, since it is difficult to indicate this on the cast (Fig. 23-8).

The appearance of the drainage is often disturbing to the patient and family. If the drainage has ceased to increase in both diameter and intensity and the color alterations with the drying process indicate that the drainage has stopped, permission may usually be obtained to add an additional roll of

plaster over the stained area before the patient is discharged.

**Positioning and turning**

Repositioning of the patient in a cast is extremely important in the redistribution of weight necessary to avoid pressure areas and skin complications. For the patient who is on bed rest during a portion of the cast therapy, repositioning is additionally significant in the prevention of those complications, such as pneumonia, usually associated with immobilization.

As a general rule, any patient in any type of cast may be repositioned prone, supine, or on either side. A turning schedule should be implemented using rotation of all of these positions, taking into account, of course, any specific requirements of positioning necessitated by certain surgical procedures or other factors. An exception to this rule is

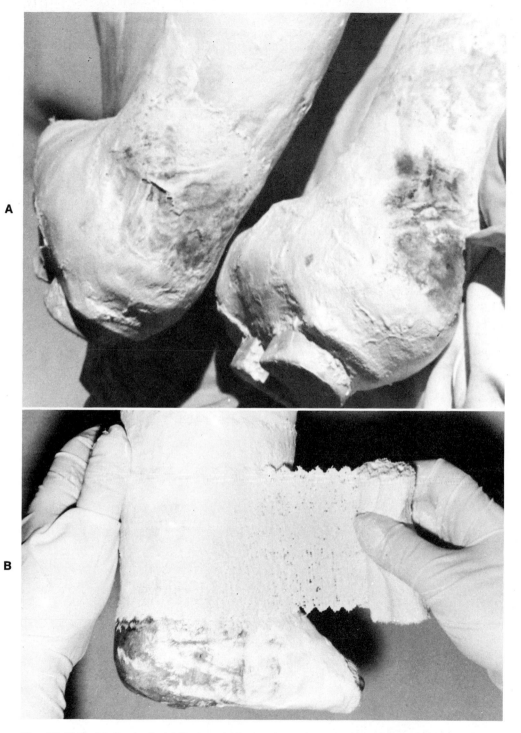

**Fig. 23-8. A,** Method of monitoring drainage through cast after surgery or traumatic injury. Circling of staining at change of each shift will appropriately designate to other personnel amount of increase that has occurred. Changes in intensity of staining should be documented on patient chart. **B,** Roll of plaster may be added over drainage if cast is dry and drainage has ceased for a sufficient amount of time. (From Hilt, N. E., and Schmitt, E. W., Jr.: Pediatric orthopedic nursing, St. Louis, 1975, The C. V. Mosby Co.)

the patient on a Bradford frame, who should only be positioned prone and supine.

The repositioning schedule will depend on the patient's history and diagnosis. Most patients can be assured skin integrity with a schedule that permits change of position every 4 hours. Those patients with a history of sensitive skin or previous skin breakdown, elderly and emaciated individuals, and those who have a diagnosis (such as myelomeningocele) compatible with anticipated skin problems, should be turned as frequently as necessary for assurance of skin integrity (every 1, 2, or 3 hours). It is advised, however, that a planned turning schedule be implemented for *all* patients rather than relying on random repositioning to be sufficient.

A consideration as important as the actual schedule of repositioning is the manner in which the patient is supported after the repositioning process. Care should be taken so that the toes, for example, are not pressing against the bed or that the edge of the cast is not pressing into the skin. Use of towel rolls and pillows will usually assure both the comfort of the patient and alleviation of potential pressure areas. As a general rule, if the patient appears uncomfortable, he probably is! Minor alterations can frequently make the difference between tolerance and intolerance of a position.

## Observation for pressure areas under cast

Regardless of the type of cast or splint that has been applied there is always the possibility that pressure areas will form under the cast. Measures are taken to avoid these problems, such as adequate padding under the plaster and proper handling of the extremity and cast during and after application, but these are not always enough to allay the problem. Muscle spasms may cause continued friction over joints; body build and amount of adipose tissue may make the patient vulnerable over a bony prominence or between skin folds; objects or toys dropped down the cast may be the source of irritation and breakdown.

The most critical nursing measure that can assist in the detection of such problems is the awareness of signs and symptoms of pressure areas under the cast. The infant, young child, or individual who is unable to verbalize the problem may show no sign other than a change in temperment, increase in fussiness or crying, or restlessness. The older child, adolescent, or adult who can communicate a problem may complain of pain or burning. Nursing personnel should carefully assess any patient with a cast or splint who complains of pain or burning, especially if the complaints are persistent and the pain occurs over a bony prominence or joint. The

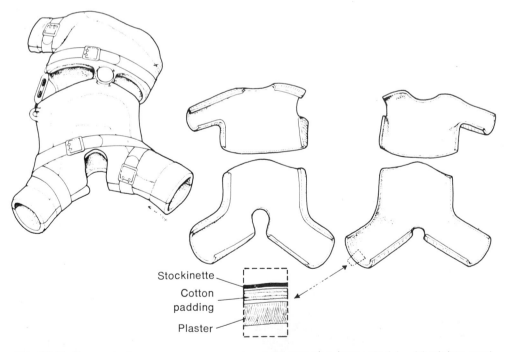

Stockinette
Cotton padding
Plaster

**Fig. 23-9.** Suspected pressure areas under cast may be inspected by bivalving cast (i.e., cutting cast in half). It may be necessary to reline cast if this is accomplished. This also allows intermittent immobilization. (From Hilt, N. E., and Schmitt, E. W., Jr.: Pediatric orthopedic nursing, St. Louis, 1975, The C. V. Mosby Co.)

pain should be noted on the chart and reported to the physician, and there should be increased monitoring of the problem and complaints. Pain medication may mask the symptoms and therefore, should be given only selectively. Complaints of pain or burning that have continued for a period of time and then suddenly cease are an even greater indication that the skin requires further evaluation. When a skin slough occurs, superficial sensation is lost and, as a result, the patient no longer complains.

The greatest difficulty in detection of a pressure area under the cast is with the patient who has decreased or no sensation. Early signs of a pressure area are almost impossible to detect and additional padding may be used for this reason. In these cases, the possibility of the area developing into a skin (or deeper tissue) slough and possible infection is great. If this happens, a fever may be noted and there may be drainage or an unusual odor from the cast. As an additional preventive measure the top of the cast should be covered with clothing or linen if food, crumbs, or small toys may fall down the cast.

When a pressure area under the cast is suspected, the physician may choose to either bivalve or "window" the cast (Fig. 23-9). In bivalving, the cast is cut into an anterior and a posterior portion; this permits examination of all of the skin under the cast. "Windowing" permits the removal of a portion of the cast over the suspect area only. The padding may then be cut and removed to inspect the skin. After this is accomplished, it is important that the padding and plaster be replaced with pressure that is equal to the remainder of the cast, or at least the area immediately surrounding the section, in an attempt to decrease the possibility of "window" edema. Depending on the purpose for the cast, and especially if it is a postoperative cast, the physician may choose to risk the possibility of a pressure area rather than jeopardize the required position to maintain the surgical correction.

### Maintaining cast clean and dry

Many problems are associated with any cast that does not stay clean and dry. Among the most common are:
1. If the cast becomes wet, it will soften and the desired position cannot be maintained or assured.
2. If the cast becomes soiled with feces or urine, an odor will develop that cannot be removed from the cast.
3. The resulting odor makes the patient undesirable to care for and to be around, and poses psychological problems.
4. Soiled and wet casts require cast changes or hospitalizations that could have been prevented.

All of these problems can be avoided by adherence to the basic guidelines given in Table 23-2. Utmost care must be taken when patients use the bedpan or urinal, and extra efforts should be made to avoid spills. In any of the above circumstances when plaster is maintained in place continuously, additional attention should be given to the skin to avoid maceration. In all cases frequent perineal care must be given.

**Split Bradford frame.** The split Bradford frame can be invaluable to the pediatric nursing staff responsible for keeping a hip spica cast dry. In the split frame the covers are placed at both ends of the frame, creating an open area at or near the center. (It should be noted that this type of frame is very different from the solid type used with children in traction.) These two frames should not be confused, since they are used in different ways. The split Bradford frame is shown in Fig. 23-10.

Not all children in a hip spica cast will require the Bradford frame; the criterion for utilization is *incontinence*. Age is often confused as a criterion for use, but a 13-year-old incontinent patient requires the frame as much as a 6-month-old infant![2, p.60]

The split Bradford frame is used with the incontinent child in a hip spica cast because it provides the continuous elevation, which, in combination with other measures, helps to maintain the cast clean and dry through the use of the law of gravity. If the purpose of the frame is to provide elevation, it is logical that the frame should be used with only the *head end* elevated.[2, p.63] Elevation of both ends of the frame to equal degrees will not assure the maintenance of a dry cast; this is another common error in the use of this type of frame. The setup of the frame is shown in Fig. 23-11, *A*.

Since the head end is elevated, the patient must be properly positioned at all times with the perineal cutout over the opening in the frame. Three buckled webbing straps are placed as follows to keep the patient from sliding on the frame:
1. Two straps are anchored at the upper end of the frame around the metal portion, one on either side.
2. Both straps are then brought under the upper canvas cover to the opening.
3. If the cast is a short leg hip spica, the straps are then secured around the thigh portion of the cast.
4. If the cast extends to the toes of one or both legs, the straps are wrapped around the metal

**Table 23-2.** Comparison of techniques for maintaining casts dry

| Type of cast | Client | Status | Nursing measures |
|---|---|---|---|
| Lower extremity casts<br>  Long leg cast<br>  Quengle cast<br>  Long leg abduction boots | Male | Continent | Careful placement of urinal<br>Use plastic around top of cast when using bedpan |
|  | Female | Continent | Use plastic around top of cast when using bedpan |
|  | Male, female, infant | Incontinent | Main plastic tucked around top of cast *at all times* (change as necessary) |
| Spinal casts<br>  Body jacket<br>  Risser casts<br>  Turnbuckle<br>  Cast<br>  Halo cast | Male | Continent | Careful placement of urinal<br>Use long plastic petals funneled into bedpan; elevate head of bed |
| Shoulder spica<br>cast | Female | Continent | Use long plastic petals funneled into bedpan; elevate head of bed |
|  | Male | Incontinent | Use condom catheter to drainage bag (change daily and as necessary)<br>Use long plastic petals funneled into bedpan; elevate head of bed |
|  | Female, infant | Incontinent | Use plastic tucked in around perineal cutout or hips at all times<br>Use diapers or waterproof pad (check every hour and change as necessary) |
| Hip spica casts<br>(all types) | Male | Continent | Careful placement of urinal<br>Use plastic petal funnel with bedpan and position shoulders higher than hips |
|  | Female | Continent | Use plastic petal funnel with bedpan and position shoulders higher than hips |
|  | Adult male | Incontinent | Use condom catheter to drainage bag (change daily and as necessary)<br>Use plastic petal funnel with bedpan and position shoulders higher than hips |
|  | Female adult | Incontinent | Use plastic petal funnel with waterproof pad at all times (change as necessary) |
|  | Infant, child, adolescent | Incontinent | Use plastic petal funnel into bedpan at all times (change every 4 hours and as necessary)<br>Maintain on split Bradford frame with head end elevated at all times |

portion of the frame at the opening and then secured around the thigh portion of the cast.

5. The third strap is placed around the child's waist and the frame.

The method of securement for the short leg hip spica cast is shown in Fig. 23-11, *B*.

For an incontinent child a plastic petal funnel into the bedpan is placed below the opening in the frame. This funnel should remain in place at all times and be changed every 4 hours. Skin and perineal care must also be provided. A few patients may be allergic to the plastic, which may cause a rash.

Changing the type of plastic will usually alleviate the reaction. If it does not, then a waterproof pad, cut in half, can be used in the same manner as the plastic funnel.

To facilitate care, safety, and security of the Bradford frame, the guidelines for the care and use of the Bradford frame should be reviewed (see Chapter 30). All personnel caring for these children should be thoroughly familiar with these guidelines. Implementation of these measures will assure the maintenance of a dry cast, a task not easily accomplished!

FRONT VIEW          BACK VIEW

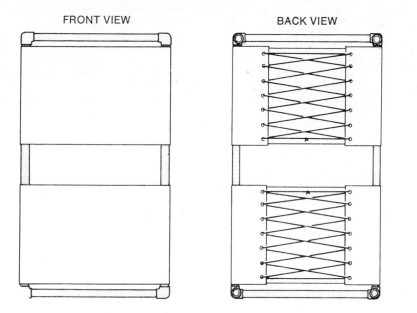

**Fig. 23-10.** Split Bradford frame utilized for incontinent children in hip spica casts. (From Hilt, N. E., and Schmitt, E. W., Jr.: Pediatric orthopedic nursing, St. Louis, 1975, The C. V. Mosby Co.)

Split Bradford frame for use with hip spica cast

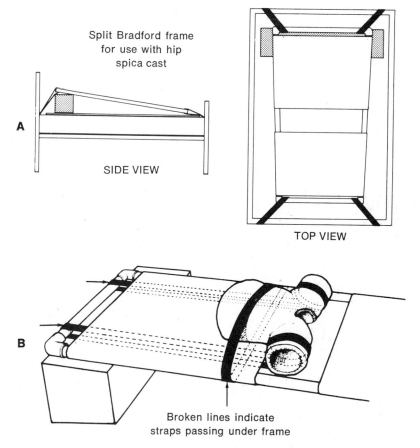

SIDE VIEW

TOP VIEW

Broken lines indicate straps passing under frame

**Fig. 23-11.** Use of split Bradford frame. **A,** Setup for split Bradford frame. **B,** Method of securing child to frame (with short leg hip spica cast). (From Hilt, N. E., and Schmitt, E. W., Jr.: Pediatric orthopedic nursing, St. Louis, 1975, The C. V. Mosby Co.)

## HOME INSTRUCTIONS
## HIP SPICA CAST WITH BRADFORD FRAME*

Your child will be going home from the hospital in a hip spica cast. It will be necessary to maintain him on a Bradford frame at all times while he is in the cast, unless otherwise specified, in order to keep the cast dry. You have already been given the instructions for making the Bradford frame. The following instructions will tell you how to take care of your child, the cast, and the frame so that he will be more comfortable for the duration of the cast therapy.

### EQUIPMENT

1. Rubbing alcohol
2. Plastic sheeting
3. Plywood to cover mattress
4. Books or magazines to elevate head of frame
5. Straps and buckles (supplied by hospital)

### Setting up frame

1. Place a piece of plywood over the mattress of the crib or bed. This will save some wear and tear on the mattress.
2. Elevate the head end of the frame _____ inches with books, magazines, or papers.
3. Strap the frame with the two straps at either end to the frame of the bed.
4. The illustrations will help you see how the frame will look.

### Daily care of frame

1. Check the canvas daily to make sure that it is tight. Tighten the straps as necessary. This prevents sagging of the covers and provides more comfort for your child and more protection for the cast.

2. Wash the plastic covers daily with warm water and soap. Be sure to dry thoroughly. This will prevent any odor. Change the plastic when necessary.
3. You will probably find that pillow cases will best cover the frame while your child is on it.
4. If the straps wear out, please replace them. Extras will be sent home with you.

### Putting child on frame

1. Put your child on the frame so that the top of the perineal cutout is just below the bottom edge of the top frame cover.
2. He will be held on the frame with three straps, which will be placed as the illustration at the end of these instructions shows. You will have an opportunity to practice this before you take your child home.

### Care of child's skin

1. Give your child a daily sponge bath. You may wash all the skin that is not covered by the cast. Be careful not to wet the cast, as this will cause softening of the cast and possible skin irritation.
2. Wash your child's perineum each time he voids or has a bowel movement. This will help keep his skin from becoming irritated.

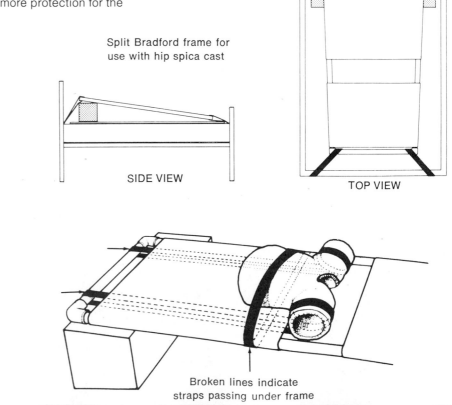

Split Bradford frame for use with hip spica cast

SIDE VIEW

TOP VIEW

Broken lines indicate straps passing under frame

*From Hilt, N. E., and Schmitt, E. W., Jr.: Pediatric orthopedic nursing, St. Louis, 1975, The C. V. Mosby Co.

3. Rub the skin around the edges of the cast with rubbing alcohol at least four times a day. This will help toughen the skin and prevent skin irritation. It is most important that *no oils, lotions, or powders* be used under the cast or around the edges—powders have a tendency to "cake," and lotions and oils will soften the skin, making it easier for the skin to break down.

4. Rub the base of the spine, heels, knees, ankles, and elbows, if exposed, with rubbing alcohol at least four times a day. These areas have a tendency to become irritated from rubbing on the bed.

5. Your child must be turned at least every 4 hours. He may be turned more frequently for comfort. This will help prevent pressure areas.

6. Each time skin care is given, check to make sure that your child can move his toes well, that he can feel his toes, and that the color of his toes is good. There should be no swelling and, if only one leg has been included in the cast, the toes should be as warm as those not in the cast.

## Care of cast

1. *Keep the cast clean and dry at all times!* If anything has accidentally spilled on the cast, keep the area uncovered until it has dried. It is most important, however, that this be avoided by covering the cast when your child is eating, drinking, etc. If the cast does become wet, it will soften, irritate the skin and not hold the leg and hip in the position in which the doctor has placed it.

2. Keep the plastic "petals" tucked well into the cast at all times and funneled into a bedpan below the frame. You will be instructed as to the best way to do this before your child goes home. These petals should be changed each time your child urinates or has a bowel movement. It is most important that these remain in place *at all times!* This will help keep the cast dry and prevent any odor.

3. Avoid letting any small items such as crumbs of food or small toys fall down the cast as they will irritate the skin. Under no circumstances should any item, such as a coat hanger, be placed down the cast to retrieve an object or to scratch the skin. Itching is a frequent complaint after one has been placed in a cast for a period of time, but the best remedy we have for this to date is to keep your child occupied.

4. When your child goes home, the edges of the cast will be covered with a stocking material or adhesive tape. Should this become loose, it should be replaced. Never put this tape over a wet area of the cast—wait until it has dried.

5. In some cases a bar will be placed between the legs of the cast. This is usually incorporated in the cast with plaster when the cast is made. It is there to stabilize the legs and positioning of your child. Please do not use this bar to turn your child as it can break off.

6. Do not put diapers totally over the perineal cutout of the cast or tuck them in. When they are wet, they will cause softening of the cast and wet the lining.

7. *Remember—keep the cast clean and dry at all times!*

## What to report to your doctor

1. Any crack or break in the cast
2. Any softening of the cast
3. Any extremely reddened areas around the edges of the cast not relieved by more frequent skin care, or any break in the skin
4. Extreme, continuous swelling of the casted toes
5. Extreme redness of the toes, especially associated with swelling
6. Blueness of the toes
7. Extreme coldness of the toes
8. Numbness of the toes or complaints of tingling or "pins and needles"
9. Continuous complaints of pain or discomfort or unexplained fussiness of your child
10. Unusual or unexplained odor from the cast
11. Temperature over 101 F (39.3 C)
12. Any severe illness such as flu or chest colds

It is most difficult for a normal, active child to be confined in a cast. It is therefore important that he be permitted to do all he possibly can for himself, but within the limitations set by your doctor. Your child can be moved on the frame and should be as often as possible, provided the head of the frame is elevated and the plastic petals are tucked in the cast. If possible, a second portable frame should be made to be used to take your child outdoors. He should be taken outdoors as often as possible, weather permitting.

TEMPERATURE: ____Yes
____No

MINI-SPICA BUG: ____Yes
____No

DOCTOR:

DOCTOR'S PHONE NUMBER:

HOSPITAL'S PHONE NUMBER:

ORTHOPEDIC NURSE SPECIALIST:

YOUR NEXT APPOINTMENT WITH YOUR DOCTOR:

SCHOOL: ____Yes
____No

SPECIAL INSTRUCTIONS: *Force fluids!*

### Care of joints not in cast

Any joint that has been immobilized for a period of time will become stiff and the muscles surrounding the joint will atrophy to a degree. By necessity, those joints incorporated within the cast undergo this process during therapy and after removal of the cast. The joints that are *not* incorporated, however, need not become stiff if range-of-motion exercises and movement activities are provided throughout cast therapy as a preventive measure. All joints not incorporated in the cast, unless contraindicated, should be considered in the plan of care. The exercises may be active, active assisted, or passive, depending on the extent of involvement or disability of the joints. Active exercise should always be encouraged when possible. Activities that promote independence and decrease the patient's feelings of boredom or immobility should also be encouraged.

### Nutritional requirements

Nutritional requirements vary depending on the degree of mobility permitted either by the physician or the type of cast. Patients may have a decreased appetite if activity is restricted or they may increase food intake if they are bored or depressed. Adequate monitoring of the diet is required and a balanced diet should always be encouraged, although sometimes this goal is difficult to achieve, especially if there is a previous history of nutritional problems or if cultural, ethnic, or religious requirements greatly affect the patient's nutritional habits.

### Bladder and kidney program

Potential bladder and kidney difficulties may be accentuated during periods of immobilization. This may not pose a high degree of concern for the patient who is immobilized in a cast for a short period of time or who is ambulatory. For the patient who is in a cast that prohibits weight-bearing or ambulation, or who requires prolonged bedrest, kidney function is likely to become sluggish. Therefore, these patients must be on forced fluids and the intake and output monitored every shift to assure adequate intake and kidney functioning. Fluids should be forced to twice the usual accepted amounts for the patient's age and body weight. In addition, it is advisable to restrict calcium intake (milk and milk products) to meals only. This helps to assure that the intake of calcium, which has a tendency to deposit in the kidney extremely rapidly and is the source of many renal calculi, is not of an amount that might contribute to potential problems with kidney function.

### Bowel program

Patients receiving weight-bearing cast therapy are often able to maintain normal bowel status. Those immobilized for prolonged periods, however, may have a tendency to become constipated. Poor nutritional status may increase the patient's usual vulnerability to this problem. Bowel movements should be monitored every shift to provide a clear indication of status. All attempts should be made to avoid impaction by giving increased amounts of roughage, juices, and so on, and, if necessary, mild laxatives or enemas. Whatever bowel program has been determined successful and necessary should be adequately documented on the care plan to avoid guesswork or unnecessary complications.

### Psychological and emotional support

Although in this chapter, we cannot elaborate all of the psychological implications of cast and splint therapy, several areas of emphasis are important. The degree of emotional and psychological adjustment to the therapy may well depend on the size of the cast, the anticipated length of therapy, and the perceived degree of immobilization inflicted upon the patient by the therapy. Precast preparation and education will influence this adjustment, as will existence of other disabilities or deformities, prior exposure to the therapy or hospitalization, and previously developed coping mechanisms for change.

Body image alterations will vary considerably from patient to patient. A usual period of adjustment is required and should be anticipated, through which patients should be supported in their efforts to cope within their limitations and abilities to merge all of these components into the adjustment process. Length of adjustment may vary, but if the adjustment period is determined to be prolonged, counseling from appropriate staff members or a mental health counselor may be appropriate. Continued reassessment of a patient's psychological status is required throughout cast therapy. (The tables in Chapter 7 will assist the reader in determining specific interventions and alleviating crisis situations.)

### Discharge instructions

Patients are frequently discharged from a facility with a cast. Statistically, most cast therapy is received in the home rather than in a medical facility. Also, care is required for the *duration* of the cast therapy. Therefore, discharge instructions should be provided before the patient goes home from the clinic or hospital and should include the following:

1. A written account of all of the required care

*Text continued on p. 503.*

## STANDARDIZED CARE PLAN: LOWER EXTREMITY CASTS

Right ☐  Short ☐
Left ☐  Long ☐
Bil. ☐  Cyl. ☐

| Problem | Outcome | Plan | Schedule | Begin | Disc. |
|---|---|---|---|---|---|
| Neurovascular compromise | Maintenance of acceptable neurovascular status | Neurovascular assessment: check pulse, edema, color, temperature, capillary filling, sensation, and motion; document<br>Notify physician if any changes | q 1 hour till _____ then<br>0400-0800-1200-<br>1600-2000-2400<br>PRN | | |
| Potential skin breakdown | Maintenance of skin integrity | Skin care with alcohol to skin around all cast edges<br>If on bedrest: skin care with alcohol to all exposed bony prominences and joints*<br>Turn q 1 hour till cast is dry then every 4 hours†<br>Petal cast when dry | 0400-0800-1200-<br>1600-2000-2400<br>0400-0800-1200-<br>1600-2000-2400<br>Prone 0400-1600<br>Supine 0800-2000<br>Left side 1200<br>Right side 2400<br>AM_____ | | |
| Potential edema* | Controlled edema or no edema* | Elevate extremity above heart level*<br>Pillows<br>Bed gatch<br>Suspension<br>Do not elevate head of bed | Continuously til<br>_____ | | |
| Potential pressure area under cast | No pressure areas under cast | Reposition as above<br>Observe for signs or complaints indicating pressure areas: burning, pain, fever, drainage | Continuously | | |
| Renal calculi† | Maintenance of kidney function with no renal calculi† | Force fluids†<br>Maintain shift intake and output record | _____ ml 7-3 shift<br>_____ ml 3-11 shift<br>_____ ml 11-7 shift<br>0700-1500-2300 | | |
| Constipation† | Maintenance of bowel function† | Promote roughage and bulk in diet†<br>Force fluids as above†<br>Obtain physician order for fecal softener, laxative, or suppository†<br>Record bowel movements† | PRN<br>PRN | | |
| Potential soiled cast* | Clean and dry cast* | Incontinent:*<br>Put plastic around top of cast<br>Continent:*<br>Put plastic around top of cast<br>Elevate head of bed | Continuously<br>When on bedpan<br>When on bedpan | | |

**Form 23-1, A**

*When appropriate.
†If nonambulatory.

## STANDARDIZED CARE PLAN: UPPER EXTREMITY CASTS

Right ☐  Short ☐
Left ☐  Long ☐
Bil. ☐  Cyl. ☐

| Problem | Outcome | Plan | Schedule | Begin | Disc. |
|---|---|---|---|---|---|
| Neurovascular compromise | Maintenance of acceptable neurovascular status | Neurovascular assessment: check pulse, edema, color, temperature, capillary filling, sensation and motion; document<br>Notify physician if any changes | q 1 hour until _____ then 0400-0800-1200-1600-2000-2400<br>PRN | | |
| Potential skin breakdown | Maintenance of skin integrity | Skin care with alcohol to skin around *all* cast edges<br>While on bedrest — skin care with alcohol to all exposed bony prominences and joints<br>Turn (expose all sides of cast) q 2 hrs. til DRY, then every 4 hours†<br>Petal cast when dry | 0400-0800-1200-1600-2000-2400<br>0400-0800-1200-1600-2000-2400<br>0400-0800-1200-1600-2000-2400<br>_____ AM | | |
| Potential edema* | Controlled edema or no edema* | Elevate extremity above heart level*<br>Pillows<br>Suspension<br>Sling<br>Do not elevate head of bed | Continuously until _____ | | |
| Potential pressure area under cast | No pressure areas under cast | Reposition as above<br>Observe for signs or complaints indicating pressure areas: burning, pain, fever, drainage | Continuously | | |
| Renal calculi† | Maintenance of kidney function with no renal calculi† | Force fluids†<br><br>Maintain shift intake and output record | _____ ml 7-3 shift<br>_____ ml 3-11 shift<br>_____ ml 11-7 shift<br>0700-1500-2300 | | |
| Constipation† | Maintenance of bowel function† | Promote roughage and bulk in diet<br>Force fluids as above†<br>Obtain physician order for fecal softener, laxative, or suppository†<br>Record bowel movements† | PRN<br><br>PRN | | |

Form 23-1, B

*When appropriate.
†When on bed-rest.

## STANDARDIZED CARE PLAN: HIP SPICA CAST

One leg ☐
1½ leg ☐
Bil. short ☐
Bil. long ☐

| Problem | Outcome | Plan | Schedule | Begin | Disc. |
|---|---|---|---|---|---|
| Neurovascular compromise | Maintenance of acceptable neurovascular status | Neurovascular assessment; (all four extremities): check pulse, edema, color, temperature, capillary filling, sensation, motion; document<br>Notify physician if any changes | q 1 hour until _____ then 0400-0800-1200-1600-2000-2400<br><br>PRN | | |
| Potential skin breakdown | Maintenance of skin integrity | Skin care with alcohol to skin around all cast edges | 0400-0800-1200-1600-2000-2400 | | |
| | | Skin care with alcohol to all exposed bony prominences and joints | 0400-0800-1200-1600-2000-2400 | | |
| | | Turn q 1 hour until cast is DRY, then every 4 hours | Prone 0400-1600<br>Supine 0800-2000<br>Left side 1200<br>Right side 2400 | | |
| | | Petal cast when dry | | | |
| Potential edema* | Controlled edema or no edema* | Do not elevate head of bed* | AM _____ | | |
| | | Ice bag to perineal area* | PRN | | |
| Potential pressure area under cast | No pressure area under cast | Reposition as above<br>Observe for signs or complaints indicating pressure areas: burning, pain, fever, drainage, etc. | Continuously | | |
| Renal calculi | Maintenance of kidney function with no renal calculi | Force fluids | _____ ml 7-3 shift<br>_____ ml 3-11 shift<br>_____ ml 11-7 shift<br>0700-1500-2300 | | |
| | | Maintain shift intake and output record | | | |
| Constipation | Maintenance of bowel function | Promote roughage and bulk in diet | | | |
| | | Force fluids as above | | | |
| | | Obtain physician order for fecal softener, laxative, or suppository | PRN | | |
| | | Record bowel movements | PRN | | |
| Potential soiled cast* | Clean and dry cast* | Incontinent:*<br> Plastic petals around perineal cutout into bedpan | Continuously | | |
| | | Maintain on split bradford frame with head end elevated | Continuously | | |
| | | Maintain position on frame with perineal cutout over opening of frame | | | |
| | | Turn prone and supine only | Cancel prior turning schedule:<br>prone-0400, supine-0800,<br>prone-1200, supine-1600,<br>prone-2000, supine-2400 | | |
| | | Continent:*<br> Plastic petals around perineal cutout into bedpan | When on bedpan | | |
| | | Elevate head of bed | When on bedpan | | |

**Form 23-1, C**

*When appropriate.

## STANDARDIZED CARE PLAN: BODY CAST

Body jacket ☐
Risser localizer ☐
Halo cast ☐

| Problem | Outcome | Plan | Schedule | Begin | Disc. |
|---|---|---|---|---|---|
| Neurovascular compromise | Maintenance of acceptable neuro-vascular status | Neurovascular assessment (*all four extremities*): check pulse, edema, color, temperature, capillary filling, sensation and motion and document<br>Notify physician if any changes | q 1 hour until _____ then 0400-0800-1200-1600-2000-2400<br><br>PRN | | |
| Cranial nerve compromise* | Maintenance of intact cranial nerve function* | Cranial nerve assessment:* check for signs or complaints of blurred vision, double vision, lateral eye movement, pupil equality and reaction, slurred speech, difficulty swallowing, drooped eyelids or mouth; document<br>Notify physician of any change | q 1 hour until _____ then 0400-0800-1200-1600-2000-2400 | | |
| Potential skin breakdown | Maintenance of skin integrity | Skin care with alcohol to skin around all cast edges<br>If on bedrest—skin care with alcohol to all exposed bony prominences and joints*<br>Turn q 1 hour until cast is dry, then q. 4 hours<br>Petal cast when dry. | 0400-0800-1200-1600-2000-2400<br>0400-0800-1200-1600-2000-2400<br>Prone 0400-1600<br>Supine 0800-2000<br>Left side 1200<br>Right side 2400<br>AM _____ | | |
| Potential pressure area under cast | No pressure areas under cast | Reposition as above<br>Observe for signs or complaints in-dicating pressure areas: burning, pain, fever, drainage | Continuously | | |
| Renal calculi† | Maintenance of kid-ney function with no renal calculi† | Force fluids†<br><br>Maintain shift intake and output record | _____ ml 7-3 shift<br>_____ ml 3-11 shift<br>_____ ml 11-7 shift<br>0700-1500-2300 | | |
| Constipation† | Maintenance of bowel function† | Promote roughage and bulk in diet†<br>Force fluids as above†<br>Obtain physician order for fecal softener, laxative, or suppository†<br>Record bowel movements† | <br><br>PRN<br>PRN | | |
| Potential soiled cast‡ | Clean and dry cast‡ | Incontinent:†<br>  Plastic petals around bottom of cast<br>Continent:†<br>  Plastic petals around bottom of cast into bedpan<br>  Elevate head of bed | Continuously<br><br>When on bedpan<br>When on bedpan | | |

**Form 23-1, D**

*Halo cast *only*.
†If nonambulatory.
‡When appropriate.

2. An explanation of all required care
3. Frequency of each component of care
4. A return demonstration of the required care
5. Verbal feedback of required care

If the instructions include all of these components the degree of compliance may be greater than frequently occurs. More often than not, when a patient returns with a soiled cast, a pressure area that has not been reported as early as desired, or a softened cast, the fault can be directly traced to inadequate discharge instructions rather than noncompliance. Patients and families will not comply with the care if they do not understand it or have not been taught exactly what their responsibilities are.

Written discharge instructions are helpful if they are both standardized and flexible enough for individualized care. Adequate written instructions should include the following:

1. Each care component
2. Explanations of procedures for each component
3. Frequency of each component of care
4. Diagrams or line drawings illustrating components of care when applicable
5. Signs and symptoms of potential problems to be reported to physician or nurse
6. Procedure of reporting potential problems or obtaining answers to questions
7. Telephone numbers of individuals to whom potential problems are to be reported
8. Any special instructions

The written instructions serve as a reminder and resource for the patient after discharge. The time and effort required to develop standardized written instructions will be justified by the decrease in complications. A sample of standardized discharge instructions is shown in the boxed material. pp. 496-497. These, of course, may be adapted to individual routines and policies accepted by the physician, nursing staff, and medical facility. Further information about patient education may be reviewed in Chapter 34.

### Documentation

Documentation of all aspects of care is required for the completion of the nursing process. The neurovascular assessment sheet (Chapter 24), orthopedic data base form and Kardex form (Chapter 6), neurologic assessment sheet (Chapter 8), and discharge instructions may be adapted to fulfill the specific needs of the orthopedic client.

**Standardized care plans.** Standardized care plans, developed and adapted to required routines and accepted policies, will assist nursing staff members in unifying necessary care. They will provide a high degree of consistency and continuity of care, which is important not only to the patient and family and the manner in which they view care during the hospitalization, but are also critical to the implementation of adequate discharge instructions. If a uniform standard of care has been used throughout the patient's hospitalization, problems associated with the implementation of discharge instructions and compliance of the same standard of care at home are considerably decreased. Examples of standardized care plans for the patient in a cast may be reviewed in Form 23-1.

### COMPLICATIONS OF CAST THERAPY

No treatment modality is without complications. The critical element in the diagnosis and treatment of complications, however, is that of early recognition of signs and symptoms, as well as the ability of nursing personnel to make judgments regarding the communication of these signs and symptoms appropriately so that early intervention may be realized. Nursing personnel should also be aware of any emergency measures that they may be required to fulfill these principles. For example, all nursing personnel should be familiar with and adept in the use of the cast saw in case it is necessary to bivalve a cast to assure neurovascular integrity (if requested to do so until the physician arrives) or split a body cast appropriately and rapidly if cardiac or respiratory arrest occurs. The most common complications of cast therapy may be reviewed in Table 23-3.

### PRINCIPLES OF CAST REMOVAL

All casts must eventually be removed. Various methods may be used to remove the cast but adherence to certain principles will facilitate the procedure and decrease any trauma that may be associated with it. The first step in the process is to adequately prepare the patient for the procedure. Cast removal may be a noisy and frightening experience even with preparation, but appropriate education should assist in allaying many of the patient's fears. At minimum, the patient should have the procedure explained. If the cast saw is being used, it should be turned on briefly to prepare the patient for the noise. Small children might be more cooperative if, after the explanation, they are provided with a set of high-frequency earphones that will reduce the amount of noise during the procedure, or earphones plugged into a cassette recorder with music or a story. Infants will be more likely to respond positively if they are brought to the plaster room or clinic hungry; the infant may then be fed while the cast

**Table 23-3.** Complications of cast and splint therapy

| Complication | Type of cast | Signs-symptoms | Treatment | Prevention |
|---|---|---|---|---|
| Peroneal nerve palsy | All casts or splints incorporating lower extremity | Pain, tingling, or paresthesia over anterior surface of affected leg and dorsilateral aspect of affected foot<br>Inability to actively dorsiflex foot<br>Drop-foot | Passive dorsiflexion exercises<br>Proper positioning<br>Possibly dorsiflexion brace for ambulation<br>Reapplication of cast or splint to alleviate source of problem | Observe for prevention of pressure over peroneal nerve<br>Proper positioning and handling during cast application<br>Avoid any potential pressure (such as indentation) over peroneal nerve |
| Compartment syndromes[3] (progressive vascular compromise) | All casts or splints incorporating upper or lower extremity | Pain—increasing and progressive in involved area<br>Pain—on passive motion<br>Paralysis—progressive<br>Paresthesias<br>Pulselessness | Relieve constriction; bivalve cast; possible reapplication<br>Elevation of the extremity<br>Possible fasciotomy | Proper positioning and handling of extremity during application<br>Early detection with recognition of signs and symptoms and initiation of treatment |
| Constrictive edema | All casts and splints | Gradual increase in swelling from vascular compromise<br>Alteration in circulatory or neurologic status | Splint—remove elastic bandage; rewrap with less tension; inspect interior for potential cause<br>Bivalve cast; cut padding; wrap with elastic bandage<br>Elevate extremity | Use care in application of padding and plaster; do not wrap too tightly<br>Observe for early signs and symptoms<br>Elevate extremity |
| Constipation/impaction | All casts if non–weight-bearing or a patient on bed rest | Inconsistent bowel movements<br>Lack of bowel movements<br>Loose bowel movements indicative of impaction | Natural alterations or additions to diet (e.g., juices, roughage)<br>Laxatives, enemas as necessary | Monitor diet<br>Monitor bowel movements<br>Individualized bowel program |
| Renal calculi | All casts if non–weight-bearing or a patient on bed rest | Flank pain—may be increasing or intermittent<br>Difficulty with urination | Report suspicion to physician<br>X-ray<br>Specific treatment determined by size and location | Force fluids to twice the usual accepted intake for age, size, and weight<br>Limit milk and milk products to meals only<br>Monitor intake and output |

**Table 23-3.** Complications of cast and splint therapy—cont'd

| Complication | Type of cast | Signs-symptoms | Treatment | Prevention |
|---|---|---|---|---|
| Pressure area or tissue breakdown at edges of or under cast | All casts and splints | Reddened areas around edge of cast<br>Pain at edge or under cast<br>Irritability, fussiness, or restlessness<br>Drainage through cast (with or without odor)<br>Elevated temperature | Notify physician<br>Bivalve or "window" cast (cutout over suspicious area)<br>Further treatment depends on findings after skin inspection | Careful application of and proper treatment of padding and plaster<br>Maintain desired position *throughout* application<br>Appropriate handling of extremity and cast with palm of hand rather than fingers<br>Observe to detect signs early |
| Pin tract infection | Halo cast; other cast if pin or wire incorporated | Erythema at pin site<br>Drainage and/or odor<br>Pin migration<br>Temperature elevation<br>Pain | Treatment depends on depth of infection; superficial infection treated with topical or oral antibiotics; deeper infection usually requires pin removal with antibiotic therapy | Appropriate pin care (see Chapter 24) if pin site exposed<br>Observe for early signs and symptoms |
| Cranial nerve impairment[1] | Halo cast | Abnormal lateral eye movements<br>Pupillary changes<br>Blurred vision<br>Diplopia<br>Difficulty swallowing<br>Difficulty with speech<br>Difficulty with tongue control | Treatment depends on severity of symptoms<br>Continue observation<br>Pin removal may be required | Observe for early signs and symptoms<br>Incorporation of signs and symptoms monitoring into neurovascular assessment |
| Superior mesenteric artery syndrome (cast syndrome) | Risser localizer cast; Risser turnbuckle cast; Halo cast (rarely) | Acute upper quadrant abdominal pain<br>Projectile vomiting<br>Possible temperature elevation from dehydration | Nothing by mouth<br>Intravenous fluids for hydration<br>Flat plate of abdomen to confirm diagnosis<br>Possible reduction of stretching due to cast application<br>Gradual increase of oral fluids after pain and projectile vomiting ceases<br>Surgical intervention may be necessary | Gradual and careful application of casts<br>Prompt documentation and reporting of symptoms |

is being removed. If crying occurs, however, logic would dictate discontinuation of the feeding to avoid increased risk of aspiration. Demonstration of the saw against the hand, if one is adept in its use, may alleviate the patient's fear of being cut and is usually a successful preparatory technique with older children, adolescents, and adults.

### Equipment

The following equipment is used to remove the cast:

1. Manual cast cutter permits cutting of the cast in circumstances when it is not advisable to use a cast saw, such as with an infant.
2. Plaster scissors are available in various sizes to cut the padding.
3. Cast saw permits cutting of the plaster. The blade is removable and should be changed often to assure efficiency. A special blade must be used for removal of a fiberglass cast. A vacuum may be attached to the saw while cutting to rid the area of dust.*
4. Cast spreader permits spreading of the cast after cutting. Cast spreaders are available in various types and sizes appropriate for all types of casts.

---

*Illustration from Hilt, N. E., and Schmitt, E. W., Jr.: Pediatric orthopedic nursing, St. Louis, 1975, The C. V. Mosby Co.

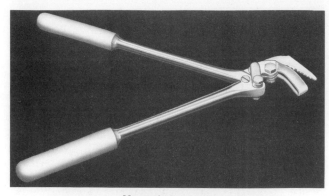

**Manual cast cutter**

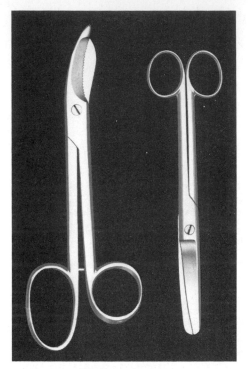

**Plaster scissors**

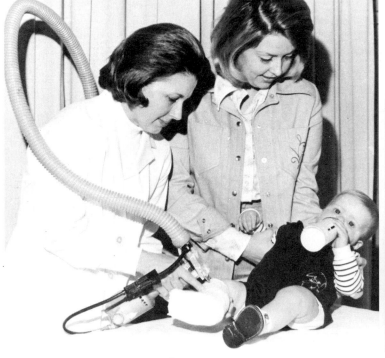

**Cast saw***

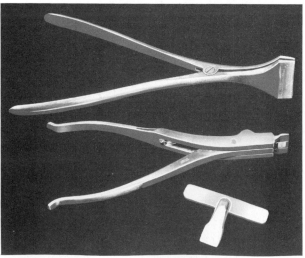

**Cast spreaders**

## Procedure

The manual cast cutter may be used to remove the cast of a small infant or to assist in the removal of a larger cast where it is difficult to position the cast saw. The scissors-like action of the manual cutter permits short cutting strokes and is, therefore, appropriate for corners or at the edges of a cast (Fig. 23-12). The padding and the plaster may be cut at the same time with the manual cast cutter; spreading of the cast and removal may then be accomplished.

The cast saw is usually the most efficient tool for cast removal. It permits the rapid cutting of plaster, but does not cut the padding at the same time. Use of the cast saw requires skill, and *if not utilized properly* it may produce abrasions or cuts in the skin. The blade is removable and should be changed often to assure efficiency. A special blade must be used for the removal of a fiberglass cast. Fig. 23-13 demonstrates the basic principles in the safe and efficient use of the cast saw. Also note the following:

1. The saw must be stabilized by either the index finger or the thumb. This will assure control of the saw. The choice of whether the index finger or thumb is used is that of the individual; some find that the thumb is more comfortable, others the index finger.
2. The saw should be used with an in-and-out motion, rather than side-to-side motion. This is crucial if cuts and abrasions are to be avoided; by the same token, safe use can be guaranteed if this principle is adhered to.
3. The cast saw should be used *only* by individuals adept in its use. All nursing personnel should be instructed in its use for emergency situations.

4. A vacuum attached to the saw can be invaluable in ridding the area of dust while cutting. It must, however, be cleaned periodically to assure maximum effectiveness and functioning.
5. All equipment should be clean and well maintained.

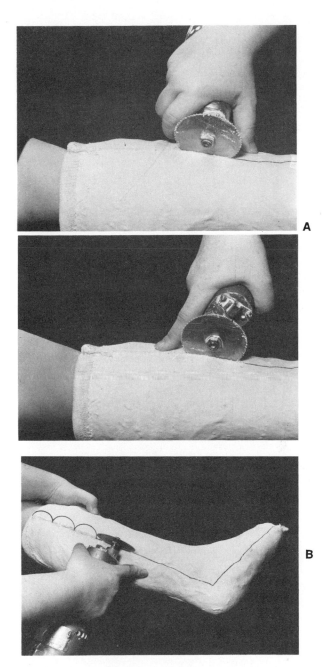

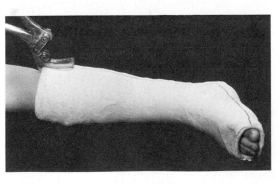

**Fig. 23-12.** Use of manual cast cutter for cast removal

**Fig. 23-13.** Principles in use of cast saw include **(A)** stabilization of saw with thumb or index finger and **(B)** use of in-and-out motion of saw.

The following procedure may be used to remove the cast; a leg cast is shown for demonstration purposes, but the same procedure applies to all cast removals.

1. Cut one side of the cast using the principles previously outlined.

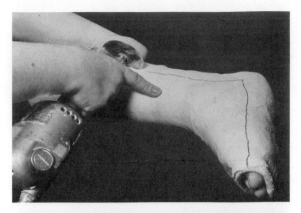

2. Both sides of the cast should be cut completely.

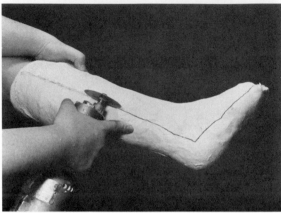

3. Spread the cast slightly at each end and cut the padding or stockinette.

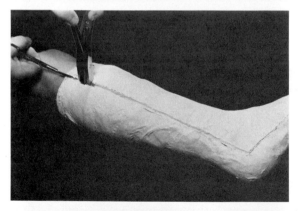

4. Spreading the cast releases some of the tension and facilitates the remainder of the procedure.

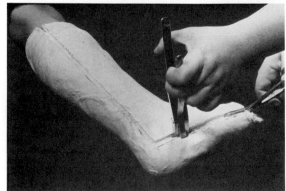

5. Spread the cast gradually (to avoid breakage) using a cast spreader.

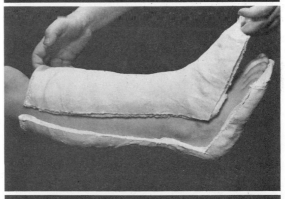

6. Cut the padding while spreading the cast.

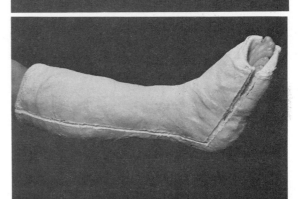

7. This procedure must be accomplished on both sides. The cast is now ready for removal.

8. Remove the anterior portion of the cast.

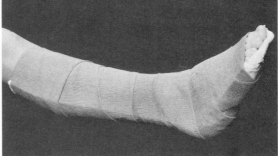

9. Unless there is a specific order from the physician to totally remove the cast, the posterior portion should be secured with an elestic bandage until the extremity has been examined by the physician.

Any extremity or portion of the body that has been incorporated in a cast for any period of time will require special care after cast removal. The skin will almost always have an exudate and it may be yellowish. The amount of exudate, which is a build-up of secretions and dead skin, will depend on the length of cast therapy. Removing this exudate and dead skin should be done gradually. The application of oil to soften it, followed by warm water soaks and bathing are usually successful. This may take several days, but this gradual approach is preferable to avoid additional skin irritation.

Handling of the extremity after cast removal is also of utmost importance, especially regarding stiff joints and muscle atrophy that develop during this type of immobilization. The extremity should be handled carefully and moved cautiously and slowly. The extremity should be supported with the palms of the hands rather than the fingertips. Gradual in-crease in this effort will depend on the reason for the cast therapy, as well as the desired progression or rehabilitation prescribed by the physician.

### Bivalving and lining

A *bivalved* cast is simply one that has been cut into two pieces, usually an anterior and posterior half. Actually, casts that have been just removed, as demonstrated above, may be said to be bivalved. The type of cast referred to in this section, however, is to be reused after removal. There are occasions when intermittent immobilization is desired after continuous cast therapy is completed. For example, a bivalve cast may be used for immobilization during rest periods or at night, to facilitate exercise programs between periods of immobilization, or to facilitate care of a complication (such as a pressure sore) when immobilization remains necessary.

To fulfill such needs, a cast may be *bivalved and lined,* that is, cut in two halves and specially prepared so that it can be removed at desired intervals. This procedure may be accomplished as follows:

1. Bivalve the cast as for any removal, except use extreme caution during the spreading process. If the cast is broken or the edges are bent, continued use may be impossible.

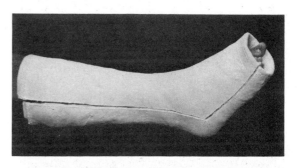

2. Remove the anterior portion of the cast with the patient in a supine position.

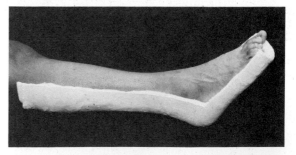

3. Secure the posterior half on the patient with an elastic bandage.

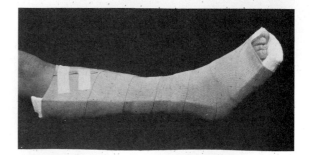

4. The anterior portion may now be prepared. Remove the padding from the plaster.

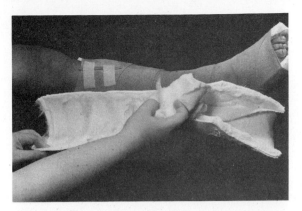

5. Inspect the interior aspect of the cast for rough areas. Ridging is likely to occur because of the manner in which the cotton padding is layered.

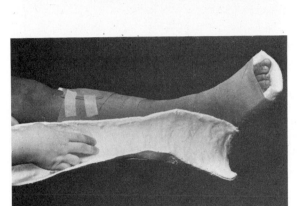

6. With an electric grinder, grind all rough spots to a smooth surface. Care should be taken not to grind through layers of plaster to the point of instability.

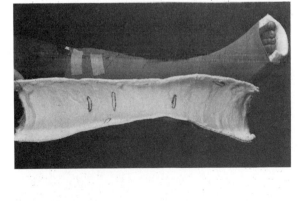

7. Bevel, or angle, the edges of the cast with a cast knife.

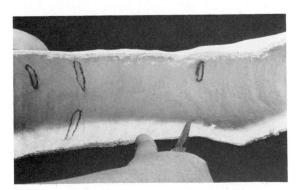

8. Place several layers of padding lengthwise over the interior aspect of the cast. Carefully apply the padding as smoothly as possible, including the joint areas of the cast.

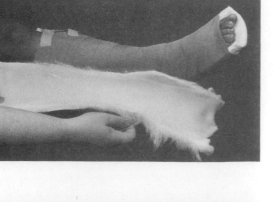

9. Excess padding that goes over the edges of the cast may be torn back to the edge surface.

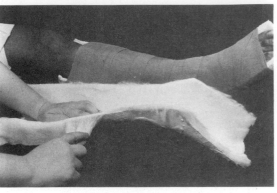

10. Place one layer of stockinette (cut lengthwise) over the cast.

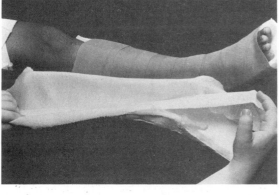

11. Tape the edges of stockinette to the exterior aspect of the cast, pulling it over the edges. Care should be taken to assure that the cotton padding remains unwrinkled and smooth, as well as secure.

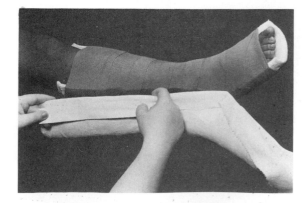

12. All edges of stockinette are now secured with tape.

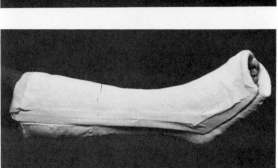

13. Replace the anterior portion of the cast on the patient, after removing the elastic bandage.

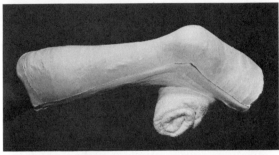

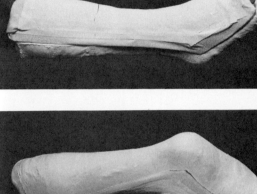

14. Manually secure both halves of the cast while the patient is turned prone; the posterior portion of the cast may then be removed.

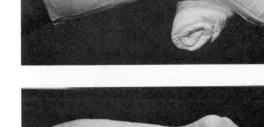

15. Secure the anterior portion of the cast on the patient with an elastic bandage.

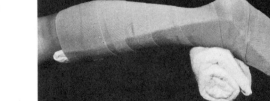

16. Repeat steps 4 through 12 of the above procedure with the posterior portion of the cast.

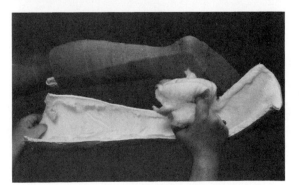

17. The posterior half of the cast has now been relined.

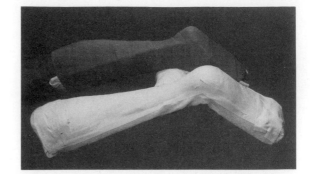

18. Using buckled webbing strap, secure a strap long enough to go around the entire cast (near the top of the cast) with tape.

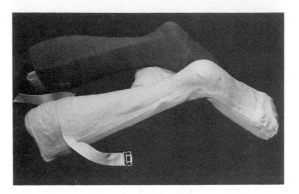

19. Secure a longer strap, with excess on the unbuckled end, and long enough to go around ankle and foot, at the level of the ankle. A third strap may be secured near the center of the cast.

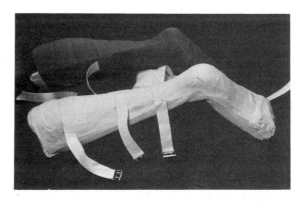

20. Remove the elastic wrap from the patient and replace the posterior portion of the cast.

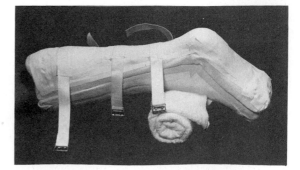

21. Securing the cast manually, turn the patient supine.

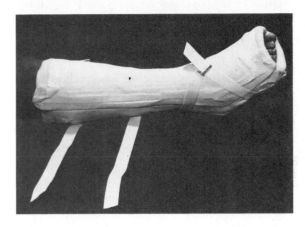

22. Using a figure-of-eight around the foot, buckle the ankle strap.

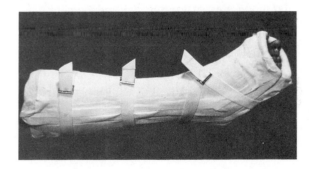

23. Buckle the upper and middle straps.

24. The bivalved and lined cast is now completed and ready for use. Note that an additional strap has been secured around the toes to assure stability.

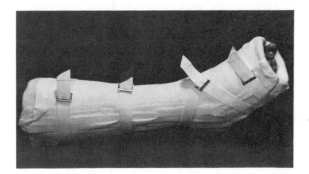

The bivalved cast has many advantages as a means of providing intermittent immobilization. One of the greatest is that of cost and longevity. A plaster cast is rather inexpensive compared to other forms of immobilization, such as orthoses, and, when used intermittently, has a relatively long lifespan if care is taken in the construction and application of the cast. There are, however, potential problems that may arise, so that the following safety measures are recommended:

1. Never remove *both* portions of the cast unless there is a specific order designating that this may be done. The actual procedure may be time consuming and, depending on the patient's status, total withdrawal of immobilization for that period of time may be detrimental.
2. During the reapplication process, be sure that the patient's skin is not being pinched by the cut edges.
3. If the cast is a leg cast, be sure that the heel is placed securely in the cast before applying the anterior portion.
4. Always use *both* halves of a bivalved cast for immobilization. Use of the posterior portion only, secured with an elastic bandage, will particularly cause problems with the patient with muscle spasms, and maintenance of the desired immobilization cannot be assured.
5. The size and amount of padding and stockinette, and the number of straps used will vary with the size of the patient and type of cast. Always use a figure-of-eight around a joint and be sure there are enough straps to properly secure the cast after reapplication.
6. After the bivalving and lining procedure has been accomplished, remove the cast, one portion at a time, and inspect the skin for potential pressure areas. If any occur, repad or grind appropriately to alleviate the problem. This inspection should be accomplished every hour until all potential pressure areas have been alleviated.

## SUMMARY

The care of the patient in a cast is not always as simple as it appears. Efforts have been made throughout this chapter to provide the reader with an adequate and thorough understanding of the application and removal process, as well as the care involved throughout cast and splint therapy. Emphasis has been placed on the necessity for a comprehensive plan of care that will alleviate complications of cast therapy or, at minimum, enable health care personnel to detect early signs and symptoms of complications so that treatment can be initiated and the possibility of permanent damage lessened.

## REFERENCES

1. Alt, P.: Care of the child in traction, ONA J **2** (1): 14-16, Jan. 1975.
2. Hilt, N. E., and Schmitt, E. W., Jr.: Pediatric orthopedic nursing, St. Louis, 1975, The C. V. Mosby Co.
3. Laucey, G. L.: Compartment syndrome, ONA J **2** (6): 148-151, June 1975.

## BIBLIOGRAPHY

Bleck, E. E., Duckworth, N., and Hunter, N.: Atlas of plaster cast techniques, ed. 2, Chicago, 1974, Yearbook Medical Publishers, Inc.
Hilt, N. E., and Schmitt, E. W., Jr.: Pediatric orthopedic nursing, St. Louis, 1975, The C. V. Mosby Co.
Larson, C., and Gould, M.: Orthopedic nursing, St. Louis, 1972, The C. V. Mosby Co.
Salib, P. I.: Plaster casting, New York, 1975, Appleton-Century-Crofts.

# 24

# Traction and suspension therapy

**NANCY E. HILT**

**SHIRLEY B. COGBURN**

Knowledge of the principles of traction and suspension therapy is fundamental to the care of all orthopedic patients. Traction therapy is one of the important adjuncts used by the orthopedic surgeon in coordinating a total care plan. It is a conservative alternative to surgical intervention. In addition, its use in conjunction with surgery preoperatively and/or postoperatively, will assure maximal benefits, positioning, alignment, and correction.

The orthopedic surgeon, as the prescriber of the patient's care, is responsible for adequate and accurate initiation of the traction therapy that will best meet the patient's needs. The responsibility for maintaining this prescription, however, is that of every health care worker who becomes even remotely involved with the patient. Nursing personnel, as the 24-hour providers and coordinators of care, assume the greatest responsibility in providing care that will not only effectively and efficiently maximize the benefits of the traction, but will also alleviate complications of traction therapy and prolonged immobilization. All other personnel, however, from the resident physician staff and therapists to the housekeeping staff, should ideally have a baseline knowledge that will permit them to observe, treat, assess, and evaluate appropriately according to their level of contact with the patient. We strongly recommend that all such personnel be provided with adequate continuing education to facilitate and implement this philosophy.

## DEFINITIONS

*Traction* is the mechanism by which a pull is placed on a part or parts of the body. *Countertraction* is a force that counteracts the direct pull of the traction, i.e., the force of the body weight on the bed. Countertraction may also be obtained by altering the angle of the body force in relation to the pull of the traction, for example, elevating the foot of the bed with "shock" blocks (Trendelenburg position). The degree of countertraction depends on the amount of force necessary to counteract the pull of the traction and, therefore, is usually accomplished in graduated degrees.

*Suspension* uses traction equipment to "suspend" a part or parts of the body but does not involve a pull. For example, suspension of an extremity may be used for postoperative control of edema.

## GENERAL TYPES

There are two basic types of traction: *skin* and *skeletal*. Skin traction is applied by exerting the pull on the body directly on the skin surface. Skeletal traction is applied by exerting the pull on the body with the use of a pin or wire directly into or through the bone.

Skin traction may be further subdivided into two types: *nonadhesive* and *adhesive*. Both types are applied with traction straps, spreading the pull over an area of the skin to decrease the patient's vulnerability to skin breakdown. In nonadhesive traction the traction strap does not adhere to the skin and usually has a soft foam backing. In adhesive skin traction a similar traction strap is used but it is made of adhesive or adherent material. Adhesive traction is used only when continuous traction is desired, whereas nonadhesive traction permits the frequent removal for facilitation of care.

Understanding these basic types of traction is the foundation for making judgments concerning daily care. If this information is known about *any* patient in *any* type of traction, reliable judgments about application and release of the traction can be made. The diagram below compares the types of traction:

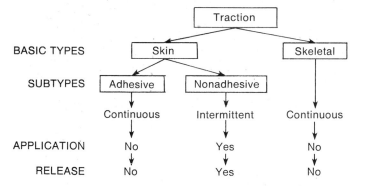

In the above diagram recommendations concerning application and release of traction are directed to all *nonphysician* personnel. For patients for whom continuous traction is prescribed the physician or resident staff should assume the responsibility, accountability, and liability for handling the affected part of the body when not in traction. Therefore, application and release of continuous tractions (adhesive skin and skeletal) should be accomplished by the physician or resident.

Some patients may have combined traction, for example, skeletal traction combined with nonadhesive skin traction. In this case skeletal traction is applied and released by the physician staff, whereas

the nonadhesive skin traction, with an appropriate order, can be applied and released by the nursing personnel.

## GENERAL USE

Traction therapy may be prescribed by the physician for a number of purposes. Its most frequent objectives include:

1. Correction of deformities
2. Gradual correction or improvement of joint contractures
3. Treatment of dislocations
4. Reduction of fractures
5. Treatment of disease processes of the musculoskeletal system
6. Preoperative and postoperative positioning and alignment
7. General immobilization of specific areas of the body

Although current use of specific types of traction for some of the above objectives is somewhat standardized, physician preference for any of the above may vary.

## GENERAL PRINCIPLES

The following are basic principles that will promote efficient, effective utilization of traction therapy and facilitate nursing care:

1. *All traction weights should be hanging free.* Ropes should not be touching any part of the bed, and the weights should not rest on any part of the bed or on the floor. Any violation of this principle decreases the amount and effectiveness of the traction.

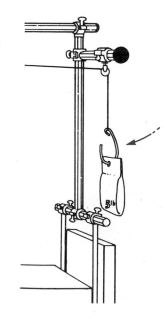

2. *Weights hanging on each part of the traction should be the specific amount ordered by the physician.* To facilitate frequent monitoring and alterations of the weights, which may be necessary on a daily basis, a traction weight record should be at the patient's bedside.

| | | TRACTION WEIGHT CHART | | | | | |
|---|---|---|---|---|---|---|---|
| **Type of traction:** | | | | | | | |
| Date | Right extremity | Left extremity | Other | Date | Right extremity | Left extremity | Other |
| | | | | | | | |
| | | | | | | | |
| | | | | | | | |
| | | | | | | | |
| | | | | | | | |
| | | | | | | | |
| | | | | | | | |
| | | | | | | | |
| | | | | | | | |
| | | | | | | | |
| | | | | | | | |
| | | | | | | | |
| | | | | | | | |
| | | | | | | | |
| | | | | | | | |
| | | | | | | | |
| | | | | | | | |
| | | | | | | | |
| | | | | | | | |
| | | | | | | | |
| | | | | | | | |
| | | | | | | | |
| | | | | | | | |
| | | | | | | | |
| | | | | | | | |

3. *All ropes should be on the center track of pulley.* Deviations will alter and decrease amount of traction.

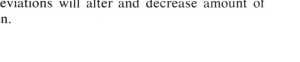

4. *All ropes should be maintained in good condition and should not be frayed.* Frayed ropes should be replaced to avoid eventual severing.

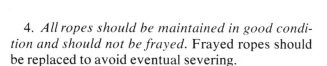

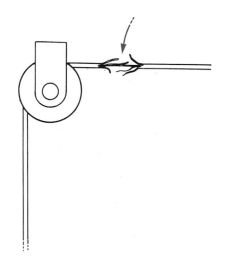

5. *Metal clips should not be used on elastic bandages*. They are a safety hazard for both patients (especially children) in traction and personnel. Paper tape may be used to secure the end of the bandage.

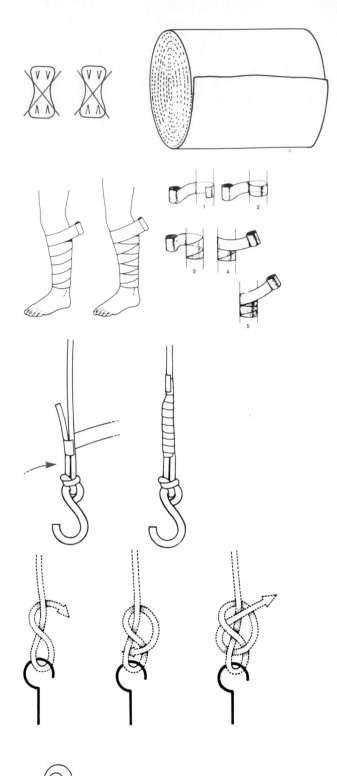

6. *Either a circular wrap or figure-of-eight wrap may be used with skin traction*. Ideally, the figure-of-eight wrap (details shown in 1 to 5) should be used because it tends to remain secure for a longer period of time; this wrap is especially recommended for children in traction. However, the number of elastic bandages required with an adult patient may be prohibitive. The wrap should always be from distal to proximal part of extremity.

7. *Tape all rope ends to the long portion above the knot*. This alleviates undesired tampering with the ropes.

8. *A slip knot should be used for all traction knots*. This knot is the best one for securing the weights.

9. *A swivel snap is used to attach the rope to any piece of equipment that will be attached directly to the patient*. This will facilitate application and removal of the traction.

10. *The line of pull is always from attachment to the patient to the first pulley.* The routing of the ropes and weights after this first pulley is merely to place them in a position that will not interfere with care or desired positioning. This line of pull determines the positioning and alignment prescribed by the physician, and is the most accurate way by which the positioning and alignment can be monitored.

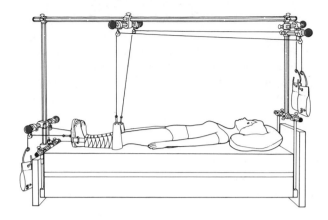

## EQUIPMENT AND TERMINOLOGY

Traction equipment and terminology can be very confusing and anxiety-provoking to health care personnel who do not fully comprehend the components and how each attaches to the other. Many different pieces of equipment are associated with traction and learning about them can seem overwhelming if they are not viewed individually.

The following are basic types of traction frames. Each consists of uprights and an overhead bar. The differences between them relate to how they are attached to the bed (the type of bed will most often dictate the type of frame used). Most equipment is made of steel or aluminum. Aluminum frames are more popular because they are lightweight, but in some cases they are not as strong as the steel frames. Steel inserts are sometimes put in the aluminum toprail to increase the strength.

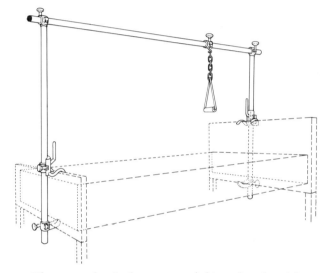

*Claw-type basic frame*—uprights at head and foot end of bed are secured by means of the claw-like attachments.

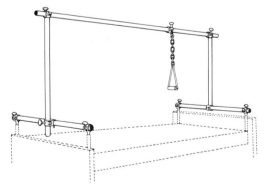

*IV-type basic frame*—uprights attach to two plain bars secured by attachments that fit into IV holders at each corner of bed.

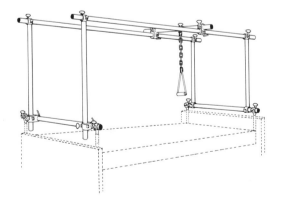

*Balkan frame*—four uprights, one at each corner and two overhead bars. Additional attachments secured to two overheads, rather than from center bar. (This frame offers more security than other two types. It may be constructed with either claw or IV attachments.)

In order to familiarize the reader with the attachments to the basic frame and how they are secured, the procedure for setting up bilateral split Russell traction is shown below. The name of the traction is not as important as the individual components comprising the entire traction set-up. All types of traction, with few exceptions, will begin with the basic overhead traction frame. For the purpose of this illustration the IV type frame has been chosen. Each component added to the frame is illustrated in detail and then shown as it is added to the other components.

Additional equipment may be used for other types of traction. The types of slings may differ according to commercial availability and preferences, and spreader bars may be used instead of footplates, but the basic principles and equipment remain unchanged. Reference may be made to the illustrations in the section that begins on p. 525 for further clarification of equipment required for specific types of traction.

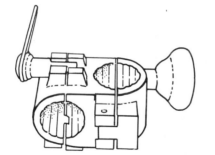

*Crossclamp*—attaches two traction bars together

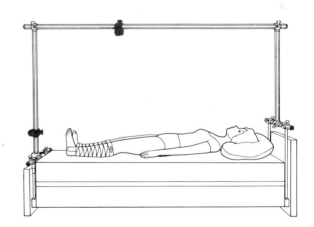

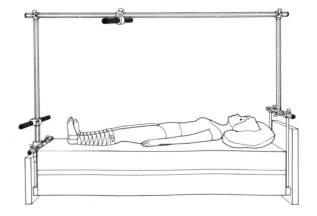

*Plain bar*—available in various sizes

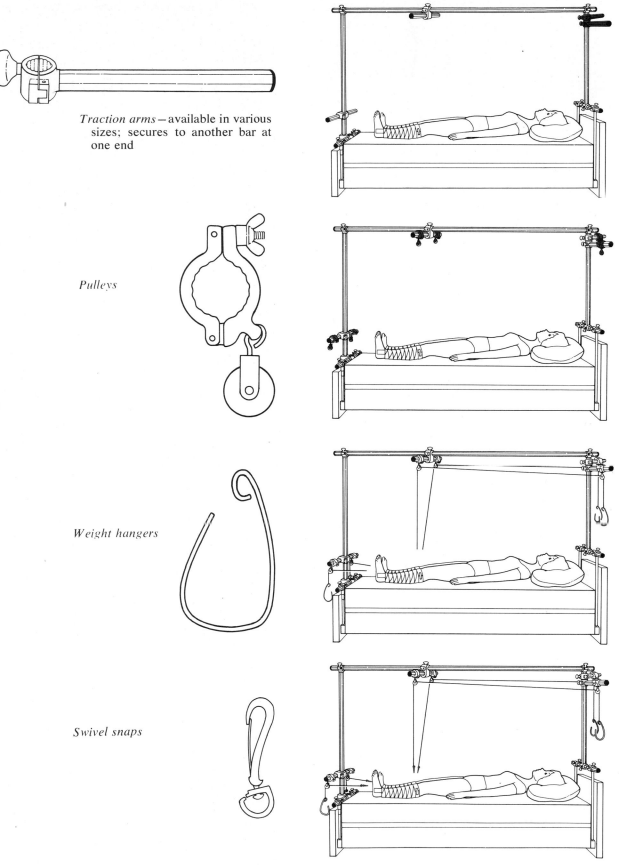

*Traction arms* — available in various sizes; secures to another bar at one end

*Pulleys*

*Weight hangers*

*Swivel snaps*

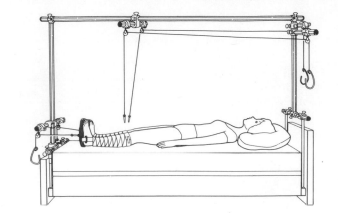

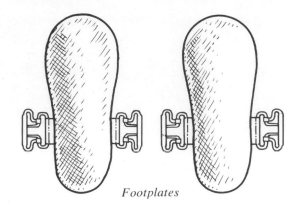

*Footplates*

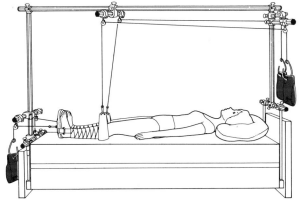

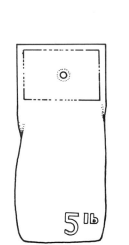

*Slings*

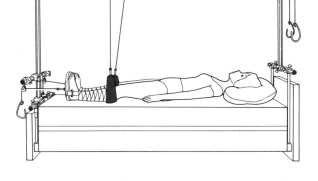

*Weights*

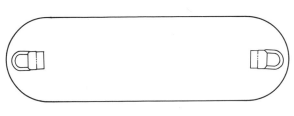

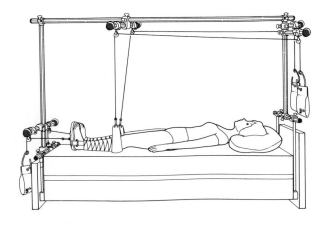

*Bumper balls*

**Type:** Split Russell traction (adhesiv
skin)*
**Use:** Congenital hip dislocation, hip
tures, postoperative immobilizatic
correction of deformities, disease p
**Notation:** May be unilateral or bilate

## SPECIFIC TYPES AND USES

The following types of traction and suspension are the most common in current use. Although the most frequent utilizations are outlined for each, there may be variations and alterations to accommodate individual preferences and needs.

### Suspensions

**Type:** Upper extremity
**Use:** Postoperative, posttraumatic, or postreduction control of edema
**Notation:** May be unilateral or bilateral (most frequently unilateral)

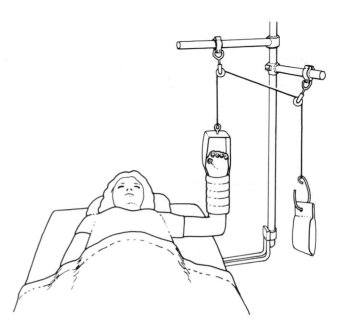

**Type:** 90-90 traction, pediatric (skel
cast or splint to facilitate positional
**Use:** Displaced fractured femur in ch
**Notation:** Usually unilateral; opposi
Buck's or split Russell for immobili:

**Type:** Lower extremity*
**Use:** Postoperative, posttraumatic, or postreduction control of edema
**Notation:** May be unilateral or bilateral

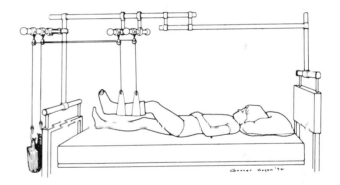

**Type:** Balanced suspension with Th
and Pearson attachment (with s
traction)
**Use:** Fractured femur, pre- or postope
tion and positioning, disease proce:
**Notation:** May be unilateral or bilater
form, this is a suspension; as sho
traction and skin traction have be
mercial splints by other names a
serve the same purpose

**Type:** Hyperextension suspension*
**Use:** Postoperative positioning of hip muscle release procedures
**Notation:** Always bilateral; long leg casts applied with rings incorporated to facilitate suspension

*Illustration from Hilt, N. E., and Schmitt, E. W., Jr.: Pediatric orthopedic nursing, St. Louis, 1975, The C. V. Mosby Co.

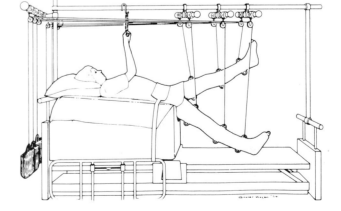

### Tractions

#### Upper extremity

**Type:** Dunlop skin tr…
**Use:** Contractures of …
zation, supracondyl…
**Notation:** May be uni…
unilateral)

**Type:** Dunlop skeleta…
or nonadhesive skin…
**Use:** Contractures of …
zation, supracondyl…
**Notation:** May be uni…
unilateral)

#### Lower extremity

**Type:** Buck's extensio…
**Use:** Hip and knee co…
operative positionin…
processes of the hip…
**Notation:** May be unil…

**Type:** Russell traction…
**Use:** Fractured femur…
correction of hip a…
tive positioning an…
cesses of the hip an…
**Notation:** May be unil…

*Illustration from Hilt,…
Pediatric orthopedic nu…
Mosby Co.

---

**Type:** Bryant traction (adhesive or nonadhesive skin)
**Use:** Fractured femur, congenital dislocation of the hip
**Notation:** Used with infants only, under 35 pounds of weight, always bilateral

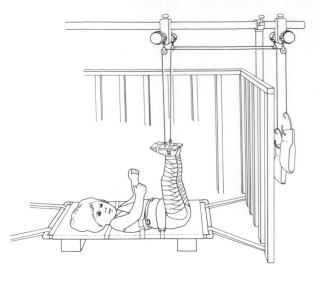

### Spinal

**Type:** Pelvic sling traction (intermittent, with pelvic girdle)
**Use:** Low back pain

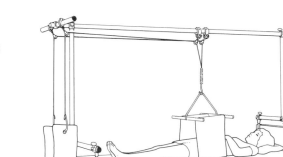

**Type:** 90-90 traction, adult (intermittent)
**Use:** Low back pain
**Notation:** Utilizes platform and may be used with or without thigh traction shown; this traction may technically be called a suspension, especially if the thigh traction is not used.

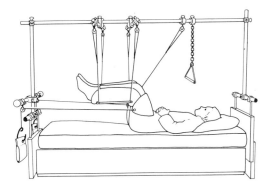

**Type:** Cotrel traction (intermittent)
**Use:** Preoperative management of scoliosis
**Notation:** Utilizes special leather head halter and pelvic girdle; exerciser attaches for special program as shown

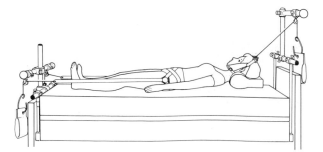

*Illustration from Hilt, N. E., and Schmitt, E. W., Jr.: Pediatric orthopedic nursing, St. Louis, 1975, The C. V. Mosby Co.

**Type:** Halo-femoral traction (skeletal)*
**Use:** Severe scoliosis
**Notation:** Traction shown here on a CircOlectric bed; regular bed or Foster frame may also be used

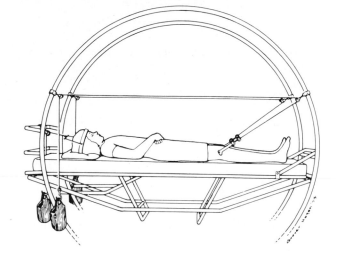

**Type:** Halo-pelvic traction (skeletal)
**Use:** Severe scoliosis
**Notation:** Traction in this case is accomplished by the tension of the outrigger (or metal apparatus shown)

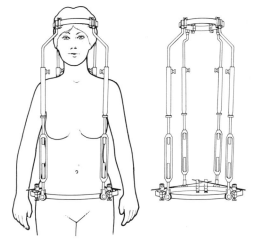

*Cervical*

**Type:** Head halter traction (nonadhesive skin)*
**Use:** Torticollis, cervical injuries, cervical disease processes
**Notation:** Head of bed usually elevated to a degree specified by physician

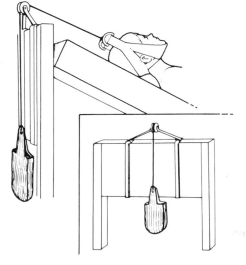

**Type:** Cervical tongs (skeletal)*
**Use:** Postoperative cervical fusions, cervical dislocations, and other injuries
**Notation:** Crutchfield tongs are shown; other types are
available.

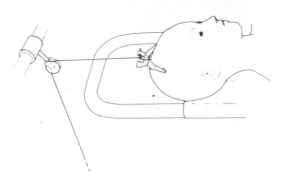

*Illustration from Hilt, N. E., and Schmitt, E. W., Jr.:
Pediatric orthopedic nursing, St. Louis, 1975, The C. V.
Mosby Co.

## PRINCIPLES OF APPLICATION

We believe that continuous traction (adhesive skin and skeletal) should be applied by the orthopedic surgeon or resident physician. The responsibility, accountability, and liability for the application should remain that of the physician. Few other health care personnel have been properly educated in other than emergency application of such types of traction, especially the handling of the extremity or area involved in a severe injury or fracture. This is not to say that some of the allied health personnel, including nursing staff with considerable experience within the specialty, do not possess the ability and skill to do so; but to assume that *all* personnel have this ability would certainly be in error. Consistency and continuity of approach, then, is

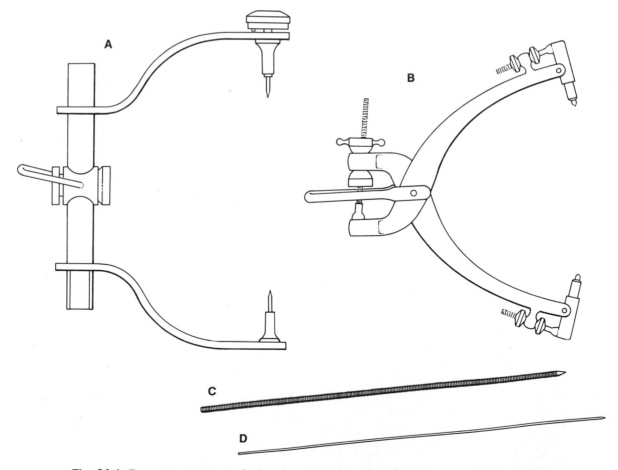

Fig. 24-1. Examples of pins and wires for skeletal traction. **A,** Vinke tongs. **B,** Crutchfield tongs. **C,** Threaded Steinman pin. **D,** Unthreaded Kirschner wire.

best assured if the physician assumes such responsibility. The acceptance of this concept also assumes that the selection process for the type of traction (adhesive or nonadhesive) has been a valid one; for example, adhesive is selected *only* for those patients who require continuous traction.

Skeletal traction is usually applied in the operating room; however, it may, of necessity, be applied in the patient's room, treatment room, or plaster room using aseptic technique. If this is done considerable attention is given to the skin preparation because of the risk of infection. The most common types of pins and wires used for skeletal traction are shown in Fig. 24-1.

Adhesive skin traction is often accompanied by complications of allergic skin reactions, blistering, and breakdown. If this occurs, traction therapy may

need to be altered. The following steps are recommended for application of adhesive traction to avoid these common skin reactions (Fig. 24-2):

1. Be sure extremity is clean.
2. Apply folded stockinette over the maleoli.
3. Spray the extremity with tincture of benzoin.
4. Roll one layer of stockinette (not wrinkled) over the extremity.
5. Apply the adhesive traction straps over the stockinette, appropriately placed for footplate or spreader bar.
6. Wrap securely with elastic bandage.
7. Attach traction straps to spreader bar or footplate.

Nonadhesive skin traction (intermittent) does not cause the skin reactions associated with adhesive skin traction and is, therefore, desirable whenever

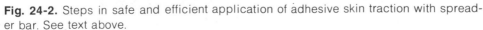

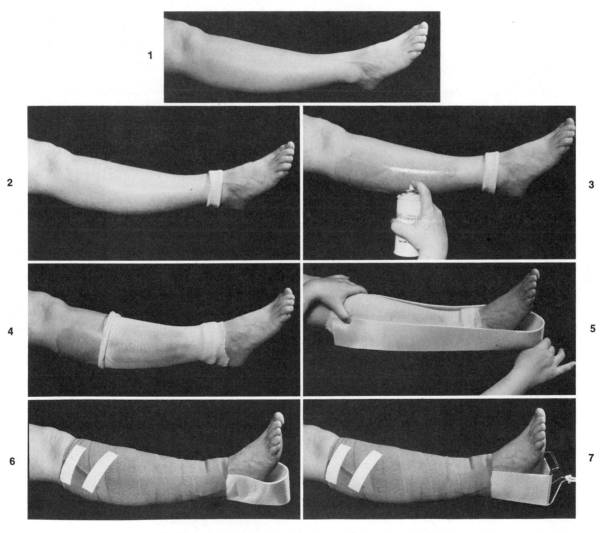

**Fig. 24-2.** Steps in safe and efficient application of adhesive skin traction with spreader bar. See text above.

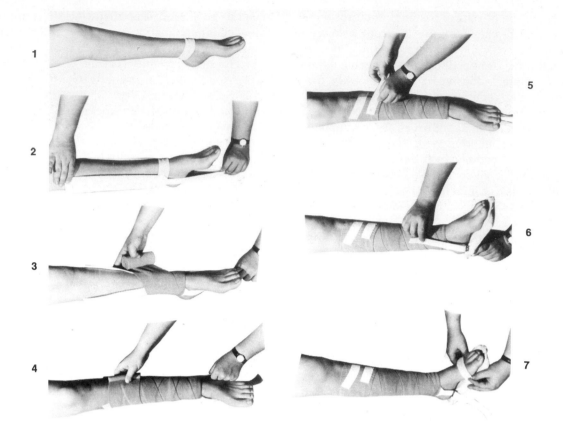

**Fig. 24-3.** Steps in safe and efficient application of nonadhesive skin traction with footplate. See text below. (From Hilt, N. E., and Schmitt, E. W., Jr.: Pediatric orthopedic nursing, St. Louis, 1975, The C. V. Mosby Co.)

the treatment will not be jeopardized by frequent removal of the traction for care. The following steps are recommended for application and reapplication of nonadhesive skin traction (Fig. 24-3):

1. Be sure extremity is clean. Apply folded stockinette over the maleoli.
2. Place the nonadhesive straps with the tapered part over the maleoli.
3. Secure the elastic bandage around the ankle.
4. Wrap the remainder of the elastic bandage, with final wrap below the knee.
5. Secure the elastic bandage with tape.
6. Attach the traction straps to the footplate or spreader bar.
7. If footplate is used, place folded stockinette over the toes and end of footplate.

All of the previously outlined basic principles of traction apply to the applications we are outlining here. The initial application of the traction straps, as shown in Figs. 24-2 and 24-3 differ depending on the use of the spreader bar or footplate. We strongly recommend using the footplate because it promotes neutral foot alignment. If the footplate is used, however, webbing strap must be sewn to the traction straps for security.

## NURSING CARE

The following standards for nursing care have been established as guidelines for personnel planning the care of the patient in traction. The majority of care is based on the premise that most complications of traction therapy are known and can be prevented; those that cannot be prevented can be detected at an early enough stage to avoid permanent tissue damage. A compilation of the care recommended and outlined may be reviewed in the standardized care plans at the end of the chapter and in Table 24-6.

### Skin care

We recommend the use of *alcohol* for skin care. Alcohol tends to toughen the skin and leaves it less vulnerable to skin breakdown. Lotions or oils soften the skin, making it more vulnerable to breakdown. Powders should not be used under the traction because they tend to cake and, in combination with skin perspiration, will be the source of increased skin irritation.

Regardless of the type of traction therapy, intermittent or continuous, skin care should be provided at least every 4 hours. This schedule should be maintained on *all* shifts. Patients who have a diagnosis of myelomeningocele, paraplegia, quadriplegia, or a known history of previous skin breakdown or sensitivity should have skin care more frequently as a preventive measure (every 2 hours during the day and every 3 hours at night). In addition, whenever a skin problem is detected the patient should be placed on a skin care schedule of every 2 or 3 hours, as necessary.

Guidelines for the actual skin care procedure will depend on the type of traction. Similarities and differences are outlined below.

**Nonadhesive skin traction.** Skin care for a patient in nonadhesive skin traction is provided *under* the traction. Since this type of traction is intermittent, it can be removed and alcohol applied under the traction straps. Reddened areas may be noted under the straps when it is removed. These areas and ridging should disappear by the time alcohol is applied and the nurse is ready to reapply the traction. The steps for reapplication of the traction are the same as for application and may be reviewed in Fig. 24-3. Again, increased redness is an indication for increasing the frequency of skin care.

**Adhesive skin traction.** Because adhesive traction is continuous, skin care should be given around the edges of the traction. Any indication that the traction is slipping should be reported to the physician and arrangements made for reapplication before spontaneous release. Reapplication of the traction should follow the guidelines outlined in Fig. 24-2.

Increased observation is required from the nursing staff for patients in adhesive traction. Because the traction is not removed routinely, the nursing staff must be able to detect skin problems at an early stage. The following signs and symptoms are likely to be exhibited if skin breakdown is occurring or has occurred, or if an allergic reaction is present:

| Signs and symptoms | Type of patient |
|---|---|
| Irritability, fussiness, crying, restlessness | Infants, young children, patients unable to communicate verbally |
| Complaints of pain or itching, scratching at edges or under the traction | All patients capable of verbal communication |

| Signs and symptoms | Type of patient |
|---|---|
| Elevated temperature; drainage through bandages; odor indicative of drainage | Signs of advanced, probably massive and infected skin breakdown in *all* patients; patients with decreased or no sensation |

Ideally, any skin breakdown should be detected early. Advanced and massive skin problems may necessitate discontinuing traction therapy.

**Skeletal traction.** Skin care for the patient in skeletal traction is focused on *pin care*. Although there is controversy regarding the care of the pin site, we offer the following guidelines. It should be understood that such care may vary according to each physician's preferences.

1. *Return from operating room:* Cleanse area around pin site with alcohol sponge; blood and prep solution may be removed. *Do not touch immediate pin site.*
2. *Ongoing care:* Do not remove crust at pin site; observe for signs of infection, such as erythema, drainage, odor, elevated temperature, and pain. Report any signs of infection to physician and document in chart.
3. If plaster is used to incorporate pin, give skin care around edges of plaster and observe for potential skin breakdown.
4. If the end of the pin is exposed, place cork over end to avoid accident and injury to patient and personnel.
5. Observe for signs of pin migration or slippage. If any noted, report to physician and document in chart.

These guidelines may be altered as necessary to meet the specific needs of the patient.

All patients in traction need increased skin care of the back, buttocks, and over the sacrum and coccyx because of their limited mobility. Alcohol is used for skin care to these areas also, which may be given at the same time as traction skin care.

## Neurovascular assessment

The frequency of neurovascular assessments is determined by the type of traction being used. The following guidelines are recommended for each type of traction:

1. **Continuous traction (adhesive skin or skeletal traction):** Every hour for the first 24 hours; if status has returned to "normal" for *that* patient, every 4 hours for the duration of the traction therapy; continue hourly assessments if status has not returned to "normal."

| NEUROVASCULAR ASSESSMENT SHEET | | | | | Patient identification | | | | | |
|---|---|---|---|---|---|---|---|---|---|---|
| **Extremity to be assessed:** | | | | | **Frequency of assessment:** | | | | | |
| Date | Time | Color | Temperature | Capillary filling | Edema | Pulse | Numbness/ tingling | Sensation | Motion | Personnel assessing |
| | | | | | | | | | | |
| | | | | | | | | | | |
| | | | | | | | | | | |
| | | | | | | | | | | |
| | | | | | | | | | | |
| | | | | | | | | | | |
| | | | | | | | | | | |
| | | | | | | | | | | |
| | | | | | | | | | | |
| | | | | | | | | | | |
| | | | | | | | | | | |
| | | | | | | | | | | |
| | | | | | | | | | | |
| | | | | | | | | | | |
| | | | | | | | | | | |
| | | | | | | | | | | |
| | | | | | | | | | | |
| | | | | | | | | | | |
| | | | | | | | | | | |
| | | | | | | | | | | |
| | | | | | | | | | | |
| | | | | | | | | | | |
| | | | | | | | | | | |
| | | | | | | | | | | |
| | | | | | | | | | | |
| | | | | | | | | | | |

*Color:* pink, pale, cyanotic

*Temperature:* warm, cool, cold

*Capillary filling:* rapid, slow, sluggish

*Edema:* present (specify degree), absent

*Numbness/tingling:* present, absent

*Sensation:* present (with or without stimuli—specify), decreased, absent

*Motion:* present, decreased, absent

REPORT ANY SIGNIFICANT CHANGE TO PHYSICIAN

Page 1

**Fig. 24-4.** Neurovascular assessment sheet. (Adapted from Hilt, N. E., and Schmitt, E. W., Jr.: Pediatric orthopedic nursing, St. Louis, 1975, The C. V. Mosby Co.)

| | Color | Temperature | Capillary filling | Edema | Pulse | Numbness/ tingling | Sensation | Motion | Comments | Personnel assessing |
|---|---|---|---|---|---|---|---|---|---|---|
| **ADMISSION NEUROVASCULAR ASSESSMENT** | | | | | | | Patient identification | | | |
| Left upper extremity | | | | | | | | | | |
| Right upper extremity | | | | | | | | | | |
| Left lower extremity | | | | | | | | | | |
| Right lower extremity | | | | | | | | | | |

*Color:* pink, pale, cyanotic

*Temperature:* warm, cool, cold

*Capillary filling:* rapid, slow, sluggish

*Edema:* present (specify degree), absent

*Numbness/tingling:* present, absent

*Sensation:* present (with or without stimuli—specify), decreased, absent

*Motion:* present, decreased, absent

*Comments:* cast, questionable status

Date of assessment

Time of assessment

Physician

Page 2

**Fig. 24-4, cont'd.** Neurovascular assessment sheet.

**Table 24-1.** Component of neurovascular assessment and descriptive terminology of results

| Major areas of assessment | Subareas of assessment | Description of result | Additional specification of result |
|---|---|---|---|
| Circulation | Color | Pink<br>Pale<br>Cyanotic | — |
| | Temperature | Warm<br>Cool<br>Cold | — |
| | Capillary filling | Rapid<br>Slow<br>Sluggish | — |
| | Edema | Present | Small amount<br>Moderate amount<br>Large amount |
| | | Absent | None |
| | Pulse | Present | Strong<br>Weak<br>Thready<br>Rate |
| | | Absent | Specify if not obtainable because area not exposed |
| Sensation | Sensation | Present | Deep or surface with stimuli (what stimuli)<br>Without stimuli |
| | | Decreased | How and where |
| | | Absent | Change from previous? |
| | Numbness/ tingling | Present | — |
| | | Absent | — |
| Motion | Motion | Present<br>Decreased<br>Absent | — |

2. **Intermittent traction (Nonadhesive skin traction):** Every 4 hours for the duration of the traction therapy; *Always 30 to 45 minutes after reapplication of traction* (if traction is being rewrapped every 2 hours, the neurovascular assessment must be accomplished every 2 hours).

The neurovascular assessment must be accomplished in its totality and documented accurately to alleviate the common legal problems associated with this aspect of care. The legal implications of neurovascular assessment are great because the resulting damage from impairment is permanent. In addition, all personnel responsible for this aspect of care should be aware that impairment of the neurovascular status can be detected early and, in most cases, permanent tissue damage can be prevented.

The components of a thorough neurovascular assessment are reviewed in Table 24-1. A neurovascular assessment flow sheet (Fig. 24-4) can be used to document the assessment.

Because neurovascular assessment is accompanied by such a vast degree of liability and legal implications, the following guidelines and cautions have been established to assist nursing personnel in avoiding errors commonly associated with this aspect of care:

1. Avoid using terminology that might be interpreted as ambiguous in the documentation of neurovascular assessment results. Examples: good, fair, poor.

2. Interpret the change in a patient's neurovascular status as the cue to increase observation; increase frequency to every 1 or 2 hours or more frequently if necessary.

3. Do not use a flashlight to accomplish the assessment during the night shift. Accuracy can be assured only if the overhead light is on. Family members staying in the patient's room should receive an adequately detailed explanation of the procedure and benefit for the patient. This, of course, should be accomplished before, not during, the night shift!

4. The patient's status prior to traction must be known so that adequate judgments can be made throughout traction therapy. If the patient's injury does not permit accurate assessment at the time of therapy, obtain as accurate information as possible from family members. Do not base the patient's neurovascular status on the diagnosis (for example, some myelomeningocele patients have sensation, as do some paraplegics).

5. Do not use the opposite extremity as an indicator of status for the extremity in traction. Many patients have "normal" differences in temperature, color, etc., between extremities. Remember that there is no "normal" for all patients; there is only a "normal" for each individual patient.

6. Always assess all five fingers and toes for sensation. Accomplish the assessment on the medial and lateral aspects of *each* finger or toe to avoid false status impressions due to nerve routing.

7. Children are not reliable in determining a sensation level. A 3-year-old will learn very rapidly that he will get stuck with a pin if he says no to some of your questions. All children under the adolescent age group should be tested with touch, pinch, or pinprick.

8. Document all components of the assessment.
9. Report all changes in neurovascular status to the physician and document the communication on the patient's chart.
10. Be aware of the permanent damage that can be avoided with accurate and complete neurovascular assessments! Also, be aware of the legal implications of adequate neurovascular assessments and their documentation!

## POSITIONING, ALIGNMENT, AND IMMOBILIZATION

The concept of maintaining proper positioning, desired alignment, and immobilization of the patient in traction is a relatively simple one. The essence of this concept lies in the purpose of traction; traction is prescribed specifically to assist in the positioning and alignment of a deformity, fracture, etc. If the maintenance of this desired positioning and alignment is not assured throughout traction therapy, the traction will not fulfill its purpose and function. Immobilization, to a degree, is the counterpart of positioning and alignment, in the sense that without immobilization, maintenance of the other two components is difficult, if not impossible.

The maintenance of these three components with the coherent and cooperative patient is preceded by proper explanation of the desired positioning and alignment. If the patient understands these components, immobilization may be obtained through voluntary cooperation. Difficulty, however, may be anticipated with the uncooperative or incoherent patient. Various types of restraints to control trunk motion and opposite extremity movement may be used to assist in this effort.

Special problems with maintenance of positioning, alignment, and immobilization also occur with infants and young children in traction. Even if they are able to understand the need for traction, immo-

bilization is difficult. To counteract the problems of traction therapy in children, we recommend using a *solid Bradford frame and restraints* specifically designed for children.

**Solid Bradford frame.** The recommended Bradford frame for use with a child in traction is the *solid* type, in which the canvas cover extends from the top to the bottom of the frame (Fig. 24-5, *A*). This type provides support for the entire body. Specific criteria may be used for selection of the Bradford frame, since not all children will require the frame. Children with whom we can anticipate difficulty in maintenance of positioning, alignment, and immobilization are:

1. All children under 5 years of age
2. Hyperactive children
3. Mentally retarded children

It is important to note that traction therapy for children over 5 years of age and for hyperactive or mentally retarded children should be attempted without the Bradford frame; it should be used only if maintenance is not obtained through other methods.[3, p.60]

The purpose of the Bradford frame is to assist in maintaining proper immobilization, positioning, and alignment by controlling the movement of the child: *it is much easier to control the child on a small area (the Bradford frame) than on a large area (the mattress).*[3, p.60]

The Bradford frame should never be placed directly on the bed; rather, it can be elevated to facilitate nursing care. In this case *both* ends of the frame are elevated. The height of elevation is not significant, provided the frame is stable, care may be easily accomplished, and both ends are elevated at an equal level. Plywood blocks may be used for elevation and a bedboard will assure stability. If countertraction is desired to assist further in maintenance of positioning, the block under the head end may be

**Table 24-2.** Use of solid Bradford frame with specific types of tractions in children

| Always used | Sometimes used | Never used |
|---|---|---|
| Bryant traction | Dunlop traction | Balanced suspension |
| | Buck's extension | Cervical traction |
| | Split Russell traction | Cervical tongs |
| | Russell traction | Cotrel traction |
| | 90-90 traction | Halo-femoral traction |
| | | Halo-pelvic traction |
| | | Hyperextension suspension |

Adapted from Hilt, N. E., and Schmitt, E. W., Jr.: Pediatric orthopedic nursing, St. Louis, 1975, The C. V. Mosby Co.

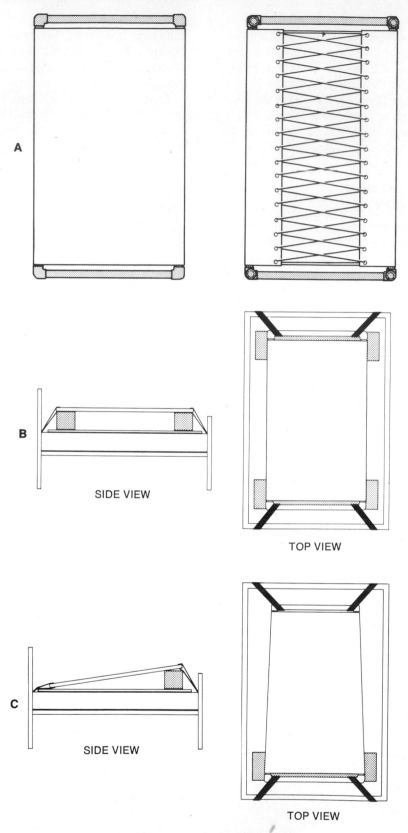

**A**

**B**

SIDE VIEW

TOP VIEW

**C**

SIDE VIEW

TOP VIEW

**Fig. 24-5. A,** Solid Bradford frame. **B,** Solid Bradford frame for use with traction. **C,** Solid Bradford frame for use with traction when counteraction is desired. (**B** and **C** from Hilt, N. E., and Schmitt, E. W., Jr.: Pediatric orthopedic nursing, St. Louis, 1975, The C. V. Mosby Co.)

**Table 24-3.** Use of restraints with children in traction

| Type of traction | Sling | Frame | Jacket | Diaper |
|---|---|---|---|---|
| Dunlop (arm), skin or skeletal | Yes (pelvic and thoracic) | No | No | No |
| Buck's extension | Yes (pelvic) | If on frame | If not on frame | No |
| Bryant | Yes (pelvic) | Yes | No | No |
| Split Russell | Yes (pelvic) | If on frame | If not on frame | If additional countertraction necessary |
| Russell | Yes (pelvic) | If on frame | If not on frame | If additional countertraction necessary |
| 90-90 | Yes (pelvic) | If on frame | If not on frame | No |
| Balanced suspension | Rarely necessary | No | Yes | No |
| Hyperextension suspension | Yes (pelvic) | No | Occasionally | No |
| Cervical, skin or skeletal | Yes (pelvic) | No | No | No |
| Cotrel | No | No | No | No |
| Halo-femoral or halo-pelvic | No | No | No | No |
| Suspension for elevation | No | No | Yes | No |
| If in doubt | Use | Use | Use | Try without |

Adapted from Hilt, N. E., and Schmitt, E. W., Jr.: Pediatric orthopedic nursing, St. Louis, 1975, The C. V. Mosby Co.

removed.[3,pp.65-66] Contraindications, however, exist for the lowering of the head end. They are (1) the patient with myelomeningocele or a shunt, (2) infants with a known regurgitation problem, and (3) children with multiple injuries, (e.g., head injury). The set-ups for both of these elevations may be reviewed in Fig. 24-5, *B* and *C*. Additional information on the Bradford frame, such as facilitation of bedmaking, etc., may be reviewed in Chapter 30. In addition, use of the solid Bradford frame for children in traction is reviewed in Table 24-2.

**Restraints.** Restraints can be useful in the management of children in traction. However, these restraints should be carefully selected and designed so that they fulfill the specific function and purpose of aiding the traction therapy and its overall objectives. The recommended restraints are shown below and in Table 24-3.

**Restraint:** Sling*
**Use:** Over pelvis to reduce pelvic motion with lower extremity traction; over thoracic and abdominal areas as countertraction with Dunlop traction
**Attachment:** Lower extremity tractions—to both sides of bedspring frame with webbing straps; Dunlop traction—to opposite side of bedspring frame; use with patient on Bradford frame (attach under frame)
**Construction:** Felt covered with stockinette; rings at ends

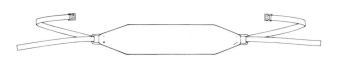

*Illustration from Hilt, N. E., and Schmitt, E. W., Jr.: Pediatric orthopedic nursing, St. Louis, 1975, The C. V. Mosby Co.

**Restraint:** Jacket*
**Use:** With any lower extremity traction to promote trunk immobilization and discourage sitting
**Attachment:** To both sides of the bedspring frame with buckled webbing straps sewn into side seams of restraint
**Construction:** Permanent press, colorful material

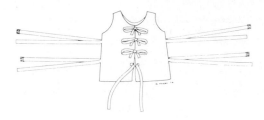

**Restraint:** Frame*
**Use:** With any lower extremity traction when child is on Bradford frame; specifically designed to attach under frame; serves same functions of trunk control and prevention of sitting as jacket restraint
**Attachment:** Webbing strap incorporated into seam and threaded through shoulder tabs; both attach under frame
**Construction:** Permanent press, colorful material

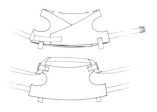

**Restraint:** Diaper*
**Use:** For countertraction with lower extremity tractions when other methods of countertraction are not effective
**Attachment:** Designed to fit over pelvic area like a diaper; rings incorporated into each of four corners, webbing strap threaded through rings and attached to top side of bedspring frame
**Construction:** Felt covered with vinyl plastic and stockinette; rings in corners
**Care alteration:** All children requiring this restraint who are incontinent should be placed on diaper checks every half hour to assist in the prevention of urinary tract infections

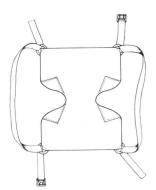

---

*Illustration from Hilt, N. E., and Schmitt, E. W., Jr.: Pediatric orthopedic nursing, St. Louis, 1975, The C. V. Mosby Co.

---

Restraints of any type, and especially for the purposes outlined here, should be used properly to maximize effectiveness and to decrease the emotional trauma usually associated with their use. The following guidelines are recommended[3, p. 136]:

1. *Use restraints at the onset of the traction therapy.* The restraints are a part of the actual therapy, but if they are not used at the outset they may not be viewed as such by the parents and child.
2. *Do not use any of the restraints as punishment!* Restraints presented here are not designed for that purpose and such use may constitute abuse.
3. *Maximize effectiveness by using a consistent approach.*
4. *Attempt to make the restraints appealing to the child.* Many of the children receiving traction therapy are not acutely ill; a stimulating environment will facilitate adjustment and recovery.
5. *Provide appropriate explanations for the child and the parents.* Avoid using the term "restraint" because of the negative connotation usually associated with it.
6. *Be sure the restraint fits properly.* Restraints that are too tight may cause skin irritation; those that are too loose will not serve their purpose.
7. *Only restrain what is necessary to accomplish the established goals and objectives.*
8. *Remove the restraints at least every 4 hours to assess skin integrity and give skin care with alcohol.*

**Table 24-4.** Recommended positions for specific types of traction

| Type | Recommended position |
|---|---|
| Lower or upper extremity suspension | Any position, provided elevation is maintained |
| Hyperextension suspension | Supine and prone, alternately; on hyperextension bed |
| Dunlop | Supine; head of bed may be slightly elevated with order from physician |
| Buck's extension | Supine and prone, alternately |
| Russell traction | Supine |
| Split Russell | Supine |
| 90-90 (pediatric) | Supine |
| Balanced suspension | Supine |
| Bryant | Supine; on solid Bradford frame with both ends elevated |
| Pelvic sling | Supine |
| 90-90 (adult) | Supine |
| Cotrel | Supine |
| Halo-femoral | Supine; supine and prone, alternately, if on mechanical turning frame |
| Halo-pelvic | Depends on apparatus; obtain physician order |
| Cervical | Supine; supine and prone, alternately, if on mechanical turning frame |

An effective adjunct to maintenance of lower extremity traction with infants and young children is to place the opposite extremity in minimal traction to assist in immobilization. Since this traction is not therapeutic, it should be nonadhesive skin traction.

The following general guidelines relate to positioning to obtain maximal benefit of traction. Specific recommendations are outlined in Table 24-4.

1. Buck's extension—may be turned prone and supine, alternately
2. Hyperextension suspension—may be turned prone and supine, alternately
3. All other traction when patient maintained on regular bed—supine only
4. Mechanical turning beds, such as the Foster frame, Stryker frame, or Circ0lectric bed, can be used to facilitate prone/supine turning schedule provided the purpose and function of traction can be maintained

All of these guidelines have been designed to facilitate maximal benefit of therapy. Patients in traction should not be tilted because it alters the alignment and desired pull of the traction. With such positioning standards and requirements, however, frequent skin care must be provided to the back, buttocks, and coccyx.

The focus of this portion of care has remained, to a great extent, on the child in traction because of the number of problems with this age group in achieving the desired quality standard of care. Our focus, however, does not by any means decrease the emphasis that should be placed on the maintenance of these same principles with the adult patient in traction. In fact, application of the principles outlined for pediatric use may be appropriate for adults who cannot maintain desired positioning, alignment, and immobilization without some assistance.

## Care of extremities not in traction

The care of the extremities not placed in traction for therapeutic purposes is neither extensive nor particularly time consuming. It is, however, frequently forgotten or considered unimportant because of the degree of care required by the extremities in traction. Motion and movement should be encouraged in the other extremities to avoid the development of stiff joints and muscle atrophy. This may be accomplished through self-help skills, the encouragement of independence, planned activities, and range of motion exercises. Range of motion exercises, active, active assisted, and passive, should be planned and implemented on a schedule appropriate for the patient's level of competence and independence. For example, those patients for whom independent exercise is not possible may be on passive or active assisted range of motion three times daily, while the more active patient may be able to accomplish active range of motion less frequently because his level of activity is increased.

## Maintenance of traction principles

The traction principles previously outlined in the chapter cannot be assumed to be achieved just because they have been assured during the initial traction application. It is essential that each of these principles be maintained throughout the duration of traction therapy; frequent monitoring is required to assure this. The following should be assessed at least once each shift:

1. Weights hanging free from the bed and not resting on the floor (usually requires more frequent monitoring)
2. Accuracy of the amount of weights
3. Ropes on center track of pulleys
4. Condition of ropes
5. Alignment and line of pull (usually requires more frequent monitoring)
6. Security (tightness) of all traction equipment

### Nutritional requirements

Nutritional requirements are not really altered for the patient in traction in comparison to the individual not undergoing traction therapy. Certain types of nutritional problems, however, may be encountered, making it necessary to monitor nutritional intake closer than usual. Appetite of the patient may be decreased because of the decreased activity level; or food intake may increase because of boredom. Individual preferences, influenced by socioeconomic level and religious, ethnic, or cultural practices, may alter or accentuate nutritional problems. Dietary counseling may be needed to maximize the healing process and recovery phase.

### Bladder and kidney program

Immobilization of any type tends to decrease the effectiveness of the kidneys. Whenever kidney function becomes sluggish, there is an increased possibility of the development of renal calculi. The most effective method of alleviating this as a potential problem is forcing fluids. All patients immobilized in traction should have a fluid intake of *twice the normal accepted intake* for the patient's size and age. Increased fluid should not be milk or milk products, since calcium has a tendency to deposit in the kidney quicker than any other substance; milk should be limited to meals only.

Intake and output should be monitored throughout immobilization. At least 8-hour shift totals are necessary to determine not only adequate fluid intake but also kidney output. Recumbent positions may pose difficulties for some patients in their ability to void and may be a predisposing factor to bladder and kidney infections. Any sign of urinary tract infection should be reported to the physician so that a culture can be obtained and treatment begun as soon as possible.

### Bowel program

As with many body systems during immobilization, bowel function may become sluggish, predisposing the patient to constipation. This predisposition may be further complicated by an improperly balanced diet and decreased roughage intake. Bowel habits should be monitored daily, with appropriate methods of facilitating bowel function through the use of natural measures (increased roughage, fruit juices, etc.), mild laxatives, or enemas to avoid impaction. An individual bowel program should be planned for each patient.

### Psychological/emotional support

It is impossible to elaborate in detail on the psychological/emotional components of care of the patient in traction within the scope of this chapter. We would like to emphasize, however, that patients need the opportunity to progress through a normal adjustment phase after initiation of traction therapy. This phase will certainly vary according to the patient's coping mechanisms, prior experience with hospitalization and traction therapy, and knowledge about traction. Repeated explanations may be necessary to assist the patient through this adjustment phase. Additional support may be required periodically throughout the therapy to assist in coping with the long-term effects of immobilization. Reassessment of the patient's psychological status will be required at intervals; often this status will be readily apparent. The tables in Chapter 7 will assist the reader in determining specific interventions that may be helpful.

### Documentation

Several forms (e.g., Neurovascular Assessment Sheet) have been shown within this and previous chapters, which facilitate accurate and efficient documentation of specific aspects of care. Although methods vary from one facility to another, the most important guideline to follow regarding documentation is that *all* care should be properly documented. Care accomplished but not documented on the patient chart is of no value in the processes of assessment and evaluation, not to mention the legal liability involved. Consider documentation the final, but no less important, step in the process of providing patient care.

Standardized care plans may serve as a guideline for patient care and when used provide for a high degree of consistency and continuity of care. It is important to note that the following standardized care plans (Form 24-1) are examples and assume the patient has *no* previous history of skin breakdown or other complications that may necessitate more frequent care. Shown here is the minimum standard of care, which must be adapted to the patient's individual needs. It may also be noted that when the traction is, for example, a combined nonadhesive and skeletal traction, components of both care plans should be used. Care plans for all three basic types of traction are provided for comparison; adaptations can be made easily.

### Discharge instructions

Although it is rare, patients are sometimes discharged with prescriptions for traction at home. Regardless of the type of traction, discharge instructions should be provided to the patient (see box, pp. 548-549). These should be accompanied by verbal instructions and demonstration.

## STANDARDIZED CARE PLAN: nonadhesive traction

| Problem | Outcome | Plan | Schedule | Begin | Disc. |
|---|---|---|---|---|---|
| Potential skin breakdown | Maintenance of skin integrity | Rewrap traction; and document | 0400-0800-1200-1600-2000-2400 and PRN | | |
| | | Skin care with alcohol under traction; document | 0400-0800-1200-1600-2000-2400 and PRN | | |
| | | Skin care with alcohol to all exposed joints or bony prominences (elbows, sacrum, coccyx, etc.); document | 0400-0800-1200-1600-2000-2400 and PRN | | |
| | | Buck's extension on regular bed or other traction on turning frame—turn entry 4 hours; document* | Prone: 0400, 1200, 2000<br>Supine: 0800, 1600, 2400 | | |
| Neurovascular compromise | Maintenance of acceptable neurovascular status | Neurovascular assessment: check pulse, edema, color, temperature, capillary filling, sensation, motion 30-45 minutes after rewrapping; document | 0430-0830-1230-1630-2030-0030 and PRN | | |
| | | Upper extremities ☐    Lower extremities ☐<br>Both ☐    Both ☐<br>Right ☐    Right ☐<br>Left ☐    Left ☐<br>All four extremities ☐ | As above | | |
| | | Notify physician of any alterations or changes | PRN | | |
| Potential malalignment of traction | Maintenance of desired positioning | Position according to diagram on bed<br>Check positioning and alignment | Even hours | | |
| Mechanical traction failure or distrubance | Maintenance of mechanics of traction | Check all ropes for fraying<br>Check all ropes to be sure they are on center tract of pulleys | 0600-1400-2200<br>0600-1400-2200 | | |
| | | Tighten all parts of equipment<br>Confirm proper numbers of weights | 0600-1400-2200<br>0600-1400-2200 | | |
| Renal calculi | Maintenance of kidney function with no renal calculi | Force fluids | _____ ml 7-3 shift<br>_____ ml 3-11 shift<br>_____ ml 11-7 shift | | |
| | | Maintain shift intake and output | 0700-1500-2300 | | |
| Constipation | Maintenance of bowel function | Promote roughage and bulk in diet<br>Force fluids as above<br>Obtain physician order for fecal softener, laxative, or suppository<br>Record bowel movements | PRN | | |
| Pressure area* under restraints | Maintenance of skin integrity under restraints* | Remove restraint and give skin care with alcohol* | 0400-0800-1200-1600-2000-2400 | | |
| Difficulty maintaining positioning (under 5 years)* | Maintenance of desired positioning* | Use solid Bradford frame*<br>Use frame restraint*<br>Elevate both ends of frame* | Continuously<br>Continuously<br>Continuously | | |

*When appropriate.

**Form 24-1, A**

## STANDARDIZED CARE PLAN: adhesive traction

| Problem | Outcome | Plan | Schedule | Begin | Disc. |
|---|---|---|---|---|---|
| Potential skin breakdown | Maintenance of skin integrity | Do not rewrap traction!<br>Skin care with alcohol around edges of traction<br><br>Skin care with alcohol to all exposed joints and bony prominences (elbows, sacrum, coccyx, etc.)<br>If on turning frame, turn*<br><br>Observe for signs or complaints of burning or itching under traction | 0400-0800-1200-1600-2000-2400<br>0400-0800-1200-1600-2000-2400<br>Prone: 0400, 1200, 2000<br>Supine: 0800, 1600, 2400<br>0400-0800-1200-1600-2000-2400 | | |
| Neurovascular compromise | Maintenance of acceptable neurovascular status | Neurovascular assessment: check pulse, edema, color, temperature, capillary filling, sensation and motion; document<br>Upper extremities     Lower extremities<br>Both ☐             Both ☐<br>Right ☐            Right ☐<br>Left ☐             Left ☐<br>All four extremities ☐<br>Notify physician of any alterations or changes | q 1 hour til ____ then<br>0400-0800-1200-1600-2000-2400<br>As above<br><br>PRN | | |
| Potential malalignment of traction | Maintenance of desired positioning and equipment | Position according to diagram on bed<br>Check positioning and alignment | Even hours | | |
| Mechanical traction failure or disturbance | Maintenance of mechanics of traction | Do not release traction!<br>Check all ropes for fraying<br>Check all ropes to be sure they are on center track of pulley<br>Tighten all parts of equipment<br>Confirm proper numbers of weights | 0600-1400-2200<br>0600-1400-2200<br>0600-1400-2200<br>0600-1400-2200 | | |
| Renal calculi | Maintenance of kidney function with no renal calculi | Force fluids<br><br>Maintain shift intake and output record | ____ ml 7-3 shift<br>____ ml 3-11 shift<br>____ ml 11-7 shift<br>0700-1500-2300 | | |
| Constipation | Maintenance of bowel function | Promote roughage in diet<br>Force fluids as above<br>Obtain physician order for fecal softener, laxative, or suppository<br>Record bowel movement | PRN | | |
| Pressure area under restraints* | Maintenance of skin integrity under restraints* | Remove restraint and give skin care with alcohol* | 0400-0800-1200-1600-2000-2400 | | |
| Difficulty maintaining positioning (under 5 years)* | Maintenance of desired positioning* | Use solid Bradford frame*<br>Use frame restraint*<br>Elevate both ends of frame* | Continuously<br>Continuously<br>Continuously | | |

*When appropriate.

**Form 24-1, B**

## STANDARDIZED CARE PLAN: skeletal traction

| Problem | Outcome | Plan | Schedule | Begin | Disc. |
|---|---|---|---|---|---|
| Potential skin breakdown | Maintenance of skin integrity | Skin care with alcohol to all exposed joints or bony prominences (elbows, sacrum, coccyx, etc.)<br>If on turning frame, TURN* | 0400-0800-1200-1600-2000-2400<br>Prone: 0400, 1200, 2000<br>Supine: 0800, 1600, 2400 | | |
| Neurovascular compromise | Maintenance of acceptable neurovascular status | Neurovascular assessment: check pulse, edema, color, temperature, capillary filling, sensation and motion; document<br>Upper extremities ☐    Lower extremities<br>  Both ☐              Both ☐<br>  Right ☐             Right ☐<br>  Left ☐              Left ☐<br>All four extremities ☐<br>Notify physician of any changes | q 1 hour til _____ then<br>0400-0800-1200-1600-2000-2400<br><br>As above<br>PRN | | |
| Cranial nerve compromise | Maintenance of intact cranial nerve function* | Cranial nerve assessment*<br>  Check for signs or complaints of blurred vision, double vision, lateral eye movement, pupil equality and reaction, slurred speech, difficulty swallowing, drooped eyelids or mouth; document<br>Notify physician of any changes | 0400-0800-1200-1600-2000-2400<br><br>PRN | | |
| Pin/wire migration | Early detection of pin/wire migration | Observe for signs or complaints of pin migration; document<br>Report any sign or suspicion of migration to physician | 0400-0800-1200-1600-2000-2400<br>PRN | | |
| Pin/wire site infection | No pin/wire infection or early detection of infection | Do not remove crust around pin site!<br>Observe sites for signs of infection: fever pain, drainage, erythema; document<br>Report any signs of infection to physician | 0400-0800-1200-1600-2000-2400<br><br>PRN | | |
| Potential malalignment of traction | Maintenance of desired positioning and alignment | Position according to diagram on bed<br>Check positioning/alignment | Even hours | | |
| Mechanical traction failure or disturbance | Maintenance of mechanics of traction | Do not release traction!<br>Check all ropes for fraying<br>Check that all ropes are on center track<br>Tighten all parts of equipment<br>Confirm proper number of weights | 0600-1400-2200<br>0600-1400-2200<br>0600-1400-2200<br>0600-1400-2200 | | |
| Renal calculi | Maintenance of kidney function with no renal calculi | Force fluids<br><br>Maintain shift intake and output record | _____ ml 7-3 shift<br>_____ ml 3-11 shift<br>_____ ml 11-7 shift<br>0700-1500-2300 | | |
| Constipation | Maintenance of bowel function | Promote roughage and bulk in diet<br>Force fluids as above<br>Obtain physic an order for fecal softener laxative or suppository<br>Record bowel movements | PRN | | |
| Pressure area under restraints* | Maintenance of skin integrity under restraints* | Remove restraints and give skin care with alcohol* | 0400-0800-1200-1600-2000-2400 | | |
| Difficulty maintaining positioning (under 5 years)* | Maintenance of desired positioning* | Use solid Bradford frame*<br>Use frame restraint*<br>Elevate both ends of frame* | Continuously<br>Continuously<br>Continuously | | |

*When appropriate.

**Form 24-1, C**

## COMPLICATIONS

Complications of traction therapy are reviewed in Table 24-5. Acute observational skills are required for the nursing personnel caring for these patients, so that complications that cannot be totally alleviated through preventive measures can be detected early. We maintain that both the detection and prevention of complications, when appropriate and applicable, are the responsibility of the providers and coordinators of 24-hour care—the nursing personnel.

---

## HOME INSTRUCTIONS: BUCK'S EXTENSION*

Your child will be going home from the hospital in traction. The following instructions are given to you now before your child is discharged so that you will be able to set up the traction. The instructions regarding putting your child in traction and the daily care of this traction will be shown to you before your child goes home. (If you do not wish to set up the traction in this manner, a metal setup can be rented or purchased. Details will be given on request.)

**Equipment needed**

1. Crossbar at foot of bed
2. Two clothesline pulleys
3. Rope
4. Weights, _____ pounds for each foot (suggestions: rocks, sand in cloth bag, window sash weights)
5. Two snappers or hooks to attach ropes to footplates
6. Rubbing alcohol
7. Thermometer

**Where obtained**

1. Lumberyard
2. Hardware store
3. Hardware store
4. Hardware store
5. Hardware store
6. Drugstore
7. Drugstore

**Equipment supplied by hospital**

1. Traction straps
2. Footplates
3. Ace bandages
4. Stockinette for toes
5. Bedpan

**Setting up traction**

1. Attach crossbar to foot of bed.
2. Attach two pulleys to crossbar _____ inches apart.
3. String rope through each pulley.
4. Attach snapper or hook to end of each rope that will be attached to footplates.
5. Attach above amount of weights to each rope at opposite end.

**Putting your child in traction**

1. Traction straps will be applied by the physician before your child is discharged if they are the type that cannot be removed. If your child is to use the removable traction straps, apply traction following the steps and diagrams below:
   a. Place the traction straps, as demonstrated by the nurse, with the broadest part of the tapered end just above the ankle.

   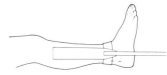

   b. Apply the Ace bandage starting just above the ankle and wrap it upward to the knee. Ace bandages should be firmly applied but loose enough so that you can easily run a finger underneath the edges at top and bottom. Secure the loose end with adhesive tape.

*From Hilt, N. E., and Schmitt, E. W., Jr.: Pediatric orthopedic nursing, St. Louis, 1975, The C. V. Mosby Co.

## HOME INSTRUCTIONS: BUCK'S EXTENSION—cont'd

c. Buckle the ends of the traction straps to the footplate. The foot should be firmly against the footplate in a normal position.

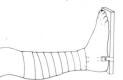

d. Place a piece of stockinette around the toes and the footplate to keep the foot from slipping off the footplate.

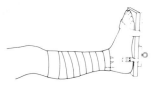

e. Attach the rope from the weights to the ring on bottom of the footplate with the snap.

### Care of your child in traction

1. Your child is to lie flat in bed at all times unless otherwise specified by your physician.
2. Turn your child from abdomen to back every 4 hours during day. Try to arrange schedule so that your child is in the position that he sleeps best at night.
3. Take the traction off every 4 hours and rewrap the Ace bandages if they are the removable type. Rub the skin under the traction straps with rubbing alcohol at this time. This will help toughen the skin and prevent it from becoming irritated. *Please do not use oils, powders, or lotions* on the skin under the traction: powders have a tendency to "cake," and oils and lotions will soften the skin, making it easier for the skin to break down.
4. Rub the base of your child's spine, heels, ankles, elbows, and knees with rubbing alcohol every 4 hours. These are the areas most likely to become irritated, since your child must spend all of his time in bed.
5. Each time skin care is given, check skin carefully for reddened areas. If any occur, give skin care more frequently to these areas. If any broken areas in the skin are noted, notify your physician.
6. Check to make sure that your child can move his toes well and can feel his toes and that the color is good. There should be no swelling. This should be checked frequently. If the toes are very hot, very

cold, very red, bluish in color, numb, or tingly, rewrap the traction; it has probably been wrapped too tightly. If rewrapping does not relieve this, let the traction off for an hour. If this does not help, notify your physician.
7. Give your child a daily sponge bath. Wash his feet well and dry them thoroughly before placing him back in traction.
8. Check at intervals
   a. Is your child flat in bed?
   b. Are the traction straps firmly attached?
   c. Are the ankle bones free from pressure?
   d. Is the Ace bandage smoothly applied and not too tight?
   e. Are the footplates in the correct normal position?
   f. Are the ropes on the pulleys?
   g. Are the weights hanging free and not resting on the floor?
   h. Can he move his toes well and feel his toes well, and is the color good? Is there any swelling?

### What to report to your doctor

1. Any reddened areas of the skin not relieved by more frequent skin care or any break in the skin
2. Tingling of the toes, swelling, blueness, or numbness not relieved by rewrapping the traction or releasing it for an hour
3. Continuous complaints of pain or discomfort or unexplained fussiness
4. Temperature above 101 F
5. Any severe illness such as flu or chest cold

It is most difficult for a normal, active child to be confined in bed in traction for any period of time. It might help if you could start to think now of some activities that might occupy him during this time. It is important that he be permitted to do all possible for himself within the limitations set by your physician.

**PHYSICIAN:**

**PHONE NUMBER:**

**HOSPITAL PHONE NUMBER:**

**ORTHOPEDIC NURSE SPECIALIST:**

**NEXT APPOINTMENT WITH PHYSICIAN:**

**SPECIAL INSTRUCTIONS:** *Force fluids!*

**Table 24-5.** Common complications caused or exacerbated by traction therapy

| Complication | Type of traction | Signs/symptoms | Treatment | Prevention |
|---|---|---|---|---|
| Peroneal nerve palsy | All lower extremity | Pain, tingling, or paresthesia over anterior surface of affected leg and dorsilateral aspect of affected foot<br>Inability to actively dorsiflex<br>Dropfoot | Passive dorsiflexion exercises<br>Proper positioning<br>Possibly dorsiflexion brace for ambulation | Observe for prevention of pressure over peroneal nerve<br>Proper placement of traction straps or elastic wrap to avoid pressure over peroneal nerve |
| Compartment syndromes[4] (progressive vascular compromise) | Dunlop traction<br>All lower extremity | Pain — increasing and progressive in involved area<br>Pain on passive motion<br>Paralysis — progressive<br>Paresthesias<br>Pulselessness | Relieve constriction; nonadhesive skin traction may be removed immediately; notify physician immediately for adhesive skin traction<br>Elevate extremity<br>Possible fasciotomy | Early detection with recognition of any of the signs and symptoms and initiation of treatment |
| Constrictive edema | All skin | Gradual increase in swelling from vascular compromise<br>Alteration in circulatory or neurologic status | Nonadhesive skin traction: rewrap with less tension<br>Adhesive skin traction: notify physician, document, arrange to have rewrapped<br>If continual problem, may choose to wrap foot in elastic wrap | Careful wrapping and rewrapping techniques with proper tension applied |
| Constipation | All | Inconsistent bowel movements<br>Lack of bowel movements<br>Loose bowel movements indicative of impaction | Natural alterations or additions to diet (juices, roughage, etc.)<br>Laxatives, enemas as necessary | Monitor diet<br>Monitor bowel movements<br>Bowel program designed for the individual patient |
| Renal calculi | All | Pain over kidney area; may be increasing or intermittent<br>Difficulty with urination | Report suspicion to physician<br>X-ray<br>Specific treatment determined by size and location | Force fluids to twice normally accepted intake for age and weight<br>Limit milk and milk products intake to meals only<br>Monitor intake and output |
| Pressure area<br>Skin necrosis<br>Allergic skin reaction[3, pp. 128-129] | All skin | Reddened areas<br>Pain or itching<br>Irritability, fussiness, or restlessness<br>Drainage through elastic wrap (with or without odor)<br>Elevated temperature | Nonadhesive skin traction:<br>  Relieve pressure<br>  Increase schedule for rewrapping<br>  Increase frequency of skin care<br>Adhesive skin traction:<br>  Notify physician<br>  Arrange to have rewrapped to assess skin integrity<br>  Document | Appropriate application and reapplication techniques<br>Frequent observation<br>Appropriate and frequent skin care |

**Table 24-5.** Common complications caused or exacerbated by traction therapy—cont'd

| | Type of traction | Signs/symptoms | Treatment | Prevention |
|---|---|---|---|---|
| Pin tract infections | All skeletal | Erythema at pin site<br>Drainage or odor<br>Pin slippage<br>Temperature elevation<br>Pain | Treatment depends on depth of infection; superficial infection treated with antibiotic therapy topically or orally; deeper infection usually requires pin removal with antibiotic therapy | Do *not* remove crust at pin site unless obvious sign of infection<br>Appropriate pin care |
| Cranial nerve impairment[2] | Cervical tongs and halo | Abnormal lateral eye movements<br>Pupillary changes<br>Blurred vision<br>Diplopia<br>Difficulty swallowing<br>Difficulty with speech<br>Difficulty with tongue control | Treatment depends on severity of symptoms; continued observation; pin removal may be required | Early detection<br>Incorporation of signs and symptoms monitoring into neurovascular assessments |
| Pulmonary embolism[1] | All types, especially in the elderly and associated with surgery or trauma | Occlusion in bifurcation of pulmonary artery:<br>May occur with or without clinical symptoms<br>Sudden onset of substernal pain, dyspnea, increasingly weak pulse, syncope, shock; may be fatal<br>Occlusion involving one or more arterial branches:<br>Lethargy, increased pulse, some degree of dyspnea with pain<br>Occlusion of pulmonary terminal arterial branches:<br>Clinical picture resembles bronchopneumonia with cough, hemoptysis, elevated temperature | Arterial blood gases, chest X-ray, lung scan, and EKG for diagnosis<br>Prevention of formation of further emboli with IV heparin, then coumadin therapy<br>Prevention of shock, hypoxia, or heart failure<br>Relief of dyspnea and pain<br>Complication of heart failure treated by digitalization<br>Emotional and psychologic support | Prophylactic anticoagulation therapy for high-risk patients<br>Dextran IV therapy; aspirin therapy<br>Antiembolic stockings<br>Active and passive exercises of lower extremities<br>Routine turning and positioning<br><br>All other nursing measures for prevention of venous stasis including earliest possible ambulation and observation for all signs and symptoms |
| Hypostatic pneumonia | All types, especially in the elderly | Elevated temperature<br>Chest pain<br>Difficulty with inspiration or expiration<br>Productive cough | Antibiotic therapy<br>IPPB<br>Turn, cough, and deep breathe every 2 hours<br>Oxygen therapy<br>Drugs for control or loosening of secretions | Turning and repositioning frequently<br>Cough and deep breathe every 2 hours<br>IPPB when indicated<br>Blow bottles, spirometer, or gloves<br>Frequent assessment of respiratory status<br>Prophylactic antibiotic therapy for high-risk patients<br>Earliest possible ambulation |

**Table 24-6.** Summary of care focuses of patient in traction

| Care focus | Type of traction | Specifications | Frequency | Rationale |
|---|---|---|---|---|
| Application/ reapplication | Adhesive skin traction | Applied by physician<br>Spray tincture of benzoin over extremity<br>Place folded stockinette over maleoli<br>Roll one layer of stockinette over extremity<br>Apply adhesive straps<br>Wrap elastic bandage | Onset of traction<br>Reapplication of traction | To decrease possibility of adhesive skin reactions |
| | Nonadhesive skin traction | Applied by physician<br>Place folded stockinette over maleoli<br>Apply traction straps (from side against skin)<br>Wrap elastic bandage | Every 4 hours<br>Every 2 hours during day, every 3 hours during night for patients having myelomeningocele, paraplegia, quadriplegia, history of sensitive skin, or reddened areas not disappearing in 15-20 minutes after removal | To maintain skin integrity |
| Skin care | All skin tractions | Use alcohol only; no lotions, oils, or powders<br>To back, buttocks, coccyx | Every 4 hours<br>Every 2 hours during day, every 3 hours during night for patients having myelomeningocele, paraplegia, quadriplegia, history of sensitive skin, or reddened areas not disappearing in 15-20 minutes after removal | To toughen skin<br>To maintain skin integrity |
| | Adhesive skin traction | Around edges of traction | | |
| | Nonadhesive traction | Under traction | | |
| Pin care | All skeletal traction | Do not remove crust<br>Observe for signs of infection, migration<br>2×2 antiseptic sponge or spray<br>(Care may vary according to physician preference) | Will vary according to physician preference | To decrease risk of infection |
| Neurovascular assessment | All tractions | Pretraction assessment (assess all components and document):<br>Color<br>Temperature<br>Capillary filling<br>Edema<br>Pulse<br>Sensation<br>Numbness/tingling<br>Motion | Before onset of traction | To establish "normal" status for individual patient<br>To detect neurovascular impairment at earliest possible time and initiate treatment |
| | Continuous traction<br>Skeletal<br>Adhesive skin | | Every 4 hours for first 24 hours; if status "normal" for that patient, every 4 hours thereafter | To facilitate early detection of neurovascular impairment as a direct result of traction application |

**Table 24-6.** Summary of care focuses of patient in traction—cont'd

| Care focus | Type of traction | Specifications | Frequency | Rationale |
|---|---|---|---|---|
| | Intermittent tractions (nonadhesive skin) | | Every 4 hours (or after each reapplication) 30-45 minutes *after* reapplication | |
| | Halo and cervical tong tractions | Pupillary reactions Lateral eye movement Blurred vision Diplopia Difficulty with speech Difficulty swallowing Difficulty with tongue control | With all neurovascular assessments | To detect cranial nerve impairment |
| Maintenance of positioning, alignment, and immobilization | All tractions | Maintain desired positioning, alignment, and immobilization | Several times per shift minimum | To obtain maximal benefit from traction |
| | | Uncooperative or incoherent patients: use appropriate restraints | As necessary | |
| | | Children in traction— Use solid Bradford frame for child under 5 years of age, mentally retarded or hyperactive | As designated in Table 24-3 | |
| | | Use restraints (sling, jacket, frame, diaper) | As designated in Table 24-4 | |
| | | Maintain positioning | As designated in Table 24-5 | |
| Extremities not in traction | All tractions | Provide activities Promote self-help independence Range of motion | As necessary | To decrease joint stiffness and muscle atrophy |
| Maintain traction principles | All tractions | Monitor weights Maintain weights hanging free Maintain ropes in center track of pulleys Check condition of ropes Maintain appropriate line of pull Maintain all equipment tight and secure | Every shift at minimum | To maintain maximal benefit and effectiveness of traction therapy |
| Nutritional requirements | All tractions | Monitor diet Encourage balanced diet Encourage juices and roughage | Every shift | To promote healing and decrease constipation |
| Bladder and kidney program | All tractions | Monitor intake and output Limit milk and milk products to meals only Force fluids to twice normally accepted amount | Every shift | To decrease infection and renal calculi |
| Bowel program | All tractions | Monitor bowel movements Juices and roughage in diet Monitor diet Laxatives and enemas as necessary to prevent impaction | Every shift | To decrease constipation |

## SUMMARY

All health care personnel should have a working knowledge of the principles of traction. This knowledge permits those responsible for prescription and c re to made adequate judgments, provide effective therapy, and decrease the length of therapeutic regimen to an absolute minimum. Consistency and continuity of approach and care are essential in the achievement of these goals and objectives.

## REFERENCES

1. Alt, P.: Care of the child in traction, O.N.A. J. **2**(1):14-16, Jan. 1975.
2. Farrell, J.: Pulmonary embolism, O.N.A. J. **2**(1):14-16, Jan. 1975.
3. Hilt, N. E., and Schmitt, W. E., Jr.: Pediatric orthopedic nursing, St. Louis, 1975, The C. V. Mosby Co., pp. 128-129.
4. Laucey, G. L.: Compartment syndrome, O.N.A. J. **2**(6):48-151, June 1975.

## BIBLIOGRAPHY

Hilt, N. E., and Schmitt, W. E., Jr.: Pediatric orthopedic nursing, St. Louis, 1975, The C. V. Mosby Co.
Larson, C., and Gould, M.: Orthopedic nursing, St. Louis, 1970, The C. V. Mosby Co.
Stewart, J. D. M.: Traction and orthopedic appliances, New York, 1975, Churchhill Livingstone.

# 25

# Pharmacologic therapeutics

D. FRANK LANDRUM

Medicinal therapeutics is a topic of interest to all health care personnel as well as to the patient. Within the scope of a single chapter it is impossible to provide detailed information for complete care of all the problems that a patient might have or develop during the hospital stay. Suffice it to say that the object here is to single out the "average" orthopedic patient who enters the hospital for observation, examination, diagnostic procedures, surgery, convalescence, and rehabilitation. Preexisting medical conditions that may complicate successful care of the patient have intentionally been disregarded. This chapter will deal with those therapeutic agents most likely to be used for those problems generally encountered. The information found here is not intended to be a complete guideline for therapy, but rather a signpost pointing the way.

## RATIONAL PRESCRIBING AND DRUG THERAPY
### Writing or dictating orders

All therapy should begin and cease with the verbal or written order of the physician; it is his or her responsibility to direct the attack on the patient's problem(s). The verbal or written orders are but tools to communicate to other health care professionals the plans for care of the patient, the therapeutic agents to be used, and how, when, how much, and why they are to be used. This makes it imperative for the physician to take care to maintain this line of communication by writing or speaking clearly to be certain that the information intended has actually been communicated. Orders for therapeutic agents should always include the following information:

1. Absolute identity of the agent (many drugs are pronounced and spelled very similarly)
2. Dosage or strength desired (practically all drugs have several strengths available)
3. Dosage form(s) authorized for use (most drugs are available in several formulations)
4. Route(s) of administration
5. Dosage schedule, including the time interval, the time to be administered if one is preferred, and any special instructions, such as after or before meals, on an empty stomach, with antacids, etc.
6. Length of time the therapy is to continue if this can be determined (many hospitals have established policies regarding the length of time agents such as controlled substances, antibiotics, and anticoagulants may be continued without review or reorder)

It is often just as important to cease therapy as to begin it; the patient's current orders should be reviewed regularly and those no longer applicable should be discontinued or revised. When one agent is ordered to replace one that was not effective, the ineffective drug should be discontinued. It is also bad practice to use abbreviations or contractions that are not authorized or recognized by the governing body of the institution or hospital being used.

### Interpreting orders

The interpretation and execution of the physician's orders are no less important than their formulation. The orders are the battle plan for attacking the patient's problems, major and minor. The nurse and pharmacist who are most likely to review, interpret, and execute these orders have the responsibility for ascertaining precisely what is intended to be done and then actually carrying out the orders. If there is any doubt as to the clarity of any of the six points mentioned above, the nurse or pharmacist should never hesitate to contact the physician to confirm the orders. With the increased potency and toxicity of today's therapeutic agents, all health care professionals should act with caution in communication, interpretation, and execution of orders to assure that the patient receives the best and safest care possible.

### BASIS FOR SELECTION OF MEDICATIONS
### Price

With the dramatic increase in health care costs and the continuing trend toward third-party payment for this care, the cost of all phases of care is being scrutinized much more carefully. As the leader of the health care team, much more responsibility will be directed toward the physician to be cognizant of the cost factors and to proceed accordingly. One method for reaching the goal of lowering costs is to be familiar with the formulary of the institution and to use those therapeutic agents if at all possible. A second method is to support a strict formulary within the institution to avoid extravagant duplication of generically or therapeutically equivalent agents. The third and perhaps most important way the physician can help control costs is by judiciously choosing the medications for patients and using those that have proved to be clinically effective over a period of time. Very often, the medications that have been on the market for many years have become much less expensive because of the competition in the market place.

Nursing personnel also have much responsibility in the area of cost management; they must take steps to prevent waste, contamination, spoilage, and pilferage of medications entrusted to their care. Proper handling, preparation, and combination of therapeutic agents can save both the patient and the institution much unnecessary expense; when questions arise, a quick review of the literature or a call to the pharmacy may clarify the situation and save dollars and time.

Good aseptic technique in the preparation or admixture of medicaments and the prompt and proper disposal of unused portions of agents intended for one-time use can also help eradicate the potentially hazardous and costly contamination of medications. The judicious review of usage rates, proper storage, and proper rotation of stocks of medications kept on the nursing unit is the most efficient method to reduce the loss to the patient and the institution of many dollars' worth of medications yearly. Proper steps should be taken to maintain the security of all medications kept on the unit whether as stock or for the patient. In large institutions, the bill for pilferage of medications often rises into the hundreds of thousands of dollars annually.

The pharmacist also must share in the responsibility for ensuring that the patient receives the finest and most efficacious therapeutic agents available at the most reasonable price possible. This can be done by maintaining strict inventory control to ensure adequate but not burdensome supplies. By buying from reputable manufacturers or suppliers on a bid or contractural basis, there can be substantial savings. Proper stock rotation and adequate security and control of the flow of medications throughout the institution can also contribute to efficiency and reduced cost.

### Patient comfort, acceptance, and compliance

The patient's condition may have a great influence on the selection of a medication by the physician. His condition may narrow the choice of routes for administration. The patient who is debilitated may be a poor candidate for intramuscular or subcutaneous injections, thus narrowing the routes available to administer a medication. If this same patient is nauseated or has diarrhea, the availability of routes is severely restricted. A thorough review of the patient and his problems should play an important role in the choice of routes of administration.

Another factor that plays an important role in the selection procedure is the availability of a suitable strength or dosage form to fit the parameters set forth. The recommended or desired dosage of a medication may not be easily achieved for an individual patient because of the dosage strength available; this is often a serious problem in dealing with pediatric patients. The more formulations (i.e., tablets, capsules, suppositories, topicals, parenterals, and oral liquids) available, the more readily can therapy be tailored to the patient's needs. All members of the health care team should make every effort to learn the strengths and dosage forms available.

Much time and effort may be wasted if the patient and family are not aware of the goals the health care team is trying to achieve. A patient who knows what the medications are intended to do, what side effects or complications may be encountered, and the ramifications involved with noncompliance is much more likely to be cooperative and compliant during therapy. It becomes the responsibility of all health care personnel to be ready with meaningful, informative, and factual answers to the questions of the patient and family concerning medications. Each member of the team should become familiar with the patient's therapeutic regimen and take care to ensure that it is executed accurately and completely. Fear of the unknown and misunderstanding the importance of the therapy should be eliminated by clear communication among the staff and by professional counseling of patients and their families.

## Appropriateness

Selecting the appropriate therapeutic agent for a specific patient may take much thought and judgment. Often preventive measures taken in formulating care plans are of greater value than treating problems after they arise. For example since many oral antibiotics have the tendency to produce severe diarrhea by destroying the normal flora in the digestive tract, it would be appropriate to take preventive measures by replacing the flora via diet (buttermilk or yogurt) or medication (Bacid or Lactinex). If the operative patient who is still receiving potent analgesics should develop a cold with a severe cough, analgesics containing codeine (a potent antitussive) or codeine alone to control both the pain and the cough would be appropriate and rational therapy. These simplified examples point toward efficiency in the use of therapeutic agents. Another example is the use of an antihistamine such as diphenhydramine (Benadryl) to control itching, since its sedative-like side effect can be of benefit also. Many agents may be used specifically for a property generally thought of as a side effect. This often reduces the number of medications required and results in a substantial savings of money to the patient and of time for all members of the health care team.

**Clinical experience.** One's own experience in dealing with patient's problems (both successful and unsuccessful) often provides the final ingredients in the selection of therapeutic agents. It is for this very reason that all health care professionals should develop good habits of scientific observation and documentation in judging the efficacy of therapeutic agents. Being cognizant of the potential interactions of medications with one another and

with foods can prevent unnecessary and potentially hazardous consequences. Many years of experience in the use of a medication with good success in a wide variety of patients gives the professional confidence and security in its use but should not preclude or exclude employing other agents should the need arise. As with any endeavor, a single dramatic experience (positive or adverse) should not determine an agent's worth in the care of all patients.

## VIEWING THE TOTAL PATIENT

While the intent of this text is to focus on the pathophysiology, problems, and care of the orthopedic patient, we must take care not to view the patient simply as a musculoskeletal system. Our patient, like all others, is a human being, and in this chapter we will deal with those problems most likely to be encountered from admission to discharge. To prevent becoming entangled in all disciplines of medical practice, we will limit our review to the following: (1) preoperative agents and adjuncts to anesthesia, (2) antiinfectives and antibiotics, (3) analgesics, (4) antiemetics and antinauseants, (5) sedatives and hypnotics, (6) muscle relaxants, (7) anticoagulants, (8) antiarthritic-antiinflammatory-antigout agents, (9) agents for the gastrointestinal tract, (10) agents for the urinary tract, (11) agents for dermatologic conditions, and (12) psychotherapeutic agents. All these areas are sources of problems that the average orthopedic patient may encounter during the diagnostic, surgical, postoperative, convalescent, and rehabilitative phases of care. It is not within the scope of this presentation to attempt to discuss all the possible complications that may develop from the multitude of underlying medical problems that might afflict the patient; therefore, the above outlined parameters will serve as an outline for this presentation.

With the scope of this presentation, we would do well to remember that the therapeutic agents presented are by no means all that are available, but are a representative sampling of those on the market. This is not intended to serve as a complete reference source, but rather as a beginning point. For this reason, the last section of this chapter points out more detailed reference sources for the health care practitioner and outlines what type of information each contains.

## PREOPERATIVE AGENTS AND ADJUNCTS TO ANESTHESIA

Preanesthetic medications are used prior to administration of anesthesia to accomplish several purposes. In general, these agents are ordered to (1) minimize anxiety with a minimum of drowsiness, (2) speed up induction without extending emergence, (3) relieve pain associated with the surgery, (4) prevent or minimize the side effects of the anesthetic agents (i.e., vomiting, bradycardia, salivation), and (5) cause amnesia for the time of the surgery. The most commonly used agents to achieve these purposes are listed in Tables 25-1 to 25-3. From time to time, many other agents may be employed for these purposes but the tables provide information on those most commonly used in medical practice.

When two or more agents are ordered preoperatively, the age-old question of compatibility arises. Complete data on compatibility are available for few drugs, but Table 25-4 is a compilation of the advisability of mixing the agents listed in the same syringe based on latest literature and information available in the manufacturers' package inserts.

## ANTIBIOTICS

All health care professionals are aware of and fear the potential problem of microbial infection of the patient and should exercise due precaution to prevent infection from occurring. The practice of good hygiene and proper aseptic techniques in the routine care of the patient can do much to prevent the possibility of infection. Special caution should be exercised in the areas of food handling, dressing changes, preparation and administration of medications (especially parenterals), handling of instruments, specimens, and drainage materials, and isolation and hand-washing techniques. Prevention is much preferred to active treatment of infection.

Antibiotic therapy generally falls into two categories: (1) prophylactic therapy and (2) therapeutic treatment of an active infection. Prophylactic therapy, especially postoperatively, is generally short-term, and usually a broad-spectrum agent is employed to afford the patient added protection from a wide range of possible pathogens. Active infections are most often treated with more specific agents for an extended period of time.

When an active infection is suspected and the decision to begin antibiotic therapy is made, the next problem is the judicious selection of the agent to be used. It would be preferable to have bacterial culture and sensitivity results before commencing therapy but this is not always practical. Even if therapy is begun before such results are obtained, cultures should be obtained before drug administration if at all possible. Here, the clinical experience and expertise of the physician should be utilized to review the "clinical picture" for hints as to the caus-

ative organism before selecting the drug to be used. Once the results of the laboratory findings are available, the treatment should be adjusted to fit the clinical findings. General criteria for selection of the proper antibiotic for the specific situation include: (1) sensitivity patterns of the infecting agent, (2) the nature of the illness being treated, (3) previous hypersensitivity reactions or serious side effects by the patient to certain drugs or classes of drugs, and (4) the cost of the drug in relation to alternative agents.

Since the advent of modern chemotherapy of infectious diseases began with the use of sulfanilamide in 1936, hundreds of antibiotics have been noted and over sixty are currently being used. The properties, antibacterial spectra, mechanisms of action, and usefulness of the agents vary widely. We have attempted to supply the basic information regarding the various systemic antibiotics, which are presented in five categories: penicillins and cephalosporins (Table 25-5), the aminoglycosides (Table 25-6), tetracyclines and chloramphenicol (Table 25-7), antifungal agents (Table 25-8), and miscellaneous agents (Table 25-9). The sulfonamides are presented in Table 25-30.

In all antibiotic therapy, it is important to do culture and sensitivity studies before, during, and after therapy and to follow the recommended usage, dosage, and precautions with respect to the agent selected. Failure to do so may result in emergence of resistant strains of pathogens, unsatisfactory results, needless cost, and severe consequences for the patient.

## ANALGESICS

Practically every patient who is institutionalized will experience some degree of pain or discomfort and most will receive an analgesic agent to alleviate that pain. Many factors should be considered to individualize treatment, such as the type and severity, the source, and the expected duration of pain; the patient's physical and psychologic reaction to pain; the patient's history of drug dependence or addiction; and the patient's natural pain threshold (ability to tolerate pain).

It is virtually impossible to accurately assess the patient's pain by any known means; therefore, all practitioners must move with caution in trying to alleviate pain. One method is to begin therapy with a mild analgesic agent, following this with an intermediate agent if the pain persists, and using narcotic analgesics only when the other agents have failed. This approach is probably as effective as any other but care should be taken to ensure that the patient is not forced to bear unnecessary pain for extended periods of time.

Since all of the potent analgesic agents, especially the narcotics, have a high addiction potential, particularly when employed for extended periods of time, it is imperative that they be employed with caution and only when necessary to control severe pain. These agents are frequently required during the immediate postsurgical period and are rightfully employed, but the patient should be examined and assessed regularly and the drug withdrawn as soon as possible.

The following categories of analgesic agents are presented: narcotic analgesics (Table 25-10), non-narcotic-nonsalicylate analgesics (Table 25-11), and salicylate analgesics (Table 25-12). Many combination analgesics are excluded in this presentation. There are literally hundreds of products that employ one or more of the agents presented in these tables in combination with other agents. All practitioners would do well to become familiar with these agents; many are safe, effective, and useful in the management of various types of pain.

## ANTIEMETICS AND ANTINAUSEANTS

Practically all patients will at some time experience nausea and/or vomiting. The problem may result from several causes, including use of general anesthetic agents, analgesic agents, or other medications, or from underlying medical causes. Regardless of the cause, this problem is both traumatic and disconcerting to the patient and should be treated with appropriate measures.

Because of the nature of this problem, the oral route may not be readily available to administer medications. For this reason, many of the agents for this purpose are available in parenteral (IM or IV use) and rectal dosage formulations. One would do well to get input from the patient in selecting the route of administration.

Certain anesthetic agents and analgesics are particularly prone to cause this problem. A potent antinauseant or antiemetic can be administered prior to induction of anesthesia and possibly repeated during surgery; postoperatively, the dosage should be adjusted to control symptoms. For the patient in severe pain (postoperatively or otherwise) who requires the use of potent analgesic agents, such as morphine or meperidine, that have a tendency to cause severe nausea or vomiting, the concomitant administration of a potent antinauseant-antiemetic would serve two purposes: (1) to control the nausea and (2) to effectively lower the dose requirements by potentiating the analgesic agent.

As with any group of potent drugs, use of antinauseant-antiemetics agents is not without hazards. Their side effects are many and serious and their usage should not be taken lightly. Care should be exercised to assure that these drugs do not mask toxic symptoms of other drugs or obscure the diagnosis of certain conditions that may cause nausea and vomiting.

Tables 25-13 and 25-14 are a starting point for using the antinauseant-antiemetic agents. Package inserts and drug reference sources should be consulted for more detailed prescribing information, specific side effects, and precautions.

## SEDATIVES-HYPNOTICS

Practically all patients during their confinement experience the problem of insomnia. This problem may result from a variety of causes including something as simple as a pillow or bed that differs from what the patient is used to, pain, muscle spasms and cramps, fear and anxiety, apprehension, indigestion, or too much daytime napping. Many of these causes may be remedied with no medication at all or by an agent that does not fit into the sedative-hypnotic category.

If there are underlying causes for the patient's insomnia, these should be dealt with before adding to the patient's medication regimen. Very often, scheduling the patient's medications so that the last dose of the day is given at bedtime precludes the necessity for administering the sedative-hypnotic agent. Many agents, such as muscle relaxants, tranquilizers, and analgesics, cause drowsiness as a side effect; thus scheduling the last dose near the bedtime hour is rational and efficient therapy. Antihistamines, muscle relaxants, and psychotherapeutic agents are frequently used for their sedative side effect to produce sleep rather than employing more potent agents with a habit-forming potential.

In the following tables are listed the commonly used sedative-hypnotics, both barbiturate (Table 25-15) and nonbarbiturate (Table 25-16). These are potent agents and should be used with due caution; most of them also have the potential to be habit-forming. The most practical approach to insomnia is to discern the cause and try to remedy it. Medication should be employed as a last resort beginning with the milder, less potent agents and progressing to more potent drugs if the problem persists.

## SKELETAL MUSCLE RELAXANTS

Many orthopedic patients encounter problems with skeletal muscle cramps or spasticity. This problem may be temporary and transient or chronic and continuous. The condition is disconcerting and painful and may seriously complicate the recovery, especially in the early postoperative stages.

Certain neuromuscular blocking agents of the current type produce very good skeletal muscle relaxation, even to the point of paralysis. These agents should be used only with *extreme* caution. This group includes tubocurarine and metocurine iodide.

Other nondepolarizing neuromuscular blocking agents are also very potent drugs and, like the curare preparations, are to be used only with great caution.

Both of the above groups are relegated primarily to use during anesthesia. In very acute situations, they could be employed in the clinical care of the patient. This, however, very rarely happens.

Most of the therapeutic agents employed as skeletal muscle relaxants act on the central nervous system; dantrolene sodium is one, however, that acts directly on the muscle itself. It should be noted that practically all of the centrally acting skeletal muscle relaxants that appear in Table 25-17 are also available in one or more combinations with a variety of analgesic agents. The health care professional should be familiar with these combinations also.

## ANTICOAGULANTS

In the postoperative orthopedic patient, especially those requiring extensive or major surgical procedures, anticoagulant therapy may be instituted for prophylaxis or prevention of extension of venous thrombosis. The available anticoagulants are well established and have been successfully used in clinical practice for many years; however, their usage requires much clinical skill, careful observation of the patient, and individualized dosage schedules to maintain each patient within the range between acceptable therapeutic activity and unacceptable hemorrhagic risk. Therapeutic use of these agents should always be accompanied by appropriate blood coagulation studies (e.g., activated partial thromboplastin time, Lee-White, whole-blood clotting time) at regular intervals and by regular examination and direct observation of the patient, since no accurate relationship can be seen between prothrombin, coagulation, and bleeding times and the onset of hemorrhage.

The potential for drug interactions with oral anticoagulants is well known. The clinical significance is not always important but each practitioner should be aware of the possibilities that exist. There are three significant types of drug-drug interactions that can alter the clinical picture regarding oral anticoagulants: (1) those that may *increase* the hypothrombinemic effect, (2) those that may *decrease* the hypothrombinemic effect, and (3) those that may potentiate the danger of hemorrhage.

Possible interactions that may potentiate the activity (increase the hypothrombinemic effect) of the oral anticoagulants may occur with the following classes of drugs:

1. Drugs interfering with availability of vitamin K
2. Drugs displacing oral anticoagulants from their protein binding sites
3. Drugs competing for degradation sites on the endoplasmic reticulum
4. Drugs suppressing activity of or reducing the level of drug-metabolizing hepatic enzymes.
5. Drugs increasing the affinity of receptor sites for oral anticoagulants
6. Steroids increasing the turnover rate of procoagulant factors.
7. Drugs decreasing the synthesis of procoagulant factors

Possible interactions that may interfere with (decrease the hypothrombinemic effect of) the activity of the oral anticoagulants may occur with these classes of drugs:

1. Drugs stimulating synthesis of procoagulant factors
2. Drugs stimulating production of drug-metabolizing hepatic enzymes
3. Certain drugs that act by as yet unknown mechanisms

Possible interactions that may potentiate the danger of hemorrhage when used with oral anticoagulants can occur with the following:

1. Certain enzymatic preparations, such as streptodornase and streptokinase
2. Drugs that impair platelet function
3. Antimetabolites and alkylating agents that decrease production of platelets and procoagulant factors
4. Antiinflammatory agents that have ulcerogenic potential.

Many endogenous factors also alter the effects of oral anticoagulants. These may include general health, radiation therapy, underlying medical conditions, heredity, and diet. Dietary changes to include or exclude foods rich in vitamin K, alcohol and fats may greatly alter the activity of oral anticoagulants.

Table 25-18 is a compilation of information concerning anticoagulant therapy, including the oral agents, fibrinolysin, heparin, and protamine sulfate, the heparin antagonist.

## ANTIARTHRITIC-ANTIINFLAMMATORY-ANTIGOUT AGENTS

Many orthopedic patients have their problems compounded by rheumatic diseases or gout. This section presents information about the medicinal agents normally used to treat these conditions with the exception of the salicylate group (which may be reviewed in Table 25-12). These agents are classified as follows: (1) antirheumatic agents: non-steroid-nonsalicylate (Table 25-19), (2) antiinflammatory agents: systemic steroids (Table 25-20), and (3) drugs for gout (Table 25-21)

Many of these agents are very potent and cause severe, irreversible, and sometimes bizarre side effects. Therapy with these agents should not be undertaken lightly by any of the health care professionals, and a thorough review of the literature is recommended before prescribing, dispensing, or administering them. Again, the patient and family should be kept informed as to the possible side effects that might be encountered.

## AGENTS FOR THE GASTROINTESTINAL TRACT

Most institutionalized patients experience some sort of gastrointestinal disturbance before their stay is completed. The type, severity, and duration of the disturbance may vary widely. Typical disturbances or complaints are spastic or "nervous" stomach, constipation, diarrhea, acid indigestion (upset stomach), and flatulence (gas or heart burn). The underlying cause of these complaints may be simple or complex. Often, the causative agent can be eliminated rather than instituting drug therapy that may be inappropriate or unnecessary.

The spastic or "nervous" stomach may be a reflection of the patient's mental status (fear and apprehension) rather than any physical problem. Regular visits by the physician to keep the patient fully informed and reassured may be just the "medicine" needed. There are many drugs that irritate the gastrointestinal tract and cannot be tolerated by some patients; here, a change to a similar alternate drug may suffice. There are also physiologic conditions that may be causing such a problem. Medication, then, is not always the correct therapy; however, if it is necessary, the agents listed in Table 25-22 (anticholinergics and antispasmodics) or products containing these agents in combination would be normally employed.

Constipation is a problem for many patients but one not necessarily solved by the use of medications. Common causes of constipation include medications (especially analgesics of opium derivation),

changes in activity level, and changes in diet and fluid intake. Often, a change in the patient's medications, increased activity during convalescence, or a modification in diet (increased roughage) or fluid intake better serves the patient's needs than ordering a laxative. There are times, however, when laxatives or stool softeners are beneficial and appropriate. Table 25-23 (laxatives and stool softeners) presents the basic agents available.

Diarrhea is another complaint that may be the result of several different causes, including medications (especially broad-spectrum antibiotic agents), changes in diet, and physiologic disturbances. Often practical measures such as adding buttermilk and yogurt to the diet and changing medications eliminate the necessity for drug therapy. In the event medication is required to control the diarrhea, Table 25-24 lists the basic compounds used in treating diarrhea; the list of products employing these in varying combinations would be almost endless. Care should also be exercised to ensure that the patient does not become dehydrated.

Acid indigestion or "heartburn" also may be caused by medications, dietary changes, or by underlying physiologic disturbances. There are many antacid products on the market that should be able to meet the requirements for practically any patient. These are found in Tables 25-25 to 25-27.

Flatulence (gas) is a common and painful complaint in institutionalized patients; air swallowing, postoperative gaseous distention, diet, or medical conditions of the GI tract may be the culprit. The excessive gas may be accompanied by distention and sharp pain. Regardless of the cause, the choices of medicinal therapy are few but generally very effective in relieving the problem (see Table 25-28).

These seven tables present the agents most frequently used to treat the most common gastrointestinal tract problems. However, in many cases medication is not the most appropriate or best solution for the patient's complaint.

## AGENTS FOR THE URINARY TRACT

Urinary tract problems seen most commonly in institutionalized patients are infection (which may be a result of instrumentation, catheterization, or urinary retention or stasis), fluid retention or overload (edema), urinary retention or incontinence (often the result of medications), and urinary pain or burning.

Table 25-29 (miscellaneous urinary tract antiinfectives) and Table 25-30 (sulfonamides and trimethoprim-sulfasoxazole) list the antibiotics and antiinfective agents commonly used in urinary tract infections. Other agents are discussed in the section of this chapter dealing with systemic antibiotics. The effectiveness of many of these agents depends on or may be enhanced by the pH of the urine; agents frequently used to alter the urinary pH are found in Tables 25-33 and 25-34. As with many other patient complaints, too much emphasis cannot be placed on prevention—strict aseptic technique should *always* be used during instrumentation or catheterization.

Fluid retention (edema) may be caused by a variety of problems and is often treated quickly and effectively with diuretics. The potency and side effects of the diuretics vary widely, thus the choice should be made on the basis of the patient's total clinical picture. The agents found in Table 25-31 should allow the physician to fit the agent to the patient's need without creating further problems caused by side effects.

Urinary retention, incontinence, burning, and pain may be secondary to infection or instrumentation and transient but are often very disturbing to the patient as well as annoying. These symptoms may be controlled by the agents listed in Table 25-32. Other agents that may be helpful can be found in Tables 25-33 and 25-34.

## AGENTS FOR DERMATOLOGIC CONDITIONS

Common dermatologic problems encountered in institutionized (especially those confined to bed) patients include chafing, drying, itching, rashes, infections, and decubitus ulcers. These may have a variety of causes, which will be discussed below. As we shall see, the use of medications may not be the solution to those patient problems either.

Rashes may be the result of medications (hypersensitivity or side effect) or allergic responses to food, soap, or other stimuli; itching very often accompanies a rash. The rash or itch may be often successfully "treated" simply by removing the causative agent. Symptomatic treatment involving systemic antihistamines or antipruritics and topical steroids (see Table 25-37) may be employed temporarily either until the causative agent is found or until therapy with a particular medication is completed or an alternate drug chosen.

Topical infections may be caused by bacteria or fungi. There are good topical antibiotics (Table 25-35) and topical antifungal agents (Table 25-36) available to treat local infections. In very severe infections where topical therapy is not sufficient, systemic antibiotic/antifungal therapy should be instituted. As in most instances, prevention should

be emphasized rather than treatment. The practice of proper aseptic technique in changing dressings, wound irrigation and cleaning, and handling of instruments, specimens, and drainage material is paramount in preventing infections. The practice of good personal hygiene and frequent handwashing by the staff and patients can reduce infection, reinfection, and cross-infection among both groups.

Chafing and drying of the skin may occur because of application of casts, immobility, or may be simply a result of the aging process. A variety of products is available to soothe these irritations. Demulcents such as glycerin, propylene glycol, polyethylene glycol, and proprietary ointment bases such as Aquaphor, Polysorb, and Unibase may be used for this purpose. Emollients (fats or oils) such as vegetable oils (olive oil, cottonseed oil, corn oil, etc.), animal fats (lanolin or wool fat) and hydrocarbons (white petrolatum and mineral oil), or products containing these agents may be used effectively as protectives and as agents to soften the skin, prevent drying, and render it more pliable. Dusting powder and mechanical protectives such as collodion preparations, zinc gelatin, and silicone derivatives may also be successfully employed to give the patient good skin care. Good hygiene is of the utmost importance.

Decubitus ulcers (bed sores or pressure sores) are caused by interruption of the blood supply to an area because of pressure and may be hastened by irritation of the skin (urine, feces, etc.), heat or moisture, and by a poor nutritional state, which increases the patient's susceptibility to tissue breakdown. Decubiti are almost always complicated by secondary infections after necrosis and ulceration have occurred. Infections may be treated by the use of topical antibiotics (Table 25-35) or by systemic antibiotics. Actual care and treatment of the decubitus ulcer should consist of: (1) debridement of necrotic tissue either surgically or by the use of enzyme preparations (see Table 25-38), (2) thorough cleansing of the lesion with mild soap solutions, normal saline, or hydrogen peroxide solution; (3) promotion of good circulation by massage, passive exercise, whirlpool, heat lamp, and stimulation of the capillary beds by agents such as Peruvian balsam; (4) proper positioning to avoid further damage to the area; (5) promoting good nutrition including ample intake of protein, vitamins, and minerals (hyperalimentation may be needed in some severely debilitated patients); (6) relieving the pressure on the area by padding bony prominences, frequent turning (preferably every 2 hours), and the use of sheepskin or an alternating air mattress or other devices; and (7) proper supportive therapy if indicated.

Decubiti are most successfully treated by prevention. Prevention measures that should be taken include: (1) proper positioning to avoid friction; (2) frequent turning (every 2 hours is preferable) to avoid undue or extended pressure on any area; (3) promotion of good nutrition by encouraging or feeding the patient; (4) promotion of good circulation; (5) maintaining good hygiene (keeping the skin clean and dry); and (6) thorough examination of the patient to detect any early signs of breakdown or necrosis. The key to prevention is to avoid extended pressure on any of the major pressure points including the iliac spine, sacrum, heels, scapula, ankles, back of the head, or any bony prominence.

## PSYCHOTHERAPEUTIC AGENTS

The two problems most likely to be encountered in the average patient requiring the use of psychotherapeutic agents are anxiety (nervousness and agitation) and depression. It would be a skilled practitioner, indeed, who could keep the patient well enough informed and gain such confidence that all the fears, doubts, and anxieties associated with hospitalization and surgery were allayed. Further, this same "miracle" would have to be repeated during the often long-term convalescent postoperative stay required for many orthopedic patients. The demanding rehabilitative training, pain, mounting medical bills, separation from the family, and the often dull-drabness of hospital routines during long-term hospitalization are some of the factors that contribute to the emotional and psychological problems often experienced by these patients. (Tables 25-39 and 25-40 list the tranquilizers most often employed.) These tables are not by any means complete. We have purposely omitted many potent agents often employed in psychotherapy by psychiatrists whose formal training in this area entitles them to use many agents that should not be employed by the surgeon or general practitioner. These tables are merely the starting point for solving the patient's problems. If the patient's problem is severe or the response to these agents is not satisfactory, it might be wise to consult a qualified psychiatrist.

## DRUG REFERENCE SOURCES FOR THE PROFESSIONAL

All health care professionals should have available an adequate drug reference library and, more importantly, take time to learn what information is available in each volume and how to locate it. Most books purported to be drug information sources also usually contain a section specifically to instruct the reader on how to use the book and what types of information it contains. One should make it a point to read this information carefully and completely as each new volume is added to the library. This type of book is usually well indexed and often cross-indexed to help the reader to use it more efficiently. Many of these books also employ charts or tables to more effectively present drug information that is of importance to all practitioners.

Below are the books we consider to comprise an effective and comprehensive drug reference library. While there is extensive overlapping of information in some of these books, each practitioner should review the type of information contained in each and select the most pertinent.

1. *AMA Drug Evaluations,* AMA Council on Drugs, American Medical Association. Information on old and new single-entity and combination drugs. General information section, discussion of groups of related drugs, brief evaluations of individual drugs. A section of detailed monographs on newer single-entity drugs. Three indexes of information: (a) indications, (b) adverse reactions, and (c) drugs.

2. *American Drug Index.* C. D. Wilson and T. E. Jones. J. B. Lippincott Company. An alphabetized cross-indexed listing of medicinals by chemical, generic, USP and NF synonyms, and brand names. Other information includes manufacturer, pharmaceutical forms, strength, size, dosages, and use.

3. *Clinical Guide to Undesirable Drug Interactions and Interferences.* S. Garb. Springer Publishing Company, Inc. A compilation of data regarding drug interactions or interferences with other drugs, foods, and diagnostic tests. The compilation is in table form and is complete with references.

4. *Current Therapy.* H. F. Conn, editor. W. B. Saunders Company. Contains concise, authoritative information on current treatment. Accurate, concise and detailed therapy of a correctly diagnosed disease state is discussed.

5. *Drugs of Choice.* W. Modell, editor. The C. V. Mosby Company. A practical guide for selection of the best drug for a particular patient's specific therapeutic problem. Includes a single alphabetical up-to-date drug index in tinted paper.

6. *Drug Treatment.* G. S. Avery, editor. Adis Press. Provides information on the use and effects of drugs in disease states, covering (a)

*Text continued on p. 569.*

**Table 25-1.** Preoperative agents: hypnotics and sedatives

| Generic name | Trade name(s) | Dosage form(s) | Strength(s) | Usual dose |
|---|---|---|---|---|
| Chlorpromazine | Chlor PZ | Tablet | 10, 25, 50, 100, 200 mg | *Adults: Oral:* 25-50 mg PO |
| | Promochel | Tablet | 25, 50, 100, 200 mg | 2-3 hr preop. *IM:* 12.5-25 |
| | Promopar | Tablet | 10, 25, 50, 100, 200 mg | mg 1-2 hr Preop. |
| | Sonozine | Tablet | 10, 25, 50, 100, 200 mg | *Children:* 0.25 mg/lb |
| | Thorazine | Tablet | 10, 25, 50, 100, 200 mg | body weight orally |
| | | Spansules | 30, 75, 150, 200, 300 mg | 2-3 hr preop or IM |
| | | Syrup | 10 mg/5 ml | 1-2 hr preop. |
| | | Suppositories | 25, 100 mg | |
| | | Concentrate | 30 mg/ml, 100 mg/ml | |
| | | Injection | 25 mg/ml-1, 2, 10 ml | |
| Diazepam | Valium | Tablet | 2, 5, 10 mg | *Adults:* 10 mg IM preop |
| | | Injection (IM or IV) | 5 mg/ml-2, 10 ml | *Children:* Dose should be adjusted according to age and size. |
| Diphenhydramine | Benadryl | Capsule | 25, 50 mg | *Adults:* 50-100 mg IM. |
| | | Elixir | 12.5 mg/5 ml | *Children:* 1.25 mg/kg IM. |
| | | Injection | 10 mg/ml-10, 3 ml | |
| | | | 50 mg/ml-1, 10 ml | |
| Droperidol* | Inapsine | Injection | 2.5 mg/ml-2, 5, 10 ml | *Adults:* 2.5-10 mg IM ½-1 hr preop. |
| | | | | *Children:* 1.0-1.5 mg/ 20-25 lb IM preop (½-1 hr). |
| Hydroxyzine pamoate | Vistaril | Capsule | 24, 50, 100 mg | *Adults:* 25-100 mg IM. |
| | | Oral suspension | 25 mg/ml | *Children:* 1.25 mg/kg IM. |
| | | Injection | 25 mg/ml-10 ml | |
| | | | 50 mg/ml-2, 10 ml | |
| Propiomazine HCl | Largon | Injection | 20 mg/ml in 1, 2 ml Ampules or Tubex | *Adults:* 20 mg with 50 mg Meperidine IM or IV pre-op. |
| | | | | *Children under 60 lbs:* 0.25 to 0.5 mg/lb body wt. |
| Pentobarbital | Nembutal sodium | Capsules | 22 mg/5 ml | *Adult:* 50-200 mg. |
| | | Gradumet | 100 mg | *Children:* 20-80 mg. |
| | | Elixir | 20 mg/5 ml | |
| | | Suppositories | 30, 50, 120, 200 mg | |
| | | Injection (IM, IV) | 50 mg/ml-2, 5, 20, 50 ml | |
| Promethazine | Fellozine | Injection | 25 mg/ml-10 ml | *Adults:* 50 mg prior to surgery. |
| | | | 50 mg/ml-10 ml | *Children:* 12.5-25 mg. |
| | Ganphen | Injection | 50 mg/ml-10 ml | |
| | Lempro-meth | Injection | 25 mg/ml-10 ml | |
| | | | 50 mg/ml-10 ml | |
| | | Tablets | 25, 50 mg | |
| | Phener-gan | Injection | 25 mg/ml-1 ml (IM, IV) | |
| | | | 50 mg/ml-1 ml (IM only) | |
| | | Tablets | 12.5, 75, 50 mg | |
| | | Syrup | 6.25 mg/5 ml or 25 mg/ 5 ml | |
| | | Suppository | 25, 50 mg | |
| | Provigan | Injection | 25 mg/ml-10 ml | |
| | | | 50 mg/ml-10 ml | |
| | Oudmite | Capsule | 50 mg | |
| | Ramsed | Tablets | 25, 50 mg | |
| | Zipan | Injection | 25 mg/ml-1, 10 ml | |
| | | Tablets | 25, 50 mg | |
| | | Syrup | 12.5 mg/5 ml | |

*Inapsine (droperidol) is a component of Innovar.

| Contraindications | Major side effects | Comments |
| --- | --- | --- |
| Comatose state; in bone marrow depression; hypersensitivity; in presence of large amounts of other CNS depressants. | Drowsiness; jaundice, hematologic disorders; cardiovascular effects; CNS effects; allergic reactions; ocular changes; endocrine disorders; autonomic reactions; neuromuscular reactions. | Also effective for nausea and vomiting; in psychotic and manic depressive states; hiccups; tetanus, acute intermittent porphyria and agitation. Safety in pregnancy has not been established. After long-term therapy cessation may cause withdrawal symptoms. |
| In children under 6 mo. old; psychoses; acute narrow angle glaucoma; hyperactivity. | CNS, GI, GU and cardiovascular disturbances; EENT and dermatologic manifestations. | May also be useful in anxiety states or to promote sleep; in cardioversion; for status epilepticus and in severe convulsing seizures and as a muscle relaxant. Note: Injection should not be mixed with other medications. |
| In premature and newborn infants; hypersensitivity; asthmatic attack; narrow angle glaucoma; prostatic hypertrophy; stenosing peptic ulcer; pyloroduodenal obstruction; concomitant use with MAO inhibitors; bladder-neck obstruction. | CNS and GI disturbances; allergic reactions; GU and circulatory problems; atropine-like side effects. | Also useful in motion sickness; allergic reactions to blood products; in anaphylaxis as adjunct to epinephrine; allergic reactions; Parkinsonism, and as bedtime sedative; use with caution with other CNS depressants; may inhibit lactation in nursing mothers. |
| Hypersensitivity. | Hypotension and tachycardia; CNS disturbances; Parkinson-like side effects; hallucinations; smooth muscle spasms. | Vital signs should be monitored routinely; usage in children under 2 and during pregnancy have not been established; this drug potentiates other CNS drugs. |
| Hypersensitivity; IV, SQ, or intraarterial injection; early pregnancy. | CNS and neurologic disturbances; anticholinergic effects | May also be useful for nausea and vomiting; bedtime sedation; to potentiate analgesics and as antianxiety agent. |
| Hypersensitivity, intra-arterial injection; use of cloudy or precipitated solution. Safety during first trimester of pregnancy has not been established. | Autonomic reactions; cardiovascular effects. | May also be used for sedation during labor. Enhances effects of CNS depressants, i.e., barbiturates and analgesics and their dose should be reduced ¼ to ½. |
| Hypersensitivity to barbiturates; porphyria (even history of). | Allergic reactions; CNS and GI disturbances; respiratory depression; thrombophlebitis; injection site pain; nerve injury adjacent to injection site. | Also useful as bedtime sedative; and for emergency control of certain acute convulsive conditions; may be habit forming; safety in pregnancy has not been established. Use with caution in conjunction with other CNS depressants and if impaired liver function is present. |
| Hypersensitivity; intra-arterial injection. | Autonomic reactions; in rare cases, blood dyscrasias. Some cardiovascular disturbances and photosensitivity | May also be used for adjunct to analgesics; motion sickness, allergic conditions, as a bedtime sedative, as antinauseant-antiemetic and to prevent allergic reactions to blood products. Use with caution in conjunction with CNS depressants. Antiemetic action may mask symptoms of undiagnosed disease. |

**Table 25-2.** Preoperative agents: adjuncts to anesthesia-analgesics

| Generic name | Trade name(s) | Dosage form(s) | Strength(s) | Usual dose |
|---|---|---|---|---|
| Meperidine | Various manufacturers | Injection | 25 mg/ml-1 ml<br>50 mg/ml-1, 30 ml<br>75 mg/ml-1, 1.5 ml<br>100 mg/ml-1, 2, 30, 30 ml | *Adults:* 50-100 mg IM or SQ 30-90 min/prior to anesthesia.<br>*Children:* 0.5-1 mg/lb IM or SQ up to adult 30-90 min/prior to anesthesia. |
| | | Tablets | 50 mg | |
| | Demerol | Injection | 25 mg/ml-0.5, ml<br>50 mg/ml-0.5, 1, 1.5, 2, 3 ml<br>75 mg/ml-1.5 ml<br>100 mg/ml-1, 2, 20 ml | |
| | | Tablets | 50/100 mg | |
| | | Elixer | 50 mg/5 ml (banana flavor) | |
| Morphine | Various manufacturers | Injection | 8 mg/ml-1ml<br>10 mg/ml-1 ml<br>15 mg/ml-1, 20 ml | *Adults:* 8-15 mg IM prior to anesthesia.<br>*Children:* 0.1 to 0.2 mg/kg IM or SQ prior to anesthesia. |
| Fentanyl | Sublimaze | Injection (IM, IV only) | 0.05 mg/ml-2, 5 ml | *Adults:* 0.05-0.1 mg IM 30-60 min prior to surgery.<br>*Children:* 2-12 yr-0.02 to 0.03 mg/20-25 lbs body wt. |
| Petazocine | Talwin | Injection (IM, IV, SQ)<br>Tablet | 30 mg/ml-1, 1.5, 2, 10 ml<br>50 mg | *Adults:* 30-60 mg IM preoperatively. |

| Contraindications | Major side effects | Comments |
|---|---|---|
| Hypersensitivity; concomitant use with MAO inhibitor. Exercise caution with other CNS depressants; in head injury and increased intracranial pressure; in asthma; and during pregnancy and lactation. | CNS, GI, GU, and cardio-vascular disturbances; allergic reactions; irritation at injection site. | Also indicated for relief of moderate to severe pain; for support of anesthesia; and for obstetric analgesia. *Note:* can cause drug dependence. Injection chemically incompatible with barbiturates. |
| Hypersensitivity; concomitant use with MAO inhibitors. Exercise caution with other CNS depressants in head injury and increased intra-cranial pressure; in asthma and during pregnancy and lactation. | CNS, GI, GU, and cardio-vascular disturbances; allergic and dermatologic reactions; pain and irritation at injection site. | Also indicated for severe pain; for sedation and hypnosis; and for dyspneic seizures of acute left ventricular failure and pulmonary edema. *Note:* may be habit forming. |
| Hypersensitivity; concomitant use with MAO inhibitors; in children under 2; in head injuries, increased intracranial pressure, and brain tumors. | CNS, GI, and cardiovascular disturbances; respiratory and neuromuscular reactions; diaphoresis. | Also indicated for analgesic action during induction and maintenance of anesthesia and for analgesia in the immediate postoperative period (Recovery Room). Individualize dose and monitor vital signs routinely. Safety in pregnancy not established. Use with caution in presence of other CNS depressants. May be habit forming. |
| Hypersensitivity; in children under 12 yr; use great caution in head injury or increased intracranial pressure. Safe use in pregnancy has not been established. | GI, CNS, and ophthalmic disturbances; hematologic, respiratory, and cardio-vascular manifestations; GU and autonomic disturbances; allergic local dermatologic problems. | May cause drug dependence. Caution should be exercised in certain respiratory conditions; impaired renal or hepatic function, myocardial infarction; biliary surgery and in patients prone to seizures. Talwin is a mild narcotic antagonist and should be used carefully in patients on methadone maintenance. |

**Table 25-3.** Preoperative agents: adjuncts to anesthesia-anticholinergics

| Generic name | Trade name(s) | Dosage form(s) | Strengths | Usual dose |
|---|---|---|---|---|
| Glycopyrrolate | Robinul | Injection (IM, IV or SQ) | 0.2 mg/ml-1, 5, 20 ml | *Adults:* 0.002 mg/lb body weight and IM 30-60 min/hr prior to induction. *Children up to 12:* 0.002 mg to 0.004 mg/lb body wt IM 30-60 min prior to induction. |
| | | Tablets | 1, 2 mg | |
| Methantheline bromide | Banthine | Injection (IM or IV) | 50 mg | *Adults:* 50-100 mg IM. *Children:* Dosage should be adjusted on the basis of age and weight. |
| | | Tablets | 50 mg | |
| Atropine sulfate | Various manufacturers | Injection | 0.3 mg/ml-1 ml 0.4 mg/ml-0.5, 1, 20, 30 ml 0.5 mg/ml-1, 3 ml 0.6 mg/ml-1 ml 1 mg/ml-1 ml 1.3 mg/ml-1 ml | *Adults:* 0.4-0.6 mg IM with preop medications. *Children:* 0.1-0.4 mg based on body weight up to 90 lb. |
| | | Tablets | 0.4 mg, 0.6 mg | |
| Scopolamine HBr | Various manufacturers | Injection (IM, IV, SQ) | 0.3 mg/ml-1 ml 0.4 mg/ml-0.9, 1 ml 0.6 mg/ml-1 ml (note: dilute for IV use) | *Adults:* 0.3-0.6 mg IM with preop medications. *Children:* 6 mo-3 yr: 0.1-0.15 mg; 3-6 yrs: 0.15 mg-0.2 mg; 6-12 yr: 0.2-0.3 mg. |
| | | Tablets | 0.4 mg, 0.6 mg | |

| Contraindications | Major side effects | Comments |
|---|---|---|
| Hypersensitivity is only absolute contraindication, but caution should be used in glaucoma, asthma, pregnancy, myasthenia gravis, coronary artery disease, congestive heart failure, hypertension and cardiac arrhythmias. | CNS, GI, and GU disturbances; allergic and dermatologic reactions; mydriasis and suppression of lactation. | May also be used intraoperatively for reversal of neuromuscular blockade as adjunctive therapy in gastrointestinal disorders, acute pancreatitis, bilary colic, and to prevent sphincter spasm caused by M.S. Note: neostigmine can be used as an antidote in cases of overdosage. Duration of action approximately 4 hours. |
| Hypersensitivity; glaucoma | Dryness of mouth; blurred vision; respiratory depression with high doses. | May also be useful in the treatment of peptic ulcer and uninhibited hypertonic neurogenic bladder; use with caution in severe cardiac disease and in elderly patients with prostate hypertrophy. |
| Hypersensitivity; glaucoma; adhesions between iris and lens of eye; asthma; obstruction, uropathy, obstructive disease of GI tract; intestinal atony, megacolon complicating ulcerative colitis, myasthenia gravis; unstable cardiovascular status or hemorrhage. Safety in pregnancy not established. | CNS, GI, and GU disturbances; allergic and dermatologic reactions; cardiovascular and visual disturbances; "dryness" due to suppression of secretions; suppression of lactation. | May be used for adjunctive therapy in peptic ulcer, irritable bowel syndrome, neurogenic bowel disturbances, spastic colon, functional GI disorders; as an antispasmodic in genitourinary spastic disorders, as a drying agent. Exercise caution in any condition that may be aggravated by anticholinergic activity of the drug. Neostigmine is antidote for overdosage. The potential for drug interactions is great, and the literature should be reviewed prior to use. |
| Hypersensitivity, glaucoma, adhesions between iris and lens of eye, asthma, obstructive uropathy, obstructive disease of GI tract; intestinal atony; Myasthenia gravis; unstable cardiovascular status or hemorrhage; megacolon complicating ulcerative colitis. Safety in pregnancy not established. | CNS, GI, and GU disturbances; cardiovascular and visual disturbances; allergic and dermatologic reactions; "dryness" due to suppression of secretions; suppression of lactation; amnesia. | Same as above. |

**Table 25-4.** Compatibility of preoperative medications mixed in same syringe

| | Atropine | Chlorpromazine (Thorazine) | Diazepam (Valium) | Diphenhydramine (Benadryl) | Droperidol (Inapsine) | Fentanyl (Sublimaze) | Glycopyrrolate (Robinul) | Hydroxyzine (Vistaril) | Meperidine (Demerol) | Methantheline (Banthine) | Morphine | Pentazocine (Talwin) | Pentobarbital (Nembutal) | Promethazine (Phenergan) | Propiomazine (Largon) | Scopolamine | Secobarbital (Seconal) |
|---|---|---|---|---|---|---|---|---|---|---|---|---|---|---|---|---|---|
| **Atropine** | C | C | X | C | C | C | | | C | | C | C | ? | C | | C | ? |
| **Chlorpromazine (Thorazine)** | C | C | X | | | | ? | C | C | | ? | C | X | C | | C | X |
| **Diazepam (Valium)** | X | X | C | X | X | X | X | X | X | X | X | X | X | X | | X | X |
| **Diphenhydramine (Benadryl)** | C | | X | C | | | | | C | | C | | X | C | X | C | X |
| **Droperidol (Inapsine)** | C | | X | | C | C | C | | | | | | | | | C | |
| **Fentanyl (Sublimaze)** | C | | X | | C | C | C | | | | | | | | | C | |
| **Glycopyrrolate (Robinul)** | | ? | X | | C | C | C | C | C | | C | C | X | | | | X |
| **Hydroxyzine (Vistaril)** | C | C | X | | | | C | C | C | | C | C | | C | | C | X |
| **Meperidine (Demerol)** | C | C | X | C | | | C | C | C | | X | X | C | | | C | X |
| **Methantheline (Banthine)** | | | X | | | | | | | C | | | X | | C | | X |
| **Morphine** | C | ? | X | C | | | C | C | | | C | X | X | C | | C | X |
| **Pentazocine (Talwin)** | C | C | X | | | | C | C | X | | X | C | ? | C | | C | C |
| **Pentobarbital (Nembutal)** | ? | X | X | X | | | | X | X | | X | ? | C | X | | ? | |
| **Promethazine (Phenergan)** | C | C | X | C | | | C | C | | | C | C | X | C | | C | X |
| **Propiomazine (Largon)** | | | X | | | | | C | | | | | | | C | | |
| **Scopolamine** | C | C | X | C | C | C | | C | C | | C | C | ? | C | | C | ? |
| **Secobarbital (Seconal)** | ? | X | X | X | | | X | X | X | | X | X | ? | X | | ? | C |

Key: C, Compatible; X, Incompatible; ?, conflicting reports regarding compatibility; blank, information regarding compatibility unavailable.

pharmacological basis of therapeutics emphasizing pharmacokinetics, (b) rational selection and usage of drugs, (c) the effect of the disease state on drug responses, and (d) drugs as a cause of disease. It has summary tables and appendices for quick reference and correlation of data.

7. *Facts and Comparisons.* E. K. Kastrup. Facts and Comparisons, Inc. Contains monographs on all available U.S. drugs (over 6,000 products) in a format to facilitate rapid comparison. The drug monographs include actions, indications, contraindications, warnings for use, drug interactions, precautions, adverse reactions (side effects), overdosage (toxicity and treatment), administration and dosage information, product listings (brand names, dosage forms, etc.), and a cost index reflecting the ratio of the average wholesale costs for equivalent quantities of different products. Products are listed by therapeutic category and are also alphabetically indexed.

8. *Hazards of Medication.* E. W. Martin. J. B. Lippincott Company. A comprehensive overview of drug interactions, incompatibilities, contraindications, and adverse effects. Features two chapters with extensive tables listing drug interferences with diagnostic laboratory test results and drug interactions with each other.

9. *Manual of Medical Therapeutics.* E. C. Boedeker, and J. H. Dauber, editors. Little, Brown & Company. A general guide to total care of the patient including specific therapy and therapeutic agents for practically all disease states.

10. *Modern Drug Encyclopedia and Therapeutic Index.* A. Jleives, editor. Dunn-Donnelley Publishing Corp. Contains factual data regarding specific medications and classes of therapeutic and diagnostic agents, and alphabetical listings (cross-indexed) with descriptive monographs under generic or trade names (prescription drugs of manufacturers who distribute nationally). Features a glossary of pharmaceutical trade name dosage forms and definitions and the following indices: therapeutic, manufacturer, and general.

11. *The Merck Index.* M. Windholz, editor. Merck and Company. Methods of preparation and properties of chemicals, drugs, and biologicals; correlation of unofficial, generic, and chemical names of compounds with chemical structures, trade names, and manufacturers. Has toxicology, basic pharmacology, and usage of the substances listed.

12. *The Merck Manual.* D. N. Holvey. Merck and Company. A manual of both diagnosis and therapy of disease states; medications are listed by generic name where possible and prescribing information is included.

13. *The Pharmacological Basis of Therapeutics.* S. Goodman and A. Gillman, et al. Macmillan Publishing Co., Inc. Pharmacology and toxicology in therapeutics with emphasis on proved, safe prototype drugs.

**Table 25-5.** Systemic antibiotics: penicillins and cephalosporins

| Generic name | Trade name(s) | Dosage form(s) | Strength | Usual dose* |
|---|---|---|---|---|
| Penicillin G, potassium | Pfizerpen | Injection | 1M, 5M, 20M U* vials | |
| | | Tablets | 200,000; 250,000; 400,000; 800,000 U | |
| | | Powder for solution | 400,000 U/5 ml | *Adults: IM or IV:* 1-80M U/day either individual doses or |
| | Genicilin | Tablets | 400,000 U | by continuous infusion based on |
| | | Powder for solution | 400,000 U/5 ml | disease state and |
| | G-Recillin | Tablet | 400,000 U | patient. *Oral:* |
| | | Powder for solution | 400,000 U/5 ml | 200,000 to 800,000 |
| | K-Cillin | Tablets | 500,000; 1,000,000 U | U q 6-8 hr depending on disease state |
| | | Powder for solution | 250,000 U/5 ml; 500,000 U/5 ml | and patient response. |
| | Kesso-Pen | Tablets | 200,000; 250,000; 400,000 U | *Children and infants:* all doses should be |
| | | Powder for solution | 200,000 U/5 ml; 400,000 U/5 ml | calculated on body wt. Usual range is |
| | Pentid | Tablets | 200,000; 400,000; 800,000 U | 25,000-90,000 U/ kg/day given in 3-6 |
| | | Powder for solution | 200,000 U/5 ml; 400,000 U/5 ml | divided doses. |
| | Palocillin | Tablet | 500,000 U | |
| | | Powder for solution | 400,000 U/5 ml | |
| | Sugracillin | Powder for solution | 125,000 U/5 ml; 250,000 U/5 ml | |
| | Various manufacturers | Injection | 200,000; 500,000, 10M U vials | |
| Penicillin G, sodium | Various manufacturers | Injection | 1,5 MU vials | |
| Penicillin G, procaine | Crysticillin | Injection | 300,000 U/ml-10 ml 500,000 U/ml-1, 2, 12 ml | *By deep IM injection Adults:* 300,000-4,800,000 U IM |
| | Diurnal-Penicillin, Readimixed | Injection | 300,000 U/ml-10 ml 500,000 U/ml-10 ml | daily as single or divided doses. |
| | Duracillin-AS | Injection | 300,000 U/ml-1, 10 ml 500,000 U/ml-2 ml 600,000 U/ml-2 ml | *Children:* dose should be calculated on wt basis and should |
| | Pfizerpen AS | Injection | 300,000 U/ml-10 ml 600,000 U/ml-1, 2 ml | range from 25,000-90,000/kg/day as a |
| | Wycillin | Injection | 300,000 U/ml-1, 10 ml | single or divided |
| | | Injection | 600,000 U/ml-1, 2, 4 ml | dose. |
| Penicillin G, benzathine | Bicillin | Injection, long acting (IM only) | 300,000 U/ml-10 ml 600,000 U/ml-1, 1.5, 2, 4 ml | *Adults:* 1.2 to 2.4 MU as single dose |
| | | Oral suspension | 150,000 U/5 ml-2 oz 300,000 U/5 ml-2 oz | *Children:* dose should be adjusted on basis of weight |
| | | Tablets | 300,000 U | approx. 50,000 U/ |
| | Permapen | Injection (IM only) | 600,000 U/ml-1, 2 ml | kg body weight as single dose. |
| Penicillin V (phenoxymethyl penicillin) | Compacillin V | Chewable wafers | 250 mg | *Adults and Children over 12:* 125-300 |
| | Pen-Vee | Tablet | 300 mg | mg q 6-8 hours for |
| | V-Cillin | Drops | 125 mg/0.6 ml | 10 days or febrile |
| | Various manufacturers | Tablets | 125, 250, 500 mg | times 2 days |
| | | Liquid | 125 mg/5 ml | |
| Penicillin V, potassium | Betapen-VK | Tablets | 250, 500 mg | *Children under 12:* calculate dose on |
| | | Powder for oral solution | 125 mg/5 ml; 250 mg/5 ml | basis of 15-50 mg/ kg daily in 3-6 |
| | Dowpen-VK | Tablets | 250, 500 mg | divided doses. |

*M U, million units.

| Contraindications | Major side effects | Comments |
|---|---|---|
| History of sensitivity to any penicillin. | Hypersensitivity reactions; GI and CNS disturbances; hematologic and renal disturbances; neuropathy; potassium poisoning (with high dose of IV potassium penicillin). Some pain or phlebitis at injection site. | *General:* Use with caution in patients having a history of allergies or asthma. Concurrent use of bacteriostatic antibiotics (tetracycline and erythromycin) may diminish the activity of the drug. Blood levels may be prolonged by administering with Probenecid. Serum levels may be raised by drugs such as aspirin and phenylbutazone, which displace it from its plasma protein binding sites.<br>*Special:* Avoid IV, intraarterial injection, or injection near or into major peripheral nerves or blood vessels to prevent neurovascular damage. This drug is not acid stable or penicillinase resistant. During prolonged therapy, periodic checks of renal, hepatic, and hematopoietic systems are recommended. Observe the patient for bacterial or fungal overgrowth. |
| History of sensitivity to any penicillin or to procaine. | Hypersensitivity reactions; pain and irritation at the injection site. | *General:* Same as above.<br>*Special:* Avoid IV, intraarterial injection, or injection into or near a major peripheral nerves or blood vessels to avoid neurovascular damage. Procaine penicillin G is neither acid stable nor penicillinase resistant. |
| History of hypersensitivity to any penicillin. | Hypersensitivity reactions; hematologic disturbances; neuropathy, nephropathy, and pain at the injection site. | *General:* Same as above.<br>*Special:* Avoid IV or intraarterial injection, or injection into or near major peripheral nerves or blood vessels to avoid neurovascular damage. Benzathine penicillin is neither acid stable nor penicillinase resistant. |
| History of hypersensitivity to any penicillin. | Hypersensitivity reactions; GI disturbances; possible hematologic and renal disturbances and neuropathy. | *General:* Same as above.<br>*Special:* Phenoxymethyl penicillin (penicillin V) is acid stable but not penicillinase resistant. |

*Continued.*

**Table 25-5.** Systemic antibiotics: penicillins and cephalosporins—cont'd

| Generic name | Trade name(s) | Dosage form(s) | Strength(s) | Usual dose |
|---|---|---|---|---|
| | Kesso-pen-VK | Tablets | 250, 500 mg | |
| | | Powder for oral solution | 125 mg/5 ml; 250 mg/5 ml | |
| | Ledevicillin-VK | Tablets | 250, 500 mg | |
| | | Powder for oral solution | 125 mg/5 ml; 250 mg/5 ml | |
| | Penapar VK | Tablets | 250, 500 mg | |
| | | Powder for oral solution | 125 mg/5 ml; 250 mg/5 ml | |
| | Pen-Vee K | Tablets | 125, 250, 500 mg | |
| | | Powder for oral solution | 125 mg/5 ml; 250 mg/5 ml | |
| | Pfizerpen-VK | Tablets | 250, 500 mg | |
| | | Powder for oral solution | 125 mg/5 ml; 250 mg/5 ml | |
| | Repen-VK | Tablets | 250, 500 mg | |
| | | Powder for oral solution | 125 mg/5 ml; 250 mg/5 ml | |
| | Robicillin VK | Tablets | 250 mg, 500 mg | |
| | | Powder for oral solution | 125 mg/5 ml; 250 mg/5 ml | |
| | Ro-Cillin VK | Tablets | 250, 500 mg | |
| | | Powder for oral solution | 125 mg/5 ml; 250 mg/5 ml | |
| | Saropen-VK | Tablets | 250 mg | |
| | | Powder for oral solution | 250 mg/5 ml | |
| | SK-Penicillin-VK | Tablets | 250, 500 mg | |
| | | Powder for oral solution | 125 mg/5 ml; 250 mg/5 ml | |
| | Uticillin VK | Tablets | 250, 500 mg | |
| | | Powder for oral solution | 125 mg/5 ml; 250 mg/5 ml | |
| | V-Cillin K | Tablets | 125, 250, 500 mg | |
| | | Powder for oral solution | 125 mg/5 ml; 250 mg/5 ml | |
| | Veetids | Tablets | 250, 500 mg | |
| | | Powder for oral solution | 125 mg/5 ml, 250 mg/5 ml | |
| Phenethicillin potassium | Maxipen | Tablet | 250 mg (400,000U) | *Adults and children over 12:* 125-250 mg PO q 6-8 hr × 10 days or until afebrile × 2 days. |
| | Syncillin | Tablet | 250 mg (400,000U) | *Children under 12:* Dosage should be calculated on basis of 12.5-50 mg/kg/day in 3 to 6 divided doses. |
| Methicillin sodium | Azapen | Injection | 1, 4, 6 g vials | *Adults:* IM: 1 g 4-6 IV: 1 g q 6 hr. |
| | Celbenin | Injection | 1, 2, 4, 6 g vials | *Infants and children:* IM: 25 mg/kg q 6 hr. |
| | Staphcillin | Injection | 1, 4, 6 g vials | IV: Because of insufficient data, there are no specific recommendations. |

| Contraindications | Major side effects | Comments |
|---|---|---|
| Hypersensitivity to any penicillin. | Hypersensitivity reactions; GI disturbances; hematologic disturbances; nephropathy; neuropathy. | *General:* Same as above.<br>*Special:* The possibility of bacterial or fungal superinfection should be noted. Phenethicillin is acid stable but not penicillinase resistant. |
| Hypersensitivity to any penicillin; safe usage during pregnancy has not been established. | Hypersensitivity reactions; GI disturbances; hematologic renal disturbances; neuropathy; pain or irritation at the injection site; phlebitis. | *General:* Same as above.<br>*Special:* The possibility of bacterial or fungal overgrowth should be noted. Methicillin is penicillinase resistant but not acid stable. May be given by IV push (slowly) after proper dilution or by IV drip in a variety of IV solutions. |

*Continued.*

**Table 25-5.** Systemic antibiotics: penicillins and cephalosporins—cont'd

| Generic name | Trade name(s) | Dosage form(s) | Strength(s) | Usual dose |
|---|---|---|---|---|
| Nafcillin sodium | Nafcil | Injection | 0.5, 1 and 2 g vials | *Adults:* IV: 500 mg-1 g q 4 hr. |
| | Unipen | Injection | 0.5, 1, g and 2 g vials | IM: 500 mg q 4-6 hr |
| | | Capsules | 250 mg | Oral: 250 mg-1 g q |
| | | Tablets | 500 mg | 4-6 hr. |
| | | Powder for oral solution | 250 mg/5 ml | *Children: IV:* no recommendations for use in infants and neonates. Children should be calculated on basis of adult dose. *IM (infants and children):* 25 mg/kg bid *Neonates:* mg/kg bid. *Oral (children and infants):* 24-50 mg/kg/ day in 4 divided doses. *Neonates:* 10 mg/kg 3-4 times daily. |
| Oxacillin | Bactocill | Capsules | 250, 500 mg | *Adults and children over 40 kg: Oral:* 50 |
| | | Injection | 1, 2, 4 g vial | mg-1 g q 4-6 hr for |
| | Prostaphlin | Capsules | 250, 500 mg | at least 5 days. |
| | | Injection | 250, 500 mg; 1, 2, 4 g vial | *Parenteral:* 250 mg-1 g q 4-6 hr. |
| | | Powder for oral solution | 250 mg/5 ml | *Children under 40 kg: Oral:* 50-100 mg/kg/day for at least 5 days. *Parenteral:* 50-100 mg/ kg/day in equal doses of 4-6 hr. *Neonates:* 25 mg/ kg/day in equal doses of 6 hr. |
| Cloxacillin sodium | Cloxapen | Capsule | 250, 500 mg | *Adults and children over 20 kg:* 250- |
| | Tegopen | Capsule | 250, 500 mg | 500 mg 2 6 hr. |
| | | Powder for oral solution | 125 mg/5 ml | *Children less than 20 kg:* 50 to 100 mg/kg/day in equal doses q 6 hr. Dose should be given on an empty stomach. |
| Dicloxacillin sodium | Dycill | Capsule | 250, 500 mg | *Adults and children over 40 kg:* 125- |
| | Dynapen | Capsule | 125, 250 mg | 500 mg PO q 6 hr. |
| | | Powder for oral suspension | 62.5 mg/5 ml | *Children under 40 kg:* |
| | Pathocil | Capsule | 250 mg | 25-50 mg/kg/day |
| | | Powder for oral suspension | 62.5 mg/5ml | in equal doses q 6 hr. Dose should be given on an empty stomach. Due to lack of data, no neonatal dose is recommended. |

| Contraindications | Major side effects | Comments |
|---|---|---|
| History of sensitivity to any penicillin; safe use during pregnancy has not been established. | Hypersensitivity reactions; GI disturbances; pain and irritation at the injection site; thrombophlebitis; possible hematologic, renal and CNS disturbances; neuropathy. | *General:* Same as above.<br>*Special:* The possibility of bacterial or fungal overgrowth should be noted. Nafcillin is both acid stable and penicillinase resistant. Nafcillin may be given by direct IV push (over 5-10 minutes) or by IV infusion when diluted in several commonly available IV solutions. |
| History of sensitivity to any penicillin; safe use in pregnancy has not been established. | Hypersensitivity reactions; GI disturbances; hematologic and renal disturbances; neuropathy; pain and irritation at injection site; thrombophlebitis. | *General:* Same as above.<br>*Special:* The possibility of bacterial or fungal overgrowth should be noted. Oxacillin is both acid stable and penicillinase resistant. Oxacillin may be given by direct IV push (over 10 minutes) or by IV drip in a variety of commonly available IV solutions. During long-term therapy, periodic assessment of renal, hepatic, and hematopoietic function should be done. |
| History of sensitivity to any penicillin; safe use during pregnancy has not been established. | Hypersensitivity reactions; GI disturbances; possible hematologic and renal disturbances and neuropathy. | *General:* Same as above.<br>*Special:* The possibility of bacterial or fungal overgrowth should be noted. Cloxacillin is both acid stable and penicillinase resistant. During long-term therapy, periodic assessment of renal, hepatic, and hematopoietic function should be done. |
| History of sensitivity to any penicillin; safe use in pregnancy has not been established. | Hypersensitivity reactions; GI disturbances; possible hematologic and renal disturbances. | *General:* Same as above.<br>*Special:* The possibility of bacterial or fungal overgrowth should be noted. Dicloxacillin is both acid stable and penicillinase resistant. During long-term therapy, periodic assessment of renal, hepatic, and hematopoietic function should be done. |

*Continued.*

**Table 25-5.** Systemic antibiotics: penicillins and cephalosporins—cont'd

| Generic name | Trade name(s) | Dosage form(s) | Strength(s) | Usual dose |
|---|---|---|---|---|
| Ampicillin | Alpen | Injection | 250, 500 mg; 1 g vials | *Adults: Oral:* 250, 500 mg q 6 h. |
| | | Capsule | 250, 500 mg | *Parenteral* doses |
| | | Powder for oral suspension | 125 mg/5 ml; 250 mg/5 ml | range from 2-16 Gm/day usually |
| | Amcill | Injection | 125, 250, 500 mg; 1 g vial | given in equal doses at 6 hr |
| | | Tablet (chewable) | 125 mg | intervals. |
| | | Capsule | 250 mg, 500 mg | *Children: Oral:* 50- |
| | | Powder for oral suspension | 125 mg/5 ml; 250 mg/5 ml | 100 mg/kg/day given in equal |
| | | Pediatric drops | 100 mg/ml | doses at 6-8 hr |
| | Ampi-Co | Capsules | 250 mg, 500 mg | intervals. |
| | | Powder for oral suspension | 125 mg/5 ml; 250 mg/5 ml | *Parenteral:* 50-250 mg/kg/day in equal |
| | Omnipen | Injection | 125, 250, 500 mg; 1, 2 g vial | doses at 6 hr intervals. |
| | | Capsules | 250, 500 mg | |
| | | Powder for oral suspension | 125 mg/5 ml; 250 mg/5 ml; 500 mg/5 ml | |
| | | Pediatric drops | 100 mg/ml | |
| | Pen-A | Injection | 250, 500 mg; 1 g vial | |
| | | Capsules | 250, 500 mg | |
| | | Powder for oral suspension | 125 mg/5 ml; 250 mg/5 ml | |
| | Penbritin | Injection | 125, 250, 500 mg; 1, 2 g vial | |
| | | Capsules | 250, 500 mg | |
| | | Powder for oral suspension | 125 mg/5 ml; 250 mg/5 ml | |
| | | Pediatric drops | 100 mg/ml | |
| | Pensyn | Capsules | 250, 500 mg | |
| | | Powder for oral suspension | 125 mg, 5 ml; 250 mg/5 ml | |
| | Polycillin | Injection | 125, 250, 500 mg; 1, 2, g vial | |
| | | Capsules | 250, 500 mg | |
| | | Powder for oral suspension | 125 mg/5 ml; 250 mg/5 ml; 500 mg/5 ml | |
| | | Pediatric drops | 100 mg/ml | |
| | | Tablet (chewable) | 125 mg | |
| | Principen | Injection | 125, 250, 500 mg; 1, 2 g vial | |
| | | Capsules | 250, 500 mg | |
| | | Powder for oral suspension | 125 mg/5 ml; 250 mg/5 ml | |
| | Saramp | Capsules | 250, 500 mg | |
| | SK Ampicillin | Injection | 500 mg vial | |
| | | Capsules | 250, 500 mg | |
| | | Powder for oral suspensions | 125 mg/5 ml; 250 mg/5 ml | |
| | | Tablet (chewable) | 100 mg/ml | |
| | Supen | Capsules | 250, 500 mg | |
| | | Powder for oral suspension | 125 mg/5 ml; 250 mg/5 ml | |
| | Totacillin | Injection | 125, 250, 500 mg; 1, 2, 4, 10 g vial | |
| | | Capsules | 250, 500 mg | |
| | | Powder for oral suspension | 125 mg/5 ml; 250 mg/5 ml | |

| Contraindications | Major side effects | Comments |
|---|---|---|
| History of hypersensitivity to any penicillin; safe usage during pregnancy has not been established. | Hypersensitivity reactions; GI disturbances; hepatic and hematologic disturbances; pain at injection site; thrombophlebitis. | *General:* Same as above.<br>*Special:* The possibility of bacterial or fungal overgrowth should be noted. Ampicillin is acid stable but not penicillinase resistant and has an extended spectrum of activity. Ampicillin may be given IM, by direct IV push (up to doses of 2 g) over 10-15 min or by IV infusion in a variety of available IV solutions. Note: With high concentrations in the urine Ampicillin may give a false positive glucose with Clinitest and Benedict's or Fehling's solutions. Therefore, Tes-Tape or Clinistix should be used. During long-term therapy, periodic assessment of renal, hepatic, and hematopoietic function should be done. |

*Continued.*

**Table 25-5.** Systemic antibiotics: penicillins and cephalosporins—cont'd

| Generic name | Trade name(s) | Dosage form(s) | Strength(s) | Usual dose |
|---|---|---|---|---|
| Amoxicillin | Amoxil | Capsules | 250, 500 mg | *Adults: Oral:* 250-50 mg q 8 hr. |
| | | Powder for oral suspension | 125 mg/5 ml; 250 mg/5 ml | *Children less than 20 kg:* 20-40 mg/kg/ |
| | | Pediatric drops | 5 mg/ml | day in equal doses at 8 hr intervals |
| | Larotid | Capsules | 250, 500 mg | |
| | | Powder for oral suspension | 125 mg/5 ml; 250 mg/5 ml | |
| | | Pediatric drops | 50 mg/ml | |
| | Polymox | Capsules | 250, 500 mg | |
| | | Powder for oral suspension | 125 mg/5 ml; 250 mg/5 ml | |
| | | Pediatric drops | 50 mg/ml | |
| Carbenicillin disodium | Geopen | Injection | 1, 2, 5, 10 g vials | *Adults: Oral:* 1 or 2 tablets q 6 hr. *IV:* 4- |
| | Pyopen | Injection | 1, 2, 5, 10 g vials | 40 g in equal doses |
| Carbenicillin Indanyl/Sodium | Geocillin | Tablet | 382 mg | at 4-6 hr intervals. *IM:* not to exceed 2 g at 4-6 hr intervals. *Children: Oral:* no recommended dose. *IM.* 50-200 mg/kg/day in divided doses q 4-6 hr preferably in the midlateral thigh. *IV:* 50-500 mg/kg/day in divided doses or by continuous drip. |
| Tricarcillin disodium | Ticar | Injection | 1, 3, 6 g vials | *Adults: IV:* 1-6 g at 3, 4, or 6 hr intervals. *IM:* not to exceed 2 g per dose at 6-8 hr intervals. *Children under 40 kg: IV:* 50-30 mg/kg/ day in divided doses every 4-8 hr. *IM:* 50-100 mg/kg/ day in divided doses q 6-8 hr. *Note:* If renal insufficiency is present all doses should be adjusted based on patient's creatinine clearance. |
| Cephalothin, sodium | Keflin | Injection | 1, 2, 4, 20g vials | *Adults:* 0.5-2g q4-6 hr; IV or deep 1M. *Infants and children:* 80-160 mg/kg daily in divided doses at 4-6 hr intervals based on patient's age and condition. *Note:* Dosage should be reduced in patients with renal impairment. |

| Contraindications | Major side effects | Comments |
|---|---|---|
| History of hypersensitivity to any penicillin; safe usage during pregnancy has not been established. | Hypersensitivity reactions; GI and hepatic disturbances; hematologic disturbances. | *General:* Same as above.<br>*Special:* The possibility of bacterial or fungal overgrowth should be noted. Amoxicillin is acid stable but not penicillinase resistant and has an extended spectrum. |
| History of hypersensitivity to any penicillin; safe usage during pregnancy has not been established. | Hypersensitivity reactions; GI disturbances; CNS and hematologic disturbances; pain at injection site; vein irritation and phlebitis; abnormal coagulation tests; hypokalemia and possible hepatic and renal disturbances. | *General:* Same as above.<br>*Special:* During long-term therapy, periodic assessment of renal, hepatic, and hematopoietic function should be done. Carbenicillin is acid stable but not penicillinase resistant and possesses an extended spectrum. *Note:* Carbenicillin may exhibit a synergistic effect with gentamicin when used in combination against *Pseudomonas* infections but should not be mixed in the same IV solution. |
| History of hypersensitivity to any penicillin; safe usage during pregnancy has not been established. | Hypersensitivity reactions; GI disturbances; CNS and hematologic disturbances; abnormalities in blood, renal, and hepatic laboratory studies; pain and irritation at injection site; vein irritation and phlebitis; hypokalemia. | *General:* Use with caution in patients having a history of allergies or asthma or those on sodium restriction. Concurrent use of bacteriostatic antibiotics (tetracycline and erythromycin) may diminish activity. Blood levels are prolonged by Probenecid. Drugs such as aspirin and phenylbutazone raise serum levels by displacing this drug from its binding sites. During long-term therapy periodic assessment of renal, hepatic, and hematopoietic functions should be done. This drug has an extended spectrum but is neither acid stable nor penicillinase resistant. Ticarcillin may exhibit a synergistic effect with gentamicin against *Pseudomonas* infections, but the two *should not be* combined in the same IV solution. |
| Hypersensitivity to any cephalosporin antibiotic. Safe usage during pregnancy has not been established. | Hypersensitivity reactions; GI disturbances; hepatic and renal disturbances; hematologic disturbances; pain with induration at IM injection site; phlebitis. | *General:* Exercise caution in patients with a history of allergies, penicillin sensitivity and renal impairment. This drug may give a false positive reaction for glucose with Clinitest tablets and Benedict's and Fehling's solutions; thus use of Tes-Tape or Clinistix is recommended. Avoid concurrent use of bacteriostatic agents. Probenecid prolongs and increases plasma levels of this drug. Concomitant use of markedly nephrotoxic agents and/or potent "loop diuretics" such as fusosemide and ethacrynic acid may enhance the possibility of nephrotoxicity. |

*Continued.*

**Table 25-5.** Systemic antibiotics: penicillins and cephalosporins—cont'd

| Generic name | Trade name(s) | Dosage form(s) | Strength(s) | Usual dose |
|---|---|---|---|---|
| Cephalothin, sodium—cont'd | | | | |
| Cephaloridine | Loridine | Injection | 250, 500 mg; 1 g vial | *Adults:* 500 mg-1 g IV or IM q 8 h<br>*Children:* 30-50 mg/kg daily in 3 divided doses at 8 hr intervals.<br>*Note:* Dosage should be reduced in patients with renal impairment. |
| Cephalexin | Keflex | Capsules<br>Tablet<br>Oral suspension<br><br>Pediatric drops | 250, 500 mg<br>1 g<br>125 mg/5 ml; 250 mg/5 ml<br>100 mg/ml | *Adults:* 250 mg-1 g PO q 6 h<br>*Children:* 25-50 mg/kg daily in divided doses q 6 hr. |
| Cefazolin sodium | Ancef<br><br>Kefzol | Injection<br><br>Injection | 250, 500 mg; 1, 5, 10 g vial<br>250, 500 mg; 1, 10 g vial | *Adults:* 0.5-1 g IV or IM q 6-8 hr.<br>*Children:* 25-100 mg/kg/day in divided doses q 6-8 hr IM or IV.<br>*Note:* Dosage should be reduced in patients with renal impairment. |
| Cephradine | Anspor<br><br><br>Velosef | Capsule<br>Oral suspension<br><br>Capsule<br>Injection<br><br>Oral suspension | 250, 500 mg<br>125 mg/5 ml; 250 mg/5 ml<br>250, 500 mg<br>250, 500 mg; 1, 2, 4 g vials<br>125 mg/5 ml; 250 mg/5 ml | *Adults: Oral:* 250-500 mg qid *Parenteral:* 2-4 g IM or IV in 4 equally divided doses.<br>*Children and infants: Oral:* 25-100 mg/kg/day in 4 equally divided doses. *Parenteral:* 50-100 mg/kg/day in 4 equally divided doses.<br>*Note:* Dosage should be reduced in patients with renal impairment. |
| Cephapirin sodium | Cefadyl | Injection (IM or IV) | 1, 2, 4, 20 g vial | *Adults:* 500 mg-1 g IM or IV q 4-6 hr.<br>*Children:* 40-80 mg/kg daily in 4 equally divided doses.<br>*Note:* Dosage should be reduced in patients with renal impairment. |

| Contraindications | Major side effects | Comments |
|---|---|---|
| | | *Special:* Cephalothin has an extended spectrum including many gram-positive and some gram-negative organisms. *Note:* Superinfections due to overgrowth of nonsusceptible organisms may occur. |
| Hypersensitivity to any cephalosporin antibiotic; safe usage during pregnancy has not been established. | Hypersensitivity reactions; GI disturbances; renal and hepatic disturbances; hematologic disturbances. | *General:* Same as above. *Special:* Cephaloridine has an extended spectrum including many gram-positive and some gram-negative organisms. |
| Hypersensitivity to any cephalosporin antibiotic; safe usage during pregnancy has not been established. | Hypersensitivity reactions; GI disturbances; renal and hepatic disturbances; hematologic disturbances. | *General:* Same as above. |
| Hypersensitivity to any cephalosporin antibiotic; safe usage during pregnancy and in prematures and infants under one mo of age has not been established. | Hypersensitivity reactions; GI and hematologic disturbances; hepatic and renal disturbances; pain at the injection site IM and thombophlebitis IV. | *General:* Same as above. |
| Hypersensitivity to any cephalosporin antibiotic; safe usage during pregnancy and in prematures and infants under 1 yr of age has not been established. | Hypersensitivity reactions; GI and hematologic disturbances; hepatic and renal disturbances; pain on IM injection and thrombophlebitis IV. | *General:* Same as above. |
| Hypersensitivity to any cephalosporin antibiotic; safe usage during pregnancy and in premature infants and those under 3 mo of age has not been established. | Hypersensitivity reactions; GI and hematologic disturbances; hepatic and renal disturbances; pain at IM and thrombophlebitis at IV injection sites. | *General:* Same as above. |

**Table 25-6.** Systemic antibiotics: the aminoglycosides

| Generic name | Trade name(s) | Dosage form(s) | Strength(s) | Usual dose |
|---|---|---|---|---|
| Amikacin sulfate | Amikin | Injection | 100, 500 mg; 1 g vial | *IM:* 15 mg/kg/day in equally divided doses q 8 or 12 hr. *IV:* Same as IM dose. *Note:* dosage should be reduced in patients with renal impairment. |
| Gentamicin | Garamycin | Injection<br>Pediatric injection | 80 mg vial; 60, 80 mg syringes; 20 mg vials | *Adults:* IM or IV: 3 mg/kg/day in 3 equal doses of 8 hr *Children:* IM or IV: 6-7.5 mg/kg/day in 3 equal doses q 8 hr. *Infants and neonates:* IM or IV: 7.5 mg/kg/day in 3 equal doses q 8 hr. *Note:* Dosage should be reduced in patients with renal impairment. |
| Kanamycin sulfate | Kantrex | Injection<br>Pediatric injection | 0.5, 1 g vial<br>75 mg vial | *Adults and children:* IM: Should not exceed 7.5 mg/kg q 12 hr. IV: Should not exceed 15 mg/kg/day and must be given slowly. |
| Neomycin sulfate | Mycifradin | Injection | 0.5 g vial | *Adults:* 15 mg/kg/day divided in 4 equally spaced doses by *IM injection only.* *Note:* Dosage should be reduced in patients with renal impairment. |
| Streptomycin | Various manufacturers | Injection | 1, 5 g vial | *Adults:* IM: 0.5-1 g bid q 6 hr. *Children:* IM: 20 to 40 mg/kg daily in divided doses q 6-12 hr. |
| Tobramycin | Nebcin | Injection<br>Pediatric injection | 80 mg vial; 60, 80 mg syringes<br>20 mg vial | *Adults, children, and older infants:* IM or IV: 3-5 mg/kg/day in equal doses q 6-8 hr. *Note:* Dose should be reduced in patients with renal impairment. |

| Contraindications | Major side effects | Comments |
|---|---|---|
| Hypersensitivity to or previous toxicity to any aminoglycoside; safe usage during pregnancy and lactation has not been established. | Ototoxicity; hypersensitivity reactions; nephrotoxicity; neurotoxic effects; pain at injection site; vein irritation. | *General:* Superinfections caused by overgrowth of nonsusceptible organisms may occur. Concurrent or sequential use with other nephrotoxic, neurotoxic, and/or ototoxic agents should be avoided if possible. *Special:* Use with potent diuretics should be avoided if possible. |
| Hypersensitivity to or previous toxicity to gentamicin or other aminoglycosides; safe usage during pregnancy has not been established. | Nephrotoxicity; neurotoxicity; hypersensitivity reactions; possible ototoxicity; pain at injection site; vein irritation. | *General:* Same as above. *Special:* Use with potent diuretics should be avoided if possible. Gentamicin has a synergistic effect with carbenicillin when used against *Pseudomonas* infections. Advanced age and dehydration may enhance toxicity. |
| Hypersensitivity or previous toxicity to kanamycin or other aminoglycosides; long-term therapy, safe usage during pregnancy have not been established. | Nephrotoxicity, neurotoxicity; hypersensitivity reactions; ototoxicity; pain and irritation at the IM injection site. | *General:* Same as above. *Special:* Use with potent diuretics should be avoided if possible. Advanced age and dehydration may enhance toxicity. Kanamycin has been used topically, intraperitoneally, and in aerosols. |
| Hypersensitivity or previous toxicity to neomycin; use in children and infants, and safe usage during pregnancy have not been established. | Nephrotoxicity; ototoxicity; neurotoxicity; hypersensitivity reactions. | *General:* Same as above. *Special:* Neomycin should be reserved for cases in which no other antimicrobial agent is effective. |
| Hypersensitivity or previous toxicity to streptomycin or other aminoglycosides; safe usage during pregnancy has not been established. | Ototoxicity; hypersensitivity reactions; neurotoxicity; hepatotoxicity; nephrotoxicity; hematologic disturbances; pain at injection site. | *General:* Same as above. *Special:* Particular caution should be used in dosing children to prevent overdosage. |
| Hypersensitivity or previous toxicity to tobramycin or other aminoglycosides; safe usage during pregnancy has not been established. | Ototoxicity, nephrotoxicity, neurotoxicity, hypersensitivity reactions, hematologic disturbances, pain at injection site, thrombophlebitis and vein irritation. | *General:* Same as above. |

**Table 25-7.** Systemic antibiotics: tetracyclines and chloramphenicol

| Generic name | Trade name(s) | Dosage form(s) | Strength(s) | Usual dose |
|---|---|---|---|---|
| Chloramphenicol | Amphicol<br>Chloromycetin | Capsule<br>Capsule<br>Oral suspension<br>Injection | 250 mg<br>50, 100, 250 mg<br>150 mg/5 ml<br>500 mg ampule; 1 g vial | *Adults:* 50-100 mg/kg/day in divided doses at 6 hr intervals. |
| | Mychel | Capsule<br>Injection | 250 mg<br>1 g vial | *Children:* 50-100 mg/kg/day in divided doses at 6 hr intervals.<br>*Note:* Dose should be reduced in patients with hepatic or renal impairment and in infants and children with immature metabolic processes. |
| Demeclocycline | Declomycin | Capsule<br>Tablet<br>Syrup<br>Pediatric drops | 150 mg<br>75, 150, 300 mg<br>75 mg/5 ml<br>60 mg/ml | *Adults:* 150 mg qid or 300 mg bid.<br>*Children:* 3 to 6 mg/lb/day in 2 or 4 divided doses. |
| Doxycycline | Doxy-II<br>Doxychol | Capsule<br>Oral suspension<br>Capsule<br>Oral suspension | 50, 100 mg<br>25 mg/5 ml<br>5, 100 mg<br>25 mg/5 ml | *Adults:* IV: 100-200 mg daily.<br>Oral: 200 mg 1st day then 100 mg daily |
| | Vibramycin | Capsule<br>Injection (IV)<br>Syrup<br>Oral suspension | 50, 100 mg<br>100, 200 mg vials<br>50 mg/5 ml<br>25 mg/5 ml | *Children under 100 lbs: IV:* 2 mg/lb day 1 then 1-2 mg/lb daily. *Oral:* 2 mg/lb day 1, then 1-2 mg/lb daily. |
| Methacycline | Rondomycin | Capsule<br>Syrup | 150, 300 mg<br>75 mg/5 ml | *Adult:* 150 mg qid or 300 mg bid.<br>*Children:* 3-6 mg/lb body weight daily divided in 2 or 4 equally spaced doses. |
| Minocycline | Minocin<br>Vectrin | Capsule<br>Injection<br>Syrup<br>Capsule<br>Syrup<br>Injection | 50, 100 mg<br>100 mg vial<br>50 mg/5 ml<br>50, 100 mg<br>50 mg/5 ml<br>100 mg vial | *Adult:* 200 mg initially then 100 mg q 12 hr or 50 mg qid.<br>*Children:* 4 mg/kg initially, then 2 mg/kg q 12 hr. |
| Oxytetracycline | Oxlopar<br>Oxybiotic<br>Oxy-Kesso-Tetra<br>Oxy-Tetrachel | Capsule<br>Capsule<br>Capsule<br>Capsule | 250 mg<br>250 mg<br>250 mg<br>250 mg | *Adult: IM:* 250-900 mg daily. *IV:* 250-500 mg up to q 6 hr.<br>*Oral:* 1-2 g daily in 4 equal doses. |

| Contraindications | Major side effects | Comments |
|---|---|---|
| History of previous sensitivity and/or toxicity to chloramphenicol; safe usage during pregnancy and lactation has not been established. | Blood dyscrasias; GI reactions; hypersensitivity reactions; neurotoxic reactions and gray syndrome in prematures and neonates. | Adequate blood studies should be done during treatment. Superinfection due to overgrowth of nonsusceptible organisms may occur. Repeated courses of the drug and use with other drugs that may cause bone marrow depression should be avoided. Parenteral form may be given IV only by direct injection or IV drip. |
| Hypersensitivity to any tetracycline; usage during last half of pregnancy and in children and infants to age of 8 years unless other suitable drugs are contraindicated. | GI disturbances; renal toxicity; hypersensitivity reactions; hematologic disturbances; dermatologic disturbances; discoloration of teeth in infants, children, and fetuses born to mothers taking this drug. | *General:* Superinfection due to overgrowth of nonsusceptible organisms may occur. Concomitant therapy with bactericidal antibiotics or with antacids should be avoided. Food and dairy products may interfere with absorption. Tetracyclines may require adjustment of anticoagulant does. *Special:* Photosensitivity may occur. |
| Hypersensitivity to any tetracycline; usage during last half of pregnancy and in infants and children to age 8 yr unless other suitable drugs are contraindicated. | GI disturbances; renal toxicity; hypersensitivity reactions; hematologic disturbances; discoloration of the teeth (permanent) during tooth development, including fetus; vein irritation with IV form. | *General:* Same as above. *Special:* Dosage and frequency of administration differs markedly from other tetracyclines. |
| Hypersensitivity to any tetracycline; usage during last half of pregnancy and in children and infants to 8 years of age unless other suitable drugs are contraindicated. | GI disturbances; renal toxicity; hypersensitivity reactions; dermatologic disturbances; hematologic disturbances; permanent discoloration of the teeth during tooth development, | *General:* Same as above. |
| Hypersensitivity to any tetracycline; usage during pregnancy and during tooth development unless other suitable drugs are contraindicated. | GI disturbances; hypersensitivity reactions; renal toxicity; dermatologic disturbances; hematologic disturbances; permanent discoloration of the teeth during tooth development; CNS disturbances; pain at injection site. | *General:* Same as above. *Special:* Photosensitivity may occur. |
| Hypersensitivity to any tetracycline; usage during pregnancy and during tooth development unless other suitable agents are contraindicated. | GI disturbances; hypersensitivity reactions; renal toxicity; dermatologic disturbances; hematologic disturbances; permanent discoloration of the teeth during tooth development;. | *General:* Same as above. *Special:* Same as above. |

*Continued.*

**Table 25-7.** Systemic antibiotics: tetracyclines and chloramphenicol—cont'd

| Generic name | Trade name(s) | Dosage form(s) | Strength(s) | Usual dose |
|---|---|---|---|---|
| | Terramycin | Capsule | 125, 250 mg | *Children:* IM: 15-25 |
| | | Tablet | 250 mg | mg/kg/day as |
| | | Syrup | 125 mg/5 ml | single or divided |
| | | Pediatric drops | 100 mg/ml | doses. *IV:* 12 mg/ |
| | | Injection (IM) | 50 mg/ml in 2, 10 | kg/day in 2 di- |
| | | | ml vials; 125 mg/ml | vided doses. *Oral:* |
| | | | in 2 ml vials | 25-50 mg/kg/day |
| | | | | in 4 equal doses. |
| Tetracycline | Achromycin | Injection (IV) | 250, 500 mg vials | *Adult: Oral:* 1-2 g |
| | | Capsule | 100, 250, 500 mg | daily in 2 or 4 equal |
| | | Injection (IM) | 100, 250 mg vial | doses. *IM:* 250 mg |
| | | Injection (IV) | 250, 500 mg vial | daily or 300 mg |
| | | Oral suspension | 250 mg/5 ml | daily in 2 or 3 |
| | | Syrup | 125 mg/5 ml | doses at 8-12 hr |
| | | Pediatric drops | 100 mg/ml | intervals. *IV:* 250- |
| | Bristacycline | Capsule | 250, 500 mg | 500 mg q 12 hr. not |
| | Centet | Capsule | 250 mg | to exceed 500 mg |
| | Cyclopar | Capsule | 250, 500 mg | q 6 hr. |
| | Fed-Mycin | Capsule | 250, 500 mg | *Children: Oral:* 25-50 |
| | G-Mycin | Capsule | 250, 500 mg | mg/kg/day in 4 |
| | Kesso- | Capsule | 250, 500 mg | equal doses. *IM:* |
| | Tetra | Syrup | 125 mg/5 ml | 15-25 mg/kg/day |
| | Lemtrex | Capsule | 250 mg | up to 250 mg daily. |
| | Maytrex | Capsule | 250, 500 mg | *IV:* 12 mg/kg/day |
| | Nortet 500 | Capsule | 500 mg | divided in 2 doses |
| | Paltet | Capsule | 250 mg | *Note:* Dosage |
| | Panmycin | Capsule | 250 mg | should be reduced |
| | | Tablet | 250, 500 mg | in patients with |
| | | Syrup | 125 mg/5 ml | renal impairment. |
| | | Pediatric drops | 100 mg/ml | |
| | | Injection (IM) | 100 mg vial | |
| | | Injection (IV) | 250, 500 mg vial | |
| | Piracaps | Capsule | 500 mg | |
| | Retet | Capsule | 250, 500 mg | |
| | | Capsule | 250, 500 mg | |
| | | Syrup | 125 mg/5 ml | |
| | Ro-Cycline | Capsule | 250, 500 mg | |
| | Sarocycline | Capsule | 250, 500 mg | |
| | SK-Tetracycline | Capsule | 250, 500 mg | |
| | | Syrup | 125 mg/5 ml | |
| | Sumycin | Capsule | 250, 500 mg | |
| | | Syrup | 125 mg/5 ml | |
| | | Tablet | 250, 500 mg | |
| | Steclin | Injection (IM) | 250 mg vial | |
| | Tetrachel | Capsule | 125, 250, 500 mg | |
| | | Tablet | 250 mg | |
| | | Syrup | 125 mg/5 ml | |
| | | Pediatric drops | 100 mg/ml | |
| | | Injection (IM) | 250 mg vial | |
| | | Injection (IV) | 500 mg vial | |
| | Tetracyn | Capsule | 250, 500 mg | |
| | | Syrup | 125 mg/5 ml | |
| | | Injection (IM) | 100, 250 mg vial | |
| | | Injection (IV) | 250, 500 mg vial | |
| | Tetramax | Capsule | 250 mg | |
| | Tetrex | Capsule | 250, 500 mg | |
| | | Syrup | 125 mg/5 ml | |
| | T-250 | Capsule | 250 mg | |
| | T-125 | Syrup | 125 mg/5 ml | |

| Contraindications | Major side effects | Comments |
|---|---|---|
| Hypersensitivity to any tetracycline; usage during pregnancy and tooth development unless other suitable agents are contraindicated. | GI disturbances; renal toxicity; hypersensitivity reactions; dermatologic disturbances; hematologic disturbances; permanent tooth development; pain and irritation at the IM injection site and vein irritation (IV form). | *General:* Same as above. |

**Table 25-8.** Systemic antibiotics: antifungal agents

| Generic name | Trade name(s) | Dosage form(s) | Strength(s) | Usual dose |
|---|---|---|---|---|
| Amphotericin B | Fungizone | Injection | 50 mg vial | 0.25 mg/kg/day initially and increased as tolerance permits up to 1.5 mg/kg/day maximum. Dose should be given by slow IV infusion over 6 hr. *Protect from light during administration.* |
| Flucytosine | Ancoban | Capsule | 250, 500 mg | 50 to 150 mg/kg/day in 4 doses at 6 hr intervals. |
| Griseofulvin | *Microsize:* | | | *Adults:* A single or divided dose of 500 mg-1 gm. |
| | Fulvicin U/F | Tablets | 125, 250, 500 mg | |
| | Grifulvin V | Tablet | 125, 250, 500 mg | *Children:* 30-50 lbs—125-250 mg daily; over 50 lbs—250-500 mg daily |
| | | Oral suspension | 125 mg/5 ml | |
| | *Microsize:* | | | |
| | Grisactin | Tablet | 500 mg | 30-50 lbs, 125-250 mg daily- |
| | | Capsule | 125, 250 mg | over 50 lbs, 250-500 mg daily. |
| | Grisowen | Capsule | 250 mg | |
| | *Ultramicrosize:* | | | |
| | Gris-PEG | Tablet | 125 mg | |
| Nystatin | Mycostatin | Tablet | 500,000 U | *Adults and children:* 400,000-1,000,000 U qid. |
| | | Suspension | 100,000 U/ml | |
| | Nilstat | Tablet | 500,000 U | *Infants:* 200,000U qid. |
| | | Suspension | 100,000 U/ml | |

| Contraindications | Major side effects | Comments |
|---|---|---|
| Hypersensitivity; safe usage during pregnancy has not been established. | GI disturbances; febrile reactions; muscle and joint pain; local venous pain at injection site with phlebitis and thrombophlebitis; hypokalemia; hematologic, renal, and hepatic disturbances; hypersensitivity reactions. | Other nephrotoxic antibiotics and antineoplastic agents should be avoided during amphotericin-B therapy. Corticosteroids, aspirin, antihistamines, mannitol, and heparin in conjunction with therapy may alleviate or lessen adverse reactions. Initial dilution requires sterile water for injection *without a preservative.* Appropriate laboratory studies should be done during therapy. *Note:* Amphotericin should be used primarily in progressive and potentially fatal fungal infections. |
| Hypersensitivity; safe usage in pregnant and lactating women and those of child-bearing age has not been established. | GI disturbances; hematologic disturbances; hepatic and renal disturbances; hypersensitivity reactions and some CNS disturbances. | Use with extreme caution in patients with bone marrow depression and renal impairment. Renal, hepatic, and hematologic functions should be closely monitored during therapy. Administering the capsules a few at a time over 15 min may reduce GI irritation (nausea and vomiting). |
| Hypersensitivity; porphyria; hepatocellular failure; safe use during pregnancy has not been established. | Hypersensitivity reactions; GI disturbances; paresthesias; proteinuria; leukopenia, and granulocytopenia. | Patients receiving long-term therapy should have periodic renal, hepatic, and hemopoietic function studies done. Photosensitivity reactions may occur. The possibility of cross-sensitivity with penicillin exists. Griseofulvin decreases the activity of *warfarin-type anticoagulants.* Barbiturates usually depress griseofulvin activity. |
| Hypersensitivity | Diarrhea; nausea; vomiting; GI distress usually associated with high doses. | This drug is not absorbed and is indicated for oral and intestinal infections caused by susceptible *Candida* species. |

**Table 25-9.** Systemic antibiotics: miscellaneous agents

| Generic name | Trade name(s) | Dosage form(s) | Strength(s) | Usual dose |
|---|---|---|---|---|
| Clindamycin | Cleocin | Capsule<br>Granules for suspension<br>Injection | 75, 150 mg<br>75 mg/5 ml<br><br>300, 600, 900 mg ampule | *Adults: Oral:* 150-450 mg q 6 hr in 2, 3, or 4 equal doses.<br>*Children: Oral:* 8-25 mg kg/day divided into 3 or 4 equal doses. *IM or IV:* 15-40 mg/kg/day divided into 3 or 4 equal doses. *Note:* Not to be given IV as a bolus. |
| Colistimethate sodium | Coly-mycin M | Injection | 20 mg vial<br>150 mg vial | *Adults and children:* 2.5-5 mg/kg/day in 2 to 4 divided doses IM or IV.<br>*Note:* Dose should be reduced in patients with renal impairment. |
| Erythromycin | Bristamycin<br>Dowmycin E<br>EES | Tablet<br>Tablet<br>Chewable tablet<br><br>Tablet<br>Pediatric drops<br>Oral suspension | 250 mg<br>250 mg<br>250 mg<br><br>400 mg<br>100 mg/2.5 ml<br>200 mg/5 ml, 400 mg/5 ml | *Adults: Oral:* 250-500 mg q 6 hr or 400 mg q 6 h of the ethylsuccinate<br>*IV:* 15-20 mg/kg/day in divided doses.<br>*Children. Oral:* 30-60 mg/kg/day in divided doses. *IV:* same as for adults. |
|  | E-Mycin<br>Erypar<br>Erythrocin | Tablet<br>Tablet<br>Tablet<br>Suppositories<br>Injection<br>Injection IM | 250 mg<br>250, 500 mg<br>125, 250, 500 mg<br>125 mg<br>0.5, 1 gm vial<br>50 mg/ml in 2, 10 ml |  |
|  | Ethril<br>Ilosone | Tablet<br>Chewable tablet<br>Capsule<br>Pediatric drops<br>Oral suspension | 250, 500 mg<br>125, 250 mg<br>125, 250, 500 mg<br>100 mg/ml<br>125 mg/ml;<br>50 mg/5 ml |  |
|  | Ilotycin | Tablet<br>Injection IV | 250 mg<br>250, 500 mg; 1 g vial |  |
|  | Kesso-Mycin<br>Pfizer-E<br>Pediamycin | Tablet<br>Tablet<br>Chewable tablet<br>Pediatric drops<br>Oral suspension | 250 mg<br>250, 500 mg<br>200 mg<br>100 mg/2.5 ml<br>200 mg/5 ml; 400 mg/5 ml |  |
|  | Robimycin<br>RP-Mycin<br>SK-Erythromycin | Tablet<br>Tablet<br>Tablet | 250 mg<br>250 mg<br>250, 500 mg |  |

| Contraindications | Major side effects | Comments |
|---|---|---|
| Hypersensitivity to clindamycin or lincomycin; safe usage during pregnancy has not been established. | Acute GI disturbances; hypersensitivity reactions; hepatic and hematologic disturbances; pain, induration, and sterile abscess at IM site; thrombophlebitis after IV infusion. | The severe colitis caused by clindamycin may be prolonged or worsened by use of antiperistaltic agents. Superinfection due to overgrowth of nonsusceptible organisms may occur. Caution should be used in patients receiving neuromuscular blocking agents, certain older patients, those having a history of GI disease and atopic individuals. If therapy is prolonged, hepatic and renal functions and blood counts should be monitored. Clindamycin may antagonize the activity of erythromycin. |
| Hypersensitivity to the drug; safe usage during pregnancy has not been established. | Neurotoxicity; nephrotoxicity; hypersensitivity reactions; pain at injection site (IM). | May be given IV by direct injection or by slow IV infusion. Exercise extreme caution when administering in presence of curariform muscle relaxants and other neurotoxic antibiotics. |
| Hypersensitivity to the drug; safe usage during pregnancy has not been established.<br><br>Estolate salt in patients with liver disease. | Hypersensitivity reactions; GI disturbances (oral); pain, abscess formation, and necrosis (IM); vein irritation (IV). | Superinfection due to overgrowth of nonsusceptible organisms may occur. The oral route is the preferred route of administration. Erythromycin activity may be antagonized by clindamycin. |

**Table 25-9.** Systemic antibiotics: miscellaneous agents—cont'd

| Generic name | Trade name(s) | Dosage form(s) | Strength(s) | Usual dose |
|---|---|---|---|---|
| Lincomycin | Lincocin | Capsule<br>Syrup<br>Injection | 250, 500 mg<br>250 mg/5 ml<br>300 mg/ml in<br>  600 mg syringe<br>  unit | *Adults:*<br>*Oral:* 500 mg q 6 or<br>  q 8 hr. *IM:* 600 mg<br>  q 12-24 hr. *IV:* 600<br>  mg-1 Gm q 8-12<br>  hr.<br>*Children: Oral:* 3060<br>  mg/kg/day in 3 or<br>  4 divided doses.<br>  *IM:* 10 mg/kg/<br>  24 hours. *IV:* 10-20<br>  mg/kg/day in<br>  divided doses q<br>  8-12 hr. |
| Polymixin<br>  B sulfate | Aerosporin | Injection | 500, 000 U<br>  vial | *Adults and children:*<br>  *IV:* 15,000-25,000<br>  U/kg/day (usually<br>  by continuous IV<br>  infusion).<br>  *IM:* 25,000-30,000<br>  U/kg/day divided<br>  and given at 4<br>  and given at 4 -6 hr<br>  intervals. *Note:*<br>  Dosage should<br>  be reduced in<br>  patients with renal<br>  impairment. |
| Vancomycin | Vancocin | Injection<br>Powder for<br>  oral use | 500 mg<br><br>10 g | *Adults: Oral:* 500 mg<br>  q 6 hr or 1 g q<br>  12 hr. *IV:* 500 mg<br>  q 6 hr or 1 g q<br>  12 hr. |

| Contraindications | Major side effects | Comments |
|---|---|---|
| Hypersensitivity to clindamycin or lincomycin; safe usage during pregnancy has not been established. | Acute GI disturbances; hypersensitivity reactions; dermatologic reactions; hepatic disturbances; cardiovascular disturbances; tinnitus; vertigo; pain (IM). | Superinfection may occur due to overgrowth of nonsusceptible organisms. The severe colitis caused by lincomycin may be prolonged or worsened by use of antiperistaltic agents. Use with caution in patients receiving neuromuscular blocking agents, certain older patients, and those having a history of GI disease. If therapy is prolonged, hepatic and renal function and blood counts should be monitored. |
| Hypersensitivity to drug; safe usage during pregnancy has not been established. | Nephrotoxicity, neurotoxicity; hypersensitivity reactions; severe pain at IM injection site. Thrombophlebitis at IV injection site. | Superinfection may occur due to overgrowth of nonsusceptible organisms. Avoid concomitant or sequential use with other nephrotoxic and/or neurotoxic agents and curariform muscle relaxants. Renal function should be monitored during therapy. |
| Hypersensitivity to the drug. | Hypersensitivity reactions; ototoxicity; nephrotoxicity; GI disturbances; pain and thrombophlebitis at the injection site. | Superinfection may occur due to overgrowth of nonsusceptible organisms. All patients should have liver and renal function studies urinalyses, and hematologic studies done periodically. |

**Table 25-10.** Narcotic analgesics

| Generic name | Trade name(s) | Dosage form(s) | Strength(s) | Usual dose |
|---|---|---|---|---|
| Meperidine | Various manufacturers | Injection | 25 mg/ml-1 ml<br>50 mg/ml-1, 3 ml<br>75 mg/ml-1, 1.5 ml<br>100 mg/ml-1, 2, 20, 30 ml | *Adults:* 50-150 mg IM, SQ, or orally q 3-4 hr prn.<br>*Children:* 0.5-0.8 mg/lb IM, SQ, or PO up to adult dose q 3-4 hr prn.<br>*Note:* Elixir should be diluted before taking. |
| | | Tablet | 50 mg | |
| | Demerol | Injection | 25 mg/ml-0.5 ml<br>50 mg/ml-0.5, 1, 1.5, 2, 3 ml<br>75 mg/ml-1.5 ml<br>100 mg/ml-1, 2, 20 ml | |
| | | Tablet | 50, 100 mg | |
| | | Elixir | 50 mg/5 ml (banana flavor) | |
| Morphine sulfate | Various manufacturers | Injection | 8 mg/ml-1 ml<br>10 mg/ml-1 ml<br>15 mg/ml-1, 2 ml | *Adults: Oral:* 5-15 mg q 4 hr. *SQ* or *IM:* 5-15 mg q 4 hr. *IV:* 2.5–15 mg diluted q 4 hr (over 4-5 minute).<br>*Children:* SQ: 0.1-0.2 mg/kg/dose. |
| | | Tablet | 10, 15, 30 mg | |
| Codeine (as sulfate or phosphate) | Various manufacturers | Injection (phosphate) | 15 mg/ml-1 ml<br>30 mg/ml-1, 20 ml<br>60 mg/ml-1 ml | *Adults:* 15-60 mg qid orally or SQ.<br>*Children:* 3 mg/kg daily in 6 divided doses. |
| | | Tablet (phosphate or sulfate) | 15, 30, 60 mg | |
| Hydromorphone | Dilaudid | Injection (HCl) | 1 mg/ml<br>2 mg/ml<br>3 mg/ml-1 ml<br>4 mg/ml | Parenteral: 2 mg IM q 4-6 hr prn. May be given SQ or IV (over 3-5 minutes). *Oral:* 2 mg q 4-6 hr prn.<br>*Rectal:* 3 mg q 6 hr prn. |
| | | Sulfate | 2 mg/ml-10, 20 ml | |
| | | Tablet | 1, 2, 3, 4 mg | |
| | | Suppository | 3 mg | |
| Oxymorphone | Numorphan | Injection | 1 mg/ml-1, 1.5, 15 ml; 1.5 mg/ml-<br><br>15 ml; 1.5 mg/ml-1, 10 ml | *Adults: SQ* or *IM:* 1-1.5 mg q 4-6 hr prn. *Rectal:* 5 mg q 4-6 hr.<br>Safety in children under 12 has not been established. |
| | | Suppositories | 5 mg | |

| Contraindications | Major side effects | Comments |
|---|---|---|
| Hypersensitivity; concomitant use with MAO inhibitors. Exercise caution with other CNS depressants, in head injury, increased intracranial pressure, in asthma, and during pregnancy and lactation. | CNS, GI, GU, and cardiovascular disturbances; allergic reactions, irritation at injection site. | Also indicated as a preoperative agent, for support of anesthesia and for obstetric analgesia at delivery. *Note:* Injection is incompatible chemically with the barbiturates. *May be habit forming.* |
| Hypersensitivity; concomitant use with MAO inhibitors. Exercise caution with other CNS depressants, in head injury, increased intercranial pressure, in asthma, and during pregnancy and lactation. | CNS, GI, GU, and cardiovascular disturbances; allergic and dermatologic disturbances; pain, and irritation at the injection site. | Also indicated for sedation and hypnosis; for dyspneic seizures or left ventricular failure and pulmonary edema; and as a preoperative agent. *May be habit forming.* |
| Hypersensitivity; exercise caution in patients with asthma and pulmonary emphysema. | CNS, GI, and cardiovascular disturbances; miosis; respiratory depression. | Also commonly used as an antitussive agent. Codeine is present in many combination analgesic products. *May be habit forming.* |
| Hypersensitivity; status asthmaticus; intracranial lesions associated with increased intracranial pressure. *Note:* Use during pregnancy should be determined by weighing possible benefits against risks. | CNS, GI disturbances; respiratory depression; hypotension; pain and local tissue irritation at injection site; induration at SQ injection site. | Dose should be individualized according to patient size and response and the severity of the pain. *May be habit forming.* |
| Hypersensitivity; usage in children under 12 years of age; acute alcoholism; bronchial asthma. | CNS and GI disturbances; respiratory depression; allergic reactions. | May be used as a preoperative medication, to support anesthesia, for obstetric analgesia, and dyspnea of acute ventricular failure and pulmonary edema. *May be habit forming.* |

*Continued.*

**Table 25-10.** Narcotic analgesics—cont'd

| Generic name | Trade name(s) | Dosage form(s) | Strength(s) | Usual dose |
|---|---|---|---|---|
| Levorphanol tartrate | Levo-Dromoran | Injection<br>Tablet | 2 mg/ml-1<br>2 mg | *Adults:* Orally or SQ: 2 mg q 4 h prn |
| Opium | Various manu-facturers<br><br>Pantopon | Tincture<br><br>Injection | 10% W/V<br><br>20 mg/ml-1 ml | *Oral:* 0.6-1.5 ml (equivalent to 6-15 mg morphine)<br>*Parenteral: Adults:* 5-20 mg IM or SQ q 4-6 h prn. |
| Anileridine | Leritine | Injection (phosphate)<br>Tablet (HCl) | 25 mg/ml-1, 2, 3 ml<br><br>25 mg | *Adults: Oral:* 25-50 mg q 4-6 hr prn. *SQ or IM:* 25-50 mg q 4-6 hr prn up to 200 mg/day. Not recommended for children under 12. |
| Alphaprodine HCl | Nisentil | Injection | 40 mg/ml-1 ml<br>60 mg/ml-1, 10 ml | Not recommended for use in children under 12.<br>*Adults: IV:* 30-60 mg as indicated. *SQ:* 3-60 mg as indicated. Not recommended for IM use. |
| Fentanyl | Sublimaze | Injection (IM and IV only) | 0.05 mg/ml-2, 5 ml | *Adults:* 0.05-0.1 mg IM or IV as indicated.<br>*Children:* 2-12 years old. 0.02-0.03 mg/20-25 lb body weight. |
| Methadone | Dolophine<br><br>Westadone | Injection<br>Tablet<br>Tablet | 10 mg/ml-1, 20 ml<br>5, 10, 40 mg<br>2.5, 5, 10, 40 mg | *Adults:* 2.5-10 mg IM, or SQ or orally q 3-4 h prn. Not recommended for use in patients under 18. |

| Contraindications | Major side effects | Comments |
|---|---|---|
| Hypersensitivity; acute alcoholism; bronchial asthma; increased intracranial pressure; respiratory depression and anoxia. | CNS and GI disturbances; respiratory depression; allergic reactions; cardiovascular disturbances; urinary retention. | Safety during pregnancy has not been established; may be used as a preoperative medication also. *May be habit forming.* |
| Bronchial asthma; narcotic idiosyncrasies; respiratory depression; hypersensitivity. Use with caution in infants, old and debilitated patients; in increased intracranial pressure, toxic psychosis, prostatic obstruction, and myxedema. | GI and CNS disturbances; respiratory and circulatory depression; GU and cardiovascular disturbances; allergic reactions. | Narcotic antagonists may be used as antidote for overdosage. *May be habit forming.* |
| Hypersensitivity; in children under 12 years old; in respiratory depression; in head injuries or brain tumors. | GI and CNS disturbances; respiratory and circulatory depression; cardiovascular disturbances; allergic responses. | May be used as preoperative medication; to support anesthesia; for obstetrical analgesic and for anxiety with dyspnea of left ventricular failure and pulmonary edema. This drug is metabolized in the liver; use with caution if liver impairment is present. *May be habit forming.* |
| Hypersensitivity; in children under 12; to relieve chronic pain; IM injection; exercise caution in presence of other CNS depressants, increased intracranial pressure; hepatic insufficiency, myxedema, alcoholism, convulsive disorders, Addison's disease, and concomitant therapy with MAO inhibitors. | CNS and GI disturbances; Urticaria and respiratory depression. | Generally indicated for use as obstetric analgesia. For urologic exams and procedures; preoperatively; for minor surgery; renal or biliary colic and for cardiovascular pain where rapid onset and short duration are desired. Should not be used for chronic pain because of short duration of action. *Note:* Nisentil is addicting. Safe usage in pregnancy has not been established. |
| Hypersensitivity; concomitant use with MAO inhibitors; in children under 2; in head injuries, increased intracranial pressure and brain tumors. | CNS, GI, and cardiovascular disturbances; respiratory and neuromuscular reactions; diaphoresis. | Generally indicated for use as preoperative medication and for analgesic action during induction and maintenance of anesthesia and for analgesia in the immediate postoperative period (recovery room). Individualize dose and monitor initial signs routinely. *May be habit forming.* |
| Hypersensitivity; use in children; exercise caution in presence of other CNS depressants, in head injury or increased intracranial pressure, asthma, and other respiratory conditions. | CNS, GI, GU, and cardiovascular disturbances; allergic reactions, pain and tissue irritation at injection site; *respiratory depression* and circulatory depression. | Indicated for relief of severe pain; detoxification and temporary maintenance of narcotic addicts. *Note: Methadone can produce drug dependence of the morphine type.* Safe use in pregnancy has not been established. Methadone may be antagonized by pentazocine. Take precautions in presence of MAO inhibitors and acute abdominal conditions. Rifampin lowers blood concentration of methadone. |

**Table 25-11.** Nonnarcotic-nonsalicylate analgesics

| Generic name | Trade name(s) | Dosage form(s) | Strength(s) | Usual dose |
|---|---|---|---|---|
| Acetaminophen | Amphenol | Suppository | 125, 300, 600 mg | *Adults:* 325 mg-650 mg 3-4 times daily. Not over 2.6 g/24 hrs. |
| | Datril | Tablet | 325 mg | |
| | | Elixir | 130 mg/5 ml (grape) | |
| | Liquiprin | Drops | 120 mg/2.5 ml (raspberry) | *Children 7-12 years:* 162.5-325 mg 3-4 times daily. Not over 1.3 g in 24 hr. |
| | Nebs | Tablet | 325 mg | |
| | | Liquid | 120 mg/5 ml (grape cream) | |
| | Neopap | Suppository | 130, 325 mg | *3-6 years:* 120 mg 3-4 times daily. Not over 480 mg in 24 hr. |
| | Phenaphen | Capsule | 325 mg | |
| | | Tablet | 325 mg | |
| | Tempra | Tablet | 325 mg | |
| | | Syrup | 120 mg/5 ml | |
| | | Drops | 60 mg/0.6 ml | |
| | Tylenol | Tablets | 325 mg | |
| | | Capsule | 500 mg | |
| | | Chewable tablet | 120 mg | |
| | | Elixir | 120 mg/5 ml (cherry) | |
| | | Drops | 60 mg/0.6 ml (cherry) | |
| | Valadol | Tablet | 325 mg | |
| | | Liquid | 120 mg/5 ml | |
| | Generically available | Tablet | 600 mg | |
| Ethoheptazine | Zactane | Tablet | 75 mg | *Adults:* 75-150 mg orally 3-4 times daily. |
| Mefenamic acid | Ponstel | Capsule | 250 mg | *Adults and children over 14:* 500 mg followed by 250 mg q 6 hr prn (with food). |
| Methotrimeprazine | Levoprome | Injection | 20 mg/ml-1, 10 ml | *Adults:* 10-20 mg IM initially, then adjust dose q 4-6 hr for relief of pain. |
| Pentazocine | Talwin | Injection (IM, IV, SQ) | 30 mg/ml-1, 1.5, 2 ml | *Adults: Oral:* 50 mg q 3-4 hr up to 600 mg daily. |
| | | Tablet | 50 mg | *Parenteral:* 30 mg IV, IM, or SQ q 3-4 up to 300 mg daily. |
| Propoxyphene HCl | Darvon | Capsule | 32, 65 mg | *Adults:* 65 mg q 4 hr prn. |
| | Dolene | Capsule | 65 mg | |
| | Harmar | Capsule | 65 mg | |
| | Progesic | Capsule | 65 mg | |
| | Propoxychel | Capsule | 65 mg | |
| | Proxagesic | Capsule | 65 mg | |
| | SK-65 | Capsule | 65 mg | |
| Propoxyphen napsylate | Darvon N | Tablet | 100 mg | *Adults:* 100 mg PO q 4 hr prn. |
| | | Suspension | 10 mg/ml | |

| Contraindications | Major side effects | Comments |
|---|---|---|
| Hypersensitivity; in patients with known glucose-6-phosphate hydrogenase deficiency. | Methemoglobinemia; hemolytic anemia; urticarial and erythematous skin reactions. | Indicated for use as analgesic and antipyretic especially in aspirin allergy, hemostatic disturbances, bleeding diatheses, and gouty arthritis. *Note:* Acetaminophen has been reported to potentiate oral anticoagulants. |
| Hypersensitivity. | Nausea; epigastric distress; dizziness. | Synthetic agent not having addiction liability. |
| Hypersensitivity; patients with ulceration or chronic inflammation of upper or lower GI tract. | GI and CNS disturbances; hematopoietic reactions; dermatologic and renal manifestations; otic, ophthalmic, and hepatic toxicity. *Causes increased need for insulin in diabetics.* | Use with caution in asthmatics; shows analgesic, antipyretic, and anti-inflammatory activity. *Administer with food.* May prolong prothrombin time. Use with caution in patients on anticoagulants. Interferes with some laboratory tests. |
| Phenothiazine hypersensitivity; in comatose states; concomitant use with antipyretic MAO inhibitors; in overdosage of CNS depressants; severe myocardial, renal, or hepatic disease; clinical hypotension and in patients under 12. Use with caution in women of childbearing potential and during pregnancy. | Orthostatic hypotension, agranulocytosis; jaundice; CNS, GI, and GU disturbances; pain, inflammation and swelling of the injection site. *Note:* This drug is a *phenothiazine* derivative and phenothiazine side effects may occur. | Indicated for analgesia; obstetric analgesia and sedation to avoid respiratory depression and as a preoperative medication. May be mixed in same syringe with atropine or scopolamine but not other drugs. Drug interactions have been reported with CNS depressant drugs, aspirin, meprobamate, reserpine, and antihypertensive agents. |
| Hypersensitivity; in children under 12 years; use great caution in head injury or intracranial pressure; safe use in pregnancy has not been established. | GI, CNS, and ophthalmic disturbances; hematologic, respiratory, and cardiovascular manifestations; GU and autonomic disturbances; allergic and local dermatologic problems. | *May cause drug dependence. Caution* should be exercised in certain respiratory conditions, impaired renal or hepatic function, myocardial infarction, biliary surgery, and in patients prone to seizures. Talwin is a mild narcotic and should be used carefully in patients on methadone maintenance. May also be used as preoperative medication and to supplement surgical anesthesia. |
| Hypersensitivity; safe use in pregnancy has not been established. Not recommended for use in children. | CNS and GI disturbances; dermatologic reactions; visual disturbances; psychoses and convulsions in very high repeated doses. | Use with caution in asthmatics; shows analgesic, antipyretic, and antiinflammatory activity. *Administer with food.* May prolong prothrombin time. Use with caution in patients on anticoagulants. Interferes with some laboratory tests. |

**Table 25-12.** Salicylate analgesics

| Generic name | Trade name(s) | Dosage form(s) | Strength(s) | Usual dose |
|---|---|---|---|---|
| Acetylsalicylic acid (aspirin) | Various manufacturers | Tablet Suppositories | 1, 1.5, 2.5, 5, 10 gr. 1, 2, 2.5, 3, 5, 10, 15, 20 gr | *Adults:* 5-10 gr orally or rectally q 3 hr prn. |
| | A.S.A. | Tablet Enseals Capsule Suppositories | 5 gr 5, 10 gr 5, 10 gr 5, 10 gr | *Children:* 1-3 gr orally or rectally q 3-4 hr prn. |
| | Ecotrin | Tablet | 5 gr | |
| | Bayer | Time-released tablet | 10 gr | |
| | Measurin | Time-released tablet | 10 gr | |
| Calcium carbaspirin | Calurin | Tablet | Equivalent to 300 mg aspirin | *Adults:* 1 or 2 tabs 1-6 times daily. *Children: 6-12:* 1 tablet 1-6 times daily. *3-6:* 1/2 tablet 1-6 times daily. |
| Choline salicylate | Arthropan | Liquid | 870 mg equivalent to 10 gr aspirin/5 ml | *Adults and children over 12:* 870 mg repeated q 3-4 hr up to 6 times daily. |
| Magnesium salicylate | Mobidin | Tablet | 600 mg | *Adults:* 600 mg tid or qid. Not recommended for children under 12. |
| Salicylamide | Various manufacturers Salrin | Tablet Tablet | 5, 10 gr 10 gr | *Adults:* 10 gr qid. Not recommended for children under 12. |
| Sodium salicylate | Various manufacturers | Injection Tablet Tablet, (enteric-coated) | 1 g/10 ml; 1.3 g/10 ml; 1.5 g/10 ml 325, 650 mg 325, 650 mg | *Adults:* 325-650 mg orally or IV q 4-6 hr prn. |

| Contraindications | Major side effects | Comments |
|---|---|---|
| Hypersensitivity. | Tinnitus; dizziness; GI upset; hypersensitivity reactions. | Has marked analgesic, antipyretic, and antiinflammatory effects. Use with caution in patients on anticoagulant therapy. May antagonize uricosuric effect of probenecid and sulfinpyrazone. Risk of GI ulceration is increased when used in presence of steroids, phenylbutazone, or alcohol. |
| Hypersensitivity to salicylates. | Tinnitus; dizziness; GI upset; hypersensitivity reactions. | More soluble with less irritation than aspirin. Has analgesic, antipyretic, and antiinflammatory effects. Use with caution in patients on anticoagulant therapy. May antagonize uricosuric effect of probenecid and sulfinpyrazone. Risk of GI ulceration is increased when used in presence of steroids, phenylbutazone, or alcohol. |
| Hypersensitivity to salicylates. | GI upset; hypersensitivity reactions; tinnitus; dizziness. | Has analgesic, antipyretic, and antiinflammatory activity. Faster acting than aspirin. May react with anticoagulants, probenecid, and sulfinpyrazone. |
| Hypersensitivity to salicylates. Advanced chronic renal insufficiency. | GI upset; hypersensitivity reactions; tinnitus; dizziness; hyperventilation; visual disturbances; occult blood loss. | Has analgesic and antiinflammatory activity. Use with caution in patients on anticoagulant therapy and in the presence of steroids, butazones, or alcohol. May antagonize action of probenecid and sulfinpyrazone. |
| Hypersensitivity to salicylates. | Drowziness; GI upset; hypersensitivity reactions; tinnitus. | Poorly absorbed from GI tract and is less effective than aspirin. Use with caution in patients on anticoagulant therapy and in the presence of steroids, butazones, or alcohol. May antagonize action of probenecid and sulfinpyrazone. |
| Hypersensitivity to salicylates. | Tinnitus; dizziness; GI upset; hypersensitivity reactions. | Less effective than an equal dose of aspirin. Use with caution in patients on anticoagulant therapy. May antagonize the uricosuric effect of probenecid and sulfinpyrazone. Use with caution in presence of steroids, butazones, and alcohol. |

**Table 25-13.** Antinauseant-antiemetic agents: single drug entities

| Generic name | Trade name(s) | Dosage form(s) | Strength(s) | Usual dose |
|---|---|---|---|---|
| Benzquinamide | Emete-cone | Injection | 50 mg/vial | *IM:* 50 mg repeated in 1 hr; then q 3-4 hr prn. *IV:* 25 mg slowly with subsequent doses IM. |
| Buclizine | Bucladin-S | Tablet | 50 mg | 50-150 mg daily |
| Chlorpromazine | Chlor-PZ | Tablet | 10, 25, 50, 100, 200 mg | *Adults: Oral:* 10-25 mg q 4-6 hr prn. |
| | Promochel | Tablet | 25, 50, 100, 200 mg | *IM or IV:* 50 mg |
| | Promopar | Tablet | 10, 25, 50, 100, 200 mg | q 3-4 hr until vomiting stops, |
| | Sonazine | Tablet | 10, 25, 50, 100 200 mg | *rectal:* 50-100 mg q 6-8 hr prn. |
| | Thorazine | Tablet | 10, 25, 50, 100 200 mg | *Children: Oral:* 0.25 mg/lb q 6-8 |
| | | Spansule | 30, 75, 150, 200, 300 mg | hr prn; *rectal:* 0.5 mg/lb q 6-8 hr prn. |
| | | Syrup | 10 mg/5 ml | *IM:* 0.25 mg/lb q 6-8 |
| | | Suppositories | 25, 100 mg | hr prn; maximum |
| | | Injection | 25 mg/ml-1, 2, 10 ml | 40-75 mg per day. |
| | | Concentrate | 30 mg/ml; 100 mg/ml | |
| Cyclizine | Marezine | Tablet (HCl) | 50 mg | *Adults: IM:* 50 mg q |
| | | Injection (lactate) | 50 mg/ml | 4-6 hr. *Rectal:* 100 mg q 4-6 hr. *Oral:* |
| | | Suppository | 50, 100 | 50 mg q 4-6 hr. *Children, 6-10: IM:* ½ adult dose. *Under 6:* ¼ adult dose. *Rectal: Over 6:* 50 mg q 4-6 hr. *Under 6:* 25 mg q 4-6 hr. *Oral: 6-10:* ½ adult dose. |
| Dimenhydrinate | Dimcrest | Injection | 50 mg/ml-10 ml | *Adult: Oral:* 50 mg q 4 hr. |
| | Dramamine | Tablet | 50 mg | *Children, 8-12:* 25-50 |
| | | Liquid (oral) | 12.5 mg/4 ml | mg tid. *Rectal:* 100 |
| | | Injection | 50 mg/ml-1, 5 ml | mg daily. *IM:* 50 mg |
| | | Suppository | 100 mg | prn. *IV:* 50 mg in 10 |
| | Reidamine | Injection | 50 mg/ml | ml saline over 2 minutes. Parenteral doses for children should be lower than oral doses. |
| Diphenidol | Vontrol | Tablet | 25 mg | *Adults: Oral:* 25 mg |
| | | Injection | 20 mg/ml-2 ml | q 4 hr prn, *IM:* 20-40 mg q 4 hr prn. *Drip IV:* 20 mg then repeat in 1 hr. and switch to alternate route. *Children: Oral:* 0.4 mg/lb up to q 4 hr. *IM:* 0.2 mg/lb up to q 4 hr (only for children 6 mo. old or over 25 lb). *IV:* not recommended for children. |

| Contraindications | Major side effects | Comments |
|---|---|---|
| Hypersensitivity; pregnancy; in children. | Autonomic and CNS effects; cardiovascular and GI disturbances; musculo-skeletal and dermatologic problems; drowsiness not common. | Drug must be reconstituted before use; IM administration preferred. |
| Hypersensitivity; during pregnancy; safe use in children not established. | Drowsiness; dryness of mouth; headache; jitteriness. | May also be useful in motion sickness and vertigo; acts at CNS level. |
| Comatose states; in bone marrow depression; presence of large amounts of CNS depressants; Hypersensitivity. | Drowsiness; jaundice; hematologic disorders; cardiovascular effects; CNS effects; allergic reactions; ocular changes; endocrine disorders; autonomic reactions; neuromuscular reactions. | Also useful in psychotic and manic depressive states; hiccups; pre- and postoperative management; tetanus; acute intermittent porphyria and agitation; safety in pregnancy has not been established; after long-term therapy may see withdrawal symptoms. |
| Hypersensitivity; pregnancy; young children. | GI, GU, and CNS disturbances; allergic reactions; auditory and visual disturbances, and cholestatic jaundice. | May be useful in motion sickness; also possesses central depressant; anticholinergic, and antispasmodic activity. |
| Hypersensitivity. | CNS depression. | May also be useful in motion sickness and vertigo; use with caution in combination with ototoxic antibiotics since it may mask ototoxicity. |
| Hypersensitivity; anuria; in pregnant or lactating women. | CNS and GI disturbances; auditory and visual hallucinations; transient lowering of blood pressure; skin rash. | May also be useful for vertigo; use with caution in conditions that may be altered by anticholinergic activity; may mask drug overdosage, i.e., Digitalis; may obscure diagnosis of some conditions; generally should be used only in hospitalized patients. |

*Continued.*

**Table 25-13.** Antinauseant-antiemetic agents: single drug entities — cont'd

| Generic name | Trade name(s) | Dosage form(s) | Strength(s) | Usual dose |
|---|---|---|---|---|
| Hydroxyzine | Atarax (HCL) | Tablet | 10, 25, 50, 100 mg | *Adults: Oral:* 25-100 mg qid. *IM:* 5-100 mg up to q 4-6 hr. |
| | | Syrup | 10 mg/5 ml | |
| | Vistaril (pamoate) | Capsule | 25, 50, 100 mg | *Children Under 6:* |
| | | Suspension (oral) | 25 mg/5 ml | *Oral:* 50 mg/day in divided doses. |
| | | Injection | 25 mg/ml-10 ml; 50 mg/ml-2, 10 ml | *Over 6:* 50-100 mg/ day in divided doses. *IM:* 0.5 mg/ lb as indicated. |
| Perphenazine | Trilafon | Tablet | 2, 4, 8, 16 mg | *Oral:* 8-16 mg daily in divided doses; reduce when nausea controlled; *IM:* 5 mg as indicated. |
| | | Repetabs | 8 mg | |
| | | Concentrate (oral) | 16 mg/5 ml | |
| | | Injection | 5 mg/ml-1 ml | |
| Prochlorperazine | Compazine | Tablet | 5, 10, 25 mg | *Adults: Oral:* 8-16 mg 3-4 times daily or 10 mg spansules q 12 hr. *rectal:* 25 mg bid. *IM:* 5-10 mg q 4 hr prn up to 40 mg daily. |
| | | Spansule | 10, 15, 30, 75 mg | |
| | | Syrup | 5 mg/5 ml | |
| | | Suppositories | 2.5, 5, 25 mg | |
| | | Concentrate | 10 mg/ml | |
| | | Injection | 5 mg/ml-2 ml, 10 ml | *Children* (not recom- mended for patients under 20 lb or 2 yr old): *Oral or rectal:* 20-29 lb 2.5 mg 1-2 times daily. 30-39 lb 2.5 mg 2-3 times daily. 40-85 lb 2.5 mg tid or 5 mg bid. *IM:* 0.06 mg/lb or single dose. |
| Promethizine | Fellozine | Injection | 25 mg/ml-10 ml 50 mg/ml-10 ml | *Adults: oral and rectal:* 25 mg repeated q 4-6 hr prn. *Injectable:* 25 mg IM or IV repeated q 4-6 hr prn. |
| | Ganphen | Injection | 50 mg/ml-10 ml | |
| | Lemprometh | Injection | 25 mg/ml-10 ml 50 mg/ml-10 ml | |
| | | Tablet | 25, 50 mg | |
| | Phenergan | Injection | 25 mg/ml-1 ml (IV or IM) | *Children: oral and injectable:* dosage should be adjusted according to age and weight of patient. |
| | | Tablet | 12.5, 25, 50 mg | |
| | | Syrup | 6.25 mg/5 ml/or 25 mg/5 ml | |
| | | Suppositories | 25, 50 mg | |
| | Provigan | Injection | 25 mg/ml-10 ml 50 mg/ml-10 ml | |
| | Qudnite | Capsule | 50 mg | |
| | Remsed | Tablet | 25, 50 mg | |
| | ZiPan | Injection | 25 mg/ml-1, 10 ml | |
| | | Tablet | 25, 50 mg | |
| | | Syrup | 12,5 mg/5 ml | |

| Contraindications | Major side effects | Comments |
|---|---|---|
| Hypersensitivity; early pregnancy; injectable form should not be given IV, SQ, or intraarterially. | CNS and neurologic disturbances; anticholinergic effects. | May also be utilized for treating anxiety and insomnia, and to potentiate analgesics; also used as an adjunct with anesthesia. |
| Hypersensitivity; drug induced CNS depression; blood dyscrasias; bone marrow depression; liver damage in children under 12. | Neuromuscular reactions; allergic reactions; autonomic reactions; other reactions. | Usage during pregnancy must be weighed (benefits against hazards); this drug may also be useful in psychotic patients and possibly in management of neuroses; this is a potent drug and the prescriber should be familiar with all hazards and side effects. |
| Hypersensitivity; drug induced CNS depression; in pediatric surgery. | Neuromuscular reactions; motor restlessness; dystonias; pseudo-Parkinsonism; persistent tardive dyskinesia; blood dyscrasias; dermatologic problems. | May also be useful in psychotic disorders, anxiety, tension, and agitation. Safe use in pregnancy not established. May mask overdose of some toxic drugs and obscure diagnosis of some conditions. This is a potent drug and should be reviewed thoroughly before being prescribed. |
| Hypersensitivity; intraarterial injection. | Autonomic reactions; in rare cases blood dyscrasias; some cardiovascular disturbances; photosensitivity. | May also be used for motion sickness, allergy, as an adjunct to anesthesia, to potentiate analgesics and as a sedative. May mask symptoms of unrecognized diseases; use with caution in conjunction with CNS depressants. |

*Continued.*

**Table 25-13.** Antinauseant-antiemetic agents: single drug entities—cont'd

| Generic name | Trade name(s) | Dosage form(s) | Strength(s) | Usual dose |
|---|---|---|---|---|
| Thiethylperazine | Torecan | Tablet<br>Injection<br>Suppositories | 10 mg<br>5 mg/ml-2 ml<br>10 mg | *Oral:* 10 mg 1-3 times daily. *Rectal:* 10 mg 1-3 times daily. *IM:* 10 mg 1-3 times daily. |
| Triflupromazine | Vesprin | Tablet<br>Suspension (oral)<br>Injection | 10, 25, 50 mg<br>5 mg/ml<br>10 mg/ml; 1 mg/1 ml syringe; 20 mg/ml 1 ml | *Adults: IV:* 1-3 mg total daily. *IM:* 5-15 mg repeated up to q 4 hr prn. *oral:* 20-30 mg total daily dose.<br>*Children: Oral:* 0.2 mg/kg up to a daily dose of 10 mg divided in 3 doses. *IM:* 0.2 to 0.25 mg/kg up to 10 mg total daily divided in 3 doses. *IV:* not recommended in children. |
| Trimetho-benzamide | Tigan | Capsule<br>Suppositories<br>Injection | 100, 250 mg<br>100, 200 mg<br>100 mg/ml-2, 20 ml vial; 2 ml syringe | *Adults: Oral:* 250 mg 3-4 times daily. *Rectal:* 200 mg 3-4 times daily. *Parenteral: IM only:* 200 mg 3-4 times daily.<br>*Children, 30-90 lb: Oral:* 100-200 mg 3-4 times daily. *Rectal:* 100-200 mg 3-4 times daily. *Parenteral:* Not recommended. *Under 30 lb: Rectal:* 100 mg 3-4 times daily. *Parenteral:* Not recommended. |

| Contraindications | Major side effects | Comments |
|---|---|---|
| Hypersensitivity to phenothiazines; pregnancy; severe CNS depression; comatose states, IV administration; use in children under 12. | Central and autonomic nervous system disturbances; hepatotoxicity; endocrine system disturbances; occasional cerebral vascular spasm and trigeminal neuralgia. All phenothiazine side effects are a possibility and the prescriber should be familiar with them as well.. | Also possibly helpful in treating vertigo; safe use following intracardiac and intracranial surgery has not been established. As with other phenothiazine derivatives, this drug may potentiate other CNS depressants. |
| Hypersensitivity; brain damage; severe CNS depression; coma; presence of blood dyscrasias; liver damage. | Central and autonomic nervous system disturbances; persistent tardive dyskinesia; metabolic and endocrine disturbances; allergic reactions; hematologic disorders; hepatotoxicity; all phenothiazine side effects should also be reviewed. | Also useful in treating psychotic disorders; this is another potent phenothiazine and caution should be exercised when it is used; safe usage during pregnancy has not been established. This drug will potentiate other CNS depressants. |
| Hypersensitivity; injectable form in children; suppositories in newborn or premature infants; known sensitivity to benzocaine and similar local anesthetics. | Hypersensitivity reactions; CNS disturbances; allergic type reactions; blood dyscrasias; Parkinson-like symptoms; visual disturbances. | Safe usage during pregnancy and lactation has not been established; antiemetic effects may impede diagnosis of some conditions and mask toxicity of some drugs; may potentiate action of other CNS depressants. |

**Table 25-14.** Antinauseant-antiemetic agents: combinations

| Generic name | Trade name(s) | Dosage form(s) | Strength(s) | Usual dose |
|---|---|---|---|---|
| Devulose, dextrose, orthophosphoric acid | Emetrol | Oral solution | | *Adults:* 15-30 ml repeated q 15 min until controlled. *Children and infants:* 5-10 ml repeated q 15 min until controlled. |
| Pyrilamine maleate, pentobarbital | Wans | Suppositories: pyrilamine/pentobarbitol Children—25 mg/30 mg Adult #1—50 mg/50 mg Adult #2—50 mg/100 mg | | *Adults:* one adult suppository q 4-6 hr. *Children, 2-12:* one child's or #1 supp. q 6-8 hr. *Under 2:* ½ above dose. Not recommended in infants under 6 mo. |
| | Emesert | Suppositories #1—25 mg/30 mg #2—50 mg/45 mg #3—50 mg/100 mg | | |
| Pyrilamine maleate, homatropine MBr, pentobarbital | Matropinal | Suppository (pyrilamine/homatropine/pentobarbital): 8/10/15 mg | | *Adults and children:* 1 or 2 metropinal or Stopp-15 supp. q 3-4 hr. *Infants:* T supp. q 3-4 hr. *Adults:* Matropinal Forte or Stopp-90 T q 4-6 hr where heavier sedation indicated. |
| | Matropinal Forte Stopp-15 Stopp-90 | 8 mg/10 mg/90 mg 8 mg/10 mg/15 mg 8 mg/10 mg/90 mg | | |

| Contraindications | Major side effects | Comments |
|---|---|---|
| None noted. | None noted. | May also be effective in morning sickness, regurgitation in infants, and motion sickness. Note: Do not dilute or give fluids prior to or 15 minutes after dose. |
| Acute intermittent porphyria; known sensitivity to barbiturates or antihistamines; previous barbiturate addiction; in infants under 6 mos.; senility; severe hepatic impairment; presence of uncontrolled pain, acute head injury or other CNS injury. | CNS, GU, and GI disturbances; cardiovascular problems; neuromuscular disturbances; blood dyscrasias; hypersensitivity reactions. | May be habit forming; use with caution in presence of other CNS depressants; caution should be exercised in use in presence of certain disorders. |
| Hypersensitivity; acute porphyria; hepatitis; severe renal disease. | Hypersensitivity reactions; CNS, GU, and GI disturbances, blood dyscrasias; cardiovascular and neuromuscular disturbances. | May be habit forming. May be helpful for conditions of smooth muscle spasm because of anticholinergic and sedative effects. |

**Table 25-15.** Sedatives and hypnotics: barbiturates

| Generic name | Trade name(s) | Dosage form(s) | Strength(s) | Usual dose |
|---|---|---|---|---|
| Phenobarbital | Various manufacturers | Tablet | 8, 15, 16, 30, 32, 65, 100 mg | *Adults:* 30-100 mg ½ to 1 hr before bedtime. |
| | Solfoton | Capsule | 16 mg | |
| | Eskabarb | Capsule | 65, 97 mg | *Children:* 8-30 mg ½ to 1 hr before bed- |
| | Various manufacturers | Time-release suppository | 8, 16, 32, 65, 100, 130 mg | time. |
| | Hypnette | Suppository | 8, 16 mg | |
| | Various manufacturers | Elixir | 20 mg/5 ml | |
| | Various manufacturers | Injection | 65 mg/ml-1, 2, 5 ml; 130 mg/ml-1, 10 ml | |
| | Luminal sodium | Injection (powder) | 130 mg | |
| | | Injection | 130 mg/ml-1 ml | |
| Mephobarbital | Mebaral | Tablet | 32, 50, 100, 200 mg | *Adults:* 32-100 mg. *Children:* 16-32 mg. |
| Amobarbital | Amytal | Tablet | 15, 30, 50, 100 mg | *Adults and children:* Adjust dosage to the individual patient. |
| | | Elixir | 22 mg/5 ml; 44 mg/ 5 ml | |
| | Amobarbital sodium | Capsule | 65, 200 mg | |
| | | Injection | 0.25, 0.5, 1 g | |
| | Amytal sodium | Capsule | 65, 200 mg | |
| | | Injection | 65, 125, 250 mg, 0.5 gm vial | |
| Aprobarbital | Alurate | Elixir | 40 mg/5 ml | *Adults:* 40-160 mg at bedtime. |
| | Verdum | Elixir | 40 mg/5 ml | |
| Butabarbital sodium | Bubartal | Tablet | 15, 30, 100 mg | *Adults:* 50-100 mg. *Children:* Dose should be deter- mined by physician according to age and weight. |
| | | Capsule | 15, 30 mg | |
| | | Elixir | 30 mg/5 ml | |
| | Buticaps | Capsule | 15, 30, 50, 100 mg | |
| | Butisol sodium | Tablet | 15, 30, 50, 100 mg | |
| | | Elixir | 30 mg/5 ml | |
| | | Repeat-action tab | 30, 60 mg | |
| | BBS | Tablet | 32 mg | |
| Talbutal | Lotsuate | Tablet | 120 mg | *Adults:* 120 mg 15-30 min before bed- time. |
| Pentobarbital | Nembutal sodium | Capsule | 30, 50, 100 mg | *Adults:* 100 mg at bed- time. |
| | | Gradumet | 100 mg | |
| | | Elixir | 20 mg/5 ml | *Children:* 50-100 mg at bedtime. |
| | | Suppository | 30, 60, 120, 200 mg | |
| | | Injection (IM, IV) | 50 mg/ml in 2, 5, 20, 50 ml | |
| Secobarbital | Seconal sodium | Elixir | 22 mg/5 ml | *Adults:* 100 mg at bedtime. |
| | | Injection (IM or IV) | 50 mg/ml 2 ml syringe; 20 ml vial | *Children:* 30-100 mg at bedtime ad- justed by age and weight. |
| | | Capsule | 30, 50, 100 mg | |
| | | Suppository | 30, 60, 120, 200 mg | |
| | | Enseals | 100 mg | |
| Hexobarbital | Sombulex | Tablet | 250 mg | *Adults:* 250-500 mg orally at bedtime. |

| Contraindications | Major side effects | Comments |
|---|---|---|
| Hypersensitivity; uncontrolled pain; known addiction potential; porphyria; respiratory disease with dyspnea or obstruction; marked hepatic or renal impairment; safe use during pregnancy and lactation has not been established. | Respiratory depression; hypersensitivity reactions; CNS disturbances; GI disturbances; megaloblastic anemia (with long-term therapy). | May be habit forming. May also be used as daytime sedative, in psychoses, as a pre- and/or postoperative sedative, and as an anticonvulsant. Barbiturates may alter effects of coumarin anticoagulants, CNS depressants, and hydrocortisone. This is a long-acting barbiturate. |
| Hypersensitivity; porphyria; impaired renal function. | CNS and GI disturbances; allergic reactions. | May be habit forming. May be used also as an anticonvulsant. Barbiturates may alter the effects of coumarin anticoagulants, CNS depressants, and hydrocortisone. This is a long-acting barbiturate. |
| Hypersensitivity; porphyria; impaired liver function; uncontrolled pain. | CNS and GI disturbances; allergic reactions. | May be habit forming. May be used also as an anticonvulsant. Barbiturates may alter the effects of coumarin anticoagulants, CNS depressants, and hydrocortisone. This is a moderate-acting barbiturate. |
| Hypersensitivity; porphyria; uncontrolled pain; impaired renal function; respiratory diseases where obstruction or dyspnea is present. | CNS and GI disturbances; allergic reactions. | Same as above. |
| Hypersensitivity; porphyria; impaired liver function; in respiratory disease where obstruction or dyspnea is present; patients with history of drug addiction; uncontrolled pain. | CNS and GI disturbances; hypersensitivity reactions. | May be habit forming. Barbiturates may alter effects of coumarin anticoagulants, CNS depressants, and hydrocortisone. This is a moderate-acting barbiturate. |
| Hypersensitivity; uncontrolled pain; known previous addiction; porphyria; respiratory disease where obstruction or dyspnea is present; marked hepatic impairment; impaired renal function. | CNS and GI disturbances; hypersensitivity reactions. | Same as above. |
| Hypersensitivity to barbiturates; porphyria (even history of); addiction; impaired liver function. | Allergic reactions; CNS and GI disturbances; respiratory depression; thrombophlebitis; injection site pain; nerve injury adjacent to injection site. | May be habit forming. May also be useful in acute convulsive conditions and as preoperative sedation. Safety in pregnancy has not been established; use with other CNS depressants. Precipitated or cloudy solutions should not be used. May alter the effects of coumarin anticoagulants, CNS depressants, and hydrocortisone. This is a short-acting barbiturate. |
| Hypersensitivity to barbiturates; parenteral form in obstetric deliveries; impaired liver function, in serious respiratory or heart disease. | Allergic reactions; CNS and GI disturbances; respiratory depression; pain at the injection site. | Same as above. |
| Hypersensitivity; to barbiturates; history of porphyria; impaired liver function; respiratory disease with dyspnea or obstruction present. | Allergic reactions; CNS and GI disturbances; respiratory depression. | May be habit forming. May also be used preoperatively with atropine when morphine is contraindicated and for postoperative sedation and in labor. Safety in pregnancy has not been established; use with caution in conjunction with other CNS depressants. May alter the effects of coumarin anticoagulants, CNS depressants, and hydrocortisone. This is an ultra-short-acting barbiturate. |

**Table 25-16.** Sedatives and hypnotics: nonbarbiturates

| Generic name | Trade name(s) | Dosage form(s) | Strength(s) | Usual dose |
|---|---|---|---|---|
| Paraldehyde | Various manufacturers | Liquid (oral or rectal) | 30 ml | *Oral or rectal:* 5-30 ml; *IM:* 5 ml; *IV:* 3-5 ml. |
| | Various manufacturers | Injection | 2, 5 ml | |
| | Paral | Liquid (oral) | 30 ml | |
| | | Capsule | 1 g | |
| | | Injection | 1 g/ml-2, 5, 10 ml | |
| Chloral hydrate | Aqua chloral | Suppository | 325, 650, 975 mg | *Adults:* Hypnotic: 500 mg-lg 15-30 minutes before bedtime. |
| | Cohidrate | Capsule | 500 mg | |
| | Felsules | Capsule | 250, 500 mg | |
| | Kessodrate | Capsule | 250, 500 mg | |
| | | Syrup | 500 mg/5 ml | *Children:* Hypnotic: 50 mg/kg body weight up to 1 g. |
| | Noctec | Capsule | 250, 500 mg | |
| | | Syrup | 500 mg/5 ml (orange) | |
| | Oradrate | Capsule | 500 mg | |
| | Rectules | Suppository | 650 mg | |
| | Somnos | Elixir | 267 mg/5 ml | |
| | Various manufacturers | Suppository | 500 mg | |
| Chloralbetaine | Beta-Chlor | Tablet | 870 mg equiv. to 500 mg chloral hydrate | *Adults:* 1 or 2 tablets 15-30 min before bedtime. |
| Triclofos sodium | Triclos | Tablet | 750 mg | *Adults:* 1500 mg 15-30 min before bedtime. |
| | | Liquid | 1.5 g/15 ml | *Children under 12:* 0.1 ml liquid per lb body weight for sleep induction in EEG (only use recommended in children). |
| Glutethimide | Doriden | Capsule | 500 mg | *Adults:* 250-500 mg at bedtime; repeat if necessary but not less than 4 hr before arising. Not recommended in children under 12. |
| | | Tablet | 125, 250, 500 mg | |
| Methyprylon | Noludar | Capsule | 300 mg | *Adults:* 200-400 mg before retiring. |
| | | Tablet | 50, 200 mg | *Children over 3 mo:* initiate therapy with 50 mg and increase up to 200 mg if necessary. |
| Ethchlorvynol | Placidyl | Capsule | 100, 200, 500, 750 mg | *Adult:* 500 mg orally at bedtime. Note: smallest effective dose should be used. |
| Ethinamate | Valmid | Capsule | 500 mg | *Adult:* 500-1000 mg orally 20 min. prior to bedtime. |
| Flurazepam HCl | Dalmane | Capsule | 15, 30 mg | *Adult:* 15-30 mg before retiring. |
| Methaqualone HCl | Parest | Capsule | 200, 400 mg | *Adult:* 150-400 mg at bedtime. |
| | Quaalude | Tablet | 150, 300 mg | *Geriatric:* smallest effective dose. |
| | Sopor | Tablet | 150, 300 mg | *Not recommended for children.* |

| Contraindications | Major side effects | Comments |
|---|---|---|
| Hypersensitivity; bronchopulmonary disease; hepatic insufficiency; gastroenteritis. | None. | *May be habit forming.* May be mixed with milk or juice to mask taste. |
| Hypersensitivity; marked hepatic or renal impairment; severe heart disease; gastritis; nursing mothers. *Note:* use with caution in pregnancy. | Gastric irritation; occasional allergic skin rashes; excitement and delirium. | *May be habit forming.* Exercise caution in patients with circulatory weakness and those on other CNS depressants. Interactions with coumarin and coumarin-related anticoagulants may occur. |
| Hypersensitivity; use with extreme caution in the presence of severe cardiac, liver, or kidney disease. | Gastric irritation; excitement. | *May be habit forming.* May also be used for preoperative sedation. Note: Beta-Chlor may interact with other medications by a variety of mechanisms; drugs include oral anticoagulants and other CNS depressants. |
| Hypersensitivity to this drug or chloral hydrate; marked renal or hepatic impairment. Exercise caution in patients with cardiac arrhythmias or severe cardiac disease. | CNS, GI, and dermatologic reactions; staggering, gait; ketonuria; reduction in total white blood cell count; excitement; delirium. | *May be habit forming.* Safety for use in pregnant or nursing mothers has not been established. May interact with oral anticoagulants to modify their action. May potentiate other CNS depressants. |
| Hypersensitivity. | Dermatologic reactions; blood dyscrasias; nausea; excitement; blurred vision; porphyria. | *May be habit forming.* Safety during pregnancy and lactation has not been established. May potentiate effects of alcohol and other CNS depressants. May alter efficacy of coumarin anticoagulants. |
| Hypersensitivity. Note: daily doses should not exceed 400 mg. | GI disturbances; headache; morning drowsiness; dizziness; skin rashes; excitation; possible blood dyscrasias. | *May be habit forming.* Not recommended for children under 3 mos. of age. Safe usage in lactation and pregnancy has not been established. May potentiate effects of alcohol and other CNS depressants. Exercise caution if hepatic or renal disorders present. |
| Hypersensitivity; porphyria; exercise caution in elderly or debilitated patients and those with impaired hepatic or renal function. | Hypersensitivity reactions; GI disturbances; hypotension; dizziness; blurred vision; thrombocytopenia; cholestatic jaundice; hangover and a variety of idiosyncratic reactions. | *May be habit forming.* Not recommended for use in children, lactating mothers, or during 1st and 2nd trimester of pregnancy. Use extreme caution in concomitant use with: CNS depressants, MAO inhibitors, coumarin anticoagulants, and tricyclic antidepressants. |
| Hypersensitivity; usage in children. | GI and dermatologic disturbances; excitement; rarely thrombocytopenic purpura. | *May be habit forming.* Safety during pregnancy and lactation has not been established. May potentiate alcohol and other CNS depressants. |
| Hypersensitivity; children under 15 years. | GI, GU, and CNS disturbances; rarely blood dyscrasias; dermatologic reactions; blurred vision; and a variety of changes in laboratory values. | *May be habit forming.* Safety during pregnancy and lactation has not been established. May potentiate effects of other CNS depressants. Note: exercise caution in elderly or debilitated patients and in presence of impaired hepatic or renal function. |
| Hypersensitivity; during pregnancy; in children. Exercise extreme caution in the presence of impaired hepatic function. | GI, dermatologic, and hematologic disturbances; neuropsychiatric reactions. | *May be habit forming.* May have some antitussive and antispasmodic activity. Metabolized in liver and excreted in urine and feces. May have addictive effects when used with other CNS depressants and/or psychotropic agents. |

**Table 25-17.** Skeletal muscle relaxants

| Generic name | Trade name(s) | Dosage form(s) | Strength(s) | Usual dose |
|---|---|---|---|---|
| Carisoprodol | Rela<br>Soma | Tablet<br>Tablet | 350 mg<br>350 mg | *Adults:* 350 mg tid and at bedtime. |
| Chlorphenesin carbamate | Maolate | Tablet | 400 mg | Initially 2 tablets tid then 1 tablet qid or less as required. |
| Chlorzoxazone | Paraflex | Tablet | 250 mg | *Adults:* 250 mg 3-4 times daily up to 750 mg 3-4 times daily<br>*Children:* 125-500 mg 3-4 times daily. |
| Dantrolene sodium | Dantrium | Capsule | 25, 50, 75, 100 mg | *Adults:* Begin with 25 mg daily, increase in increments of 25 mg up to 100 mg qid as necessary.<br>*Children:* use same approach as in adults with basis of 1 mg/kg body weight. |
| Diazepam | Valium | Tablet<br>Injection (IM or IV) | 2.5, 10 mg<br>5 mg/ml-2, 10 ml | *Adults:* 2-10 mg 2-4 times daily<br>*Children under 6:* 50 mg/day in divided doses.<br>*Over 6:* 50-100 mg/day in divided doses. |
| Meprobamate | Equanil<br><br><br><br>Miltown | Tablet<br>Coated tablet<br>Capsule<br>Oral suspension<br>Tablet<br>Injection | 200, 400 mg<br>400 mg<br>400 mg<br>200 mg/5 ml<br>200, 400, 600 mg<br>400 mg/5 ml ampule | *Adults: Oral:* 1200-1600 mg daily in divided doses.<br>*IM:* 400 mg q 3-4 hr.<br>*Children: 6-12: Oral:* 100-200 mg 2-3 times daily. *IM:* ½ adult dose.<br>*Infants: IM:* 125 mg q 6 hr. |
| Metaxalone | Skelaxin | Tablet | 400 mg | *Adults and children over 12:* 800 mg 3 or 4 times daily. |
| Methocarbamol | Robaxin<br><br>MethoCarb<br>Metho-500 | Tablet<br>Injection (IV or IM)<br>Tablet<br>Tablet | 500, 750 mg<br>100 mg/ml-10 ml<br>500, 750 mg<br>500 mg | *Injection: IV:* 1 mg IV push or in fusion.<br>*IM:* 500 mg in each hip up to q 8 hr.<br>*Oral: Adults:* 1.5 gm qid initially, then 1 gm qid or 750 mg q 4 hr or 1.5 gm tid. |
| Orphenadrine citrate | Norflex<br><br>X-Otag | Tablet<br>Injection<br>Injection | 100 mg<br>30 mg/ml-2 ml<br>30 mg/ml-10 ml | *Oral:* 100 mg in AM and PM<br>*Injection:* IV or IM repeated q 12 hr. |
| Quinine sulfate | Various manufacturers | Capsule | 3, 5 grains (200, 325 mg) | *Adults:* 5 or 10 grains at bedtime for leg cramps. |

| Contraindications | Major side effects | Comments |
| --- | --- | --- |
| Hypersensitivity; acute intermittent porphyria; usage in children under 12. | CNS and cardiovascular disturbances; allergic and idiosyncratic reactions; GI disturbances, and hematologic reactions. | May have addictive effect if used with alcohol, CNS depressants, or psychotropic drugs; use caution in patients with impaired liver or kidney function. |
| Hypersensitivity; use in children; in hepatic dysfunction. | Hypersensitivity reactions; CNS disturbances; GI distress; hematopoietic disturbances. | Has not been proved efficacious for muscle spasticity; safe use in pregnancy has not been established. May impair mental and physical abilities such as operating machinery or driving. |
| Hypersensitivity. | CNS and GI disturbances; allergic responses; may cause drug-induced hepatitis. | Safe usage in pregnancy has not been established. Occasionally causes discoloration of urine. |
| Active hepatic disease; hypersensitivity. | CNS and GI disturbances; neurologic and cardiovascular disturbances; urogenital and dermatologic problems; hepatobiliary toxicity. | Safe usage in children under 5 not established nor in pregnant women; may evoke a photo-sensitivity reaction. Use caution if impaired pulmonary function present; may have drug interaction with estrogens and tranquilizing agents; does not act on CNS but directly on the muscle. |
| In children under 6 mo; psychoses; acute narrow angle glaucoma; hypersensitivity. | CNS, GI, GU, and cardiovascular disturbances; EENT and dermatologic manifestations. | Is also useful for anxiety; as a preoperative medication, cardiospasm, for status epilepticus and in severe convulsive seizures. *Note:* injection should not be mixed with other medications. |
| Hypersensitivity; acute intermittent porphyria. | CNS, cardiovascular, and GI disturbances; allergic and idiosyncratic reactions; hematologic disturbances. | May also be useful for anxiety states and/or to promote sleep. *Note:* causes exacerbation of porphyric symptoms. Use with caution with alcohol. CNS depressants, and psychotropic agents. |
| Hypersensitivity; impaired renal or hepatic function; in patients with known tendency toward drug-induced or other anemias. | GI and CNS disturbances; allergic response; liver damage; hematologic disturbances. | Safety in children under 12; during pregnancy and/or lactation is not established. May give false-positive Benedict's test. |
| Known or suspected renal impairment; hypersensitivity. | *Oral:* CNS and GI disturbances; allergic manifestations. *Injectable:* CNS and GI disturbances; thrombophlebitis; sloughing and pain at injection site; cardiovascular and ophthalmic complaints. | May interfere with lab tests for 5-HIAA and VMA; safe usage in children under 12 or during pregnancy and lactation not established. |
| Hypersensitivity; glaucoma; pyloric or duodenal obstruction; peptic ulcer; prostatic hypertrophy; obstruction of bladder neck; cardiospasm; myasthenia gravis. | CNS and cardiovascular disturbances; GI, GU, and ophthalmic manifestations; dermatologic problems. | May have drug reaction with propoxyphene and these should not be given concomitantly. |
| Women of childbearing potential; pregnancy; sensitivity; glucose-6-phosphate dehydrogenase deficiency; and serious heart disease. | CNS and GI disturbances; otic and dermatologic manifestations; renal and cardiovascular disturbances. | Reversible thrombocytopenic purpura may occur. Of value as an antimalarial; muscle relaxant. Action is directly on skeletal muscle fiber. *Note:* Has some quinidine-like action on the heart. |

**Table 25-18.** Anticoagulants

| Generic name | Trade name(s) | Dosage form(s) | Strength(s) | Usual dose |
|---|---|---|---|---|
| Anisindione | Miradon | Tablet | 50 mg | 300 mg day 1, 200 mg day 2, 100 mg day 3, then 25-250 mg maintenance daily. |
| Dicumarol | Various manufacturers | Tablet<br>Capsule | 25, 50, 100 mg<br>25, 50, 100 mg | 200-300 mg day 1 then 25-200 mg daily if prothrombin activity 25% or more of normal. |
| Acenocoumarol | Sintrom | Tablet (double-scored) | 4 mg | 16-28 mg day 1, 8-16 mg day 2, 2-10 mg daily for maintenance. |
| Diphenadione | Dipaxin | Tablet | 5 mg | 20-30 mg day 1, 10-15 mg day 2, 3-5 mg maintenance. |
| Fibrinolysin | Thrombolysin | Injection | 50,000 U | 50,000-100,000 U/hr by IV drip for 1-6 hr. daily for 3-4 days; dosage should be individualized and followed with anticoagulant therapy. |
| Heparin sodium | Various manufacturers | Injection primarily for SQ and IV use | 1000 U/ml-1, 10, 30 ml; 5000 U/ml 1, 10 ml; 7500 U/ml-1 ml; 10,000 U/ml-1, 45, 10 ml; 15,000 U/ml-ml; 20,000 U/ml-1, 2, 4, 5, 10 ml; 40,000 U/ml-1, 2, 4, 5, 10 ml | *SQ:* initially 10,000-20,000 U, then q 8 h, 8-10,000 U or q 12 h, 12-20,000 U<br>*IV:* initially 10,000 U, then 5-10,000 q4-6h Cont. Inf: 2-40,000 U/day in 1 L solution. |
| Phenindione | Hedulin<br>Danilone<br>Eridione | Tablet | 50 mg | 500 mg day 1, 100 mg daily as maintenance. |
| Phenprocoumon | Liquamar | Tablet | 3 mg | Induction 24 mg; maintenance 0.75 to 6 mg daily |
| Protamine sulfate | Various manufacturers | Injection | 10 mg/ml-5, 25 ml ampules; 50 mg powder with 5 ml ampule of diluent | Not to exceed 50 mg protamine in any 10-hr. period. Each mg neutralizes 90 U lung or 115 U intestinal heparin. |
| Warfarin potassium | Athrombin | Tablet | 5, 10 mg | Initial 40-60 mg maintenance 2.5-10 mg. |
| Warfarin sodium | Coumadin<br><br>Panwarfin | Tablet<br>Injection<br>Tablet | 2, 2.5, 5, 7.5, 10, 25 mg<br>50 mg vial with 2 ml vial of diluent<br>2, 2.5, 5, 7.5, 10, 25 mg | Initially 40-60 mg; maintenance 2-10 mg orally, IM, or IV. |

| Contraindications | Major side effects | Comments |
|---|---|---|
| Hemophilia, thrombocytopenic purpura; leukemia; with bleeding tendency; open wounds; impaired hepatic or renal function; severe hypertension; acute nephritis; subacute bacterial endocarditis; hypersensitivity. | Dermatitis; colors urine red-orange; watch for agranulocytosis; jaundice; nephropathy, diarrhea; urticaria, and fever. | Safe use in pregnancy not established. Vitamin K is specific antidote; potential for drug interactions is great. Therapy should be controlled by daily prothrombin time determinations. |
| Active bleeding; subacute bacterial endocarditis; hypersensitivity. | Hemorrhage; dermatologic reactions; GI and hematologic disturbances; colors urine red-orange; nephropathy. | Anticoagulant effect altered by many drugs, disease states and many other factors; adjunct dosage based on prothrombin time; safe usage in pregnancy has not been established. |
| Hypersensitivity; active bleeding; subacute endocarditis. | GI and GU disturbances; hematologic problems; allergic type reactions; nephropathy and red-orange urine. | Therapy should be determined by periodic prothrombin times; safe use in pregnancy not established; activity altered by many drugs, foods, and other factors. |
| Hypersensitivity; active bleeding; subacute bacterial endocarditis. | GI and GU disturbances; hematologic disturbances; allergic type reactions; nephropathy; discoloration of urine. | Same as above |
| Presence of hemorrhagic diathesis or hypofibrinogenemia. | Febrile reaction with other accompanying symptoms; hypertension; flushing; chest and abdominal pain. | Contains no preservative and is unstable in solution. Should be used within 2 hr. Do not use NaCl as diluent and do not shake solution. May be used intraarterially in thrombosed arteries. |
| Hypersensitivity; active bleeding or bleeding tendencies; severe hepatic, renal, or biliary disease; subacute bacterial endocarditis; threatened abortion; visceral carcinoma; during and immediately after major surgery of eye, brain, and spinal cord. | Bleeding from overdosage; thrombocytopenia; osteoporosis; alopecia; allergic reactions. | Test doses may be advisable before beginning therapy; drug interactions may occur with aspirin, ACTH, insulin, corticosteroids, digitalis, tetracyclines, nicotine, and antihistamines. |
| Hypersensitivity; active bleeding; subacute bacterial endocarditis. | GI and GU disturbances; hematologic and hepatic reactions; allergic responses; dermatologic responses and discoloration of the urine. | Therapy should be determined by periodic prothrombin times; safe use in pregnancy has not been established; activity may be altered by many drugs and other factors. |
| Hypersensitivity; active bleeding; subacute bacterial endocarditis. | GI and GU disturbances; hematologic and hepatic reactions; allergic responses; dermatologic reactions; discoloration of the urine. | Safety during pregnancy has not been established; therapy should be determined by periodic prothrombin times; activity may be altered by many drugs, foods, and other factors. |
| Safety in pregnancy not established. | Cardiovascular disturbances are most prominent. | Antidote for heparin overdosage; has anticoagulant effect alone. |
| Active bleeding; open wounds; visceral carcinoma; GI ulcers; severe liver or kidney disease; uncontrolled hypertension; subacute bacterial endocarditis; patients with recent eye, brain, or spinal cord surgery; Vitamin K deficiency. | Hemorrhage and resulting problems. | Safe use during pregnancy and lactation not established; activity is altered by diet, many drugs, and disease states; dosage should be altered according to prothrombin time. |
| Same as above. | Same as above. | Same as above. |

618 Treatment alternatives

**Table 25-19.** Antirheumatic agents: nonstearoid-nonsalicylates

| Generic name | Trade name(s) | Dosage form(s) | Strength(s) | Usual dose |
|---|---|---|---|---|
| Indomethacin | Indocin | Capsule | 25, 50 mg | Smallest effective dose for individual patient should be used. *Adult:* 25-50 mg 2-3 times daily. |
| Phenylbutazone | Butazolidin | Tablet | 100 mg | Smallest effective dose for the individual patient for shortest period of time should be used. *Adult dose:* 300-600 mg daily in 3-4 equal doses. |
| | Azolid | Tablet | 100 mg | |
| Phenylbutazone with antacids | Butazolidin Alka | Capsule | 100 mg* | |
| | Azolid-A | Capsule | 100 mg* | |
| Oxyphenbutazone | Tandearil | Tablet | 100 mg | Smallest effective dose for patient for the shortest period of time should be used. *Adult dose:* 300-400 mg daily in 3-4 equally divided doses. |
| | Oxalid | Tablet | 100 mg | |
| Ibuprofen | Motrin | Tablet | 300 and 400 mg | *Adults:* 300-400 mg orally tid or gid. Dosage should be tailored to individual patient. |
| Fenoprofen calcium | Nalfon | Capsule | 300 mg | *Adults:* 600 mg 4 times daily. Dosage should be adjusted to individual patient. Should be given 30 min before or 2 hr after meals unless GI distress is observed. |
| Naproxen | Naprosyn | Tablet | 250 mg | *Adults:* 250 mg orally bid. Dosage should be adjusted to individual patient. |

*With aluminum hydroxide gel and magnesium trisilicate.

| Contraindications | Major side effects | Comments |
|---|---|---|
| GI lesions; allergy to aspirin or indomethacin; pregnancy; usage in children under 14. | GI and CNS reactions; hepatic and hematologic reactions; eye and ear reactions; hypersensitivity reactions; cardiovascular, renal, dermatologic reactions. | Nonsteroid drug with antiinflammatory, antipyretic, and analgesic properties; should be given at meals; with food, or with antacids. Indomethacin is likely to interact with probenecid and anticoagulants. |
| Use in children under 14 yr; use in senile patients; GI lesions or ulceration; concomitant therapy with anticoagulants and other potent chemotherapeutic agents; history or presence of: drug allergy, blood dyscrasias; renal, hepatic, or cardiac dysfunction; hypertension; thyroid disease; systemic edema; polymyalgia rheumatica and temporal arteritis. | GI and hematologic reactions; allergic reactions; fluid and electrolyte disturbances; hepatic and renal disturbances; CNS and cardiovascular reactions; metabolic, otic, and ocular disturbances. | Should always be given with food or milk or the antacid combination used. *This is a potent drug with a potential for severe or fatal side effects and should be used with extreme caution.* Should be used with extreme caution if at all in pregnant women or nursing mothers. This drug potentiates the action of insulin, sulfanylurea, and sulfanamide-type agents. Phenylbutazone is a nonhormonal anti-arthritic antiinflammatory agent with antipyretic, analgesic, and uricosuric properties. |
| Use in children under 14 yr; use in senile patients; GI lesions or ulcerations; concomitant therapy with anticoagulants and other potent chemotherapeutic agents; history or presence of: drug allergy, blood dyscrasias, renal, hepatic, or cardiac dysfunction; hypertension; thyroid disease; systemic edema; polymyalgia rheumatica, and temporal arteritis. | GI and hematologic-reactions; allergic reactions; fluid and electrolyte disturbances; hepatic and renal disturbances; CNS and cardiovascular reactions; metabolic, otic, and ocular disturbances. | Should always be given with food or milk or an antacid. *This is a potent drug with a potential for severe or fatal side effects and should be used with extreme caution.* Should be used with extreme caution if at all in pregnant women or nursing mothers. This drug potentiates the action of insulin, sulfonylurea, and sulfonamide-type agents. Oxyphenbutazone is a nonhormonal antiarthritic antiinflammatory agent with antipyretic, analgesic, and uricosuric properties. |
| Hypersensitivity; hypersensivity to aspirin or other nonsteroidal antiinflammatory agents | GI and CNS disturbances; dermatologic and hematologic reactions; cardiovascular disturbances; audio and visual disturbances. | Use extreme caution in patients with GI conditions. Safe usage in pregnant women, nursing mothers and children has not been established. Possible drug interactions may occur with aspirin and coumarin-type anticoagulants. May be given with meals or milk to minimize GI upset. |
| Hypersensitivity; hypersensitivity to aspirin or other nonsteroidal antiinflammatory drugs. | GI and CNS disturbances; dermatologic and hematologic reactions; cardiovascular disturbances. | Safe use in pregnant women, nursing mothers, children and patients with impaired hearing has not been established. Use with extreme caution in patients with GI conditions. Drug interactions may occur with phenobarbital, coumarin-type anticoagulants, and other drugs that are albumin bound. |
| Hypersensitivity; hypersensitivity to aspirin or other nonsteroidal antiinflammatory drugs. | GI and CNS disturbances; dermatologic reactions; audiovisual disturbances; cardiovascular and hematologic disturbances. | Safe use in pregnant women, nursing mothers, and children has not been established. Use with caution in patients with GI conditions or impaired renal function. This drug may interact with coumarin-type anticoagulants and other albumin-bound drugs; it also may alter the results of certain lab studies. |

*Continued.*

**Table 25-19.** Antirheumatic agents: nonstearoid-nonsalicylates—cont'd

| Generic name | Trade name(s) | Dosage form(s) | Strength(s) | Usual dose |
|---|---|---|---|---|
| Gold sodium thiomalate | Myochrysine | Injection | 10 mg/ml-1 ml<br>25 mg/ml-1 ml<br>50 mg/ml-1, 10 ml<br>100 mg/ml-1 ml | *Adults:* weekly injections as below: injection 1, 10 mg; injection 2, 25 mg; injection 3-16 or 20, 50 mg.<br>*To be given IM* 6 to 8 wk may be required to note improvements. |
| Aurothioglucose | Solganal | Injection (suspension) | 50 mg/ml-10 ml | *Adults:* Weekly injections as below: dose 1, 10 mg; doses 2 and 3, 25 mg; subsequent doses, 50 mg.<br>*Children:* 6-12 yr: $\frac{1}{4}$ the adult dose governed by body weight.<br>*To be given IM.* |
| Gold sodium thiosulfate, sodium thiosulfate | | Injection | 50 mg/5 ml-5 ml | *Adults:* Weekly injections as below: week 1, 5 mg, 25 mg weekly until 500-1000 mg total dose given.<br>*To be given IM.* |
| Tolmetin sodium | Tolectin | Tablet | 200 mg | *Adults:* 200 mg tid with one dose on arising and one at bedtime. Dosage should be adjusted to each individual patient. |
| Hydroxy-chloroquine sulfate | Plaquenil sulfate | Tablet | 200 mg | *Adults:* 400-600 mg daily with a meal or glass of milk. |

| Contraindications | Major side effects | Comments |
|---|---|---|
| Severe toxicity from previous use of gold or heavy metals; severe debilitation; systemic lupus erythematosus; Sjogren's syndrome in rheumatoid arthritis. Save use in pregnancy has not been established. | Cutaneous or dermatologic reactions; renal and hematologic reactions; mucous membrane reactions; nitritoid and allergic reactions; GI distress; alopecia; reactions involving the eye. | Gold compounds should be only one part of a complete program of therapy. Greatest benefit occurs in the early active stages of the disease. Before each injection, blood counts and urinalysis should be done. Use with extreme caution in patients having: marked hypertension, previous liver or kidney disease; hypersensitivity to medications; history of blood dyscrasias caused by drug sensitivity. |
| Severe diabetes; renal disease; marked hypertension; hepatitis; heart failure; pregnancy; history of agranulocytic angina; hemorrhagic diathesis; patients with blood dyscrasias; recent radiation; urticaria; eczema; colitis. | Skin and mucous membrane reactions; hematologic reactions; GI reactions; toxic hepatitis. | Urine examinations and complete blood counts should be done at 2-week intervals; the patient should be questioned regarding side effects and examined prior to each injection. |
| History of toxic reactions to gold or heavy metals; disseminated lupus erythematosus; tuberculosis; presence of anemia or blood dyscrasias; impaired liver or kidney function; chronic skin disorders; pregnancy. | Skin and mucous membrane reactions; peripheral neuritis; blood dyscrasias; encephalitis. | Urinalyses and blood counts should be done routinely during therapy; patients should avoid exposure to sunlight or artificial ultraviolet light. May also be used for discoid lupus erythematosus. |
| Hypersensitivity; hypersensitivity to aspirin or other nonsteroidal antiinflammatory drugs. | GI and CNS disturbances; dermatologic and hematological reactions; cardiovascular disturbances; tinnitus. | Safe use in pregnant women, nursing mothers, and children has not been established. Use with caution in patients with GI conditions or impaired renal function. Metabolites of this drug may give positive tests for proteinuria. |
| Hypersensitivity; long-term therapy in children; retinal or visual field changes attributable to any 4-aminoquinoline compound. | CNS and GI disturbances; ocular reactions; dermatologic and hematologic reactions. | May also be useful in lupus erythematosus and malaria. Use with extreme caution in pregnant women, children, patients with psoriasis, porphyria, and hepatic disease. Patients on long-term therapy should be monitored closely. |

**Table 25-20.** Antiinflammatory agents' systemic steroids

| Generic name | Trade name(s) | Dosage form(s) | Strength(s) | Usual dose |
|---|---|---|---|---|
| Corticotropin (ACTH) | Acthar | Injection | U/vial | Dosage should be adjusted to patient and condition. Short-term administration in acute episodes of rheumatic disorders is usual. |
| | Various manufacturers | Injection | 20 U/ml-2, 10 ml<br>40 U/ml-5 ml<br>80 U/ml-5 ml | |
| Corticotropin repository | HP Acthar Gel | Injection | 40 U/ml-1, 5 ml<br>80 U/ml-1, 5 ml | |
| | Cortigel-40 | Injection | 40 U/ml-5 ml | |
| | Cortigel-80 | Injection | 80 U/ml-5 ml | |
| | Cortrophin Gel | Injection | 40 U/ml-1, 5 ml<br>80 U/ml-5 ml | |
| Corticotropin zinc | Cortrophin Zinc | Injection | 40 U/ml-5 ml | |
| Cortisone acetate | Cortone | Tablet<br>Injection (for IM use) | 5 mg, 25 mg<br>25 mg/ml-20 ml<br>50 mg/ml-10 ml | Lowest dose that provides adequate relief. |
| Hydrocortisone | Cortef | Tablet<br>Injection (IM)<br>Suspension | 5, 10, 20 mg<br>50 mg/ml-5 ml<br>10 mg/ml-4 oz. | *Oral:* begin with 20-40 mg daily and increase to smallest amount that gives the desired relief.<br>*Parenteral:* $\frac{1}{3}$-$\frac{1}{2}$ oral dose q 12 h. |
| | Hydrocortone | Tablet<br>Injection (IM, SQ, IV) | 10, 20 mg<br>50 mg/ml-2, 10 ml | |
| | SoluCortef | Injection (IM or IV) | 100 mg-2, 10 ml<br>25 mg-2 ml<br>500 mg-4 ml<br>1 gm-8 ml | |
| Methylprednisolone | Medrol | Tablet<br>Medule (sustained action capsule) | 2, 4, 16 mg<br>2, 4 mg | *Oral:* initial daily dose from 4-48 mg.<br>*Parenteral: Adult:* initial dose from 10-40 mg.<br>*Children and infants:* Not less than 0.5 mg/kg every 24 hr. Dosage should be adjusted to disease state and patient's response. |
| | Depo Medrol | Injection | 20 mg/ml-5 ml<br>40 mg/ml-1, 5, 10 ml<br>62.5 mg/ml-2, 8, 16 ml vials | |
| Prednisone | Delta-Dome | Tablet | 5 mg | Initial dosage may vary from 5 to 60 mg/day. Dosage requirements vary and must be individualized on basis of disease state and patient's response. |
| | Deltasone | Tablet | 2.5, 5, 10, 20, 50 mg | |
| | Fernisone | Tablet | 5 mg | |
| | Lisacort | Tablet | 5 mg | |
| | Meticorten | Tablet | 1 mg, 5 mg | |
| | Orasone | Tablet | 1, 5, 10, 20 mg | |
| | Paracort | Tablet | 5 mg | |
| | Pred-5 | Tablet | 5 mg | |
| | Prednicen-M | Tablet | 5 mg | |
| | Servisone | Tablet | 5 mg | |
| | Sterapred | Tablet | 5 mg | |

| Contraindications | Major side effects | Comments |
|---|---|---|
| Scleroderma; osteoporosis; systemic fungal infections; ocular herpes simplex; recent surgery; history or present peptic ulcer; congestive heart failure; hypertension; sensitivity to proteins of porcine origin; hypersensitivity. Conditions accompanied by primary adrenocortical insufficiency or adrenocortical hyperfunction; IV use except for diagnostic testing. | Fluid and electrolyte disturbances; allergic reactions; endocrine and metabolic disturbances; musculoskeletal and GI reactions; dermatologic and ophthalmic disturbances; cardiovascular and neurologic disturbances. | Safe usage in pregnancy has not been established. Use with caution in ulcerative colitis, diverticulitis, peptic ulcer, not reversible. ACTH should be adjunctive and not sole therapy. Use with caution in diabetes; abscess; pyogenic infections, diverticulitis, renal insufficiency and myasthenia gravis. Drug interactions may occur with aspirin, insulin, and oral hypoglycemic agents. |
| Hypersensitivity; systemic fungal infection. | Fluid and electrolyte disturbances; allergic reactions; endocrine and metabolic disturbances; musculoskeletal and GI reactions; dermatologic and ophthalmic disturbances; neurologic reactions; psychological and/or physiological dependency; pigmentation changes. | Safe usage in pregnancy has not been established. Use with caution in ocular herpes simplex, ulcerative colitis, diverticulitis, peptic ulcer, renal insufficiency, hypertension, osteoporosis, and myasthenia gravis. Large oral doses should be given with food, milk, or antacids. Drug interaction may occur with aspirin, phenytoin, phenobarbital, and coumarin-type anticoagulants. |
| Hypersensitivity; systemic fungal infections. | Fluid and electrolyte disturbances; allergic reactions; endocrine and metabolic disturbances; dermatologic and ophthalmic disturbances; musculoskeletal and GI reactions; neurologic reactions; psychic derangements. | Safe usage in pregnancy has not been established. Use with caution in ulcerative colitis, diverticulitis, peptic ulcer, renal insufficiency, hypertension, osteoporosis, and myasthenia gravis. Large oral doses should be given with food, milk, or antacids. |
| Hypersensitivity; systemic fungal infections. | Same as above. | Same as above. |
| Hypersensitivity; systemic fungal infections. | Fluid and electrolyte disturbances; metabolic and endocrine disturbances; dermatologic and ophthalmic reactions; musculoskeletal reactions; GI and neurologic disturbances; psychic derangements. | Safe usage in pregnant women, nursing mothers, and women of childbearing potential has not been established. Use with caution in herpes simplex, ulcerative colitis, diverticulitis, peptic ulcer, renal insufficiency, hypertension, osteoporosis, and myasthenia gravis. Large oral doses should be given with food, milk, or antacids. |

*Continued.*

**Table 25-20.** Antiinflammatory agents: systemic steroids—cont'd

| Generic name | Trade name(s) | Dosage form(s) | Strength(s) | Usual dose |
|---|---|---|---|---|
| Prednisolone | Various manufacturers | Tablet | 1, 2.5, 5 mg | *Oral:* Initial dose may range from 5-60 mg daily. *Parenteral: IM:* 4-60 mg per day. Not recommended for IV use. Dosage requirements vary and must be individualized on basis of disease state and patient's response. |
| | Delta-Cortef | Tablet | 5 mg | |
| | Durapred | Injection | 100 mg/ml-10 ml | |
| | Fernisolone | Tablet | 5 mg | |
| | | Buffered tablet | 5 mg | |
| | | Injection | 25 mg/ml-1 ml | |
| | Hydeltrasol | Injection | 200 mg/ml-2, 5 ml | |
| | Meticortelone | Injection | 25 mg/ml-5 ml | |
| | Prednis | Tablet | 5 mg | |
| | Predoxine | Tablet (buffered) | 5 mg | |
| | Ropredlone | Tablet | 1, 5 mg | |
| | | Injection | 25 mg/ml-10 ml | |
| | | | 50 mg/ml-10 ml | |
| | | | 100 mg/ml-10 ml | |
| | Sterane | Tablet | 5 mg | |
| | | Injection | 25 mg/ml-5 ml | |
| | Savacort-50 | Injection | 50 mg/ml-10 ml | |
| | Savacort-100 | Injection | 100 mg/ml/10 ml | |
| Triamcinolone | Aristocort | Tablet | 1, 2, 4, 8, 16 mg | *Oral:* Initial daily dose range is 8-16 mg. *Parenteral: Not for IV use. IM:* 40 mg 1 week. Dosage requirements vary and must be individualized on basis of disease state and patients response. |
| | | Syrup | 2 mg/5 ml | |
| | | Injection, forte | 40 mg/ml-1, 5 ml | |
| | Cenocort | Injection, forte | 40 mg/ml-5 ml | |
| | Cino-40 | Injection | 40 mg/ml-5 ml | |
| | Kenacort | Tablet | 1, 2, 4, 8 mg | |
| | | Syrup | 4 mg/5 ml | |
| | Kenalog-40 | Injection | 40 mg/ml-1, 5, 10 ml | |
| | Rocinolone | Tablet | 4 mg | |
| Meprednisone | Betapar | Tablet | 4 mg | Initial dose may vary from 8-60 mg/day. Dosage should be adjusted to disease state and patient's response. |
| Paramethasone acetate | Haldrone | Tablet | 1, 2 mg | Initial dose may vary from 2 to 24 mg/day. Dosage should be adjusted to disease state and patient's response. |
| Fluprednisolone | Alphadrol | Tablet | 1.5 mg | Initial dose may vary from 2.5 to 30 mg per day. Dosage should be adjusted to disease state and patient's response. |
| Dexamethasone | Decadron | Tablet | 0.25, 0.5, 0.75, 1.5, 4 mg | *Adults:* initial dose may vary from 0.75 mg to 9 mg daily. *Children:* approximately 0.2 mg/kg/24 hr in oral divided doses. Dosage should be adjusted to disease state and patient's response. |
| | | Elixir | 0.5 mg/5 ml | |
| | | Injection | 4 mg/ml-1, 5, 25 ml | |
| | Deronil | Tablet | 0.75 mg | |
| | Dexameth | Tablet | 0.75 mg | |
| | Dexone | Tablet | 0.5, 0.75, 1.5, 4 mg | |
| | Gamma corten | Tablet | 0.75 mg | |
| | Hexadrol | Tablet | 0.5, 0.75, 1.5, 4 mg | |
| | | Elixir | 0.5 mg/5 ml | |
| | | Injection | 4 mg/ml-1, 5 ml | |
| Betamethasone | Celestone | Tablet | 0.6 mg | *Oral:* 0.6 to 7.2 mg daily. *Parenteral:* 1 ml (6 mg) initial dose. Dosage should be adjusted to disease state and patient's response. |
| | | Syrup | 0.6 mg/5 ml | |
| | Celestone soluspan (not for IV use) | Injection | 6 mg/ml-5 ml | |

| Contraindications | Major side effects | Comments |
|---|---|---|
| Hypersensitivity; systemic fungal infections. | Same as above. | Same as above. |
| Hypersensitivity; systemic fungal infections. | Same as above. | Same as above. |
| Same as above. | Same as above. | Same as above. |
| Same as above. | Same as above. | Same as above. |
| Same as above. | Same as above. | Same as above. |
| Same as above. | Same as above. | Same as above. |
| Same as above. | Same as above. | Same as above. |

**Table 25-21.** Drugs for gout

| Generic name | Trade name(s) | Dosage form(s) | Strength(s) | Usual dose |
|---|---|---|---|---|
| Allopurinol | Zyloprim | Tablet | 100, 300 mg | *Adults:* Dosage ranges from 200-600 mg daily in single or divided doses. *Children, 6-10 yrs:* up to 300 mg daily. *Under 6:* up to 150 mg daily. |
| Colchicine | | Injection (IV) Tablet Granules | 1 mg/2 ml-2 ml 0.6, 0.5 mg 0.5 mg | *IV:* 2 mg then 0.5 mg q 6 h until response achieved. *Oral:* 1 to 1.2 mg, then 0.5-0.6 mg qid until pain relieved or diarrhea ensues. |
| Probenecid | Benemid | Tablet | 0.5 g | *Adults:* 0.25 g orally bid for 1 wk. then 0.5 gm bid thereafter. *Children, 2-14 yr:* Initial dose 25 mg/kg body weight. Maintenance dose 40 mg/kg body weight per day in divided doses. |
| Sulfinpyrazone | Anturane | Tablet Capsule | 100 mg 200 mg | *Initial dose:* 200-400 mg daily in two divided doses. *Maintenance:* 400 mg daily in two divided doses. |

| Contraindications | Major side effects | Comments |
|---|---|---|
| Hypersensitivity; in nursing mothers; and in children except for hyperuricemia secondary to malignancy. Safe usage in pregnancy has not been established. | Dermatologic and GI disturbances; vascular and hematopoietic reactions. Neurologic and ophthalmic disturbances; drug idiosyncrasy reactions. | Periodic liver and renal function studies and complete blood counts should be done. In patients being treated with colchicine/antiinflammatory agents, these drugs should be continued while allopurinol dosage is adjusted. Fluid intake should be encouraged. There is the possibility of drug interactions with iron salts, mercaptopurine, azathioprine, dicumarol, and the uricosuric agents. |
| Hypersensitivity. | GI disturbances; dermatologic and hematologic reactions; muscular weakness; alopecia; peripheral neuritis. | Use with extreme caution in aged or debilitated patients. Reduce dosage if weakness, anorexia, nausea, vomiting, or diarrhea occurs. Thrombophlebitis may occur at injection site. |
| Hypersensitivity; in children under 2 yr; blood dyscrasias; uric acid kidney stones. | GI symptoms; hypersensitivity reactions; urinary frequency; nephrotic syndrome; hepatic necrosis; hematologic disturbances; headache; sore gums. | Therapy should not begin until an acute gouty attack has subsided. Dosage requirements may be increased in renal impairment. Use with caution in patients with history of peptic ulcer. Certain problems may be prevented by alkalizing urine and increasing fluid intake. Drug interactions may occur with salicylates, sulfa drugs, indomethacin, and rifampin. May give a false positive in Benedict's test. |
| Hypersensitivity; active peptic ulcers; concomitant therapy with salicylates. Safe usage during pregnancy has not been established. | GI disturbances; dermatologic and hematologic reactions. | Should be given with food, milk, or antacids. Periodic blood counts and assessment of renal function are advised. Alkalinization of the urine and adequate fluid intake are advised. May interact with sulfanamides, insulin, salicylates, coumarin-type anticoagulants and the hypoglycemic sulfonylurea agents. |

**Table 25-22.** Anticholinergics and antispasmodics

| Generic name | Trade name(s) | Dosage form(s) | Strength(s) | Usual dose |
|---|---|---|---|---|
| Adiphenine HCl | Trasentine | Tablet | 75 mg | *Adults:* 75-150 mg tid (before meals) *Children:* adjust dosage according to age and weight. |
| Anisotropine methylbromide | Valpin-50 | Tablet | 50 mg | *Adults:* 50 mg tid |
| Belladonna alkaloids | Various manufacturers | Tincture | | *Adults:* 0.4-0.8 mg q 12 hr or 0.2-0.4 mg tid or qid. |
| | Prydon | Spansule | 0.4, 0.8 mg | |
| Clindium bromide | Quarzan | Capsule | 2.5, 5 mg | *Adults:* 2.5 mg tid or qid before meals and at bedtime. |
| Dicyclomine HCl | Bentyl | Injection | 10 mg/ml-2, 10 ml | *Adults:* 10-20 mg tid or qid. |
| | | Capsule | 10 mg | *Children:* 10 mg tid or qid. |
| | | Tablet | 20 mg | *Infants:* 5 mg tid or qid. |
| | Dibent | Injection | 10 mg/ml-2, 10 ml | |
| | | Tablet | 20 mg | |
| | Nospaz | Injection | 10 mg/ml-2, 10 ml | |
| | | Tablet | 10, 20 mg | |
| | | Liquid | 10 mg/5 ml | |
| | Or-tyl | Injection | 10 mg/ml-10 ml | |

| Contraindications | Major side effects | Comments |
|---|---|---|
| Glaucoma; obstructive GI disorders; obstructive uropathy; ulcerative colitis; myasthenia gravis; hypersensitivity | GI and CNS disturbances; "drying" effects; ocular disturbances; cardiac and renal disturbances. | *General:* Safe usage during pregnancy and lactation has not been established. In presence of high environmental temperature, heat stroke, may occur. *Special:* Has an anesthetic action on buccal mucosa (tablets should not be chewed). Use with caution in patients with hepatic or renal disease, cardiac conditions, hyperthyroidism, autonomic neuropathy, hiatal hernia. |
| Glaucoma; obstructive uropathy; obstructive GI disorders; severe ulcerative colitis; myasthenia gravis; paralytic ileus; intestinal atony; toxic megacolon; and hypersensitivity. | GI and CNS disturbances; "drying" effects; ocular disturbances; cardiac and renal disturbances; allergic reactions; impotency. | *General:* Same as above. *Special:* Use with caution in patients with hepatic or renal disease, autonomic neuropathy, ulcerative colitis, hiatal hernia, hyperthyroidism, or heart conditions. |
| Hypersensitivity; glaucoma; advanced hepatic or renal disease; pyloric or bladder neck obstruction; prostatic hypertrophy; obstructive GI disorders; myasthenia gravis. | GI and CNS disturbances; "drying" effects; ocular disturbances; cardiac and renal disturbances. | *General:* Same as above. *Special:* Use with caution in elderly patients and those with autonomic neuropathy, hyperthyroidism, heart conditions, hepatic or renal disease. |
| Hypersensitivity to anticholinergic drugs; obstructive GI disorders; glaucoma; obstructive uropathy; paralytic ileus; intestinal atony; myasthenia gravis; unstable cardiovascular status; severe ulcerative colitis; toxic megacolon. | GI and CNS disturbances; "drying" effects; ocular disturbances; cardiac and renal disturbances; allergic reactions; impotency. | *General:* Same as above. *Special:* Use with caution in elderly patients and those with autonomic neuropathy, hepatic or renal disease, heart conditions, prostatic hypertrophy, hyperthyroidism, hiatal hernia, and ulcerative colitis. |
| Obstructive uropathy; myasthenia gravis; obstructive GI disorders; paralytic ileus; unstable cardiovascular status; intestinal atony; severe ulcerative colitis; toxic megacolon; hypersensitivity. | Same as above. | *General:* Same as above. *Special:* Use with caution in patients with glaucoma, prostatic hypertrophy, hepatic or renal disease, hiatial hernia, hyperthyroidism, heart conditions, autonomic neuropathy, and ulcerative colitis. |

*Continued.*

**Table 25-22.** Anticholinergics and antispasmodics—cont'd

| Generic name | Trade name(s) | Dosage form(s) | Strength(s) | Usual dose |
|---|---|---|---|---|
| Diphemanil methylsulfate | Prantal | Tablet<br>Repeat action tablet | 100 mg<br>100 mg | *Adults:* 100-200 mg q 4-6 hr initially, then 50-100 mg q 4-6 hr. Repetabs: 100-200 mg q 8 hr. |
| Hexocyclium methylsulfate | Tral | Tablet<br>Gradumet | 25 mg<br>50, 75 mg | *Adults:* 25 mg qid, before meals and at bedtime. *Long-acting form:* 50 mg bid before lunch and at bedtime. Not for use in children. |
| Hyoscyamine sulfate, levorotatory | Anaspaz<br>Cysto-spaz<br><br>Levsin<br><br><br><br><br>Levsinex | Tablet<br>Tablet<br>Tablet (SR)<br>Tablet<br>Elixir<br>Drops<br>Injection<br><br>SR capsule | 0.125 mg<br>0.15 mg<br>0.375 mg<br>0.125 mg<br>0.125 mg/5 ml<br>0.125 mg/1 ml<br>0.25 mg/ml-1, 10 and 30 ml<br>0.375 mg | *Adults:* 0.125-0.25 mg tid or qid or 0.375 mg. SR form q 12 hr. *Children, 2-10 yr:* ½ adult dose. *Infants, up to 2 yr:* ¼ adult dose. |
| Isopropamide iodide | Darbid | Tablet | 5 mg | *Adults:* 5 mg bid q 12 hr. Not for use in children under 12. |
| Mepenzolate bromide | Cantil | Tablet<br>Liquid | 25 mg<br>25 mg/5 ml | *Adults:* 25-50 mg qid with meals and at bedtime. Not recommended for use in children. |
| Methixene HCl | Trest | Tablet | 1 mg | *Adults:* 1 or 2 mg tid. No dosage established for children. |

| Contraindications | Major side effects | Comments |
|---|---|---|
| Glaucoma; myasthenia gravis; obstructive uropathy; obstructive GI disorders; toxic megacolon; unstable cardiovascular status; paralytic ileus; intestinal atony; hypersensitivity. | GI and CNS disturbances; "drying" effects; ocular disturbances; cardiac and renal disturbances; allergic reactions; impotency. | *General:* Same as above.<br>*Special:* Safe usage in women of childbearing potential and in children has not been established. Use with caution in elderly patients and those with hiatal hernia, ulcerative colitis, prostatic hypertrophy, hyperthyroidism, hepatic or renal disease, and heart conditions. |
| Same as above. | Same as above. | *General:* Same as above.<br>*Special:* Use with caution in patients having hepatic or renal disease, hiatal hernia, ulcerative colitis, autonomic neuropathy, hyperthyroidism, and heart conditions. |
| Same as above. | GI and CNS disturbances; "drying" effects; ocular disturbances; cardiac and renal disturbances; allergic reactions. | *General:* Same as above.<br>*Special:* Use with caution in patients with cardiac conditions, hyperthyroidism, autonomic neuropathy, and hepatic or renal disease. |
| Hypersensitivity; myasthenia gravis; obstructive uropathy; obstructive GI disorders; glaucoma; severe ulcerative colitis; intestinal atony; toxic megacolon; unstable cardiovascular status. | GI and CNS disturbances; "drying" effects; ocular disturbances; cardiac and renal disturbances; allergic responses; impotency. | *General:* Same as above.<br>*Special:* Safe usage in women of childbearing potential has not been established. Iodine content suppresses uptake of $I^{131}$ and may alter PBI test results. Use with caution in elderly patients or those with cardiac conditions, hepatic or renal disease, hyperthyroidism, autonomic neuropathy, and ulcerative colitis. |
| Hypersensitivity; myasthenia gravis; glaucoma; obstructive uropathy; obstructive GI disorders; unstable cardiovascular status; paralytic ileus; intestinal atony; severe ulcerative colitis; toxic megacolon. | Same as above. | *General:* Same as above.<br>*Special:* Use with caution in patients having hyperthyroidism, cardiac conditions, hypertension, autonomic neuropathy, hepatic or renal disease, and ulcerative colitis. |
| Hypersensitivity; obstructive uropathy; obstructive GI disorders; myasthenia gravis; glaucoma; intestinal atony; unstable cardiovascular status; toxic megacolon. | Same as above. | *General:* Same as above.<br>*Special:* Safe usage in women of childbearing potential has not been established. Use with caution in elderly patients or those with hepatic or renal disease, hyperthyroidism, cardiac conditions, ulcerative colitis, autonomic neuropathy, and hiatal hernia. |

*Continued.*

**Table 25-22.** Anticholinergics and antispasmodics—cont'd

| Generic name | Trade name(s) | Dosage form(s) | Strength(s) | Usual dose |
|---|---|---|---|---|
| Methscopolamine | Pamine (bromide) | Tablet | 2.5 mg | *Oral:* Tablet 2.5 mg ½ hr. before meals 2.5-5 mg at bedtime. SR capsule: 5 mg q 8-12 hr. |
| | Paraspan (nitrate) | SR capsule | 5 mg | |
| Oxyphen-cyclimine HCl | Daricon | Tablet | 10 mg | *Adults:* 5-10 mg bid or tid. Not for use in children under 12. |
| | Gastrix | Tablet | 10 mg | |
| Oxyphenonium bromide | Antrenyl | Tablet | 5 mg | *Adults:* Initially 10 mg qid then reduced according to response. Not for use in children. |
| Propantheline bromide | Giquel | Tablet | 15 mg | *Adult: Oral:* 7.5 to 15 mg tid with meals and 15-30 mg at bedtime. *Adult: Parenteral:* initially 30 mg or more IM or IV q 6-8 h, then reduced according to response to ½ above dose. |
| | Pro-Banthine | Tablet | 7.5, 15 mg | |
| | | Injection | 30 mg vial | |
| Thiphenamil | Trocinate | Tablet | 100, 400 mg | *Adults:* 400 mg initially and repeated in 4 hr. Not for use in children. |
| Tridihexethyl chloride | Pathilon | Tablet | 25 mg | *Adult: Oral:* 25-50 mg 3-4 times daily, or, 75 mg SR form q 12 hr. *Parenteral:* 10-20 mg q 6 hr. IV, IM, or SC |
| | | Sequel | 75 mg | |
| | | Injection | 10 mg/ml-1 ml | |

| Contraindications | Major side effects | Comments |
|---|---|---|
| Glaucoma; myasthenia gravis; obstructive uropathy; obstructive GI disorders; intestinal atony; unstable cardiovascular status; severe ulcerative colitis; toxic megacolon. | CNS and GI disturbances; "drying" effects; ocular disturbances; cardiac and renal disturbances; allergic reactions. | *General:* Same as above.<br>*Special:* Use with caution in patients with autonomic neuropathy, hepatic or renal disease, cardiac disease, ulcerative colitis, hyperthyroidism, hiatal hernia, and prostatic hypertrophy. |
| Same as above. | Same as above; impotency. | *General:* Same as above.<br>*Special:* Safe usage in children has not been established. Use with caution in elderly patients and those with hepatic and renal disease, autonomic neuropathy, ulcerative colitis, hiatal hernia, hyperthyroidism, cardiac disease, hypertension, and prostatic hypertrophy. |
| Same as above; hypersensitivity; | Same as above. | *General:* Same as above.<br>*Special:* Safe usage in children has not been established. Use with caution in patients with hepatic or renal disease, cardiac disease, chronic lung diseases, autonomic neuropathy, ulcerative colitis, hyperthyroidism, hiatal hernia, and prostatic hypertrophy. |
| Glaucoma; obstructive GI disorders; obstructive uropathy; unstable cardiovascular status; hiatal hernia; toxic megacolon; myasthenia gravis. | CNS and GI disturbances; "drying" effects, ocular disturbances, cardiac and renal disturbances; allergic reactions; impotency. | *General:* Same as above.<br>*Special:* Safe usage in children has not been established. Use with caution in patients with hepatic or renal disease, cardiac diseases, autonomic neuropathy, ulcerative colitis, hyperthyroidism. |
| Obstructive uropathy; obstructive GI disorders; intestinal atony; severe ulcerative colitis; toxic megacolon; myasthenia gravis. | No typical symptoms have been reported. | Safe usage during pregnancy and in children has not been established. Thiphenamil HCl is a potent anti-spasmodic and smooth muscle relaxant which also has a local anesthetic action on contact with mucous membranes. |
| Glaucoma; myasthenia gravis; obstructive uropathy; obstructive GI disorders intestinal atony; severe ulcerative colitis; unstable cardiovascular status; toxic megacolon. | CNS and GI disturbances; "drying" effects; ocular disturbances; cardiac and renal disturbances; allergic reactions; impotency. | Safe usage during pregnancy and lactation or in women of childbearing potential and children has not been established. In the presence of high environmental temperatures heat stroke may occur. Use with caution in patients with autonomic neuropathy, ulcerative colitis, hepatic or renal disease, hiatal hernia, hyperthyroidism, cardiac disease, prostatic hypertrophy, early evidence of ileus. |

**Table 25-23.** Laxatives and stool softeners

| Generic name | Trade name(s) | Dosage form(s) | Strength(s) | Usual dose |
|---|---|---|---|---|
| Bisacodyl | Various manufacturers | Tablet | 5, 10 mg | *Oral:* 5-15 mg. *Rectal:* 10 mg. |
| | Biscolax | Tablet | 5 mg | |
| | | Suppository | 10 mg | |
| | Ban-O-Lax | Tablet | 5 mg | |
| | Dulcolax | Tablet | 5 mg | |
| | | Suppository | 10 mg | |
| | Fleet Biscodyl | Tablet | 5 mg | |
| | | Suppository | 10 mg | |
| | Laxadan | Supule | 10 mg | |
| | Theralax | Tablet | 5 mg | |
| | | Suppository | 10 mg | |
| Casanthranol | Peristim Forte | Capsule | 90 mg | *Adults:* 90 mg at bedtime. Not recommended for children. |
| Cascara sagrada | Various manufacturers | Tablet | 120, 325 mg | 120-360 mg at bedtime. 1 ml at bedtime. 5 ml at bedtime. |
| | | Fluid extract | | |
| | | Aromatic fluid extract | | |
| Castor oil | Various manufacturers | Capsule | 0.62, 2.5 ml | *Adults:* 15-60 ml. |
| | | Liquid | | *Children:* 5-15 ml. |
| | Alphamul | Emulsion | 60% castor oil | *Infants:* 1-5 ml. |
| | Neoloid | Emulsion | 36.4% castor oil | |
| Danthron | Dorbane | Tablet | 75 mg | *Adults:* 137.5-150 mg with evening meal. |
| | Modane | Tablet | 37.5, 75 mg | *Children:* Dosage should be calculated according to age and given at evening meal. |
| | | Liquid | 37.5 mg/5 ml | |
| Dioctyl calcium sulfosuccinate | Surfak | Capsule | 50, 240 mg | *Adults:* 240 mg daily until bowel movements are normal. *Children:* 50-150 mg daily. |
| Dioctyl sodium sulfo-succinate | Afko-Lube | Capsule | 100 mg | *Adults and older Children:* 50-200 mg daily. |
| | | Syrup | 20 mg/5 ml | |
| | Bu-Lax | Capsule | 100, 250 mg | *Children,* 6-12 yr: 40-120 mg daily. |
| | Colace | Capsule | 50, 100 mg | *Children,* 3-6 yr: 20-60 mg daily. |
| | | Solution | 10 mg/ml | *Infants:* (under 3 yr): 10-40 mg daily. |
| | | Syrup | 20 mg/5 ml | |
| | Colax | Capsule | 250 mg | |
| | Comfolax | Capsule | 100 mg | |
| | Dilax | Capsule | 100, 250 mg | |
| | Diomedicone | Tablet | 50 mg | |
| | Diosuccin | Capsule | 100, 250 mg | |
| | Disonate | Capsule | 60, 100, 240 mg | |
| | | Solution | 10 mg/ml | |
| | | Syrup | 20 mg/5 ml | |
| | Doctate | Capsule | 100 mg | |
| | | Tablet | 300 mg | |
| | Doss-300 | Capsule | 300 mg | |
| | Doxinate | Capsule | 60, 240 mg | |
| | | Solution | 50 mg/ml | |
| | DSS | Capsule | 50, 100 mg | |
| | Laxinate | Capsule | 100 mg | |
| | Modane-Soft | Capsule | 120 mg | |
| | Molatoc | Capsule | 100 mg | |
| | Parlax | Syrup | 20 mg/5 ml | |
| | Regul-Aid | Capsule | 100 mg | |
| | | Syrup | 20 mg/5 ml | |
| Magnesium citrate solution | Various manufacturers | Oral solution | 10 oz bottles | *Adults:* 200 ml Not recomended for children. |

| Contraindications | Major side effects | Comments |
|---|---|---|
| Acute abdominal symptoms requiring surgery. | Abdominal cramps. | Tablets should be swallowed whole and not taken within 1 hr. of antacids or milk. Frequent or continued use may lead to laxative dependence. |
| Abdominal pain or other symptoms of appendicitis. | Nausea; cramping or pain; rash; diarrhea. | Frequent or continued use may lead to laxative dependence. |
| Abdominal pain or other symptoms of appendicitis. | Abdominal cramps; nausea. | Same as above. |
| Abdominal pain or other symptoms of appendicitis; pregnancy. | Cramps or griping. | Same as above. |
| Abdominal pain; nausea; vomiting; or other signs or symptoms of appendicitis. | Overdosage may cause griping; may appear in milk of nursing mothers producing catharsis in the baby; brownish temporary staining of mucosa with prolonged use. | May color alkaline urine pink. Hypokalemia may impair the effectiveness of Danthron. Frequent use may result in laxative dependence. |
| None known. | Occasional GI disturbances; rashes have occurred. | Surfactants such as Dioctyl (calcium or sodium) sulfosuccinate should not be administered with mineral oil; they may cause absorption and subsequent lipoid pneumonia. *Note:* Effects on stools may not be seen for several days |
| Abdominal pain or other symptoms of appendicitis. | Cramps; nausea. | Frequent or continued use may lead to laxative dependence. |

*Continued.*

**Table 25-23.** Laxatives and stool softeners—cont'd

| Generic name | Trade name(s) | Dosage form(s) | Strength(s) | Usual dose |
|---|---|---|---|---|
| Methylcellulose derivatives | Cologel | Liquid | 450 mg methyl-cellulose/5 ml | *Adults:* 5-20 ml tid with water. |
| | Hydrolose | Syrup | 985 mg methyl-cellulose/5 ml | *Adults:* 15 ml AM and PM with water. *Children:* 5-10 ml AM and PM with water. |
| | Mucilose | Flakes | | *Flakes:* 1-2 tsp. in liquid bid. |
| | | Granules | | *Granules:* 1-2 tsp. with liquid bid. |
| Milk of magnesia (magnesium hydroxide) | Various manufacturers | Suspension | | 15-30 ml |
| Mineral oil | Various manufacturers | | | *Adult:* 15-45 ml at bedtime. |
| | Agoral Plain | Emulsion | | *Adult:* 15-30 ml at bedtime. *Children over 6 yr:* 10-20 ml at bedtime. |
| | Kondremul Plain | Emulsion | Heavy mineral oil, 55% | *Adults:* 15 ml at bedtime. *Children over 6 yr:* 5-10 ml at bedtime. |
| | Neo-Caltol | Jelly | | *Adults:* 5-10 ml at bedtime. *Children:* 5 ml daily. |
| | Petrogalar, Plain | Suspension | Mineral oil, 65% | *Adults:* 15 ml at bedtime. *Children over 6 yr:* 5 ml at bedtime. |
| Phenolphthalein | Chocolax | Chewable tablet | 32.4 mg | 60-200 mg at bedtime. |
| | Evac-U-Gen | Chewable tablet | 81 mg | |
| | Evac-U-Lax | Chewable tablet | 80 mg | |
| Poloxamer 188 | Polykol | Capsule | 250 mg | 500-750 mg daily as single or in divided doses for not more than 5 days. |
| Senna | Black draught | Tablet | 180 mg senna | *Adults:* 2 tablets, ¼-1 tsp granules. Not recommended for children. |
| | | Granules | 66.2% senna | |
| | Senokot | Tablet | 187 mg senna | *Adults:* 1 suppository at bedtime. |
| | | Granules | 326 mg/tsp | *Children over 60 lbs:* 1 tablet, ¼-½ tsp granules, or ½ suppository at bedtime. |
| | | Suppos. | 652 mg senna Conc. | |
| Senna extract | Black draught | Syrup | 20% | *Adults:* 7.5-15 ml at bedtime. |
| | Casafru | Syrup | | *Children: 5-10 yr:* 5-10 ml at bedtime. *1-5 yr:* 2.5-5 ml at bedtime. |
| | Senokot | Syrup | 218 mg/5 ml | |
| Sodium phosphate | Phospho-Soda | Oral solution | 18 g sodium phosphate, 48 g sodium biphosphate 100 ml | 2-40 ml in cold water. |
| Psyllium preparations | Effersyllium | Powder | | *Adults:* 1 tsp to 1 Tbsp tid for several days. |
| | Hydrocil, Plain | Powder | | *Children over 6:* approximately ½ adult dose. |
| | Konsyl | Powder | | |
| | LA Formula | Powder | | |
| | Metamucil | Powder | | |
| | Modane Bulk | Powder | | |
| | Mucillium | Powder | | |
| | Rogacillium | Powder | | |
| | Sibdin | Powder | | |
| | Syllact | Powder | | |

| Contraindications | Major side effects | Comments |
|---|---|---|
| Intestinal obstruction; fecal impaction. | Nausea. | Several days may be required to restore regularity with this drug. |
| Abdominal pain or other symptoms of appendicitis. | Cramps and nausea. | Frequent or continued use may lead to laxative dependence. |
| In infants and young children; pregnancy. | May prevent or slow absorption of oil-soluble vitamins. | Should be taken only at bedtime. Prolonged use should be avoided. Use with caution in bedridden or aged patients. *Note:* Surfactants may cause absorption of mineral oil, possibly resulting in lipoid pneumonia. |
| Abdominal pain or other symptoms of appendicitis. | Rash; abdominal cramps. | Frequent or continued use may result in laxative dependence. |
| None known. | Occasional GI disturbances. | Several days of therapy may be required before full stool-softening effect is apparent. Surfactants may cause absorption of mineral oil resulting in lipoid pneumonia. |
| Abdominal pain or other symptoms of appendicitis. | Abdominal cramps. | Frequent or continued use may lead to laxative dependence. |
| Abdominal pain or other symptoms of appendicitis; usage in children under 6. | Abdominal cramps; nausea. | Same as above. Most effective when taken on empty stomach. |
| Intestinal obstruction; fecal impaction. | Nausea. | Psyllium preparations may also be used in diarrhea to help form bulk and in weight control to cause a "full" sensation in the stomach. Several days may be required to restore regularity with this drug. |

**Table 25-24.** Antidiarrheal agents

| Generic name | Trade name(s) | Dosage form(s) | Strength(s) | Usual dose |
|---|---|---|---|---|
| *Bacterial cultures:* | | | | |
| Lactobacillus acidophilus | Bacid<br>Dofus | Capsule<br>Tablet | 200,000 viable organisms per tablet | 2 capsules bid.<br>1 daily before meals with water. |
| Lactobacillus, acidophilus, L. bulgaricus | Lactinex | Tablet<br>Granules | | 4 tablets or 1 packet tid or qid with food, milk, or juice. |
| Belladonna alkaloids | Various manufacturers | Tincture<br>Powder | 10% wt/vol | *Adults:* 0.4 to 0.8 mg of alkaloids q 12 hr or prn. |
| Bismuth subgallate | Devrom | Chewable Tablet | 200 mg | 1-2 tablets 3 times daily after meals. |
| Diphenoxylate with atropine sulfate | Lomotil | Tablet<br>Liquid | Diphenoxylate, 2.5 mg; atropine sulfate, 0.025 mg/tab or 5 ml | *Adults:* 2 tabs or 10 ml liquid qid.<br>*Children:* 0.3 to 0.4 mg/kg/day of diphenoxylate in divided doses. |
| | Lonox | Tablet | Diphenoxylate, 2.5 mg; atropine sulfate, 0.025 mg | |
| Kaolin pectin suspension | Kaopectate<br>Pargel<br>Pectocel | Suspension<br>Suspension<br>Suspension | | 60-120 ml prn. |
| Loperamide HCl | Imodium | Capsule | 2 mg | Initial dose of 4 mg, then 2 mg after each unformed stool up to 16 mg daily. |
| Opium alkaloids | Various manufacturers | Tincture<br>Camphorated tincture (paregoric) | 10% wt/vol<br>20 mg/5 ml | *Tincture:* 0.6-1.5 ml prn.<br>*Paregoric:* 5 ml prn. |

| Contraindications | Major side effects | Comments |
|---|---|---|
| None reported. | None reported. | Must be refrigerated. |
| Hypersensitivity; glaucoma; advanced hepatic or renal disease; obstructive uropathy; prostatic hypertrophy; myasthenia gravis; obstructive GI disorders. | GI and CNS disturbances; "drying" effects; ocular disturbances; cardiac and renal disturbances. | Safe usage during pregnancy and lactation has not been established. In the presence of high environmental temperatures, heat stroke may occur. Use with caution in elderly patients and those with heart conditions, hepatic or renal disease, hyperthyroidism, and autonomic neuropathy. |
| Use in children under 3 years of age; high fever. | High doses or prolonged use may cause heavy metal (bismuth) poisoning. | May be chewed or swallowed whole. Should be protected from light and moisture. May cause coating and discoloration of the tongue or darkening of the stool—both of which are harmless and temporary. |
| In children under 12 years of age; hypersensitivity; jaundice; diarrhea associated with treatments using clindamycin and lincomycin. | Atropine (anticholinergic) effects; CNS disturbances; GI disturbances; respiratory depression; pruritis; neurologic disturbances. disturbances. | Safe usage during pregnancy and lactation has not been established. Use with caution in patients with hepatic disease and in young children. In cases of overdosage, naloxone HCl may be used. At high doses, addiction could theoretically occur. Diphenoxylate should not be used concomitantly with MAO inhibitors and in general potentiates the depressant action of barbiturates, alcohol, and tranquilizers. |
| None reported. | Nausea. | Shake well before using and give full therapeutic doses after each loose BM. |
| Known hypersensitivity; in patients in whom constipation is to be avoided; diarrhea associated with broad-spectrum antibiotic therapy. | GI disturbances; CNS disturbances; skin rash. | Safe usage during pregnancy and lactation and in children under 12 years of age has not been established. |
| Bronchial asthma; narcotic idiosyncrasies; respiratory depression; hypersensitivity. | GI and CNS disturbances; respiratory and circulatory depression; cardiovascular and renal disturbances; allergic reactions. | May be habit forming. Use with caution in infants, old and debilitated patients, in increased intracranial pressure, toxic psychosis, prostatic obstruction, myxedema. |

**Table 25-25.** Antacids: single agents

| Generic name | Trade name(s) | Dosage form(s) | Strength(s) | Usual dose |
|---|---|---|---|---|
| Aluminum hydroxide gel | Alu-Cap | Capsule | 475 mg | 300-600 mg 5-6 times daily, between meals and at bedtime. |
|  | Alu-Tab | Tablet | 600 mg |  |
|  | Amphojel | Tablet | 300, 600 mg |  |
|  |  | Oral suspension | 320 mg/5 ml* |  |
|  | Dialume | Capsule | 500 mg. |  |
| Aluminum phosphate gel | Phosphaljel | Oral suspension |  | 15-30 ml q 2 hr between meals and at bedtime. |
| Dihydroxy-aluminum aminoacetate | Robalate | Chewable tablet | 500 mg | 0.5-1 gm p̄ c and at bedtime or as needed. Tablets should be chewed well before swallowing. |
| Aluminum carbonate | Basaljel | Capsule |  | Capsule or tablet: 1 or 2 prn. |
|  |  | Tablet |  |  |
|  |  | Oral suspension |  | Suspension: 1 or 2 tsp prn. |
|  |  | Extra-strength suspension |  | Extra-strength suspension: $\frac{1}{2}$-1 tsp prn. |
| Magnesium oxide | Various manufacturers | Capsule | 140 mg | 250 mg with water or milk prn. |
|  |  | Tablet | 250, 400, |  |
| Magaldrate | Riopan | Chewable tablet | 650 mg | 400-800 mg, preferably taken between meals and at bedtime. |
|  |  | Tablet | 400 mg |  |
|  |  | Oral suspension | 400 mg |  |
|  |  |  | 400 mg/5 ml |  |
| Calcium carbonate | Various manufacturers | Tablet | 650 mg | 1 g with water 4-6 times daily. |
|  | Mellamint | Tablet | 420 mg |  |
| Sodium bicarbonate | Various manufacturers | Tablet | 325, 650 mg | 0.3-2 g prn. |

| Contraindications | Major side effects | Comments |
|---|---|---|
| Concomitant therapy with tetracycline derivatives. | Constipation. | Aluminum hydroxide may decrease the absorption of warfarin and quinidine. |
| Same as above. | Constipation. | Aluminum phosphate gel is useful when therapy is complicated by pancreatic insufficiency or diarrhea. |
| Same as above. | Constipation. | |
| Same as above. | Constipation. | Aluminum carbonate may also be used to prevent the formation of urinary phosphatic stones. |
| Same as above. | Diarrhea. | Use with caution in patients with renal insufficiency. |
| Concomitant therapy with tetracycline derivatives; advanced renal failure. | | Use with caution in patients with renal insufficiency. |
| Concomitant therapy with tetracycline derivatives. | Constipation. | |
| Use in patients on restricted or low-sodium diets. | Systemic alkalosis. | Sodium bicarbonate is absorbed and chronic use may lead to systemic alkalosis. |

**Table 25-26.** Antacids: combinations

| Trade name | Antacid ingredients | Dosage form(s) | Usual dose |
|---|---|---|---|
| Aludrox | Aluminum hydroxide gel, magnesium hydroxide | Suspension<br>Tablet | 10 ml prn.<br>2 tablets prn. |
| A-M-T | Aluminum hydroxide gel, magnesium trisilicate | Suspension<br>Tablet | 5-10 ml qid.<br>2 tablets 5-6 times daily. |
| Camalox | Aluminum hydroxide, magnesium hydroxide | Suspension<br>Chewable tablet | 10-20 ml up to qid.<br>2-4 tablets up to qid. |
| Creamalin | Aluminum hydroxide, magnesium hydroxide | Suspension<br>Chewable tablet | 10-20 ml up to qid.<br>2-4 tabs up to qid. |
| Delcid | Aluminum hydroxide, magnesium hydroxide | Suspension | 5 ml qid. |
| Ducon | Aluminum hydroxide, magnesium hydroxide, calcium carbonate | Suspension | 40-60 ml daily in divided doses. |
| Gelusil | Aluminum hydroxide, magnesium trisilicate | Suspension<br>Chewable tablet | 10 ml or more prn.<br>2 tablets prn. |
| Gelusil-M | Nonreactive aluminum hydroxide, magnesium hydroxide, magnesium trisilicate plus alginates | Suspension | 5-10 ml prn.<br>1 or 2 tablets prn. |
| Kolantyl | Magnesium hydroxide, Aluminum hydroxide | Gel<br>Chewable tablet<br>Chewable wafer | 5-20 ml qid.<br>1 or 2 qid.<br>1 to 4 qid. |
| Kudrox | Aluminum hydroxide magnesium carbonate | Suspension<br>Chewable tablet | 5 ml qid. |
| Maalox | Aluminum and magnesium hydroxide | Suspension<br>Chewable tablet #1<br>Chewable tablet #2 | 10-20 ml qid.<br>2-4 qid.<br>1-2 qid. |
| Malcogel | Aluminum hydroxide, magnesium trisilicate | Liquid | 5 to 10 ml.<br>5-6 times daily. |
| Titralac | Calcium carbonate, glycine | Liquid<br>Tablet | 5 ml prn.<br>2 or more prn. |
| Trisogel | Aluminum hydroxide, magnesium trisilicate | Liquid<br>Capsule | 10 ml or more prn; 3-5 capsules prn. |
| WinGel | Aluminum and magnesium hydroxide | Liquid<br>Chewable tablet | 5-10 ml qid.<br>1 or 2 qid. |

| Contraindications | Major side effects | Comments |
|---|---|---|
| Concomitant therapy with tetra-cycline derivatives. | | Use with caution in patients with renal insufficiency. |
| Same as above. | | Same as above. |
| Same as above. | | Same as above. |
| Same as above. | | Same as above. |
| Same as above. | Nausea, vomiting, and diarrhea. | Same as above. |
| Same as above. | May cause diarrhea. | Same as above. |
| Same as above. | | Same as above. |
| Same as above. | | Same as above. |
| Concomitant therapy with tetra-cycline derivatives. | | Same as above. |
| Same as above. | | Same as above. |
| Same as above. | | Same as above. |
| | | None. |
| Same as above. | | Same as above. |
| | May cause constipation. | |
| Concomitant therapy with tetra-cycline derivatives. | | Use with caution in patients with renal insufficiency. |
| Same as above. | | Same as above. |

**Table 25-27.** Antacids with additional agents

| Trade name | Antacids | Other ingredients | Dosage form(s) | Usual dose |
|---|---|---|---|---|
| Gaviscon Foamtab | Aluminum hydroxide gel Magnesium trisilicate Sodium bicarbonate | Alginic acid | Chewable tablet (not to be swallowed whole) | 2-4 qid. |
| Maalox Plus | Aluminum and magnesium hydroxides | Simethicone | Suspension Chewable tablet | 10-20 ml qid. 2-4 qid. |
| Mylanta | Aluminum and magnesium hydroxide | Simethicone | Suspension Chewable tablet | 5-10 ml qid. 1 or 2 prn. |
| Mylanta II | | | Suspension Chewable tablet | 5-10 ml qid. 1 or 2 qid. |
| Oxaine-M | Alumina gel, milk of magnesia | Oxethazine | Suspension | *Adults:* 5-10 ml qid. Not recommended for children. |
| Silain-Gel | Aluminum and magnesium hydroxide | Simethicone | Suspension | 10 ml prn. |

**Table 25-28.** Antiflatulents

| Generic name | Trade name(s) | Dosage form(s) | Strength(s) | Usual dose |
|---|---|---|---|---|
| Dexpanthenol, choline bitartrate | Ilopam choline | Tablet | 50 mg dexpanthenol 25 mg choline bitartrate | *Adults:* 2 or 3 tablets 3 times daily. |
| Charcoal, activated | Various manufacturers | Tablet Capsule | 10 gr 10 gr | *Adults:* 2-6 tablets or capsules after meals. |
| Simethicone | Mylicon | Chewable tablet Drops | 40, 80 mg 40 mg/0.6 ml | *Adults:* 40-100 mg after each meal and at bedtime. |
| | Silain | Chewable tablet | 50 mg | |

| Contraindications | Major side effects | Comments |
|---|---|---|
| Concomitant therapy with tetracycline derivatives. | High doses for extended periods may cause systemic alkalosis. | Do not exceed recommended dosages. Use with caution in patients with renal insufficiency and those on sodium restricted diets. |
| Same as above. | | Simethicone relieves pain from gas. Use with caution in patients with renal insufficiency. |
| Same as above. | | Same as above. |
| Known hypersensitivity; concomitant therapy with tetracycline derivatives. | With high doses, dizziness, faintness, or drowsiness may occur. | Oxethazaine has a topical anesthetic effect. Do not exceed recommended dosage. This product may mask symptoms of gastrointestinal carcinoma. |
| Concomitant therapy with tetracycline derivatives. | | Simethicone relieves pain from gas. Use with caution in patients with renal insufficiency. |

| Contraindications | Major side effects | Comments |
|---|---|---|
| None known. | Increased frequency of bowel movements. | Hypokalemia may impair effectiveness. Do not administer until 1 hr after succinylcholine and 12 hr after neostigmine or other enterokinetic drugs. |
| None known. | None reported. | Tablets may be chewed or allowed to dissolve in the mouth and followed by water. |
| None known. | None reported. | Tablets should be thoroughly chewed before swallowing. |

**Table 25-29.** Urinary tract antiinfectives: miscellaneous agents

| Generic name | Trade name(s) | Dosage form(s) | Strength(s) | Usual dose |
|---|---|---|---|---|
| Nalidixic acid | NegGram | Caplet<br>Oral suspension | 250, 500 mg, 1 g<br>250 mg/5 ml | *Adults:* 1 g qid<br>*Children over 3 months:* 55 mg/kg/day in 4 equally divided doses. Not for children under 3 months of age. |
| Oxolinic acid | Utibid | Tablet | 750 mg | One tablet twice daily for 2 weeks. |
| Nitrofurantoin | Cyantin<br>Furadantin<br><br><br>Furalan<br>J-Dantin<br>Parfuran<br>Sarodant<br>Various manufacturers<br>Macrodantin (macrocrystals) | Tablet<br>Tablet<br>Oral suspension<br>Injection<br>Tablet<br>Tablet<br>Tablet<br>Tablet<br>Capsule<br><br>Capsule | 100 mg<br>50, 100 mg<br>25 mg/5 ml<br>180 mg (sodium salt)<br>50, 100 mg<br>50, 100 mg<br>50 mg<br>50 mg<br>50, 100 mg<br><br>25, 50, 100 mg | *Adults: Oral:* 50-100 mg qid.<br>*Parenteral: patients over 120 lb:* 150 mg in at least 150 ml liquid bid.<br>*Patients under 120 lb:* 3 mg/lb/day in 2 equal doses.<br>*Children:* 5-7 mg/kg/day in divided doses qid. |
| Methenamine Mandelate salts |  | Tablet | 0.5 g | *Adults:* 1 Gm qid |
|  | Mandalay | Tablet | 0.5 g | *Children, 6-12 yrs:* 0.5 gm qid, *under 6 yrs:* dose should be based on body wt. |
|  | Mandelanine | Tablet<br>Oral suspension<br>Granules for reconstitution | 0.25, 0.5, 1 g<br>0.25 g/5 ml<br>0.5 g/5 ml<br>0.5, 1 g<br>Packets |  |
|  | Mandelets<br>Prov-U-Sep<br>Renelet | Tablet<br>Tablet<br>Tablet | 0.5, 1 g<br>0.5 gm<br>0.5, 1 g | Hippurate:<br>*Adults:* 1 Gm bid.<br>*Children:* 0.5 Gm bid. |
| Hippurate salt | Hiprex<br>Urex | Tablet | 1 g |  |
| Sulfosalicylate salt | Hexalet | Tablet | 0.5, 1 g |  |
| Methylene blue | M-B Tabs<br>Urolene Blue | Tablet<br>Tablet | 65 mg<br>65 mg | 65 mg 2-3 times daily with water |

| Contraindications | Major side effects | Comments |
|---|---|---|
| Hypersensitivity; history of convulsive disorders; safe usage during the first trimester of pregnancy and in children under 3 months old has not been established. | CNS and visual disturbances; GI disturbances; allergic reactions; rare hematologic disturbances. | May enhance the effects of oral anticoagulants warfarin and bishydroxy-coumarin. Nalidixic acid may give false positive for glucose with Clinitest tablets and Benedict's or Fehling's solutions; use of Clinistix or Tes-Tape is recommended. Photosensitivity may occur. Use with caution in patients with liver disease, epilepsy, or cerebral arteriosclerosis. |
| Known hypersensitivity; history of convulsive disorders; in nursing mothers and infants; safe use during pregnancy has not been established. | CNS and GI disturbances; hepatic and hematologic disturbances; allergic-type reactions. | Oxolinic acid has CNS-stimulant properties and concomitant use with other CNS-stimulant type drugs should be avoided. It may enhance effects of oral anticoagulants, warfarin and bihydroxycoumarin. Use with caution in patients with severe renal impairment. |
| Hypersensitivity; in infants under 3 months of age; in pregnant patients at term; in patients with anuria, oliguria, or significant renal impairment. | GI and neurologic disturbances; hematologic and dermatologic reactions; pulmonary sensitivity reactions; hypersensitivity reactions; alopecia; pain at injection site (IM). | Safe usage of this drug during pregnancy and lactation or of the parenteral form in children under 12 years of age has not been established. Superinfections of pseudomonas may occur. Diluents without preservatives should be used in preparing parenteral form. Oral dosage may be given with food or milk to minimize gastric upset. |
| Hypersensitivity; renal insufficiency; liver disease; severe dehydration; the sulfosalicylate salt in patients sensitive to salicylates. Concomitant use with sulfonamides. | GI disturbances; dysuria, skin rash. | Acidification of the urine must be maintained for the action of methenamine preparations to occur; ammonium chloride or ascorbic acid may be used. Safe use of the hippurate salt during early pregnancy is not established. Liver function should be monitored when using the hippurate salt. |
| Hypersensitivity; renal insufficiency. | GI disturbances; bladder irritation; fever with large doses. | Discolors the urine (and sometimes stool) blue-green. Continued administration may cause anemia. May also be used as an antidote for cyanide poisoning and for treatment of methemoglobinemia. |

**Table 25-30.** Urinary tract antiinfectives: sulfonamides and trimethoprim-sulfusoxazole

| Generic name | Trade name(s) | Dosage form(s) | Strength(s) | Usual dose |
|---|---|---|---|---|
| Sulfacytine | Renoquid | Tablet | 250 mg | *Adults:* Initially 500 mg then 250 mg qid for 10 days. Do not use in children under 14 years old. |
| Sulfadiazine | Coco-Diazine<br>Various<br>  manufacturers | Oral suspension<br>Injection<br>Tablet | 500 mg/5 ml<br>250 mg/amp.<br>325, 500 mg | *Adults: Oral:* 2-4 g initially, then 2-4 g daily in divided doses.<br>*Parenteral:* 100 mg/kg/24 hours in 4 divided doses by slow IV infusion.<br>*Children: Oral:* 150 mg/kg/24 hours divided into 4-6 doses. Parenteral-same as adult dose. |
| Sulfameter | Sulla | Tablet | 500 mg | *Patients over 100 lb or 12 yr:* 1.5 g first day then 500 mg q 24 hr. Not recommended for children under 12 years. |
| Sulfamethizole | Proklar<br><br>Sulfstat<br>  Forte<br>Thiosulfil<br><br>Urifon | Tablet<br>Oral suspension<br>Tablet<br><br>Tablet<br>Oral suspension<br>Tablet | 500 mg<br>500 mg/5 ml<br>500 mg<br><br>250, 500 mg<br>250 mg/5 ml<br>500 mg | *Adults:* 0.5-1.0 Gm tid or qid.<br>*Children over 2 mo:* 30-45 mg/kg/24 hr in 4 equal doses. |
| Sulfamethoxazole | Gantanol | Tablet<br>Oral suspension | 0.5 g<br>0.5 g/5 ml | *Adults:* 2 g initially then 1 g bid or tid.<br>*Children or infants over 2 mo:* 50-60 mg/kg/initially then 25-30 mg/kg bid up to 75 mg/kg/24 hr. |
| Sulfamethoxy-<br>  pyridazine | Midicel | Tablet<br>Oral suspension | 500 mg<br>0.5 g/5 ml | *Adults:* 1 g initially then 0.5 g qd or 1 gm qod.<br>*Children:* 30 mg/kg initially then 15 mg/kg daily up to 0.5 g daily. |
| Sulfisoxazole | Gantrisin<br><br><br><br>J-Sul<br>Lipo Gantrisin<br>Rosoxol<br>SK-Soxazole<br>Soxomide<br>Sulfalar | Tablet<br>Syrup<br>Pediatric<br>  Suspension<br>Injection<br>Tablet<br>Emulsion<br>Tablet<br>Tablet<br>Tablet<br>Tablet | 500 mg<br>500 mg/5 ml<br>500 mg/5 ml<br><br>400 mg/ml-5, 10 ml<br>500 mg<br>1 g/5 ml<br>500 mg<br>500 mg<br>500 mg<br>500 mg | *Adults: Oral:* 2.4 g initially then 4-8 g/24 hr in 4-6 divided doses<br>*Children: Oral:* 150 mg/kg/day in 4 to 6 equal doses, first dose ½ of 24 hr dose.<br>*Parenteral:* Same as adult dose, subcutaneous or IV. |
| Trimethoprim,<br>  sulfamethoxazole | Bactrim<br><br><br><br><br>Septra | Tablet<br><br><br>Oral suspension<br>Tablet<br><br>Oral suspension | Trimethoprim sulfa-<br>  methoxazole:<br>  80 mg/400 mg;<br>  160 mg/800 mg<br>40 mg/200 mg/5 ml<br>80 mg/400 mg; 160<br>  mg/800 mg<br>40 mg/200 mg/5 ml | *Adults:* 160 mg/800 mg q 12 hr for 10-14 days.<br>*Children:* 8 mg/40 mg per kg/24 hr in 2 divided doses for 10 days. Reduce dosage if renal impairment present. |

| Contraindications | Major side effects | Comments |
|---|---|---|
| Hypersensitivity to any of the sulfonamide; in infants less than 2 mo old; in pregnancy at term and in nursing mothers; porphyria. | GI disturbances; allergic reactions; blood dyscrasias; CNS disturbances; renal reactions. | *General:* Blood counts and urinalyses should be done periodically. Fluid intake should be encouraged during therapy. Use with caution in patients with impaired renal or hepatic function, allergies, or bronchial asthma. Avoid concomitant use with methenamine, PABA, and its derivatives. *Special:* Safe usage during pregnancy has not been established. |
| Same as above. | Hypersensitivity reactions; GI disturbances; CNS and hematologic disturbances; renal reactions; alopecia is possible. | *General:* Same as above. *Special:* None. |
| Hypersensitivity to any of the sulfonamide derivatives; marked hepatic or renal impairment; in pregnancy at term or in nursing mothers; porphyria. | Hypersensitivity reactions; hematologic and renal disturbances; hepatotoxicity; neuropsychiatric disturbances; GI disturbances. | *General:* Same as above. *Special:* Because of slow excretion resulting in prolonged high blood levels, lower doses at extended intervals are employed. Hepatic function tests should be done periodically. |
| Hypersensitivity to any of the sulfonamide derivatives; in infants less than 2 mo old; in pregnancy at term or in nursing mothers; porphyria. | Hypersensitivity reactions; GI and CNS disturbances; hematologic disturbances; renal disturbances. | *General:* Same as above. *Special:* May discolor the skin and/or alkaline urine orange-yellow color. It has been reported to increase the half life of phenytoin. Renal function studies should be done periodically. |
| Same as above. | Allergic reactions; hematologic disturbances; GI and CNS disturbances; renal disturbances | *General:* Same as above. *Special:* Liver function studies should be done periodically. |
| Hypersensitivity to any of the sulfonamide derivatives; in infants under 2 mo old; in pregnancy at term and in nursing mothers; porphyria. | Allergic reactions; hematologic disturbances; GI and CNS disturbances; renal disturbances. | *General:* Same as above. *Special:* Use with caution in patients with blood dyscrasias. Due to slow excretion resulting in prolonged high blood levels, lower doses at extended intervals are employed. |
| Hypersensitivity to any of the sulfonamide derivatives; advanced kidney disease; in infants under 2 mo old; in pregnancy at term; in nursing mothers; porphyria. | Hematologic disturbances; allergic reactions; GI and CNS disturbances; renal disturbances; irritation at the injection site (subcutaneous). | *General:* Same as above. *Special:* None. |
| Hypersensitivity to trimethoprim or any of the sulfonamide derivatives; during pregnancy and while nursing; in infants under 2 mo old; advanced kidney disease; porphyria. | Same as above. | *General:* Same as above. *Special:* None. |

**Table 25-31.** Diuretics

| Generic name | Trade name(s) | Dosage form(s) | Strength(s) | Usual dose |
|---|---|---|---|---|
| Bendroflume-thiazide | Naturetin | Tablet | 2.5, 5, 10 mg | 5 mg daily usually taken in morning. |
| Benzthiazide | Aquapres | Tablet | 50 mg | 50-150 mg daily either in the morning or divided into morning and evening doses. |
| | Aquastat | Tablet | 50 mg | |
| | Aquatag | Tablet | 25, 50 mg | |
| | Exna | Tablet | 50 mg | |
| | Hy-drine | Tablet | 50 mg | |
| | Lemazide | Tablet | 25, 50 mg | |
| | Proaqua | Tablet | 50 mg | |
| | S-Aqua | Tablet | 50 mg | |
| | Urazide | Tablet | 50 mg | |
| Chlorothiazide | Diuril | Tablet | 250, 500 mg | *Adult:* IV or orally: 0.5-1.0 g qd or bid. *Children:* Oral: 10 mg/lb/day in 2 doses. *IV:* Use in children and infants not generally recommended. |
| | | Oral suspension | 250 mg/5 ml | |
| | | Injection | 500 mg/vial | |
| | Ro-Chlorozide | Tablet | 250, 500 mg | |
| Chlorthalidone | Hygroton | Tablet | 50, 100 mg | 50-100 mg daily, on alternate days, or 3 times weekly as single dose in morning with food. |
| Cyclothiazide | Anhydron | Tablet | 2 mg | *Adults:* 1 or 2 mg daily in the morning. |
| Ethacrynic acid | Edecrin | Tablet | 25, 50 mg | *Adults:* Oral: 50-100 mg daily in the morning. *Parenteral:* usually 50 mg IV over several minutes in urgent conditions. *Children:* 25 mg initially and increased increments until maintenance dose reached. *Parenteral:* Pediatric use is not recommended. |
| | | Injection | 50 mg/vial | |
| Furosemide | Lasix | Tablet | 20, 40 mg | *Adults:* Oral: 20-80 mg as single dose preferably in AM. *Parenteral:* 20-40 mg or more IM or IV over 1-2 min. *Children:* Oral: 2 mg/kg as a single dose. *Parenteral:* 1 mg/kg IM or IV as single dose. |
| | | Injection | 10 mg/ml-2, 10 ml | |
| | | Oral suspension | 20 mg/5 ml | |

| Contraindications | Major side effects | Comments |
|---|---|---|
| Anuria; hypersensitivity to this or other sulfonamide derivatives. | GI disturbances; CNS and hematologic reactions; hypersensitivity; dermatologic reactions; cardiovascular reactions; musculoskeletal reactions. | Use with caution during pregnancy and in patients with impaired renal or hepatic function, allergies, and bronchial asthma. Hypokalemia may occur. May alter various laboratory test results and may interact with other antihypertensive agents, adrenergic blocking agents, corticosteroids, and curariform drugs. |
| Same as above. | Same as above. | Same as above. |
| Same as above. | Same as above. | Same as above. |
| Same as above. | Same as above. | Same as above. |
| Same as above. | GI disturbances; CNS and hematologic reactions; hypersensitivity; dermatologic reactions; cardiovascular disturbances; musculoskeletal reactions. | Same as above. |
| Anuria; oral or parenteral use in infants; during pregnancy and lactation. | GI disturbances; renal and hepatic disturbances; hematologic and carbohydrate metabolism disturbances; allergic and CNS reactions. | Use with caution in patients with advanced cirrhosis of the liver. Hypokalemia may occur. Ethacrynic acid alters activity and/or toxicity of a number of drugs including oral anticoagulants, antihypertensive agents and aminoglycoside antibiotics. Not to be injected IM or subcutaneously because of pain. |
| Anuria; hypersensitivity; in women of childbearing potential except in life-threatening situations. | GI disturbances; renal and hepatic disturbances; allergic reactions; CNS disturbances; ototoxicity; local irritation and pain at injection site IM or IV. | Hypokalemia may occur. Patients with sulfonamide sensitivity may show allergic reactions to furosemide. Furosemide alters activity or toxicity of a number of drugs including salicylates, antihypertensive agents, digitalis glycosides, aminoglycoside antibiotics, lithium preparations, cephaloridine, pressor amines, and curariform drugs. |

*Continued.*

**Table 25-31.** Diuretics—cont'd

| Generic name | Trade name(s) | Dosage form(s) | Strength(s) | Usual dose |
|---|---|---|---|---|
| Hydrochlorothia-zide | Diucen-H | Tablet | 50 mg | *Adults:* 25-200 mg daily. |
| | Esidrix | Tablet | 25, 50 mg | *Infants and children:* |
| | Hydro-Diuril | Tablet | 25, 50 mg | 1 mg/lb daily in |
| | Hydromal | Tablet | 50 mg | 2 doses. |
| | Hydro-Z-50 | Tablet | 50 mg | |
| | Lexor | Tablet | 50 mg | |
| | Oretic | Tablet | 25, 50 mg | |
| | Ro-Hydrazide | Tablet | 25, 50 mg | |
| | Thiuretic | Tablet | 25, 50 mg | |
| Hydroflume-thiazide | Diucardin | Tablet | 50 mg | *Adults:* 25-200 mg daily |
| Methyclo-thiazide | Aquatensen | Tablet | 5 mg | *Adults:* 2.55 10 mg once daily. |
| | Enduron | Tablet | 2.5, 5 mg | *Note:* maximum effective single dose is 10 mg. |
| Metolazone | Zaroxolyn | Tablet | 2.5, 5, 10 mg | *Adults:* 5-10 mg once daily. |
| Polythiazide | Renese | Tablet | 1, 2, 4 mg | *Adults:* 1-4 mg daily. |
| Quinethazone | Hydromox | Tablet | 50 mg | *Adults:* 50-100 mg daily in a single dose. |
| Spironolactone | Aldactone | Tablet | 25 mg | *Adults:* Initially 100 mg daily in divided doses. *Children:* 1.5 mg/lb body weight |
| Triamterene | Dyrenium | Capsule | 50, 100 mg | Dosage should be titrated to the patient's needs. *Adults:* 100 mg bid after meals initially. |
| Trichlor-methiazide | Diurese | Tablet | 4 mg | *Adults:* 2-4 mg daily. |
| | Naqua | Tablet | 2, 4 mg | |
| | Metahydrin | Tablet | 2, 4 mg | |

| Contraindications | Major side effects | Comments |
|---|---|---|
| Anuria; hypersensitivity to this or any other sulfonamide derivatives. | GI disturbances; CNS and hematologic disturbances; hypersensitivity reactions; cardiovascular, renal, and musculoskeletal disturbances. | *General:* Use with caution in patients with impaired renal or hepatic function, allergies, and bronchial asthma. Hypokalemia may occur. Thiazides may alter various laboratory test results and also interact with other antihypertensive agents, adrenergic blocking agents, corticosteroids, lithium compounds, and curariform drugs. *Special:* Use with caution during pregnancy. |
| Same as above. | Same as above. | *General:* Same as above. *Special:* Same as above. |
| Same as above. | Same as above; dermatologic reactions. | *General:* Same as above. *Special:* Same as above. |
| Anuria; hepatic coma or precoma; hypersensitivity to this or any other sulfonamide derivative; pregnancy. | Same as above. | *General:* Same as above. *Special:* Not recommended for use in pediatric patients. |
| Anuria; hypersensitivity to this or any other sulfonamide derivative. | Same as above. | *General:* Same as above. *Special:* Use with caution during pregnancy. |
| Anuria; hypersensitivity to this or any other sulfonamide derivative; pregnancy; progressively impaired renal function. | Same as above. | *General:* Same as above. Special: None. |
| Anuria; acute renal insufficiency; hyperkalemia; progressive impairment of renal function; safe usage in pregnancy has not been established. | GI and CNS reactions, dermatological reactions; gynecomastia; impotence; androgenic effects. | Hyperkalemia may occur. Spironolactone potentiates the action of other antihypertensive drugs. May be used in initial diagnostic testing for primary hyperaldosteronism. |
| Severe or progressive kidney disease or dysfunction; severe hepatic disease; hypersensitivity; patients with hyperkalemia. | GI disturbances; allergic responses; photosensitivity. | Hyperkalemia may occur. Safe usage during pregnancy has not been established. Triamterene may potentiate antihypertensive agents. |
| Anuria; hypersensitivity to this or any sulfonamide derivative. | GI and CNS reactions; dermatologic-hypersensitivity, and musculoskeletal reactions; hematologic and cardiovascular disturbances. | Hypokalemia may occur. May alter various laboratory test results and also interact with other antihypertensive agents, adrenergic blocking agents, corticosteroids, lithium compounds, and curariform type drugs. Use with caution during pregnancy and in patients with impaired renal or hepatic function, allergies, and bronchial asthma. |

**Table 25-32.** Urinary tract antispasmodics and analgesics

| Generic name | Trade name(s) | Dosage form(s) | Strength(s) | Usual dose |
|---|---|---|---|---|
| Ethoxazene HCl | Serenium | Tablet | 100 mg | *Adults:* 100 mg tid before meals. *Children under 8:* 100 mg bid before meals. |
| Phenazo-pyridine HCl | Azo-Standard | Tablet | 100 mg | *Adults:* 200 mg tid after meals. |
| | Azo-Stat | Tablet | 200 mg | |
| | Di-Azo | Tablet | 100 mg | |
| | Phenyl-Idium | Tablet | 100, 200 mg | |
| | Pyridium | Tablet | 100, 200 mg | |
| | Urodine | Tablet | 100 mg | |
| Flavoxate | Urispas | Tablet | 100 mg | *Adults and Children over 12:* 100-200 mg tid or qid. |
| Oxybutynin | Ditropan | Tablet | 5 mg | *Adults:* 5 mg bid or tid, maximum 5 mg qid. *Children over 5:* 5 mg bid maximum 5 mg tid. |

**Table 25-33.** Urinary alkalinizers

| Generic name | Trade name(s) | Dosage form(s) | Strength(s) | Usual dose |
|---|---|---|---|---|
| Potassium citrate, citric acid | Polycitra | Syrup | 1100 mg potassium citrate, 334 mg citric acid/5 ml | *Adults:* 15-30 ml in water after meals and at bedtime. *Children:* 5-15 ml in water. |
| Potassium citrate, sodium citrate, citric acid | Polycitra | Syrup | 550 mg potassium citrate, 500 mg sodium citrate, 334 mg citric acid/5 ml | *Adults:* 15-30 ml diluted with water after meals and at bedtime. *Children:* 5-15 ml diluted with water after meals and at bedtime. |
| | Polycitra-LC | Solution | Same as syrup | |
| Sodium bicarbonate | Various manufacturers | Tablet | 325, 650 mg | 325 mg to 2 g up to 4 times daily. |
| Sodium citrate, citric acid | Bacitra | Liquid | 500 mg sodium citrate, 300 mg citric acid/5 ml | *Adults:* 10-30 ml in water after meals and at bedtime. *Children:* 5-15 ml in water after meals and at bedtime. |

| Contraindications | Major side effects | Comments |
|---|---|---|
| Uremia, severe liver disease; chronic glomerulonephritis; in pyelonephritis, pregnancy, GI disturbances. | Occasional GI disturbances. | Colors urine orange or red. Use with caution in all GI conditions (analgesic). Safe usage during pregnancy has not been established. |
| Renal insufficiency. | Same as above. | Colors the urine reddish-orange. Safe usage during pregnancy has not been established. |
| Pyloric or duodenal obstruction; obstructive intestinal lesions or ileus; achalasia; GI hemorrhage; obstructive uropathies of lower urinary tract. | GI and CNS disturbances; dermatologic and cardiovascular disturbances; visual disturbances; dry mouth. | Safe usage during pregnancy and in children and infants has not been established. Use with caution in patients with suspected glaucoma. |
| Glaucoma; partial or complete GI obstruction; paralytic ileus; intestinal atony of elderly or debilitated; obstructive uropathy; severe colitis; myasthenia gravis; unstable cardiovascular status in acute hemorrhage; megacolon; toxic megacolon complicating ulcerative colitis; in children under 5 years. | GI and CNS disturbances; allergic reactions; ocular disturbances; anticholinergic reactions; suppression of lactation; impotence. | Safe usage during pregnancy has not been established. May produce drowsiness and/or blurred vision. Use with caution in high environmental temperature and in the presence of diarrhea. |

| Contraindications | Major side effects | Comments |
|---|---|---|
| Severe renal impairment with oliguria or azotemia; hyperkalemia; acute dehydration; anuria; heat cramps; severe myocardial damage; untreated Addison's disease; and adynamia episodica; hereditaria. | Hyperkalemia; systemic; alkalosis; GI disturbances. | Useful when sodium salts are undesirable or contraindicated. Use with caution in patients with low urinary output. Should be diluted with water and given after meals to minimize GI side effects. *Note:* Contains 2 mEq K+/ml. May enhance the effectiveness of aminoglycoside antibiotics and solubility of sulfonamides. |
| Severe renal impairment; hyperkalemia; acute dehydration. | Same as above. | May enhance effectiveness of aminoglycoside antibiotics and the solubility of sulfonamides. Dilution with water and taking after meals may minimize GI side effects. *Note:* contains 1 mEq each of Na+ and k+ per ml. |
| Use in patients on restricted or low sodium diets. | Systemic alkalosis; GI disturbances. | May enhance effectiveness of aminoglycoside antibiotics and solubility of the sulfonamides. May also be used as gastric antacid. |
| Use in patients on restricted sodium intake. | GI disturbances; hyperpnea; convulsions. | May enhance effectiveness of aminoglycoside antibiotics and the solubility of sulfonamides. Use with caution in patients with cardiac failure hypertension, impaired renal function, toxemia of pregnancy and pulmonary or peripheral edema. *Note:* contains I mEq Na+/ml. |

**Table 25-34.** Urinary acidifiers

| Generic name | Trade name(s) | Dosage form(s) | Strength(s) | Usual dose |
|---|---|---|---|---|
| Ammonium biphospate, sodium Biphosphate and sodium acid pyrophosphate | Phos-Phaid | Tablet 0.5 g (regular and enteric coated) | (190 mg ammonium phosphate; 200 mg sodium biphosphate; 110 mg sodium acid pyrophosphate) 0.5 g (½ of above formula) | 1 Gm followed by 1 glass of water qid. |
| Ammonium chloride | Various manufacturers | Tablet  Tablet, enteric coated | 0.5 g  0.5 g | 0.5-1 g q 2-3 hr. |
| Ascorbic acid (vitamin C) | Various manufacturers | Tablet  Capsule Syrup Drops | 50, 100, 250, 500 mg; 1 Gm 250, 500 mg 500 mg/5 ml 100 mg/1 ml | *Adults:* 250 mg-1 g qid. |
| Potassium acid phosphate | K-Phos | Tablet | 500 mg | 1 g with full glass of water qid. |

**Table 25-35.** Topical antibiotics

| Generic name | Trade name(s) | Dosage form(s) | Strength(s) | Usual dose |
|---|---|---|---|---|
| Bacitracin | Baciquent Various manufacturers | Ointment Powder for solution | 500 U/g 50,000 U/vial | Apply to affected area 3 or 4 times daily. |
| Chloramphenicol | Chloromycetin | Cream | 1% | Apply to affected areas 3 or 4 times daily after cleansing. |
| Erythromycin | Ilotycin | Ointment | 1% | Apply to affected areas 3 or 4 times daily. |
| Gentamicin | Garamycin | Cream Ointment | 0.1% 0.1% | Apply small amount to affected areas 3 or 4 times daily. |
| Neomycin | Myciguent Various manufacturers | Cream Ointment Powder | 0.5% 1.5% 0.5 g sterile; 10, 50, 100 g nonsterile. | Apply to affected areas 3 or 4 times daily. |
| Penicillin | Various manufacturers | Ointment | 5000 U/g | Same as above. |
| Tetracycline | Achromycin | Ointment | 3% | Same as above. |

| Contraindications | Major side effects | Comments |
|---|---|---|
| None indicated. | GI disturbances; | Enteric-coated tablets may eliminate GI disturbances. Use with caution in severe renal damage. May enhance or assure effectiveness of antibacterials requiring an acid medium. |
| Severe renal impairment; severe hepatic failure. | GI disturbances; systemic acidosis with large doses. | May be used in treatment of systemic alkalosis; also has mild diuretic effect. May enhance the effectiveness of certain antiinfectives. |
| None known. | May cause some GI irritation. | Ascorbic acid is one of the essential vitamins in man. May interfere with effectiveness of disulfiram. High intake of ascorbic acid has been shown to aid in fracture and wound healing. May enhance or assure effectiveness of antibacterials requiring an acid medium. |
| Renal insufficiency; Addison's disease; severe hepatic failure. | Laxative effect. | May enhance or assure effectiveness of antibacterials requiring an acid medium. Administration should be followed with adequate fluid intake. |

| Contraindications | Major side effects | Comments |
|---|---|---|
| Hypersensitivity; not for otic use if eardrum is perforated, or ophthalmic use. | Hypersensitivity reactions. | Severe infections may require systemic antibiotics. Prolonged use may result in secondary infections due to overgrowth of nonsusceptible organisms, especially fungi. |
| Hypersensitivity. | Hypersensitivity reactions including bone marrow hypoplasia (with prolonged use). | Same as above. |
| Same as above. | Hypersensitivity reactions. | Same as above. |
| Same as above. | Hypersensitivity reactions; possible photosensitization. | Same as above. If irritation occurs, discontinue use. |
| Same as above. | Hypersensitivity reactions; nephrotoxicity and/or ototoxicity if absorption occurs. | Same as above. |
| Same as above. | Hypersensitivity reactions. | Same as above. |
| Same as above. | Same as above. | Same as above. |

**Table 25-36.** Topical antifungal agents

| Generic name | Trade name(s) | Dosage form(s) | Strength(s) | Usual dose |
|---|---|---|---|---|
| Acrisorcin | Akrinol | Cream | 2 mg/g | Apply small amount to affected areas bid, morning, and evening. Continue for at least 6 weeks. |
| Amphotericin B | Fungizone | Cream<br>Lotion<br>Ointment | 30 mg/g<br>30 mg/ml<br>30 mg/g | Apply liberally to candidal lesions 2-4 times daily. |
| Clotrimazole | Lotrimin | Cream<br>Solution | 1%<br>1% | Massage into affected areas and surrounding skin areas bid, morning and evening. |
| Haloprogin | Halotex | Cream<br>Solution | 1%<br>1% | Apply liberally to affected areas twice daily for 2-3 weeks. |
| Iodochlor-<br>hydroxyquin | Mycoquin<br>Vioform | Cream<br>Cream<br>Ointment<br>Powder | 3%<br>3%<br>3% | Apply to affected areas 2-4 times daily. |
| Miconazole nitrate | Micatin | Cream | 2% | Cover affected areas twice daily, morning and evening |
| Nystatin | Mycostatin | Cream<br>Ointment<br>Powder | 100,000 U/g<br>100,000 U/g<br>100,000 U/g | Apply to the affected areas bid or tid until healing complete. |
| Tolnaftate | Aftate<br><br><br><br>Tinactin | Gel<br>Powder<br>Powder (aerosol)<br>Liquid<br>Gel<br>Powder<br>Powder (aerosol)<br>Solution | 1%<br>1%<br>1%<br>1%<br>1%<br>1%<br>1%<br>1% | Apply small quantities twice daily for 2-3 weeks. |
| Triacetin | Enzactin<br><br><br>Fungacetin | Aerosol<br>Cream<br>Powder<br>Liquid<br>Ointment | 15%<br>250 mg/g<br>33.3%<br>30%<br>25% | Apply twice daily to affected areas after cleansing and drying. |
| Undecylenic acid derivatives | Blis-To-Sol<br>Caldesene<br>Cruex<br><br><br><br>Desenex | Gel<br>Powder<br>Aerosol<br>Powder<br>Squeeze bottle<br>Ointment<br><br><br>Powder<br><br><br>Powder (aerosol)<br><br><br><br>Soap<br>Solution | 5% undecylemic acid<br>10% calcium unde-cyclenate<br>10% calcium unde-cylenate<br>10% calcium unde-cylenate<br>10% calcium unde-cylenate<br>5% Undecylenic acid, 20% zinc unde-cylenate<br>2% undecylinic acid 20% zinc unde-cylenate<br>20% undecylenic acid 20% zinc unde-cylenate<br>2% undecylenic acid<br>2% hexachlorophene 10% undecylenic acid | Apply to affected area gently after thorough cleansing. |

| Contraindications | Major side effects | Comments |
|---|---|---|
| Sensitivity to any component. | Pruritis; blisters; burning; eruptions; hives. | Do not use around the eyes. Discontinue use if irritation or sensitization occurs. Recommended only for tinea versicolor. |
| Same as above. | Local irritation with burning, pruritis. | Discontinue use if hypersensitivity reactions occur. Recommended for infections caused by *Candida (Monilia)* species. |
| Same as above. | General irritation of the skin including erythema, blistering, peeling edema, pruritis, urticaria. | Safe usage during pregnancy has not been established. Not for ophthalmic use. Discontinue use if irritation or sensitivity develops. Clotrimazole is a broad spectrum antifungal agent. |
| Same as above. | Local irritation with burning or vesicle formation; increased maceration, pruritis, or exacerbation of preexisting lesions. | Safe usage during pregnancy has not been established. Keep out of eyes. Discontinue use if sensitization or irritation occurs. |
| Idiosyncrasy to iodine; tuberculosis, vaccinia, varicella, or other viral infections of the skin. | Local irritation; may stain hair or fabric. | Not for ophthalmic use. Discontinue use if irritation or sensitization occurs. May be absorbed and interfere with thyroid function tests. May also interfere (false positive) with ferric chloride test for phenylketonuria. |
| Hypersensitivity to any of the components. | Irritation, burning, and maceration. | Avoid introduction into the eyes. Discontinue use if sensitization or irritation occurs. |
| Same as above. | Virtually nontoxic and nonsensitizing. | Discontinue use if irritations or hypersensitivity occurs. |
| Same as above. | Virtually nontoxic; sensitization or local irritation may occur. | Discontinue use if irritation or hypersensitivity occurs. Keep out of the eyes. |
| Same as above. | Local irritation. | Prevent contact with rayon fabrics and cover treated areas. Use with caution in persons with impaired circulation, including diabetics. |
| Hypersensitivity to any components; pustular or severely broken skin. | Local irritation. | Keep away from eyes and mucous membranes. These products have both antibacterial and antifungal action. Use with caution in patients with impaired circulation, including diabetics. |

**Table 25-37.** Topical steroids

| Generic name | Trade name(s) | Dosage form(s) | Strength(s) | Usual dose |
|---|---|---|---|---|
| Betamethasone | Celestone | Cream | 0.2% | Apply thin film 1-3 times daily. |
| Betamethasone benzoate | Benisone | Cream | 0.025% | |
| | Fluobate | Gel | 0.025% | |
| | | Cream | 0.025% | |
| | | Gel | 0.025% | |
| | | Lotion | 0.025% | |
| Betamethasone dipropionate | Diprosone | Cream | 0.05% | |
| | | Ointment | 0.05% | |
| Betamethasone valerate | Valisone | Aerosol | 0.15% | |
| | | Cream | 0.1% | |
| | | Lotion | 0.1% | |
| | | Ointment | 0.1% | |
| Dexamethasone | Aeroseb-Dex | Aerosol | 10 mg/90 g | Apply to affected areas 3-4 times daily. |
| | Decaspray | Aerosol | 10 mg/90 g | |
| | Decaderm | Gel | 0.1% | |
| | Hexadrol | Cream | 0.04% | |
| Dexamethasone phosphate | Decadron | Cream | 0.1% | |
| Flumethasone pivalate | Locorten | Cream | 0.03% | Same as above. |
| Fluocinolone acetonide | Fluonid | Cream | 0.01, 0.025% | Apply sparingly to affected areas 3-4 times daily. |
| | | Ointment | 0.025% | |
| | | Solution | 0.01% | |
| | Synalar | Cream | 0.01, 0.025, 0.2% | |
| | | Ointment | 0.025% | |
| | | Solution | 0.01% | |
| | Squemol | Cream | 0.025% | |
| Fluocinonide | Lidex | Cream | 0.05% | Massage small amount into affected area 3-4 times daily. |
| | | Ointment | 0.05% | |
| | Topsyn | Gel | 0.05% | |
| Fluorometholone | Oxylone | Cream | 0.025% | Apply to affected area 3-4 times daily. |
| Flurandrenolide | Cordran | Cream | 0.025, 0.05% | Apply to affected area 2-3 times daily. |
| | | Lotion | 0.05% | |
| | | Ointment | 0.025, 0.05% | |
| | | Tape | 4 $\mu$g/cm² | |
| Halcinonide | Halog | Cream | 0.1% | Rub gently into affected areas 2-3 times daily. |

| Contraindications | Major side effects | Comments |
| --- | --- | --- |
| In vaccinia and varicella; hyper-sensitivity. | Burning; itching; irritation and dryness of skin; hypo-pigmentation; folliculitis; hypertrichosis; acneform eruptions. | *General:* Discontinue use if irritation develops. In the presence of infection steroid therapy should be stopped until infection is adequately con-trolled. *Special:* Safe use during pregnancy has not been established. |
| In vaccinia and varicella; in herpes simplex; in fungal infections; tuberculosis of the skin; hypersensitivity. | Same as above. | *General:* Same as above. *Special:* Same as above. |
| In vaccinia and varicella; hyper-sensitivity. | Same as above. | *General:* *Special:* Infection may occur when using the occlusive dressing technique. |
| Hypersensitivity; vaccinia and varicella. | Burning, itching, irritation, dryness of skin; hypopig-mentation; hypertrichosis; folliculitis; and acneform eruptions. | *General:* Same as above. *Special:* Use caution when employing occlusive dressing technique. Safe usage during pregnancy has not been established. |
| Same as above. | Same as above. | *General:* Same as above. *Special:* Safe use during pregnancy has not been established. |
| Same as above. | Same as above. | *General:* Same as above. *Special:* Same as above. |
| Same as above. | Same as above. | *General:* Same as above. *Special:* Safe use during pregnancy has not been established. Use caution when the occlusive dressing technique is employed. |
| Hypersensitivity; vaccinia and varicella; for ophthalmic use. | Acneform eruptions; hypo-pigmentation; striae; skin atrophy; folliculitis; hyper-trichosis; secondary infec-tion; burning, itching, irri-tation, and dryness of skin. | *General:* Same as above. *Special:* Same as above. |

*Continued.*

**Table 25-37.** Topical steroids—cont'd

| Generic name | Trade name(s) | Dosage form(s) | Strength(s) | Usual dose |
|---|---|---|---|---|
| Hydrocortisone | Acticort | Lotion | 1% | Apply to affected areas 3 or 4 times daily. |
| | | Gel | 0.25% | |
| | Aeroseb-HC | Spray | 0.5% | |
| | Cetacort | Lotion | 0.125, 0.25, 0.5, 1% | |
| | Cort-Dome | Cream | 0.125, 0.25, 0.5, 1% | |
| | | Lotion | Same as cream | |
| | Cortril | Ointment | 1% | |
| | Dermacort | Cream | 1% | |
| | | Lotion | 0.5% | |
| | Eldecort | Cream | 1, 2.5% | |
| | | Lotion | 0.5% | |
| | Epicort | Lotion | 0.5, 1% | |
| | HC Cream | Cream | 0.5, 1% | |
| | Heb-Cort | Cream | 0.25, 0.5, 1% | |
| | Hi-Cor | Cream | 2.5% | |
| | Hexaderm | Cream | 0.5% | |
| | Hytone | Cream | 0.5, 1, 2.5% | |
| | | Lotion | 0.5, 1% | |
| | | Ointment | 0.5, 1, 2.5% | |
| | Microcort | Lotion | 0.5% | |
| | Nutracort | Cream | 0.25, 0.5, 1% | |
| | | Lotion | 0.25, 0.5, 1% | |
| | | Gel | 1% | |
| | Relecort | Cream | 0.25, 0.5, 1% | |
| | Texacort | Scalp lotion | 1% | |
| Hydrocortisone acetate | Cortef | Ointment | 1, 2.5% | |
| | Hydrocortone | Ointment | 1% | |
| Methylprednis-olone acetate | Medrol | Ointment | 0.25, 1% | Apply to affected areas 3-4 times daily. |
| Prednisolone | Meti-Derm | Cream | 0.5% | Same as above. |
| | | Aerosol 0.5% | | |
| Triamcinolone acetonide | Aristocort | Cream | 0.025, 0.1, 0.5% | |
| | | Ointment | 0.1, 0.5% | |
| | Aristocort -A | Cream | 0.1, 0.5% | |
| | | Ointment | 0.1% | |
| | | Spray | 17 mg/15 g | |
| | Aristoderm | Foam | 0.1% | |
| | Aristogel | Gel | 0.1% | |
| | Kenalog | Cream | 0.025, 0.1, 0.5% | |
| | | Lotion | 0.025, 0.1% | |
| | | Ointment | | |
| | | Spray | 0.025, 0.1, 015% (3 sec delivers 0.2 mg) | |
| | Tramacin | Cream | 0.025, 0.1, 0.5% | |

| Contraindications | Major side effects | Comments |
|---|---|---|
| Hypersensitivity; in vaccinia and varicella. | Same as above. | *General:* Same as above.<br>*Special:* Same as above. |
| Hypersensitivity; in vaccinia and varicella. | Hypopigmentation; acneform eruptions; folliculitis; hypertrichosis; burning, itching, irritation, and dryness of the skin. | *General:* Same as above.<br>*Special:* Same as above. |
| Same as above. | Same as above.<br><br>Same as above, and skin atrophy; striae; miliaria; secondary infection. | *General:* Same as above.<br>*Special:* Same as above.<br>*General:* Same as above.<br>*Special:* Same as above. |

**Table 25-38.** Topical enzymes

| Generic name | Trade name(s) | Dosage form(s) | Strength(s) | Usual dose |
|---|---|---|---|---|
| Collagenase | Collagenase ABC | Ointment | 250 U/g | Apply daily or qod after proper cleaning and preparation of the lesion, including application of antibiotics when indicated. |
| | Santyl | Ointment | 250 U/g | |
| Fibrinolysin and desoxyribonuclease | Elase | Dry powder | Fibr./Des: 25/20,000 U/vial | Apply to the lesion 1-3 times daily after proper cleansing, preparation, and cover with non-adhering dressing. |
| | | Ointment | 20 U/20,000 U/30 g | |
| Papain | Panafil | Ointment | 10% papain with 1% urea and 0.5% chlorophyll derivatives. | Apply directly to lesion once or twice daily and cover with gauze. |
| | Panafil White | Ointment | 10% papain with 10% urea. | |
| Streptokinase-streptodornase | Varidase | Injection | 100,000 U streptokinase and at least 25,000 U of streptodornase-vial. | All treatment should be individualized. For local application only where adequate drainage is possible. |
| | | Combination package | 1 vial + 15 ml jar of 4.5% carboxymethylcellulose jelly | |
| Sutilains | Travase | Ointment | 82,000 U/g | Apply in thin layer extending $1/4$-$1/2$ inch beyond area to be debrided 3-4 times daily and cover with loose wet dressings. |
| Trypsin | Granulex | Aerosol | 0.1 mg trypsin, 72.5 mg balsam Peru, and 650 mg castor oil/0.82 ml | Apply a minimum of twice daily, coating the wound thickly but not excessively. |

| Contraindications | Major side effects | Comments |
|---|---|---|
| Hypersensitivity. | None have been noted when used as directed. | Enzymatic activity is decreased by detergents, hexachlorophene, and heavy metal ions such as mercury, and silver. Cleansing of the site should be done with saline, hydrogen peroxide, or Dakin's solution. Ointment should be applied only to the lesion; surrounding normal skin may be protected by Lasser's paste. Enzyme activity may be stopped by application of Burrow's solution, USP. |
| History of hypersensitivity to any of the components; parenteral use. | Local hyperemia. | Successful results depend more on frequency of application than on the amount of ointment used. Necrotic debris should be flushed away so that the enzyme can be applied directly to the substrate. |
| Hypersensitivity to any of the components. | Itching or stinging sensation. | Hydrogen peroxide should not be used in conjunction with papain since it may inactivate the enzyme. At each dressing change, accumulated liquefied necrotic material should be flushed away with a mild cleansing solution. |
| The presence of active hemorrhage; hypersensitivity. | Pyrogenic reaction; allergic reactions. | Not intended for use on fibrous tissues, mucoproteins, or collagens. Prepared solutions should be refrigerated. Antibiotics such as penicillin, tetracycline, streptomycin, and dihydrostreptomycin can be mixed with solutions or the prepared jelly. |
| Pregnancy; fungating neoplastic ulcers; exposed major nerves or nervous tissue; wounds communicating with major body cavities. | Transient pain; paresthesias; bleeding; dermatitis. | Optimal activity requires moist environment. If infection is present, appropriate antibiotic therapy should be initiated. Detergent and antiseptic compounds such as nitrofurazone, iodine, hexachlorophene, and benzalkonium chloride may render the substrate indifferent to the action of the enzyme. Compounds containing heavy metal ions interfere directly with enzyme activity. Avoid contact with eyes. |
| Hypersensitivity to any of the components; use on fresh arterial clots. | Local irritation. | Avoid contact with eyes or nostrils. This combination acts to remove wound debris, stimulate blood flow to the area, to improve healing, and to reduce pain and odor. |

**Table 25-39.** Psychotherapeutic agents: antianxiety agents

| Generic name | Trade name(s) | Dosage form(s) | Strength(s) | Usual dose |
|---|---|---|---|---|
| Chlordiazepoxide | Librium | Capsule | 5, 10, 25 mg | *Adults:* 5-25 mg 2-4 |
| | | Injection | 100 mg/5 ml | times daily. |
| | Libritabs | Tablet | 5, 10, 25 mg | *Children:* 5 mg 2-4 |
| | SK-Lygen | Capsule | 5, 10, 25 mg | times daily. |
| Chlormezanone | Trancopal | Tablet | 100, 200 mg | *Adults:* 100-200 mg 3-4 times daily. |
| | | | | *Children:* 50-100 mg 3-4 times daily. |
| Clorazepate di-potassium | Tranxene | Capsule | 3.75, 7.5, 15 mg | *Adults:* 30 mg/day. |
| | Tranxene-SD | Tablet | 22.5 mg | |
| | Tranxene-SD half-strength | Tablet | 11.25 mg | |
| Diazepam | Valium | Tablet | 2, 5, 10 mg | *Adults:* 2-10 mg 2-4 |
| | | Injection IM/IV | 5 mg/ml in 2, 10 ml | times daily. |
| | | | | *Children:* 1-2.5 mg 3-4 times daily. |
| Doxepin | Adapin | Capsule | 10, 25, 50 mg | *Adults:* 25 mg 3 times |
| | Sinequan | Capsule | 10, 25, 50, 100 mg | daily. |
| | | Oral concentrate | 10 mg/ml | |
| Hydroxyzine HCl | Atarax | Tablet | 10, 25, 50, 100 mg | *Adults:* 25-100 mg |
| | | Syrup | 10 mg/5 ml | 4 times daily. |
| | | | | *Children under 6:* 50 mg/day in divided doses. |
| | | | | *Over 6:* 50-100 mg/day in divided doses. |
| Hydroxyzine pamoate | Vistaril | Capsule | 25, 50, 100 mg | *Oral:* Same as above. |
| | | Oral suspension | 25 mg/5 ml | *Adults:* IM: 50-100 |
| | | Injection | 25 mg/ml in 1 ml | mg up to every 4-6 |
| | | | 50 mg/ml in 2, 10 ml | hours. |
| | | | | *Children:* 0.5 mg/lb as indicated. |
| Meprobamate | Various manufacturers | Tablet | 200, 400, 600 mg | *Adults:* 1200-1600 mg daily in divided |
| | Equanil | Tablet | 200, 400 mg | doses. |
| | | Coated Tablet | 400 mg | *Children 6-12:* 100- |
| | | Capsule | 400 mg | 200 mg 2-3 times |
| | | Oral Suspension | 200 mg/5 ml | daily. |
| | Miltown | Tablet | 200, 400, 600 mg | |
| | Meprospan | SR Capsule | 200, 400 mg | |
| Oxazepam | Serax | Capsule | 10, 15, 30 mg | *Adults:* 10-40 mg 3-4 |
| | | Tablet | 15 mg | times daily. |
| | | | | *Children:* dosage not established for children 6-12 years. |
| Tybamate | Tybatran | Capsule | 125, 250, 350 mg | *Adults:* 750-2000 mg daily in divided doses. |
| | | | | *Children 6-12:* 25-35 mg/kg/day in 3-4 equally divided doses. |

| Contraindications | Major side effects | Comments |
|---|---|---|
| Use in children under 6; psychoses; acute narrow-angle glaucoma. | CNS, GI, GU, and cardio-vascular disturbances; EENT and dermatological manifestations. | Injection is very painful when given IM. |
| Hypersensitivity. | CNS, GI, GU disturbances; dermatological and neuro-logical involvement. | Onset of action within 15-30 minutes and of up to 6 hrs. duration; drowsiness may be marked. |
| Not recommended for patients under 18; psychoses; acute narrow-angle glaucoma. | CNS, GI, GU, and cardio-vascular disturbances; EENT and dermatological manifestations. | Note: Lower doses may be indicated in elderly or debilitated. |
| In children under 6 months; psychoses; acute narrow-angle glaucoma. | Same as above. | Also useful for muscle spasm, preoper-ative medication, cardioversion, and status epilepticus and severe convul-sive seizures. |
| Hypersensitivity; glaucoma; tendency toward urinary reten-tion; in children under 12 years old; concomitant use of MAO inhibitors and acute post-recovery phase p̄ MI. | CNS, cardiovascular and neurological disturbances; anticholinergic effects; allergic responses; GI dis-turbances; hematologic and endocrine involvement; withdrawal symptoms. | Also useful as antidepressant. |
| Previous hypersensitivity; early pregnancy. | CNS, neurologic distur-bances, anticholinergic effects. | Also useful for nausea and vomiting; bedtime sedation. |
| *Oral:* Same as above. *IM:* not for IV, SQ, or intraarterial injection. | Same as above. | Also useful for nausea and vomiting; bedtime sedation; adjunct to anesthe-sia, and to potentiate analgesics. |
| Hypersensitivity; acute intermittent porphyria; usage in children under 6. | CNS, cardiovascular and GI disturbances; allergic and idiosyncratic reactions; hematologic involvement. | Also useful for muscle relaxant to promote sleep. Causes exacerbation of porphyric symptoms. |
| In children under 6; hypersensi-tivity; psychoses; acute narrow-angle glaucoma. | CNS, GI, GU, and cardio-vascular disturbances; EENT and dermatologic manifestations. | Dosage should be increased with caution in older patients. |
| Hypersensitivity; acute inter-mittent porphyria; usage in children under 6 years of age. | CNS, cardiovascular, GI dis-turbances; allergic and idiosyncratic reactions. | Avoid abrupt cessation of therapy; safe use in pregnancy and lactation not established. |

**Table 25-40.** Psychotherapeutic agents: antidepressant agents

| Generic name | Trade name(s) | Dosage form(s) | Strength(s) | Usual dose |
|---|---|---|---|---|
| Amitriptyline HCl | Elavil | Tablet<br>Injection<br>Injection | 10, 25, 50, 75, 100, 150 mg<br>10 mg/ml-10 ml | *Adults: Oral:* 75-150 mg daily at bedtime or in divided doses; *IM:* 20-30 mg tid |
| | Endep | Tablet | 10, 25, 50, 75, 100 mg | |
| Desipramine HCl | Norpramin<br>Pertofrane | Tablet<br>Capsule | 25, 50 mg<br>25, 50 mg | *Adults:* 50 mg 3 times daily up to 200 mg daily in divided doses. |
| Doxepin HCl | Adapin<br>Sinequan | Capsule<br>Capsule<br>Oral concentrate | 10, 25, 50 mg<br>10, 25, 50, 75, 100 mg<br>100 mg/1 ml | *Adults:* 25 mg 3 times daily. |
| Imipramine CHl | Janimine<br>Presamine<br>Tofranil | Tablet<br>Tablet<br>Tablet<br>Injection IM | 10, 25, 50 mg<br>10, 25, 50 mg<br>10, 25, 50 mg<br>25 mg/2 ml | *Oral:* 75-200 mg/day in divided doses. *Adolescent and geriatric:* 30-40 mg/day. *IM:* up to 100 mg daily. |
| Imipramine pamoate | Tofranil-PM | Capsule | 75, 100, 125, 150 mg | 75-150 mg daily. For maintenance in 1 dose preferably at bedtime. |
| Isocarboxazid | Marplan | Tablet | 10 mg | 30 mg daily |
| Nortriptyline HCl | Aventyl | Capsule<br>Oral liquid | 10, 25 mg<br>10 mg/5 ml | 25 mg 3 or 4 times daily. |
| Phenelzine sulfate | Nardil | Tablet | 15 mg | *Adult:* 15 mg tid initially, then reduce to 15 mg daily or every other day. |
| Protriptyline HCl | Vivactil | Tablet | 5, 10 mg | *Adults:* 15-40 mg daily divided into 3-4 doses. |
| Tranylcypromine | Parnate | Tablet | 10 mg | *Adults:* 20-30 mg daily. |

| Contraindications | Major side effects | Comments |
|---|---|---|
| Not recommended for children under 12; hypersensitivity; acute recovery phase after MI; concomitant use of MAO inhibitors. | CNS, cardiovascular, allergic, and gastrointestinal disturbances; neurologic problems; anticholinergic effects; hematologic and endocrine involvement; withdrawal symptoms. | Also useful in anxiety; adequate therapeutic effect may take up to 30 days; sedatives effect may be utilized by giving single dose at bedtime. |
| Not recommended for children under 6 except for enuresis hypersensitivity; acute recovery phase after MI; concomitant use of MAO inhibitors. | Same as above. | Useful in children for enuresis. |
| Not for children under 12; hypersensitivity; acute recovery phase after MI; concomitant use of MAO inhibitors; concomitant intake of alcohol. | Same as above. | Also useful in anxiety. |
| Not recommended for children under 6 except in enuresis; hypersensitivity; acute recovery phase MI; concomitant use of MAO inhibitors. | CNS, cardiovascular, neurologic, GI disturbances; anticholinergic effects; allergic responses; hematologic and endocrine involvement; withdrawal symptoms. | Also useful in childhood enuresis. |
| Not recommended for children; hypersensitivity; acute recovery phase with MI; concomitant use of MAO inhibitors. | Same as above. | Sedative effect may be utilized by giving single dose at bedtime. |
| Hypersensitivity; pheochromocytoma; congestive heart failure; liver disease; patients taking guanethidine; concomitant use of sympathomimetic substances. | Orthostatic hypotension; cardiac rate and rhythm disturbances; GI upset; CNS disturbance. | For use in patients where tricyclic antidepressants contraindicated; clinical effect may require 3-4 weeks. |
| Not recommended for children, hypersensitivity; acute recovery phase with MI, concomitant use of MAO inhibitors. | CNS, cardiovascular, neurologic, GI disturbances; anticholinergic effects; allergic response; hematologic and endocrine involvement; withdrawal symptoms. | Dosage may be lowered for elderly and adolescent patients. |
| Hypersensitivity; pheochromocytoma; congestive heart failure; liver disease; concomitant use of guanethidine or tricyclic compounds. | Orthostatic hypotension; cardiac, CNS, and GI disturbances. | If the condition is not controlled in 3-4 weeks, further therapy is useless. |
| Not recommended for children; hypersensitivity; acute recovery phase with MI; concomitant use of MAO inhibitors. | CNS, cardiovascular, neurologic, GI disturbances; anticholinergic effects; allergic responses; hematologic and endocrine involvement; withdrawal symptoms. | Anticholinergic effects very pronounced; elderly patients' dose should be lowered and/or cardiovascular symptoms monitored closely. |
| Hypersensitivity; pheochromocytoma; congestive heart failure; liver disease; concomitant use of guanethidine or tricyclic compounds. | Orthostatic hypotension; cardiac, CNS and GI disturbances. | Therapeutic improvement may be seen in 48 hours up to 3 weeks. |

**BIBLIOGRAPHY**

1. Kastrup, E. K., Boyd, J. R., and Gifford, S.: Facts and comparisons. St. Louis, 1977, Facts and Comparisons, Inc.
2. Goodman, L. S., Gillman, A., Gillman, A. G., and Koelle, G. B.: The pharmacological basis of therapeutics, ed. 5, New York, 1975, Macmillan Publishing Co., Inc.
3. Baker, C. E., Jr.: Physicians' desk reference, ed. 31, Oradell, N. J., 1977, Medical Economics Co.
4. Miller, M. E., and Sachs, M. L.: About bedsores, Philadelphia, 1974, J. B. Lippincott Co.
5. Osol, A., and Hoover, J. E.: Remington's pharmaceutical sciences, ed. 15, Easton, Pa., 1975, Mack Publishing Co.
6. *AMA Drug Evaluations,* ed. 3, Littleton, Mass., 1977, Publishing Sciences Group, Inc.
7. *Handbook of Nonprescription Drugs,* ed. 5, Washington, D.C., 1977, American Pharmaceutical Association.
8. Conn, H. F.: Current therapy. Philadelphia, 1977, W. B. Saunders Co.
9. Martin, E. W., Alexander, S. F., Farage, D. J., and others: Hazards of medication, Philadelphia, 1971, J. B. Lippincott Co.
10. King, J. C.: Guide to parenteral admixtures, St. Louis, 1970, Cutter Laboratories, Inc., (Continual update).

# 26

# Infection: prevention, detection, and control

**MARGARET M. MARTIN**

The current concept of infection control as a comprehensive program now required of health care facilities has evolved from a decade of epidemiologic studies linking the patient, the infecting microorganisms, their mode of transmission, and the environment as factors that determine the occurrence of infection. Perhaps the greatest progress has been made in recognizing the individual department and team members as the key factors in the prevention, detection, and control of infection. It is truly a challenge to personnel of all disciplines to recognize their responsibility and contribution to infection control and the implications during routine daily patient care activities. Orthopedic health care professionals' understanding, compliance, and conscientious efforts throughout daily patient care and facility maintenance safeguard not only the patients, but themselves as well.

The term *infection control* represents such a growing collection of topics, theories, concepts, and controversial issues that the reader will undoubtedly discover areas untouched in this chapter. The intent here is to provide a basic understanding of infection control as a program that deals with prevention, detection, and control of infection within the scope of the orthopedic specialty. Topics and discussions have been arbitrarily chosen to provide an overview of hospital-acquired infections in the surgical orthopedic patient. Reference material listed at the conclusion will provide a more in-depth review for the interested reader.

The control of infection is appropriately placed in this text as a treatment alternative when we consider that to control infection is quite often an *option* of health care personnel! Personnel of all disciplines must be acquainted with the scope of an infection control program and its significance to their individual responsibilities and practices. No one individual, unit, department, or service is capable of ensuring adequate control of infection without cooperation of all concerned.

The major components of an infection control program, when dealt with individually, warrant a full chapter in themselves. The following overview is intended to define and highlight the key areas of concern for any infection control program, whether viewed from the administrative, committee, departmental, or patient unit level. (See boxed material on p. 672.) The purpose of such a program is to provide for the prevention, control, and investigation of potential and existing infections and related problems through multidisciplinary cooperation.

---

**COMPONENTS AND HIGHLIGHTS OF INFECTION CONTROL PROGRAM**

| Major components | Descriptive highlights | Major components | Descriptive highlights |
|---|---|---|---|
| Infection committee | Responsible for overseeing and coordinating all aspects of the program; providing surveillance of potential and existing problems. Promotion of a preventive and corrective program designed to minimize these hazards. | Isolation policy and procedure | The containment of potential pathogenic microorganisms without unnecessary restraints on patients or personnel. |
| Infection surveillance | Detection and analysis of the incidence and cause of infections among patient population; identification and isolation of "transmittable" disease processes among patient and employee population. | Microbiology laboratory | Proper collection and transportation of specimens, and interpretation of results; laboratory consultation in patient treatment and identification of epidemiologically unique strains of bacteria. |
| Employee health and hygiene | Surveillance and management of employees' exposure to communicable disease and employee health conditions deemed transmittable to patient population; handwashing practices; basic hygiene as related to safe health care delivery, including dress code. | Antibiotic utilization | Selective and controlled use of antimicrobial agents for restriction of unnecessary opportunistic microorganisms capable of causing clinically significant disease. |
| Policy and procedure (written) | As related to all departmental practices for care of patients, equipment, and facility systems; *ineffective unless enforced.* | Community referral and resources | Communication of reportable disease and infectious agents to state health departments; patient referral for community follow-up; investigative assistance from state health departments; patient referral for community follow-up; investigative assistance from state health departments and centers for disease control. |
| Environmental control | Housekeeping practices, including trash and linen handling; ventilation system maintenance; refrigeration, ice, and incubation system maintenance; selective microbiologic sampling of the animate and inanimate environment; traffic control. | Continuing education | The key to a successful continuing education program is employee understanding of the principle behind infection control policies and procedures. |

---

## NORMAL FLORA, PATHOGENS, AND SUSCEPTIBLE PATIENT

Understanding the basic concepts of *contamination, colonization,* and *infection* is perhaps the key to appreciating and knowledgeably practicing infection control measures. It is difficult to comprehend, or even define, the multitude of routes contributing to the contamination and colonization of patients and personnel in the daily activities of health care. Obviously, control measures must be directed toward the prevention of contamination, colonization, and the accumulation of microorganisms capable of causing infection.

It is universally accepted that every person must be considered to harbor potentially pathogenic (disease-producing) organisms. Health care personnel must acquire a basic understanding of the role of normal flora, their own and that of the patient, as a potential source of infection. Although healthy individuals harbor heavily concentrated areas of bacteria considered as normal, nonpathogenic flora, these same organisms under changed conditions can be reclassified as opportunistic pathogens capable of causing infection within the host or when transferred from the host to a susceptible individual. If the patient's resistance or natural immunity is

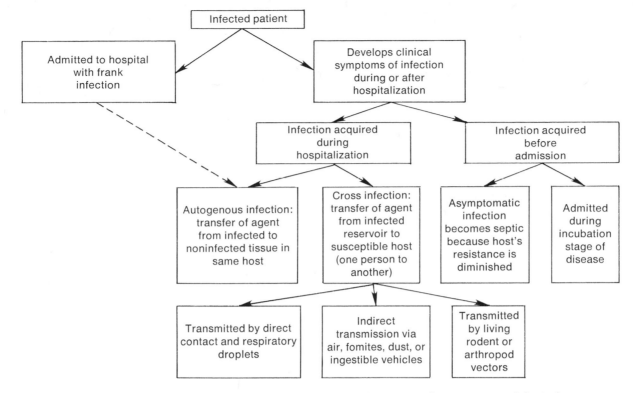

**Fig. 26-1.** Classification of hospital infection situations according to source. Adapted, with permission, from *Hospital, Journal of the American Hospital Association,* Vol. 44, no. 3, February 1, 1970, p. 126.

compromised in some way, the balance may be upset, resulting in autogenous infection. It is not known just what factors prevent resident bacteria (normal flora) from multiplying uncontrollably on the skin, in mucous membranes, or in the gastrointestinal, respiratory, and the genitourinary tracts and tissues in healthy individuals, although certainly immunologic factors and the coexistence of the bacterial agents themselves play a key role.

Development of infection evolves around three major factors:

1. Inoculum size (number of organisms encountered during exposure)
2. Virulence (ability of the organisms to initiate and maintain infection in the host)
3. Susceptibility of the host (patient's ability to respond to the invading organisms)

This interrelationship is most commonly represented by the following equation:

$$\frac{\text{No. of organisms} \times \text{Virulence}}{\text{Degree of susceptibility}} = \text{Infection}$$

The degree of susceptibility of infection will vary with respect to not only the inoculum size and virulence, but also with local and systemic resistance

factors, age, and general health condition. Orthopedic surgical patients are particularly vulnerable to infection since the body's main barriers to infection (skin, respiratory and urinary tracts, and circulatory system) are invaded by foreign bodies such as instruments, catheters, drains, and prosthetic implants. The following is an oversimplified version of the full progression from contamination to infection. The progression may be from any one point, not necessarily occurring in the order shown here:

1. Contamination (existence)
2. Transient colonization (residence)
3. Persistent colonization (residence)
4. Invasion (localized involvement)
5. Dissemination (widespread involvement)

Normal skin generally accepts a transient rather than persistent colonization for several days after contamination. Perineal and nasal areas are more likely to consistently harbor potential pathogens. The spread of such normal flora organisms is primarily by direct contact, thus placing emphasis on good hygiene and handwashing for all personnel before, during, and after patient care.

It is clear then that the source of infection in the institutionalized patient may stem from the patient's own resident bacteria or organisms transmitted to him, acquired either in the community or health care facility environment. Fig. 26-1 depicts the various sources of infections for the hospitalized patient.

The following discussions of prevention, detection, and control are intended as a guide to further reading and, most important, to encourage the reader to scrutinize the policies, procedures, practices, and quality of in-service education within the health care institution.

## PREVENTION OF INFECTION

Many infections acquired by the hospitalized orthopedic patient may be related to specific lapses in technique during daily care, surgical procedures, environmental control, etc. Awareness of factors predisposing to infection can greatly reduce the incidence of these "preventables." It must be noted, however, that in the majority of patients who develop infection there is no clear evidence of cross contamination, leaving only speculation as to the endogenous (from within) or exogenous (from without) origin of the infection.

### Hygiene

The rationale for good hygienic practices for patient and personnel is simply to reduce the number of microorganisms and the chances of infection. The accumulation of organic material provides an excellent breeding ground for the growth of many organisms present on the body. Many routine procedures such as perineal care, tracheotomy site care, skin preps, catheter insertion site care, and even patient bathing are a means of preventing the build-up of potential pathogens. Good personal hygiene on the part of all health care personnel protects the staff and the patient from unnecessary contamination. Continual attention to cleanliness of fingernails, hair, and uniforms, and the avoidance of habits such as hand-to-face contact are pertinent examples.

### Handwashing

Handwashing is recognized as the single most effective means of preventing cross-contamination among patients and personnel, and, unfortunately, it is one of the most neglected patient care practices. Emphasis should be placed on the availability of facilities and the thoroughness of routine handwashing. Degerming is accomplished primarily through mechanical action and through thorough rinsing, the "killing power" of the soap used being secondary. Personnel must be willing to note and

correct infractions of handwashing practices if the first step in controlling infection is to be taken.

### Hydrotherapy

Hydrotherapy is an area of major concern in infection control as well as an important adjunct to orthopedic care. Physical therapy departments must enforce rigid tank cleaning procedures between patient treatments and at the end of the day. Use of disposable plastic liners for the smaller tanks and bathtubs enhances control of cross-contamination between patients and reduces the time-consuming task of tub and tank cleaning between patients. Patients with open lesions, draining wounds, or clean granulating tissue are prime candidates for the lined tank or tub but should be restricted from the large pool. Liners *do not* alleviate the need for tank agitator cleaning/disinfection between patients. Both patient unit and physical therapy personnel carry a responsibility for communication of patient infection status and the knowledge of infection control measures in both areas.

### Most prevalent sites of acquired infections

Urinary tract infections, bacterial pneumonias, bacteremias, and wound infections constitute the majority of acquired infections on most surgical services. Their prevention and treatment involve many theories, principles, practices, and techniques too complex and often controversial to be dealt with here. Major areas of concern for the prevention of these infections are reviewed in Table 26-1.

How ironic that the more susceptible the patient, the more likely the need for therapeutic measures noted for their potential to contaminate. All direct care personnel (physician, nurse, assistant, therapist, and technician) carry a significant responsibility for the prevention of infection through their knowledge of the pathophysiologic systems, their techniques, and their understanding of the modes of spread and containment of infection. All disciplines must identify their responsibilities for the prevention of infection and strictly adhere to accepted policies.

### Postoperative wound management

Measures for the prevention of infection in the surgical wound must begin in the preoperative stage and continue until the wound is sealed and well granulated. Although clean surgical wounds are primarily referred to here, spontaneous infection requiring surgical intervention and the dirty wound associated with trauma must receive equal attention for the prevention of contamination. At no time

**Table 26-1.** Key preventive measures to lessen incidence of acquired infections

| Type of infection | Preventive measures |
|---|---|
| Urinary tract | *Routine*<br>Adequate fluid intake; avoid bladder distention; avoid unnecessary catheterization<br>*Closed drainage catheterization*<br>Strict adherence to asepsis during catheter insertion; routine perineal hygiene and meatal cleansing; proper taping of catheter; maintain collection bag below bladder level at all times; handwashing before and after handling catheter systems; portal aspiration for fresh specimen collection |
| Respiratory tract | *Preoperatively*<br>Patient instruction for postoperative breathing techniques<br>*Postoperatively and for immobilized patient*<br>Vigorous pulmonary regimen to avoid fluid accumulation: (1) cough, (2) deep breathing, (3) positioning (also for prevention of aspiration), (4) activity<br>*Suctioning*<br>Aseptic technique with sterile catheter and irrigating fluid; avoid traumatizing mucosa<br>*Equipment*<br>Respiratory therapy and anesthesia equipment includes nebulization, humidification, IPPB, and mechanical ventilating equipment<br>In-use maintenance: Sterility of solutions, medications, and equipment for aerosolization; reservoirs emptied completely, rinsed, and refilled with sterile solution; breathing circuit changed every 24 hours; individual circuit restrictions for individual patient<br>Processing: Thorough removal of particulate matter prior to final cleaning; selective use of disinfection and sterilization agents for nondisposables; thorough rinsing or aeration |
| Surgical wounds | *Preoperative*<br>Avoid unnecessary patient colonization through short preoperative hospitalization; initial skin preparation; mechanical and antiseptic<br>*Operative*<br>Final skin antisepsis and draping; adequate overall environmental cleanliness and disinfection of suite between cases and terminally preventive maintenance (includes air-handling system)<br>Surgical team: Restriction of personnel with active infection unless under proper treatment; acceptable hygienic practices; proper hand scrub practices and attire, including glove and mask changes as needed; traffic control. Maintain sterility of irrigation fluids and equipment<br>Basic preventive operative measures: Gentle tissue handling; careful suturing; evacuation of hematomas; preservation of blood supply; elimination of dead space; provision for drainage when indicated; thorough removal of necrotic tissue |

*Continued.*

**Table 26-1.** Key preventive measures to lessen incidence of acquired infections—cont'd

| Type of infection | Preventive measures |
| --- | --- |
|  | *Postoperative*<br>Close observation for indications of complications; aseptic technique for wound care; assure sterility of any irrigating solutions and equipment; defined responsibility for wound management |
| Other wounds: Includes infections from percutaneous puncture for diagnostic and therapeutic purposes (i.e., medication injection and fluid aspiration) | Eliminate possibility of contaminated medications, syringes, and needles; provide adequate skin antisepsis before injection |
| Primary bacteremia: Includes any category of organism introduced via *intravenous or intra-arterial vascular system as a result of diagnostic or therapeutic measures* | *Maintain sterility of solutions and medications being infused*<br>1. Use strict aseptic techniques for reconstitutions of medications, dyes, anesthetics, etc., by trained personnel<br>2. Use single dose units<br>3. Discard solutions if opened and not used<br>4. Scrutinize all fluids for possible contamination before use<br>*Maintain sterility of delivery system*<br>1. Avoid contamination of the system from hands, improper handling of tubing, etc.<br>2. Restrict use of stopcocks and CVP manometers; restrict use of catheter/needle hubs for obtaining blood specimens.<br>3. Regulate changing of solution containers and delivery of tubing.<br>4. Use proper skin antisepsis and disinfection of injection ports.<br>*Maintain percutaneous insertion sites (areas considered an open wound with foreign body)*<br>1. Skin preparation preceding a traumatic insertion.<br>2. Securely anchor needle/catheter hub; cover insertion site with light dressing<br>3. Inspect and redress insertion site a minimum of every 2 days<br>4. Avoid prolonged cannulation |

should the assumption be made that techniques can be relaxed if infection is already well established. Strict aseptic techniques must be employed to prevent additional contamination, which may be of a more virulent strain.

Bacterial contamination can occur during the time that the wound is open until postoperatively when a protective fibrin seal has formed between the approximated wound edges. This fibrin crust provides an isolation barrier to the wound below unless (1) moisture softens the seal allowing bacterial migration from the wound surface into the wound, (2) organisms have been trapped under or within the seal, or (3) the crust is mechanically re-moved. The type of wound and the adequacy of the healing process will dictate the operative wound care. The routine postoperative wound care period is critical to the prevention of infection until a proper seal is formed with good healing process below. Aseptic techniques should be observed when changing wound dressings, administering pin care, irrigating the wound, packing, or removing sutures until the wound is well approximate and sealed. Handwashing is essential before and after dressing changes; gloves and mask should be worn throughout the procedure. Soiled dressings should be placed in a plastic or wax-lined bag before discarding to prevent contact or airborn transmission of

**Table 26-2.** Dressing techniques

| Procedure | Special | Standard |
|---|---|---|
| Handwashing, before | Necessary | Necessary |
| Gloves (2 sets) | Necessary | Not necessary |
|    Change between removal of soiled dressing and application of new dressing | | |
| Gown | Necessary | Not necessary |
|    Need not be sterile, unless advisable to prevent cross-infection of extensive burns or wounds | | |
| Mask | Necessary | Not necessary |
| Sterile equipment | Necessary | Necessary |
| Double-bag technique for soiled dressings and equipment | Necessary | Necessary |
| No-touch technique | Necessary | Necessary |
| Handwashing, terminal | Necessary | Necessary |

Adapted from Center for Disease Control, Public Health Service: Pub. No. 76-8314, Washington, D.C., 1975, U.S. Government Printing Office.

any organism present. The dressing itself must provide adequate protection and absorption to prevent skin breakdown.

Dressing technique should be outlined for both the routine and infected wound. A more rigid protocol (as shown in Table 26-2) should be used for all extensive wound infections.

Delegation of responsibility for wound management is critical to quality patient care, regardless of the method preferred by the individual surgeon. An example is given below:

1. The first dressing change should be the responsibility of the physician. If there is excessive drainage, the dressing should be reinforced and the physician immediately notified.
2. Interval dressing changes should be done or ordered by the physician.
3. Agreement should be reached as to any skin prep for each dressing change.
4. The physician should be notified of any changes in the condition of the wound; all observations should be charted.
5. The physician should be responsible for ordering specific wound care irrigations, packing etc.
6. The incision should be examined by the physician before the patient is dismissed from the hospital.

## DETECTION OF INFECTION

Early detection of an infectious process can, in many cases, prevent extensive health impairments, lengthy hospitalization, financial drain, and even death. Assessment for developing infection must be an ongoing process of anticipation, recognition, communication, and prompt action if indicated.

*Anticipation* of an infectious process can often minimize the impact, and postpone or prevent its development. Personnel must recognize potential sites of infection, the patient's propensity to infection, and be familiar with the organisms (normal flora) most likely to be involved. This will be accomplished if *all* personnel:

1. Understand the pathophysiology of the primary disease process
2. Are aware of deficiencies in the patient's local and systemic defense mechanisms:
   a. Impaired immunologic and physiologic mechanisms
   b. Drug therapy regimen (antibiotic, steroid, chemotherapy)
   c. Procedures instituted (assistive ventilatory measures, X-ray therapy, instrumentation such as bladder catheterization and venous cannulation)
3. Know the patient's history
   a. Previous bouts of infection
   b. Recent surgical procedures and instrumentation
   c. Recent drug therapies

Personnel should *recognize* and be suspicious of any change in the clinical course, such as:

1. General malaise
2. Temperature elevation pattern; chills
3. Tachycardia
4. Hyperventilation
5. Elevated blood pressure
6. Localized pain
7. Erythema, warmth, and swelling
8. Serous or purulent exudates
9. Tenacious, foul-smelling sputum
10. Cough, pleuritic chest pain
11. Costavertebral tenderness (flank pain)

Any rise in body temperature, sudden spike, persistent low grade, or intermittent fever may indicate an underlying infection and should be thoroughly investigated. The infection process responsible for the febrile reaction may or may not be clinically apparent, thus making the fever pattern itself an important diagnostic tool. Bacteriologic cultures of suspect areas should be done to rule out or identify pathogenic organisms.

Verbal and written *communication of observations* should be initiated when there is the slightest indication of developing infection. Observations should be relayed both on the medical chart and among health team members (such as during shift reporting and patient rounds). Descriptive terminology may be important to early detection or used as a comparative basis later in the clinical course. For example, notation of pain should be identified further as localized, diffuse, sharp, dull, burning, etc. urine and sputum defined by consistency, color, odor; wounds by appearance, type, amount and odor of drainage.

### Culturing for microorganisms

Microbiologic culturing is a frequent adjunct to the diagnosis and treatment of infection, but meaningful results depend on proper collection, transportation, processing, and interpretation. Indications for patient culturing include the following:

1. To identify unknown or suspect organisms as causative agents of suspected or confirmed disease process
2. To establish appropriate antibiotic therapy through antimicrobial sensitivity testing
3. To document existing organisms for future reference, such as culturing new patients who are suspected of harboring highly resistant organisms capable of causing further infection in that patient and spreading to other patients and personnel

If adequate attention is not given to proper specimen collection techniques, insufficient or misleading information may result in an erroneous etiologic diagnosis and misdirected antimicrobial therapy. Likewise, delays in transport and processing of specimens may lead to unwanted multiplication or death of organisms present. A few general rules apply to all specimens being collected and transported for culture.

1. The culture results are only as good as the technique employed in the collection.
2. Appropriate clinical information must accompany the specimen to facilitate proper laboratory processing. For example, notations should be made as to whether the patient is on antibiotics and if so, what type; urine should be labeled as either clean catch or catheterized; the type and location of wounds should be noted.
3. Care must be taken to avoid contamination of the specimen by using only sterile equipment and aseptic technique.
4. Specimens must represent the infectious process itself, not surrounding flora: (a) Choose the material most likely to reflect the disease process. (b) Avoid contamination with patient's own normal flora.
5. Specimens should be obtained *before* antimicrobial therapy has been initiated when possible to avoid the suppression or destruction of pathogens.
6. Appropriate specimen containers should be used for the collection and transportation of specimens to maintain viability of pathogens and to avoid contamination.
7. All specimens should be transported to the laboratory promptly.

The physician should be responsible for ordering or collecting wound cultures in the following instances:

1. All new admissions with drainage from surgical wound sites, unless recently documented by a laboratory from a referring facility.
2. All patients with new drainage from wound sites, particularly those patients who are to be discharged when there is question of developing irritation.
3. When there is change in the amount, consistency, or odor of the drainage.

Selected references at the end of this chapter offer the reader detailed information on specimen collection, transportation, processing, and interpretation of multiple anatomic sites and physiologic systems.

### Wound specimen collection and interpretation of results

Pertinent information can be readily derived from the microscopic examination of a gram stain in conjunction with the culture results or by itself. Significant information gleaned from the gram stain includes the type of organism (gram negative rods, gram positive cocci, etc.) and the quality of the specimen, such as the presence of many polymorphonuclear cells indicating an active inflammatory process.

Wound culturing will be briefly discussed below primarily because all too often the literature assumes this as a responsibility of the experienced surgeon when, unfortunately, this important procedure often is delegated or left to personnel who may lack proper training in specimen collection.

**Specimen collection at wound site.** Specimen collection may be accomplished by various methods which, in order of preference (yield or meaningful results), include: (1) tissue biopsy, (2) needle aspiration, and (3) swabbing. The method employed must be chosen according to the clinical condition of the wound (deep or superficial, purulent or nonpurulent) and the organisms being sought (e.g., aerobic, anaerobic, fungi). Although the use of sterile swabs is usually the most rapid and practical method, it is frequently limited in its representation of the organisms present because of the inherent risk of swab contamination with organisms in the immediate surrounding area. With all methods, an effort must be made to avoid unnecessary contamination when approaching the specific site to be cultured. The wound site should be initially cleaned (wiped) with sterile gauze to remove superficial drainage accumulation which may contain numerous contaminating organisms from the patient's skin, saturated dressings, and the environment. The most active area of inflammation, usually the advancing border, should be the site of aspiration or swabbing rather than the central "pooling" area of purulent material, which will likely contain excessive debris. A sterile swab (two swabs should be made and submitted to the laboratory) should be pressed and rotated against the selected site for extraction of tissue fluid or drainage. Needle aspiration should be done in a still "sealed off" pocket of fluid in the selected area. A sterile intravenous catheter attached to a syringe may provide a less traumatic approach in deeper wounds where visibility is poor.

When culturing deep tissue where anaerobic and aerobic organisms may be infecting in concert (synergistic action) care must be taken to preserve the air-sensitive anaerobes by immediately transporting the capped aspirating syringe or swab (in sterile tube) to the laboratory. Preferably, a culture caddy with pre-reduced holding media for swabs or "gassed out" vials for aspirated fluid should be available at the time of collection to provide a more stable environment (increased $CO_2$). Wound culturing should be done *before* local irrigation with antiseptic solutions and preferably before antibiotic therapy is initiated.

**Culture report interpretation.** The interpretation of culture results from all sites and sources requires a working knowledge of microorganisms and their interrelationship with the patient. Organisms recovered from a clinical specimen may be representative of contamination, normal, or transient flora of the patient as well as the culprit pathogens in the area. Consideration must, therefore, be given to the effects of the variable host factors, underlying disease process, and any therapeutic measures affecting the selection or depression of specific organisms. Findings suggestive of the presence of infection often include the presence of many polymorphonuclear leukocytes on smear (usually reported as "many polys") and large numbers of organisms seen on smear or culture showing predominance of a single type. An absence of these "markers" may be indicative of a noninvasive colonization contamination resulting from a poorly collected specimen or sterility of the culture site. Personnel must guard against reacting to the names of reported organisms and instead evaluate their significance from that specific site.

Culture results may represent simple colonization, local invasion, or a generalized invasion leading to systemic involvement. Bacterial growth in a wound, therefore, must be interpreted with caution since the clinical state of the wound most often provides the criterion for therapy modification. Tissue changes will reflect invasion on a localized or deep level as opposed to heavy colonization of the surface wound.

## CONTROL OF INFECTION

The control of existing infections may be accomplished through the judicious use of isolation or precautionary measures. Personnel of all disciplines must realize, however, that the *undiagnosed* infectious process can be a greater hazard. Colonization of patients or personnel may occur without apparent infection, and infectious diseases are not always identified as being "communicable." Handwashing, uncompromised aseptic techniques, and thorough environmental sanitation procedures are a must in any case.

### Determining need for isolation or precautionary measures

The individual patient's situation must be of primary concern when considering the need for isolation or precautionary measures and selecting the appropriate category.

The patient's situation should be assessed for the following variable factors:

1. Microbiology and epidemiology of the infectious process
2. Extent of the disease process

3. Extent of direct patient care required (by nursing staff and other department personnel)
4. Effective treatment in progress
5. Staffing and facilities available (nursing staff assignments)
6. Types of patients on unit (degrees of susceptibility)
7. Patient's physiologic needs

Any patient on isolation/precaution measures must be periodically assessed with consideration to the above factors. A change in any one factor may create a need for modification of the type of measures employed. This flexibility is the key to achieving maximal patient care and adequate containment of the infectious process with limited restriction to patient and staff.

When an infectious disease process requiring isolation is suspected, appropriate isolation precautions must be instituted until diagnosis is confirmed or ruled out.

## RESPONSIBILITY AND AUTHORITY

The *attending physician* should be responsible for promptly ordering the appropriate category of isolation/precaution when an infectious process deemed transmittable is suspected or diagnosis confirmed.

The *nurse* in charge should be responsible for ensuring that isolation measures are initiated and maintained and for informing and educating the patient and family. Both the patient and family must understand the reasons for such measures. Instruction should include proper handwashing techniques; use of gowns, gloves, and masks when applicable; caring for the patient's personal items; and visiting regulations. Every effort should be made to make the patient feel accepted, not rejected.

The nurse is responsible for initiating appropriate precautionary measures for a patient suspected of having an infectious process if the physician is not available or has not done so. If the attending physician does not order appropriate isolation measures, the nurse in charge should seek consultation on this matter from infection control personnel. The attending physician should be notified as soon as possible if isolation measures are instituted by someone other than himself or physicians attending that patient.

*Infection control personnel* should be available for consultation to all patient care departments regarding specific problems in the initiation and interpretation of isolation procedures and the epidemiology of infecting organisms.

*All hospital personnel* must assume a personal sense of responsibility in complying with isolation procedures and for tactfully calling observed infractions to the attention of offenders. Any major or consistent minor infractions should be reported to infection control personnel.

Once the type of isolation to be employed has been decided upon, discussion of the patient situation and measures to be carried out should be held during each shift report, with special staff conferences, if necessary. Consistency in interpretation of the patient's disease process and in approach to patient care is vital to the effectiveness of the measures. Guidelines for the following sections should be available, explained, and enforced:

1. Responsibility and authority.
2. Determining the need for isolation/precaution measures
   a. Patient assessment
   b. Suspected infectious process
3. Recommended measures for each isolation/precaution category (strict, protective, respiratory, full wound, modified wound, enteric, excretion, blood, and secretion)
4. Isolation facilities
5. Isolation cart and supplies
6. Handwashing
7. Double-bagging method
8. Use of gowns, mask, gloves
9. Initiation of isolation/precaution measures
10. Departmental responsibilities
    a. Disposal of trash
    b. Disposal of linens
    c. Removing equipment and supplies
    d. Cleaning the isolation room (daily and terminal)
    e. Food service for patients on isolation
    f. Portable X-ray equipment
    g. Portable diagnostic equipment (ECG, EEG)
    h. Collecting laboratory specimens
    i. Death
    j. Visiting regulations
    k. Transporting the isolation patient
11. Termination of isolation/precautions (discharge, transfer, discontinuation)
12. Additional guidelines tailored for special care areas such as operating room, recovery room, diagnostic and procedure areas, and physical therapy.

## INFECTION SURVEILLANCE AND INVESTIGATION

A system for routine and special monitoring of infections of all types must be established for the orthopedic service if there is to be continuity of infection control within the patient care unit and throughout the entire patient care facility. Although "preventable" infections may first be noted or diagnosed on the patient care unit, their occurrence may reflect infection control problems in other areas such as in the operating room, physical therapy, or special procedure area.

Although infection incidence data collection, analysis and investigative measures for all services are the designated responsibility of the infection committee and surveillance personnel, the orthopedic health care team members have an inherent responsibility for early detection, and reporting of infection in addition to providing quality patient care. The orthopedic team should be aware of and concerned with the incidence and type of infection on their service and the microorganisms responsible for each type of infection. This baseline data should be available through the infection surveillance personnel and reviewed with them to assure proper interpretation.

An active monitoring program for potential and existing infection problems requires full cooperation and communication between surveillance and orthopedic team personnel. The routine collection of data and related observations will provide for rapid identification of any developing or existing infection control problems. Once it has been established that "preventable" infections are occurring, the degree of cooperation from all departments and personnel involved will determine the expediency and effectiveness of investigative and corrective measures to be taken. All disciplines involved must be willing to collaborate in a review of their practices and procedures pertaining to the area of concern. Cultures of the environment, patients, and personnel may provide pertinent investigative data but should be done under the direction or supervision of trained surveillance personnel.

## SUMMARY

The goals of an infection control program for the orthopedic service should be the same as those for the entire health care facility: *to promote a preventive and corrective program designed to minimize infection hazards and to provide for the detection of potential and existing infection problems.* Structured continuing education and supervision of personnel involved with the orthopedic service (including all associated disciplines) are critical to the coordination of infection control as it relates to daily patient care activities. Personnel at all levels must be able to acknowledge that potential infection problems exist and should be encouraged to participate in formulating and enforcing practices of prevention and control.

## BIBLIOGRAPHY

1. American College of Surgeons: Control of infections in surgical patients, Philadelphia, 1976, J. B. Lippincott Co.
2. American Hospital Association: Infection control in the hospital, ed. 3, Chicago, 1974, The Association.
3. Artz, C. P.: Infections in surgery. In Artz, C. P., and Hardy, J. D., editors: Management of surgical complications, ed. 3, Philadelphia, 1975, W. B. Saunders Co.
4. Bartlett, R. C.: Control of hospital-associated infections. In American Society for Microbiology: Manual of clinical microbiology, ed. 2, Washington, D.C., 1974, The Society.
4a. Bennett, J. V., and Brachman, P. S., editors: Hospital infections, Boston, 1979, Little, Brown & Co.
5. Center for Disease Control: Isolation techniques for use in hospitals, ed. 2, Pub. No. 76-8314, Washington, D.C., 1975, Public Health Service.
6. Cluff, L. F., and Johnson, J. E.: Clinical concepts of infectious diseases, Baltimore, 1972, The Williams and Wilkins Co.
7. Gardner, P, and Provine, H. H.: Manual of acute bacterial infections—early diagnosis and treatment, Boston, 1975, Little, Brown and Co.
8. Hampton, O. P.: Complications of common fractures. In Artz, C. P. and Hardy, J. D., editors: Management of surgical complications, ed. 3, Philadelphia, 1975, W. B. Saunders Co.
9. Polk, H. C., and Stone, H. H., editors: Hospital acquired infections in surgery, Baltimore, 1977, University Park Press.
10. Hunt, T. K.: Wound complications. In Management of surgical complications.
11. Isenberg, H. D., and Painter, B. G.: Indigenous and pathogenic microorganisms of man. In American Society for Microbiology: Manual of clinical microbiology ed. 2, Washington, D.C., 1974, The Society.
12. Stevens, J.: Infections of bones and joints. In Meltzer, W., editor: Orthopedics, New York, 1976, Harper and Row, Inc.

# 27

# Pain: evaluation and intervention

KATHLEEN G. WALLACE

Pain is the most common reason a person seeks medical care.[7,p.508] Health care personnel must deal almost daily with patients in pain. The pain caused by orthopedic conditions and interventions is among the most difficult to manage.

Variations in pain are quite large, from chronic pain of rheumatoid arthritis to acute postoperative pain from spinal fusion or total joint replacement. In the postoperative period the clinician must consider pain originating from cutaneous and visceral origins, as well as pain originating from the periosteum or joint capsule. When dealing with a patient with chronic pain, the clinician must be cognizant not only of the physical problems causing the pain but also the behavioral problems that often occur.

Knowing the origin of pain is not enough in any setting. The clinician must be skilled in many pain relief measures. Bochank[15,p.337] found that the method most found frequently used by nurses to relieve pain was administration of narcotics. It is

this narrow view of pain relief held by many caregivers that can lead to overuse or underuse of drugs. Health care professionals are taught the antithesis of this action in their formal education, yet something changes their behaviors when they are in a practice situation. The goal of this chapter is to acquaint the reader with information relative to pain that will increase understanding and thereby improve the care of the orthopedic patient in pain.

In this chapter pain is considered as both a physiologic and psychologic phenomenon. I feel it is better to have one malingerer go unnoticed than to have patients suffer needlessly. Emphasis is placed on the ability of nursing professionals to understand, assess, and evaluate pain, although we recognize that an understanding of pain is necessary for all health care professionals.

## DEFINITION OF PAIN

Defining pain is somewhat difficult. Pain has been described as the perception of noxious stimuli or the distressing sensations that result from tissue damage. Perhaps the most useful definition is that suggested by Margo McCaffery: Pain is "whatever the experiencing person says it is and exists whenever he says it does."[16,p.29] This definition relieves the health professional of "proving" that pain exists and it uses the patient's understanding and complaints as a beginning point for treatment.

Health professionals seem to have problems dealing with the patient who is suffering with pain and has no discovered physiologic reason for it. These patients quickly become labeled as "malingerers," "crocks," and untreatables. The answer to these patients' problems is usually to send them to a psychiatrist. Every health professional should keep in mind that our diagnostic armamentarium is not so exact that physical pathology cannot be missed with myelography or venography. It is a rare patient who does not have a psychogenic overlay to the physical experience of pain. This leaves the professional with a two-fold responsibility to work with both the psyche and soma as one to relieve suffering.

## ANATOMY AND PHYSIOLOGY OF PAIN
### Pain theories

**Specificity theory.** Probably the most easily understood and often quoted theory of pain is the *specificity theory* developed by Von Frey in the late 1800s.[23,pp.11-13] This theory suggests that pain is picked up in the periphery and sent to the spinal column through the dorsal horn and is transmitted via the anterolateral spinothalamic tracts to the thalamus. Von Frey's theory has been criticized because it proposes that certain stimuli are picked up only by certain nerve endings (for example, pain is transmitted only by nerve fibers designated for pain; cold is transmitted only by fibers for cold). This theory has also been criticized because it does not allow for perception of pain on the cortical level. As we now know pain perception is not merely limited to thalamic and dorsal column input, but these stimuli *plus* the individual's past and present experiences, emotional situation, motivations, and drives. Another criticism of the Von Frey theory is that he was not accurate when he placed all skin sensations into the four categories of warm, cold, touch, and pain.[23,pp.11-14]

**Substances thought to control and cause pain.** The actual cause of pain at the peripheral level is poorly understood. It is thought that bradykinin and histamine may be two of the substances that can cause pain.[8,p.579] Bradykinin is a polypeptide that is split off from globulin when cells are damaged. Histamine is a substance released by mast cells when damage occurs to the lining of blood vessels. Along with substances that cause pain, naturally occurring analgesics have been discovered.

Substances called enkephalins (two derivatives are methionine and leucine) have been identified as pentapeptides similar in action to morphine but in some experiments ten times as potent.[12,p.459] Endorphins have also been isolated from the pituitary gland of animals, and researchers have demonstrated that there are three different derivatives of this morphometic substance.[3,pp.630-632] Alpha, beta, and gamma endorphins have been identified; beta endorphin seems to be the strongest in terms of morphomimetic properties. One can only speculate what this particular discovery will mean. Will pain relief be afforded in humans by merely triggering

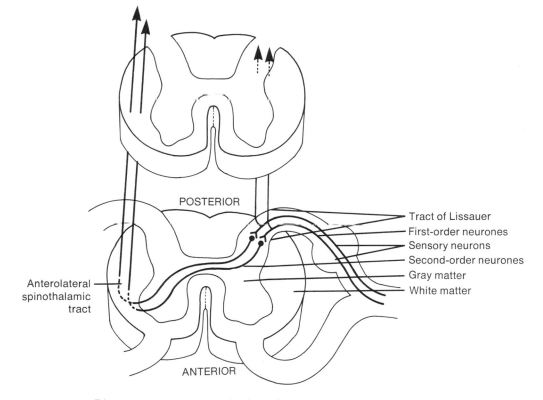

**Fig. 27-1.** Diagram of basic organization of spinal cord. Sensory nerves transmit their impulses initially through dorsal column, then synapse and cross over to anterolateral tract and ascend spinal column to thalamus, reticular formation, and cortex.

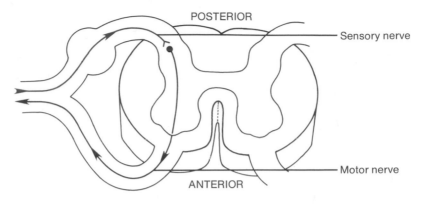

POSTERIOR

Sensory nerve

ANTERIOR

Motor nerve

**Fig. 27-2.** Diagram of reflex arc, which allows individual to react quickly to noxious stimuli.

the pituitary to send out its own opiate for pain relief?

Once histamine or other substances are released, the sensation of pain travels to two types of fibers: fast-conducting, small, delta, type A fibers and slow-conducting type C fibers. These fibers then transmit pain to the dorsal root ganglion. These nerve fibers then ascend or descend one to three segments in the tract of Lissauer (Fig. 27-1).

At varying points the fibers synapse with second-order neurons in the posterior horns of the gray matter. The second-order neurons then form the anterolateral spinothalamic tract and ascend to the reticular formation and the thalamus. At the thalamus nerves synapse again and form third-order neurons and these disperse to various areas of the brain, such as the cortex and hypothalamus.

Pressure and touch fibers end at the same area of the thalamus that pain fibers do and one wonders if this in itself is not an important mechanism for understanding how nonnoxious stimuli, such as touch, can induce intense pain in certain unexplained syndromes, such as causalgia.

**Reflex arc.** Involved in our reactions to pain is an immediate reaction to the stimulus itself. The immediate reaction is carried over the reflex arc (Fig 27-2). Sensory nerve fibers enter the dorsal horn of the spinal column and synapse with motor neurons in the anterior horn. This anatomic arrangement allows the individual to move quickly on the touch of some noxious stimulus. Together with the reflex arc, the messages to move away from noxious stimuli are sent via efferent fibers from the brain.

**Emotional component of pain.** One of the problems with all of the classical anatomic considerations of pain is that the emotional component is not considered. The classic study by Beecher[1,pp.1609-1613] with wounded soldiers during World War II brings to light the importance of this emotional component. Dr. Beecher, an anesthesiologist, was serving in the Army in Italy during World War II and noted that only one out of three of the wounded soldiers wanted morphine for pain relief. In contrast, patients at Massachusetts General Hospital, many of whom had the same type of surgery as the soldiers, did not obtain relief of their pain with even large doses of morphine. What was the difference Beecher was seeing in these patients? The soldiers realized that they would not have to return to the battlefield and therefore were euphoric. The patients in the hospital, however, viewed their injuries as catastrophic. Beecher concluded that it was this difference in *perception* that brought about the difference in the need for pain relieving drugs.

**Gate control theory.** Melzack and Wall have proposed the gate control theory of pain[23,pp.11-37] and have introduced the idea that pain travels by small afferent excitatory fibers from the periphery of the body to the spinal cord. Cells in the spinal cord, called the *substantia gelatinosa* (Fig. 27-3), receive this impulse. The substantia gelatinosa is located in the dorsal horn (gray matter) and traverses the entire length of the spinal cord. The substantia gelatinosa contains a physiologic gate that can prevent or allow transmission of information to the anterolateral spinothalamic tract.

This gate can be triggered to operate by another nerve fiber from the periphery called the large-diameter, cutaneous, afferent nerve fiber. This large-diameter fiber can cause the gate to close and override the impulses from the small nerve fiber. Some of the impulses carried by the large-diameter fibers

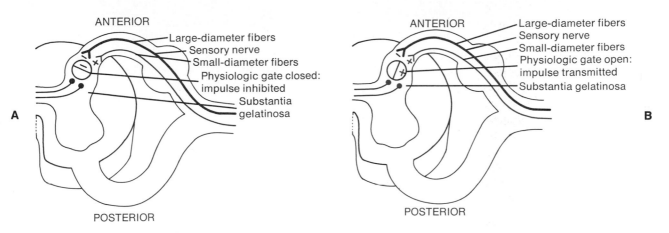

**Fig. 27-3.** Physiologic gate. **A,** Pain impulse blocked by closed gate. **B,** Pain impulse transmitted through open gate. Sensation is then transmitted to second-order neurons.

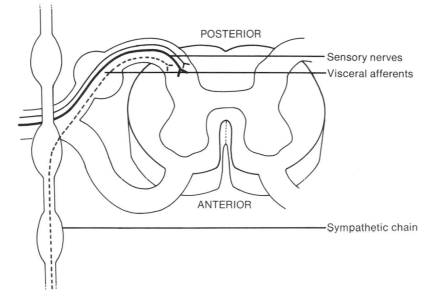

**Fig. 27-4.** Diagram demonstrating a theory of referred pain in which visceral and sensory afferents have some type of "interaction," which allows transmission of impulse back through sensory fiber to cause pattern of "referred" pain.

are those triggered by rubbing or scratching the painful area. It is theorized that the large afferent nerves carry a positive charge and the small nerves carry a negative charge; positive charges "close" the gate and negative charges "open" the gate.

This theory deals with other methods of inhibition and transmission as well. Melzack and Wall believe that the gate can be opened or closed by *descending* information from the cortex. In other words, past experiences, drives, and motivations allow the gate to open or close.[23,pp.11-37] This theory would explain what Beecher could not explain—

how do an individual's feelings influence the perception of pain.

**Pattern theories.** Pattern theories are also important to understanding pain. Many researchers have discovered and written about various patterns of pain. For example, mild or moderate pain can be decreased or eliminated by vibration whereas severe pain will be increased by vibratory movements (rubbing).[22,p.110] In causalgic pain a mere touch may elicit severe pain, although vigorous massage is not painful.

Nordenboos notes that pain intensity increases

when the area of pain enlarges. The reverse can be true, as well. A small area can be triggered and it becomes stinging and painful; however, when the whole area is subjected to a certain temperature, there is no pain.[22,pp.111,112]

Goldscheider's pattern or summation theory proposes that the particular patterns of nerve impulses that evoke pain are produced by the summation of skin sensory input at the dorsal horn cells. Summation occurs in two cases: when the total output of stimuli reaches a critical level and when there is a pathologic state, there is an increase in the number of impulses.[22,p.140]

Weddell and Sinclair theorize that alterations in firing patterns of nerves distinguish what pain is transmitted.[22,p.140] The nerves that conduct pain are alike, but their firing patterns and the area of skin tissue covered will make a difference in the pain transmitted.

Livingston's theory adds much to the understanding of phantom limb pain.[21,p.63-68,22,p.142] He claims that the damaged neurons from the amputation set up abnormal impulse reactions in the dorsal horn of the spinal column. These nerves send impulses reverberating in other directions in the dorsal and lateral areas of the spinal tract. The reverberations send messages to adjacent cells and cause autonomic reactions (e.g., sweating, jerking movements). Those reactions increase the pain stimuli and the pattern cycle is then established.

Referred pain (Fig. 27-4) is another phenomenon seen in patients with visceral pain problems. Visceral afferent nerves apparently use the sympathetic fibers to reach the sensory nerve pathway at the dorsal root.[31,pp.54-55] When the pain is transmitted, there is some type of energy interaction that allows transmission of impulse back through the sensory fiber, which causes a strange pattern of pain.

One of the typical tests for referred pain is to press on the "referred" pain site. When this pressure is exerted, the same pattern of pain is evoked as if the visceral defect were touched.

*Application.* Some of the direct applications of these theories are summarized here: All people have the same threshold for pain but people perceive pain differently. Tolerance for pain therefore varies greatly among individuals.

Past experiences, anxiety, and motivations will greatly affect the experience of pain. The gate control theory gives the clinician the theoretical rationale for attempting to reduce anxiety by providing preoperative instruction and counseling in order to influence postoperative pain.

Referred pain is a poorly understood but readily acknowledged pattern. The classic example is seen in patients who have gallbladder problems. Instead of pain in the epigastric area, the patient may complain of right scapular pain.

### Cultural aspects

Pain is not only the most frequent reason someone seeks help but it is also a greatly feared sensation. Some authors state that it is second only to the fear of death. Fear and anxiety can often heighten the pain experience.[20,p.257]

Pain perception is also affected by cultural influences. Zborowski,[33] a well-known sociologist who has studied the cultural component of pain reactions, studied individuals whose parents and grandparents were from Irish, Jewish, Italian, and American descent. He found that patients of Anglo-Saxon and Irish heritage expressed fewer complaints of pain and that patients of Italian and Jewish descent verbalized their pain fully. Anxiety and worry were frequently expressed by Jewish patients. The Old Americans, even though preoccupied with pain, were reluctant to seek relief and delayed seeking medical attention. The Old Americans and Irish withdrew from others when in pain rather than complain.

This study points out the importance of considering the patients' cultural values when assessing pain behavior. Cultural values often clash between caregiver and patient. When health professionals value stoicism and the patient values empathy and much discussion or expression of pain, the problems of pain relief are colored by subjective feelings and values. The health professional must be able to see beyond his or her own feelings and treat the patient objectively.

### ASSESSMENT OF PAIN (Table 27-1)

Probably the first area of assessment the clinician should investigate is: Given a particular set of circumstances, should the patient experience pain? For example, if the patient has head pain following a particular procedure, was it the result of the procedure or lack of food for many hours? Patients can suffer needlessly or have manifestations of complications go unrecognized because of failure to assess this simple point.

Next, assessment of the patient's previous, present, and future perceptions of pain should be investigated. Some have questioned whether this focus on pain will heighten the patient's present pain experience, but this has not been the case.[18,pp.1224-1227] The history of previous pain should also include the

**Table 27-1.** Pain assessment

| Area of assessment | How to assess | Comments |
|---|---|---|
| Expectation of pain | Does area involved contain nerve endings? Do you expect pain with this procedure/illness/problem? | If no expectation of pain, does pain represent a complication? |
| Location and pattern | Nature of disease process: Referred pain? Triggered from another area in body? Where is trigger zone? Pain constant, intermittant, rhythmic? What tissues are damaged? | Does the pain stay localized? Does it occur in different joints (e.g., rheumatoid arthritis; sciatic pain is typically referred down to back of knee)? *Visceral:* patient quiet and withdrawn; pain described as dull, aching; patient holds or splints area affected *Cutaneous:* patient restless; rubs part affected; described as burning, piercing, stinging pain *Periosteum:* behavior variable, often like visceral behavior; pain described as boring, aching, deep |
| Duration | | |
| Acute | Number of hours postop or posttrauma? Exacerbation or disease? Painful diagnostic procedure? | Patient restless; crying out behaviors in the immediate postop period |
| Chronic | Length of painful experience | Often see quiet, withdrawn behavior; depression can be a problem; often manifest controlling behavior in an attempt to control disease; coping behaviors often nondemanding of patient |
| | Type of disease process: usually painful? progressive? slow? fatal? nonfatal? stage? | |
| Intensity | Ask patient to label pain as mild, moderate, severe | In all situations; comfort measures and reduction of fatigue Mild pain: relief measures should include distraction, nonnarcotic analgesics Moderate pain: cognitive dissonance, narcotic and nonnarcotic analgesics Severe pain: waking imagined analgesia; narcotics |

patient's methods of coping with the experience. This information can be utilized in the management of the present pain, if the coping mechanisms are appropriate.

Cultural influences are also important in understanding a patient's reaction to pain. Does the patient's behavior bear out his or her cultural orientation? Does this influence the clinician's response?

The caregiver should also assess the patient's communication of pain. McCaffery[17, pp. 20-22] labels the nonverbal expressions of pain as:

1. Vocalizations, such as moaning and groaning
2. Facial expressions
3. Gestures, such as holding one's side, a clenched fist, or rubbing a painful area

McCaffery[17, pp. 27-44] also describes the important physical data the nurse should collect about the pain experience:

1. Occurrence of pain (not to be confused with other phenomena)
2. Intensity: small or large area of pain, associated tenderness, increase or decrease with movement, pressure, anxiety, worse at certain periods of the day
3. Location: visceral, cutaneous, periosteal, referred, joint capsule
4. Duration: days, hours, months, years
5. Pattern: stinging, burning, pricking, aching, referred; caused by light touch or pressure; rhythmicity of pain; other associated stimuli

such as triggering of parasympathetic or sympathetic nervous system

6. Past experiences: first real experience with pain (often these individuals are frightened); chronic pain (person may remain silent so as not to be rejected)

7. Meaning the pain has for the patient: synonymous with punishment; religious interpretations (the Bible cites many examples of the "good, long-suffering" individual); does the patient think the illness is worse because of pain

## Types of pain

One of the next areas to assess is the nature of the pain the patient is experiencing. Is the pain acute or chronic? Not only will pain relief measures be different but also health care personnel may see a difference in the patient's behavior.

**Acute pain.** Acute pain usually occurs immediately after trauma or surgical intervention. External stimuli (light, noise, distractions) should be at a minimum and fatigue should be avoided in these patients. Health care personnel should awaken the patient only when essential care is given; two or three interventions (treatments, medications, and turning) can perhaps be done at the same time.

Several investigators have found that patients over age 50 need less analgesia than do younger patients.[13,p.257] There are conflicting data concerning gender differences in need for analgesia between males and females.

Acute pain occurring in the first 24 to 48 hours after surgery is often difficult to relieve, and it is a mistake to tell the patient that drugs will totally relieve the pain. It is also false to assume that all patients suffer acute pain after surgery. For example, in one study investigators found that 23% did not require analgesia.[25,p.107] (Unfortunately, this article does not address the problem of bone and joint surgery.) Acute pain in the person with orthopedic problems originates from the periosteum, joint surfaces, and arterial walls. Muscle pain accompanying bone surgery results from muscle ischemia rather than "muscle tension."[14,p.553]

**Chronic pain.** The chronic pain of rheumatoid arthritis or low back pain syndrome has different characteristics from acute pain. It is often of less intensity than acute pain but is of long duration. The person with long-standing pain may be quiet and stoical about the experience and often must endure the pain without benefit of drugs because of the nature of the disease and the fear of addiction. The person with chronic pain may cease to display autonomic signs of pain such as increased pulse and rapid respiration because these reactions cannot be sustained for long periods.[16,p.29]

Another hallmark of persons with chronic pain is their need to control their surroundings. Since many of these individuals cannot control their disease, they seek to control others and their environment. These patients are often labeled "uncooperative" or "manipulative."

Chronic pain can be complicated by multiple treatment modalities. For instance, scarring, continuing psychologic stress, and medication can complicate the pain picture. One author suggests that individuals with chronic pain begin to focus on the pain exclusively. This focus eliminates interaction with friends, family, and any other environmental stimuli so that the individual lives in a world of pain only.[30,pp.130-134]

**Character of pain.** Another area to assess is the character of the pain. Again, this will help determine relief measures and help identify some expected behaviors. McCaffery[17,pp.29-30] describes the person with visceral pain as very quiet, holding himself still, perhaps drawn up in the fetal position. Thus visceral pain seems to have a "depressing" effect on the individual. On the other hand the person experiencing the bright, pricking, stinging pain associated with cutaneous fiber damage may rub the painful areas and seem restless.

**Intensity.** It can be helpful to have the patient describe the pain in terms of degrees—mild, moderate, or severe. Although pain measurement is subjective, it can give the practitioner a clue as to the intervention necessary. It also communicates to the patient that there is concern and treatment for varying levels of discomfort and that there is no need to inflate or pretend pain for treatment or attention.

Mild pain might be best relieved by comfort measures and distraction (television, visitors, crossword puzzles). These measures take very little effort on the part of nurse or patient.

If the patient describes the pain as moderate, drugs as well as comfort measures may be used, and active patient-nurse interaction and distraction techniques will also be needed. One such method is cognitive dissonance in which the nurse asks the patient to reflect on some pleasant experiences, happenings, or events. The patient can describe these experiences out loud and make conversation about them. This takes energy on the part of both parties but can be quite successful.

For patients in severe pain the nurse may try decreasing environmental stimuli and employing comfort measures, purposeful interaction, narcotic analgesics, and "waking imagined analgesia" (WIA).

[17,pp.170-176] McCaffery describes waking imagined analgesia as concentrating on a pleasant "feeling" experience rather than events. The patient describes a pleasant sensation such as lying in the warm sand surrounded by cool ocean water. It may help if the patient discusses this out loud so that the nurse or other professional can encourage the conversation.

**Tolerance.** Tolerance for pain is another factor about which the nurse should be informed. McCaffery states that the person who has undergone many surgeries actually has a decreased tolerance for pain.[17,p.55] The assumption that a person who has undergone a similar surgery previously is better able to tolerate pain may not be valid.

## Other factors influencing pain perception (Table 27-2)

Other factors contributing to an increase or decrease in pain include temperature, fatigue, anxiety, and the presence or absence of external stimuli.

Pain often increases in a cold room because the person tightens his muscles and draws up his legs and arms. However, local application of cold on a swollen joint may decrease swelling and, therefore, pain.

Fatigue is another factor that increases the perception of pain. Coping with pain becomes increasingly difficult as the patient becomes more fatigued. The patient will seek less and less strenuous methods of pain relief as he or she becomes more tired.

Past experiences may increase or decrease the person's perception of pain. For example, if the person was able to effectively cope with pain in the past, those same factors may help in dealing with pain again. If past experiences were negative, however, and the patient lost hope, or became anxious or fearful, they may not help reduce present pain.

Anxiety as a factor in pain perception is frequently discussed in the literature.* Anxiety seems to increase muscle tension and sympathetic activity (heart rate, sweating), which may increase physical suffering as well.

Sensory restriction, according to McCaffery, may increase pain because of a lack of distracting factors.[16,p.29] However, overstimulation may also contribute to increased pain if the patient copes best with acute pain in a quiet environment. Overstimulation may cause fatigue or anxiety, thus increasing the pain experienced.

Religious beliefs may be effective in helping the patient decrease pain or increase tolerance if the

*See refs. 4, pp. 36-14; 15, p. 337; 29, pp. 82, 85.

**Table 27-2.** Factors influencing pain experience

| Factor | Influence on pain |
|---|---|
| Cold | |
| Room temperature below 20 C (68 F) | May increase |
| Local application | May decrease |
| Heat | |
| Room temperature above 27 C (80 F) | Increase or decrease |
| Local application | Decrease |
| Fatigue | Decreases tolerance |
| Past pain experience | |
| Positive | Increases tolerance |
| Negative | Decreases tolerance |
| Anxiety | Increase pain perception; may motivate search for appropriate coping mechanisms |
| Sensory restriction | Increase pain if person cannot cope with additional stimuli; decrease pain for introspective person |
| Increased environmental stimuli | Increases pain if person fatigued; Decreases pain if patient distracted |
| Religious beliefs | |
| Positive connotation to pain | Decrease |
| Negative connotation to pain | Increase |
| Age | Influence unclear; decreased demand for analgesics may occur over age 50 |
| Sex | |
| Male | US culture—taught not to complain or be emotionally demonstrative; often less expression of pain |
| Female | US culture—may demonstrate feelings, cry, moan, etc., without rejection |
| Culture | |
| Old American | Value stoicism and suffering in silence |
| Italian | Verbalize pain freely; likely to share feelings with others |
| Jewish | Verbalize pain freely; anxious about pain |
| Irish | Do not verbalize pain; prefer to be alone when in pain |

pain is seen as necessitating self-discipline or as a cleansing mechanism for past transgressions. Both of these usually have very positive connotations and may well decrease the patient's perceptions of pain. On the other hand, religious beliefs may increase perception of pain if the patient sees this as "punishment" and relates the severity of pain with the seriousness of any transgressions or faults. If the patient begins to feel guilty about past wrongdoings, both anxiety and pain may increase.

## PAIN IN ORTHOPEDIC CONDITIONS
(Table 27-3)

With the basic assessment of pain accomplished, the health professional should investigate other physical factors. The physical conditions discussed here are those most commonly experienced by orthopedic patients.

### Infection

One of the most feared complications of orthopedic injury or surgery is infection. The pain associated with infection is usually described as "hot," throbbing pain. The health professional will recognize the appearance of infection by the redness, heat, swelling, and pain at the site. The pain results from swelling of the involved tissues, as well as the release of toxic substances from the damaged tissues. (see discussion on bradykinin and histamine). Relief measures for localized infection include antibiotic therapy as appropriate, ice to reduce swelling, elevation of the limb, and distraction.

**Osteomyelitis.** Infection may become chronic as in the case of osteomyelitis. Contaminated wounds such as those resulting from compound fractures often lead to osteomyelitis. The pain associated with this type of infection is exceedingly acute. The patient can barely tolerate movement of any kind. Buck's traction (5 lbs) on an injured leg can be of great benefit for the relief of pain. Opiates given at regular intervals and an hour before dressing changes may help somewhat, but for some persons even with medication the pain associated with dressing changes is almost unbearable. During this time it helps some patients to practice cognitive dissonance by concentrating on some pleasant time in the past. Talking aloud to the nurse or doctor during the procedure may help.

Pain in osteomyelitis is from several sources. Deep, boring pain of the periosteum occurs when sequestra leaves the bone and attempts to exit the body. Cutaneous pain occurs from the sequestrum

**Table 27-3.** Typical types of pain seen in orthopedic conditions

| Condition | Causative factors | Pain relief measures |
|---|---|---|
| Infection | | |
| Soft tissue | Bacteria, typically *Staphylococcus, Streptococcus, Pseudomonas;* pain from pressure on nerve endings; swelling; toxic substances | Local application of ice; aspirin; later warm soaks, antibiotics; pain managed by distraction, elevation of limb |
| Bone | Bacteria, typically *Staph; Strep Pseudomonas;* pain from elevation of periosteum when sequestra leaves bone; pain perception increases with multiple surgeries; depression | Traction; cast therapy; opiates; cognitive dissonance; sometimes amputation only method of relief and cure |
| Ischemia | Peripheral vascular disease; pain may result from hypoxic tissues, toxic substances released by damaged cells, arterial spasm | By-pass surgery with Dacron graft; rest limb; liberal use of narcotics; embolectomy is appropriate; amputation; avoid heat application |
| | Claudication; pain from hypoxic tissues | Periods of rest whenever pain occurs |
| | Pressure from casts; occlusive dressings | Bivalve cast; elevate limb; remove dressings |
| | Decubitus ulcers (from pressure on casts, bed); pain caused by hypoxic tissues; no pain if nerve damage is severe | Window or bivalve cast to check area of complaint and relieve pressure; massage reddened area, if appropriate; relieve pressure on area by turning or ambulating |
| | Compartment syndrome; pain from accumulation of blood under fascia layers causing pressure and ischemia | Bivalve cast; elevate limb; surgical intervention to relieve pressure |

**Table 27-3.** Typical types of pain seen in orthopedic conditions—cont'd

| Condition | Causative factors | Pain relief measures |
|---|---|---|
| Muscle spasm | Cause of pain related to injured area and constant pressure of contracted muscle and increase in lactic acid(?) | Back muscle spasm—firm mattress; bed boards; 90-90 traction; hip flexion; William's position; in case of fracture Buck's traction |
| Muscle sprain | Tearing of ligaments and joint capsule | Rest joint; elevation of limb; ice to reduce swelling |
| Muscle strain | Change of osmotic pressure within muscle cells; some ischemia may contribute to pain; overuse of muscle | Rest area; ice; elevation of limb |
| Muscle injury (blow) | Injury to muscle by blunt instrument | Nonnarcotic analgesic; ice, then heat |
| Muscle tension | Splinting; holding muscle in one position too long; may also cause headache | Back rub; repositioning; exercise when appropriate; range of motion; decrease anxiety, if possible |
| Incisional pain | Damage to sensory nerves of joint capsule, periosteum, muscle and skin; damage may be caused by cutting, tearing, or pressure created by surgical instruments | Narcotics; comfort measures (back care, careful turning, bath); early movement and ambulation for muscle stiffness and soreness; when moving patient keep limb supported; keep back straight and use turning frame to decrease pain and maintain alignment. |
| Causalgia | Damage or alternation of large, afferent nerve fibers; severence of large peripheral nerve; violent amputation by gunshot wound, etc. | Avoid soft touch to the limb; avoid emotional upsets; sympathectomy, central or local; nerve blocks |
| Phantom pain | More likely to occur if there was pain in the amputated part prior to the amputation; cause (?), pattern of pain imprinted on CNS; may be affected by descending information from the cortex, information (sensory) from the periphery and/or information already imprinted on the CNS | Performing pleasant activity with the affected limb which might stimulate large afferent nerve activity; increasing sensory input (even noxious stimuli); decreasing stimuli (local anesthetic); psychotherapy; chordotomy and rhizotomy are generally unsuccessful |
| Intractable pain | Neoplasm; hysterical reactions; undiagnosed problems | *Neoplasm*—repair of fracture, radiation; nerve blocks; chordotomy; oral and parenteral narcotics; narcotic cocktail; psychologic manipulations; distraction; cognitive dissonance; WIA; hypnosis *Hysterical reactions*—pain clinics; behavior modification; psychotherapy; nerve blocks |
| Chronic low back pain | Pressure on nerve roots, scar tissue pressing on nerve roots; herniated nucleus pulposus; other causes | Williams position; exercises to strengthen back musculature; distraction; use of proper body mechanics; bedrest; bed boards; firm mattress; comfort measures; weight reduction; traction; surgical procedures (disc removal, fusion, neurectomy, rhizotomy); dorsal column stimulator |
| Pain associated with myelography | Cause suspected to be related to tearing of arachnoid covering and resultant leakage of CSF into extra arachnoid space | Keep body flat (no pillow) 6-8 hours following myelogram (Pantopaque, iodine dyes); keep room dark; apply ice to head; narcotics offer little relief once headache occurs; force fluids to reestablish fluid volume |

pushing through muscle and subcutaneous tissue. Pain from inflammation occurs when the condition becomes chronic. In addition, the individual often has been through multiple surgical procedures and extended hospitalizations. Therefore, the pain is often enhanced because of depression and a decreased tolerance. The patient may have the added burden of threatened amputation as well. As discussed previously, psychic disturbances can play a significant role in perception of pain; the person with osteomyelitis is no exception.

### Ischemic pain

Ischemia may result from peripheral vascular disease (caused by diabetes, atherosclerosis, or arteriosclerosis), obstruction of blood flow caused by constricting casts, pressure from the bed or a body part, or lack of blood flow resulting from surgical trauma or accidental injury.

**Peripheral vascular disease.** One of the most outstanding features of arterial occlusive disease is pain, which may go completely unrelieved even with liberal use of narcotics. The pain of an embolus completely occluding an artery is abrupt and severe.[2, p. 569] The cause is thought to be related to arterial spasm or ischemia.

The patient with peripheral vascular disease may experience pain only in exercise. This pain occurs when the metabolic demands for oxygen are greater than the amount that can be supplied by the blood vessels. This pain is typically relieved by rest whereas pain resulting from total occlusion is not.

Relief measures for arterial disease are usually not successful without some type of surgical intervention. Bypass surgery with dacron graft may be done or embolectomy may be attempted in some cases. Amputation is often the only solution to the problem.

**Cast pressure.** Determining whether the ischemic pain is caused by surgical intervention or pressure from a cast is difficult. Rather than being diffuse as with trauma, the pain often becomes localized; the patient can point out a particularly uncomfortable area. Swelling below the cast, negative blanching sign, decreased movement of the extremity, a very red or very pale extremity, and a cool or very warm extremity are signs of occlusion of arterial or venous flow. Opiates are seldom effective when the pain is caused by a tight cast or dressing. The best method of relief is to bivalve the cast. Relief will be almost immediate and the patient will often drop off to sleep from sheer exhaustion. Every nurse who cares for othopedic patients must understand the procedure for bivalving a cast.

Pain that progresses to numbness is a critical sign that nerve damage may have occurred. The numbness may indicate damage done during surgery or in the postoperative period. The cast should be changed or windowed to allow visualization of the part in question. Elevating the limb may decrease the swelling and thus decrease the pressure and pain. If the pressure area is allowed to continue without removing the cast, permanent damage to the extremity may occur or decubitus ulcers may form under the cast.

Signs and symptoms of decubitus ulcers include pain, a tingling sensation, or numbness of the part. Often the area of ischemia is red at first; later, if ischemia continues the area becomes blue-red and the turgor of the skin becomes reduced. If the area does not become perfused at this time, the skin appears abraded. If the wound is left unattended, the skin layers will continue to necrose and sensation disappears. The wound will no longer be painful, although necrosis will continue through skin and muscle to the bone. If the casted limb is observed and assessed regularly, this damage should never occur. It is far better to reapply a cast bivalved in error than to have pressure areas develop.

### Compartment syndrome

Diagnosing the pain associated with compartment syndrome is difficult. The cause of this pain is thought to be blood and serous drainage collecting under the fascia of the traumatized area resulting in edema and restricted blood flow in the extremity.[5] The patient develops unbearable pain in the affected extremity. Often there will be deteriorating neurovascular signs in the extremity involved but this is not always true. If the nurse or physician notes the pain is unrelieved by usual doses of narcotics and there are neurovascular signs of complication, the cast should be bivalved, the extremity elevated, and physician in charge notified. Sometimes surgical intervention is necessary to relieve this serious, painful complication.

### Muscle spasm and muscle tension

Muscle spasm often occurs following a sprain, strain, or fracture as well as postoperatively. Low back pain, another common problem, is often accompanied by muscle spasm. Muscle spasm is thought to be a protective, splinting action of the muscle. It is the continuous contraction over the injured part, which supposedly accounts for the pain associated with the spasm. Many times relief of the muscle spasm will bring about much relief of the injured area. Traction can often relieve pain of muscle spasm associated with fractures. A firm supportive mattress as well as flexion of knees and hips will relax back muscles and cause a decrease in muscle spasm of the back.

**Sprains and strains.** *Sprains* result from tearing of ligaments and capsule fibers. The associated pain is relieved by resting the joint, elevation, and treating it with ice to reduce the swelling.[5,p.442]

A *strain* is overuse of muscles during some strenuous activity. Hannington-Kiff describes the cause of this pain as the result of "increased water in the muscle cells owing to the osmotic effect of the accumulated metabolites of anaerobic metabolism which follows a period of relative ischemia."[9,p.110] Rest of the involved extremity and application of cold help reduce discomfort.

**Blows.** When direct blows occur to muscles or tendons there can be varying amounts of discomfort. Injury to the belly of the muscle is less painful than injury at the origin or insertion site of the muscle.[5,p.443]

Pain caused by blows to the muscle can often be relieved by nonnarcotic analgesics. Application of ice may cause vasoconstriction and therefore decrease bleeding and resultant swelling that may contribute to pain.

**Muscle tension.** This pain can be the cause of headache pain, and it can result in the stiffness from splinting muscles to avoid postoperative pain. Patients may experience this pain when malpositioned in bed. Often unknowingly patients "hold" themselves in one position, which results in sore and fatigued muscles. Anxiety may also make an individual tense his muscles, and the result can often be pain associated with muscle tension. Patients often clench their jaws or fists or arch their backs when in pain. The muscle tension caused by these activities can increase the original pain and thus contribute to suffering.

## Incisional pain

Like all other types of surgery, orthopedic surgery produces cutaneous and muscular pain. In addition, the individual may have trauma to a joint capsule or the periosteum. Patients describe this discomfort as deep, boring, unrelenting pain.

**Drug therapy.** A large dose of morphine will often relieve pain of this origin. However, meperidine is frequently ordered for orthopedic patients, and because the dose is not large enough the patient usually suffers. Meperidine's duration of action is only 2 to 4 hours and 50 mg of meperidine is equal to about 5 mg of morphine. Therefore, meperidine must be ordered in larger amounts (for example,

100 mg every 2 to 3 hours) in order to provide adequate relief. We believe that patients who undergo orthopedic surgery should receive morphine instead of meperidine. Morphine is usually ordered in the correct dosage (10 mg) at 3 to 4 hour intervals. The duration action is 4 to 5 hours and, therefore, these patients get adequate pain relief.[11,p.256]

*Tolerance.* Many health care workers do not understand the problem of drug tolerance. Tolerance to opioids is defined as a shortened duration of action and decreased intensity of relief as well as a decreased manifestation of other side effects of the drug with continued use.[107] An orthopedic patient might well require many doses of narcotics during a long postoperative course; therefore some tolerance will develop. This fact does *not* mean the patient is an addict. It merely means that an expected phenomenon is taking place. The nurse and physician should consult each other and decide with the patient where he is in the recovery phase. Perhaps the most appropriate intervention is to increase the dose and shorten the interval between doses in order to provide relief.

The physician may decide to discontinue administration of the narcotic analgesic and substitute another drug. One mistake commonly made is to give the patient pentazocine (Talwin). Pentazocine is a weak opioid antagonist and patients who have been on opioids will experience withdrawal.[11,pp.276-277] Along with the physiologic effects of withdrawal, patients may experience hallucination and nightmares with pentazocine. To avoid these effects the drug should not be administered until 1 to 2 days after the opioid is discontinued.[11,pp.276-277]

*Placebos.* Many health care professionals seem to have no compunction when using this device. Unfortunately, what many nurses do not realize is that approximately 30% of clients who receive placebos will have pain relief for a time.[9,p.41] The relief afforded by placebo is only evidence that the psyche plays a powerful role; it does *not* "prove" the patient does not have pain. Nurses, physicians, and therapists use the "placebo" of their presence and interaction every day, and this distraction may also relieve a patient in pain for a time. This method does not "prove" the patient is feigning pain, yet, when a nurse uses normal saline injection and convinces the patient it will relieve pain, it becomes a measurement tool for diagnosing psychogenic or pretended pain. What nurses do not realize is that they are using themselves and the patient's trust and belief that he will be helped as the placebo. I wonder how many patients suffer because of the misguided use of a placebo.

**Positioning.** Principles of positioning are also important in relieving incisional pain. While splinting the incision is helpful in reducing pain in abdominal surgery, careful handling of the affected limb in orthopedics is essential. The injured part should be lifted as a whole with support given to the joints. This principle is the same as log-rolling the patient after spinal surgery.

Many patients who undergo joint replacement surgery have suffered pain resulting from rheumatoid arthritis, avascular necrosis, or osteoarthritis. Some patients are so relieved from the dull, aching, unrelenting pain of arthritis that the incisional and bone pain after surgery are not particularly devastating. Most patients, however, have acute pain especially when turned. Careful elevation of the limb on pillows or other supportive devices helps to reduce pain in these joints. Also, careful handling of the affected limb during repositioning can make the turning experience more comfortable. Having one person handle the affected limb exclusively reduces any chance of rough or jerky movement. Enlisting the patient's help in positioning, of course, is also needed to assure smooth turning or repositioning. Usually the patient knows the best way to move in terms of comfort, and the nurse and physician know the best way to move in terms of protecting the operated or traumatized area. Therefore, a team approach with the patient functioning as a full member is optimal for the patients comfort and safety.

### Causalgia

Causalgic pain is thought to be caused by damage or alteration of large afferent nerve fibers or by partial severance of a large peripheral nerve.[9,p.75;24, pp.100-109] One theory is that there is some type of interaction (electrical) between different types of nerve fibers so that sympathetic fibers interact in some way with unmyelinated sensory nerves. The damaged sensory nerves at the periphery may carry large volleys of pain and at the cord level interact with sympathetic fibers, thus causing the sympathetic fibers to be involved in the pain causation. This theory may explain why interruption of sympathetic pathways stops causalgic pain.[9,p.75]

Hannington-Kiff notes that emotional trauma may trigger the recurrence of causalgia.[9,p.75] Causalgia is often the result of violent injury to a limb such as occurs in auto accidents or gunshot wounds. Medical treatment usually consists of sympathectomy, local anesthetic blocks, or local sympathectomy. Actual treatment for causalgia is left to the physician but nursing personnel should be aware that emotional upsets and touch of the affected limb may cause this phenomenon to occur.

### Phantom limb pain

Phantom limb pain is a curious pain problem. The pain is perceived as occurring in an absent limb following amputation. Phantom limb pain is more likely to occur if the limb had some painful condition prior to the amputation.[9,p.75;20,p.680] The cause of this problem is not fully understood but Livingston's theory offers a viable explanation (cited in Melzack[22,p.142]). Livingston's reverberating circuit theory suggests that in the injured limb the small afferent nerves set up a pain pattern in the spinal cord which later can be triggered by descending information from the brain, incoming pain from the peripheral sensory nerves, and sympathic interactions as noted in causalgia. The reverberating circuit is described as a pain reaction that is imprinted on the central nervous system. If this theory is correct, it would easily explain why neurectomies, rhizotomies, and chordotomies do not alter the painful reaction. Also, by projecting the gate control theory onto the reverberating circuit theory, one can easily see that severing a nervous tract would not alleviate the pain since there are so many factors that open and close the physiologic "gate."

The phantom limb problem is a multimodal problem that must be dealt with in a multimodal treatment plan. Treatment must involve reducing painful input from the periphery, decreasing descending painful information from the cortex and perhaps interruption of nerve pathways. Melzack[21,pp.63-68] describes the treatment as:

1. Performing activity that will stimulate large afferent nerve fibers (pleasant stimuli)
2. Increasing sensory input, even noxious stimuli (e.g., injection of salt solution into the amputation site)
3. Decreasing stimuli to the amputation site through local anesthetic
4. Treating the patient's problems to attempt to inhibit the descending nerve tract information

### Intractable pain

Another pain problem that occurs occasionally is intractable pain. It is seen in patients with metastatic disease to bones, primary bone tumors, and sometimes low back pain syndromes.

**Metastatic disease.** In treating pain associated with neoplastic conditions, it is important to realize that with the advent of chemotherapy (antimetabolites, etc.), these patients will live longer than individuals who did not have the benefit of chemotherapy; therefore, reconstruction may be necessary to relieve pain. Hip-pinning, fusion, and stabilizing bones with plates and screws do much to relieve pain and also improve function. Other neurologic manipulations can be performed to relieve pain when orthopedic interventions are not enough. Procedures such as chordotomies will relieve this pain, and radiation to the affected area will often give temporary relief as well.

*Drug therapy.* Some authorities recommend waiting and attempting other methods of pain relief before resorting to narcotics as a primary method for pain relief.[6;9,p.40] Narcotics tend to confuse the thought processes or put the patient to sleep. In the case of terminal neoplastic conditions, sometimes there are no other alternatives. The health professional should keep in mind the principles of tolerance and dependence, if narcotics are the chief modality employed for pain relief; however, use of injectable narcotics becomes a problem when the patient becomes cachexic. Some institutions have begun using a "cocktail" to help solve this problem. Hannington-Kiff recommends a combination of diamorphine, morphine, and cocaine in a sweetened base.[9,p.40] Oral methadone syrup also useful in cachexic patients. Methadone has a long duration of action and has some cumulative effects as well. In England various mixtures of heroin, chlorpromazine, and cocaine are used with good success.

*Psychologic methods.* Some of the other treatments for intractable pain use the psyche to help close the gate to sensory input. Such activities as cognitive dissonance, "waking imagined analgesia", simple distraction, relaxation, and comfort measures that offer pleasant stimuli all can be employed to assist in decreasing intractable pain sensation.

**Low back pain.** One of the most difficult pain problems to deal with in the orthopedic setting is the patient with low back pain syndrome. Nurses and physicians are empathetic to the person who has obvious pathology, but when myelography or venography does not demonstrate disease or damage, the individual becomes easily labeled. Weiner wrote an excellent description of the interactions on an orthopedic unit when patients must "prove" their pain.[32,pp.508-516]

*General relief measures.* The following are methods to relieve pain that every orthopedic clinician should know:

1. William's position, with hips and knee joints flexed at 90 degree angle
2. Exercises to strengthen back muscles, such as situps with head resting on chest, pelvic tilt, etc.
3. Use of bed boards and a firm mattress
4. Proper body mechanics
5. Bedrest
6. Distraction from pain (occupational therapy, recreational therapy, interpersonal interaction, TV, radio, reading, etc.)
7. Comfort measures
8. Weight reduction
9. Traction
10. Surgical procedures (discectomy, laminectomy, fusion, neurectomy, or more drastic chordotomy, rhizotomy)

Another important part of the treatment is understanding the clinician's own feeling about these patients.[32,pp.508-516] Does the clinician value stoicism? Does the clinician have to *see* pathology to be empathetic to patients in pain? What is the clinician's pattern of response to these patients? Does the clinician give out negative nonverbal and verbal signals to these patients that will interrupt therapeutic communication and perhaps encourage "doctor-shopping"?

*Dorsal column stimulator.* There has been limited success with the use of the dorsal column stimulator in the treatment of low back pain. A laminectomy is required to insert electrodes into the dorsal column at the interdural space. Studies suggest, however, that over time, the effectiveness of dorsal column stimulation decreases.[19,p.195] This instrument should be used only when there is obvious pathology and there is no evidence of hypochondriasis, hysteria, or depression. It should not be used on patients involved in legal battles for compensation.

## Myelography

Providing relief from the headache of myelography can be a real challenge. If the headache becomes protracted, the individual may experience nausea and vomiting as well. The headache after myelography may result from tearing of the arachnoid covering by the puncture needle which introduces the dye. This tearing then allows cerebrospinal fluid (CSF) to leak out of the subarachnoid space into the extra-arachnoid space. Many physicians recommend that the patient force fluids, which will replace the volume CSF lost during the procedure. It is important to keep the patient's body flat after myelogram since this may help decrease the possibility of headache. A dark room sometimes also helps. Narcotics seem to provide little relief. It is hoped that new contrast media that does not have to be removed and that causes little meningeal irritation will be passed through clinical trials. Some of these drugs are being tested and may be in general use in the not-too-distant future.

## PAIN RELIEF EVALUATION

While treating the patient with pain, it is necessary to assess the efficacy of the interventions instituted. This evaluation should be an ongoing task. McCaffery points out that the clinician should not suggest another pain relieving measure when beginning a single maneuver since this suggests that the clinician does not place great value on the original measure.[18,pp.1224-1227] There must be adequate written goals for pain relief in order to begin and complete evaluation appropriately. The first area of evaluation probably should be with the patient: Did the patient feel there was adequate pain relief? Did the patient rest or become more functional? Was the patient satisfied with the intervention(s)? (Sometimes the goal is attained but not in a way consistent with the patient's desires. For example, the patient may wish pain relief but does not want to be somnolent. If the nurse administers a high dose of morphine the goal of pain relief will be achieved, but the patient may sleep for hours.) Were different modalities of treatment relied upon? (We know that there is a physical and psychologic overlay to all pain; has the clinician used both modalities in pain relief?) Has the clinician taught the patient some of the pain relieving measures so that these can be performed independently?

If the clinician has noted a physiologic response to pain (for example, altered blood pressure and pulse during the pain experience), these parameters can be evaluated during the experience and the aftermath.[2,p.282] However, interpreting pain should not be done solely on the basis of respiratory alteration, since this activity is under voluntary control as well as autonomic.

The efficacy of a pain relief action may be difficult to evaluate, as it is not always practical to use it several times for the same patient. Instead it may be possible to evaluate a certain nursing approach based on the response of several patients. Obviously, different people react differently to pain, but if one particular action seems to work well, its use should be continued.

Clinicians should also be aware of their own placebo effect. In a study done by McBride, it was reported that nurses seldom use themselves and their communication skills to help relieve a patient's pain.[15,p.337] Physicians are often criticized for not spending time with their patients even though both nurses and physicians know the importance of the psyche in pain perception, interpretation, and reaction.

When evaluation takes place, there is always the prospect of discovering negative findings. The patient may *not* have been helped because of inadequate doses of medication, too long a time interval between medication doses, inadequate original assessment of the pain problem, or inadequate preparation of the patient for a painful experience; perhaps, too, the patient may "need" the pain for emotional or psychologic reasons. It is a frustrating experience to try many modalities of pain relief and be unsuccessful. However, because pain results from so many factors, it is impossible to pinpoint one cause of failure. It is probably inappropriate to try to evaluate or search for *one* reason for failure to effect pain relief since the cause of pain is multimodal. Failure to effect pain relief is sometimes a signal that there is significant pathology present which may have been missed. For example, the patient with a compound fracture who is casted may complain bitterly of pain despite use of morphine and other pain relief measures. This complaining often signals ischemia; the patient needs immediate surgical intervention or bivalving the cast.

## SUMMARY

It is unfortunate that such a widespread problem as pain has not been considered for research more often. In recent years there seems to be a revival of interest in the subject of pain, both in understanding its mechanisms and in management of symptoms.

This chapter has attempted to cover basic information about pain; it is impossible to cover the entire subject here. The reader is directed to the bibliography for a broader perspective of the subject. Pain is one of the subjective realities with which clinicians frequently must deal. Adequate knowledge of pain physiology and theory, as well as common treatment modalities is essential to deliver intelligent, competent health care.

## REFERENCES

1. Beecher, H. K.: Relationship of significance of wound to pain experience, J.A.M.A. **161**(17):1609-1613, Aug. 25, 1956.
2. Beland, I., and Passos, J.: Clinical nursing, New York, 1975, Macmillan, Inc.
3. Bloom, F., Segal, D., Ling, D., and Guillemin, R.: Endorphins: Profound behavioral effects in rats suggest new etiological factors in mental illness, Science **194**(4265):630-632, 1976.
4. Bruegel, M. A.: Relationship of preoperative anxiety to perception of postoperative pain, Nurs. Res. **20**(1): 26-31, 1971.
5. Buckwalter, K. C., and Buckwalter, J. A.: Pain associated with orthopedic conditions. In Jacox, A. K., editor: Pain; A sourcebook for nurses and other

health professionals, Boston, 1977, Little, Brown and Co.

6. Collins, J.: A doctor looks at pain. In Jacox, A. (Chair): Advances in the management of pain. Symposium presented at the Second National Conference on Cancer Nursing, St. Louis, May 9-10, 1977.
7. Drakontides, A. B.: Drugs to treat pain, Am. J. Nurs. **74**(3):508, Mar. 1974.
8. Guyton, A. C.: Textbook of medical physiology, ed. 4, Philadelphia, 1971, W. B. Saunders Co.
9. Hannington-Kiff, J.: Pain relief, Philadelphia, 1974, J. B. Lippincott Co.
10. Jaffe, J. H.: Drug addiction and drug abuse. In Goodman, L. S., and Gilman, A., editors: The pharmacological basis of therapeutics, New York, 1975, Macmillan, Inc.
11. Jaffe, J. H., and Martin, W. R.: Narcotic analgesics and antagonists. In Goodman, L. S., and Gilman, A., editors: The pharmacological basis of therapeutics, New York, 1975, Macmillan, Inc.
12. Leybin, L., Pinsky, C., and others: Intraventribular Met 5-enkephalin causes unexpected lowering of pain threshold and narcotic withdrawal signs in rats, Nature **264**(5585):459, Dec. 1976.
13. Loan, W. B., and Morrison, J. D.: The incidence and severity of postoperative pain. In Weisenberg, M., editor: Pain: Clinical and experimental perspectives, St. Louis, 1975, The C. V. Mosby Co.
14. Luckmann, J., and Sorensen, K.: Medical-surgical nursing, Philadelphia, 1974, W. B. Saunders Co.
15. McBride, M. A.: Nursing approach, pain, and relief: An exploratory experiment, Nurs. Res. **16**(4):337, Fall 1967.
16. McCaffery, M.: Intractable pain, Nursing 73, Nov. 1973, p. 29.
17. McCaffery, M.: Nursing management of the patient with pain, Philadelphia, 1972, J. B. Lippincott Co.
18. McCaffery, M., and Moss, F.: Nursing intervention for bodily pain, Am. J. Nurs. **67**(6):1124-1127, June 1967.
19. McDonnell, D.: Surgical and electrical stimulation methods for relief of pain. In Jacox, A. K., editor: Pain: A sourcebook for nurses and other health professional, Boston, 1977, Little, Brown & Co.
20. Melzack, R.: How acupuncture can block pain. In Weisenberg, M., editor: Pain: Clinical and experimental perspectives, St. Louis, 1975, The C. V. Mosby Co.
21. Melzack, R.: Phantom limbs, Psychology Today, Oct. 1970, pp. 63-68.
22. Melzack, R.: The puzzle of pain, New York, 1973, Basic Books, Inc.
23. Melzack, R., and Wall, P. D.: Gate control theory of pain. In Soulairac, A., Cahn, J., and Carpentier, J., editors: Pain: Proceedings of the International Symposium on Pain, London, 1971, Academic Press.
24. Noordenboos, W.: Pain, Amsterdam, 1959, Elsevier.
25. Papper, E., Brodie, B. B., and Rovenstine, E. A.: Postoperative pain: Its use in the comparative evaluation of analgesics, Surgery **32**:107, 1952.
26. Pasnau, R. O., and Pfefferbaum, B.: Psychologic aspects of postamputation pain, Nurs. Clin. N. Am. **11**(4):680, Dec. 1976.
27. Shapiro, R.: Myelography, Chicago, 1975, Yearbook Medical Publishers.
28. Steel, J.: A nurse looks at pain. In Jacox, A. (Chair): Advances in the management of pain. Symposium presented at the Second National Conference on Cancer Nursing, St. Louis, May 9-10, 1977.
29. Sternbach, R. A.: Pain: A psychophysiological analysis, New York, 1968, Academic Press.
30. Swanson, D. W.: Less obvious aspects of chronic pain, Postgrad. Med. **60**(5): 130-134, 1976.
31. Wall, P. D.: Physiological mechanisms involved in the production and relief of pain. In Bonica, J., Procacci, P., and Pagni, C. A., editors: Recent advances on pain, Springfield, Ill., 1972, Charles C Thomas, Publisher.
32. Weiner, C.: Pain assessment on an orthopedic unit, Nurs. Outlook. **23**(8):508-516, Aug. 1975.
33. Zborowski, M.: People in pain, San Francisco, 1969, Jossey-Bass.

## BIBLIOGRAPHY

Beecher, H. K.: Relationship of significance of wound to pain experienced, Journal of the American Medical Association, August 25, 1956, 161, 1609-1613.

Engel, G. L. "Psychogenic Pain and the Pain Prone Patient", American Journal of Medicine, 1959, 26(6), 899-918.

Jacox, A. K.: Pain: a sourcebook for nurses and other health professionals. Boston; 1977, Little, Brown and Co.

McCaffery, M.: Nursing management of the patient with pain, Philadelphia, 1972, J. B. Lippincott Co.

McCaffery, M. and Hart, L. "Undertreatment of Acute Pain with Narcotics", American Journal of Nursing, October 1976, 76(10), 1586-1591.

Melzack, R.: The puzzle of pain, New York, 1973, Basic Books, Inc.

Melzack, R., and Wall, P. D.: Gate control theory of pain. In Soulairac, Cahn, A. J., and Carpentier, J. eds.: Pain: Proceedings of the international symposium on pain, Baltimore; 1972, The Williams & Wilkins Co.

Merskey, H., and Spear, F. G.: Pain: psychological and psychiatric aspects, London, 1967, Balliere, Tindall and Cassel.

Sternbach, R. A.: Pain: a psychophysiological analysis, New York, 1968, Academic Press.

# 28

# Therapy: physical and occupational

**BEVERLY A. GRYTH**

**LAURA K. VOGTLE**

Therapy as provided by the occupational and physical therapist is a valuable adjunct in the treatment of orthopedic conditions. The therapists, along with the nursing staff and the orthopedist, are part of the orthopedic team who provide treatment (restoration techniques) for existing problems and prevention, if possible, of further difficulties. Therapy services are provided at the request and in cooperation with the physician. The range of these services varies greatly depending on the specific conditions being treated. In this chapter we will outline the following general principles, which, ultimately, all the goals and objectives of therapy programs:

1. Prevention of deformity
2. Treatment of preexisting deformity, including use of positioning and devices
3. Evaluation and treatment for functional independence
4. Promotion of activities of daily living

In each case it is important to know the patient, and the medical and family history before a judgment is made concerning which preventive or corrective techniques will be followed. Knowing the contraindications to treatment is necessary as well; what is an indication in one diagnosis may be contraindicated in another. In this chapter we cannot include all indications or contraindications; however, we will provide some general techniques and procedures in the prevention and control of deformities prevalent in orthopedic disabilities.

The methods of prevention or treatment—active or passive exercises, range of motion, weightbearing activities, positioning—are chosen depending on the patient's diagnosis and the therapist's assessment of the patient. In making the assessment the therapist uses several standard tests with forms for documentation and follow-up evaluation (see box, p. 700). These include *manual muscle testing,* in which each muscle or muscle group is tested against resistance and against gravity. There are five grades from normal to zero. The grade given the muscle will determine the type of exercise or functional activity chosen for treatment. *Joint range of motion* is evaluated to determine the actual degree of active or passive motion in relation to full or normal range of each joint. By using these tests for strength and range of motion the therapist can also determine if there are areas of pain on movement or sensory changes. Documentation is important as a means of showing changes resulting from therapy and to assist in the determination of goals, short- or long-term, in the care of the patient.

## PREVENTION OF DEFORMITY

Prevention of possible deformity or contractures is especially important when muscle strength varies throughout the trunk or in any of the extremities as a result of spasticity, congenital, bony, or muscular abnormalities, trauma, or neurologic changes, either motor or sensory. Prevention can be achieved through positioning, exercise, and range of motion exercises.

## Positioning

Positioning is most important in prevention of deformities. Splinting can be used to achieve elongation of the strong muscle in opposition to a weak or absent muscle, or to correct a flail segment of an extremity, such as dropfoot or wrist deviation (Fig.

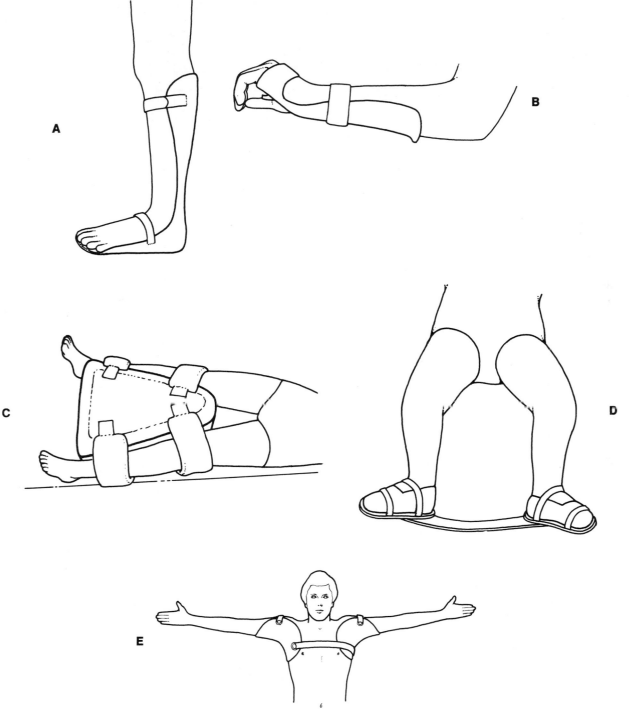

**Fig. 28-1.** Devices that assist in prevention of deformity. **A,** Dropfoot splint. **B,** Wrist cock-up splint. **C,** Abduction pillow. **D,** Dennis-Brown splint. **E,** Airplane splint.

# University of Virginia Hospital
## Muscle Examination*

| Name |
| --- |
| History no. |

Diagnosis _____  Dr. _____

Age _____  Date of onset _____  Date of Birth _____

| | | | | Left | | Trunk and Legs | | | | Right | | |
| --- | --- | --- | --- | --- | --- | --- | --- | --- | --- | --- | --- | --- | --- |
| | | | | Date | | | | | | Date | | | |
| | | | | | | | | | | | | | |
| | | | | | | | | | | | | | |
| | | | | | | **Neck** | Flexors | | | | | | |
| | | | | | | | Extensors | | | | | | |
| | | | | | | **Trunk** | Dorsal extensors | | | | | | |
| | | | | | | | Lumbar extensors | | | | | | |
| | | | | | | | Abdominals, upper | | | | | | |
| | | | | | | | Abdominals, lower | | | | | | |
| | | | | | | | Transversalis | | | | | | |
| | | | | | | | Quadratus lumborum | | | | | | |
| | | | | | | **Hip** | Gluteus maximus | | | | | | |
| | | | | | | | Ilio psoas (flexor) | | | | | | |
| | | | | | | | Sartorius | | | | | | |
| | | | | | | | Tensor fascia lata | | | | | | |
| | | | | | | | Gluteus medius (abductor) | | | | | | |
| | | | | | | | Hip adductors | | | | | | |
| | | | | | | | Inward rotators (hip) | | | | | | |
| | | | | | | | Outward rotators (hip) | | | | | | |
| | | | | | | **Knee** | Quadriceps | | | | | | |
| | | | | | | | Hamstrings, Inner | | | | | | |
| | | | | | | | Hamstrings, Outer | | | | | | |
| | | | | | | **Ankle** | Gastrocnemius | | | | | | |
| | | | | | | | Anterior tibial (invertor) | | | | | | |
| | | | | | | | Posterior tibial (invertor) | | | | | | |
| | | | | | | | Peroneus longus (evertor) | | | | | | |
| | | | | | | | Peroneus brevis (evertor) | | | | | | |
| | | | | | | | Peroneus tertius | | | | | | |
| | | | | | | **Toes** | Extensor digitorum longus | | | | | | |
| | | | | | | | Extensor digitorum brevis | | | | | | |
| | | | | | | | Extensor hallucis longus | | | | | | |
| | | | | | | | Flexor digitorum longus | | | | | | |
| | | | | | | | Flexor digitorum brevis | | | | | | |
| | | | | | | | Lumbricales | | | | | | |
| | | | | | | | Flexor hallucis longus | | | | | | |
| | | | | | | | Flexor hallucis brevis | | | | | | |
| | | | | | | **Deformities** | Back | | | | | | |
| | | | | | | | Hip | | | | | | |
| | | | | | | | Knee | | | | | | |
| | | | | | | | Ankle and foot | | | | | | |

N—Normal: full range against heavy resistance    P—Poor: full range with gravity eliminated
G—Good: full range against some resistance    T—Trace: perceptible contraction
F—Fair: full range against gravity    O—Zero: no contraction
*Used with permission of University of Virginia Hospital.

| Left Arm | | | | | Name | | Right Arm | | | | |
|---|---|---|---|---|---|---|---|---|---|---|---|
| | | | | | **Shoulder** | Deltoid, Anterior | | | | | |
| | | | | | | " Middle | | | | | |
| | | | | | | " Posterior | | | | | |
| | | | | | | Latissimus dorsi | | | | | |
| | | | | | | Trapezius, Upper | | | | | |
| | | | | | | " Middle | | | | | |
| | | | | | | " Lower | | | | | |
| | | | | | | Serratus anterior | | | | | |
| | | | | | | Rhomboids | | | | | |
| | | | | | | Inward rotators, shoulder | | | | | |
| | | | | | | Outward rotators, shoulder | | | | | |
| | | | | | | Pectoralis major, sternal | | | | | |
| | | | | | | Pectoralis major, clavicular | | | | | |
| | | | | | **Elbow** | Biceps | | | | | |
| | | | | | | Brachioradialis | | | | | |
| | | | | | | Triceps | | | | | |
| | | | | | **Wrist** | Supinators | | | | | |
| | | | | | | Pronators | | | | | |
| | | | | | | Flexor carpi ulnaris | | | | | |
| | | | | | | Flexor carpi radialis | | | | | |
| | | | | | | Palmaris longus | | | | | |
| | | | | | | Extensor carpi ulnaris | | | | | |
| | | | | | | Extensor carpi radialis | | | | | |
| | | | | | **Fingers** | Flexor profundus 1 | | | | | |
| | | | | | | " 2 | | | | | |
| | | | | | | " 3 | | | | | |
| | | | | | | " 4 | | | | | |
| | | | | | | Flexor sublimis 1 | | | | | |
| | | | | | | " 2 | | | | | |
| | | | | | | " 3 | | | | | |
| | | | | | | " 4 | | | | | |
| | | | | | | Extensor digitorum communis 1 | | | | | |
| | | | | | | " 2 | | | | | |
| | | | | | | " 3 | | | | | |
| | | | | | | " 4 | | | | | |
| | | | | | | Lumbricales 1 | | | | | |
| | | | | | | " 2 | | | | | |
| | | | | | | " 3 | | | | | |
| | | | | | | " 4 | | | | | |
| | | | | | | Dorsal interossei | | | | | |
| | | | | | | Abductor digiti minimi | | | | | |
| | | | | | | Palmar interossei | | | | | |
| | | | | | **Thumb** | Abductor pollicis longus | | | | | |
| | | | | | | Abductor pollicis brevis | | | | | |
| | | | | | | Adductor pollicis | | | | | |
| | | | | | | Flexor pollicis longus | | | | | |
| | | | | | | Flexor pollicis brevis | | | | | |
| | | | | | | Opponens policis | | | | | |
| | | | | | | Extensor pollicis longus | | | | | |
| | | | | | | Extensor pollicis brevis | | | | | |
| | | | | | **Deformities** | Shoulder | | | | | |
| | | | | | | Elbow | | | | | |
| | | | | | | Wrist | | | | | |
| Left Arm | | | | | | Fingers | Right Arm | | | | |

28-1, *A* and *B*). An abductor pillow (28-1, *C*) is useful for maintaining hip abduction in opposition to strong or spastic hip adductors. Splinting is used most often during times of inactivity such as nap time, or it may be used full time, if necessary, if the patient is to remain in bed or immobile. The infant who has undergone frequent cast changes for correction of congenital foot deformities (clubfoot or metatarsus adductus) may wear a Denis-Browne splint (Fig. 28-1, *D*) or reverse-last shoes to maintain correction and prevent recurrence of the deformity. The splint may be used day and night while the child is nonambulatory and continued at night once weightbearing activities are begun.

Bracing (orthoses) can accomplish static and dynamic positioning. The dynamic splint provides a function not present in the unsplinted joint or extremity. It is more commonly used in hand splints (for example, a wrist-driven flexor hinge splint to provide for grasp in the flail hand).

Static splinting is usually considered to be primarily for maintenance or correction of a position. Examples of static splints are the airplane splint (Fig. 28-1, *E*) to prevent axillary contractures and a posterior shell (Fig. 28-1, *A*) for prevention of footdrop. A long leg (knee-ankle-foot) orthosis (Fig. 28-2) with or without the pelvic band can provide prolonged stretch for tightened muscles (especially hamstrings and gastroc-soleus) and maintain range of motion of knee and ankle. It also provides a dynamic component for weightbearing. (Weightbearing may be ambulation unassisted or with crutches or use of a standing table or other assistive devices; all types offer change of position, which helps to prevent complications.)

Probably the most important factor in prevention of contractures and deformities is frequent position changes, (i.e., prone to supine to sitting to standing to ambulation). All position changes applicable to the individual are used. Long periods of static positioning are *not* preventive or corrective.

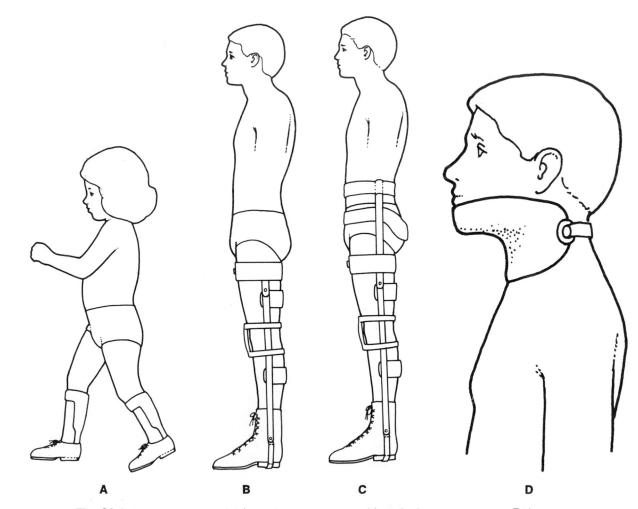

**Fig. 28-2.** Devices that assist in maintenance of position. **A,** Short leg braces. **B,** Long leg braces. **C,** Long leg braces with pelvic band. **D,** Cervical collar.

## Exercise

Prevention of deformity can be achieved by exercise. Active exercise is performed by the individual while passive exercise is accomplished by the therapist or other personnel. Strengthening exercises are especially valuable in contracture and deformity prevention when there is asymmetrical muscle strength. Active or active resistive exercise is a means of strengthening the weakened muscle, which gives more symmetrical movement of the joint. Well chosen mobility exercises can assist in reducing muscle tone (spasticity) and therefore reduce the deformities resulting from spasticity. In the individual with increased muscle tone, proper positioning during both waking and sleeping hours is more critical than an itemized exercise program.

## Range of motion

Range of motion, which is used by the occupational and physical therapist for patient assessment, is also useful in preventing contractures and maintaining joint motion and mobility. Table 28-1 shows the positioning for active antigravity or gravity-eliminated exercises that accomplish range of motion of upper and lower extremities.

*Text continued on p. 708.*

**Table 28-1.** Range-of-motion exercises

**Upper extremity: Shoulder**

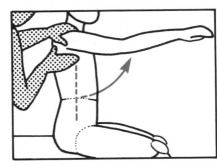

**Flexion:** Sitting; shoulder at side, then raised to 90° angle; antigravity

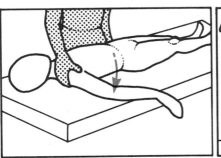

**Abduction:** Supine; arm at side, then lift to 90° to body; gravity eliminated

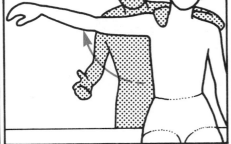

**Abduction:** Sitting; arm at side, then lift arm level with shoulder; antigravity

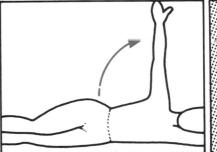

**Abduction:** Side-lying; arm at 90° angle to shoulder; antigravity

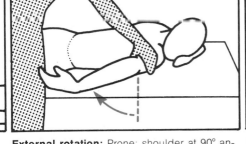

**External rotation:** Prone; shoulder at 90° angle to trunk, elbow parallel to trunk with palm flat on table; with elbow flexed, move palm 180° until it rests with dorsum of hand flat

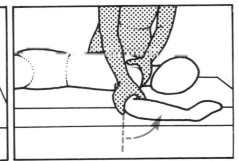

**Internal rotation:** Reverse of external rotation

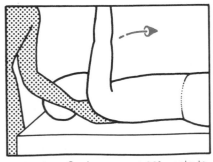

**Adduction:** Supine; arm at 90° angle to body, then move arm over midline of body

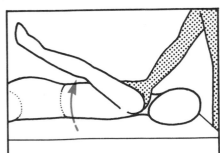

**Extension:** Prone; arms flat at side, then raise to about 70°

*Continued.*

**Table 28-1.** Range-of-motion exercises—cont'd

**Upper extremity: Elbow**

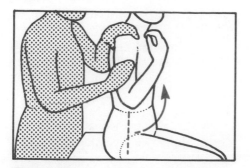

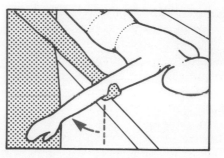

**Flexion:** Sitting; arm hanging at side, then lift arm as far as it will go (160°); antigravity

**Extension:** Prone; arm bent at elbow over edge of table or bed, then straighten at elbow

**Upper extremity: Forearm/wrist**

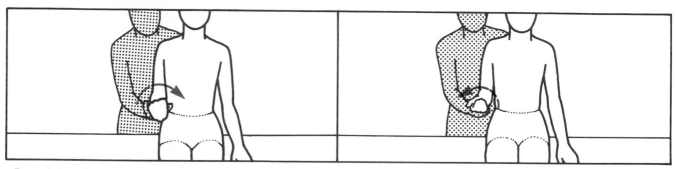

**Pronation-supination:** Sitting; arm flat at side, elbow bent at 90°, palm facing down; then turn palm over, maintaining elbow at side, until palm faces upward; reverse procedure

**Upper extremity: Wrist**

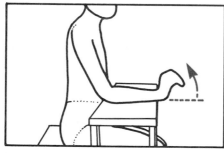

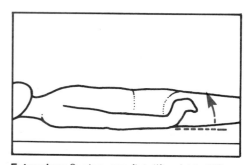

**Extension:** Sitting; elbow bent; lift wrist to 90°

**Extension:** Supine; arm flat; lift wrist to 90°

**Lower extremity: Hip**

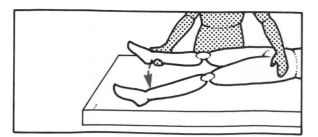

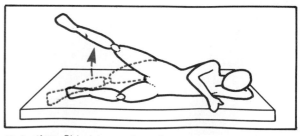

**Abduction:** Supine; gravity eliminated

**Abduction:** Side-lying; antigravity

**Table 28-1.** Range-of-motion exercises—cont'd

**Lower extremity: Hip—cont'd**

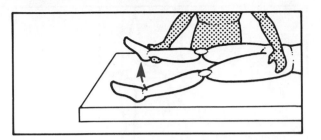

**Adduction:** Supine; gravity eliminated

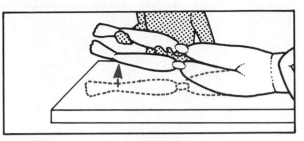

**Adduction:** Side-lying antigravity

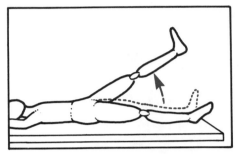

**Flexion:** Supine; straight leg raising; antigravity

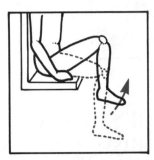

**Flexion:** Sitting; knee flexion of 90°, then pull knee toward chest; antigravity

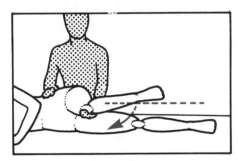

**Flexion:** Side-lying; gravity eliminated

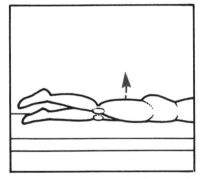

**Extension:** Prone; raise leg backward; antigravity

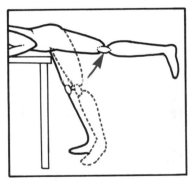

**Extension:** Prone; flex hip over table, then raise leg; antigravity

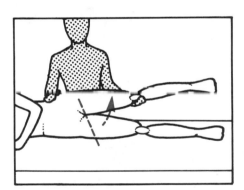

**Extension:** Side-lying; gravity eliminated

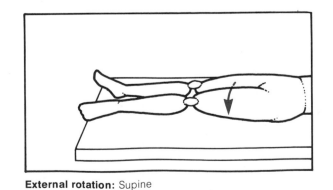

**External rotation:** Supine

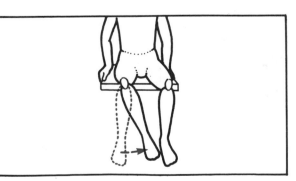

**External rotation:** Sitting

*Continued.*

**Table 28-1.** Range-of-motion exercises—cont'd

**Lower extremity: Hip—cont'd**

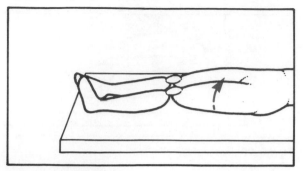

**Internal rotation:** Supine

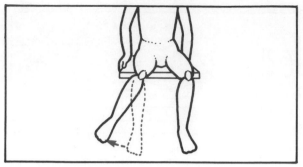

**Internal rotation:** Sitting

**Lower extremity: Knee**

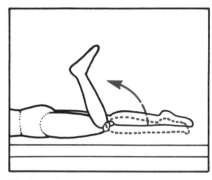

**Flexion:** Prone; antigravity

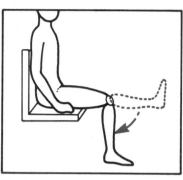

**Flexion:** Sitting; gravity eliminated

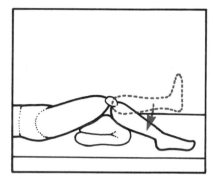

**Flexion:** Supine; roll or pillow under knee

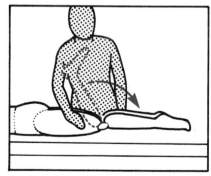

**Extension:** Prone; gravity assisted

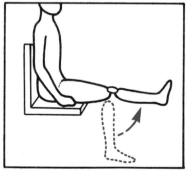

**Extension:** Sitting; antigravity

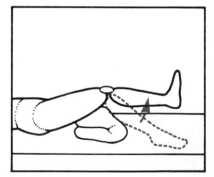

**Extension:** Supine; roll or pillow under knee

**Lower extremity: Ankle**

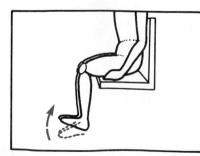

**Dorsiflexion:** Sitting; antigravity

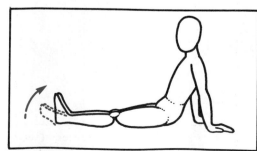

**Dorsiflexion:** Supine; gravity eliminated

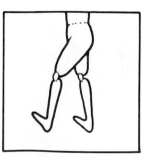

**Dorsiflexion:** Heel walking; antigravity

**Table 28-1.** Range-of-motion exercises—cont'd

**Lower extremity: Ankle—cont'd**

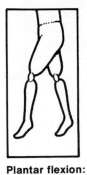 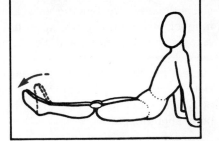 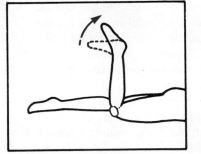 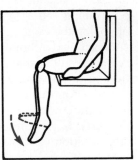

**Plantar flexion:** Toe walking

**Plantar flexion:** Supine

**Plantar flexion:** Prone; antigravity

**Plantar flexion:** Sitting; gravity assisted

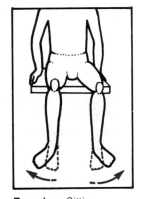 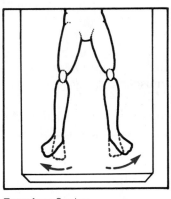

**Eversion:** Sitting

**Eversion:** Supine

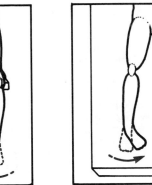 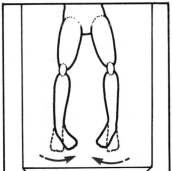

**Inversion:** Sitting

**Inversion:** Supine

**Lower extremity: Toe**

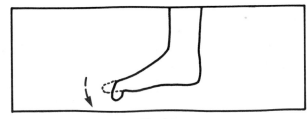 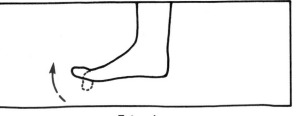

**Flexion**

**Extension**

## TREATMENT OF PRE-EXISTING DEFORMITIES

If deformity or contractures are present because of tight masculature rather than bony deformity, positioning and active exercise working the muscle opposing the contracture are useful in reducing the contracture; without treatment permanent deformity may result. Table 28-2 gives suggestions for positioning and exercise to reduce the most common types of contractures.

Treatment for contractures of the hand other than the wrist have not been included in the table. Specific positioning for the hand varies widely with the type of injury or condition, and contraindications are numerous. Several good references on treatment of hand injuries are available in the literature. Care of hand deformities should be carried out only by an experienced therapist with the supervision of a qualified physician.

Active exercises (those done *by* not *to* the individual), are a means of maintaining joint motion and muscle strength. There are several types of exercises, determined by the muscle activity, to accomplish this goal.

*Isometric* exercise consists of contracting the muscle in a fixed position—not moving the body segment through a range of motion. Quadriceps setting is an example of isometric exercise and is an excellent way to maintain quadriceps strength while immobilized in a long leg cast and provide free knee motion at the time of cast removal.

*Isotonic* exercise refers to contraction of a muscle resulting in movement through the joint range of motion. Resistance can be added to isometric or isotonic exercise manually or by application of weights as progressive resistive exercise for strengthening. Systematic increases in weight or number of repetitions are accepted methods of increasing muscle strength and endurance.

Push-ups, sit-ups, deep-breathing, stair-climbing, ambulation, and other weightbearing activities assist in maintaining strength and range of motion, provided they are done correctly and with good body alignment.

### Children vs adults

While many of the same principles are used in both adult and pediatric conditions, the method of approaching the patient is different because of the differences in perception. While an adult can understand the reasons for exercise or positioning, a child is not as easily convinced of the benefits of such measures. Creativity on the part of staff working with children can smooth over reluctance on the part of the young patient. Range of motion or strengthening exercises can be converted into games, particularly when more than one child is involved. Role modeling using a favorite doll or stuffed animal is also helpful. Competition with staff can be used effectively in certain instances as well. It is important not to set up a win-lose situation with the patient, however, since this often results in an ongoing power struggle.

**Table 28-2.** Positioning and exercise for treatment of deformities and contractures

| Deformity/contracture | Positioning | Exercise |
| --- | --- | --- |
| **Upper extremity** | | |
| Shoulder adduction | Side-lying on affected side with arm positioned overhead<br>Supine or prone with shoulder in 90° of abduction and externally rotated; elbow may be flexed; airplane splint (see Fig. 28-1, *E*) may be used when prescribed; foam wedge may be used under arm to maintain position | Passive movement: patient supine, arm by side; move through abduction<br>  Support arm at or just above elbow while placing other hand above shoulder joint to stabilize<br>Full range (180°)<br>  If full range not attainable, move to point of pain, hold briefly, then return<br>  For active exercise use same exercise in sitting position to allow for gravity resistance |
| Internal rotation | Supine with arm abducted and externally rotated<br>If full range not attainable pillow under forearm may be used<br>Foam wedge may be used to maintain position | Passive movement: patient supine with shoulder abducted, elbow flexed, and internally rotated.<br>  Forearm is moved from full internal rotation to point of pain<br>Active movement: patient prone with shoulder abducted and elbow flexed over edge of bed<br>  Arm actively brought to full external rotation or as far as possible |

**Table 28-2.** Positioning and exercise for treatment of deformities and contractures—cont'd

| Deformity/contracture | Positioning | Exercise |
|---|---|---|
| Elbow flexion | Supine or prone with arm extended by side<br>Posterior shell splint may be used to maintain range or serial casting or splinting used to increase range | Prone with shoulder abducted, elbow flexed over edge of bed<br>  Passive range: one hand above elbow joint and one below; move to point of pain<br>  Active range: same without stretching resistance below elbow |
| Pronation contracture | Posterior shell with elbow flexed and supinated | Elbow flexed and firmly at side in pronation; one hand to stabilize at elbow, one to turn just above wrist; turn to point of pain |
| Wrist flexion | Wrist cock-up splint or platform (Fig. 28-1, B) | Stabilize above wrist; hold in palm of hand; bring to point of pain |
| Lateral flexion of head (torticollis) | Head in midline when supine<br>Neck conformer or soft collar may be used (Fig. 28-2, D)<br>Side-lying toward side of pull | Head brought from midline to one side, then the other |
| Head flexion | Supine with no pillow<br>Supine with pillow under shoulders instead of head | Prone, head lifted to extension |

**Lower extremity**

| Deformity/contracture | Positioning | Exercise |
|---|---|---|
| Hip flexors | Prone; use pillow under abdomen if necessary to reduce lumbar lordosis<br>For children: prone on scooter board or tilt cart (Fig. 28-3, A and B)<br>Standing: standing brace or standing table (Fig. 28-3, C and D) | Active hip extension while prone<br>Active hip extension over edge of table<br>Passive stretch of hip flexors<br>Walking and standing |
| Hip adductors | Abductor pillow while sleeping or anytime patient is in bed (Fig. 28-1, C)<br>Abductor splint: bar attached to shoes with hips held in abduction; can be worn as night splint<br>Abduction bar between casts: most often used following hip surgery, especially hip adductor release | Active antigravity abductor strengthening in side-lying position.<br>Active abductor strengthening while supine; gravity eliminated<br>Passive stretch or ROM of abductors<br>Standing on prone board with abduction pummel or standing in casts with abductor bar |
| Knee flexion (hamstrings) | Posterior splint from ankle to hip with knee pad or wrapped on with Ace bandage; used as night splint and if not ambulatory and sitting most of day<br>Long leg brace with knee joint locked except during exercise (Fig. 28-2, B)<br>Prolonged stretch into extension while prone<br>Wedging casts with frequent changes | Quadriceps setting every hour<br>Active knee extension through range of motion possible<br>Weight bearing stressing knee extension<br>Weight bearing with long leg brace if patient wears a long leg orthosis<br>Weight bearing in standing table or brace<br>Passive hamstring stretch |
| Knee extension: quadriceps; (often occurs following long-term casting in full-length lower extremity casts) | Sitting in chair or over edge of table, increasing flexion as tolerated; keep thigh supported on table or chair<br>Prone with lower leg and ankle supported; gradually increase knee flexion as tolerated<br>Footboard | Active knee flexion (hamstring) exercise<br>Passive knee flexion with gentle stretch<br>Tricycle or bicycle riding, depending on age of individual<br>Stair climbing |
| Plantar flexors: gastrocnemius and soleus | Plaster cast posterior splint with ankle at 90°; used as night splint; may be held in position with Ace bandage<br>Ankle-foot orthosis with ankle joint set at neutral (Fig. 28-2, A) | Active dorsiflexion<br>Walking up ramps and inclines<br>Weight bearing to include standing and ambulation (heels must be on ground)<br>Stretch of heelcord: passive by PT or member of family; by patient leaning forward to wall, keeping heels flat on floor<br>Heel walking |
| Dorsiflexors: anterior tibial | Ankle-foot orthosis; can be worn as night splint or all day<br>Cast application | Toe walking<br>Active plantar flexion<br>Passive ROM<br>Ambulation and standing while feet are casted |

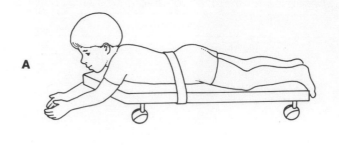

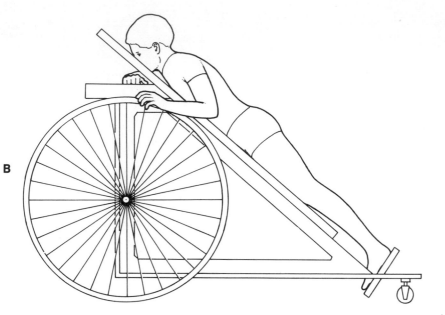

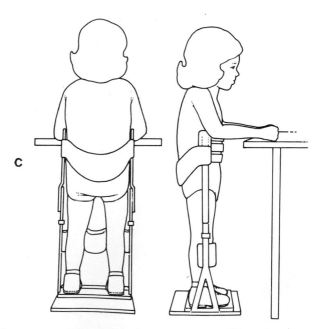

**Fig. 28-3.** Equipment used for weight bearing, ambulation, or mobilization. **A,** Scooter board. **B,** Tilt cart. **C,** Standing (parapodium) brace.

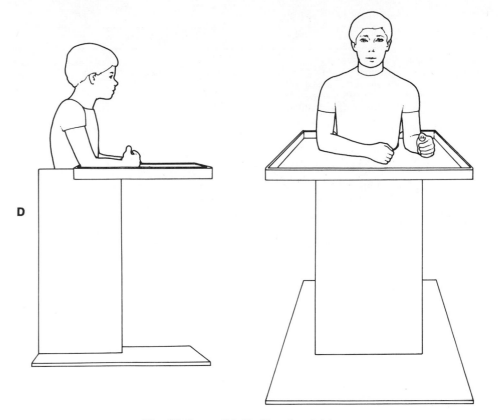

D

**Fig. 28-3, cont'd. D,** Standing table.

## EVALUATION FOR FUNCTIONAL INDEPENDENCE

A priority of occupational and physical therapy is to establish the individual's functional skills, and, if these are lacking, to develop the means to achieve the highest possible functional ability in order to reach the goal of independence. The same level of independence is not available to all individuals but decisions need to be made regarding the level anticipated and the program plan for achievement of the goal. Table 28-3 is an outline of some of the functional activities to be evaluated and placed in the training program if needed and if possible within the realm of the disability. Again the therapist and other staff members need to know the patient before determining the training program.

### Ambulation

The patient's need for gait training and assistive devices may be temporary or permanent depending on the condition being treated. Casting following trauma or surgery may require nonweightbearing or partial weightbearing for a limited period of time. In some of the congenital or traumatic situations, however, assistive devices and an altered gait pattern may become a permanent mode of mobility.

The crutch gait pattern used will depend on the patient's diagnosis and physical and functional abilities. The most common crutch gaits (Fig. 28-4) are:

1. 3-point gaits—crutches used with involved leg (usually progress to full weightbearing; more frequently a temporary gait pattern used by patients with casting)
   a. Nonweightbearing on involved leg
   b. Touch-down gait—touching floor with involved leg
   c. Partial weightbearing—some weight placed on individual leg
2. 4-point gait—provides stability by using legs and crutches individually
3. 2-point gait—uses one crutch with opposite leg
4. Swing-to or swing-through gait—used most frequently by paraplegic patients of any age; patients usually wear braces and propel themselves by swinging entire body below the waist to or through the crutches.

## ACTIVITIES OF DAILY LIVING

While exercises, passive range of motion, and positioning are important in maintaining optimal function in the hospitalized patient, routine self-

**Table 28-3.** Components of evaluation of functional skills

| Functional skill | Components |
|---|---|
| Head control and sitting balance | Supported by chair or brace<br>Unsupported by devices but using hands or arms for balance<br>Unsupported, no assistive devices<br>Long sitting<br>Cross-legged sitting (tailor-fashion)<br>Side sitting<br>Protective and righting abilities in sitting position |
| Mobility (independent or assisted) | Sitting-standing-ambulation<br>Sitting-standing-sitting<br>Transfers from wheelchair to toilet, bed, or chair<br>From prone or supine to sitting position<br>Lying or sitting on floor–kneeling-standing |
| Standing balance | Unsupported, no assistive devices<br>Supported with crutches, canes, or walker; bracing (long leg orthosis, ankle-foot orthosis, trunk orthosis); standing table, standing brace<br>Protective responses while standing |
| Ambulation | Independent, no assistive devices<br>Independent with devices (orthosis, crutches, canes)<br>Supervised ambulation without manual assistance with or without devices<br>Manual assistance with or without devices |

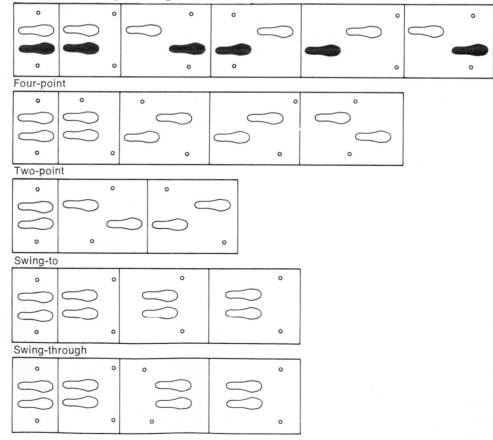

**Fig. 28-4.** Crutch gaits. (From Hilt, N. E., and Schmitt E. W., Jr.: Pediatric orthopedic nursing, St. Louis, 1975, The C. V. Mosby Co.)

care activities provide another means of achieving this goal. When patients are encouraged to do as much as possible in taking care of their needs, they are able to realize what their bodies are capable of and how to make the most of their potential. Equally important is the boost to the patient's self-concept gained by independence. Some simple suggestions for facilitating independence in feeding, dressing, hygiene, and toileting are given below, as well as ideas for appropriate adaptive equipment.

## Feeding

When broken down into components, the skills necessary for feeding include (1) head control, (2) trunk control, (3) at least partial use of one upper extremity, (4) enough oral control to allow jaw opening and closing, chewing, and swallowing, and (5) visual-motor coordination to allow for hand-to-mouth movements. By discussing each component individually, we will present some common problems and solutions.

**Head and trunk control.** Many patients are confined to bed in casts or traction or are otherwise immobilized. In these circumstances, the patient often cannot even be elevated to a sitting position in the bed. Whenever possible, the prone position is preferable to supine. This allows the patient to see the tray and to bring food up to his mouth without spilling it on himself as often occurs when supine. An adjustable bedside table can be placed within easy reach of the patient who is lying prone propped on his elbows. In the case of a CircOlectric bed or Stryker frame, food can be placed underneath or in front of the patient.

Patients who are confined to the flat, supine position can have their head supported by pillows or a wedge to allow better visualization of the tray. An adjustable bedside table positioned as low as possible places food within reach. The recessed trays available in most hospitals allow for food to be scooped even though it is on the same horizontal plane as the patient.

The patient who can be elevated to a sitting position in bed obviously should be elevated for all meals. Asymmetries in trunk or extremity control can cause slipping to the side. Elevating the bed to 75 instead of 90 degrees can alleviate this. Propping a flail arm on the bed table or on pillows will do the same.

Whenever possible, the patient should be encouraged to eat in a chair rather than in bed. A lap tray or bedside table provides a stable surface to eat from. Positioning in the chair is critical for the patient with incomplete or asymmetrical control of

trunk. The patient who is not stable in a sitting position will not be able to feed himself comfortably. Seat inserts or lateral supports should be provided by the therapist when indicated.

**Partial use of upper extremity.** A patient with at least partial use of one upper extremity can be fully independent in eating. The range of commercially available adapted utensils is considerable. In Table 28-4 some of the simpler devices and practical applications are indicated. In addition, overhead slings and balanced forearm orthoses are often used to provide hand placement in the individual without shoulder function. These devices are usually fitted by an occupational therapist who also trains the patient in their use.

**Oral function.** Assessment of oral function is done by a licensed speech pathologist. Soft food can facilitate independent eating in the patient who cannot chew or who has difficulty in swallowing.

**Visual-motor control.** This can be a particular problem in head trauma victims, and in patients with long-term degenerative diseases such as multiple sclerosis or chronic conditions such as cerebral palsy. Minor incoordination can usually be managed by adjustment in the speed of eating. Greater difficulties can be treated by continuing therapy programs.

A word of caution regarding assistive devices. The patient should use only devices that are necessary. Gadgetry can be carried to extremes, causing the patient to be dependent on tools that are not needed.

## Dressing

This area would be more applicable to the long-term hospital patient. Even if dressing is confined to a regular change of night clothes, it represents an important part of daily care. Even an individual without lower extremity control or use of only one side of the body can and should be independent in dressing.

**Bed-confined patients.** The individual who is not in traction or immobilized can use some simple techniques to be independent. Patients who are able to sit should have no difficulty in dressing. Lack of trunk control can be compensated for by using side-to-side rolling to dress the lower extremities (Fig. 28-5, C). If the patient cannot roll independently, side rails or a strap attached to the side boards can be used.

**Hemiplegic patient.** Standard dressing techniques for the hemiplegic are demonstrated in Fig. 28-5, A and B. It is critical that the patient have adequate balance to sit before trying these techniques. If the

**Table 28-4.** Adapted eating utensils

| Utensil | Indications |
|---------|-------------|
| Built up handles | Weak grasp caused by intrinsic minus hand; limitation in metacarpal-phalangeal PIP and DIP joint flexion; absent or poor thumb use; median nerve injury causing weak finger flexion |

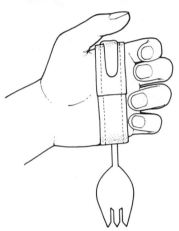

| | |
|---------|-------------|
| Swivel utensils (often built up as well) | Limitation in elbow supination or wrist mobility |
| Long-handled utensils or iced tea spoon | Limitation in elbow or shoulder flexion; elbow or shoulder weakness; rigid or immobile neck and trunk with elbow and shoulder weakness or limitation |
| Orthotic cuff | Absent grasp |

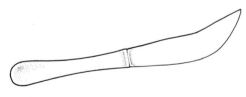

| | |
|---------|-------------|
| Rocker knife | Use of one hand only |

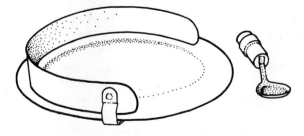

| | |
|---------|-------------|
| Plate guard, deep plate | Use of one hand only; incorrdination; intention tremor; poor grasp |

patient does not have good balance he or she should be seated in a chair with arms and have supervision throughout the procedure.

In addition to specific techniques, there are also commercially available devices to assist in dressing. These devices are primarily special fasteners (i.e., button aids, Velcro, zipper rings, etc.). Size of clothing and quality of fabric can also affect the ease with which a patient dresses. Using clothing one size larger than normally worn is helpful for the per-

son learning to dress independently. Knit fabrics have more give and stretch over immobile or stiff joints.

**Toileting**

Creative solutions for the bedridden patient in this area are nonexistent. The bedpan remains the major solution to toileting for patients in casts or confined to bed.

The individual who can sit or ambulate has a few

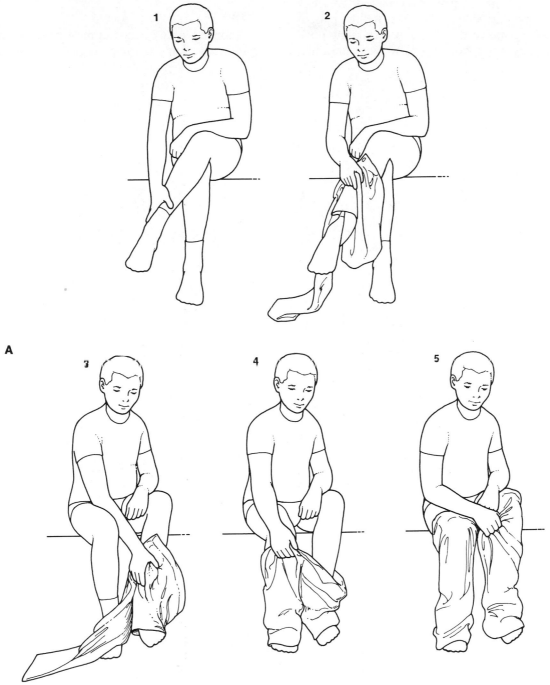

**Fig. 28-5. A** and **B,** Dressing techniques for hemiplegic patient.

*Continued.*

more options available. Commode chairs are an alternative for the patient who can be transferred out of bed but cannot ambulate to the bathroom. Many of these are equipped with casters, which should be either locked or removed before the patient is transferred as a safety precaution.

Aids in the bathroom are fairly basic. The patient who is lacking mobility at the hips or knees can use a raised toilet seat. A safety bar placed to the side of the seat may provide lateral stability for the patient with unstable trunk control. Wall or floor bars can be placed on either side of the toilet for the patient who needs assistance in pulling to a standing position. There are a few commercially available toilet seats for patients with adductor tightness, thus providing a wide base of support for the most comfortable sitting.

Patients with Risser casts, halo casts, neck conformers, or with limited spine mobility may have difficulty cleansing themselves after a bowel movement. Several more common varieties of long-handled reachers are pictured in Fig. 28-6. Simple devices such as these may make a major difference in independence in the bathroom.

### Hygiene

Sponge bathing is sometimes the only method of bathing available to the patient in traction or a body

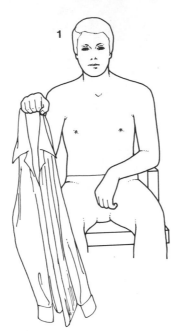
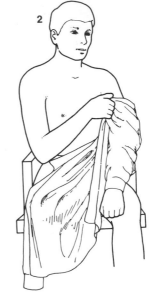
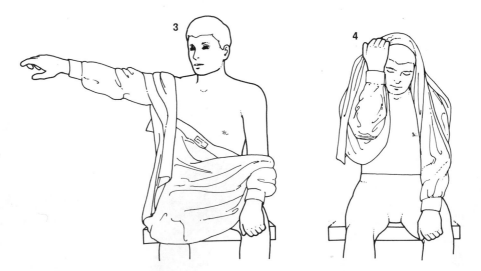

**Fig. 28-5, cont'd. B,** Dressing techniques for hemiplegic patient.

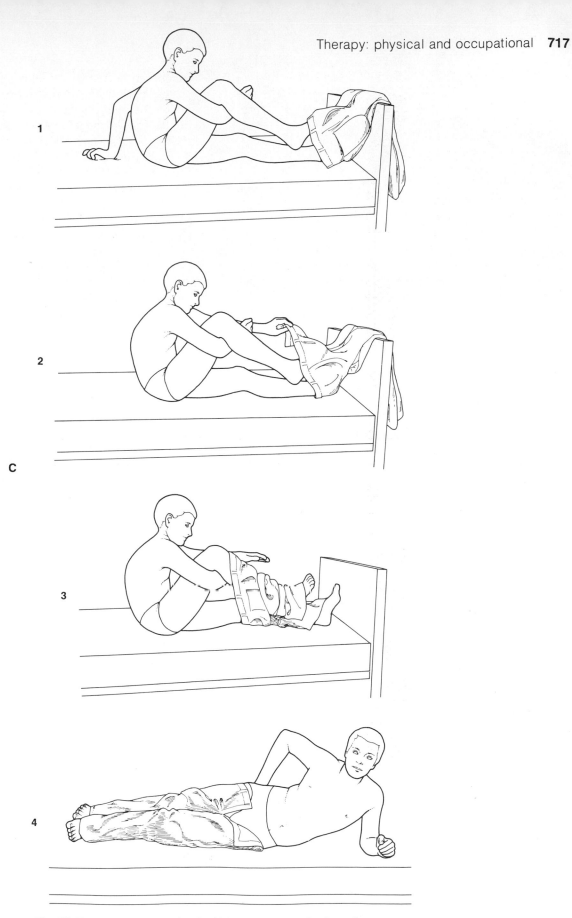

**Fig. 28-5, cont'd. C,** Dressing techniques for paraplegic patients.

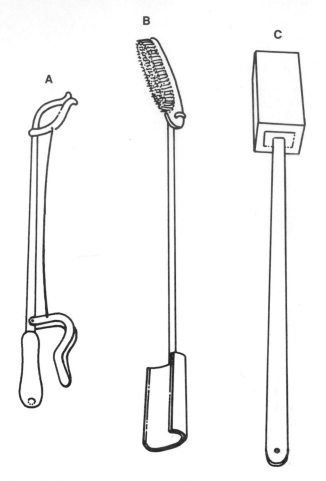

**Fig. 28-6.** Devices to assist with personal hygiene. **A,** Long-handled grasper. **B,** Long-handled brush. **C,** Long-handled sponge.

cast. The patient should be encouraged to do as much as possible. Easy access to soap, basin, towels, and washcloth is imperative. Patients who can be elevated are better able to reach their legs than individuals who are flat.

Encouragement of self-care early in the treatment of individuals with the use of only one hand or one side can facilitate independence when this patient is out of bed. Learning to bathe and care for a non-

functional extremity should begin early in the recovery period. Bath mitts (commercially available) which slip over one hand often have a place for soap in the mitt. This eliminates the awkwardness of trying to grasp a wet bar of soap with one hand. Another device is "soap on a rope" which can be slipped around the neck and is easily accessible.

In hospitals where shower and tub are available to patients, a few simple devices can make life easier for both staff and patients. A chair placed in the shower provides a stable seat for those who cannot stand. Rubber mats on the floor of the shower and tub should be mandatory safety precautions. Bars at chest height in the tub and shower assist the person who needs stability in rising up. Tub seats for bath tubs are available at most hospital supply companies. Those with backs are more useful for a larger variety of patients. This kind of seat allows the person without lower extremity control to transfer in and out of the tub with minimal or no aid. Persons who have restricted reach may benefit from long-handled utensils that allow access to feet or back.

To summarize briefly, independence in activities of daily living provides a further outlet for the patient to deal with altered function. This can be a valuable adjunct to exercise in maintaining muscle function and range of motion. Most important, it allows patients some control over their body in a situation where others (physicians, nurses) may have temporary control. It also provides a boost to self-esteem.

## SUMMARY

Functional independence can take many different avenues depending on diagnosis, functional abilities, motivation, and socioeconomic situation, to mention only a few of the influences on the individual. The goal of both occupational and physical therapy is to help each individual function as independently as possible within his or her environment. This may mean, for some patients, that wheelchair independence is preferable if ambulation can be accomplished only with assistance.

# 29

# Surgical procedures

**E. WILLIAM SCHMITT, Jr.**

This chapter presents a guide to the many operative procedures within the realm of orthopedics. Tables 29-1 through 29-7 give the indications, approach, complications, and usual postoperative course of the procedures listed.

A number of factors guide the orthopedic surgeon in making the decision to proceed with an operative procedure. There may be several variations of one type of operative procedure; the one selected depends on the clinical setting and the patient's status. Usually, the operative procedure is preceded by conservative, nonoperative treatment although in certain instances surgery will be the treatment of choice. Likewise, the surgeon may use a variety of surgical approaches.

There are basic complications common to all procedures, whether emergency or elective surgery. Sepsis is a continual threat that may complicate an exposure of the joint (arthrotomy), leading to a septic joint or, when it involves a bony structure, osteomyelitis. Both of these problems are formidable postoperative complications. Any time an osteotomy or corrective incision of the bony structure is performed to regain corrective alignment in an extremity failure of healing may occur (pseudoarthrosis) or delayed union may complicate the convalescent period. This may also occur where end-to-end bony healing is desired. Certain procedures in bony structures are predisposed to this and these are noted throughout the tables. Likewise, postoperative malalignment or loss of correction is a complication common to similar procedures.

Although there are certain basic principles that each physician will follow in postoperative management, details of treatment may vary from individual to individual. The tables in this chapter cannot begin to enumerate the many possible methods utilized with each surgical procedure but does lay out the general principles involved in the postoperative phase.

Certain basic principles are applied to each operative procedure. It is generally accepted that the patient, regardless of the procedure, may need to use various external support devices, such as crutches, a cane, orthoses, etc., to assist with mobilization prior to and after discharge from the hospital. These devices are usually used until the postoperative goals have been reached and satisfactory stability and control of the extremity or spine have been achieved together with bony union. Certain periods of immobilization may need to be prolonged until postoperative healing is satisfactory or adequate muscular control in tone has been obtained. This time factor may vary highly from patient to patient. The postoperative phase is the variable time factor in the patient's convalescence. Immobilization of a joint or extremity after a period of rest or protection may require continued external support until these goals can be reached.

Whenever a deformity, particularly a flexion contracture of longstanding is corrected, sudden or operative alignment to the corrected position may lead to neurovascular loss. This is likewise a potential complication in those procedures in which the proximity of these structures lend themselves to injury. The procedures which particularly possess this likelihood have been mentioned.

**Table 29-1.** Surgical procedures of the neck, shoulder, and upper arm

| Procedure | Indications | Approach | Complications | Postoperative management |
|---|---|---|---|---|
| Arthrodesis of shoulder | Otherwise unreconstructable instability<br>Symptomatic degenerative arthritis<br>Persistent sepsis<br>Paralytic deformity | Lateral or posterior | Pseudoarthrosis | Spica cast 8 to 12 weeks with additional immobilization until osseous union evident |
| Open reduction of humeral shaft fractures | Displaced humeral shaft fractures not amenable to conservative measures | Lateral | Nonunion<br>Loss of reduction<br>Radial nerve palsy | Long arm cast or posterior splint 6 to 12 weeks; thereafter, gradual range of motion |
| Open reduction, internal fixation of proximal humeral fracture, or fracture dislocation of shoulder | Irreducible proximal humeral fracture, dislocation of shoulder | Anterior | Adhesive capsulitis with loss of range of motion<br>Nonunion<br>Recurrent dislocation<br>Axillary nerve palsy (results in deltoid paralysis leading to loss of abduction at shoulder) | Early mobilization, working to gain improvement of range of motion |
| Release of sternocleidomastoid muscle for torticollis (wryneck) | Surgical correction for persistent torticollis | Transverse incision of proximal and distal aspects of SCM muscle | Interruption of nerve supply to scapular muscles with resultant weakness, winging of scapula | Early range of motion with or without use of postoperative brace or Minerva cast |
| Transfer of latissimus dorsi–teres major of shoulder (Sever-l'Episcopo procedure) | Paralytic loss of abduction and external rotation of shoulder | Anterior or posterior | Neurologic loss resulting in loss of pre-existing abduction at shoulder or flexion at elbow | Shoulder in spica cast with arm in abduction, flexion, and external rotation for 3 to 6 weeks; thereafter, orthosis in similar position until rehabilitation complete |
| Reconstruction of Sprengel's deformity (congenital elevation of scapula) | Functional lack of shoulder elevation secondary to congenital elevation of scapula | Posterior scapula | Neurovascular embarrassment of upper extremity | Variable; use either sling immobilization or single leg spica cast with skeletal traction on scapula; thereafter, mobilization and range-of-motion exercises of upper extremity |
| Steindler flexorplasty of elbow | Paralytic weakness of flexion of elbow with functional wrist and hand flexors | Medial | | Immobilization in long arm cast for 2 weeks; protective immobilization for another 6 weeks |
| Synovectomy of shoulder | Persistent and chronic synovial thickening without destructive articular signs | Anterior | Axillary nerve palsy (loss of abduction)<br>Subluxation of shoulder | Early range-of-motion exercises as clinical status permits |
| Tenorrhaphy of rotator cuff | Symptomatic persistent laceration of rotator cuff limiting abduction of shoulder | Anterior | Adhesive capsulitis of shoulder with loss of motion<br>Recurrent rupture with loss of active abduction of shoulder | Early mobilization in sling with pendulum and active range-of-motion exercises as clinical status permits, particularly at 3 weeks postoperatively |

**Table 29-2.** Surgical procedures of the elbow and forearm

| Procedure | Indications | Approach | Complications | Postoperative management |
|---|---|---|---|---|
| Arthrodesis of elbow | Symptomatic degenerative arthritis; persistent sepsis Unreconstructable instability Paralytic deformity | Posterolateral | Pseudoarthrosis with loss of position Ulnar nerve palsy | Immobilization in long arm cast for 8 weeks or until osseous union is evident |
| Bone graft to radius or ulna | Nonunion of radius or ulna following trauma or osteotomy | Medial or lateral | Persistent nonunion Bony fusion between radius and ulna | Immobilization as necessary, usually 3 to 6 months, until bony union is solid |
| Fasciotomy of forearm | Volkmann's ischemic contracture of forearm | Volar (forearm) | Recurrence of pathologic condition | Immobilization in early phases in functional position; thereafter, early motion as clinical status allows |
| Incision of extensor origin of elbow | Persistent and recurrent tennis elbow | Lateral | | Active, early motion |
| Open reduction of radial head | Displaced radial head fracture, particularly in young person | Lateral | Loss of reduction Nonunion | Motion at 3 to 6 weeks postoperatively with removal of K wire fixation; thereafter, gradual range of motion |
| Radial head excision or prosthetic replacement | Comminuted radial head neck fracture Degenerative arthritis of radioulnar joint Angular or congenital anomaly with bony protuberance subject to repeated trauma | Lateral | Radial nerve palsy Distal radioulnar pain with proximal radial migration Radial neck subluxation | Early range of motion as clinical status allows |
| Reduction of supracondylar fracture of elbow | Comminuted or displaced condylar fracture of elbow not responding to nonoperative measures | Posteromedial or lateral | Radial and ulnar nerve palsy Volkmann's ischemic contracture of forearm musculature Loss of reduction Nonunion | Posterior splint with removal of internal fixation device; healing time 6 to 12 weeks |

**Table 29-3.** Surgical procedures of the hand and wrist

| Procedure | Indications | Approach | Complications | Postoperative management |
|---|---|---|---|---|
| Adductor tenotomy of thumb or flexor release of thumb-in-palm deformity | Thumb-in-palm deformity in spastic patients | Volar or palmar | Recurrence of deformity Weakness of thumb flexion | Usually associated with other tendon transfer; mobilization begun as other transfer allows |
| Arthrodesis of interphalangeal or metacarpal phalangeal joints | Nonreconstructable instability of joint for congenital or posttraumatic deformity Painful arthritis not amenable to other reconstructive procedures | Dorsomedial | Nonunion Loss of position | Immobilization by intraarticular K wires, dressing, or splints for 4 to 6 weeks |
| Arthrodesis of wrist | Chronic and symptomatic instability Symptomatic degenerative arthritis unreconstructable by other means | Dorsal | Median and ulnar nerve palsy Vascular impairment Pseudoarthrosis with loss of position | Immobilization in long or short arm cast until osseous union evident, usually 8 to 10 weeks |
| Carpal tunnel release (volar compression of median nerve) | Symptomatic compression of median nerve at wrist | Volar | Recurrent symptoms Median nerve injury | Immobilization until comfortable; early range of motion; use of hand to comfort |
| Flexor tendon laceration repair | Laceration of flexor tendons | Volar | Flexion contracture with loss of function and failure to perform satisfactory functional flexion | Varies highly but usually early motion in acute flexion; orthotic devices for at least 3 to 6 weeks |
| Open reduction of dislocation of thumb carpophalangeal joint | Injury as noted with disruption of ligamentous stability and failure to respond to nonoperative measures | Lateral to involved joint | Recurrent dislocation Instability Painful neuroma | Immobilization with either intraarticular wire for 3 to 6 weeks and bulky dressing or cast; splint immobilization for same period; wire suture may be removed at 3 to 6 weeks |
| Phalangeal collateral ligament injury repair | Rupture of phalangeal collateral ligament requiring open repair | Medial or lateral | Recurrent instability Loss of motion | Immobilization for 3 to 6 weeks; wire suture removed at 3 to 6 weeks |
| Syndactyly release | Deforming syndactyly of fingers | Dorsal and medial | Loss of skin Neurovascular interruption Recurrence of skin webs | Immobilization with bulky dressing until skin and graft sites healed |

**Table 29-4.** Surgical procedures of the hip and upper leg

| Procedure | Indications | Approach | Complications | Postoperative management |
|---|---|---|---|---|
| Release of abduction contracture of hip (Ober and Yount procedure) (proximal and distal releases) | Abduction contracture of hip, symptomatic | Anterolateral (proximal); lateral (distal) | Recurrence of contracture | Immobilization for 3 to 6 weeks in spica cast with leg in adduction or on hyperextension bed, alternating flexion and extension with limbs adducted to further stretch muscular components of iliotibial tract, may be maintained for 2 to 3 weeks; thereafter, active physiotherapy program |
| Above-knee amputation | Neurologic, vascular, or posttraumatic injury necessitating amputation<br>Congenital anomalies necessitating amputation<br>Tumors<br>Malignant or chronic sepsis necessitating amputation | Transverse | Loss of skin flap with bony overgrowth in young persons | Immobilization in rigid plaster dressing or prosthesis as clinical status allows |
| Adductor tenotomy and anterior branch obturator neurectomy | Adduction deformity of hip in patients with spasticity | Medial | Persistent abduction of hip | Hip spica cast or bilateral long leg cast in abduction for 6 to 10 weeks; abduction strengthening; mobilization with external support as necessary |
| Arthrodesis of hip | Unilateral unreconstructable symptomatic degenerative arthritis or instability of hip<br>Chronic sepsis<br>Unilateral hip disease in young with major loss of bony elements | Lateral or anterolateral | Pseudoarthrosis<br>Sciatic palsy<br>Symptomatic knee instability<br>Low back pain | Immobilization as necessary in spica cast until osseous union is complete, usually 3 to 6 months |
| Femoral shortening | Equalization of limb lengths in mature individual | Lateral femoral | Pseudoarthrosis<br>Femoral fracture | Internal fixation, particularly intramedullary rod fixation; protective weight bearing for 12 to 14 weeks until osteotomy site heals |
| Hindquarter amputation | Neurologic, vascular, or posttraumatic loss necessitating amputation<br>Congenital anomalies necessitating amputation<br>Malignant tumors<br>Chronic sepsis necessitating amputation | Anterior and posterior | Sepsis<br>Loss of skin flap | Ambulation in prosthesis as clinical status allows |
| Iliopsoas recession of hip | Internal rotation during gait secondary to spasticity | Anterior | Flexion weakness of hip | Bedrest with an occasional immobilization in hip spica cast 3 to 6 weeks; ambulation as clinical status allows |
| Innominate osteotomy of hip (Salter, Pemberton, Chiari, Steel, Southerland procedures) | Persistent lack of acetabular development or subluxation of hip<br>Neuromuscular subluxation of hip<br>Subluxation of hip secondary to Legg-Perthes disease | Anterolateral | Loss of position postoperatively with recurrent subluxation<br>Pin migration | May be internally fixed with threaded or smooth pins, which are usually removed 6 to 12 weeks postoperatively; spica cast 6 to 12 weeks; thereafter, progressive ambulation with external support as necessary |

Surgical procedures **723**

**Table 29-4.** Surgical procedures of the hip and upper leg—cont'd

| Procedure | Indications | Approach | Complications | Postoperative management |
|---|---|---|---|---|
| Mold arthroplasty of hip | Degenerative arthritis of hip, particularly young patients not suitable for total hip reconstruction<br>Postseptic degenerative arthritis | Anterior or lateral | Heterotrophic bone formation with secondary loss of motion<br>Avascular necrosis of bone within cup necessitating revision | Crutches for 6 to 9 months, cane for additional 6 months; requires extensive patient cooperation and extensive exercise program |
| Open reduction or capsulorrhaphy of congenital dislocation of hip | Dislocation of hip in patient unsuitable for or failing to respond to nonoperative management | Anterior | Recurrent dislocation<br>Avascular necrosis of capital femoral epiphysis<br>Femoral nerve palsy (weakness of quadriceps muscle) | Immobilization in spica cast, traction, or abduction brace for 6 to 12 weeks; thereafter, progressive range of motion and ambulation with external support as necessary |
| Open reduction of femoral fractures | Femoral shaft fractures requiring open reduction | Lateral femoral | Nonunion or delayed union with loss of reduction<br>Shortening of extremity<br>Postoperative thrombophebitis | Internal fixation device; ambulation tolerated with touchdown gait until union apparent, usually 3 months postoperatively |
| Open reduction and internal fixation of proximal femoral fractures | Intertrochanteric or pretrochanteric fractures of proximal femur not amenable to closed treatment | Lateral | Delayed union or nonunion or loss of reduction<br>Postoperative thrombophlebitis<br>Pulmonary complications in elderly | Ambulation allowed with crutches as tolerated, usually with touch-down gait on involved side until union apparent at 3 months; internal fixation device may need to be removed in the young 1 to 2 years postoperatively |
| Proximal temoral osteotomy | Correct angular deformity<br>Degenerative arthritis in young patient with satisfactory motion<br>Realignment of femur to maintain acceptable alignment with acetabulum | Lateral | Loss of correction<br>Pseudoarthrosis | Depends on age of patient; may necessitate immobilization postoperatively in spica cast; older patients with satisfactory internal fixation may only need crutches until osteotomy site is healed |
| Replacement prosthesis for femoral neck fracture | Femoral neck fracture not amenable to open reduction or internal fixation, particularly in elderly patients<br>Avascular necrosis of femoral head | Anterolateral or posterior | Loosening of prosthesis<br>Increase in symptoms of osteoarthritis<br>Dislocation of prosthesis | Bedrest until postoperative situation stable; thereafter, ambulation with external support; early mobilization to prevent postoperative phlebitis and pulmonary complications |
| Southwick biplane femoral osteotomy | Slipped capital femoral epiphysis with unsatisfactory posterior and medial displacement of capital femoral epiphysis | Lateral | Femoral shortening<br>Loss of motion<br>Loss of position<br>Pseudoarthrosis | Bedrest until postoperative situation stable; thereafter, ambulation with external support; early mobilization to prevent postoperative phlebitis and pulmonary complications |
| Transfer of iliopsoas muscle to greater trochanter | Paralytic loss of abduction of hip with or without paralytic subluxation-dislocation | Anterior | Recurrent dislocation<br>Heterotrophic bone formation<br>Femoral nerve palsy | Immobilization in spica cast for 6 to 10 weeks; thereafter, exercise program to retain transfer with external support and ambulation |
| Varus osteotomy of femur | Valgus deformity of femur | Lateral | Relative femoral shortening<br>Pseudoarthrosis | Immobilization in spica cast (proximal) or long leg cast (distal), depending on age of individual and internal fixation device used; usual healing time 12 weeks |

**Table 29-5.** Surgical procedures of the knee and lower leg

| Procedure | Indications | Approach | Complications | Postoperative management |
|---|---|---|---|---|
| Arthrodesis of knee | Symptomatic and otherwise non-reconstructable degenerative arthritis of knee; Chronic sepsis; Chronic and symptomatic instability of knee | Medial parapatellar | Nonunion; Sepsis; Loss of correction | Immobilization in cylinder cast or other external support for 8 to 12 weeks or until osseous union is complete; Charnley compression apparatus may be utilized for 6 to 12 weeks |
| Below-knee amputation | Neurologic, vascular, or post-traumatic losses necessitating amputation; Congenital anomalies necessitating amputation; Malignant tumors; Chronic sepsis necessitating amputation | Transverse, below knee | Skin loss; Phantom limb pain | May be fitted with temporary prosthesis; early immobilization cast to be followed by patellar tendon-bearing or other prosthesis to assist ambulation |
| Eggers procedure of knee | Flexion deformity of cerebral palsy | Posterior popliteal | Recurrence of deformity | Symptomatic splinting until postoperative symptoms allow active exercise program |
| Epiphysiodesis of distal femur–proximal tibia | Equalization of limb lengths by epiphyseal arrest | Medial and lateral | Incomplete arrest of epiphysis leading to either angular deformity or continued growth of extremity | Cylinder or long leg cast for 3 to 6 weeks; progressive motion and weight bearing as limb strength improves |
| Excision of Baker's cyst of knee | Painful recurrent synovial cyst of knee | Posteromedial | Recurrence of lesion | Ambulation to tolerance as symptoms allow |
| Extension osteotomy of distal femur | Correction of flexion deformity of distal femur | Lateral | Distal neurovascular loss caused by stretch phenomenon resulting from correction of deformity; Pseudoarthrosis; Recurrence of flexion deformity | Plaster or other immobilization until osseous unicn, usually 10 to 12 weeks |
| Excision of loose body of knee | Symptomatic osteocartilaginous loose body of knee | Medial or lateral parapatellar | Recurrence of loose bodies | Immobilization as necessary for symptoms; thereafter, rehabilitation of quadriceps muscle and progression in gait as clinical status allows |
| Open reduction of patellar fracture | Displaced or comminuted fracture; Symptomatic chondromalacia of patella | Transverse | | Immobilization for 6 to 8 weeks in cylinder cast until fusion is stable or patella ligament heals; thereafter, progressive range of motion and quadriceps rehabilitation |
| Open reduction of supracondylar fracture of femur | Displaced supracondylar fracture of femur not responding to non-surgical measures, particularly if fracture line extends to intra-articular surface of distal femur | Lateral or medial | Loss of reduction; Nonunion; Femoral shortening | Plaster immobilization with weight bearing possible at 2 to 6 weeks postoperatively; immobilization may need to be continued for 6 to 12 months |
| Open reduction of tibia, with or without intramedullary fixation | Fracture of tibia necessitating open reduction | Posteromedial or posterolateral (dependent on internal fixation device utilized) | Delayed union or nonunion; Loss of reduction; Extremity shortening | |
| Patellectomy | Irreparable fracture of patella; Degenerative arthritis of patella or patellofemoral joint; Chronic sepsis | Median parapatellar | Loss of motion; Persistent pain; Disruption of quadriceps mechanism | Quadriceps exercises soon after surgery with immobilization; usually cylinder cast for 6 weeks |
| Patelloplasty | Painful chondromalacia of patella | Median parapatellar | Progressive degenerative process of patellofemoral joint; Loose bodies; Recurrent pain | Early immobilization is allowed with quadriceps setting |
| Posterior capsulotomy of knee | Capsular contracture of knee leading to flexion deformity | Medial and lateral or single bayonet incision | Distal neurovascular loss caused by correction or deformity or surgical injury | Immobilization in plaster cast or external support with progression for 7 to 14 days; thereafter, active motion and |

| Procedure | Indications | Approach | Complications | Postoperative management |
|---|---|---|---|---|
| Proximal tibial osteotomy | Single compartment osteoarthritis<br>Angular deformity of tibia | Media or lateral | Peroneal palsy, secondary to varus osteotomy of proximal tibia | protection with use of night braces or splints<br>Immobilization until healed at 10 to 12 weeks postoperatively |
| Quadricepsplasty for recurrent dislocation of patella (Green, Goldthwait, Hauser procedures) | Recurrent symptomatic subluxation or dislocation of patella | Median parapatellar | Recurrent medial or lateral subluxation of patella with symptomatic chondromalacia | Immobilization in cylinder or long leg cast for 6 to 8 weeks with quadriceps exercises instituted early postoperatively; if Hauser procedure performed screw fixation may need to be removed at 3 to 12 months postoperatively |
| Repair of medial or lateral collateral ligaments | Traumatic interruption of collateral ligaments | Medial or lateral parapatellar with possible posterior medial lateral approach | Persistent instability<br>Posttraumatic arthritis | Immobilization in long or cylinder cast 8 to 12 weeks, with braces for any persistent instability |
| Soleus neurectomies | Spastic equinus deformity secondary to clonus | Posterior popliteal | Calcaneal gait (lack of pushoff) | Active dorsiflexion and activity to improve plantar muscles |
| Stapling of distal femur–proximal tibial epiphysis | Curtailment of epiphyseal growth<br>Equalize limb lengths or correct angular deformities through medial or lateral application of staples | Medial or lateral | Complete arrest of epiphysis<br>Loss of staple position | Immobilization in cylinder or long leg cast for 3 to 6 weeks with ambulation as strength improves |
| Synovectomy of knee | Persistent synovial thickening or effusion with chronic inflammatory disease without articular destruction | Usually medial parapatellar | Loss of motion with recurrence of disease | Usually early motion is possible; manipulation of knee under anesthesia not uncommon at 2 to 3 weeks postoperatively; immobilization as necessary |
| Tenorrhaphy of patella or quadriceps tendon of knee | Rupture or laceration of quadriceps tendons | Medial parapatellar | Loss of continuity with lack of extension of knee<br>Knee flexion contracture | Immobilization in long leg cylinder cast for 6 to 8 weeks; progressive range of motion and active extension of the knee with quadriceps exercises; external support necessary until rehabilitation complete |
| Tibial grafting for nonunion | Nonunion of tibia | Posterior or medial | Persistence of nonunion | Immobilization until healing satisfactory; 6 to 12 months of immobilization in weight-bearing cast not unusual |
| Tibial lengthening | Limb lengthening to equalize limb length, out of range for epiphysiodesis alone, particularly in paralytic situation | Lateral or medial | Neurovascular compromise<br>Angular deformity<br>Pseudoarthrosis | Place in distraction device postoperatively and lengthen 0.08 to 0.9 cm daily; 3 to 6 months in long leg casts; secondary bone grafting not unusual |
| Tibial osteotomies | Correction of tibial angular or rotational deformity | Anterolateral; anteromedial | Anterior compartment syndrome<br>Pseudoarthrosis<br>Peroneal palsy (more likely to occur with varus osteotomies) | Immobilization in long leg cast for 6 weeks; additional immobilization in long leg or short leg cast for 6 to 8 weeks |
| Total knee replacement | Symptomatic degenerative arthritis of knee with varus or valgus malalignment | Medial or lateral parapatellar | Extension sepsis necessitating amputation<br>Loosening of prosthetic components | Immobilization with external support in early phases until strength and motion improve |
| Transfer of hamstring tendons | Paralytic loss of quadriceps extension of knee | Medial and lateral | Lack of active extension caused by weakening of transferred muscles | Immobilization in plaster cast or other external devices for 3 to 6 weeks with nighttime management in same; setting of transferred muscles during first 6 weeks of postoperative phase; use of external support as necessary |
| Transfer of pes anserinus for rotatory instability of knee (Slocum procedure) | Medial rotatory instability of knee | Medial parapatellar | Persistent rotatory instability of knee | Immobilization in long leg cast 6 to 12 weeks; thereafter, support by brace if indicated |

**Table 29-6.** Surgical procedures of the ankle and foot

| Procedure | Indications | Approach | Complications | Postoperative management |
|---|---|---|---|---|
| Arthrodesis of ankle | Symptomatic degenerative arthritis of ankle<br>Paralytic deformity of ankle with lack of active control<br>Chronic sepsis or instability | Anterior or anterolateral | Pseudoarthrosis<br>Recurrence of deformity or loss of position | Immobilization in plaster or external device for 6 to 12 weeks until union complete; ambulation with external device as needed |
| Bunionplasty (McBride, Keller, Mayo, Lapitus, Mitchell, Joplin procedures) | Correction of painful hallux valgus (bunion) | Medial or lateral to great toe | Recurrence of deformity<br>Hallux varus deformity<br>Clawing of great toe<br>Hallux rigidus (rigid first metatarsophalangeal joint) | Immobilization in plaster cast, usually short leg, walker, or varied plaster immobilization for 3 to 6 weeks; progressive range of motion thereafter |
| Dwyer osteotomy of os calcis | Varus deformity of os calcis secondary to clubfoot, paralytic, or cavus deformity | Medial or lateral | Skin loss of wound (medial)<br>Nonunion<br>Recurrence of deformity | Short or long leg cast for 6 weeks; night brace and shoe corrections post-immobilization |
| Extraarticular subtalar arthrodesis (Green-Grice procedure) | Valgus deformity of hindfoot | Lateral | Fibrous ankylosis of graft<br>Donor site fracture<br>Loss of correction<br>Overcorrection with varus deformity of hindfoot | Immobilization in long leg cast for 6 to 10 weeks; additional immobilization for 4 to 6 weeks in short leg cast; progressive ambulation with or without night braces depending on age of patient |
| Excision of interdigital neuroma (Morton's neuroma) | Painful interdigital neuroma | Dorsal web space | Recurrence of neuroma<br>Interruption of digital neurovascular supply | Nonspecific; ambulation as tolerated |
| Interphalangeal joint fusion of toe | Hammer toe or other flexion deformity of distal phalanges | Dorsolateral or medial | Pseudoarthrosis<br>Recurrence of deformity | Intramedullary wire fixation 3 to 6 weeks; immobilization 4 to 6 weeks; ambulation as tolerated |
| Lengthening of achilles tendon (heel-cord lengthening) or posterior capsulotomy | Correction of equinus deformity | Posteromedial | Calcaneal gait (lack of pushoff or toe-off component in gait)<br>Skin loss | Immobilization in long leg cast for 3 weeks; additional immobilization for 3 weeks in short leg or long leg cast; further use of night brace may be necessary in young |
| Open reduction of bimalleolar fracture of ankle | Fractures of medial or lateral malleoli | Medial and lateral malleolar | Nonunion<br>Subluxation of tibiotalar joint | Immobilization for 8 to 12 weeks; removal of internal fixation devices as indicated |
| Open reduction of congenital vertical talus | Congenital vertical talus (congenital convex pes valgus deformity) | Medial | Recurrence of deformity<br>Persistent hindfoot valgus or forefoot abduction | Usually K-wire fixation at talonavicular joint for 6 weeks with plaster immobilization; long leg cast 10 to 12 weeks; thereafter, period of orthotic support at night and corrective shoe additions |
| Percutaneous plantar fasciotomy | Cavus foot deformity<br>Forefoot adduction | Medial plantar | Delayed wound healing<br>Interruption of flexor hallux longus<br>Interruption of plantar medial neurovascular bundle | Short leg cast in dorsiflexion and eversion for 4 to 6 weeks |

**Table 29-6.** Surgical procedures of the ankle and foot—cont'd

| Procedure | Indications | Approach | Complications | Postoperative management |
|---|---|---|---|---|
| Posteromedial release of foot | Hindfoot varus and forefoot adduction secondary to residuals of clubfoot in young child | Posteromedial | Skin loss along incision Recurrence of deformity Severe planovalgus foot Neurovascular loss | Immobilization in long leg or short leg cast for 10 to 12 weeks; postoperative orthosis and corrective shoe additions to maintain correction until postoperative status is stable |
| Resection calcaneal-navicular osseo-cartilaginous bar (hindfoot coalition) | Painful hindfoot coalition (calcaneal navicular or talocalcaneal osseocartilaginous bar) limiting hindfoot motion | Lateral or medial | Recurrence with talonavicular arthritis | Immobilization in short leg cast; thereafter, progressive range of motion and mobilization exercises |
| Syme amputation of foot | Neurovascular, congenital, or posttraumatic status necessitating amputation of forefoot | Transverse | Loss of skin flap Higher amputation secondary to original process | Ambulation as soft tissue status dictates; may need revision or prosthesis to allow for satisfactory ambulation |
| Talectomy | Persistent equinus and clubfoot Severe deformities secondary to congenital vertical talus | Dorsomedial or lateral | Recurrence of talar growth Recurrence of deformity | K-wire fixation through distal tibia from plantar aspect of foot for 6 to 12 weeks with immobilization in short leg or long leg cast for 12 weeks; short leg brace for maintenance of correction |
| Tarsal tunnel release | Tarsal tunnel syndrome | Medial | Interruption of neurovascular structures at ankle | Ambulation to tolerance after surgical procedure with external support as necessary for comfort |
| Tenorrhaphy of achilles tendon | Rupture or laceration of calcaneus | Posteromedial | Calcaneal gait Lack of pushoff or toe off in gait | Immobilization in short or long leg cast for 6 weeks; heel lift in early ambulatory phases after cast immobilization discontinued |
| Transfer of flexor extensor tendon of foot and ankle | Paralytic weakness or deformity secondary to inherent weakness | Dependent on tendon transfer | Recurrence of weakness because of failure of transfer | Immobilization or short leg cast for 3 to 6 weeks; begin exercises of transfer of new position between 5 days to 4 weeks postoperatively |
| Transfer of long toe extensors to metatarsal necks | Paralytic weakness or deformity secondary to inherent weakness | Dependent on tendon transfer | Recurrence of weakness because of failure of transfer | Immobilization or short leg cast for 3 to 6 weeks; begin exercises of transfer of new position between 5 days to 4 weeks postoperatively |
| Triple arthrodesis of foot | Stabilization of hindfoot prior to tendon transfer Correction of varus or valgus deformity of hindfoot in patient with mature foot Correction of cavus deformity of foot (excessively high arch) | Lateral | Pseudoarthrosis, particularly of talonavicular joint, symptomatic with loss of correction | Immobilization in long leg or short leg cast for 14 to 16 weeks; non-weight bearing during most of convalescent phase |

**Table 29-7.** Surgical procedures of the spine

| Procedure | Indications | Approach | Complications | Postoperative management |
|---|---|---|---|---|
| Anterior spinal fusion | Progressive scoliosis<br>Traumatic instability<br>Symptomatic degenerative or developmental disease of spine | Anterior or thoraco-abdominal | Pseudoarthrosis<br>Neurologic deficit<br>Failure to maintain correction | Orthotic or plaster immobilization for 6 to 12 months; progressive ambulation as possible postoperatively |
| Anterior spinal fusion with Dwyer cable instrumentation | Scoliosis with lack of posterior elements, such as in myelomeningocele without kyphosis | Anterior | Neurologic deficit<br>Retroperitoneal infection<br>Pseudoarthrosis with loss of correction | Bedrest or immobilization in Risser cast for 6 to 12 months |
| Anterior spinal fusion with fibular strut graft | Kyphosis with lack of posterior elements, particularly kyphosis and myelomeningocele | Anterior, usually thoraco-abdominal | Fracture with pseudoarthrosis of fibular graft and loss of correction<br>Neurologic deficit in neurologically intact spine | Bedrest or immobilization in Risser cast for 6 to 12 months |
| Excision of nucleus pulposus | Herniation of nucleus pulposus producing disabling disease or neurologic deficit | Posterior | Permanent neurologic loss<br>Recurrent symptomatic nerve root fibrosis | Usually early ambulation, dependent on severity of disease and neuromuscular function of patient |
| Harrington rod instrumentation and posterior spinal fusion | Progressive or severe scoliosis<br>Comminuted vertebral fracture | Posterior | Pseudoarthrosis<br>Failure of instrumentation and loss of correction<br>Postoperative paraplegia from distraction<br>Superior mesenteric artery syndrome | Special bed or plaster shell immediately postoperatively; ambulatory immobilization in Risser cast for 6 to 12 months |
| Osteotomy of spine | Flexion deformity of spine secondary to chronic arthritis | Posterior spinal | Paraplegia with loss of bladder or bowel function<br>Pseudoarthrosis | Plaster or orthotic immobilization for 6 months to 1 year |
| Posterior spinal fusion | Congenital scoliosis, posterior spinal instability<br>Progressive or severe kyphosis, congenital kyphosis<br>Progressive scoliosis<br>Degenerative disease of spine | Posterior | Postoperative neurologic deficit<br>Pseudoarthrosis | Bedrest until stable followed by 6 to 9 months immobilization in Risser cast |
| Spinal fusion: anterior cervical | Degenerative disc disease<br>Degenerative osteoarthritis of cervical spine with or without neurologic deficit<br>Cervical instability with loss of posterior elements | Anterior cervical | Pseudoarthrosis<br>Neurologic deficit or loss of quadriceps and paraplegia<br>Loss of bladder or bowel control<br>Rupture of esophagus<br>Vascular impairment | Orthotic plaster device for 12 to 16 weeks until healing complete |
| Spinal fusion: lumbar | Degenerative osseous spinal disease with instability | Posterior spinal | Neurologic deficit<br>Pseudoarthrosis | Usually 6 months of convalescence with or without immobilization with orthotic plaster device |

## SUMMARY

Many orthopedic surgical procedures and variations thereof are used within the scope of current orthopedic practice. Presented here in tabular form are the most frequently used procedures. It is advisable for all health care personnel to become familiar with these most common procedures. In some circumstances additional detailed information regarding the procedures themselves may be required; it is suggested that the reader refer to the sources given in the Bibliography when this is necessary. Any variations in indications and management will often be reflective of physician preference; the orthopedic surgeon is in these cases the reader's most reliable resource for unanswered questions.

## BIBLIOGRAPHY

Crenshaw, A. H., editor: Campbell's operative orthopaedics, ed. 5, St. Louis, 1971, The C. V. Mosby Co.

Ferguson: Orthopedic surgery in infancy and childhood, Baltimore, The Williams & Wilkins Co.

Goldstein, L. A., and Dickerson, R. C.: Atlas of orthopaedic surgery, St. Louis, 1974, The C. V. Mosby Co.

Tachdjian, M. O.: Pediatric orthopedics, Philadelphia, 1972, W. B. Saunders Co.

# PART SEVEN

# Equipment

# 30

## Special beds and frames

**PATSY A. GETZ**

Special beds and frames are important adjuncts in the management of immobilized patients. Basic to the treatment of any patient who needs recumbency is a firm surface providing support to maintain a bed posture that mimics anatomic standing posture.

The human body is not a static, inert mass, but a dynamic, living organism that suffers atrophy, contracture, deformity, and skin deterioration when proper consideration is not given its dynamic nature. Most special beds and frames have been designed to minimize or eliminate the complications or hazards of prolonged bedrest and to facilitate the nursing care of the immobilized patient.

The purpose of this chapter is to present a survey of the specialty equipment presently available for management of a patient who requires a period of recumbency. No attempt is made to discuss all available beds and frames for, indeed, there are probably as many modalities available as there are orthopedists.

## HISTORICAL SURVEY

Modalities for immobilizing a patient with a musculoskeletal problem are illustrated in textbooks dating from Greek, Roman, and Egyptian civilizations.

There is dead medical literature and there is live one. The dead is not all ancient, and the live is not all modern.
(Oliver Wendell Holmes)

The above quotation is found on the frontispiece of Edgar M. Bick's Source Book of Orthopaedics,[3] published in 1937, which cites the treatment of spinal deformities from the writings of Hippocrates. All methods of treatment began with "extension on a flat surface." Galen (131-201 AD) studied Hippocratic texts and added considerably to the body of knowledge in the treatment of fractures. "It should be kept in mind that exercise strengthens and inactivity wastes."[3,p.8] Treatment of spinal curvature in the seventh century as recorded by Paul of Aegina (625-690 AD) continued to follow the Greek teachings, especially the need for "prolonged recumbency with the patient strapped firmly to the table or board."[3,p.26]

Because of Arabian cultural influence during the Middle Ages, emphasizing topical application of oils and salves for healing, few orthopedic surgical advances were recorded until the eleventh century when the study of anatomy and its influence on surgery were revived. Monastic hospitals and university centers of medical education were established in Europe and were instrumental in the transition into the Renaissance period.

During the fourteenth century Guy de Chauliac at the University of Montpellier used weights and pulleys for traction. He describes ". . . a mattress bed on which the patient sleeps, and if it is necessary let it be perforated so that he may go to stool."[3,p.32] Did the origin of the Bradford frame or CircOlectric bed come from this description?

Special extension beds were designed by Venel (eighteenth century) and Heine (nineteenth century) for the management of spinal tuberculosis and scoliosis. The bed by Heine was constructed so that "longitudinal traction could be extended on the spinal column from the head to the lower extremities during long periods of supine recumbency."[3,p.309]

An English practitioner, Robert Chessher (1750-1831), used a type of traction with a plane similar in effect to convex, or hyperextension, frames used in later years for the treatment of spine diseases and injuries.[3,p.170]

According to Bick, later in the nineteenth century modern methods of fracture treatment began with another Englishman, Hugh Owen Thomas (1843-1891), a surgeon and pioneer in brace-making. His theory of "enforced, uninterrupted, and prolonged" rest justified the end-fracture healing.[3,p.167] His rest theory was later challenged by a Frenchman, Just Lucas-Champonniere (1843-1913), who placed emphasis on "early application of movement" as a preventive measure against the deformities and disabilities that resulted with the Thomas method of treatment.[3,p.197] Lucas-Champonniere also observed that slight movement at the fracture site stimulated, through a process of irritation, early growth of callus. Functional position and exercise during bedrest and shorter periods of immobilization were emphasized.

Early mobilization along with the use of plaster of paris (1852, by Mathysen), the advent of surgical asepsis (1861, by Cooper and 1877, by Lister), and the discovery of X-ray (1895, by Roentgen) contributed to outcomes that returned the injured industrial workers to work earlier.

The treatment of fractures as practiced by Sir Robert Jones (1857-1933), a nephew of H. O. Thomas, had a profound influence on the practice of modern orthopedics in Europe and America. Jones advocated early reduction of fractures, a practice aided by the advent of anesthesia (mid 19th century) and X-ray control. He also redefined the term fracture to include the resultant damage to soft tissues surrounding the break in continuity of the bone. According to Bick, Jones "must be counted among the great teachers of modern orthopedic surgery."[4,p.29] As director of orthopedics of the British army during World War I, his influence was felt by the American military physicians.

In the United States, Louis Bauer (1814-1898), who has been called the "real founder of the Ameri-

can school of orthopedics,"[10,p.130] was a strong advocate of prolonged recumbency as a necessity for relief of weightbearing in the treatment of "caries" of the spine. Bauer used a special bed or frame to maintain proper positioning. According to Shands, Bauer recommended the use of "a water bed which both yields to and supports all parts of the body and exposes more in particular to exceptional pressure."[16,p.22] He was highly critical of his contemporaries, Lewis Sayre, Henry Davis, James Knight, and Charles F. Taylor, for their ambulatory management of spinal problems with plaster of paris, suspension apparatuses, and braces.

In the latter nineteenth century, Edward H. Bradford, of Boston, challenged the center of American orthopedics in New York through his work for crippled children. He established the first orthopedic ward at the Boston City Hospital.[8,p.6] According to Sir Arthur Keith, Bradford was "the chief link between the old school and the new school of orthopaedics."[10,p.182] Shands states that Bradford "undoubtedly did more for the crippled child than any other one orthopaedic surgeon of the early days."[14,p.182] To provide long periods of recumbency in the treatment of pediatric spinal conditions, he developed the Bradford frame in 1893. An excellent teacher at Harvard Medical School and prolific contributor to orthopedic literature, Bradford probably made his most lasting contribution with the development of the frame which bears his name.[14,p.182]

In 1911 Hibbs performed the first spinal fusion. Later that same year, Albee described a method of spinal fusion using an autogenous bone graft from the tibia. In 1922 Kleinbeng devised a different type of fusion advocating preoperative traction on a convex frame in order to obtain an optimal posture for the surgical procedure.

Thus operative as well as nonoperative treatment of spinal conditions called for the use of special frames, attached to a regular hospital bed. The Bradford frame, bent at the thorax, was prevalent in the treatment of scoliosis during the 10 years from 1920 to 1930.

In 1936 Homer H. Stryker, an orthopedist and inventor, from the University of Michigan, developed a device for turning a patient on a frame. His description was published in *The Journal of American Medical Association* in 1939.[16,p.1732] In the article, a photograph shows the frame, suspended 1 foot above a standard mattress, clamped to the head and foot of the bed. Also pictured is a "portable" frame that could be lifted onto a stretcher. The basic design of the portable frame was later mounted onto four legs with casters and became the Stryker turning frame used in many hospitals today.

The earliest dated picture of the Foster bed is one dated January 16, 1944. Information concerning the development of the Foster bed is sketchy before 1947-1948, at which time the bed was first marketed by G. Hyde Chick Co. Basically, the bed consists of two convex Bradford frames that can be turned on a horizontal axis to allow supine and prone positions while maintaining immobilization of the spine.

The CircOlectric (COL) bed was designed by Homer H. Stryker in the 1960s as a vertical turning bed to facilitate positioning of severely injured patients. The COL bed is more versatile than the horizontal frames and its use is not limited to orthopedic and neurosurgical patients. The COL bed is useful for patients with chronic illnesses to help combat the consequences of long-term recumbency. In selected cases the CircOlectric bed is helpful in preparing a long-term patient for the transition from recumbency to ambulation. By utilizing the COL bed as a tilt table several times each day the patient regains standing balance without using strength and energy to get to a sitting position on the side of the bed. Some physicians use the circular or vertical turning frame for patients following hip or back surgery or for controlled weightbearing to provide early ambulation when sitting is contraindicated.

The search through yesterday's texts confirms Oliver Wendell Holmes' belief that "the dead [literature] is not all ancient, and the live is not all modern." The clinical challenges of immobilization are not new, and many of the methods to prevent the complications of recumbency have their roots in the experiences of our forebearers.

Analysis of the past reveals that the role of prolonged rest in orthopedic management and the role of early mobilization "are not as mutually contradictory as they seem . . ."[4,p.290] As Bick states: "The value of enforced and uninterrupted rest *as long as it is required* is incontrovertible; the value of mobilization *at the earliest safe opportunity* is equally so."[4,p.290] Clinical judgment is needed to determine the time factor involved for each.

## CURRENT BEDS AND FRAMES
### Standard orthopedic bed

Management of many patients with orthopedic problems can be accomplished without special beds or frames. The quality of the mattress and the type of bed are important considerations in selecting the beds to be used on an orthopedic unit.

For many years at Emory University Hospital, Atlanta, Georgia, cotton mattresses (without in-nersprings) and bedboards were used for orthopedic patients on bedrest for treatment of low back pain or for long-term traction therapy. Since 1965, that institution has used orthopedic mattresses made of 4- to 5-inch virgin (polyurethane) foam. Used with a bedboard, the foam mattress gives a firm, evenly distributed support for a bedfast patient.

A desirable but not easily obtainable feature of an orthopedic bed is one that will allow countertraction when a patient in continuous lower extremity traction elevates his head. In most hospital beds when the patient is in semi-Fowler's position, the fulcrum changes and the desired amount of countertraction is lost. The end result is that the patient often slips down in bed, the traction apparatus comes in contact with the foot of the bed and full effectiveness of traction is compromised. Higher shock blocks (for nonelectric beds) or increased Trendelenburg (for electric beds) is needed to ensure continuous, uncompromised traction.

Two other features needed for an orthopedic bed include a trapeze bar and siderails so that the patient can assist in positioning himself in bed. The patient can learn how to assist in turning from side to side and, unless contraindicated, how to raise his torso off the mattress by grasping the trapeze bar, bending the hips and knees, thus pushing himself up in bed.

The nursing staff must be cognizant of the need for the patient to use special features of the hospital bed, but they must also remember that the patient needs to learn how to get in and out of bed without the use of the trapeze bar and siderails. Part of dismissal planning for the patient includes learning to manage activities without special equipment unless it is needed and available at home.

One safety feature of an orthopedic bed that is of particular importance is the locking mechanism. Generally, caster locks are not very satisfactory in providing stability when the patient is getting in or out of the bed. There is now a bed on the market with a central braking and steering lock. A brake pedal locks all four casters rendering the bed more stable.

### Bradford frame

Proper and frequent use of Bradford frames can alleviate two major problems—keeping hip spica casts clean and providing immobilization of children in traction. The frames are available commercially or may be constructed by the engineering department of most hospitals (Fig. 30-1).

The split Bradford frame is used for an incontinent patient in a hip cast. Age is not a factor in the

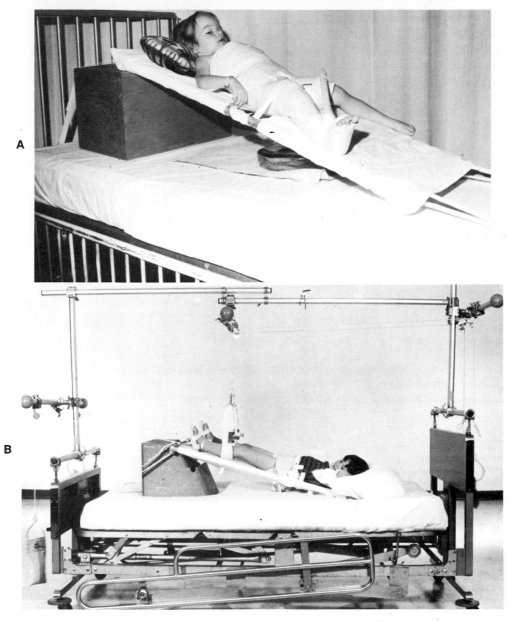

**Fig. 30-1. A,** Use of split Bradford frame with child in hip spica cast. Note elevation of head end of frame and straps securing frame and patient. **B,** Use of solid Bradford frame with child in split Russell traction. Note elevation of foot end of frame to obtain additional countertraction. Pelvic sling restraint and frame restraint are used to maintain proper immobilization and good body alignment. (From Hilt, N. E., and Schmitt, E. W., Jr.: Pediatric orthopedic nursing, St. Louis, 1975, The C. V. Mosby Co.)

clinical use of the split frame; *incontinence* is the most important criterion. An older, retarded child who is incontinent can benefit from the use of the split frame as well as an infant or a recently "potty trained" toddler. Proper use of the frame helps to keep the cast dry and clean. The head end of the Bradford frame is elevated on a plywood block so that when the child urinates, the urine will not run under the case in the area of the buttocks. Careful consideration is given to protecting the cast by directing the flow of urine with the use of plastic petals around the perineal cutout as described in Chapter 23.

The frame is secured to the bed frame by 1 inch webbing strap at each corner. The plywood block should provide 30 to 45 degrees of angulation, depending on the size of the frame (small frame, 6 inches; medium frame, 8 inches; large frame, 10 inches). If postoperative perineal edema occurs it may be necessary to lower the frame for 36 to 48 hours until the edema begins to subside. The child is secured to the frame with three buckled webbing straps. The anterior and posterior edges of the perineal cutout should be at the level of the bottom edge of the cephalad canvas.

The clinical indication for the use of the solid Bradford frame is continuous traction. Age (under 5 years), retardation, and hyperactivity are three criteria used to select children in traction who can benefit by being immobilized in the smaller area of the frame rather than on a large mattress.

The solid frame is secured to the bed frame with buckled webbed straps, and countertraction is obtained by placing a plywood box at the end opposite the direction of the traction. If countertraction is not needed, both ends of the frame are elevated on blocks. Restraints are necessary to maintain the child in proper alignment with the traction apparatus. The types of restraints are presented in Chapter 24.

Nursing care guidelines for the patient on a Bradford frame are outlined below.

### GUIDELINES FOR NURSING CARE OF PATIENT ON A BRADFORD FRAME*

**A. Types of Bradford frames**
   1. Split.
   2. Solid.

**B. Use**
   1. Split: with children in hip spica casts; to maintain dry cast.
   2. Solid: with children in traction; to aid in immobilization and maintenance of desired alignment and positioning.
   3. Principles of use
      a. Split: law of gravity.
      b. Solid: area of body control.

**C. Clinical indications**
   1. Split: incontinence, *not* age.
   2. Solid: age (under 5 years); hyperactivity and retardation, if unable to immobilize by other methods.

**D. Advantages**
   1. Split
      a. Provides for appropriate elevation to maintain dry cast.
      b. May be used to mobilize child.

---

*By N. E. Hilt. Illustrations (with exception of solid frame) from Hilt, N. E., and Schmitt, E. W., Jr.: Pediatric orthopedic nursing, St. Louis, 1975, The C. V. Mosby Co., pp. 57-67.

   2. Solid
      a. Provides for maintenance of immobilization, desired alignment, and positioning.
      b. May be used for countertraction.

**E. Disadvantages**
   1. May be considered unsafe if frame not adequately secured to bed.
   2. May be considered unsafe if patient not adequately secured to frame.
   3. Will not be effective if elevation not appropriate.
   4. Will not be stable if bedboard not used over mattress.
   5. Split and solid types are *not* interchangeable.

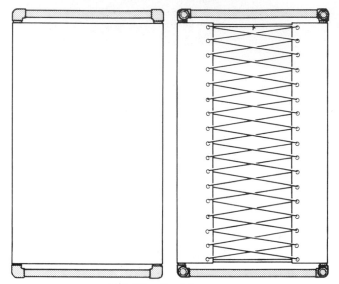

**Solid Bradford frame**

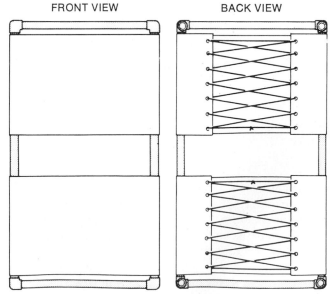

FRONT VIEW                          BACK VIEW

**Split Bradford frame**

## F. Procedural notes and safety factors

1. Measure patient and choose appropriate size frame (head of patient not resting on metal portion of frame). Common sizes (inches) appropriate for most children are small, 13 × 30; medium, 16 × 42; large, 18 × 50.
2. Confirm appropriate type for designated use.
3. Construct appropriate type and size Bradford frame.
   a. Split:
      (1) Obtain metal rectangular frame of designated size.
      (2) Obtain two canvas covers for appropriate size frame (small, medium, large); eyelets in back seam as shown.
      (3) Place canvas covers appropriately at either end of the frame; will have an opening of approximately 4 to 6 inches in center.
      (4) Secure canvas covers in place with rope, elastic fasteners, or springs; be sure covers are taut.
   b. Solid
      (1) Obtain metal rectangular frame of designated size.
      (2) Obtain one canvas cover for appropriate size frame (small, medium, large); eyelets in back seam as shown.
      (3) Place canvas cover appropriately over metal frame; will extend from end to end.
      (4) Secure canvas cover in place with rope, elastic fasteners, or springs; be sure that cover is taut.
4. Prepare bed on which Bradford frame will be set up and utilized:
   a. Strip bed of all linen.
   b. Place bedboard on mattress for stability.
   c. Make bed, placing appropriate linen over bedboard and mattress.
      (1) Place one drawsheet at upper end of board and mattress.
      (2) Place second drawsheet at lower end of board and mattress.
      (3) Place rubber drawsheet, vinyl plastic, or waterproof pads over center section of bed.
      (4) Place third drawsheet over center section of bed.
5. Set up designated Bradford frame to maintain principles of utilization:
   a. Place plywood or similar blocks on bed for elevation
      (1) Split: always elevate head end of frame; block will be placed under head of frame and foot end will rest on bed; degree of elevation required will depend on presence or absence of perineal edema *and* size of child.
      (2) Solid: both ends of frame are elevated to an equal degree; blocks of equal height are placed under head and foot end of frame;

degree of elevation insignificant as long as nursing care is facilitated.
      (a) Countertraction: foot end only will be elevated; block is placed under foot end of frame, with head end resting on bed; degree of elevation will depend on amount of countertraction desired.
      (b) Contraindications to lowering head end of solid Bradford frame: patients with myelomeningocele with shunt; infants with known regurgitation problem; multiple injuries (e.g., head, abdominal injury).
   b. Place Bradford frame on appropriate blocks for elevation.
   c. Secure Bradford frame to bed with four buckled webbing straps, one at each corner; secure to spring frame of bed.
   d. Bradford frame set-ups. (See illustration on p. 736).
6. Provide for patient comfort, security, and facilitation of continuous nursing care:
   a. Place foam pad (i.e., egg crate foam) over canvas on set up Bradford frame.
   b. Place tie sheets over foam and canvas covers.
   c. Place and secure patient on frame:
      (1) Split: secure patient on the Bradford frame with three buckled webbing straps as shown.

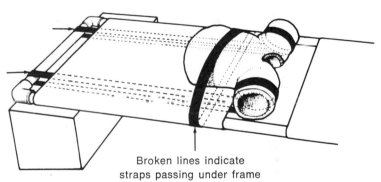

Broken lines indicate
straps passing under frame

      (2) Solid: secure patient on Bradford frame with frame restraint. Traction and additional restraints (see Chapter 24) chosen to assist in maintenance of desired alignment and positioning will secure child on frame.

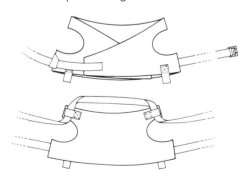

**GUIDELINES FOR NURSING CARE OF PATIENT
ON A BRADFORD FRAME—CONT'D**

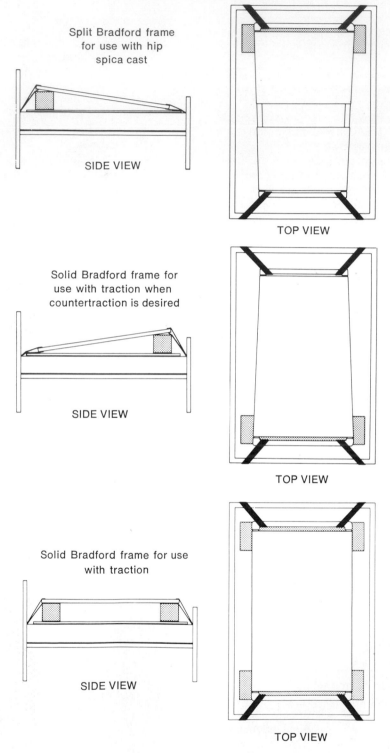

Split Bradford frame
for use with hip
spica cast

SIDE VIEW

TOP VIEW

Solid Bradford frame for
use with traction when
countertraction is desired

SIDE VIEW

TOP VIEW

Solid Bradford frame for use
with traction

SIDE VIEW

TOP VIEW

**Bradford frame set-ups**

## Hyperextension (Schwartz) bed

In pediatric orthopedics, the hyperextension (Schwartz) bed (Fig. 30-2) is used to maintain correction and to increase range of motion of the hip(s) following an operative muscle release procedure. The bed may be purchased or converted from a regular hospital bed. Removal of the regular mattress and the addition of three half mattresses allows enough height to permit alternating prone and supine positions with concomitant alternating flexion and extension of the hips. The bilateral casted extremities are suspended over the lower half of the bed with rings and traction apparatus. The position of the hips is alternated at 2-hour inter-

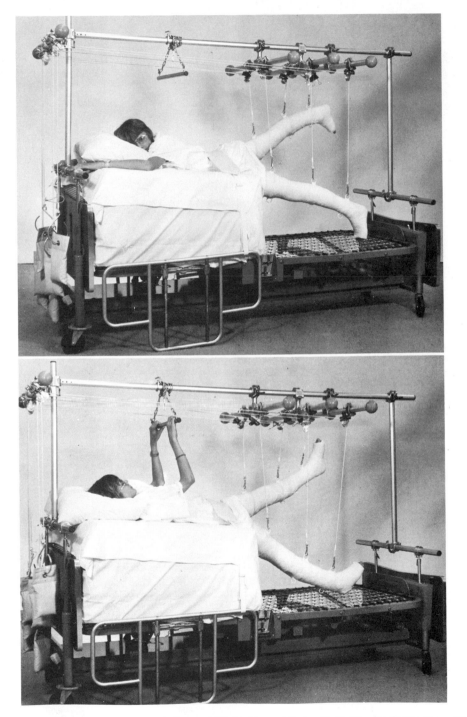

**Fig. 30-2.** Hyperextension bed. (From Hilt, N. E., and Schmitt, E. W., Jr.: Pediatric orthopedic nursing, St. Louis, 1975, The C. V. Mosby Co.)

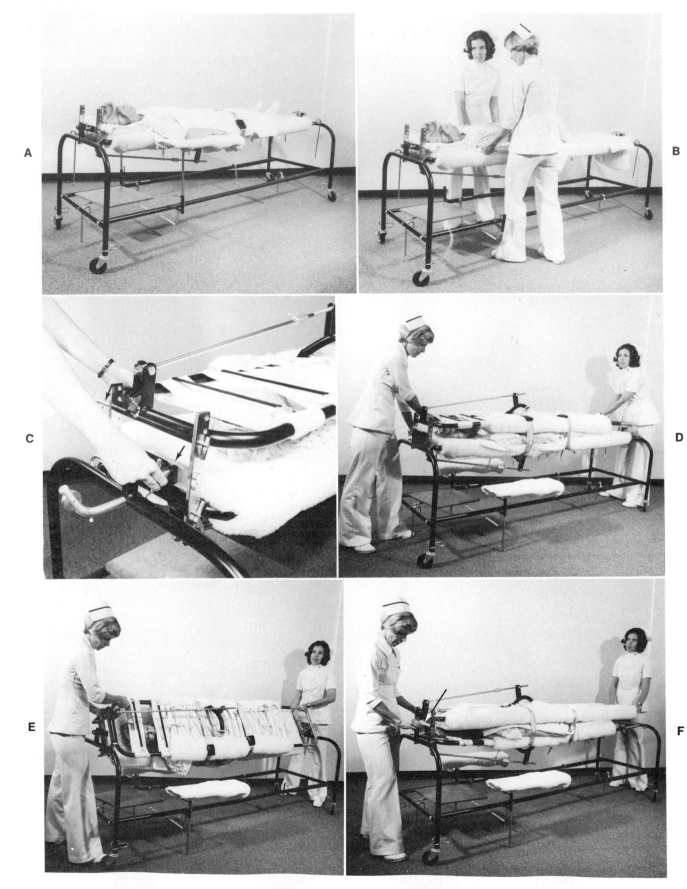

**Fig. 30-3.** For legend see opposite page.

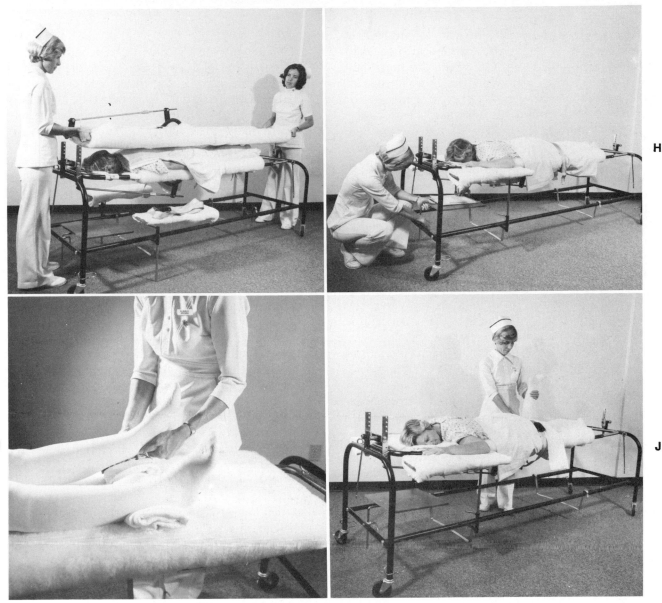

**Fig. 30-3.** Foster Bed. Foster reversible bed may be utilized for horizontal alteration of position from prone to supine. The steps of turning process are as follows. **A,** Patient supine on Foster frame. Note that safety strap or belt is utilized to secure patient and arms are appropriately supported with arm boards. **B,** Before turning patient each time, it is important to position patient appropriately on frame. Utilization of drawsheet underneath patient may assist. **C,** After anterior frame is placed over patient and secured with pin *(upper arrow),* frame should be secured with one hand while turning key is turned and released *(lower arrow). Two or three restraining straps* are used to secure patient between frames. **D,** With anterior frame secured, positioning of hands denotes beginning of turning process. Note that two safety straps are in place to secure patient. **E,** Patient is then turned with one individual at one end of frame and another assisting at other end. *Two individuals* are always used for this process. **F,** When patient is prone, frames are held securely while turning key *(arrow)* is tightened securely. **G,** Both straps are removed, and posterior frame is lifted off after removing both upper pins, which secure posterior frame. Care must be taken to assure that *only* pins to top frame are removed. **H,** Armboards are appropriately placed for support and comfort of patient. Reading board or table is then placed under patient. Again note that patient in prone position is also secured by safety belt. **I,** It is advantageous when patient is supine to appropriately and adequately elevate heels off frame to avoid pressure. Sheepskin (or synthetic sheepskin) will also assist in alleviating skin irritation; it is recommended that entire length of both frames be lined routinely. **J,** It is recommended that patient on Foster frame, as with any immobilized patient, be exercised periodically to avoid contractures and promote adequate range of motion for all joints.

vals. Abduction and adduction can be controlled by the position of the pulleys. Restraints are needed to maintain the child in position so that the horizontal gluteal folds are even with the bottom edge of the stacked mattresses.[8,p.55] (See Chapter 24 for restraints.)

### Foster bed

As stated earlier, the Foster bed, first used in the 1940s, consists of two Bradford frames mounted on a castered base and secured, with locking bars to the head and foot end assemblies. The assembly at each end is attached to the rotary bearing mechanism permitting horizontal turning. Supine and prone positions can be accomplished while maintaining proper immobilization and alignment (Fig. 30-3).

The Foster bed is the only horizontal turning frame that permits hyperextension as well as traction at each end of the frame. Also, either end of the bed can be elevated to provide countertraction.

The Foster bed is used today in posttraumatic management of patients with spinal instability, with or without cord damage, and in the management of the postoperative patient with multilevel spinal fusion when weightbearing or ambulation is contraindicated. The Foster bed is also used in many scoliosis centers for halo-femoral traction, preparatory to spinal procedures with Harrington rods and Dwyer instrumentation. This preoperative technique permits stretching of the paravertebral soft tissues on the concavity of the curve prior to operative correction and fusion.

Ackerman[1,pp.1114-1116] describes a technique for maintaining continuous cervical traction in flexion for selected patients with unstable cervical neck problems. An outrigger attachment for the Foster bed maintains a constant angle in the supine and prone positions.

Advantages of this horizontal turning bed include a convenient storage rack at the base of the bed and the availability of three sizes (child, $66\frac{1}{2} \times 30\frac{1}{2} \times 31$ inches; standard, $89 \times 30\frac{1}{2} \times 31$ inches; and extra long, $95-101 \times 30\frac{1}{2} \times 31$ inches). Also, the patient and the nursing staff have a choice of which direction the bed will be rotated.

The weight of each frame is approximately 20 pounds. The bed can be turned by one person; however, to ensure safety of the patient and the welfare of the nursing staff, turning by two staff members is recommended. Also, two safety straps are needed to guard against the margin of human error. A pillow is placed over the patient's lower legs to prevent movement during the turning.

The Foster bed, as is true of all special beds and frames, is not custom made. The length of canvas must be adjusted to correspond with the size of the patient so that correct ankle posture can be maintained when the patient is prone. Also, the relative position of the patient on the posterior frame must correspond so that when the bedpan portion is released, the patient's buttocks will not sag and compromise the alignment of the lumbosacral spine. The anatomic landmark is the level of the trochanters, which should be at the level of the bottom edge of the torso canvas in order to prevent hyperextension of the lumbosacral spine. A turn sheet under the patient's torso is recommended to adjust movement up or down the frame without danger of improper alignment.

Other safety factors to be considered in giving nursing care to the patient on the Foster bed include precautions to prevent tugging on IV tubing and the catheter tube. The tubing should be placed at the head and foot ends of the frame before rotating the frames. If the patient has thoracotomy tubing, the frames should be rotated *toward* the chest tube side.

A patient who is recovering from anesthesia or is heavily sedated should have a safety strap secured at the thigh level to help prevent turning or falling.

A patient on the Foster bed should be encouraged to do as many bed exercises and activities as medical management permits. The prone position with the use of the reading board permits the patient to feed himself as well as to participate in personal hygiene. Massage of the forehead and chin area toughens the skin and increases the patient's tolerance of the prone position. On rare occasions, a patient with claustrophobia does not tolerate being "sandwiched" between the frames. However, if the rotating of the bed is handled in a well-organized and skillful way, minimizing the "sandwiching" time, the fear of being in tight places can be alleviated.

Immobilization for weeks or months on a horizontal turning frame is a difficult experience for the patient. Diversional activities help to fight boredom and despondence. Prism glasses are helpful for TV and reading. Frequent sensory stimulation with patient-staff interaction, discussions, and games helps the patient to cope with inactivity. Weather permitting, "sunbathing" in the courtyard or solarium is a welcome diversion.

Nursing care guidelines for the patient on a Foster bed are outlined below.

## GUIDELINES FOR NURSING CARE OF PATIENT ON A FOSTER BED

### A. Clinical indications

1. Pre- and postoperative management of patient with scoliosis.
2. Posttraumatic management of patient with spinal instability, with or without cord damage.
3. Posttraumatic management of vertebral fracture when hypertension is indicated.
4. Management of postoperative patient with spinal fusion when weight bearing or ambulation is contraindicated.
5. Use of halo or halo-femoral traction as well as traction with Crutchfield or Venke tongs.
6. Management of patient who requires cervical *flexion* traction (by adapting bed with a special attachment).
7. Management of severely burned patient.

### B. Advantages

1. Permits change of position without altering torso alignment (supine-prone).
2. Has pulley attachments at each end of frame for head or femoral traction.
3. Head or foot end of bed may be elevated to provide countertraction.
4. Each frame may be adjusted with turnbuckle to provide hypertension.
5. Patient has choice of which direction he or she will be turned.
6. Has storage rack for frame.
7. Sizes available (inches):
   Child: 66½ × 30½ × 31
   Standard: 89 × 30½ × 31
   Extra long: 95 × 30½ × 31

### C. Disadvantages

1. Requires two staff members, one at each end of bed, for turning.
2. Weight of each Bradford frame is 20 pounds.
3. Patient with claustrophobia may not tolerate being "sandwiched" between frames.

### D. Procedure and safety factors

1. Whenever possible, introduce Foster bed to patient and family by turning patient on bed.
2. Measure patient and adjust length of canvas to correspond with the patient's size.
   a. Lower edge of trunk section of posterior canvas corresponds to trochanteric level so that when bedpan section is removed buttocks does not sag (prevents hyperextension of lower back).
   b. When patient is prone, lower edge of leg section corresponds to area superior to malleolus level so that correct ankle posture is maintained.

| Procedure | Safety factors |
|---|---|
| **Preparation** | |
| 1. Lock casters of bed. | Two staff members, one at each end of the bed are required (at least one RN). |
| 2. Remove or lower armboards. | |
| 3. Lower reading board. | |
| 4. Drape patient with pillow and remove top linens. | Turnsheet (length of patient's torso) may be necessary if patient needs to be moved toward head or foot end of frame. |
| 5. Place pillow lengthwise over patient's lower leg. | Pillow prevents shifting during turn. |
| 6. Check position of all tubes. Place them at head or foot end of frame. | If indwelling catheter is present, bridge with foam blocks (18 × 5 × 3 inches) to keep pressure off catheter. If unable to thread tube to head or foot end of frame (e.g., chest tubes), prepare to turn toward tubing. |
| 7. Place frame over patient and secure with locking pins. | If patient is being turned to prone position, adjust face sections above brow level and at chin level. Insert pins in opposite direction of anticipated turn. |
| 8. Secure head end first. | To ensure level frame, place foot end pin at same level with head end pin. Distal ends of pins (safety right angle joints) adjacent to frame locking bars prevent removal of "wrong" pins. |
| 9. Place safety belt at elbow level. | *Two* safety belts *prevent* accidents. Include arms if patient does not have control of arms. |
| 10. Place safety belt at thigh level. | Secure safety straps to prevent shifting during turn. |
| 11. If patient has control of upper extremities, have patient clasp arms around frame. | Each staff member double checks position of lock pin. |
| **Turning** | |
| 1. Staff member at head end turns T handle (safety lock) while second staff member steadies frames. | Make sure patient knows direction of turn. |

| Procedure | Safety factors |
|---|---|
| 2. Each staff member places both hands on frames opposite direction frames are to be turned. | |
| 3. On command of staff member at head end, frames are turned horizontally. | Turn at safe, even rate. |
| 4. Release hands only when frames are in locked position (counterclockwise turn of T handle). | |

**Care after turning**

| Procedure | Safety factors |
|---|---|
| 1. Remove safety belts. | Store on frame that is removed. |
| 2. Remove pins of uppermost frames. | Thread pins in loops of pins engaged in frame-locking bar. |
| 3. Remove top frame. | Store on storage rack. |
| 4. Remove lower leg pillow. | |
| 5. Check position of all tubes. | Ensure proper position of tubing. |
| 6. Place one safety belt at thigh level as reminder for patient. | Patients recovering from anesthesia or requiring narcotics must be observed frequently. Patients with lower extremity spasm may require padded straps over knees. |
| 7. Prone position | |
| a. Check position of headband sections. | Observe for proper trunk alignment. Use turnsheet if adjustment is needed. |
| b. Adjust padded armboards toward head end. | Level of armboards depends on shoulder posture. |
| c. Adjust reading board. | |
| d. Place flat towels or foam pieces under shoulders if necessary to prevent forward drop of shoulder girdle. | Shoulders properly positioned will enhance chest expansion. |
| e. Check ankle posture (feet should be free with ankle in neutral position). | Prevents plantar flexion and tight heel cords. |
| f. Encourage self-care such as personal grooming, oral hygiene, and feeding while patient is prone. | |

| Procedure | Safety factors |
|---|---|
| g. Diversional activities such as reading, writing, art work. | |
| h. If medically feasible, active knee flexion and ankle circumduction are encouraged while patient is prone. | Prevents hazards of long-term recumbency. |
| i. Deep breathing and coughing are programmed at regular intervals. | Splinting of the abdomen by the frame enhances coughing. |
| 8. Supine position | |
| a. If medically feasible, place small pillow to support head and cervical contour. | |
| b. Adjust armboards toward foot end. | Level of armboards depends on shoulder posture. |
| c. Clamp foot support in place with ankles in neutral position. | *Caution:* With sensory denervation avoid pressure of foot support against feet. Use foot support to keep linens off toes. |
| d. Place foam bridge to support heel contour and to free heel from mattress. | Prevents heel decubitus ulcers. |
| e. Observe forehead and chin areas for erythema. Massage with silicone cream or alcohol to toughen skin. | Additional padding of bands may be indicated before patient is turned prone again. Observe for pressure areas. |
| f. Encourage self-care and diversional activities. Prism glasses permit reading and TV viewing. | Isometric exercises such as quadriceps setting and gluteal setting maintain muscle tone. Active assistance or passive ROM as directed |
| 9. Keep written schedule planned with patient and posted at bedside. | |

NOTE: Nursing care of the patient with halo-femoral traction is essentially the same as suggested in the above procedure.

Special considerations must be given to the following:

1. Use one head band only (to support the halo ring).
2. Adequately support shoulders without pressure of the frame on the upper arms anteriorly.

3. Adjust length of canvas to accommodate McCarroll bows on the anterior frame (when patient is prone).
4. Maintain diligent pin site care and observation.
5. Record at bedside daily schedule of weights applied to head and femurs.
6. Observe other principles of traction such as checking ropes and pulleys to minimize friction.

## Stryker wedge turning frame

The Stryker wedge turning frame (Model 124) (Fig. 30-4) is a newer model of the original Stryker turning frame. It is constructed of lightweight aluminum mounted at the head end to the base by two posts: anterior for the prone frame and posterior for the supine frame. Each frame is secured to its corresponding post by a knurled nut. The foot ends of the frames are secured by resting on crossbars within a ring which, when closed, secures the patient between the frames. The ring has two handles to permit turning of the patient by one person. The ring is released for turning when the red knob (turning lock) is pulled. Rotation of the frames is prevented by a safety pin at the head end of the frames. The safety pin is pulled prior to releasing the ring by pulling the red knob.

The design of the bed is unique in that the crossbars are wedge shaped; that is, the patient always turns toward the apex of the wedge formed by the crossbars. The lower frame always locks when it is horizontal and level. The ring may then be unlocked and opened for removal of the upper frame. Half of the circle may be removed for exercises, but closure of the circle is recommended for added security. The armboards may be turned up as siderails at night. Prior to rotating the frame, the armboards and the reading table must be lowered to prevent arm injury. The armboards can be adjusted toward the head end to support the arms when the patient is prone or toward the foot end to support the arms when the patient is supine.

The bedpan shelf is adjustable but must be lowered to allow free rotation of the frames. The bedpan section can be released for elimination purposes. However, the relative position of the patient needs to be considered. As with all horizontal turning frames, the level of the trochanters must be aligned with the bottom edge of the torso canvas to prevent hyperextension of the lumbosacral spine when the bedpan portion of the frame is open.

Although designed for one person to operate, most institutions recommend that two people turn the patient. Also, two safety belts are needed, espe-

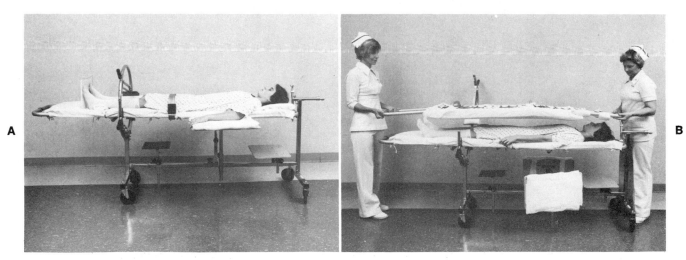

**Fig. 30-4.** Stryker frame. Stryker wedge frame is a redesign of the original Stryker frame. The major advantage of the Stryker wedge frame is its ability to permit turning of the patient by one individual. Despite this as an advantage, liability and safety within a health care facility dictates that *two individuals* be present and assist with the turning process. The following are steps of the turning process. **A,** Patient is positioned supine on Stryker wedge frame. Note that safety belt is in place, arms are supported by attached arm boards, and foot board (designed to attach to frame) is utilized for positional purposes. **B,** Circular portion of frame has been opened, and anterior frame is being placed over patient. Foot board has been removed, and arm boards have been lowered for turning process.

*Continued.*

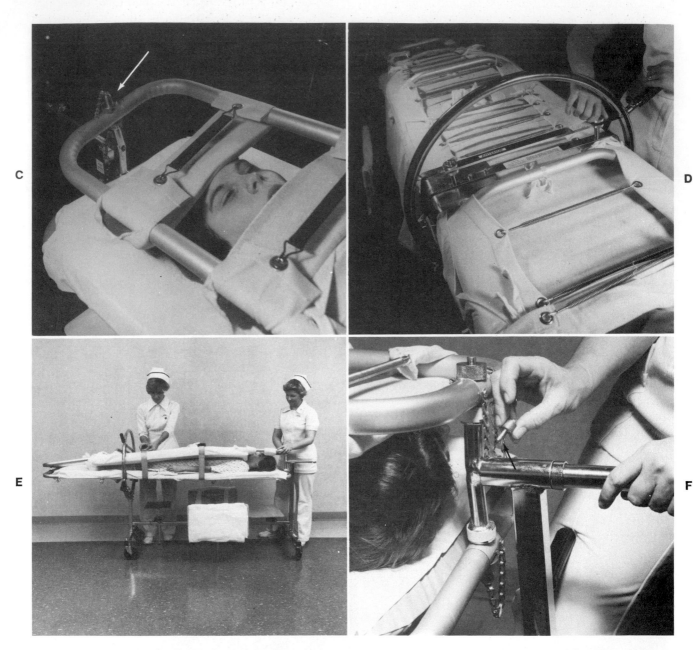

**Fig. 30-4, cont'd. C,** Anterior frame is positioned with forehead band and anterior portion of large canvas to approximately shoulder level. Chin band (as shown) is optional. Turning pin *(arrow)* has been tightened securely. **D,** Circle has been enclosed to secure anterior frame and position secured by tightening screws on crossbar. Ideally, this adjustment is accomplished during the teaching process prior to actual placement of patient on frame. This adjustment provides for custom fitting. **E,** Two safety straps secure patient between anterior and posterior frames. **F,** Safety pin at head of bed *(arrow)* is removed to permit entire frame to turn. **G,** Release pin *(arrow)* at circle is released to permit circular portion of frame, which secures both anterior and posterior frame, to be mobile. Firm grasp should be maintained on frame at this time. **H,** With pin released, frame and patient are turned utilizing handles on circular portion of frame. **I,** The safety pin is replaced at the head of bed *(arrow)*. **J,** Anterior portion of circle is open, and safety straps are removed. **K,** Screw at head of frame is removed, and posterior portion of frame is lifted off. **L,** Patient is prone. Note safety strap in place, feet over edge of canvas, arm boards in place for comfort and support, table in place for utilization, and bridging of knees.

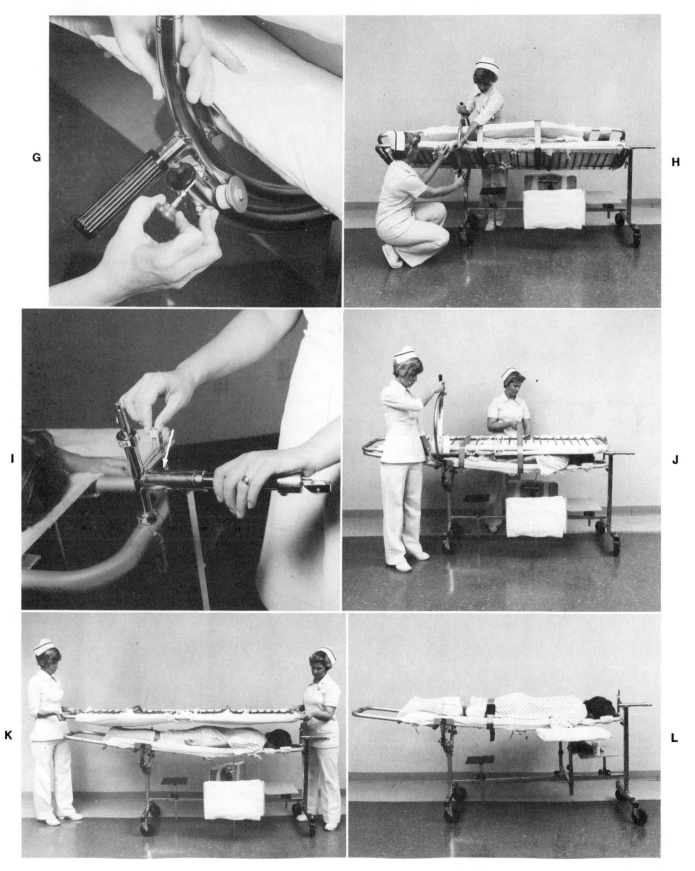

**Fig. 30-4, cont'd.** For legend see opposite page.

*Continued.*

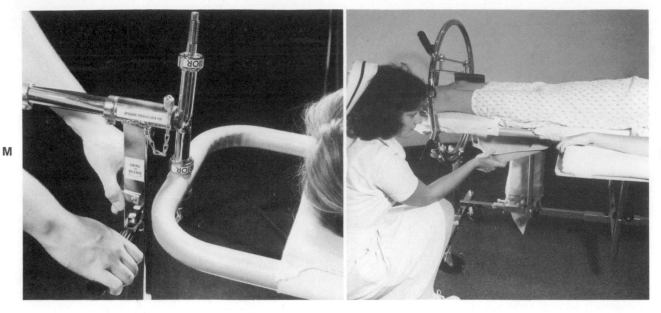

**Fig. 30-4, cont'd. M,** Adjustment for raising or lowering frame is shown at head of bed. **N,** As with many turning frames, placement of bedpan may be easily accomplished with opening near center of frame.

cially if the patient does not have complete control of the extremities.

The Stryker wedge frame is not recommended if hyperextension of the spine is required or if lower extremity traction is needed. Like the Foster bed, clinical indications for the use of the frame include immobilization for patients with unstable spines, postoperative management of multilevel spinal fusions, and management of severe burn patients.

The frame comes only in one size. The only adaptation to accommodate extremes in body build is an adjustable crossbar of the anterior circle. By turning the knurled nuts of the crossbar up or down, a snug fit can be obtained for a small patient or a more comfortable fit obtained for a large patient. If the crossbar is properly adapted the patient is held firmly between the frames without the addition of pillows or extra "stuffing."

Loose linen and catheter tubes can become entrapped in the ring during rotation of the frames if careful attention is not given to removal of excess top covers and to placement of the catheter tubing between the patient's legs with the drainage bag at the foot end of the bed.

The elevation lock of the wedge is useful for elevating the head end of the anterior frame when the patient is prone. In the immediate postoperative period, it is also useful to elevate the head end of the frame, anterior or posterior, to increase pulmonary expansion by decreasing visceral pressure on the diaphragm.

When a patient is in halo or tong cervical traction the elevation lock provides countertraction up to a maximum of 7 inches. The Stryker literature includes a chart to determine the elevation needed for countertraction according to the weight of the patient and the amount of pull of the traction weight.

Specific nursing care measures for a patient on a horizontal frame are outlined below.

### GUIDELINES FOR NURSING CARE OF PATIENT ON STRYKER WEDGE FRAME

**A. Clinical indications**
  1. Postoperative management of patient following spinal fusion when weightbearing or ambulation is contraindicated.
  2. Posttraumatic management of patient with spinal instability, with or without cord damage.
  3. Cervical traction with use of skin traction (cervical halter) or skeletal traction (Crutchfield or Venke tongs).

**B. Advantages**
  1. Designed for turning by one person (institutional policy may require turning by *two* staff members).
  2. Lighter in weight than Foster bed.
  3. Size of patient accommodated by adjusting knurled nuts on crossbar of anterior circle.
  4. For larger patient, base of main frame may be extended to permit more comfortable fit.
  5. Has safety pin at head end to prevent unplanned rotation if turning knob is pulled.
  6. Wedge mechanism provides security for patient because frame always rotates toward apex, or narrow side of wedge.

7. Lower frame automatically locks when it is horizontal and level.

### C. Disadvantages

1. Unable to provide stable lower extremity traction.
2. Unable to provide spinal hyperextension.
3. Not useful for halo-femoral traction.
4. Loose linen and catheter tubing can become entrapped in ring if careful attention is not given to removing excess top linen before turning.
5. Patient with claustrophobia may not tolerate being "sandwiched" between frames.

### D. Procedure and safety factors

1. If medically feasible, demonstrate Wedge to patient and family by turning patient on frame. If patient is unable to be placed on frame before surgery, demonstrate mechanism, including safety factors, by permitting patient to observe a staff member (or another patient) being rotated on frame.
2. Measure patient and adjust canvas to correspond with patient's size.
   a. Lower edge of trunk section of posterior canvas corresponds to trochanteric level so that when bedpan section is removed, buttocks does not sag (prevents hyperextension of lower back).
   b. When patient is prone, lower edge of leg section corresponds to area superior to malleolus level so that correct ankle posture is maintained.
3. Check to ensure that posterior frame is secured to posterior post and that anterior frame is secured to anterior post. (Turning handles are always on left side of patient, and patient is always rotated toward right side.)

| Procedure | Safety factors |
|---|---|
| **Preparation** | |
| 1. Lock casters of frame. | Two staff members are preferred to ensure safety. |
| 2. Lower armboards. | Remove any obstructions. |
| 3. Clear and lower reading board and bedpan rack. | To protect patient's arms. |
| 4. Drape patient with pillow case over loin area and remove top linens. | Turnsheet (length of patient's torso) may be necessary if patient requires being moved up or down on frame. |
| 5. If indwelling catheter is present, bridge with 3 × 5 × 18 inch foam blocks. | To ensure proper drainage by keeping pressure off catheter. |
| 6. Check position of all tubes. Whenever possible, thread tubing laterally to head or foot end of frame. | |

| Procedure | Safety factors |
|---|---|
| 7. Place frame over patient and secure with knurled nut at head end and with closure of ring. *Recheck* knurled nut after closure of ring. | If turning to prone position, adjust head sections above brow level and at chin level. |
| 8. Place safety belt at elbow level. If patient has control of upper extremities, have patient clasp arms around frame. | *Two* safety straps prevent falls and injury to extremities. Include arms under safety strap if patient does not have control of arms. |
| 9. Remove safety pin at head end of frame. Place one safety belt at thigh level. | Secure safety straps to prevent shifting during turn. |
| **Turning** | |
| 1. Recheck tube positions and excess linen that may become entangled in ring turning mechanism. | |
| 2. Pull (turning lock) knob and rotate frame by grasping turning handles. | Second staff member assists with tubing. Frame automatically locks after turning if it is level and horizontal. |
| **Care after turning** | |
| 1. Remove safety belts. | |
| 2. Unlock and open ring and release knurled nut. | |
| 3. Remove top frame and close circle, or ring. | |
| 4. Check position of all tubes. | Avoid obstruction or kinking of tubing. |
| 5. Place one safety belt over thigh level. | Patients recovering from anesthesia or requiring narcotics must be observed frequently. |
| 6. Supine position | |
| a. Support normal contour of neck with small pillow or foam. | Not necessary with halo traction. |
| b. Adjust foot support. | Prevent heel cord tightening. *Caution:* With sensory denervation, avoid pressure of foot support against plantar surface of feet. Use foot support to keep top linens off toes. |
| c. Place flat towel or foam bridge to free heels from mattress. | Prevent heel decubiti. |

| Procedure | Safety factors |
|---|---|
| d. Check skin for pressure areas. Massage bony prominences, including forehead and chin. | |
| e. Encourage self-care and diversional activities. Prism glasses permit reading and TV viewing. | If part of the therapeutic plan, ROM and isometric exercises. |
| 7. Prone position | |
| a. Check position of headband sections. | Observe for proper trunk alignment. Use turnsheet if adjustment is needed. |
| b. Adjust padded armboards toward head end. | Level of armboards depends on shoulder posture. |
| c. Adjust reading board. | |
| d. Place flat towels or foam pieces under shoulders if necessary to prevent forward drop of shoulder girdles. | Shoulders properly positioned will enhance chest expansion. |
| e. Check ankle posture (feet should be free with ankle in neutral position). | Prevents plantar flexion and tight heel cords. |
| f. Encourage self-care such as personal grooming, oral hygiene, feeding while patient is prone. | |
| g. Diversional activities such as reading, writing, art work. | |
| h. If medically feasible, active knee flexion and ankle circumduction are encouraged while patient is prone. | Prevention of hazards of long-term recumbency. |
| i. Deep breathing and coughing are programmed at regular intervals. | Splinting of abdomen by frame enhances coughing. |
| j. When patient is prone, elevate head end 2 or 3 inches by freeing latch underneath black handle at patient's heel and raising lock tab. | |
| 8. Keep written schedule planned with patient and posted at bedside. | |

## CircOlectric bed

Some of the clinical indications for the vertical turning bed and the versatility of the Stryker CircOlectric (COL) (Fig. 30-5) bed have been presented earlier in the chapter. A photostory of the CircOlectric bed by Gordon[6,pp.42-62] is useful for staff and family education.

The posterior mattress of the COL bed (model 460) is 30 inches wide and permits side-lying as well as supine or prone posture. The model 360, manufactured until 1965, is 26 inches wide. The posterior and anterior sections are equipped with adjustable footboards.

The anterior frame is secured to the posterior mattress by tightening the stud nut on the stud at each e..d of the frame. The head end stud should be secured first. The anterior frame footboard is adjusted gently against the patient's feet and the stud nut is tightened on the foot end stud. Next, the forehead and chin supports are slid to just above the brow level and just below the lower lip level. The distance between the frames is adjusted by pulling the adjusting knobs on the anterior support bar and lowering the anterior frame until it rests on the patient's chest. Once this has been set, it is not necessary to adjust it each time the patient is prone. Casters should be checked to be sure they are locked. The knobs are released and the frame tested to make sure the pins are engaged in the notches. After the safety belts and arm slings are secured, the patient is ready to be rotated.

The electric motor (1725 rpm) is operated by a control switch that consists of a toggle switch (*up* rotates the bed face forward, *down* rotates the bed backward) and a lever button. Release of the lever button stops the rotation. The control switch clamps onto the ring or circle when not in use.

If power failure or control switch malfunction should occur, the COL bed can be operated manually by a hand crank inserted into the control box. The control box is under the metal panel at the head end of the bed. The crank is stored in the metal panel. For safety reasons, the crank is an essential part of the COL bed.

Smith[15] and co-workers in 1975 cautioned practitioners about the complications resulting from use of the COL bed for patients with unstable spines. Roberts and Curtiss[13] in 1970 also issued a warning about the dangers of the vertical turning bed in the management of these patients. Smith and co-workers have demonstrated that the amount of weight borne by the patient's feet, on the average, is 90% of the body weight. These authors conclude

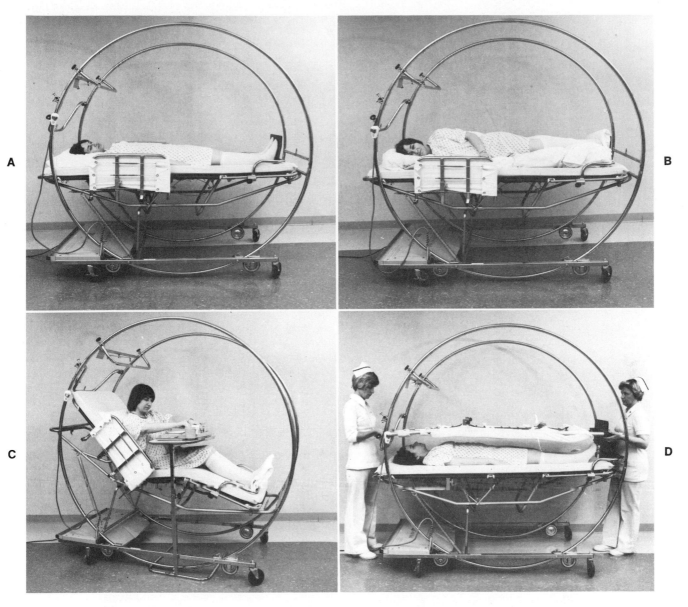

**Fig. 30-5.** CircOlectric bed. The CircOlectric bed is electronically controlled and permits vertical alteration of position from prone to supine. Its versatility permits other changes of position as shown. Again, because of liability and safety involved within health care settings, it is recommended that two individuals be present and assist during the turning process. The following are steps in the turning process. **A,** Patient is supine on CircOlectric bed. Note that footboard is in place and arm boards may serve as safety side rails. It is recommended that bed remain unplugged except during turning process. **B,** Patient is side lying. Note abundant use of pillows to support body in proper alignment. This is only turning frame that permits side lying, due to width of posterior mattress. **C,** CircOlectric bed is adjustable and permits sitting to varying degrees. Note that knees are flexed slightly and footboard is utilized to maintain appropriate position. **D,** Anterior frame is placed over patient and appropriately adjusted to begin turning process.

*Continued.*

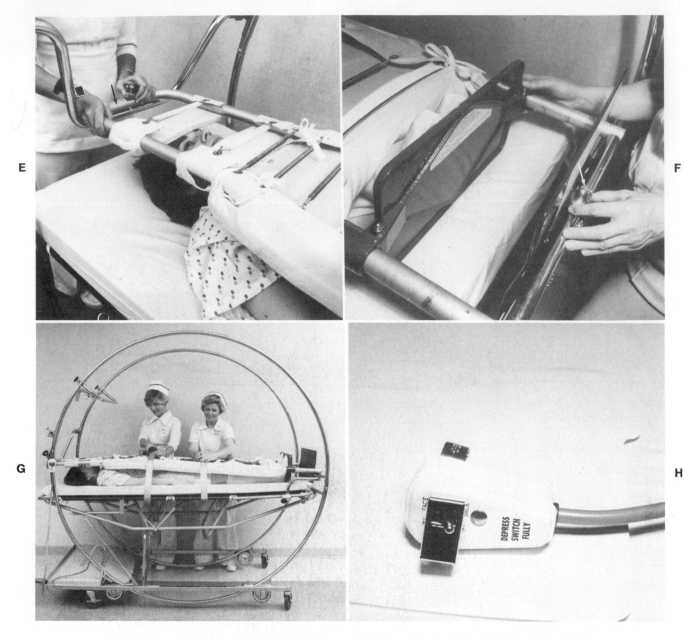

**Fig. 30-5, cont'd. E,** Screw at head of frame is secured. Note that forehead band is appropriately adjusted; anterior portion of canvas should come to just above shoulders. Chin band (shown) is optional for comfort. **F,** Screw at foot of bed is secured after footplate is adjusted. **G,** Two safety straps are utilized and secured. Bed may now be plugged into electrical outlet. **H,** Hand control is shown.

that if the patient's spine is not stable enough for standing posture, a horizontal rather than a vertical turning frame should be used.

Another disadvantage of the COL bed mentioned by Smith[15] is the development of "CircOlectric feet." A patient without protective sensation can get decubiti from the pressure of the footboard against the feet and from the posterior mattress resting on the heels when prone. These pressure complications can be prevented if the staff gives thoughtful consideration to eliminating the pressure on the dorsum of the feet by releasing the footplate after turning the patient prone and repositioning the footplate before turning the patient supine. The COL instruction booklet includes a technique of gatching the posterior mattress after putting the pa-

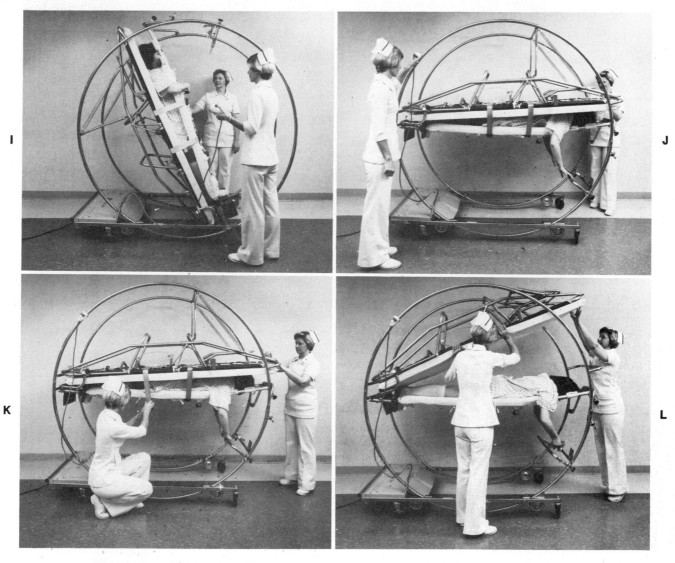

**Fig. 30-5, cont'd. I,** When all screws and footplate are properly secured, patient is turned. It is recommended, unless otherwise designated by physician, that turning be continuous process. **J,** When patient is prone, hand control may be attached to bed, and bed may be unplugged from electrical outlet. **K,** Safety straps are loosened, and screw at head of bed on posterior frame is removed. Note that this is *only* screw removed when prone. **L,** Posterior frame is then secured under safety latch provided at top of bed.
*Continued.*

tient in the prone position in order to eliminate pressure on the patient's heels.

An additional hazard is the height of the frame. A COL bed has no high-low mechanism. An elderly patient, a postanesthesia patient, or a heavily sedated patient must be observed carefully and frequently. A safety belt is secured around the patient at the thigh level to prevent falls. A body holder or re-

straint may be indicated if patients who are not responsible for their behavior.

For a patient who is not permitted to have the posterior frame gatched, a good practice is to remove the gatch levers and tape them to the aluminum horizontal frame of the bed.

The COL bed has many safety features. In addition to the caster locks, which stabilize the bed

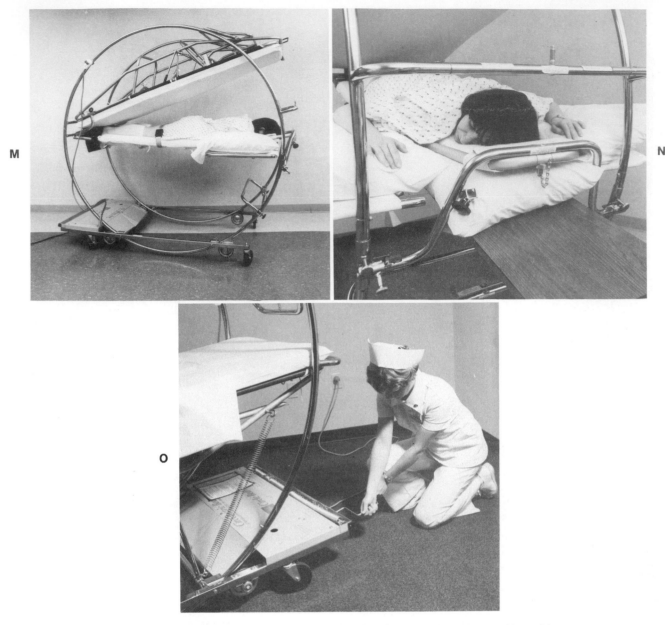

**Fig. 30-5, cont'd. M,** Patient is then secured with safety strap in prone position with arm boards in place for support and comfort. **N,** Note utilization of pillow on overbed table for comfort. Forehead strap or padded faceplate may also be utilized for positioning when patient is prone. **O,** Hand crank may be utilized at head of bed to permit position alteration and turning during power failures or electrical malfunction.

when it is being operated, there are permanent stops to prevent the bed from rotating beyond 210 degrees. There are two stops that can be engaged by levers to prevent the bed from being rotated past the sitting position (on the right side of the base) and to prevent the bed from being rotated past the standing position. These stops are used when the anterior frame is *not* used, that is, when the patient is placed in a sitting or standing posture.

To use the bed for standing or preparation for ambulation (Fig. 30-6) the nurse puts the anterior frame in place and stops the bed at the standing position for a short time. The patient's cardiovascular response to the upright posture must be carefully monitored. When the patient tolerates standing between the frames for 5 to 10 minutes, he or she is ready for standing without the front support of the frame. The patient then progresses to standing with

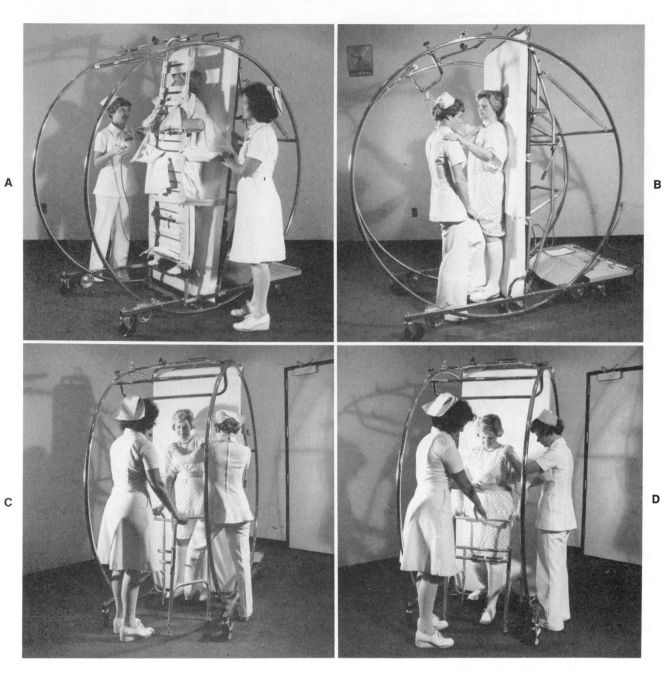

**Fig. 30-6.** The CircOlectric bed utilized to promote an upright position and ambulation. **A,** Bed may be utilized to promote upright position with anterior frame in place for security. This is frequently a gradual process. Note utilization of arm slings for support. **B,** Establishment of upright position without anterior frame. Note support is provided by nurse by bracing patient's knee to provide stability. This support is frequently necessary during initial stages of ambulation. **C,** Transition from CircOlectric bed to walker. Note manner in which one nurse stabilizes walker while additional nurse stabilizes patient by bracing of lower extremity and by general support. **D,** Patient is able to step off footplate onto floor with assistance of nurses and walker. Note the use of safety belt around waist of patient.

safety belts at the knee and waist. When the gluteal and quadriceps muscles are strong enough to control the hips and knees, the patient is ready to stand without the torso resting against the posterior mattress. The grab bar should be placed within easy reach. Well-planned progression of activities helps the patient achieve this goal.

The operating manual has instructions regarding use of the bedpan. For most patients, a standard fracture or orthopedic pan is used, and the patient is rolled onto the pan. COL beds can be adapted by using 3- to 4-inch polyurethane foam mattresses, thus eliminating the bedpan apertures. The posterior mattress is made firmer with a medium $3/8$ inch plywood square between the vinyl and the springs. The anterior arm support bracket reinforces the anterior frame.

Other features of the CircOlectric bed include adjustable footboards, overbed table, siderails/arm supports, and an adjustable face piece. Some traction apparatus, such as halo-femoral, cervical, and Buck's extension, can be managed on the COL bed. With the weights hung at the head of the bed by a series of clamps and pulleys, the patient may be placed prone without interrupting continuous traction.

When cervical traction is used, an additional weight of 5 pounds is necessary during the turn to account for the weight of the patient's head; this weight must be removed after the vertical turn is completed.

Transferring the patient via chairlift or litter is a very smooth, efficient procedure with a COL bed. The most important step is to attach the counterbalance sleeve over the head end stud. The grab bar is removed so that it will not interfere with the straight swing of the chains from the swivel bar.

One of the greatest advantages of the CircOlectric bed is that it enhances patient comfort during the position changes that are essential for the severely traumatized patient or during the immediate postoperative period following orthopedic surgery. The COL bed also permits a patient who has had hip surgery to stand with controlled weight-bearing and to progress to ambulation without having to sit first during the immediate postoperative period. Elderly patients can be mobilized using COL rather than risking the consequences of 5 to 7 days of bedrest.

## NURSING GUIDELINES FOR NURSING CARE OF PATIENT ON A CIRCOLECTRIC BED

### A. Clinical indications
1. Facilitation of bed positioning for the severely injured patient with multiple fractures or burns.
2. Posttraumatic management of the patient with spinal instability with or without cord damage.
3. Pre- and postoperative management of the patient with scoliosis.
4. Utilization of halo or halo-femoral traction as well as traction with other types of cervical skeletal traction.
5. Immediate postoperative management of the patient following hip or back procedure for early ambulation when sitting is contraindicated.
6. In selected long-term cases, facilitation of patient's transition from recumbency to standing and progressive ambulation.

### B. Advantages
1. Permits side-lying as well as supine and prone bed posture.
2. Designed for turning by one person (although institutional policy may require turning by two staff members).
3. Permits standing posture for patient who is required to remain on long-term recumbency and thus aids in prevention or complications such as orthostatic hypotension, osteoporosis, and other problems related to immobilization.
4. Adjustable components (footboard, anterior support bar) accommodate for weight and height of patients.
5. Patient can operate the bed providing some degree of participation in tilting the frame. (NOTE: sitting and standing stops should be engaged if patient operates bed independently).
6. Bed can be operated manually with a hand crank in event of power failure.
7. Provides excellent sitting posture for patient's participation in activities such as mealtimes and using bedpan.
8. Transfer sling or litter provides safe and efficient transfer to chair or stretcher. (CAUTION: grab bar must be removed for transfer procedures.)

### C. Disadvantages
1. Unable to provide lower extremity balanced suspension traction.
2. Unable to provide spinal hyperextension.
3. Height of bed is not adjustable.
4. Unsafe for unattended patient who is confused, hyperactive, or not responsible for own behavior.
5. May be contraindicated if patient's spinal instability does not permit weight bearing to 90% of total body weight.
6. Patient with claustrophobia may not tolerate being "sandwiched" between frames.

### D. Procedure and safety factors
1. If medically feasible, demonstrate COL bed to patient and family by turning patient on bed.

2. Measure patient and adjust anterior canvas and head and chin bands to correspond with height of patient.
3. Utilize adjustable facepiece rather than head and chin bands if immobilization of cervical spine is desired or necessary. (See CircOlectric bed operating manual).
4. Ensure expertise of staff members by orienting each to all features, including safety stops and hand crank, of COL bed. Have each staff member participate in demonstration and practice session so that he or she knows sensation of being turned on bed.
5. Have mechanical and electrical components checked by orthopedic technician or engineering department before bed is placed in service.

| Procedure | Safety factors |
|---|---|
| **Preparation** | |
| 1. Lock casters of bed. | Two staff members required (at least one RN) |
| 2. Remove armboards. | |
| 3. Disengage safety stop levers. | In addition to standing and sitting safety stop levers, there are permanent stops that do not permit full 360° rotation. |
| 4. Move posterior footboard to neutral position at foot of bed. (NOTE: on 1977 COL bed posterior footboard is *removed* for turning procedure.) | |
| 5. Place anterior frame over patient, securing head end stud nut first. | |
| 6. Adjust anterior footboard against patient's feet by depressing spring-loaded buttons. | To ensure stability of footboard to make sure buttons are engaged in appropriate holes. |
| 7. Secure floor end stud nut. | |
| 8. Lower anterior frame to patient by pulling adjusting pins out to allow frame to slide down rings and to lock in place into corresponding holes when pins are released. | Once this adjustment is made according to patient's size it is not necessary to make adjustment each time patient is prone. |
| 9. Check position of headbands (foot headband above brow | Chin band and uppermost anterior frame mattress must not |

| Procedure | Safety factors |
|---|---|
| level and chin band over chin) and make sure shoulders will be well supported. | press against anterior neck. |
| 10. Place patient's arms in arm slings. | Optional for patient who has good control of arms. |
| 11. Secure frame with two safety belts. | One safety belt across pelvis and one belt across thigh level. |
| **Turning** | |
| 1. Check security of stud nuts before rotating bed. | |
| 2. Check position of tubing. | Second staff member holds urinary drainage tubing clear of rings. |
| 3. Grasp operating controls, push toggle switch (face), and press lever until patient is in head-down position. Release of lever stops bed instantly. | Staff member operating control box places hand on patient's shoulder to give confidence and support to patient. |
| 4. Remove safety belts. | |
| 5. Raise posterior mattress off patient by removing head end stud nut. | |
| 6. Secure posterior frame overhead, pull safety bar forward until bar locks frame in position. | With patient in head-down posture, the safety bar is within better reach. |
| 7. Level anterior frame by snapping toggle switch down (back) and pressing lever. | |
| 8. Reposition IV and catheter tubing. | Avoid kinking or obstruction of tubing. |
| 9. Prone position a. Place one safety belt over thigh level. | Patients recovering from anesthesia or requiring narcotics must be observed frequently. |
| b. Check head and neck posture. | |
| c. Place folded towels under shoulders to prevent forward drop of shoulder girdles. | Shoulders properly positioned will enhance chest expansion. |
| d. Adjust armboards, padded with pillows. | |

| Procedure | Safety factors |
|---|---|
| e. Place folded towel above patellae. | Prevents pressure areas on patellae. |
| f. Check ankle posture (ankles should be in neutral position). | If patient has motor ability, encourage active ankle range of motion. |
| g. To alleviate pressure on heels, gatch posterior frame. | CAUTION: for patient who lacks protective sensation of the feet, move footboard away from feet. |
| | CAUTION: for patient with sensory deficit, relieve pressure from heels by gatching posterior frame. |
| | *Remember:* reposition footboard before turning to supine position. |
| h. Promote self-care activities such as oral hygiene and eating by placing overbed table between rings and within reach of patient. | |
| i. Encourage deep-breathing and coughing exercises while prone. | With head end of anterior frame and splinting of abdomen by frame, coughing is enhanced. |
| 10. Supine position | |
| a. Reverse procedure to turn patient to supine position. | |
| b. If medically feasible, place small pillow to support head and cervical contour. | |
| c. Adjust padded footboard for support. | CAUTION: Footboard flush against patient's feet is contraindicated with spastic paralysis or insensitive feet. |
| d. Place side rail on each side. | |
| e. Observe forehead and chin areas for erythema. | Additional padding of bands may be indicated before patient turned to prone position. |
| f. If patient is high risk for decubiti, bridge bony prom- | Areas to observe closely include ankles, knees, anterior and |

| Procedure | Safety factors |
|---|---|
| inences to relieve pressure. | superior iliac spines, scapulae, sacrum, and trochanters. |
| g. If medically feasible, encourage active ROM of shoulders, hips, knees, and ankles. | Isometric exercises such as quadriceps and gluteal setting maintain muscle tone. |
| h. Keep written turning schedule planned with patient and posted at bedside. | COL bed facilitates turning but does not diminish need for frequent turning. |

**Transfer to wheelchair**

| Procedure | Safety factors |
|---|---|
| 1. Place transfer sling over patient's back (sling is marked *Head end*). | Two staff members are required for transfer procedure. |
| 2. Turn patient supine and remove anterior frame. | *Lock* casters before rotating bed. |
| 3. Place counterbalance spring sleeve over head end stud. | CAUTION: counterbalance spring *must* be engaged for transfer procedure. |
| 4. Have patient flex hips and knees so that chain hooks can be easily attached to swivel bar. | CAUTION: grasp bar must be removed for transfer procedure. |
| 5. Gatch bed by releasing gatch lever. | |
| 6. Rotate bed with operating control box (toggle switch up, *face*) until patient is clear of mattress. | Free safety stop levers for free rotation of bed. |
| 7. Rotate swivel bar so that patient is facing mattress. | |
| 8. Position wheelchair under patient and continue rotation of bed until patient is seated in wheelchair. | |
| 9. Detach chain hooks from swivel bar. | Reverse procedure for returning patient to bed. |

**Transfer by litter**

| Procedure | Safety factors |
|---|---|
| 1. Lock casters. | Stryker litter is necessary for litter transfer. |
| 2. Attach counterbalance sleeve to head end stud. | CAUTION: counterbalance spring assembly *must* be used for transfer. |
| 3. Rotate bed so that mattress is vertical. | |
| 4. Fasten chain clamps to head end of litter. | |
| 5. With stretcher and its removable litter between | |

**Procedure**

circles or rings, attach chain assembly to swivel bar.

6. As COL bed is rotated toward *back* by one person, second staff member supports foot end of litter.

7. Person operating bed removes stretcher and then continues to rotate bed until litter is resting on mattress.

8. Remove chain assembly from swivel bar and detach chains from litter.

9. Turn patient to position in order to remove litter from bed.

**Safety factors**

If medically feasible, patient may be turned from side to side to remove litter. CAUTION: patient with unstable spine may not be permitted to turn side to side.

### Using bedpan

1. Remove bedpan plug by pulling the plastic cord.

2. Place bedpan in position between plastic cords.

3. Place patient in sitting position by releasing gatch levers and rotating mattress (toggle switch up, *face*).

If sitting is contraindicated, patient may be turned onto fracture pan.

NOTE: For some patients with back or hip problems, sitting posture may be contraindicated. Therefore the gatch levers are removed and taped on the horizontal support bars beneath the posterior mattress. Also the firmness of the posterior mattress is reinforced by placing a piece of ⅜ inch plywood between the springs and the vinyl cover of the posterior frame.

### Other specialty beds

**Nelson patient handling device.** Another special bed designed to place the patient in a standing posture is the Nelson Patient Handling Device. The Nelson bed will also place the patient in a chair posture. Further information can be obtained from the manufacturer, W. H. McMills, Inc., Palo Alto, California.

**Keane Roto Rest.** The Roto Rest Treatment Table (Fig. 30-7) was designed by Frank Keane, a physician in Ireland. Based on the theory that stasis and akinetics are the causes of many clinical problems of the immobilized patients, Keane developed a mechanical means of giving the recumbent patient mobility. The bed rotates on a horizontal axis from 62 degrees on each side at 4.5 minute intervals. Personal hygiene to the back and perineum and exercise of the extremities can be accomplished by releasing a series of hatches on the underside of the bed. The electric motor is silent and can be stopped for meals and treatments in any of the ten locking positions. Continuous cervical or lower extremity traction is possible by using the apparatus at the head or the foot end of the bed.

Presently there are two models of Keane's kinetic table. The Mark I is designed for management of

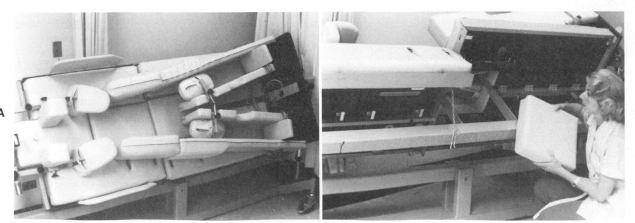

**Fig. 30-7.** Keane Roto Rest bed. **A,** Bed is turned 60° to right. **B,** Pelvic hatch is open for placement of bedpan. (From Valentin, L.: Kinetic nursing and the Roto Rest bed, O.N.A.J. **4**(3):62-65, 1977.)

the critically ill or multiple trauma patient. A smaller table, the Mark III, is available for long-term bedrest or severely disabled patients.

**Other devices.** Several other types of beds are available commercially, such as the water bed, the mud bed, the air fluidized bed. Some of these devices are listed in Tables 30-1 and 30-2 at the end of this chapter. These beds are designed primarily to prevent or treat decubitus ulcers in the management of long-term bedridden patients.

### Preventive maintenance

Preventive maintenance of the equipment is an important consideration. In some institutions, the maintenance or engineering departments assume responsibility for keeping the beds in good working order. In others, the central service departments maintain the beds. In large medical centers, specialized orthopedic technicians are trained to inspect and service the specialty equipment. Generally, the patient on the bed is charged a fee for initial servicing and preparation of the bed plus a daily fee. The installation and daily fees are determined on the basis of usage and expected life of the apparatus.

### STAFF EDUCATION

One of the most crucial factors in enhancing the patient's adjustment and acceptance of a special bed, as well as ensuring the patient's safety, is the level of expertise demonstrated by the nursing staff. The patient's fears and apprehensions are minimized if the staff members are knowledgeable about the special bed and skillful in operating it. The patient who has confidence in the staff's ability to use the bed and to make adaptations to ensure increased safety and comfort fares much better on the bed.

Demonstration and practice sessions are the best way to educate staff members. Each person who gives nursing care to a patient on a turning frame should have the opportunity to be turned on the frame. Role-playing is an excellent way to gain appreciation of the detailed adaptations, such as placing foam pads under the patients shoulders when prone to maintain proper alignment and increase pulmonary expansion. Operating manuals are helpful to staff and to patients and their families, but they are adjuncts only. Experience is the best teacher.

A sound hospital policy is to have *two* staff members, including an experienced registered nurse, assisting with the vertical or horizontal turning of the patient. Unfortunate incidents must be prevented. Two persons can check each other and remind each other of the need for checking the tubing, position-

ing the safety straps, and the many mechanical details that are essential for safe and effective turning.

Placing the adult or adolescent patient on the bed prior to surgery for a demonstration is an important step in preparing the patient for weeks or months of immobility on the bed or frame. Using a Bradford frame at the onset of treatment is easier for a child to accept than waiting until problems arise.

For the trauma patient, preplanning or orientation to the frame may not be possible. However, using brochures or photographs or having the patient observe another patient or a staff member being turned is a good way to help the patient understand the mechanics of the bed and the need for the apparatus and to allay any apprehensions about the device.

None of the frames and beds are custom built; adjustment of the canvas to fit the patient's body size and build is another important step in preparing the bed for the patient and the patient for the bed.

In some areas of the country, the Wedge, Foster, or CircOlectric bed can be rented for extended immobilization at home, which shortens the hospital stay and reduces medical costs. Home management of patients who have had multilevel spinal fusions (thoracolumbar or lumbosacral) has been very satisfactory. A van-type ambulance will accommodate the length and height of the Wedge frame with special lashing of the frame to stabilize it. CircOlectric beds require a floor-to-ceiling measurement of at least 84 inches. COL beds have been used well in a mobile home. Patient and family education, along with referral to the home health care agency, is the key to successful home management of the patient on a turning frame or bed. Several days before discharge, a family member should participate in rotating the frame or bed so that he or she can safely handle the apparatus. Written instructions, along with a copy of the manufacturer's manual, reinforce the learning process.

### SPECIAL NURSING CARE CONSIDERATIONS
### Exercise

Bed exercises that may be appropriate for the patient include deep-breathing and coughing with blow glove exercises, full active range of motion to shoulders, gluteal setting and quadriceps setting (isometric) exercises, active circumduction of ankles, internal rotation of the hips, and active flexion of the knees when the patient is prone.

If the patient is quadriplegic or paraplegic, all involved joints should be taken through ROM exercises at least once a day. Positioning of the extremities in functional posture includes use of the foot frame to prevent heel cord (drop foot) contracture and deformity. The upper extremities are positioned at intervals with the shoulders abducted and externally rotated to prevent frozen shoulders. Resting or cock-up splints may be prescribed by the physician and made by the therapist to prevent wristdrop and loss of thumb-finger apposition. Prolonged faulty positioning, at rest or in activity, is the cause of contracture and deformity.

## Turning schedules

Turning schedules vary according to the patient and condition. Of course, a patient with cord damage who lacks protective sensation requires more frequent observation of skin tolerance to pressure and more frequent turning. Even 2 hours may be too long for a thin quadriplegic or for an obese patient who has sensation but moist, warm skin surfaces rubbing together in the gluteal fold. Each patient is considered individually, and a specific turning schedule is programmed based on specific needs.

## Prevention of osteoporosis and kidney stones

Consideration of demineralization of the long bones as well as generalized osteoporosis as consequences of long-term recumbency requires that the patient's plan of care include adequate hydration (adult: 3000 ml/day) and measures to maintain an acid urine to help prevent kidney stones and urinary tract infections. Alkaline urine is a good medium for stone formation and bacterial growth. Dietary measures that ensure acid urine include certain foods such as cranberries, prunes, limited citrus intake, and limited daily allowance of milk, cheese and other dairy products. The physician may prefer to give ascorbic acid daily during the period of recumbency for urine acidity.

## Bladder and bowel management

The trend today with cord-damaged patients is toward intermittent catheterization. With this program, fluids are restricted to 100-150 ml per hour during the day. In the evening (7 to 10 PM.) fluids are restricted to 300/ml, bringing the total fluid allotment to 1800 to 2100 ml per day. The patient is catheterized regularly at intervals that permit the bladder to fill to optimal capacity yet prevent overdistention. Extreme care is taken in technique to prevent urinary tract infections.

Constipation is avoided if careful assessment of the patient's usual bowel habit is considered and regularity established. The use of stool softeners, mild laxatives, nutritional adjuncts such as prune juice and roughage, and, if needed, glycerine suppositories at periodic intervals will prevent the misery of constipation or impaction. Most of all, careful and consistent monitoring by a concerned and thoughtful nurse will prevent this age-old misery for the long-term recumbent patient.

## Prevention of decubitus ulcers

A chapter on special beds and frames in orthopedics is not complete without a discussion of the prevention of decubitus ulcers. A decubitus ulcer is the most discouraging of all the complications of immobility. The health care team cannot prevent the occurrence of some of the consequences of recumbency and inactivity, such as pulmonary embolism, but nurses *can* prevent pressure sores.

The scope of the problem is well known. Not only is the patient with a decubitus ulcer having to cope with a long-term health problem, but also the length of the hospital stay is doubled or tripled, and the goal-directed program for rehabilitation is interrupted. Activities are confined to a bed or guerney, progression to wheelchair activities or ambulation seems far removed from the reality of turning schedules, dressing changes, debridement, and sometimes surgical procedures. The cost of this unfortunate, unpleasant, and depressing complication is estimated to be as much as $15,000.[35]

The term *decubitus* is of Latin derivation, meaning "lying down." Because decubiti may and do occur when an area of the patient's body surface is subjected to pressures other than the bed or mattress, a more appropriate term is *pressure sore* or *pressure necrosis*. The term "pressure necrosis" is even more meaningful when the pathophysiology is understood.

Medical and nursing literature is replete with articles about the etiology, prevention, and treatment of pressure sores. Reliable and valid research results have been published, but all too often the research has been based on inadequate sampling without control of variables. However, some impressive research has been accomplished in the etiology, progression of ulceration, and factors that influence the tissue breakdown.[2]

One must understand the effects of pressure on living tissue and the consequences of duration as it relates to intensity of pressure before learning how pressure sores can be prevented. The following outline is based on Berecek's[2] article:

1. Normal intercapillary pressure in arterioles is 32 mm Hg; in venules, 15 mm Hg.
2. In a recumbent position, if the pressure were evenly distributed over the surface area being

supported, the pressure would be less than ⅓ pound per square inch (or approximately 17 mm Hg).

3. In a supine position, the highest points of pressure are the sacrum, the buttocks, and the heels (40 to 60 mm Hg for a healthy person with ideal body weight).

4. In a prone position, the pressure on knees and chest is up to 50 mm Hg.

5. Body weight affects pressure distribution:
   a. For the thin person, recumbent, peak pressures are higher than for normal and obese persons recumbent.
   b. For the thin person, sitting, there are sharper gradients and higher peaks of pressure.
   c. For the obese person, sitting, there is very high pressure over larger areas.

6. According to two independent studies by Husain and Kosiak,[9] when pressure is 60 to 70 mm Hg, the critical time interval is 1 to 2 hours for normal and denervated tissue.

7. Reactive hyperemia is a normal response to circulatory embarrassment to tissue through a mechanism of restoring nutrients by increasing the blood flow.

8. If pressure is not relieved within 1 to 2 hours, irreversible changes occur, which result in tissue necrosis, or a pressure sore.

9. Pressure sores can be classified as two types[7]: superficial (benign) and deep (malignant). Ischemic changes occur in the deep tissues that are not clinically or grossly identifiable until the skin is involved.

In summary the etiology of pressure necrosis is as follows:

Miller and Sachs[11] present an excellent photographic essay to demonstrate how skin under pressure looks. Patients were photographed from below a transparent surface so that the effects of pressure—ischemia and reactive hyperemia—could be visualized. Every member of the nursing staff should have access to this book.

Berecek[2, p. 166] lists the following factors that predispose a patient to pressure sores:

1. Physical factors
   a. Pressure (compression)
   b. Shearing force
   c. Heat (fever)
   d. Moisture
   e. Friction
   f. Hygiene
2. Nutrition
   a. General undernutrition
   b. Specific nutritional deficiencies (protein, ascorbic acid)
3. Anemia
4. Infection
5. Movement (mobility)

With the knowledge of what factors contribute to the formation of pressure necrosis, the nurse can assess each patient and determine if he or she is highly susceptible to decubiti. The most important assessment includes careful inspection, monitoring of the skin surfaces, and determination of measures within the plan of care to prevent pressure sores.

Orthopedic patients who are considered highly predisposed to pressure sores include patients with:

1. Severe trauma, immobilized in traction, casts, braces

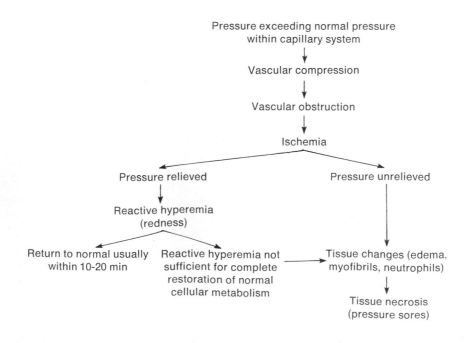

2. Denervation or peripheral nerve involvement with loss of motor and sensory function; spasticity
3. Moderately severe to severe rheumatoid arthritis (or other collagen diseases) with vasculitis
4. Geriatric problems, including undernutrition, immobility, atherosclerosis, senility, and lack of motivation.
5. Incontinence
6. Postoperative immobilization, especially multilevel spinal fusion

After careful assessment of the patient's susceptibility to skin breakdown, the nurse must determine what plans can be implemented to preserve the integrity of the skin. The options are many; so many that to survey them is beyond the scope of this chapter. The market is flooded with products designed to protect the skin. For most of the products (mechanical devices, softwares, alternating pressure pads, gel pads, foam, waterbeds, mattresses, topical applications, and oral agents) research findings are not conclusive. Many times a nurse in good faith selects a product only to discover that the patient's reddened area continues to progress to ulceration.

Selection of adjunctive measures is often not aggressive enough. A high risk patient should be afforded the best product available. However, unless the patient receives diligent and frequent nursing care, pressure sores will not be prevented.

In orthopedic nursing practice there are unique problems that compound the danger of skin breakdown. One of the most significant problems, of course, is enforced recumbency with application of external fixation devices such as casts and traction. With skin traction, the unique factor is the shearing force caused by improperly applied traction apparatus. In addition, some nursing measures, such as positioning and helping patients with the bedpan, may be improperly executed. To reduce friction and shearing forces, which are more destructive to the tissues than pressure itself, a turn sheet that includes the entire torso should be used. Also, as soon as possible the patient should be taught the technique of pulling up in bed by *lifting* his trunk with the aid of a trapeze bar.

The orthopedic bedpan is a necessary evil. Shearing forces in the sacral region can be avoided by turning the patient onto the pan. When the patient is turned to remove the pan, the buttocks are cleansed with mild soap and water, dried thoroughly, and inspected, and a silicone vanishing cream is massaged into the skin to protect against moisture and soiling.

A fallacy of turning schedules is that the schedules are not based on the needs of the individual patient. For a patient with severe rheumatoid arthritis and vasculitis that resulted in an above knee amputation, for example, turning every 2 hours is not enough. To prevent hip flexion tightness and to protect the sacrum and trochanters this patient should be prone for 45 minutes three times a day with the heel and malleolus elevated off the mattress at all times with the use of a 1-inch wedge of foam that supports the belly of the calf muscle. Wearing a sock or heel protector reduces friction as the patient moves in bed. Heel protectors help reduce friction but they do not alleviate pressure unless they are used with a foam wedge to keep the heels off the bed.

The effect of shearing force on the deeper sacral tissue is well described by Berecek[2,p.163] Clinically, the effect of this phenomenon is observed through inspection of the undermining, which lies deep within the opening of the crater of a sacral decubitus. This precaution applies to innervated as well as denervated tissue. To avoid this force, the angle of Fowler's position is limited to 30 degrees, and, unless contraindicated, the knees are bent 5 to 10 degrees to prevent the patient from sliding toward the foot of the bed.

After each position change the skin areas over bony prominences and skin fold areas are inspected for the presence of reactive hyperemia. If redness is present the nurse observes the length of time necessary for the redness to disappear. If the time of hyperemia exceeds 10 to 20 minutes, pressure is alleviated by alternative positioning or by "bridging."

"Bridging" is an old nursing technique that is sound in principle. Rehabilitation centers have renewed this technique in the nursing care of the patient with paraplegia or quadriplegia. In the past bridging was done with pillows; now quality polyurethane foam blocks or custom-made 3- or 4-inch foam pads are cut with an electric knife. Problem areas, such as the ischium or the sacrum, can be made pressure free by beveled cut-outs. This is an inexpensive, effective way to protect bony prominences.

*Guidelines for Skin Care* by the Craig Institute, Denver, is comprehensive for teaching spinal cord injured patients how to protect their skin from injury or pressure. It is of interest that bridging is recommended rather than expensive mechanical devices. Patients often must increase skin tolerance so that a regular mattress at home will be suitable. For the wheelchair patient, ischial pressure can be relieved by doing sit-ups and weight shifting. This technique is helpful on an orthopedic unit also.

Another factor that is often encountered in orthopedics is nutritional deficiency. Healing does not take place when the patient is in negative nitrogen balance, which occurs when the patient has a protein deficient diet or when an unusual amount of protein is lost. The geriatric patient, for example, may be despondent or anorexic. Prompt referral to the clinical nutritionist for high protein, high calorie supplements, including a prescription for ascorbic acid, will aid in reversing the process. A family conference to determine the patient's food preferences may also be helpful.

One of the most helpful mechanical devices for the long-term, recumbent orthopedic patient is the Lapidus pad, designed by man who spent several months on bedrest following trauma. The Lapidus pad has several features that are superior to alternating air mattresses. The pressure exerted on the body surface by the air columns changes every 15 seconds. In addition, there are many small pinholes in the trunk portion of the mattress through which air flows. The mattress is covered with a 1-inch foam pad so that moisture from perspiration seeks a lower level through the porous foam and is dryed by the air flow. Another desirable feature of the Lapidus pad is a smaller pad that can be placed under a draining wound to protect the foam pad. This pad can be disconnected from the air compressor motor and washed at the lavoratory, dried, and replaced as often as needed.

Another specific product developed within recent years is the Lotus water mattress, a clear vinyl mattress filled with 130 to 150 pounds of water and placed on a hospital mattress. It provides a displacement effect to eliminate high pressure points over bony prominences. Because the weight of the patient's trunk displaces water toward the foot end of the bed, the patient's heels and malleoli must be bridged to eliminate the increased pressure. The Lotus provides a cooling effect to decrease heat and moisture of perspiration for the long-term recumbent patient. Another advantage is that this system can be purchased for home use for approximately $50.

Clinically, water flotation is more beneficial in prevention of pressure necrosis than in treatment of pressure sores. As soon as the patient becomes more mobile and can participate in the rehabilitation process, it is important to transfer the patient to a regular mattress, using bridging to protect potential problem skin areas. This step, as mentioned previously, better prepares the patient for increased skin tolerance.

Current topical therapy, including enzymatic debridgement, is surveyed by Vasconez who concludes that "no study has demonstrated healing with a specific topical agent unless that treatment included control of infection, debridement of dead tissue, and decrease of pressure."[18] Vasconez agrees with Morgan[12] that studies in the treatment with topical agents "lack adequate controls and undoubtedly nursing care is superior because of the interest of physicians and nurses."

Vasconez's monograph presents an excellent discussion of surgical management of pressure sores in patients with spinal cord injury. Surgical debridement and the use of split-thickness grafts, obtained from skin with sensation, when possible, are described and illustrated. Areas of grafting include the occiput, scapula, elbow, anterior iliac spine, knee, sacrum, trochanters, the ischium, ankle, and foot.

Newer avenues of approach to the prevention and treatment of pressure sores are being researched. Temperature and pressure sensors, nerve grafting to provide protective sensation, and air support (levitation) are among the research efforts of today.

## SUMMARY

In this chapter we have surveyed from a historical point of view the special beds and frames designed for immobilized patients with musculoskeletal problems. Each of the designs is the result of the inventor's attempt to prevent the complications of prolonged immobilization and to facilitate nursing care while the patient is bedridden.

Presently, the most widely used specialty beds and frames include the Bradford frame, the hyperextension bed, the Foster frame, the Stryker wedge frame, and the CircOlectric bed. Because the patient's welfare and safety depend on the expertise of the practitioners responsible for care, a guideline for each of the most commonly used beds has been included. A guideline coupled with an experienced clinical teacher or role model will enhance the nursing management of the patient was well as allay the apprehensions of the patient and family.

Of all the hazards of long-term recumbency, the development of a decubitus ulcer, or pressure necrosis, is perhaps the most discouraging. Of all the devices used as adjunctive measures, none is a panacea. The common denominator of all the devices is the nurse who recognizes the need for prompt intervention with proper selection of the devices or methods for the patient who is at risk for skin breakdown. None of the methods replaces the need for expertise and diligence in the care of patients who are predisposed to tissue breakdown.

## REFERENCES

1. Ackerman, E. A.: Cervical traction in flexion, J. Bone Joint Surg. **54-A:**1114-1116, July, 1972.
2. Berecek, K. H.: Etiology of decubitus ulcers, Nurs. Clin. North Am. **10:**157-170, Mar. 1975.
3. Bick, E. M.: Source book of orthopaedics, ed. 1, Baltimore, 1937, The Williams & Wilkins Co.
4. Bick, E. M.: Source book of orthopaedics, ed. 2, Baltimore, 1948, The Williams & Wilkins Co.
5. Edberg, E. L., Gerney, J., and Stauffer, E. S.: Prevention and treatment of bedsores, Phys. Therapy **53:**246, Mar. 1973.
6. Gordon, J.: CircOlectric beds, Nursing 77, pp. 42-47, Feb. 1977.
7. Groth, K. E. In Berecek, K. H.: Etiology of decubitus ulcers, Nurs. Clin. North Am. **10:**157-170, Mar. 1975.
8. Hilt, N. E., and Schmitt, E. W., Jr.: Pediatric orthopedic nursing, St. Louis, 1975, The C. V. Mosby Co.
9. Husain, T., and Kosiak, M., as cited by Berecek, K. H.: Etiology of decubitus ulcers, Nurs. Clin. North Am. **10:**164, Mar. 1975.
10. Keith, A.: Menders of the maimed, London, 1919, Oxford University Press.
11. Miller, M. E., and Sacks, M. L.: About bedsores, Philadelphia, 1974, J. B. Lippincott Co.
12. Morgan, E. J.: Topical therapy of pressure sores, Surg. Gynecol. Obstet. **141:**945, 1975.
13. Roberts, J. B., and Curtiss, P. H., Jr.: Stability of the thoracic and lumbar spine in traumatic paraplegia following fracture or fracture dislocation, J. Bone Joint Surg. **52A:**1115-1130, 1970.
14. Shands, A. R., Jr.: The early orthopaedic surgeons of America, St. Louis, 1970, The C. V. Mosby Co.
15. Smith, T. K., Whitaker, J., and Stauffer, E. S.: Complications associated with the use of the circular electrical turning frame, J. Bone Joint Surg. **57A:**711, 1975.
16. Stryker, H. H.: A device for turning the frame patient, J.A.M.A. **113:**1731-1732, 1939.
17. Valentin, L.: Kinetic nursing and the Roto-Rest bed, ONAJ **4**(3):62-65, Mar. 1977.
18. Vasconez, L. O., Schneider, W. J., and Jurkiewicz, M. J.: Pressure sores; a monograph of current problems in surgery, Chicago, 1977, Year Book Medical Publishers, vol. XIV(4), Apr. 1977.

## BIBLIOGRAPHY

Ackerman, E. A.: Cervical traction in flexion, J. Bone Joint Surg. **54-A:**1114-1116, July 1972.
Altshuler, A., Meyer, J., and Butz, M.: Even children can learn to do clean catheterization, Am. J. Nurs. **77**(1): 97-101, Jan. 1977.
Berecek, K. H.: Etiology of decubitus ulcers, Nurs. Clin. North Am. **10**(1):157-170, Mar. 1975.
Berecek, K. H.: Treatment of decubitus ulcers, Nurs. Clin. North Am. **10**(1):171-210, Mar. 1975.
Bergstrom, D.: Rehabilitation nursing. In Licht, S.: Rehabilitation and medicine, Vol. X, Baltimore, 1968, Waverly, Press, Inc.
Bick, E. M.: Source book of orthopaedics, ed. 1, Baltimore, 1937, The Williams & Wilkins Co.
Bick, E. M.: Source book of orthopaedics, ed. 2, Baltimore, 1948, The Williams & Wilkins Co.
Blount, W. P., and More, J. H.: The Milwaukee Brace, Baltimore, 1973, The Williams & Wilkins Co.
Boardman, J.: New treatment for decubitus ulcers, ONAT **2**(3):60, Mar. 1975.
Champion, V. L.: Clean technique for intermittent self-catheterization, Nurs. Res. **25:**13-18, Jan.-Feb. 1976.
Coombs, R. M.: Supporting patients on air; an answer to pressure sores, Nurs. Mirror, **142:**45, 1976.
Dinsdale, S. M.: Decubitus ulcers: Role of pressure and friction in causation, Arch. Phys. Med. Rehab. **55:**147, 1974.
Edberg, E. L., Cerney, J., and Stauffer, E. S.: Prevention and treatment of bedsores, Phy. Therapy **53:**246, Mar. 1973.
Fischer, B. H.: Topical hyperbaric oxygen treatment of pressure sores and skin ulcers, Lancet **2:**405, 1969.
Gordon, J. E.: CircOlectric beds, a photostory, Nursing 77 Feb. 1977, pp. 42-47.
Craig Rehabilitation Institute: Guidelines for home: Skin Care, Englewood, Colo., 1976.
Harvin, J., and Hargest, T.: The air fluidized bed: A new concept in the treatment of decubitus ulcers, Nurs. Clin. North Am. **5:**181-187, 1970.
Hilt, N. E.: Bradford frame, use in pediatric nursing care, ONAJ **1:**10-15, Jan. 1974.
Hilt, N. E., and Schmitt, E. W. Jr.: Pediatric orthopedic nursing, St. Louis; 1975, The C. V. Mosby Co.
Kavchak-Keyes, M. A.: Four proven steps for preventing decubitus ulcers, Nursing 77, Sept. 1977, pp. 58-61.
Keane, F. X.: Roto-rest, Paraplegia **7:**254-258, Feb. 1970.
Keith, A.: Menders of the maimed, London, 1919, Oxford University Press.
Kelley, T. A. Jr.: Rehabilitation of the spinal cord injured patient. In Rothman, R. H., and Simeone, F. A.: The spine, Philadelphia; 1975, W. B. Saunders Co.
Kosiak, M.: Etiology and pathology of decubitus ulcers, Arch. Phys. Med. **40:**62-69, 1959.
Love-Mignogna, S.: Scoliosis, Nursing 77, May 1977, pp. 50-55.
Miller, M. E., and Sachs, M. L.: About bedsores, Philadelphia, 1974, J. B. Lippincott Co.
Orthopedic Nurses' Association, Inc.: Circolectric bed (audiovisual). ONA, Inc., 1938 Peachtree Road, N. W., Atlanta, Georgia 30309
Orthopedic Nurses' Association, Inc.: Wedge Stryker Frame (audiovisual). ONA, Inc., 1938 Peachtree Road, N. W., Atlanta, Georgia 30309.
Osgood, R. B.: The evolution of orthopaedic surgery, St. Louis; 1925, The C. V. Mosby Co.
Patterson, T. D., Roberts, J. M., and Cantrell, D.: Scoliosis, RN **39**(11):51-80, Nov. 1976.
Rao, D. B.: Management of dermal and decubitus ulcers, Drug Therapy, Oct. 1976, pp. 26-31.
Rao, D. B., and others: Collagenase in the treatment of

dermal and decubitus ulcers, J. Am. Geriat. Soc. **23:**22, Jan. 1975.

Roach, L. B.: Skin changes in dark skin, Nursing 72 **2:**19, Nov. 1972.

Roberts, J. B., and Curtiss, P. H., Jr.: Stability of the thoracic and lumbar spine in traumatic paraplegia following fracture or fracture dislocation, J. Bone Joint Surg. **52-A**Test, 1970

Rubin, Ch. F., and others: Auditing the decubitus ulcer problem, Am. J. Nurs. **74**(10):1820-1821, Oct. 1974.

Senf, H. R.: Caring for the patient in the CircOlectric bed, Am. J. Nurs. Feb. 1960. Reprint.

Shands, A. R., Jr.: The early orthopaedic surgeons of America, St. Louis; 1970, The C. V. Mosby Co.

Shea, J. D., and Merlino, A.: Decubiti classified, Patient Care **8:**236, 1974.

Skinner, G.: Nursing care of the patient on a Stryker frame, Am. J. Nurs. **46:**288-292, May 1946.

Smith, T. K., Whitaker, J., and Stauffer, E. S.: Complications associated with the use of the circular electrical turning frame, J. Bone Joint Surg. **57A:**711, July 1975.

Spence, W. and others: Gel support for prevention of decubitus ulcers, Arch. Phys. Med. Rehab. **28:**292-299, 1967.

Stryker, Corp.: CircOlectric bed operating manual. Available from Stryker Corp., 420 Alcott Street, Kalamazoo, Michigan 49001.

Stryker, H. H.: A device for turning the frame patient, J.A.M.A. **113:**1731-1732, 1939.

Valentin, L.: Kinetic nursing and the Roto-Rest bed, ONAJ4(3):62-65, Mar. 1977.

Vasconez, L. O., Schneider, W. J., and Jurkiewicz, M. J.: Pressure sores, a monograph of current problems in surgery, Chicago, 1977, Year Book Medical Publishers, Inc.

Verhonick, P.: Clinical investigations in nursing, Nurs. Forum, **10:**80-88, 1971

Wallace, G. and Hayter, J.: Karaya for chronic skin ulcers, Am. J. Nurs. **6:**1094, June 1974.

Yucel, V. E., and Basmajian, J. V.: Decubitus ulcers: Healing effect of an enzymatic spray, Arch. Phys. Med. Rehab. **55:**517-518, Nov. 1974.

# 31

# Orthotics and shoes

**NANCY E. HILT**

Terminology
Fitting, measurements, and design
Types
Care of orthotic devices
Shoes
Summary

An *orthosis* is "a force system that is designed to control, correct, or compensate for a deformity, deforming forces, or absent forces".[2,p.13]

The term *orthosis* is gradually replacing the term *brace;* in many cases, however, they are still used synonymously. Orthoses, either alone or in combination with other treatment modalities, are frequently used to treat musculoskeletal diseases, disorders, or deformities. The prescription of an orthotic device is written by the orthopedic surgeon or physiatrist. The actual construction of the orthosis is done by the *orthotist*, a specialist in brace construction.

An orthotic device may serve one or several purposes in the total comprehensive care program. The most common are to (1) prevent a deformity, (2) correct a deformity, (3) assist in the restoration of a lost function, (4) replace a lost function, and (5) permit function not otherwise achievable.

Orthotic devices are usually constructed of a combination of metals (steel, aluminum), leather, various plastics, synthetic fabrics, and plaster. The type of materials chosen depends on the specific purpose of the device and are a part of the prescription.

## TERMINOLOGY

The terminology associated with the use and prescription of orthotic devices has changed frequently over the past decade as the art and science of orthotic construction has become much more precise and specialized. Specific body markings (bony landmarks, surface markings, and points of reference or pressure) are usually used to communicate details of the prescription to the orthotist. These are reviewed in Table 31-1.

*Text continued on p. 778.*

**Table 31-1.** Body markings used for orthotic prescription[3,p.98]

| Conventional longitudinal lines | Reference points | Pressure points |
|---|---|---|
| Posterior axillary line | Seventh cervical spinous process | Occiput |
| Scapular line | First cervical spinous process | Costal |
| Median vertebral line | Acromion and spinous process of acromion | Olecranal |
| Median or midsternal line | Tuberculum majus humeri | Metacarpal |
| Parasternal line | Twelfth dorsal vertebra spinous process | Phalanx |
| Midclavicular line | Spinous process of fifth lumbar vertebra | Ilium |
| Anterior axillary line | Sacrococcygeal joint | Sacrum |
| | Femoral condyles and articular line | Ischium |
| | Malleoli | Subtrochanteric |
| | Acromion and head of humerus | Achillic |
| | Clavicle | Sternal |
| | Suprasternal notch | Pubic |
| | Manubrium | Trochanteric |
| | Ensiform cartilage | Condylar |
| | Head of radius | Patellar |
| | Iliac crest | Metatarsal |
| | Anterior superior spine of ilium | Condylicus humeri |
| | Head of fibula | Styloideus |
| | | Metacarpal |
| | | Metacarpophalangeal of thumb |

TECHNICAL ANALYSIS FORM                    LEFT UPPER LIMB

Name_____ No._____ Age_____ Sex_____

Date of Onset_____ Cause _____

Occupation_____ Present Upper-Limb Equipment_____

Diagnosis_____

Hand Dominance:      Right ☐   Left ☐

Status of other upper limb:      Normal ☐      Impaired ☐

1.   Ambulatory status:       Normal ☐      Impaired ☐      Walking Aid ☐

2.   Wheelchair ☐    Sitting Position:    Stable ☐   Unstable ☐   Reclined ☐   Upright ☐
     Sitting Tolerance:      Normal ☐      Limited ☐      Duration_____
     Propulsion:      Manual ☐      Motor ☐      Dependent ☐

3.   Cognition:      Normal ☐      Impaired ☐

4.   Endurance:      Normal ☐      Impaired ☐

5.   Skin:      Normal ☐      Impaired ☐

6.   Pain ☐          Location_____

7.   Vision:      Normal ☐      Impaired ☐

8.   Coordination:   Normal ☐   Impaired ☐      Function:   Normal ☐   Compromised ☐
                                                              Prevented ☐

9.   Motivation:      Good ☐      Fair ☐      Poor ☐

10.  Associated impairments: _____

————————————————————————— LEGEND —————————————————————————

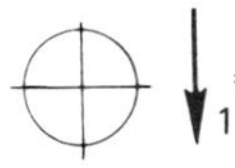

| | |
|---|---|
| ↓1 = Direction of Translatory Motion *(Grade 1,2 or 3)* | |
| 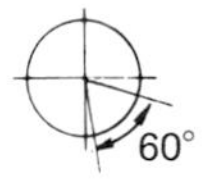 60° = Abnormal Degree of Rotary Motion | |
| 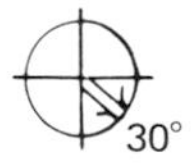 30° = Fixed Position | 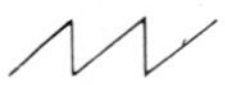 |
| /\/\ = Fracture | |

Volitional Force (V)
N  = Normal
G  = Good
F  = Fair
P  = Poor
T  = Trace
Z  = Zero

Hypertonic Muscle (H)
N  = Normal
M  = Mild
Mo = Moderate
S  = Severe

Sensation
☐ N = Normal
▓ = Hypesthesia
▨ = Paresthesia
▩ = Anesthesia

Proprioception (P)
N  = Normal
I  = Impaired
A  = Absent

D  = Distension or Enlargement

**Fig. 31-1.** Technical analysis form: left upper limb. (From American Academy of Orthopaedic Surgeons: Atlas of orthotics, St. Louis, 1975, The C. V. Mosby Co.)

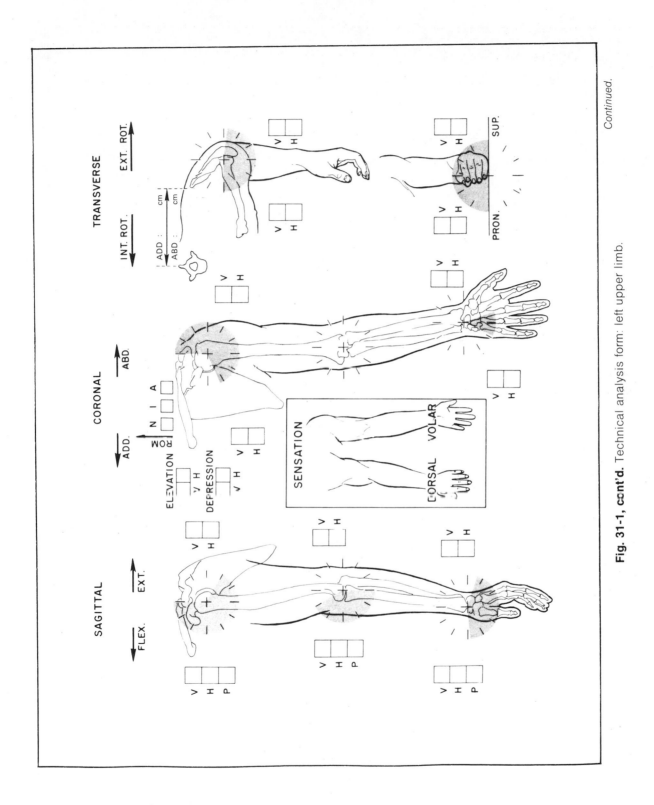

**Fig. 31-1, cont'd.** Technical analysis form: left upper limb.

Continued.

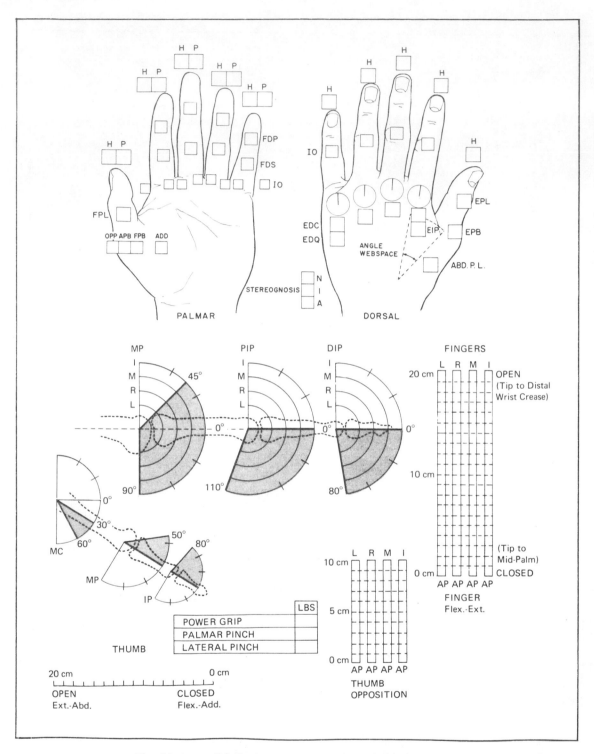

**Fig. 31-1, cont'd.** Technical analysis form: left upper limb.

Summary of Functional Disability _____

_____

_____

_____

_____

_____

Treatment Objectives:    Prevent/Correct Deformity ☐      Improve Function ☐

                  Relieve Pain ☐      Other _____

### ORTHOTIC RECOMMENDATION

| UPPER LIMB | | FLEX | EXT | ABD | ADD | ROTATION Int. | ROTATION Ext. | AXIAL LOAD |
|---|---|---|---|---|---|---|---|---|
| SEWHO | Shoulder | | | | | | | |
| EWHO | *Humerus* | | | | | | | |
| | Elbow | | | | | | | |
| | Forearm | | | | | (Pron.) | (Sup.) | |
| WHO | Wrist | | | (RD) | (UD) | | | |
| HO | Hand | | | | | | | |
| Fingers 2-5 | MP | | | | | | | |
| Fingers 2-5 | PIP | | | | | | | |
| Fingers 2-5 | DIP | | | | | | | |
| Thumb | CM | | | | | (Opposition) | | |
| Thumb | MP | | | | | | | |
| Thumb | IP | | | | | | | |

REMARKS:

_____         _____

Signature                        Date

KEY:  Use the following symbols to indicate desired control of designated function:

    F = FREE    — *Free* motion.

    A = ASSIST    — Application of an external force for the purpose of increasing the range, velocity, or force of a motion.

    R = RESIST    — Application of an external force for the purpose of decreasing the velocity or force of a motion.

    S = STOP    — Inclusion of a static unit to deter an undesired motion in one direction.

    v = Variable    — A unit that can be adjusted without making a structural change.

    H = HOLD    — Elimination of all motion in prescribed plane (verify position).

    L = LOCK    — Device includes an optional lock.

**Fig. 31-1, cont'd.** Technical analysis form: left upper limb.

TECHNICAL ANALYSIS FORM        SPINE

Name_____ No._____ Age____ Sex____ Weight_____ Height_____

Diagnosis_____ Occupation _____

Present Orthotic Equipment _____

_____

      Ambulatory ☐        Non Ambulatory ☐     Wheelchair ☐

Standing Balance:    Normal ☐      Impaired ☐     Walking Aid _____

Sitting Position:      Stable ☐       Unstable ☐     Reclined ☐     Upright ☐

Sitting Tolerance:    Normal ☐      Limited ☐

MAJOR IMPAIRMENTS

A.  Structural:    No Impairment ☐

     1.    Bone:    Osteoporosis ☐     Fracture ☐     Level _____

                  Other _____

     2.    Disc Space: (Describe)_____

                 _____

     3.    Alignment:  Scoliosis ☐     Kyphosis ☐    Lordosis ☐

B.  Sensory:   No Impairment ☐

     1.    Anesthesia ☐     Location _____

     2.    Pain ☐      Location _____

C.  Upper Limb:  No Impairment ☐

     1.    Amputation ☐ _____

     2.    Other_____

D.  Lower Limb:  No Impairment ☐

     1.    Limb Shortening:  Right ☐     Left ☐    Amount _____

     2.    Hip Contracture ☐     Ankylosis ☐    Flexion ☐    Degree _____

           Adduction ☐     Degree_____;    Abduction ☐    Degree_____;

           Extension ☐     Degree_____

     3.    Major Motor Loss ☐    Location _____

     4.    Sensation:  Anesthesia ☐    Location_____;

           Hypesthesia ☐    Location _____

           Pain ☐     Location _____

E.  Associated Impairments:_____

     _____

**Fig. 31-2.** Technical analysis form: spine. (From American Academy of Orthopaedic Surgeons: Atlas of orthotics, St. Louis, 1975, The C. V. Mosby Co.)

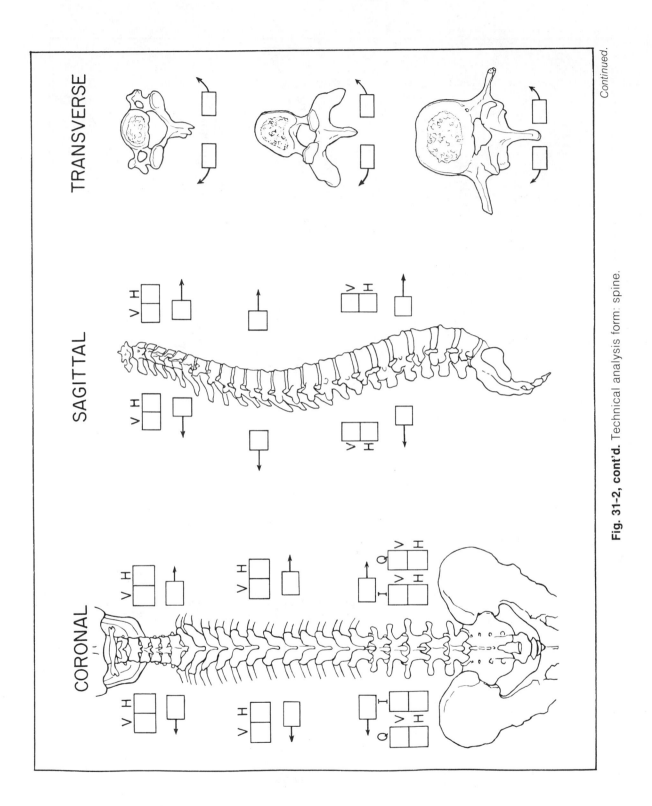

*Continued.*

**Fig. 31-2, cont'd.** Technical analysis form: spine.

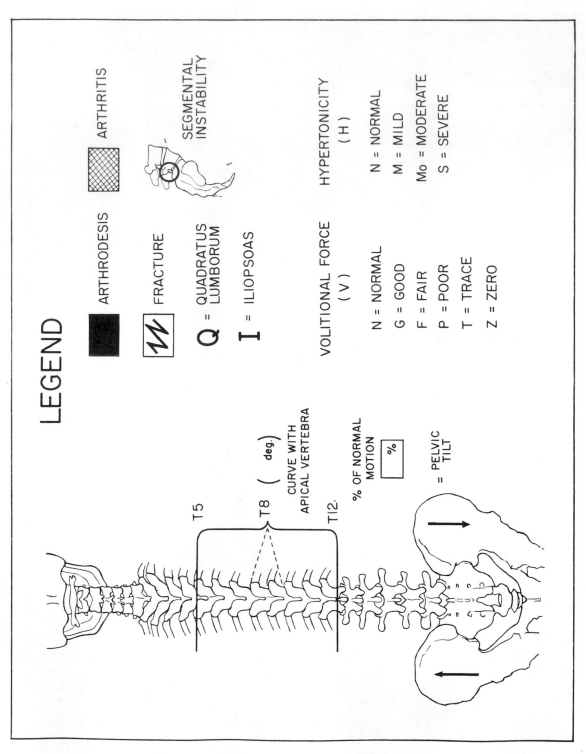

**Fig. 31-2, cont'd.** Technical analysis form: spine.

Summary of Functional Disability: _____

_____

_____

Treatment Objectives:

Spinal Alignment ☐          Motion Control ☐

Axial Unloading ☐           Other _____

_____

### ORTHOTIC RECOMMENDATION

| SPINE | | FLEX | EXT | LATERAL FLEXION | | ROTATION | | AXIAL LOAD |
|---|---|---|---|---|---|---|---|---|
| | | | | R | L | R | L | |
| CTLSO | Cervical | | | | | | | |
| TLSO | Thoracic | | | | | | | |
| LSO | Lumbar | | | | | | | |
| | (Lumbo sacral | | | | | | | |
| SIO | Sacroiliac | | | | | | | |
| | | | | | | | | |

**REMARKS:**

_____

KEY:  Use the following symbols to indicate desired control of designated function:

F = FREE      – Free motion

A = ASSIST    – Application of an external force for the purpose of increasing the range, velocity, or force of a motion.

R = RESIST    – Application of an external force for the purpose of decreasing the velocity or force of a motion.

S = STOP      – Inclusion of a static unit to deter an undesired motion in one direction.

v = Variable  – A unit that can be adjusted without making a structural change.

H = HOLD      – Elimination of all motion in prescribed plane: specify position, e.g. in degrees or (+) (–).

L = LOCK      – Device includes an optional lock.

_____

Signature

_____

Date

**Fig. 31-2, cont'd.** Technical analysis form: spine.

TECHNICAL ANALYSIS FORM                    LOWER LIMB

Name_____ No._____ Age_____ Sex_____

Date of Onset_____ Cause_____

Occupation_____ Present Lower-Limb Equipment_____

Diagnosis_____
_____
_____

Ambulatory ☐        Non-Ambulatory ☐

MAJOR IMPAIRMENTS:
A.  Skeletal
 1.  Bone and Joints:    Normal ☐    Abnormal_____
 2.  Ligaments:    Normal ☐    Abnormal ☐    Knee: AC ☐   PC ☐   MC ☐   LC ☐
                                              Ankle: MC ☐   LC ☐

 3.  Extremity Shortening:   None ☐     Left ☐     Right ☐
     Amount of Discrepancy:   A.S.S.-Heel_____   A.S.S.-MTP_____   MTP-Heel_____

B.  Sensation:   Normal ☐    Abnormal ☐
 1.  Anaesthesia ☐    Hypaesthesia ☐    Location:_____
     Protective Sensation:    Retained ☐    Lost ☐
 2.  Pain ☐    Location:_____

C.  Skin:   Normal ☐    Abnormal:_____

D.  Vascular:   Normal ☐    Abnormal ☐    Right ☐    Left ☐

E.  Balance:   Normal ☐    Impaired ☐    Support:_____

F.  Gait Deviations:_____
_____

G.  Other Impairments:_____

——— LEGEND ———

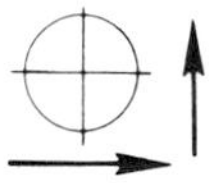

⊕↑ = Direction of Translatory Motion

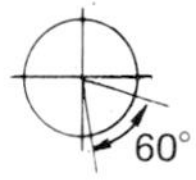

⊕60° = Abnormal Degree of Rotary Motion

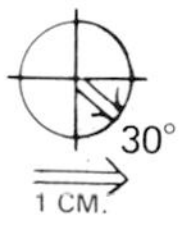

⊕30° →1 CM. = Fixed Position

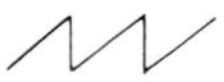

〰 = Fracture

Volitional Force (V)
N = Normal
G = Good
F = Fair
P = Poor
T = Trace
Z = Zero

Hypertonic Muscle (H)
N = Normal
M = Mild
Mo = Moderate
S = Severe

Proprioception (P)
N = Normal
I = Impaired
A = Absent

D = Local Distension or Enlargement

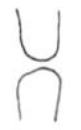

= Pseudarthrosis

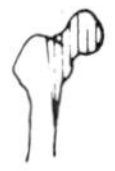

= Absence of Segment

**Fig. 31-3.** Technical analysis form: lower limb. (From American Academy of Orthopaedic Surgeons: Atlas of orthotics, St. Louis, 1975, The C. V. Mosby Co.)

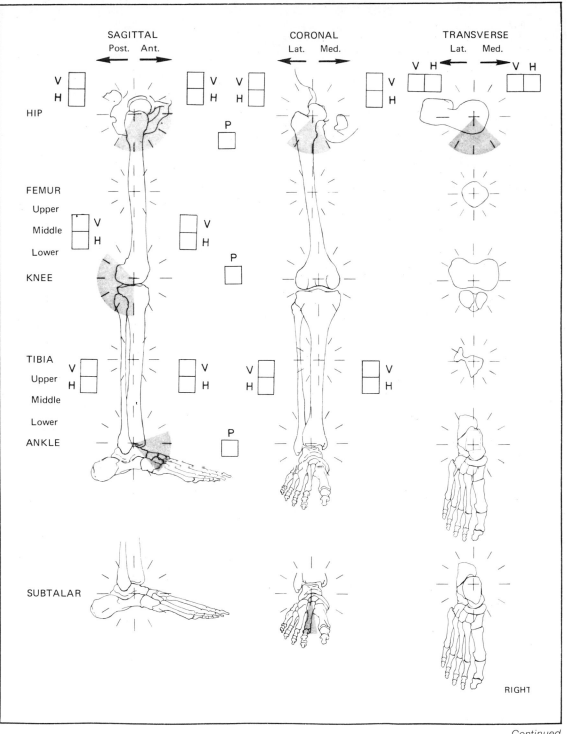

**Fig. 31-3, cont'd.** Technical analysis form: lower limb.

*Continued.*

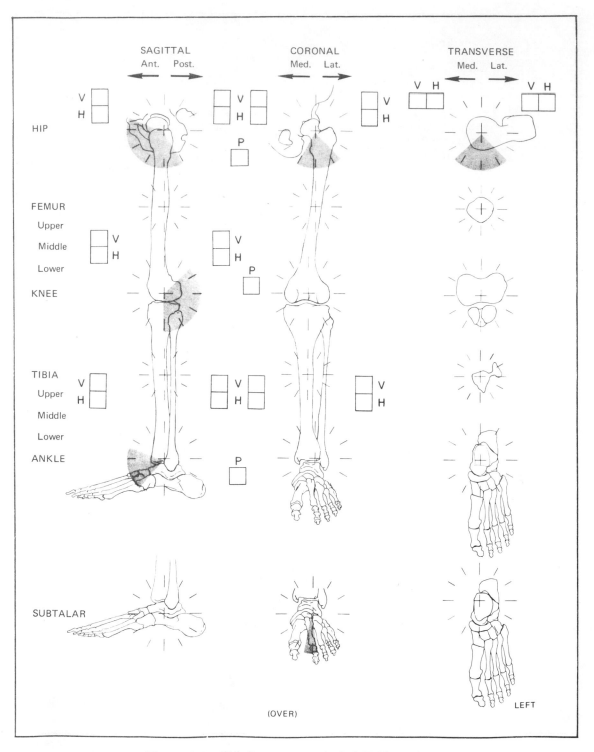

**Fig. 31-3, cont'd.** Technical analysis form: lower limb.

Summary of Functional Disability _____

_____

_____

_____

_____

_____

Treatment Objectives:

Prevent/Correct Deformity ☐     Improve Ambulation ☐

Reduce Axial Load        ☐     Fracture Treatment ☐

Protect Joint             ☐     Other _____

### ORTHOTIC RECOMMENDATION

| LOWER LIMB | | FLEX | EXT | ABD | ADD | ROTATION Int. | ROTATION Ext. | AXIAL LOAD |
|---|---|---|---|---|---|---|---|---|
| HKAO | Hip | | | | | | | |
| KAO | Thigh | | | | | | | |
| | Knee | | | | | | | |
| AFO | Leg | | | | | | | |
| | Ankle | (Dorsi) | (Plantar) | | | | | |
| | Subtalar | | | | | (Inver.) | (Ever.) | |
| FO Foot | Midtarsal | | | | | | | |
| | Met.-phal. | | | | | | | |

**REMARKS:**

_____    _____

                         Signature                          Date

KEY:   Use the following symbols to indicate desired control of designated function:

F = FREE      — *Free* motion.

A = ASSIST    — Application of an external force for the purpose of increasing the range, velocity, or force of a motion.

R = RESIST    — Application of an external force for the purpose of decreasing the velocity or force of a motion.

S = STOP      — Inclusion of a static unit to deter an undesired motion in one direction.

v = Variable   — A unit that can be adjusted without making a structural change.

H = HOLD      — Elimination of all motion in prescribed plane (verify position).

L = LOCK      — Device includes an optional lock.

**Fig. 31-3, cont'd.** Technical analysis form: lower limb.

The terms used in the description and prescription of orthotic devices relate to the anatomic area involved and the desired motion of the involved joints. Abbreviations for the anatomic area are used and are relatively standardized (e.g., long leg brace, knee-ankle orthosis and KAO mean the same). Note that the specific anatomic area is named when the term *brace* is used; the joints covered by the brace are named when the term *orthosis* is used.[2,pp. 4-5] Desired joint motion is communicated through specific terminology relating to the degree and type of control available:

**free** motion that is unregulated in a specific direction.

**assist** application of an external force to increase the range, velocity, or force of a specific motion.

**resist** application of an external force to decrease the range, velocity, or force of a specific motion.

**stop** design that prevents motion in a specific direction.

**variable** design that can be adjusted at the level of joint control.

**hold** design that eliminates a motion in a specified plane.

**lock** design to include an optional lock, which may be used periodically.

## FITTING, MEASUREMENT, AND DESIGN

Orthotic devices are comprised of three parts: (1) the frame, (2) materials that cover and pad, and (3) elements that suspend or attach one component to another. Although there are many standardized types of braces, each is custom designed and made to fulfill the individual patient's needs. For the most useful orthoses, measurements are taken to provide a custom fit. In some cases, such as with the Milwaukee brace, a mold (plaster) is used to contour a portion of the brace (in this case the pelvic girdle). Information relevant to the construction, purpose, measurements, and objectives are provided the orthotist in detail to facilitate construction and achievement of purpose and objectives. This composite is usually transformed onto a form, which then becomes the foundation for a blueprint of the orthotic device (Figs. 31-1 to 31-3).

The design of all orthotic devices includes a three-point pressure system; some have more than one such system (see Fig. 31-4). Inclusion of this system as a necessary part of orthotic construction was first described in 1939 by Jordan who stated that the *supportive forces of a brace which are applied from three directions, "must be active and should be distributed over adequate surfaces or divided into a number of single units, the sum of which is equal in degree and direction to the desired or main force."*[3,p.97] This principle, applied to orthotic design, is mainly responsible for the control of motion.

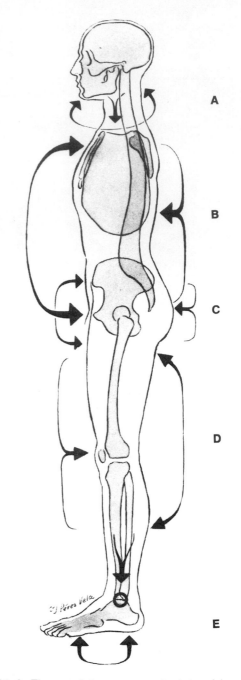

**Fig. 31-4.** Three-point-pressure principle of brace design (as described by Jordan). **A,** Braces designed to support neck require supporting forces of brace to be applied on chin, on occiput, and to base of neck. **B,** Three components in trunk corset consist in two backward thrusts, one sternal and one iliac, and forward thrust over dorsal spine. **C,** In iliofemoral region backward thrusts are applied over ilium and proximal end of femur, while forward thrust applies over sacrum. **D,** Thrusts for lower limb are as follows: over thigh and leg in forward direction; over knee, backward thrust. **E,** Upward thrust applies over two points of foot sole; downward thrust on talocruralis complex. (From Tohen, A.: Manual of mechanical orthopaedics, Springfield, Ill., 1973, Charles C Thomas, Publisher.)

**Table 31-2.** Selected upper extremity orthotics[1,2]

Metacarpal bar: Prevention of MP joint
  hyperextension

Outrigger splint, dynamic hand splint:
  Variable degrees of force applied; permits
  stretching; frequently used with arthritis

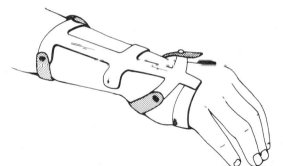

Wrist-hand orthosis, long opponens splint:
  Wrist stabilization

Finger-driven Rancho orthosis (used with
  spring and external power): Mobile arm
  support; wrist immobilization; provides
  positioning for grasp motion

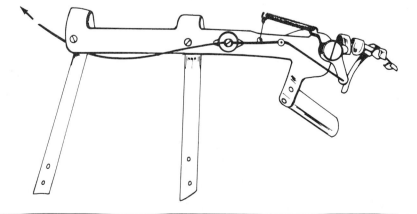

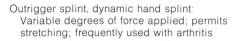

Illustrations from Bunch, W., and Keagy, R.: Principles of orthotic treatment, St. Louis, 1976, The C. V. Mosby Co.

**Table 31-3.** Selected cervical and spinal orthotics[1,2]

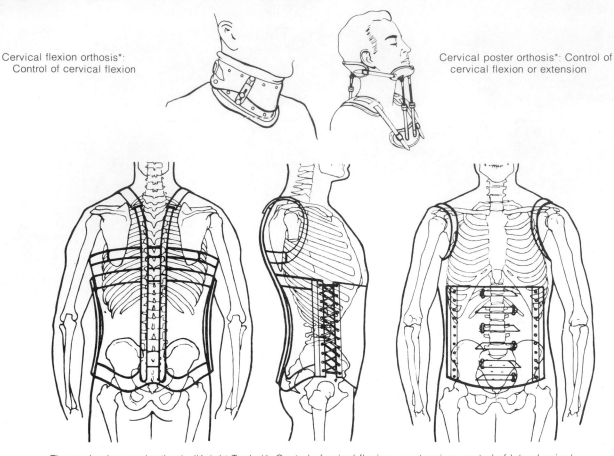

Cervical flexion orthosis*: Control of cervical flexion

Cervical poster orthosis*: Control of cervical flexion or extension

Thoracolumbosacral orthosis (Knight-Taylor)*: Control of spinal flexion or extension; control of lateral spinal motion

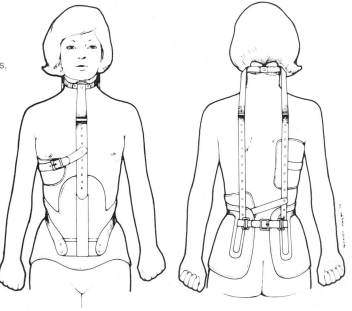

Milwaukee brace†: Correction of spinal scoliosis, lordosis, kyphosis

*Illustrations from A.A.O.S.: Atlas of orthotics: Biomechanical principles and application, St. Louis, 1975, The C. V. Mosby Co.
†Illustrations from Hilt, N. E., and Schmitt, E. W., Jr.: Pediatric orthopedic nursing, St. Louis, 1975, The C. V. Mosby Co.

**Table 31-4.** Selected lower extremity orthotics[1,2]

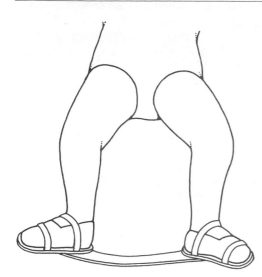

Denis Browne splint: Maintains hip flexion; maintains hip abduction

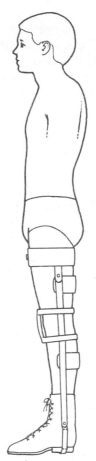

Short leg orthosis: Maintains support; stabilizes ankle motion

Long leg orthosis: Maintains support; provides for joint motion and stability for ambulation

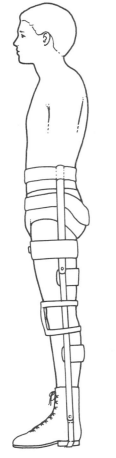

Long leg orthosis with pelvic band: Provides for controlled motion, possible ambulation, and stability for paralyzed patient

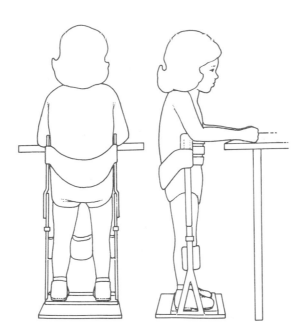

Parapodium: Maintains stability and support for upright position; provides limited mobility

## TYPES

There are many types of orthoses that are used for a variety of deformities. Although it is not possible in one chapter to review all types and options available, the major types are outlined in Tables 31-2 to 31-4. These tables provide the reader with an overview of some of the major types of orthoses. The Bibliography provides a more comprehensive review.

## CARE OF ORTHOTIC DEVICES

As is true with most equipment, the anticipated longevity of an orthotic device is often proportionate to the degree of care it receives. The specific care of an orthotic device will be dependent on the materials used for construction. Plastic materials require daily washing with warm water and a mild soap. Leather requires periodic cleaning as well. Metal portions of the device should be kept clean, and all moving parts must be lubricated periodically to maintain maximum mobility. All specific aspects of care should be reviewed with the patient or family. However, the care outlined should be consistent with treatment and therapy goals; for example, a patient should not be instructed to remove the orthosis daily for care if this is contrary to treatment goals.

## SHOES

Special shoes are frequently used as an adjunct to orthotic therapy and, in some cases, they are the only component of treatment. The shoes prescribed may be corrective or nonadaptive but sturdily constructed commercial shoes. Common adaptations for children's shoes include: wedges, high tops, arch supports, modified lasts, and lifts (Fig. 31-5).

Although adult modification may also be similar, they are frequently more supportive than corrective. In all cases, when shoe modifications or inserts are prescribed, appropriate fitting is important, as is appropriate shoe sizing.

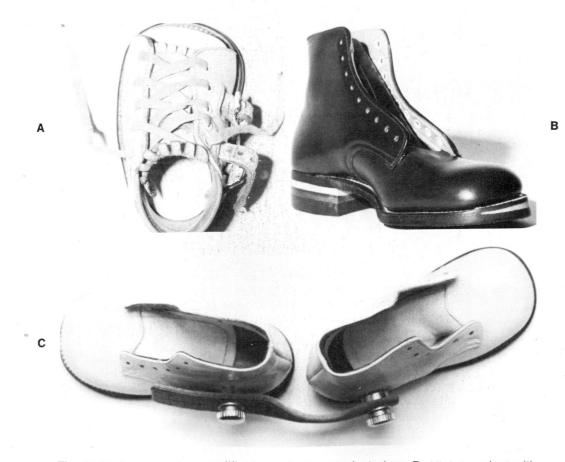

**Fig. 31-5.** Common shoe modifications. **A,** Reverse-last shoe. **B,** High-top shoe with wedges. **C,** Freidman counterstrap with high-top shoes. (From Hilt, N. E., and Schmitt, E. W., Jr.: Pediatric orthopedic nursing, St. Louis, 1975, The C. V. Mosby Co.)

## SUMMARY

Orthotic devices are used frequently for the correction of deformity, support and maintenance of desired alignment, and positioning. All personnel should be thoroughly familiar with the type, purpose, and care of a patient's orthotic device.

## REFERENCES

1. American Academy of Orthopaedic Surgeons: Atlas of orthotics: Biomedical principles and application, St. Louis, 1975, The C. V. Mosby Co.
2. Bunch, W., and Keagy, R.: Principles of orthotic treatment, St. Louis, 1976, The C. V. Mosby Co.
3. Jordan, as cited by Tohen, A.: Manual of mechanical orthopaedics, Springfield, Ill., 1972. Charles C Thomas, Publisher.

## BIBLIOGRAPHY

American Academy of Orthopaedic Surgeons: Atlas of orthotics: Biomechanical principles and application, St. Louis, 1975, The C. V. Mosby Co.

Anderson, M. H., editor: A manual of lower extremities orthotics, Springfield, Ill. 1972, Charles C Thomas, Publisher.

Bloomberg, M.: Orthopedic braces: rationale, classification and prescription, Philadelphia, 1964, J. B. Lippincott Co.

Blount, W. P., and More, J. H.: The Milwaukee brace, Baltimore, 1973, The Williams & Wilkins Co.

Bunch, W., and Keagy, R.: Principles of orthotic treatment, St. Louis, 1976, The C. V. Mosby Co.

Percy, J., and Hislop, H.: Principles of lower extremity bracing. Washington, D.C., 1973, American Physical Therapy Association.

Tohen, A.: Manual of mechanical orthopaedics Springfield, Ill. 1975, Charles C Thomas, Publisher.

# 32

# Prosthetics

NANCY E. HILT

*Prosthetics* is the science and art of the designing, fitting, and constructing an artificial limb replacement. Although in its strictest interpretation a "prosthesis" is the replacement of any part of the body (such as the total hip prosthesis used for internal replacement), we limit its use here to mean a limb replacement for extremity amputations.

Amputation may be congenital, the result of mechanical injury, or a surgical alternative to progressive malignant processes or neurovascular compromise. If the amputation is the result of congenital abnormality or injury, revision may be necessary to maximize functional or ambulatory goals. An amputation becomes the "treatment of choice" only when a disease process cannot be controlled or arrested by other means. In these cases the amputation may be a life-saving measure. In malignant disease such surgery may offer comfort, increased function, and potential longevity not possible through other treatment modalities. With neurovascular compromise and infection, improved function is probably of greatest significance in the decision to amputate as a choice of treatment.

## LEVELS OF AMPUTATION

The level of amputation depends on the specific process or deformity for which the procedure is being accomplished. The terminology used for the levels of amputations is relatively descriptive and may be categorized as follows:

| Upper extremity | Lower extremity |
|---|---|
| Partial hand | Partial foot |
| Transcarpal | Transmetatarsal |
| Wrist disarticulation | Syme's type (foot) |
| Long below-elbow | Medium or standard below-knee |
| Medium below-elbow | |
| Short below-elbow | Short below-knee |
| Very short below-elbow | Very short below-knee |
| Elbow disarticulation | Knee disarticulation |
| Standard above-elbow | Long above-knee |
| Short above-elbow | Medium below-knee or mid-thigh |
| Shoulder disarticulation | Short above-knee |
| Forequarter amputation | Very short above-knee |
| | Hip disarticulation |
| | Hemipelvectomy |

These levels of amputations are shown in Fig. 32-1. All are potential candidates for prosthetic appliances.

## FITTING OF PROSTHESIS

The fitting of a prosthesis may be accomplished either immediately following surgery or after healing has taken place. If done immediately after surgery, the prosthesis is a temporary one and permanent fitting is done after stump shrinkage and complete healing have occurred.

The following considerations are of great significance in determining the ability of a permanent prosthesis to provide optimal function and performance:[2,pp.61-72]

1. Maintenance of optimal length and tension of remaining musculature, with consideration of all transferred musculature existing in the stump
2. Minimization of edema
3. Maintenance of optimal posture and mobility in the stump and proximal joints
4. Use of a temporary prosthesis immediate following surgery or as soon thereafter as possible
5. Recognition of the biomechanical factors involved with pressure distribution and maintenance of skin integrity.

Each of these above considerations is important in obtaining a stump with maximum power, strength,

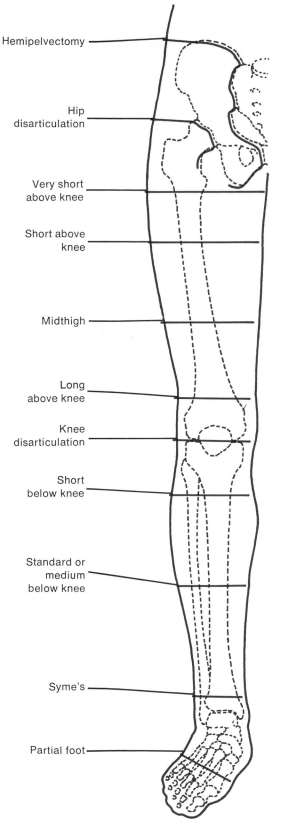

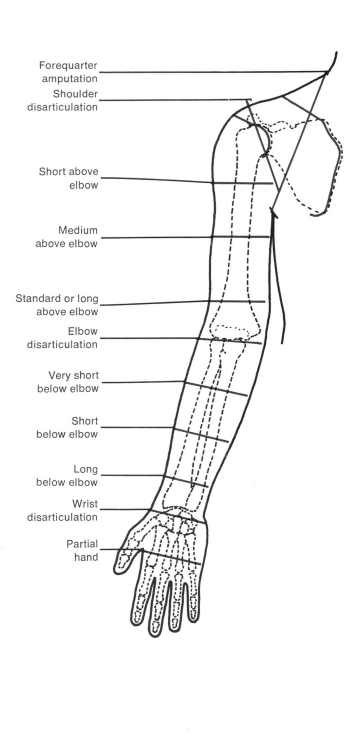

**Fig. 32-1.** Terminology associated with upper and lower extremity levels of amputation.

**Table 32-1.** Comparison of normal extremity structure and function with prosthetic replacement[2, pp. 77-78]

| Normal extremity structure/function | Function | Prosthetic replacement |
|---|---|---|
| Skeletal structure (bone) | Strength | Replacement accomplished easily |
| | Support | Replacement accomplished easily |
| Joints | Proprioception | Replacement impossible |
| | Sense of orientation in space | Replacement impossible |
| Muscular structure | Motion | Motion easily accomplished with mechanical pivot or hinge joint |
| | Motor function | Replacement accomplished successfully |
| | Shock absorber | Replacement impossible |
| Sensation | Stabilization | Replacement partially accomplished with joint blocks |
| | Tactile | Replacement impossible |
| Dexterity | Proprioception | Replacement to a limited degree |
| | Dexterity | Replacement to a limited degree |

and mobility — essential components for successful prosthetic fitting and use. The maintenance of skin integrity and prevention of contracture deformities cannot be over-emphasized. In most cases, temporary prosthetic fittings have proved extremely useful in the achievement of early function, psychological adjustment to the amputation, and, to a degree, have decreased associated phantom pain.

Lower extremity prostheses replace function and simulate cosmesis much more successfully than upper extremity prostheses. In general, upper extremity prostheses cannot replace fine movements associated with the hand, are more cumbersome, and are more difficult to use than lower extremity prostheses. Some components of normal extremity structure and function are easier to replace than others; a comparison is given in Table 32-1.

## CONSTRUCTION OF PROSTHESIS

The materials used in the construction of prostheses offer specific advantages and disadvantages in their ability to conform, support, and replace lost function. The most commonly used materials are given below. The specific combination of materials used in the prescription of a prosthesis is determined on an individual basis, according to the needs of the patient and the desired outcome related to functional goals. A temporary prosthesis is designed to be simply functional and economical.

**Plastics.** Plastic materials are currently in widespread use as a prosthetic component because they are economical, mold easily, are heat and moisture resistant, and can match skin tones well. They are also easy to clean. Plastics are available in varying thicknesses and compositions, which provides tremendous flexibility in their use.

**Wood.** Wood is less extensively used since the advent of plastic materials but still offers some fine qualities. Wood has low thermal and sound conductivity, and is vibration and shock absorbent. Although skin tones cannot be matched as well with wood as with plastic, wood is useful because it is extremely lightweight.

**Leather.** Leathers are most commonly used for their flexible molding qualities. However, they lack the strength offered by other materials and require metal reinforcement in some cases. Leather is also difficult to clean.

**Metals.** Aluminum alloys offer resistance required for certain components of prosthetic construction. Metal is used especially for joint parts, bands, and bars needed for strength and mobility.

## TYPES OF PROSTHESES

Specific options are available with upper and lower extremity prostheses. To facilitate review of some of these, Tables 32-2 and 32-3 relate them to the level of amputation. It should be emphasized again that the options shown are, in many cases, interchangeable and custom designed to meet specific needs and goals. The objective here is to familiarize the reader both with some of the types of prostheses available to the amputee and current prosthetic trends.

## PROSTHESIS AND STUMP CARE

Prosthetic care is part of the patient's training in the use of the prosthesis. The training program will vary depending on the level of amputation and type of prosthesis.

**Care of prosthesis.** For patients with a lower extremity prosthesis emphasis is placed on achievement of ambulatory goals through gradual progression of standing balance to assisted gait to independent gait. An upper extremity prosthesis requires mastery of control and function, which is

**Table 32-2.** Selected prosthetic options available for upper extremity amputations[1,3]

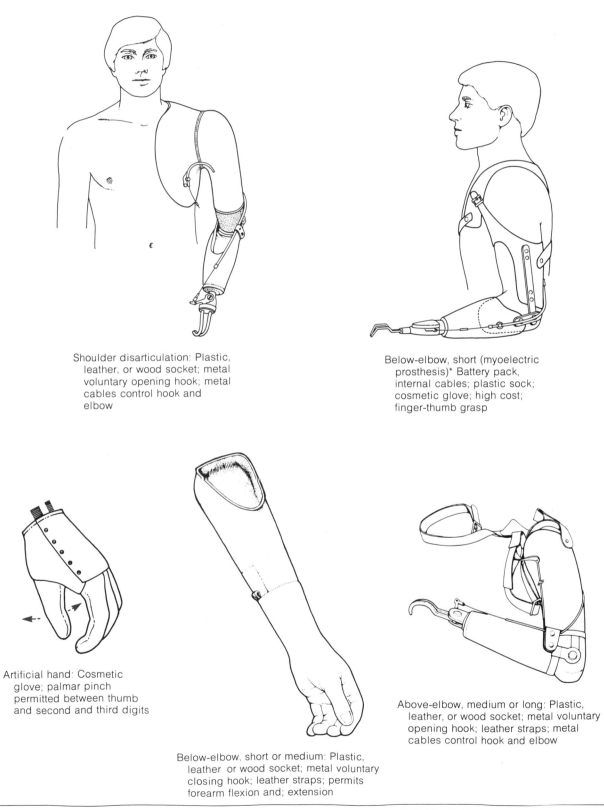

Shoulder disarticulation: Plastic, leather, or wood socket; metal voluntary opening hook; metal cables control hook and elbow

Below-elbow, short (myoelectric prosthesis)* Battery pack, internal cables; plastic sock; cosmetic glove; high cost; finger-thumb grasp

Artificial hand: Cosmetic glove; palmar pinch permitted between thumb and second and third digits

Below-elbow, short or medium: Plastic, leather or wood socket; metal voluntary closing hook; leather straps; permits forearm flexion and; extension

Above-elbow, medium or long: Plastic, leather, or wood socket; metal voluntary opening hook; leather straps; metal cables control hook and elbow

*Illustration from Hilt, N. E., and Schmitt, E. W.: Pediatric orthopedic nursing, St. Louis, 1975, The C. V. Mosby Co.

**Table 32-3.** Selected prosthetic options available for lower extremity amputations*

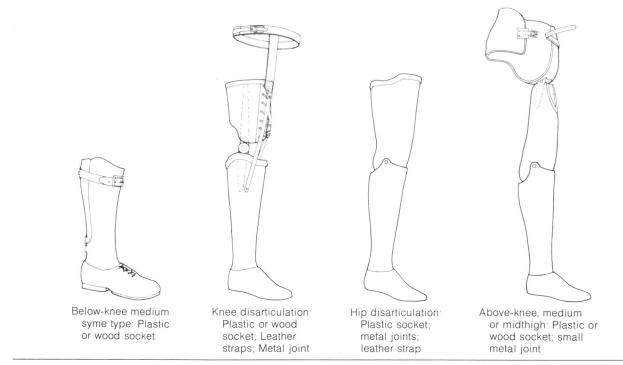

| Below-knee medium syme type: Plastic or wood socket | Knee disarticulation: Plastic or wood socket; Leather straps; Metal joint | Hip disarticulation: Plastic socket; metal joints; leather strap | Above-knee, medium or midthigh: Plastic or wood socket; small metal joint |

*Illustrations from Hilt, N. E., and Schmitt, E. W.: Pediatric orthopedic nursing, St. Louis, 1975, The C. V. Mosby Co.

usually more time-consuming and often more frustrating. Encouragement and support are extremely important during this training phase.

Care of the prosthesis may vary slightly depending on the materials used in construction. Since plastic materials are the most frequently used, the following guidelines are offered for these specific types for patient education in the care of their prosthesis:

1. Wash prosthesis (especially socket) *daily* with a mild soap and water. Dry thoroughly; it is best to allow the prosthesis to dry overnight.
2. Follow the manufacturer's instructions for maintenance and lubrication.
3. Condition of shoes should be checked frequently and altered when necessary.
4. Artificial hands, hooks, and gloves may be sensitive to temperature extremes or chemicals, so avoidance is advocated.
5. Malfunctions, even minor ones, should receive prompt attention and adjustment or repair.

Adherence to these guidelines will contribute to increased longevity of the prosthesis.

**Stump care.** The major emphasis should be placed on maintenance of skin integrity. Any skin breakdown may act as a tremendous deterrent to achieving functional and adjustment goals; it can represent a setback in the total therapeutic program. Rubbing alcohol over the end of the stump (after it is healed) several times a day will assist in toughening the skin and decreasing potential skin breakdown. Powders and lotions should be avoided. The stump should be washed well daily and thoroughly dried. Bandages or socks should be changed daily or more frequently if there is excessive perspiration. External compression should be used to prevent edema and maintain shape; alterations of shape or size of the stump will be a source of potential pressure. Considerable time and effort must be spent in educating the patient concerning everything required to achieve all the goals in these specific areas of care.

## SUMMARY

Using a prosthesis is always a traumatic event to the patient and even under the best of circumstances, adjustment requires encouragement, support, and education. The more the patient knows about the prosthesis and care, the more readily he or she can learn to deal with the associated problems. Personnel who care for the patient with a prosthesis must be thoroughly familiar with the specific components and functional abilities of the prosthesis. The orthopedic surgeon or prosthetist should be consulted whenever necessary.

## REFERENCES

1. Bender, L. F.: Prostheses and rehabilitation after arm amputation, Springfield, Ill., 1974, Charles C Thomas, Publisher.
2. Mital, M., and Pierce, D. S.: Amputees and their prostheses, Boston, 1971, Little, Brown & Co.
3. Tohen, A.: Manual of mechanical orthopaedics, Springfield, Ill., 1973, Charles C Thomas, Publisher.

## BIBLIOGRAPHY

Aitken, G. T., editor: The child with an acquired amputation, National Academy of Sciences, Washington, D.C., 1970.

Bender, L. F.: Prostheses and rehabilitation after arm amputation, Springfield, Ill., 1974, Charles C Thomas, Publisher.

Burgess, E., Romano, R., and Zettl, J.: The management of lower extremity amputations, Prosthetic and Sensory Aids Service, Veterans Administration, Washington, D.C., 1969.

Burgess, E., Traub, J., and Wilson, A. B.: Immediate postsurgical prosthetics in the management of lower extremity amputees, Prosthetic and Sensory Aids Service, Veterans Administration, 1967.

Dumbleton, J. H., and Black, J.: An introduction to orthopaedic materials, Springfield, Ill., 1975, Charles C Thomas, Publisher.

Gleane, J. A. E.: Moulds and casts for orthopaedic and prosthetic appliances, Springfield, Ill., 1972, Charles C Thomas, Publisher.

Mital, M., and Pierce, D. S.: Amputees and their prostheses, Boston, 1971, Little Brown & Co.

Tasberg, W. A.: Upper and lower extremity prostheses, Springfield, Ill., 1962, Charles C Thomas, Publisher.

Tohen, A.: Manual of mechanical orthopaedics, Springfield, Ill., 1973, Charles C Thomas, Publisher.

Wilson, A. B. Jr.: Limb prosthetics, Huntington, N.Y., 1976, Robert E. Kreign Publishing Company.

# 33

# Assistive devices

NANCY E. HILT

Devices aiding activities of daily living
Devices aiding in sitting, standing, movement, and mobilization
Devices aiding and supporting motion and ambulation
Devices facilitating hand grasp, thumb-finger opposition and hand/finger exercises
Devices supporting or immobilizing joints
Summary

The term *assistive device* is used in this chapter to mean any type of equipment, supportive or otherwise, that assists the orthopedic patient to maintain, improve, or resume maximal functioning. These devices may maintain position, replace altered levels of functioning, assist in maintenance of activities of daily living, promote mobilization, ambulation, or exercise, etc. In many cases a single device may help the patient achieve more than one objective.

This chapter is organized according to the major objectives the devices aid in achieving. Only major indications of use for each device are outlined because the primary purpose is to familiarize the reader with available devices. Only the most frequently used devices are included because of the vastness of the topic. Special beds, frames, orthotic devices, shoes, and prosthetics are reviewed in the preceding chapters and are, therefore, not discussed here, although they could be defined as assistive devices.

All devices should be selected carefully to assure that they will accomplish the designated purpose. Some categories of devices may require some trial and error accompanied by considerable persistence from both the patient and health care personnel. Throughout this period it is important that the patient's potential be recognized. Regardless of whether the device is supportive or substitutive, success or failure may well depend on this persistence.

The devices reviewed below constitute a tremendous cost to the patient, especially since some patients need several devices. Those prescribed by a physician for short-term or temporary use do not pose a major problem, although because of their limited use the least expensive method of achieving the objective should be chosen. Those prescribed or recommended for long-term or multiple use may pose problems depending on the patient's insurance coverage and socioeconomic level. Other avenues can also be explored to obtain the desired devices; for example, various organizations may be willing to fund some of the cost. In many cases, a device can be constructed at home rather than purchased. Patients should be instructed as to any available alternatives.

## DEVICES AIDING ACTIVITIES OF DAILY LIVING

Of all the assistive devices available, those that aid in the performance of activities of daily living are probably the most important. If patients are able to maintain a high degree of independence in caring for themselves, serious psychological problems may be avoided or at least lessened. Devices listed in this section permit the patient to continue daily activities despite the absence of specific physiological functions. The most common of these devices are designed to fulfill specific objectives in the following areas:

1. Communication
2. Continence
3. Dressing
4. Eating and food preparation
5. Grooming and bathing
6. Toileting

### Communications

**prism or Televue glasses**  permit reading, viewing television, and other activities when patient is recumbent.
**pencil/pen holder**  aids handwriting when finger flexion and fine hand motor coordination are lacking.
**page turner**  assists with reading for patient who lacks fine hand control or motion necessary for page turning.
**hearing aids**  help to replace or restore lost hearing or amplify remaining function.

## Continence

**indwelling catheter** used in selective cases for absent bladder control.

**conduit and ostomy appliances** for collection of urine and feces following bladder and bowel diversion procedures.

**external urinary devices** used as an alternative to indwelling catheter.

## Dressing (Fig. 33-1)

**elastic shoelaces** for patients who are unable to put shoes on; permits tie shoes to be slipped on and off without tying.

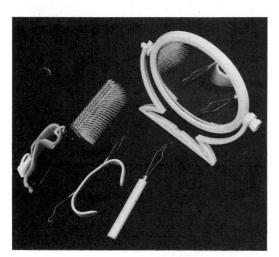

**Fig. 33-1.** Devices to assist in grooming and dressing. (From Boroch, R. M.: Elements of rehabilitation in nursing: an introduction, St. Louis, 1976, The C. V. Mosby Co.)

**long-handled shoehorn** for patients who are unable to flex the trunk enough to put shoes on.

**button aids** for patients who have limited dexterity and are unable to perform fine control movements necessary to manipulate buttons.

**zipper aids** for patients who have limited dexterity and are unable to perform the fine movements necessary to manipulate zippers.

NOTE: Dressing techniques may also assist some patients in the maintenance of an independent status (see Chapter 28).

## Eating and food preparation (Fig. 33-2)

**cutting board with suction cup** for patients who are unable to prepare food with unstable chopping or slicing surface.

**cup with grasp handle** for children and adults whose grasp strength will not permit holding a cup or glass.

**straw holder** for children and adults unable to control or use their hands.

**spill-proof drinking cup** for children and adults unable to maintain control required to keep cup upright.

**plate with suction cup** for children and adults unable to control stability of the plate while eating.

**plate with food guard** for children or adults unable to control movements enough to maintain food on the plate.

**long-handled utensils** for children and adults unable to flex the arm enough to eat with utensils of normal length.

**moldable-handled utensils** for children or adults who do not have the ability to grasp small handles; this type will permit flexible molding of the handle to the patient's specific need.

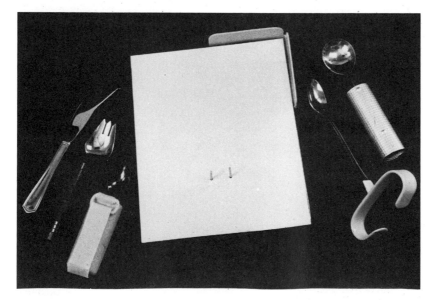

**Fig. 33-2.** Devices to assist in food preparation and eating. (From Boroch, R. M.: Elements of rehabilitation in nursing: an introduction, St. Louis, 1976, The C. V. Mosby Co.)

**utensils with hand attachments**   for patients who do not have the ability to maintain grip on utensils.

**homemade bulky handles for utensils**   for patients who do not have the ability to grasp small handles.

## Grooming and bathing
### (Figs. 33-1 and 33-3)

**adjustable neck mirror**   for patients who do not have full cervical range of motion or who are not able to stand to use mirrors at normal height.

**comb handle**   for patients who do not have full shoulder and arm range of motion.

**long-handled toothbrush**   for patients who do not have full elbow flexion.

**toothbrush with built-up handle**   for patients who do not have the ability to maintain grasp of small handle.

**toothbrush with hand grip**   for patients who do not have the ability to maintain grasp.

**nail brush with suction cups**   for patients who cannot use a nail brush in the usual manner; this permits stabilization of the brush on the sink for use.

**soap mitt**   for patients unable to maintain grasp.

**bathtub safety rails or grips**   for patients who cannot get in and out of the tub safely without assistance.

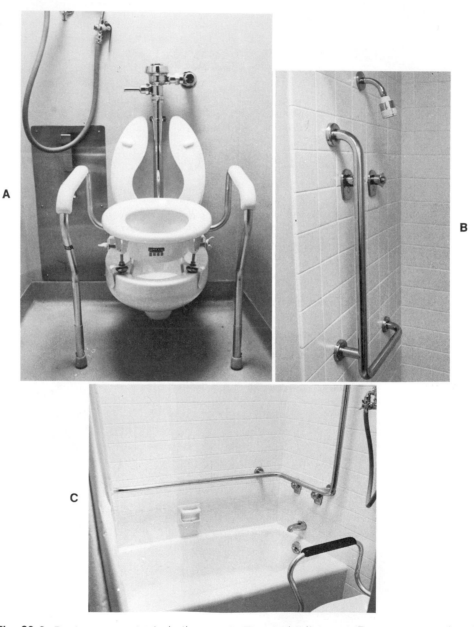

**Fig. 33-3.** Devices to assist in bathroom. **A,** Elevated toilet seat. **B** and **C,** Safety hand grasps for shower and tub. (From Boroch, R. M.: Elements of rehabilitation in nursing: an introduction, St. Louis, 1976, The C. V. Mosby Co.)

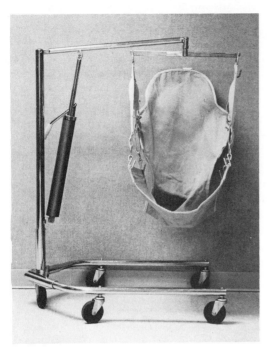

**Fig. 33-4.** Portable hydraulic lift. (From Boroch, R. M.: Elements of rehabilitation in nursing: an introduction, St. Louis, 1976, The C. V. Mosby Co.)

### Toileting (Fig. 33-3)

**commode chair**   for patients who are unable to use a regular bathroom because of immobility or difficulty with equipment.

**toilet guardrail**   provides additional stability.

**elevated toilet seat**   for patients who are unable to sit on a toilet of the usual height.

## DEVICES AIDING IN SITTING, STANDING, MOVEMENT, AND MOBILIZATION

Many assistive devices are available to help patients sit, stand, move, and become mobile. All these devices are extremely useful when appropriately prescribed to facilitate independence. Of those most commonly used, both within the home and in institutional settings, are the following:

1. Chair-table
2. Hydraulic lift
3. Infant walker
4. Scooter board
5. Stand-in table
6. Support seats or seat inserts
7. Tilt table
8. Wheelchair

The uses and indications for many of these devices are self-evident. *Stand-in tables* can be adjusted in height and they provide upright support (see Fig. 28-3, *D*). *Seat inserts* are often custom designed to fulfill the specific positional needs of the patient. These are most often used by infants and

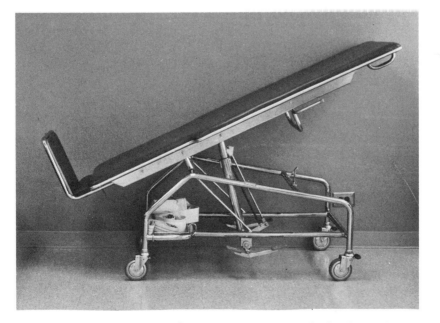

**Fig. 33-5.** Tilt table. (From Boroch, R. M.: Elements of rehabilitation in nursing: an introduction, St. Louis, 1976, The C. V. Mosby Co.)

children, although they may be extremely useful as well for adults.

The *hydraulic lift* (Fig. 33-4) is available commercially for both institutional and home use. Although many of the designs are portable, they can be permanently installed. They are extremely useful for transferring patients from a bed to a wheelchair, from a bed to a stretcher, or from a wheelchair to a tank, tub, or pool. Most of these lifts are designed to decrease the manual exertion required from those assisting with the transfer process, and they are most useful for those patients who have limited ability to assist in this effort.

The *tilt table* (Fig. 33-5) permits gradual vertical change of position, often for increasing periods of time. They may be constructed of wood or metal with padding, and are commercially available or may be individually constructed.

A *wheelchair* (Fig. 33-6) can provide independent mobilization when ambulation is not required, desired, or possible. It also provides an alternative for the ambulatory patient in situations where ambulation may not be feasible or advisable, as in large crowds. For self-mobilization upper extremity strength is extremely important. Gradual use of a wheelchair will help the patient and specific strengthening exercises develop the necessary strength. Several options are available for the person who must use a wheelchair permanently. Custom-designed wheelchairs with all the appropriate attachments and comfort devices tremen-

dously increase the potential of the wheelchair itself. Use of a wheelchair as the mode of transportation in public areas is becoming less of a problem with the current laws requiring access to buildings.

## DEVICES AIDING AND SUPPORTING MOTION AND AMBULATION

The types of devices commonly used to support motion and ambulation are *canes, crutches, walkers,* and *orthoses.* Orthoses (see Chapter 32) contribute to the support and stability required for ambulation. Additional stability can be provided by specific types of canes, crutches, or walkers for patients who are unable to maintain the stability necessary for independent ambulation. A degree of strength and muscle power is required even with this assistance to provide for an acceptable gait pattern. The choice of a cane, crutches, or walker will depend on the degree of assistance required. Minimal assistance will be provided with a cane, while a walker provides maximal assistance.

Various types of canes are available; the most popular provides a single support system and is constructed of wood or metal. Some are adjustable in height. The patient is usually taught to use the cane on the side opposite the affliction to provide a wide base of support during the phase of ambulation that requires weightbearing on the side with the least amount of strength. When additional support is required a multiple pedestal type cane (Fig. 33-7) may be used.

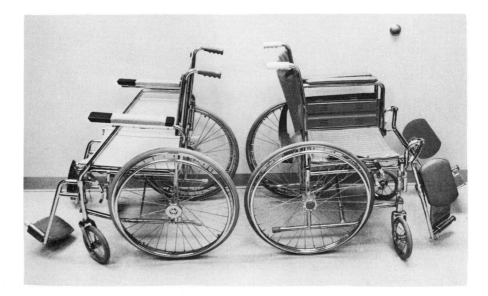

**Fig. 33-6.** Wheelchairs. Many wheelchairs are custom designed for long-term use. Removable armrests are an option. (From Boroch, R. M.: Elements of rehabilitation in nursing: an introduction, St. Louis, 1976, The C. V. Mosby Co.)

The three most common types of crutches are *axillary*, *forearm*, and *trough* (Fig. 33-8). The most frequently used are axillary crutches, which are usually constructed of wood, but metal ones are also available. These are for temporary use, while the forearm and trough crutches are more often prescribed when permanent use is anticipated. Both the forearm and trough types are constructed of metal and are adjustable in height.

A walker (Fig. 33-9) is prescribed for patients with limited ability to propel themselves during ambulation. It provides a much broader base of support and stability than a cane or crutches, permitting a more stable gait. Most walkers are made of aluminum because it is lightweight.

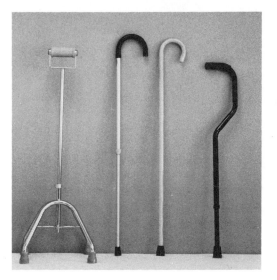

**Fig. 33-7.** Various canes to assist in stability and ambulation. (From Boroch, R. M.: Elements of rehabilitation in nursing: an introduction, St. Louis, 1976, The C. V. Mosby Co.)

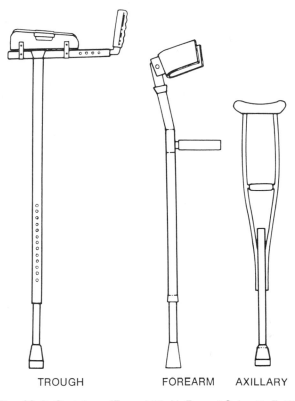

TROUGH    FOREARM    AXILLARY

**Fig. 33-8.** Crutches. (From Hilt, N. E., and Schmitt, E. W., Jr.: Pediatric orthopedic nursing, St. Louis, 1975, The C. V. Mosby Co.)

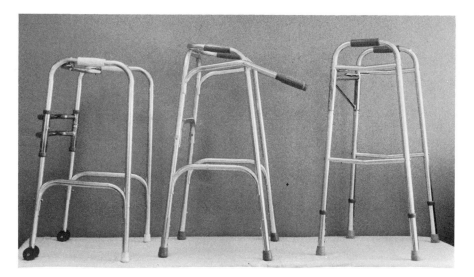

**Fig. 33-9.** Walkers. *Left to right:* front wheel, stair, conventional. (From Boroch, R. M.: Elements of rehabilitation in nursing: an introduction, St. Louis, 1976, The C. V. Mosby Co.)

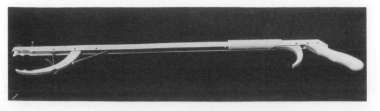

**Fig. 33-10.** "Helping Hand" grasper. (From Boroch, R. M.: Elements of rehabilitation in nursing: an introduction, St. Louis, 1976, The C. V. Mosby Co.)

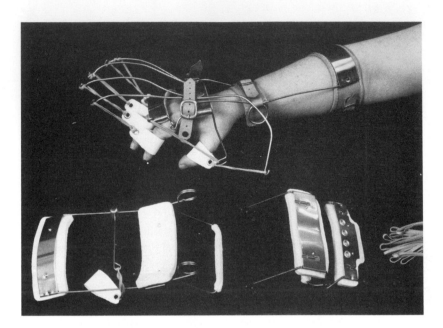

**Fig. 33-11.** Hand splints for exercise. (From Boroch, R. M.: Elements of rehabilitation in nursing: an introduction, St. Louis, 1976, The C. V. Mosby Co.)

## DEVICES FACILITATING HAND GRASP, THUMB-FINGER OPPOSITION, AND HAND/FINGER EXERCISES

The grasp function of the hand, as well as the thumb-finger opposition, affects the patient's ability to perform many of the fine movements required for activities of daily living. In addition, the overall strength and flexibility of the hand have great effect as well. When function is weak, an assistive device may be used to replace the fine movements required to pick up and grasp objects and, to limited degrees, promote other activities (Fig. 33-10). All of these devices require a degree of muscular function and are not useful if function or strength is totally absent; all require a degree of power for utilization. Few devices exist that will totally promote fine movement in the performance of tasks such as sewing, although many traditional objects may be adapted or built up to enhance the patient's limited function.

During the early rehabilitation phases, mainte-nance of the hand in the functional position is critical to the patient's overall potential and anticipated rate of progression. Neglect of this principle can be a tremendous deterrent to achievement of goals related to hand function. Functional position of the hand can be maintained with devices such as a hand roll, plaster splint, plastic splint, etc. A variety of commercial hand splints are available that will simultaneously promote maintenance of functional positioning and encouragement of exercise of the fingers (Fig. 33-11). Varying degrees of correction of specific deformities may also be obtained with some of these splints, but they are prescribed most frequently when motion is desired and the potential for function is recognized.

## DEVICES SUPPORTING OR IMMOBILIZING JOINTS

During all phases of treatment and rehabilitation support or immobilization of one or more joints may

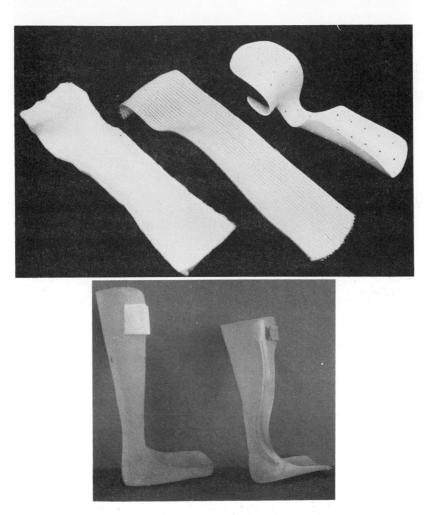

**Fig. 33-12.** Splints for supporting or immobilizing joints of the arm *(top)* or leg *(bottom).* (From Boroch, R. M.: Elements of rehabilitation in nursing: an introduction, St. Louis, 1976, The C. V. Mosby Co.)

be necessary, either intermittently or continuously. Indications for supportive and immobilization joint devices include:

1. Prevention of deformity
2. Prevention of contracture
3. Prevention of subluxation or dislocation
4. Correction of deformity
5. Maintenance of correction of deformity
6. Promotion of comfort and decrease of pain
7. Prevention of mobilization friction of a joint
8. Protection of a joint

With an appropriate prescription of a specific type of equipment or device several objectives may be achieved. The degree and the length of immobilization depend on the specific objective to be achieved and the progression or rate with which the device accomplishes those objectives.

The most common types of devices used to immobilize or support a joint are (Fig. 33-12):

1. Plaster cast
2. Fiberglass or synthetic cast
3. Plaster splints
4. Fiberglass or synthetic splints
5. Commercial plastic splints
6. Commercial splints (already constructed)
7. Orthoses
8. Slings

The cost-effectiveness of the type of device chosen should be taken into consideration in relation to the anticipated achievement of the objectives and the length of use anticipated.

**SUMMARY**

Assistive devices are extremely important in helping patients reach treatment objectives and to recognize their capabilities. All avenues of restoration of function should be explored for each patient. Health care personnel can assist the patient and family to adapt as much equipment as possible to decrease the cost associated with this equipment, especially when several devices are needed. The patient should be given appropriate and adequate instructions for all assistive devices being used.

## BIBLIOGRAPHY

Boroch, R. M.: Elements of rehabilitation in nursing: an introduction, St. Louis, 1976, The C. V. Mosby Co.

Copeland, K. Aids for the severely handicapped, New York, 1974, Grune & Stratton, Inc.

Hilt, N. E., and Schmitt, E. W. Jr.: Pediatric orthopedic nursing, St. Louis, 1975, The C. V. Mosby Co.

Kennedy, J. M.: Orthopaedic splints and appliances, London, 1974, Balliere, Tindalle and Cassell, Ltd.

Larson, C., and Gould, M.: Orthopedic nursing, St. Louis, 1978, The C. V. Mosby Co.

Robinault, I. P., editor: Functional aids for the multiply handicapped, New York, 1973, Harper and Row.

Rosenberg, C.: Assistive devices for the handicapped, Atlanta, 1968, American Rehabilitation Foundation and the National Medical Audiovisual Center.

Stewart, J. D.: Traction and orthopaedic appliances, New York, 1975, Churchill Livingstone.

# PART EIGHT

# Adjuncts to care

# 34

# Client education

**MARSHA BRANDON**

A newly diagnosed diabetic was hospitalized to be regulated on insulin. Diligently the nurse had gone to the client's room each day and talked to the client about diabetes, insulin, and injections. On the day of his dismissal the client demonstrated an insulin injection into an orange extremely well. The client was dismissed only to be readmitted a few days later with a blood sugar of 272. The nurse was puzzled. Before his dismissal the client had been well regulated and his blood sugar was 156. While assessing the client the nurse asked if he had been administering his insulin. The client replied, "Yes. Each morning I inject 24 units of insulin into an orange."

This is a common anecdote often used as an amusing ice breaker before a speech. Unfortunately, it is an all-too-true example of today's client education.

Was this client's education inadequate? What should have been taught? How should it have been taught? How could the nurse have determined if the client comprehended what has been taught? These are questions which this chapter proposes to answer.

The purpose of this chapter is to instruct the reader of the development of education plans for client education. This chapter will also supply the reader with basic lesson plans to be used as refer-ences for the most common needs of client educa-tion.

## WHO IS THE CLIENT?

The term *client* has been used intentionally in this chapter. This is to indicate that the recipient of edu-cation is not always the patient. The family very often is the client to be taught in addition to the pa-tient. This is especially true in orthopedics because so often the patient is immobilized. There is a ten-dency in pediatric orthopedics to teach the family *rather than* the patient. Sometimes this is necessary because of the age of the child. Whenever possible, however, the patient and the family should be in-cluded in the education plan.

At times a health team member is the client to be taught. Communication among members, may be excellent and each member may understand the patient's educational needs. However, if one mem-ber does not have the knowledge or the ability to follow through with the teaching plan, his or her understanding of the educational needs is of no value to the patient.

## WHO IS THE TEACHER?

This question could be posed to 100 different people and we would receive 100 different answers. The most common of which would be, "Not I! I am a nurse," or "Not I! I am a therapist."

Realistically, anyone who is in contact with the client is a teacher. One does not have to march to-ward a client armed with a written lesson plan in order to teach. Incidental learning may take place anytime someone does something for or says some-thing to a client. Direct learning may also occur but, again, the teacher does not have to be armed with a written plan. However, the goal that the teacher wants to accomplish at this meeting with the client may be only one component of the education plan. A planned design is needed for this learning to be a result of an educational process.

The health team member who is in initial contact with the client is probably the most effective teach-er, since these first instructions usually form the basis for future learning. Consequently, each time a health team member meets a client, knowledge may be communicated and behavior modified, making teachers of all the health team.

## WHAT IS CLIENT EDUCATION?

Providing information and explanation is often considered to be client education. However, information and explanation are *components* of education. Information is possessed knowledge; explanation is communicating this knowledge so that it is understandable. Information and knowledge work together; for example, when a person is hyperventilating, he is told to rebreathe into a paper bag to increase the $CO_2$ content in his body. The *knowledge* (increased air in the lung with $CO_2$ being "blown off") and the *communication* of what to do and why results in the appropriate action. A client may receive information and explanation separately or combined; however, neither is education.

Education is a dynamic process of behavior modification. It is a process because it is the utilization of the information and explanation. Education is planned to result in a new insight or method of doing something: a new behavior may be learned or an old behavior may be adapted. If this change in behavior is to occur, it must be designed to be real and meaningful to the learner—something that, when acquired, will be useful. This process can be stated as:

Information + Explanation + Planned design = Education

## WHY IS CLIENT EDUCATION NECESSARY?

It has already been stated that the purpose of education is to bring about a change in behavior, but for what reason and to what end is this desired? Education helps the client maintain the level of wellness achieved. This may be a task such as the skillful application of a brace, or a feeling, such as acceptance of one's body image after an amputation.

Education helps clients to assess their progress and set new goals so that they are able to work realistically toward what they know they can and should accomplish. Education gives the client an incentive.

## WHAT SHOULD THE CLIENT ACCOMPLISH?

The answer to this question constitutes the objective of a client education plan. The development of objectives is the first step in the education plan. Unfortunately, persons who are "nonteachers" often believe they must go back to school to learn how to develop objectives. An objective is simply a goal—what the client should be able to do after the teaching takes place.

Stating the objective in a meaningful way is most important. As Mager states, an objective should succeed in communicating the teacher's intent.[3,p.10]

The most confusing factor is usually selecting the most descriptive terms for writing the objective. These terms may be divided into levels of accomplishment. The descriptions are arranged from the most basic behavior to the most complicated behavior to be accomplished. An example of such progression is: The client will be able to (1) identify, (2) describe, (3) analyze, and (4) create. Any term used to describe a measurable behavior is appropriate.

The descriptive behavioral term will determine what action is expected of the client. The remaining components of an objective are the conditions under which the action is to be performed and the extent to which the performance is expected.[3,p.12] For example, after reading the booklet on cast care and without reference materials, the client will be able to identify three of the five indicators of poor circulation of an extremity in a cast. This objective has the action (identify), the condition (after reading the booklet), and the extent of performance (three out of five indicators).

## WHEN AND WHERE DOES CLIENT EDUCATION START?

Client education should start with the first encounter with a health team member. Too often client education consists of last minute instructions given a client as he walks through the door waving goodbye. At the initial meeting with a client the health team member should begin planning an education program that will lead to maximal understanding and functioning.

Caution must be taken when initiating client education to be sure that clients are not bombarded with instruction. They must be given time simply to adapt. Basic information is the first step in alleviating a client's anxiety, which will enable him or her to absorb and retain future instruction.

Education should start at the client's level of knowledge, which should be assessed in the initial interview. After the client's ability has been determined, an education program can be designed with relevant terminology and performance objectives.

## WHAT SHOULD BE TAUGHT?

Generally, the material to be taught is considered *content*. Content then becomes facts or knowledge that is transferred from one person to another. Remember that "knowledge keeps no better than fish"[4,p.4]; using the knowledge vitalizes the content.

Determination of the content to be taught is the second phase of the development of an educational plan. Content should be determined by the type and amount of knowledge and its use that will enable the client to attain the performance objective. Content is the bridge that spans from the client's knowledge base to where he or she desires to be. The amount of time available for client education will also determine how much can be taught. Time and materials available may allow only basic knowledge to be transferred to the client. However, this time factor may be overcome by using the various teaching strategies discussed later in this chapter. Regardless of the content taught, the health team members' involvement, enthusiasm, and motivation will add the dynamic sphere to education.

## HOW SHOULD THE CLIENT BE TAUGHT?

The manner or method of teaching is called a *teaching strategy*. The development or selection of the teaching strategy is the third phase in the development of an education plan.

The most important factor to remember when making this selection is the appropriateness of the strategy. The strategy should be appropriate to the client's level of learning, the teacher, the objective, and the setting.

Exactly how people learn has not been determined, yet learning takes place by different ways and at different speeds. Psychologist Carl Rogers believes that self-discovered learning is the most significant kind. The old adage that experience is the best teacher may be true; however, in the health field, experience may prove to be more detrimental than helpful to the client. For example, a person who has herniated a disc because he bent down rather than stooped to pick up a heavy object has learned what not to do. Unfortunately, this lesson was learned *after* the damage has been done.

Self-discovery is just one teaching strategy. Lectures can be used to give a large amount of information in a short period of time. Discussion allows for interaction between teacher and learner since the learner is free to question. Role playing allows the person to take on the role of another and become cognizant of a different point of view. Gaming is a strategy especially useful with children. This strategy uses a game format as the vehicle for the transferance of knowledge. For example, to encourage a child in a Risser cast to deep breathe, the nurse can fill two blow bottles with colored water and have a race with the child. The person who moves the largest amount of water with one breath is the winner.

Two components to be included in any teaching strategy are *reinforcement* and *closure*. Reinforcement of learning increases motivation by increasing one's self-esteem. Often reinforcement will add consistency to learning. Closure is a form of reinforcement. It may be used as a review of all information taught. Closure provides an opportunity for learners to gain information they had missed and to clarify what they may have misunderstood.

## IS THE CLIENT EDUCATED?

Evaluation is the last phase in the development of an education plan. To determine if the client has learned what was intended and if the objective has been met, evaluation must take place. Evaluation serves as a measurement and assessment of the client's knowledge level and ability after he or she has been taught. It measures how well the objective has been accomplished, if indeed at all. Evaluation should serve to encourage the client to set new objectives or revise old ones.

Evaluation need not be a lengthy, highly scholarly endeavor. It should just help client and teacher recognize what learning has taken place and to assess the client's level of understanding and learning at that time. The best way to do this is simply to ask the client to review the lesson to determine if the pertinent information has been acquired. Asking the client if he or she understands or has any questions not only "opens the door" for a client who may be inhibited to ask questions, but also determines the clarity and effective design of that explanation.

Various methods can be used to evaluate the attainment of objectives. A well-constructed quiz is one. When using this method it is important to review the examination with the client and use it as a learning tool It is also important to give positive feedback to clients to avoid creating a threatening atmosphere.

Demonstration is a method that does not require that the client use verbal or written ability. This will enable the quality of the action to be evaluated.

When deciding upon the method, manner of presentation, and time of evaluation, the teacher should frequently refer to the objective. This is the guiding light by which the client has been directed; evaluate this and only this. Do not expect the client to learn something that is not the objective of the lesson.

## REFERENCE EDUCATION PLANS

To assist the reader in developing education plans, some examples of basic plans follow. These plans can be considered "mini" plans, since they contain only one objective. They are a basic component of a larger, more complete education plan. These plans are only examples; each plan must be adapted so that it will be appropriate for the specific needs of an individual client and be consistent with established standards of care policies and procedures accepted by the specific setting. Additional detailed information for education plans may be found in the chapters that review this care (i.e., Chapter 23, Cast and splint therapy; Chapter 24, Traction and suspension therapy).

**Education plan:** Adequate circulation
Objective: After the lesson the client will be able to identify all of the discussed indicators of poor circulation.
Content: Any part of the body experiencing poor circulation or restraint of blood flow may demonstrate one or all of the following indicators:
  1. Change in skin color.
     a. Cyanosis (blueness) indicates pooling of venous blood.
     b. Pallor indicates a lack of arterial blood.
     c. Change in color may also be observed in the mucous membrane of the mouth or eyelids.
  2. Change in blanching of nail bed. When the nail is pressed near the cuticle, it should turn white, then pink when the pressure is released.
     a. Color may return too slowly. This indicates a restriction of arterial blood flow, which prohibits oxygenated blood from reaching the nail.
     b. Color may return too quickly. This indicates a restriction in venous flow, which prohibits the blood from being pushed from the nail.
  3. Change in temperature of the skin. The skin is usually cool or cold if circulation is inadequate.
  4. Change in sensation—numbness.
  5. Change in size—swelling and edema.
Teaching strategy: Discussion, demonstration, pictures.
Evaluation: Ask the client to name all the indicators of poor circulation discussed.

**Education plan:** Alleviating edema
Objective: After the lesson the client will be able to demonstrate using pillows, the methods discussed to alleviate edema of an extremity.
Content: 1. Position the extremity above the level of the heart.
  2. Position the extremity on pillows that comfortably fit the contour of the extremity.
  3. Position the pillows in graduating steps of elevation. Each pillow should be placed beneath and about one half the length of two previous pillows moving toward the proximal end of the extremity.
  4. The most edematous part of the extremity should be highest.
  5. Positioning the extremity at heart level will prevent further edema, but will not alleviate existing edema.
Teaching strategy: Discussion, demonstration.
Evaluation: Ask the client to demonstrate the elevation of an extremity using pillows as discussed.

**Education plan:** Cast care[5, pp. 82-105]
Objective: After the lesson the client will be able to identify all of the discussed factors necessary for adequate care of a cast.
Content: 1. Keep the cast on soft surfaces until it is dry. Handle the wet cast with palms of the hands only. Reposition frequently to facilitate drying.
  2. Keep the cast dry. If the cast is plaster, moisture will cause it to dissolve. It may be necessary to protect a child's cast from urine. This may be done by the insertion of plastic petals that may then be funneled into a bedpan.
  3. Avoid hitting the cast against a hard surface. This force could cause the cast to crack. There may be cracks inside the cast that are not visible. Crumbs of plaster from these cracks may cause skin irritation.
  4. Do not put powder under the cast. It will accumulate, causing skin irritation and decreased body secretions.
  5. Do not scratch under the cast with breakable or sharp objects. These may be lost in the cast or cause puncture wounds. If itching

occurs, use a hair dryer set on cool to blow underneath the cast.

6. Observe the skin around the edges of the cast for redness denoting irritation. Also check for any burning under the cast. This may be a sign of skin irritation.
7. Check sensory, motor, and circulatory status of the extremity.
8. Keep the cast clean and dry. This is necessary to avoid cast changes and jeopardizing the position.

Teaching strategy: Discussion, demonstration, pictures.
Evaluation: Ask the client to verbally name the discussed factors of cast care.

**Education plan:** Traction care
Objective: The client will be able to identify all the discussed factors necessary for adequate care of traction.
Content: 1. Stay in straight alignment with the line of pull. This does not mean that the body will always be straight with the traction. However, the extremity in traction must remain straight. This will maintain the desired position.
2. Keep the weights hanging free to maintain maximum traction.
3. Keep the ropes free. Anything touching the traction apparatus decreases tension and therefore decreases traction.
4. Observe the skin for redness indicating irritation. Also observe sensory-motor and circulatory status.
5. Apply the traction apparatus, such as a Sayre sling, correctly to assure proper traction. Continuous tractions (adhesive skin and skeletal) should not be released.

Teaching strategy: Discussion, demonstration, pictures.
Evaluation: Ask the client to name all of the discussed factors of traction care. If the client is to apply the traction apparatus, demonstration of this would be an appropriate evaluation method. However, this would necessitate a second objective in this plan.

**Education plan:** Brace care
Objective: After the lesson, the client will be able to identify all of the discussed factors necessary for adequate care of a brace.
Content: 1. No brace is completely comfortable. Adjustment to it will come with proper application and time.
2. Observe for skin irritation. Also observe sensory-motor and circulatory status.
3. Keep the brace clean. Clean and oil the hinges. Clean the vinyl parts with a damp cloth. This will keep the brace in working condition and make it more comfortable.
4. Keep the brace in proper alignment when not in use. This will avoid any twisting or misalignment of the brace.[1,p.175]
5. Check the condition of the brace before applying to ascertain its condition for reasons of safety.[1,p.175]

Teaching strategy: Discussion, demonstration.
Evaluation: Ask the client to name all of the discussed factors of adequate brace care. If the client has the brace, demonstration of its application would be an appropriate evaluating method. However, this would necessitate a second objective in this plan.

**Education plan:** Body mechanics
Objective: After this lesson, the client will be able to demonstrate the proper body mechanics discussed and demonstrated to reduce stress on the body when lying, standing, lifting, and moving an object.
Content: 1. Keep the body on the same plane as the pelvis. This will necessitate stooping rather than bending.
2. Keep the feet apart. This gives a broad base of support.
3. Pull rather than push. This allows the pull of gravity and the body weight rather than just muscle to accomplish the task.
4. Lie in bed in the same straight position as standing. Support the extremities. This will alleviate muscle pull and strain.[2,pp.6-7]

Teaching strategy: Discussion, demonstration, pictures.
Evaluation: Ask the client to demonstrate the proper position for lying, standing, lifting, and moving an object.

## SUMMARY

Today's health care system is based on curative measures. The increasing population, increasing numbers of people seeking health care, and the more sophisticated methods of diagnosing make prevention of illness the aim of the future health care system. No longer is it enough to make people well; preventive measures must be used to keep people from becoming ill or experiencing recurring illnesses.

Education is the foundation on which this preventive design must be based. Each client receiving health care should also receive some education. Client education is an integral part of health care and it should begin as soon as the client enters the health care system.

Every health team member is a teacher to the client, and each bit of information or explanation is a component of education. This information, when given in a planned design, comprises education. To develop this design four phases are necessary:

1. Setting objectives — what is to be accomplished
2. Developing content — what is to be taught
3. Developing a teaching strategy — how it is to be taught
4. Evaluation — what the client learned

Education is a dynamic process of behavior modification. It is a challenge to each member of the health care team to vitalize this educational process. The information, explanation, and planned design will be the most utilized, but the caring and respectful manner in which information is given will be most remembered by the client.

## REFERENCES

1. Brunner, L., and others: Textbook of medical-surgical nursing ed. 2, Philadelphia; 1970, J. B. Lippincott, Co.
2. Larson, C. B., and Gould, M. L.: Orthopedic nursing, ed.9, St. Louis, 1978, The C. V. Mosby Co.
3. Mager, R. F.: Preparing instructional objectives, Belmont, Calif., 1962, Fearon Publishers.
4. Parker, J. C., and Rubin, L. J.: Process as content.
5. Hilt, N. E., and Schmitt, E. W., Jr.: Pediatric orthopedic nursing, St. Louis, 1975, The C. V. Mosby Co.

## BIBLIOGRAPHY

Bizze, M. L.: Learning theories for teachers, ed. 2, New York; 1971, Harper and Row.

Brunner, L., and others: Textbook of medical surgical nursing, ed. 2, Philadelphia; 1970, J. B. Lippincott Co.

deTornyay, R.: Strategies for teaching nursing, New York, 1971, John Wiley and Sons, Inc.

Heidgerhem, L. E.: Teaching and learning in schools of nursing, ed. 3, Philadelphia; 1965, J. B. Lippincott Co.

Hilt, N. E., and Schmitt, E. W., Jr.: Pediatric orthopedic nursing, St. Louis, 1975, The C. V. Mosby Co.

Hyman, R. T.: Ways of teaching ed. 2, Philadelphia; 1974, J. B. Lippincott Co.

Larson, C. B., and Gould, M.: Orthopedic nursing ed. 9, St. Louis; 1978, The C. V. Mosby Co.

Mager, R. F.: Preparing instructional objectives, Belmont; Texas, 1962, Fearon Publishers.

Mager, R. F., and Pipe, P.: Analyzing performance problem or 'You really oughta wanna', Belmont; Texas, 1970, Fearon Publishers, Inc.

Parker, J. C., and Rabin, L. J.: Process as content, Chicago; 1966, Rand McNally College Publishing Co.

Postman, N., and Weingartner, C.: Teaching as a subversive activity, New York; 1969, Dell Publishing Co.

Read, D. A., and Greene, W. H.: Creative teaching in health, ed. 2, New York; 1975, Macmillan Publishing Co.

Reilly, D. E.: Behavioral objectives in nursing: Evaluation of learner attainment, New York; 1975, Appleton-Century-Crofts.

Rogers, C.: Personal thoughts on teaching and learning, Improv Coll Univ Teach 6(1):7-8, 1958.

# 35

# Multidisciplinary care of the multiply handicapped

E. DENNIS LYNE

KATHRYN M. VEDDER

Any initial statement concerning treatment for the multiply handicapped, both adult and child, must include the high priority for coordinated care, both inside and outside the medical environment. The goals of the multidisciplinary care team include:

1. Assessment of each patient by defining past, present, and anticipated problems
2. Establishment of individualized goals and objectives for each person in their own environment
3. Development, coordination, implementation, and reevaluation of the comprehensive plan
4. Documentation and evaluation of care outcome

Without a clearly defined statement of goals and constant reevaluation of the dynamic milieu of the multiply handicapped, comprehensive treatment cannot be fully achieved. Many articles have attempted to deal with the subject, and it is impossible in this brief chapter to cover the entire range of adult and childhood conditions requiring this approach. To focus our attention, we have chosen to deal with one particular entity as our model—myelodysplasia. It is our feeling that myelodysplasia epitomizes many of medical, social, and emotional problems multiply handicapped persons face.

Material is available pertaining to coordinated care of the person with myelodysplasia.[1-4,7-9,11] From the hospital's point of view, the medical care should not submerge the individual's uniqueness for the sake of "conform now, be well later."[10,p.811] On the other side of the coin, the family's concern tends to focus primarily on the physical aspects of the illness. The social and emotional effects of a chronic condition have less impact but nevertheless play an equally important role, especially in later life.[5,p.98] Therefore, with myelodysplasia we are dealing with a multiplicity of physical, social, and emotional crises both inside and outside the hospital, all of which must be dealt with by a multidisciplinary team.

## OUTPATIENT CARE

As stated by Bunch,[3] one approach in the treatment of myelodysplasia is to have the patient seen in various specialty clinics. However, this approach frequently produces frustration and annoyance because of lack of communication among the specialists; it also tends to ignore the other areas of health care that the child must have. This chapter presents some advantages and disadvantages of multidisciplinary care, with a major focus on outpatient care and more limited attention on inpatient care.

### Organization

First, it should be stated quite clearly that when a professional is working on a team, he or she is responsible primarily to the team and not to his or her specialty in the traditional sense. Without this primary allegiance to the team, the team's efforts can be seriously undermined. We strongly recommend that the authority of the multidisciplinary team be equal or superior to the various divisions and departments from which the team members are drawn. If this is not the case, some department personnel may simply refuse to cooperate in multidisciplinary care cases, or the team may be ineffective because participants do not have the potential for positive input. Encouraging the parents' dependence on specific established departments, or simply not finding adequate personnel for staffing are other overt ways the team can be made ineffective.

If the multidisciplinary team does not have the necessary authority, a "star system," comes to the fore. This ensures that the existing system will remain paramount and undermines the entire structure of the clinic. This is not to say that the individual departments should not have input into the ultimate direction, time, and structure of the clinic, but one department should not have the power to completely destroy the working arrangement among other departments represented by otherwise agreeable staff. As Horowitz[6] states, the team should make decisions not according to bureaucratic rules but in conformity with the best and independent judgment of the professionals most familiar with the patient's situation.

### Physical setting

The multidisciplinary team should work in a completely independent functioning clinic. All necessary equipment and space should be immediately available in this clinic or close by. The unit should not have to depend on sending the patient to another floor for a test that is likely to be needed. The unit's uniqueness depends upon efficiency yet overall comprehensiveness; once the patient leaves the unit for testing there is a tendency to lose control. The isolation should not be so complete as to divorce the multidisciplinary care clinic from the actual hospital, but it must be largeley self-contained to promote the needed level of staff communication. Above all, the clinic must govern itself, and such authority promotes continual internal scrutiny and policy review.

### Funds

Though some federal and state funding may be available, it is our firm belief that the hospital must undertake the responsibility for funding the basic unit. Our personal experience has shown that with a decrease in individual visits leading to increased time/space utilization, physician time, and paramedical personnel utilization, such a unit can easily become economically self-sustaining.

One reason for the insistence on basic hospital funding is to initiate total commitment by the administration to the responsibility for such a unit. The downfall of many multidisciplinary clinics can be traced directly to a lack of commitment on the part of the hospital administration. If financial responsibility is sidetracked and confused by restrictive third-party funding, active participation by the administration is easily side-stepped.

In the funding of such a clinic it is most advantageous to have a set budget that includes time paid for physician and paramedical personnel. This adds to the permanence and status of the team, which now no longer has to rely upon the emotional commitment of the staff, but has a financial commitment on the part of the participants and their departments. We consider this latter type of commitment most necessary.

### Physical setup

As stated above, the unit should be physically independent. We prefer the central core type of plan. In this respect we are in complete agreement with Bunch.[3] There should be a separate room for each child. The staff members should come to see him, rotating on an efficient basis. When one try to "rotate" the child through various rooms to see specialists, the result is much less efficient in terms of the physician's time. Use of the staff member's time is sometimes questioned in any case, but it has been our experience that the physicians' time is actually better utilized when they are free to move from room to room.

To ensure that each child is seen by each staff member, a simple checklist attached to the door of each room suffices. These lists can be made out by the coordinator ahead of time. During clinic time, it is best to have available a large space in the clinic area for both occupational and physical therapy where exercises, etc., can be initiated and reviewed with the parent. It is considered advantageous, but not a necessity, to have the pediatrician see the child first, since he or she is the generalist with an overall view of the child's needs. During the initial interview by the pediatrician (each visit, or first visit only), various staff members can be brought in when this seems desirable.

### Personnel

Although Ames and Schut[1,p.466] have written about a clinic staffed with two physicians and several paramedical staff members, we feel that at least four primary physicians should be involved in myelodysplasia care: a pediatrician, neurosurgeon, orthopedic surgeon, and urologist. While the pediatrician can often screen for various specialty problems, the specialists themselves should be involved in each child's care. The time-honored principle of knowing the patient and family before surgery should be emphasized to the surgeons. Paramedical personnel still constitute the majority of the team and should include staff members from nursing, physical therapy, occupational therapy, social service, special education, and psychology. All paramedical personnel must be assured of adequate input in deciding the team's function and objectives. In many cases they are the primary care participants.

Choosing personnel requires long and arduous sorting. The attitudes of the successful team member, as stated by Horowitz, are[6]:

1. Dedication to a common goal
2. Willingness to share treatment of a patient
3. Receptive outlook
4. Flexibility
5. Willingness to learn
6. Willingness to accept and abide by decisions made by consensus

Equally important, according to Horowitz,[6] is the attitude of the professional toward the group. This must involve (1) respect, (2) confidence in each colleague's goodwill, and (3) confidence in each colleague's competence. These attitudes are more easily obtained in the paramedical personnel. Physicians, unfortunately, are taught in most medical centers to be self-reliant and in many cases are egotistical about their own attitudes. *Egotism is defeating to a team.* In our experience we had little problem integrating paramedical personnel but had to change some medical personnel before a functioning team was established. Surgeons, particularly, tend to be individualistic and often tend to reject a decision made by consensus. As emphasized previously, the team must have the ability to go to the various departments represented and request personnel changes. This can only be done if the team is constituted on an *equal* basis among the various departments.

This clinic can be extended to include the patient's community if these health professionals and community members can be trained by clinic personnel. There must be adequate communication between clinic personnel and both medical and school personnel in the child's community.

### Team leadership

The team is directed by a limited hierarchy with a defined leader who needs not only imagination and ability to make decisions, but also must have a measure of status within the complex organization.

Ideally, the team leader should be a generalist, preferably a pediatrician with a thorough knowledge of all aspects of the disease, although a knowledgeable specialist may be an excellent director. The major prerequisite may be likened to that of a benevolent dictator who has the unique quality of being able to take an overall view of the child's management without becoming obsessed with his or her own specialty or abilities in total child care. Many physicians cannot function within this concept because of habit; therefore, the team leader must be carefully chosen. As stated previously, the team leader must have the power through the group to represent the group within the traditional structure of authority in the hospital. Through the team leader, the team must have an equal voice in the hospital power structure with the various departments and divisions involved. It should also be emphasized again that no division or department should have the ability to destroy the function and work of other departments or divisions who are cooperating adequately in providing interdisciplinary care.

The team leader's position should be adequately defined within the administrative apparatus of the hospital before the team is even started. Authority that comes only from goodwill and a hearty handshake will eventually be dissipated, leading to the dissolution of a clinic.

It is also important to emphasize that the child's primary care belongs to the *team* rather than to the specialists involved. Each member of the team must realize that an efficient clinic is not measured by patients seen per hour, but by the advantages to the patient of the clinic approach. When a child has a specific procedure performed on another service, it should be with the clear understanding that the child is still under the direct supervision of the team, and that team decisions have precedence over further nonemergency procedures. This concept will pose problems until other departments realize that the child has many other problems, some of which may be more pressing than those that they have defined. An excellent example is the child who needs an elective ileal diversion, but may have a serious iron deficiency anemia or may, for emotional reasons, be unable to handle the idea of an external appliance at the present time. This is not to say that emergency life-saving procedures should not be undertaken immediately, but this policy provides a safeguard against elective procedures being done at an inopportune time.

### Coordination outside clinic

Staff meetings are mandatory after each clinic, be they monthly or weekly. The team leader should be responsible for coordination of such meetings, but he or she can delegate authority to paramedical personnel. Adequate preparation must be made beforehand by informing the participating staff of the subjects to be discussed. Community personnel should be included whenever possible when individual children are discussed. Whether these staff meetings are directly connected with the clinic, as advocated by Bunch,[3] or held at another time more convenient for the personnel involved, is inconsequential. The number of patients seen per clinic often decides the time, since a full day spent in clinic can leave the participants too tired to hold a productive staff meeting. Needless to say, a staff meeting should be a command performance for all members of the team, as only at this time can true interdisciplinary discussion of the child be undertaken. Though the combined clinic provides some opportunity for individual interchange between the various personnel, this has a tendency to be anecdotal, random, and haphazard, and is therefore not adequate to meet the needs of the patient.

## INPATIENT CARE

In-hospital care for the multiply handicapped is an entire subject in itself and will be discussed in this chapter only briefly. Several important principles should be emphasized. First, the inpatient care philosophy should not differ from outpatient care philosophy; therefore, the team's approach is paramount in coordinating such inpatient care. It should be constantly emphasized that when the patient is in the hospital, primary responsibility for care still rests with the team. Staff meetings are equally necessary to coordinate inpatient care and to arrange for adequate follow-up care upon discharge. All members of the team should be immediately aware when a patient is admitted on an emergency basis.

When the patient is electively admitted, all members of the team should be adequately informed beforehand and coordination of necessary procedures to be done outside the primary admission service should be prearranged. In balancing this, it should be remembered that the desire to test in all areas on a single admission can often confuse and sometimes anger the patient and family. This can be as detrimental as neglect of necessary testing.

Second, we emphasize that many of the principles outlined are appropriate for inpatient care as well as outpatient. It must be remembered, however, that the entire experience is that of a continuum and, for the most part, begins and ends in the outpatient area. Communication between members of the team in the inpatient and outpatient area is essential.

### Parental input

Input from the child's parents is essential. The parents should be made to realize that they have a voice in the care of their child and that they will be listened to. Ignoring the parents' emotional and intellectual ability to contribute can lead to disenchantment, patient loss, and a high failure rate in return visits. The parents should be encouraged to form groups inside the hospital and to hold group therapy and discussion sessions.

Parents should also be encouraged to join groups such as the Spina Bifida Association. However, it is important that Spina Bifida Association chapters are or become independent of any one hospital or particular multidisciplinary care unit. Many times the conclusions that parents reach independently are extremely valuable in the ultimate care of their child and children with similar problems. These groups often provide a good sounding board and they may produce new ideas that can be applied to patient management. If the parents' group becomes totally dependent upon the medical personnel at the hospital, they eventually merely mouth the feelings of the individual medical members of the team. Much will then be lost in terms of individual ability to cooperate and build a team.

During parent meetings, it should be emphasized that controversy and variation in treatment should be freely and openly discussed both with the specialized personnel and among the parents themselves. Question-and-answer periods should be encouraged. Fixed lectures should be short and concise, leaving time for the parents to express their own anxieties and opinions.

### Coordinator

A coordinator is necessary for the day-to-day function of the inpatient team. Though the team leader can assume overall responsibility, this solution is a costly waste of the physician's time if he or she is to be responsible for the bookkeeping aspects of care. A nonphysician coordinator, functioning as the primary input unit, seems to be an excellent and advisable solution. There is no one specialty from which this coordinator must come, but the person should be both a responsible and efficient administrator and knowledgeable enough in the various areas of treatment to handle preliminary problems and immediately contact the necessary personnel to when expert advice is needed. The coordinator has to be extremely mature with an outlook of self-confidence, and be able to efficiently and pleasantly handle complicated emotional and medical problems. The coordinator becomes the central core for administration of the team.

## CONCLUSION

It should be understood that the topic presented lends itself to a diversity of opinion as to approach. The approach presented has been successful in our experience, but the resources available to implement this complex approach are often not available.

In this chapter we have discussed the creation of an interdisciplinary clinic for the care of myelodysplasia. Adapting this basic clinic plan to management of other multiply handicapping problems, such as cerebral palsy, has been relatively easy in our experience. The clinic approach can also be used in the treatment of other orthopedic problems, such as arthritis. Personnel and emphasis may shift accordingly, depending on the age of the patients and various aspects of the disease, deformity, or process. What may be readily ascertained from this discussion is that the inter- or multidisciplinary approach is not only preferable to other approaches, but frequently necessary to accomplish optimal standards of care for the orthopedic patient. Emphasis here has been placed on the physical, political, and financial structure of the clinic approach and the associated pitfalls that frequently act as deterrents to the function of the approach.

In summary, it should be said that the team, whether viewed from an outpatient or inpatient setting, should be multidisciplinary in both medical and paramedical personnel, with equal status among the participating members and within the complex hospital structure. The community should be brought in as an equal contributing partner, as should the patients and their families. Until there is total cooperation and understanding among families, patients, and cooperating hospital personnel, optimal care cannot be given to the patient. If one group or another becomes dominant, the patient's care will be warped in one area at the expense of overall care. Initial construction of a multidisciplinary team is both emotionally and physically draining, but a well functioning multidisciplinary team eventually becomes a thing of beauty both for the participants and the patient. We hope and believe that the future of the care of the multiply handicapped is represented in the multidisciplinary approach, and we encourage active group pressure in order to bring this about.

## REFERENCES

1. Ames, M. D., and Schut, L.: Results of treatment of 1971 consecutive myelomeningoceles—1963 to 1968, Pediatrics **50:**466, 1972.
2. Bluestone, S. S., and Deaver, G. G.: Habilitation of the child with spinal bifida and myelomeningocele, J.A.M.A. **161:**1248, 1956.
3. Bunch, M. H., and others: Modern management of myelomeningoceles, St. Louis, 1972, Warren H. Green.
4. Eckstein, H. B., and MacNab, G. H.: Myelomeningocele and hydrocephalus. The impact of modern treatment, Lancet **1:**842, 1966.
5. Glaser, H. H., Lynn, D. B., and Harrison, G. S.: Comprehensive medical care for handicapped children, Am. J. Dis. Child. **102:**98, 1961.
6. Horowitz, J. J.: Team practice and the specialist, Springfield, Ill., 1970, Charles C Thomas, Publisher.
7. Kilfoyle, R. M.: Myelodysplasia, Ped. Clin. North Am. **14:**419, 1967.
8. Menelaus, M. B.: The orthopedic management of spina bifida cystica, Edinburgh, 1971, E. & S. Livingstone.
9. Smith, E. D.: Spina bifida and the total care of spinal myelomeningocele, Springfield, Ill., 1965, Charles C Thomas, Publisher.
10. Sorensen, K. M., and Amis, D. B.: Understanding the world of the chronically ill, Am. J. Nurs. **67:**811, 1967.
11. Tzimas, N., and Badell-Ribera, A.: Orthopedic and habilitation management of patients with spina bifida and myelomeningocele, Med. Clin. Am. **53:**502, 1969.

# APPENDIX

# Normal laboratory values

## ABBREVIATIONS USED IN TABLES

| | | | |
|---|---|---|---|
| < | = less than | mIU | = milliinternational unit |
| > | = greater than | mOsm | = milliosmole |
| dl | = 100 ml | m$\mu$ | = millimicron |
| g | = gram | mU | = milliunit |
| IU | = international unit | ng | = nanogram |
| kg | = kilogram | pg | = picogram |
| L | = liter | $\mu$Eq | = microequivalent |
| mEq | = milliequivalent | $\mu$g | = microgram |
| mg | = milligram | $\mu$IU | = microinternational unit |
| ml | = milliliter | $\mu$l | = microliter |
| mM | = millimole | $\mu$U | = microunit |
| mm Hg | = millimeters of mercury | U | = unit |

**Table A-1.** Normal leukocyte count in peripheral blood*

| Age | Leukocyte count (cells/mm³) | | Leukocyte count, SI units (cells × 10⁹/l)† | |
|---|---|---|---|---|
| | Average | 95% range‡ | Average | 95% range |
| At birth | 18,100 | 9,000-30,000 | 18.1 | 9.0-30.0 |
| 12 hr | 22,800 | 13,000-38,000 | 22.8 | 13.0-38.0 |
| 24 hr | 18,900 | 9,400-34,000 | 18.9 | 9.4-34.0 |
| 1 wk | 12,200 | 5,000-21,000 | 12.2 | 5.0-21.0 |
| 2 wk | 11,400 | 5,000-20,000 | 11.4 | 5.0-20.0 |
| 4 wk | 10,800 | 5,000-19,500 | 10.8 | 5.0-19.5 |
| 2 mo | 11,000 | 5,500-18,000 | 11.0 | 5.5-18.0 |
| 4 mo | 11,500 | 6,000-17,500 | 11.5 | 6.0-17.5 |
| 6 mo | 11,900 | 6,000-17,500 | 11.9 | 6.0-17.5 |
| 8 mo | 12,200 | 6,000-17,500 | 12.2 | 6.0-17.5 |
| 10 mo | 12,000 | 6,000-17,500 | 12.0 | 6.0-17.5 |
| 12 mo | 11,400 | 6,000-17,500 | 11.4 | 6.0-17.5 |
| 2 yr | 10.600 | 6,000-17,000 | 10.6 | 6.0-17.0 |
| 4 yr | 9,100 | 5,500-15,500 | 9.1 | 5.5-15.5 |
| 6 yr | 8,500 | 5,000-14,500 | 8.5 | 5.0-14.5 |
| 8 yr | 8,300 | 4,500-13,500 | 8.3 | 4.5-13.5 |
| 10 yr | 8,100 | 4,500-13,500 | 8.1 | 4.5-13.5 |
| 12 yr | 8,000 | 4,500-13,500 | 8.0 | 4.5-13.5 |
| 14 yr | 7,900 | 4,500-13,000 | 7.9 | 4.5-13.0 |
| 16 yr | 7,800 | 4,500-13,000 | 7.8 | 4.5-13.0 |
| 18 yr | 7,700 | 4,500-12,500 | 7.7 | 4.5-12.5 |
| 20 yr | 7,500 | 4,500-11,500 | 7.5 | 4.5-11.5 |
| 21 yr | 7,400 | 4,500-11,000 | 7.4 | 4.5-11.0 |

(From Miale, J. B.: Laboratory medicine: hematology, ed. 5, St. Louis, 1977, The C. V. Mosby Co.)

*Data from Albritton, 1952.

†To convert the WBC in traditional units (cells/mm³) to SI units (cells/L), the number in thousands is multiplied by 10⁹ (e.g., 10,600/mm³ = 10.6 × 10⁹/L). To convert the WBC in SI units to traditional units the number is expressed in thousands (e.g., 10.6 × 10⁹/L = 10.6 thousands/mm³).

‡Average value ±2 SD.

**Table A-2.** Normal values for red corpuscles at various ages

| Age | Red cell count (millions/mm³) | Hemoglobin (g/100 ml) | Vol packed RBC (ml/100 ml) | Corpuscular values* | | | |
|---|---|---|---|---|---|---|---|
| | | | | MCV (cu $\mu$) | MCH ($\gamma\gamma$) | MCHC (%) | MCD ($\mu$) |
| First day | 5.1 ± 1.0 | 19.5 ± 5.0 | 54.0 ± 10.0 | 106 | 38 | 36 | 8.6 |
| 2-3 days | 5.1 | 19.0 | 53.5 | 105 | 37 | 35 | |
| 4-8 days | 5.1 | 18.3 ± 4.0 | 52.5 | 103 | 36 | 35 | |
| 9-13 days | 5.0 | 16.5 | 49.0 | 98 | 33 | 34 | |
| 14-60 days | 4.7 ± 0.9 | 14.0 ± 3.3 | 42.0 ± 7.0 | 90 | 30 | 33 | 8.1 |
| 3-5 mo | 4.5 ± 0.7 | 12.2 ± 2.3 | 36.0 | 80 | 27 | 34 | 7.7 |
| 6-11 mo | 4.6 | 11.8 | 35.5 ± 5.0 | 77 | 26 | 33 | 7.4 |
| 1 yr | 4.5 | 11.2 | 35.0 | 78 | 25 | 32 | 7.3 |
| 2 yr | 4.6 | 11.5 | 35.5 | 77 | 25 | 32 | |
| 3 yr | 4.5 | 12.5 | 36.0 | 80 | 27 | 35 | 7.4 |
| 4 yr | 4.6 ± 0.6 | 12.6 | 37.0 | 80 | 27 | 34 | |
| 5 yr | 4.6 | 12.6 | 37.0 | 80 | 27 | 34 | |
| 6-10 yr | 4.7 | 12.9 | 37.5 | 80 | 27 | 34 | 7.4 |
| 11-15 yr | 4.8 | 13.4 | 39.0 | 82 | 28 | 34 | |
| Women | 4.8 ± 0.6 | 14.0 ± 2.0 | 42.0 ± 5.0 | 87 ± 5 | 29 ± 2 | 34 ± 2 | 7.5 ± 0.3 |
| Men | 5.4 ± 0.8 | 16.0 ± 2.0 | 47.0 ± 5.0 | 87 ± 5 | 29 ± 2 | 34 ± 2 | 7.5 ± 0.3 |

(From Wintrobe, M. M.: Clinical hematology, ed. 6, Philadelphia, 1967, Lea & Febiger.)
*MCV, mean corpuscular volume; MCH, mean corpuscular hemoglobin; MCHC, mean corpuscular hemoglobin concentration; MCD, mean corpuscular diameter.

**Table A-3.** Serology

| Test | Normal value |
|---|---|
| Antibovine milk antibodies | Negative |
| Antideoxyribonuclease (ADNAase) | <1:20 |
| Antinuclear antibodies (ANA) | <1:10 |
| Antistreptococcal hyaluronidase (ASH) | <1:256 |
| Antistreptolysin-O (ASO) | <160 Todd units |
| Australia antigen | See hepatitis-associated antigen |
| *Brucella* agglutinins | <1:80 |
| Coccidioidomycosis antibodies | Negative |
| Cold agglutinins | <1:32 |
| Complement, C'3 | 100-170 mg/dl |
| C-reactive protein (CRP) | 0 |
| Fluorescent treponemal antibodies (FTA) | Nonreactive |
| Hepatitis-associated antigen (HAA or HBAg) | Negative |
| Heterophile antibodies | <1:56 |
| *Histoplasma* agglutinins | <1:8 |
| Latex fixation | Negative |
| *Leptospira* agglutinins | Negative |
| Ox cell hemolysin | <1:480 |
| Rheumatoid factor | |
|   Sensitized sheep cell | <1:160 |
|   Latex fixation | <1:80 |
|   Bentonite particles | <1:32 |
| Streptococcal MG agglutinins | <1:20 |
| Thyroid antibodies | |
|   Antithyroglobulin | <1:32 |
|   Antithyroid microsomal | <1:56 |
| *Toxoplasma* antibodies | <1:4 |
| *Trichina* agglutinins | 0 |
| Tularemia agglutinins | <1:80 |
| Typhoid agglutinins | |
|   O | <1:80 |
|   H | <1:80 |
| VDRL | Nonreactive |
| Weil-Felix (Proteus OX-2, OX-K, and OX-19 agglutinins) | Four-fold rise in titer between acute and convalescent sera |

(From Tilkian, S. M., Conover, M. B., and Tilkian, A. G.: Clinical implications of laboratory tests, ed. 2, St. Louis, 1979, The C. V. Mosby Co.)

**Table A-4.** Gastric fluid

| Test | Normal value |
|---|---|
| Fasting residual volume | 20-100 ml |
| pH | <2.0 |
| Basal acid output (BAO) | 0.6 mEq/hr |
| Maximal acid output (MAO) after histamine stimulation | 5-40 mEq/hr |
| BAO/MAO ratio | <0.4 |

(From Tilkian, S. M., Conover, M. B., and Tilkian, A. G.: Clinical implications of laboratory tests, ed. 2., St. Louis, 1979, The C. V. Mosby Co.)

**Table A-5.** Hematology

| Test | Normal value |
|---|---|
| Blood volume | Male: 69 ml/kg<br>Female: 65 ml/kg |
| Coagulation factors | |
|   Factor I (fibrinogen) | 0.15-0.35 g/100 ml |
|   Factor II (prothrombin) | 60-140% |
|   Factor V (accelerator globulin) | 60-140% |
|   Factor VII-X (proconvertin-Stuart) | 70-130% |
|   Factor X (Stuart factor) | 70-130% |
|   Factor VIII (antihemophlic globulin) | 50-200% |
|   Factor IX (plasma thromboplastic cofactor) | 60-140% |
|   Factor XI (plasma thromboplastic antecedent) | 60-140% |
|   Factor XII (Hageman factor) | 60-140% |
| Coagulation tests | |
|   Bleeding time (Ivy) | 1-6 min |
|   Bleeding time (Duke) | 1-3 min |
|   Clot retraction | ½ the original mass in 2 hr |
|   Dilute blood clot lysis time | Clot lyses between 6 and 10 hr at 37° C |
|   Euglobin clot lysis time | Clot lyses between 2 and 6 hr at 37° C |
|   Partial thromboplastin time (PTT) | 60-70 sec |
|     Kaolin activated | 25-37 sec |
|   Prothombin time | 12-14 sec |
|   Venous clotting time | |
|     3 tubes | 5-15 min |
|     2 tubes | 5-8 min |
|   Whole blood clot lysis time | None in 24 hr |
| Complete blood count (CBC) | |
|   Hematocrit | Male: 40-54%<br>Female: 38-47% |
|   Hemoglobin | Male: 13.5-18.0 g/dl<br>Female: 12.0-16.0 g/dl |
|   Red cell count | Male: $4.6\text{-}6.2 \times 10^6/\mu l$<br>Female: $4.2\text{-}5.4 \times 10^6/\mu l$ |
|   White cell count | $4500\text{-}11,000/\mu l$ |
| Erythrocyte indices | |
|   Mean corpuscular volume (MCV) | $82\text{-}98\ \mu^3$ (fl) |
|   Mean corpuscular hemoglobin (MCH) | 27-31 pg |
|   Mean corpuscular hemoglobin concentration (MCHC) | 32-36% |
| Haptoglobin | 100-300 mg/100 ml |
| Hemoglobin $A_2$ | 1.5-3.5% |
| Hemoglobin F | <2% |
| Osmotic fragility | (see table below) |

| % NaCl | % Lysis (fresh) | % Lysis (after 24 hr incubation at 37°C) |
|---|---|---|
| 0.20 | 97-100 | 95-100 |
| 0.30 | 90-99 | 85-100 |
| 0.35 | 50-95 | 75-100 |
| 0.40 | 5-45 | 65-100 |
| 0.45 | 0-6 | 55-95 |
| 0.50 | 0 | 40-85 |
| 0.55 | | 15-70 |
| 0.60 | | 0-40 |
| 0.65 | | 0-10 |
| 0.70 | | 0-5 |
| 0.75 | | 0 |

| Test | Normal value |
|---|---|
| Plasma volume | Male: 39 ml/kg<br>Female: 40 ml/kg |
| Platelet count | 200,000-350,000/mm |
| Platelet function tests: | |
|   Clot retraction | 50-100% at 2 hr |
|   Platelet aggregation | Full response to ADP, 1-epinephrine, and collagen |
|   Platelet factor 3 | 35-57 sec |
| Reticulocyte count | 0.5-1.5%<br>$25,000\text{-}75,000$ cells/$\mu l$ |
| Sedimentation rate (ESR) (Westergren) | Men under 50 yr: <15 mm/hr<br>Men over 50 yr: <20 mm/hr<br>Women under 50 yr: <20 mm/hr<br>Women over 50 yr: <30 mm/hr |
| Viscosity | 1.4-1.8 times water |

| White blood cell differential (adult) | Mean percent | Range of absolute counts |
|---|---|---|
| Segmented neutrophils | 56% | (1800-7000/$\mu l$) |
| Bands | 3% | (0-700/$\mu l$) |
| Eosinophils | 2.7% | (0-450/$\mu l$) |
| Basophils | 0.3% | (0-200/$\mu l$) |
| Lymphocytes | 34% | (1000-4800/$\mu l$) |
| Monocytes | 4% | (0-800/$\mu l$) |

(From Tilkian, S. M., Conover, M. B., and Tilkian, A. G.: Clinical implications of laboratory tests, ed. 2, St. Louis, 1979, The C. V. Mosby Co.)

**Table A-6.** Whole blood, serum, and plasma (chemistry)

| Test | Material | Normal value | Special instructions |
|------|----------|--------------|----------------------|
| Acetoacetic acid | | | |
|   Qualitative | Serum | Negative | |
|   Quantitative | Serum | 0.2-1.0 mg/dl | |
| Acetone | | | |
|   Qualitative | Serum | Negative | |
|   Quantitative | Serum | 0.3-2.0 mg/dl | |
| Adrenocorticotropic hormone (ACTH) | Plasma | 15-70 pg/ml | Place specimen on ice and send promptly to lab |
| Albumin, quantitative | Serum | 3.2-4.5 g/dl (salt fractionation) <br> 3.2-5-6 g/dl by electrophoresis <br> 3.8-5.0 g/dl by dye binding | |
| Alcohol | Serum or whole blood | Negative | |
| Aldolase | Serum | Adults: 1.3-8.2 U/dl <br> Children: Approximately 2 times adult levels <br> Newborn: Approximately 4 times adult levels | |
| Alpha-amino acid nitrogen | Plasma | 3.0-5.5 mg/100 mg/dl | |
| $\delta$-Aminolevulinic acid | Serum | 0.01-0.03 mg/dl | |
| Ammonia | Blood | 80-110 $\mu$g/dl | Collect with sodium heparinate; specimen must be delivered packed in ice and analyzed immediately |
| Amylase | Serum | 4-25 U/ml | |
| Arginiosuccinic lyase | Serum | 0-4 U/dl | |
| Arsenic | Whole blood | <3 $\mu$g/dl | |
| Ascorbic acid (vitamin C) | Plasma <br> Whole blood | 0.6-1.6 mg/dl <br> 0.4-1.5 mg/dl | Analyze immediately |
| Barbiturates | Serum, plasma, or whole blood | Negative <br> Coma level: phenobarbital, approximately 10 mg/dl; most other drugs, 1-3 mg/dl | |
| Base excess | Whole blood | Male: −3.3 to +1.2 <br> Female: −2.4 to +2.3 | |
| Base, total | Serum | 145-160 mEq/L | |
| Bicarbonate | Plasma | 21-28 mM/L | |
| Bile acids | Serum | 0.3-3.0 mg/dl | |
| Bilirubin | Serum | Up to 0.4 mg/dl (direct or conjugated) <br> Total: 0.7 mg/dl <br> Newborns total: 1-12 mg/dl <br> Indirect is total minus direct | |
| Blood gases | | | |
|   pH | | 7.38-7.44 arterial <br> 7.36-7.41 venous | |
|   $P_{CO_2}$ | | 35-40 mm Hg arterial <br> 40-45 mm Hg venous | |
|   $P_{O_2}$ | | 95-100 mm Hg arterial | |
| Bromide | Serum | Toxic level: 17 mEq/L | |
| BSP (sulfobromophthalein) (5 mg/kg) | Serum | <5% retention after 45 min | |
| Calcitonin | Plasma | Undetectable in normals <br> >100 pg/ml in medullary carcinoma | |
| Calcium | Serum | Ionized: 4.2-5.2 mg/dl <br>   2.1-2.6 mEq/L or <br>   50%-58% of total <br> Total: 9.0-10.6 mg/dl <br>   4.5-5.3 mEq/L <br> Infants: 11-13 mg/dl | |
| Carbon dioxide ($CO_2$ content) | Whole blood, arterial | 19-24 mM/L | |
| | Plasma or serum, arterial | 24-30 mEq/L <br> 20-26 mEq/L in infants (as $HCO_3$) | |
| | Whole blood, venous | 22-26 mM/L | |
| | Plasma or serum, venous | 24-30 mM/L | |
| $CO_2$ combining power | Plasma or serum, venous | 24-30 mM/L | |
| $CO_2$ partial pressure ($P_{CO_2}$) | Whole blood, arterial <br> Whole blood, venous | 35-40 mm Hg <br> 40-45 mm Hg | |

(From Tilkian, S. M., Conover, M. B., and Tilkian, A. G.: Clinical implications of laboratory tests, ed. 2, St. Louis, 1979, The C. V. Mosby Co.)

**Table A-6.** Whole blood, serum, and plasma (chemistry)—cont'd

| Test | Material | Normal value | Special instructions |
|---|---|---|---|
| Carbonic acid | Whole blood, arterial | 1.05-1.45 mM/L | |
| | Whole blood, venous | 1.15-1.50 mM/L | |
| | Plasma, venous | 1.02-1.38 mM/L | |
| Carboxyhemoglobin (carbon monoxide hemoglobin) | Whole blood | Suburban nonsmokers: <1.5% saturation of hemoglobin<br>Smokers: 1.5-5.0% saturation<br>Heavy smokers: 5.0-9.0% saturation | |
| Carotene, beta | Serum | 40-200 $\mu$g/dl | |
| Cephalin cholesterol flocculation | Serum | Negative to 1+ after 24 hours<br>2+ or less after 48 hours | |
| Ceruloplasmin | Serum | 23-50 mg/dl | |
| Chloride | Serum | 100-106 mEq/L | |
| Cholesterol, total | Serum | 150-250 mg/dl (varies with diet and age) | |
| Cholesterol, esters | Serum | 65-75% of total cholesterol | |
| Cholinesterase | Erythrocytes | 0.65-1.00 pH units | |
| Psuedocholinesterase | Plasma | 0.5-1.3 pH units<br>8-18 IU/L at 37% C | |
| Citric acid | Serum or plasma | 1.7-3.0 mg/dl | |
| Congo red test | Serum or plasma | >60% after 1 hour | Severe reactions may occur if dye is injected twice; check patient's record |
| Copper | Serum or plasma | 100-200 $\mu$g/dl | |
| Cortisol | Plasma | 8 A.M.: 5-25 $\mu$g/dl<br>8 P.M.: <10 $\mu$g/dl | |
| Creatine | Serum or plasma | 0.6-1.5 mg/dl | |
| Creatine phosphokinase (CPK) | Serum | Males: 5-55 mU/ml<br>Females: 5-35 mU/ml | |
| Creatinine | Serum or plasma | 0.6-1.2 mg/dl | |
| Creatinine clearance (endogenous) | Serum or plasma and urine | Male: 123 ± 16 ml/min<br>Female: 97 ± 10 ml/min | |
| Cryoglobulins | Serum | Negative | Keep specimen at 37°C |
| Doriden (Glutethmide) | Serum | 0 | |
| Electrophoresis, protein | Serum | | |

| | | *Percent* | *g/dl* |
|---|---|---|---|
| | Albumin | 52-65 | 3.2-5.6 |
| | Alpha 1 | 2.5-5.0 | 0.1-0.4 |
| | Alpha 2 | 7.0-13.0 | 0.4-1.2 |
| | Beta | 8.0-14.0 | 0.5-1.1 |
| | Gamma | 12.0-22.0 | 0.5-1.6 |

| Test | Material | Normal value | Special instructions |
|---|---|---|---|
| Ethanol | Blood | 0.3-0.4%, marked intoxication<br>0.4-0.5%, alcoholic stupor<br>0.5% or over, alcoholic coma | Collect in oxalate and refrigerate |
| Fats, neutral | Serum or plasma | 0-200 mg/dl | |
| Fatty acids | | | |
| Total | Serum | 9-15 mM/L | |
| Free | Plasma | 300-480 $\mu$Eq/L | |
| Fibrinogen | Plasma | 200-400 mg/dl | |
| Fluoride | Whole blood | <0.05 mg/dl | |
| Folate | Serum | 5-25 ng/ml (bioassay) | |
| | Erythrocytes | 166-640 ng/ml (bioassay) | |
| Galactose | Whole blood | Adults: none<br>Children: <20 mg/dl | |
| Gammaglobulin | Serum | 0.5-1.6 gm/dl | |
| Gastrin | Plasma | 0-200 pg/ml | |
| Globulins, total | Serum | 2.3-3.5 g/dl | |
| Glucose, fasting | Serum or plasma | 70-110 mg/dl | Collect with heparin-fluoride mixture |
| | Whole blood | 60-100 mg/dl | |
| Glucose tolerance, oral | Serum or plasma | Fasting: 70-110 mg/dl<br>30 min: 30-60 mg/dl above fasting<br>60 min: 20-50 mg/dl above fasting<br>120 min: 5-15 mg/dl above fasting<br>180 min: fasting level or below | Collect with heparin-fluoride mixture |
| Glucose tolerance, IV | Serum or plasma | Fasting: 70-110 mg/dl<br>5 min: Maximum of 250 mg/dl<br>60 min: Significant decrease<br>120 min: Below 120 mg/dl<br>180 min: Fasting level | Collect with heparin-fluoride mixture |
| Glucose-6-phosphate dehydrogenase (G-6-PD) | Erythrocytes | 250-500 units/$10^9$ cells<br>1200-2000 mIU/ml of packed erythrocytes | |
| $\gamma$-Glytamyl transpeptidase | Serum | 2-39 U/L | |
| Glutathione | Whole blood | 24-37 mg/dl | |

*Continued.*

**Table A-6.** Whole blood, serum, and plasma (chemistry)—cont'd

| Test | Material | Normal value | Special instructions |
|---|---|---|---|
| Growth hormone | Serum | <10 ng/ml | |
| Haptoglobin | Serum | 100-200 mg/dl as hemoglobin binding capacity | |
| | | Qualitative: Negative | |
| Hemoglobin | Serum or plasma | Quantitative: 0.5-5.0 mg/dl | |
| Hemoglobin | Whole blood | Female: 12.0-16.0 g/dl | |
| | | Male: 13.5-18.0 g/dl | |
| Hemoglobin $A_2$ | Whole blood | 1.5-3.5% of total hemoglobin | |
| $\alpha$-Hydroxybutyric dehydrogenase | Serum | 140-350 U/ml | |
| 17-Hydroxycortico-steroids | Plasma | Male: 7-19 $\mu$g/dl | Perform test immediately or freeze plasma |
| | | Female: 9-21 $\mu$g/dl | |
| | | After 25 USP units of ACTH | |
| | | IM: 35-55 $\mu$g/dl | |
| Immunoglobulins | Serum | | |
| IgG | | 800-1600 mg/dl | |
| IgA | | 50-250 mg/dl | |
| IgM | | 40-120 mg/dl | |
| IgD | | 0.5-3.0 mg/dl | |
| IgE | | 0.01-0.05 mg/dl | |
| Insulin | Plasma | 11-240 $\mu$IU/ml (bioassay) | |
| | | 4-24 $\mu$U/ml (radioimmunoassay) | |
| Insulin tolerance | Serum | Fasting: Glucose of 70-110 mg/dl | Collect with heparin-fluoride mixture |
| | | 30 min: Fall to 50% of fasting level | |
| | | 90 min: Fasting level | |
| Iodine | | | |
| Butanol extraction (BEI) | Serum | 3.5-6.5 $\mu$g/dl | Test not reliable if iodine- |
| Protein bound (PBI) | Serum | 4.0-8.0 $\mu$g/dl | containing drugs or radio-graphic contrast media were given prior to test |
| Iron, total | Serum | 50-150 $\mu$g/dl | Hemolysis must be avoided |
| Iron-binding capacity | Serum | 250-410 $\mu$g/dl | |
| Iron saturation, percent | Serum | 20-55% | |
| Isocitric dehydrogenase | Serum | 50-250 U/ml | |
| Ketone bodies | Serum | Negative | |
| 17-Ketosteroids | Plasma | 25-125 $\mu$g/dl | |
| Lactic acid | Blood | 0.6-1.8 mEq/liter | Draw without stasis |
| Lactic dehydrogenase (LDH) | Serum | 80-120 Wacker units | |
| | | 150-450 Wroblewski units | |
| | | 71-207 IU/L | |
| Lactic dehydrogenase isoenzymes | Serum | Anode: $LDH_1$ 17-27% | |
| | | $LDH_2$ 27-37% | |
| | | $LDH_3$ 18-25% | |
| | | $LDH_4$ 3-8% | |
| | | Cathode: $LDH_5$ 0-5% | |
| Lactic dehydrogenase (heat stable) | Serum | 60-120 U/ml | |
| Lactose tolerance | Serum | Serum glucose changes are similar to those seen in a glucose tolerance test | |
| Lead | Whole blood | 0-50 $\mu$g/dl | |
| Leucine aminopeptidase (LAP) | Serum | Male: 80-200 Goldbarg-Rutenburg units/ml | |
| | | Female: 75-185 Goldbarg-Rutenburg units/ml | |
| Lipase | Serum | 0-1.5 Cherry-Crandall | |
| | | 2 U/ml or less | |
| Lipids | Serum | | |
| Total | | 450-1000 mg/dl | |
| Cholesterol | | 120-200 mg/di | |
| Triglycerides | | 40-150 mg/dl | |
| Phospholipids | | 9-16 mg/dl as lipid phosphorus | |
| Fatty acids | | 190-420 mg/dl | |
| Neutral fat | | 0-200 mg/dl | |
| Lipoprotein electro-phoresis | | 40-150 mg/dl | |
| Lithium | Serum | Toxic level 2 mEq/L | |
| | | Therapeutic level: 0.5-1.5 mEq/L | |

**Table A-6.** Whole blood, serum, and plasma (chemistry)—cont'd

| Test | Material | Normal value | Special instructions |
|---|---|---|---|
| Long-acting thyroid-stimulating hormone (LATS) | Serum | None | |
| Luteinizing hormone (LH) | Plasma | Male: <11 mIU/ml<br>Female: midcycle peak >3 times base line value<br>    Premenopausal: <25 mIU/ml<br>    Postmenopausal: >25 mIU/ml | |
| Macroglobulins, total | Serum | 70-430 mg/dl | |
| Magnesium | Serum | 1.5-2.5 mEq/L<br>3.0 mg/dl | |
| Methanol | Blood | 0 | May be fatal as low as 115 mg/100 ml; collect in oxalate |
| Methemoglobin | Whole blood | 0-0.24 g/dl<br>0.4-1.5% of total hemoglobin | |
| Mucoprotein | Serum | 80-200 mg/dl | |
| Nonprotein nitrogen (NPN) | Serum or plasma<br>Whole bood | 20-35 mg/dl<br>25-50 mg/dl | |
| 5 Nucleotidase | Serum | 0.3-3.2 Bodansky units | |
| Ornithine carbamyl transferase (OCT) | Serum | 8-20 mIU/ml | |
| Osmolality | Serum | 280-295 mOsm/L | |
| Oxygen | | | |
|    Pressure ($P_{O_2}$) | Whole blood, arterial | 95-100 mm Hg | |
|    Content | Whole blood, arterial | 15-23 vol % | |
|    Saturation | Whole blood, arterial | 96-100% | |
| Parathyroid hormone | Plasma | <10 $\mu$l equiv/ml | Keep blood on ice, or plasma must be frozen if sent a distance |
| pH | Whole blood, arterial<br>Whole blood, venous<br>Serum or plasma, venous | 7.35-7.45<br>7.36-7.41<br>7.35-7.45 | |
| Phenylalanine | Serum | Adults: 0-2.0 mg/dl<br>Newborns (term): 1.2-3.5 mg/dl<br>Male total: 0.13-0.63 sigma U/ml<br>Female total: 0.01-0.56 sigma U/ml<br>Prostatic: 0-0.7 Fishman-Lerner U/dl | |
| Phosphatase, acid | Serum | 0-1.1 U/ml (Bodansky)<br>1-4 U/ml (King-Armstrong)<br>0.13-0.63 U/ml (Bessey-Lowry)<br>1.4-5.5 U/ml (Gutman-Gutman)<br>0-0.56 U/ml (Roy)<br>0-6.0 U/ml (Shinowara-Jones-Reinhart) | Hemolysis must be avoided; perform test without delay or freeze specimen |
| Phosphatase, alkaline, | Serum total | Adults: 1.5-4.5 U/dl (Bodansky)<br>4-13 U/dl (King-Armstrong)<br>0.8-2.3 U/ml (Bessey-Lowry)<br>15-35 U/ml (Shinowara-Jones-Reinhart)<br>Children: 5.0-14.0 U/dl (Bodanksy)<br>3.4-9.0 U/dl (Bessey-Lowry)<br>15-35 U/dl (King-Armstrong) | |
| Phospholipid phosphorus | Serum | 8-11 mg/dl | |
| Phospholipids | Serum | 150-380 mg/dl | |
| Phosphorus, inorganic | Serum | Adults: 1.8-2.6 mEq/L<br>3.0-4.5 mg/dl<br>Children: 2.3-4.1 mEq/L<br>4.0-7.0 mg/dl | Separate cells from serum promptly |
| Potassium | Plasma | 3.8-5.0 mEq/L | |
| Primidone (Mysoline) | Serum | Therapeutic level, 4-12 $\mu$g/ml | |
| Prolactin | Serum | 2-15 ng/ml | AM sample |
| Proteins | Serum | | |
|    Total | | 6.0-8.4 g/dl | |
|    Albumin | | 3.5-5.0 g/dl | |
|    Globulin | | 2.3-3.5 g/dl | |

*Continued.*

**Table A-6.** Whole blood, serum, and plasma (chemistry)—cont'd

| Test | Material | Normal value | Special instructions |
|---|---|---|---|
| Protein fractionation | Serum | | |
| Protoporphyrin | Erythrocytes | 15-50 $\mu$g/dl | |
| Pyruvate | Whole blood | 0.3-0.9 mg/dl | |
| Renin activity | Plasma | Supine: 1.1 ± 0.8 ng/ml/hr | EDTA tubes on ice<br>Normal diet |
| | | Upright: 1.9 ± 1.7 ng/ml/hr | |
| | | Supine: 2.7 ± 1.8 ng/ml/hr | Low sodium diet |
| | | Upright: 6.6 ± 2.5 ng/ml/hr | |
| | | Diuretics: 10.0 ± 3.7 ng/nl/hr | Low sodium diet |
| Salicylates | Serum | Negative<br>Therapeutic level: 20-25 mg/dl | |
| Sodium | Plasma | 136-142 mEq/L | |
| Sulfate, inorganic | Serum | 0.5-1.5 mEq/L<br>0.9-6.0 mg/dl as $SO_4$ | Hemolysis must be avoided |
| Sulfhemoglobin | Whole blood | Negative | |
| Sulfonamides | Serum or whole blood | Negative | |
| Testosterone | Serum or plasma | Male: 400-1200 ng/dl<br>Female: 30-120 ng/dl | |
| Thiocyanate | Serum | Negative | |
| Thymol flocculation | Serum | Uo to 1+ in 24 hours | |
| Thyroid hormone tests | Serum | *Expressed as* *Expressed as*<br>*thyroxine* *iodine* | |
|   $T_4$ (by column) | | 5.0-11.0 $\mu$g/dl 3.2-7.2 $\mu$g/dl | |
|   $T_4$ (by competitive binding Murphy-Pattee) | | 6.0-11.8 $\mu$g/dl 3.9-7.7 $\mu$g/dl | |
|   Free $T_4$ | | 0.9-2.3 ng/dl 0.6-1.5 ng/dl | |
|   $T_3$ (resin uptake) | | 25-38 relative % uptake | |
|   Thyroxine-binding globulin (TBG) | | 15-25 $\mu$g/dl (expressed as $T_4$ uptake) | |
| Thyroid-stimulating hormone (TSH) | Serum | 0.5-3.5 $\mu$U/ml | |
| Transaminases | | | |
|   GOT | Serum | 10-40 U/ml | |
|   GPT | Serum | 1-36 U/ml | |
| Triglycerides | Serum | 10-190 mg/dl | |
| Urea nitrogen | Serum | 8-25 mg/dl | |
| Urea clearance | Serum and urine | Maximum clearance: 64-99 ml/min<br>Standard clearance: 41-65 ml/min<br>  or more than 75% of normal clearance. | |
| Uric acid | Serum | 3.0-7.0 mg/dl | |
| Vitamin A | Serum | 0.15-0.6 $\mu$g/ml | |
| Vitamin A tolerance | Serum | Fasting: 15-60 $\mu$g/dl<br>3 hr or 6 hr after 5000 units vitamin A/kg:<br>  200-600 $\mu$g/dl<br>24 hr fasting values or slightly above | Administer 5000 units vitamin A in oil per kg body weight |
| Vitamin $B_{12}$ | Serum | Male: 200-800 pg/ml<br>Female: 100-650 pg/ml | |
| Unsaturated vitamin $B_{12}$ binding capacity | Serum | 1000-2000 pg/ml | |
| Vitamin C | Plasma | 0.6-1.6 mg/dl | Collect with oxalate and analyze within 20 min |
| Xylose absorption | Serum | 25-40 mg/dl between 1 and 2 hr; in malabsorption, maximum approximately 10 mg/dl<br>Dose<br>  Adult: 25 g D-xylose<br>  Children: 0.5 g/kg D-xylose | For children administer 10 ml of a 5% solution of D-xylose per kg of body weight |
| Zinc | Serum | 50-150 $\mu$g/dl | |
| Zinc sulfate turbidity | Serum | <12 units | |

**Table A-7.** Urine

| Test | Type of specimen | Normal value | Special instructions |
|------|------------------|--------------|----------------------|
| Acetoacetic acid | Random | Negative | |
| Acetone | Random | Negative | |
| Addis count | 12-hr collection | WBC and epithelial cells: 1,8000,000/12 hr | Rinse bottle with some neutral formalin; discard excess |
| | | RBC: 500,000/12 hr | |
| | | Hyaline casts: 0-5000/12 hr | |
| Albumin | | | |
|   Qualitative | Random | Negative | |
|   Quantitative | 24 hr | 10-100 mg/24 hr | |
| Aldosterone | 24 hr | 2-26 $\mu$g/24 hr | Keep refrigerated |
| Alkapton bodies | Random | Negative | |
| Alpha-amino acid nitrogen | 24 hr | 100-290 mg/24 hr | |
| $\delta$-Aminolevulinic acid | Random | Adult: 0.1-0.6 mg/dl | |
| | | Children: <0.5 mg/dl | |
| | 24 hr | 1.5-7.5 mg/24 hr | |
| Ammonia nitrogen | 24 hr | 20-70 mEq/24 hr | Keep refrigerated |
| | | 500-1200 mg/24 hr | |
| Amylase | 2 hr | 35-260 Somogyi units per hour | |
| Arsenic | 24 hr | <50 $\mu$g/L | |
| Ascorbic acid | Random | 1-7 mg/dl | |
| | 24 hr | >50 mg/24 hr | |
| Bence Jones protein | Random | Negative | |
| Beryllium | 24 hr | <0.05 $\mu$g/24 hr | |
| Bilirubin, qualitative | Random | Negative | |
| Blood, occult | Random | Negative | |
| Borate | 24 hr | <2 mg/L | |
| Calcium | | | |
|   Qualitative (Sulkowitch) | Random | 1 + turbidity | Compare with standard |
|   Quantitative | 24 hr | Average diet: 100-250 mg/24 hr | |
| | | Low calcium diet: <150 mg/24 hr | |
| | | High calcium diet: 250-300 mg/24 hr | |
| Catecholamines | Random | Epinephrine <20 $\mu$g/24 hr | |
| | 24 hr | Norepinephrine <100 $\mu$g/24 hr | |
| Chloride | 24 hr | 110-250 mEq/24 hr | |
| Chorionic gonadotropin | First morning voiding | 0 | Specific gravity should be at least 1.015 |
| Concentration test (Fishberg) | Random after fluid restriction | Specific gravity: >1.025 | |
| | | Osmolality: >850 mOsm/L | |
| Copper | 24 hr | 0-100 $\mu$g/24 hr | |
| Coproporphyrin | Random | Adult: 50-250 $\mu$g/24 hr | Use fresh specimen and do not expose to direct light; preserve 24 hr urine with 5 g $Na_2CO_3$ |
| | 24 hr | Children: 0-80 $\mu$g/24 hr | |
| Creatine | 24 hr | Under 100 mg/24 hr or less than 6% of creatinine | |
| | | Pregnancy: up to 12% | |
| | | Children: up to 30% of creatinine | |
| Creatinine | 24 hr | 15-25 mg/kg of body weight/24 hr | |
| Cystine, qualitative | Random | Negative | |
| Cystine and cysteine | 10 ml | 0 | |
| Diacetic acid | Random | Negative | |
| Epinephrine | 24 hr | 0-20 $\mu$g/24 hr | |
| Estrogens, total | 24 hr | Male: 5-18 $\mu$g/24 hr | Keep refrigerated |
| | | Female | |
| | |   Ovulation: 28-100 $\mu$g/24 hr | |
| | |   Luteal peak: 22-105 $\mu$g/24 hr | |
| | |   At menses: 4-25 $\mu$g/24 hr | |
| | |   Pregnancy: up to 45,000 $\mu$g/24 hr | |
| | |   Postmenopausal: 14-20 $\mu$g/24 hr | |
| Estrogens | 24 hr | Nonpregnant, mid-cycle | |
|   Fractionated | | | |
|   Estrone (E1) | | 2-25 $\mu$g/24 hr | |
|   Estradiol (E2) | | 0-10 $\mu$g/24 hr | |
|   Estriol (E3) | | 2-30 $\mu$g/24 hr | |

(From Tilkian, S. M., Conover, M. B., and Tilkian, A. G.: Clinical implications of laboratory tests, ed. 2, St. Louis, 1979, The C. V. Mosby Co.)

*Continued.*

**Table A-7.** Urine—cont'd

| Test | Type of specimen | Normal value | Special instructions |
|------|------------------|--------------|----------------------|
| Fat, qualitative | Random | Negative | |
| FIGLU (N-formi-minoglutamic acid) | 24 hr | <3 mg/24 hr<br>After 15 g L-histidine:<br>    4 mg/8 hr | |
| Fluoride | 24 hr | <1 mg/24 hr | |
| Follicle-stimulating hormone (FSH) | 24 hr | Follicular phase 5-20 IU/24 hr<br>Mid-cycle 15-60 IU/24 hr<br>Luteal phase 5-15 IU/24 hr<br>Menopausal 50-100 IU/24 hr<br>Men 5-25 IU/24 hr | |
| Fructose | 24 hr | 30-65 mg/24 hr | |
| Glucose | | | |
|   Qualitative | Random | Negative | |
|   Quantitative | 24 hr | 0.5-1.5 g/24 hr | |
|   Copper-reducing substances | | | |
|     Total sugars | | Average: 250 mg/24 hr | |
|     Glucose | | Average: 130 mg/24 hr | |
| Gonadotropins, pituitary (FSH and LH) | 24 hr | 10-50 mouse uterine units/24 hr | |
| Hemoglobin | Random | Negative | |
| Homogentisic acid | Random | Negative | |
| Homovanillic acid (HVA) | 24 hr | <15 mg/24 hr | |
| 17-Hydroxycortico-steroids | 24 hr | Male: 5.5-14.5 mg/24 hr<br>Female: 4.9-12.9 mg/24 hr<br>Lower in children<br>After 25 USP units ACTH, IM:<br>    a 2- to 4-fold increase | Keep refrigerated |
| 5-Hydroxyindole-acetic acid (5-HIAA) | 24 hr | 2-9 mg/24 hr (women lower than men) | Some muscle relaxants and tranquilizers interfere with test |
| 5-Hydroxyindolacetic acid, quantitative | 24 hr | <9 mg/24 hr | |
| Indican | 24 hr | 10-20 mg/24 hr | |
| Ketone bodies | Random | Negative | Fresh, keep cool |
| 17-Ketosteroids | 24 hr | Age   Males   Females<br>10   1-4 mg   1-4 mg<br>20   6-21 mg   4-16 mg<br>30   8-26 mg   4-14 mg<br>50   5-18 mg   3-9 mg<br>70   2-10 mg   1-7 mg | |
|   Androsterone | | Male: 2.0-5.0 mg/24 hr<br>Female: 0.8-3.0 mg/24 hr | |
|   Etiocholanolone | | Male: 1.4-5.0 mg/24 hr<br>Female: 0.8-4.0 mg/24 hr | |
|   Dehydroepiandro-sterone | | Male: 0.2-2.0 mg/24 hr<br>Female: 0.2-1.8 mg/24 hr | |
|   11-Ketoandro-sterone | | Male: 0.2-1.0 mg/24 hr<br>Female: 0.2-0.8 mg/24 hr | |
|   11-Ketoetio-cholanolone | | Male: 0.2-1.0 mg/24 hr<br>Female: 0.2-0.8 mg/24 hr | |
|   11-Hydroxyandro sterone | | Male: 0.1-0.8 mg/24 hr<br>Female: 0.0-0.5 mg/24 hr | |
|   11-Hydroxyetio-cholanolone | | Male: 0.2-0.6 mg/24 hr<br>Female: 0.1-1.1 mg/24 hr | |
| Lactose | 24 hr | 12-40 mg/24 hr | |
| Lead | 24 hr | <100 μg/24 hr | |
| Magnesium | 24 hr | 6.0-8.5 mEq/24 hr | |
| Melanin, qualitative | Random | Negative | |
| 3-Methoxy-4-hydroxy-mandelic acid | 24 hr | 1.5-7.5 mg/24 hr (adults)<br>83 μg/kg/24 hr (infants) | No coffee or fruit two days prior to test |
| Mucin | 24 hr | 100-150 mg/24 hr | |
| Myoglobin | | | |
|   Qualitative | Random | Negative | |
|   Quantitative | 24 hr | <1.5 mg/L | |

**Table A-7.** Urine—cont'd

| Test | Type of specimen | Normal value | Special instructions |
|---|---|---|---|
| Osmolality | Random | 500-800 mOsm/L | May be lower or higher, depending on state of hydration |
| Pentoses | 24 hr | 2-5 mg/kg/24 hr | |
| pH | Random | 4.6-8.0 | |
| Phenolsulfonphthalein (PSP) | Urine, timed after 6 mg PSP IV | | |
| | 15 min | 20-50% dye excreted | |
| | 30 min | 16-24% dye excreted | |
| | 60 min | 9-17% dye excreted | |
| | 120 min | 3-10% dye excreted | |
| Phenylpyruvic acid, qualitative | Random | Negative | |
| Phosphorus | Random | 0.9-1.3 g/24 hr | Varies with intake |
| Porphobilinogen | | | |
| Qualitative | Random | Negative | |
| Quantitative | 24 hr | 0-2.0 mg/24 hr | |
| Potassium | 24 hr | 40-80 mEq/24 hr | Varies with diet |
| Pregnancy tests | Concentrated morning specimen | Positive in normal pregnancies or with tumors producing chorionic gonadotropin | |
| Pregnanediol | 24 hr | Male: 0-1 mg/24 hr | Keep refrigerated |
| | | Female: 1-8 mg/24 hr | |
| | | Peak: 1 week after ovulation | |
| | | Pregnancy: 60-100 mg/24 hr | |
| | | Children: Negative | |
| Pregnanetriol | 24 hr | Male: 1.0-2.0 mg/24 hr | Keepr refrigerated |
| | | Female: 0.5-2.0 mg/24 hr | |
| | | Children: <0.5 mg/24 hr | |
| Protein | | | |
| Qualitative | Random | Negative | |
| Quantitative | 24 hr | 10-100 mg/24 hr | |
| Reducing substances, total | 24 hr | 0.5-1.5 mg/24 hr | |
| Sodium | 24 hr | 80-180 mEq/24 hr | Varies with dietary ingestion of salt |
| Solids, total | 24 hr | 55-70 g/24 hr | |
| | | Decreases with age to 30 g/24 hr | |
| Specific gravity | Random | 1.016-1.022 (normal fluid intake) | |
| | | 1.001 1.035 (range) | |
| Sugars (excluding glucose) | Random | Negative | |
| Titrable acidity | 24 hr | 20-50 mEq/24 hr | Collect with toluene |
| Urea nitrogen | 24 hr | 6-17 gm/24 hr | |
| Uric acid | 24 hr | 250-750 mg/24 hr | Varies with diet |
| Urobilinogen | 2 hr | 0.3-1.0 Ehrlich units | |
| | 24 hr | 0.05-2.5 mg/24 hr or 0.5-4.0 Ehrlich units/24 hr | |
| Uropepsin | Random | 15-45 units/hr | |
| | 24 hr | 1500-5000 units/24 hr | |
| Uroporphyrins | | | |
| Qualitative | Random | Negative | |
| Quantitative | 24 hr | 10-30 $\mu$g/24 hr | |
| Vanillylmandelic acid (VMA) | 24 hr | Up to 9 mg/24 hr | |
| Volume, total | 24 hr | 600-1600 ml/24 hr | |
| Zinc | 24 hr | 0.15-1.2 mg/24 hr | |

**Table A-8.** Cerebrospinal fluid

| Test or constituent | Normal value | Special instructions |
|---|---|---|
| Albumin | 10-30 mg/dl | |
| Albumin/globulin ratio | 1.6-2.2 | |
| Calcium | 2.1-2.9 mEq/L | |
| Cell count | 0.8 cells/$\mu$l | |
| Chloride | Adult: 118-132 mEq/L | These values are invalidated |
| | Child: 120-128 mEq/L | by admixture of blood |
| Colloidal gold curve | 0001111000 | |
| Globulins | | |
|   Qualitative (Pandy) | Negative | |
|   Quantitative | 6-16 mg/dl | |
| Glucose | 45-75 mg/dl | |
| Lactic dehydrogenase (LDH) | Approximately $\frac{1}{10}$ of serum level | |
| Protein | | |
|   Total CSF | 15-45 mg/dl | |
|   Ventricular fluid | 8-15 mg/dl | |
| Protein electrophoresis | | |
|   Pre-albumin | 4.1 ± 1.2% | |
|   Albumin | 62.4 ± 5.6% | |
|   Alpha 1 globulin | 5.3 ± 1.2% | |
|   Alpha 2 globulin | 8.2 ± 2.0% | |
|   Beta globulin | 12.8 ± 2.0% | |
|   Gamma globulin | 7.2 ± 1.1% | |
| Xanthochromia | Negative | |

(From Tilkian, S. M., Conover, M. B., and Tilkian, A. G.: Clinical implications of laboratory tests, ed. 2, St. Louis, 1979, The C. V. Mosby Co.)

**Table A-9.** Miscellaneous

| Test | Specimen | Normal value |
|---|---|---|
| Bile, qualitative | Random stool | Negative in adults; positive in children |
| Carcinoembryonic antigen (CEA) | Plasma | 0-2.5 ng/ml, 97% healthy nonsmokers |
| Chloride | Sweat | 4-60 mEq/L |
| Clearances | Serum and timed urine | |
|   Creatinine, endogenous | | 115 ± 20 ml/min |
|   Diodrast | | 600-720 ml/min |
|   Inulin | | 100-150 ml/min |
|   PAH | | 600-750 ml/min |
| Diagnex blue (tubeless gastric analysis) | Urine | Free acid present |
| Fat | Stool, 72 hr | Total fat: <5 g/24 hr and 10-25% of dry matter or <4% of measured fat intake in 3 days |
| | | Neutral fat: 1-5% of dry matter |
| | | Free fatty acids: 5-13% of dry matter |
| | | Combined fatty acids: 5-15% of dry matter |
| Immunologic tests | | |
|   Alpha-fetoglobulin | Blood | Abnormal if present |
|   Alpha 1 antitrypsin | Blood | 200-400 mg/100 ml |
|   Antinuclear antibodies | Blood | Positive if detected with serum diluted 1:10 |
|   Anti-DNA antibodies | Blood | <15 units/ml |
|   Bence-Jones protein | Urine | Abnormal if present |
|   Complement, total hemolytic | Blood | 150-250 U/ml |
|   C3 | Blood | 55-120 mg/100 ml |
|   C4 | | 20-50 mg/100 ml |
| Immunoglobulins | | |
|   IgG | Blood | 1140 mg/100 ml Range 540-1663 |
|   IgA | | 214 mg/100 ml Range 66-344 |
|   IgM | | 168 mg/100 ml Range 39-290 |
|   Viscosity | | 1.4-1.8 |
| Nitrogen, total | Stool, 24 hr | 10% of intake or 1-2 gm/24 hr |
| Sodium | Sweat | 10-80 mEq/L |
| Synovial fluid | | |
|   Glucose | | Not less than 20 mg/100 ml lower than simultaneously drawn blood sugar |
|   Mucin | | Type 1 or 2 |
| Trypsin activity | Random, fresh stool | Positive (2+ to 4+) |
| Thyroid $^{131}$I uptake | | 7.5-25% in 6 hr |
| Urobilinogen | | |
|   Qualitative | Random stool | Positive |
|   Quantitative | Stool, 24 hr | 40-200 mg/24 hr |
| | | 30-280 Ehrlich units/24 hr |

(From Tilkian, S. M., Conover, M. B., and Tilkian, A. G.: Clinical implications of laboratory tests, ed. 2, St. Louis, 1979, The C. V. Mosby Co.)

# Glossary*

**abduction** motion in which part moves away from defined line (i.e., midline of body).

**abrasion** injury in which skin has been scraped off.

**abscess, Brodie's** chronic, localized abscess, usually caused by staphylococcus of low virulence.

**acetylcholine** chemical thought to fill synaptic vesicles at axional termination of neuron; it is believed that release of this substance at synapses activates postsynaptic membrane of another neuron, muscle fiber, or gland cell.

**acheiria** absence of hand.

**achondroplasia** most common type of dwarfism, resulting from developmental abnormality of enchondral ossification in which there is failure of normal ossification of long bones but not of flat bones of the hands and feet.

**aclasis, diaphyseal** relatively uncommon hereditary disease of generalized skeletal system, characterized by multiple exostoses or bony protrusions.

**acrocephalosyndactylism** rare condition of unknown etiology affecting head, hands, and feet primarily with characteristic craniofacial appearance in combination with partial or complete syndactylism.

**acromegaly** hypersecretion of growth hormones produced by anterior lobe of pituitary gland, resulting in gradual bony thickening; this adult form corresponds to gigantism in children.

**activities for daily living** those skills required for the promotion of independence in feeding, dressing, hygiene, and toileting.

**adactylia** absence of digit.

**adduction** motion in which part moves toward defined line (i.e., midline of body).

  **forefoot** deformity in which distal portion of foot is deviated toward midline of body.

**adenosine triphosphate (ATP)** compound composed of sugar, nitrogen, phosphorus, and adenosine; breakdown of this compound provides energy for many cellular processes.

**ADL** *see* **activities for daily living.**

---

*Entries of more than one word are listed according to the principal word, generally the noun; i.e., *benign chondioblastoma* is listed as *condroblastoma, benign.* Cross references are given where necessary.

**amelia** absence of limb.

**amphiarthrosis** type of articulation in which articulating bony surfaces are separated by cartilage.

**amphiarthrotic** slightly moveable type of joint, having cartilage in between bones.

**amyotonia congenita** *see* **atrophy, infantile muscular.**

**analgesia, waking imagined** conscious effort to experience pleasant sensation during painful experience.

**anisomelia** inequality of leg lengths; very common orthopedic problem caused by variety of conditions.

**angioma** single or multiple, highly vascular lesions that may involve any part of bone; multiple lesions are known as angiomatosis of bone.

**angiosarcoma of bone** malignant lesion of vascular origin which infiltrates the healthy areas surrounding the primary site and metastasizes very early.

**ankylosis** limitation or restriction of normal range of motion caused by tissue alterations in or out of joint cavity.

**anteversion** *see* **femoral torsion.**

**aphalangia** absence of one or more phalanges.

**aphasia** impairment or loss of the capacity to use words as symbols of ideas; not associated with a defect in the mechanics of speaking; of organic origin secondary to central nervous system lesion.

**apodia** absence of foot.

**arm** upper extremity.

  **force** *Referring to motion:* perpendicular distance from fulcrum to line of action of force.

  **weight or resistance** perpendicular distance from fulcrum to the line of action of the weight.

**arteriography** radiographic technique permitting visualization of arterial structures of specific area by injection of a radiopaque dye.

**arthritis** inflammation of joint resulting in structural damage.

  **gouty** hereditary, metabolic disorder characterized by sodium urate crystals within the joint spaces.

  **hemophiliac** destruction of joint from repeated and excessive hemorrhage into joint structures resulting from hemophilia (a hereditary disease of the blood occurring in males and transmitted by females).

  **infectious** pyogenic arthritis.

  **pyogenic** inflammation of synovial lining of joint caused by pus-forming organism.

**rheumatoid** chronic inflammatory systemic disease of unknown etiology characterized by destruction and proliferation of synovial membrane, resulting in joint destruction, ankylosing, and deformity.

**rheumatoid juvenile** chronic inflammation of joint structures having its onset during the childhood years; systemic reaction more severe than adult form; similar appearances in deterioration of the joint structures.

**septic** pyogenic arthritis.

**suppurative** pyogenic arthritis.

**traumatic** inflammatory joint disease resulting from traumatic injury.

**arthrodesis** surgical fusion of joint.

**arthrodia** *see* Joint, gliding.

**arthrography** radiographic technique permitting ization of joint by injection of air or radiopaque dye.

**arthrogryposis multiplex congenita** extremely disabling condition of unknown cause characterized by multiple congenital contractures of joints, particularly hips, knees, elbows, and wrists; results from incomplete fibrous ankylosis of involved joints.

**arthroplasty** operative creation of a new joint replacing stiff, ankylosed, painful, or nonfunctional joint.

**arthroscopy** diagnostic tool permitting visualization of internal joint structures through utilization of an arthroscope; most frequently used to visualize knee joint.

**arthrotomy** operative exploration of joint.

**aspiration**

**bone marrow** diagnostic procedure which permits microscopic examination of bone marrow obtained through needle aspiration.

**joint** diagnostic procedure accomplished by inserting needle into synovial capsule of joint for purpose of withdrawing fluid for microscopic examination or relief of pain.

**assessment**

**neurovascular** process of continued or intermittent evaluation of circulatory, sensory, and motor components of status and function.

**nursing** process by which nurse collects and compares data to an accepted standard and from this makes determination of need for nursing intervention.

**ataxia, Freidreich's** hereditary or familial disorder involving primarily posterior columns of spinal cord; progressive in nature, with ataxia, weakness of the lower extremities, and a characteristic gait.

**atrophy** wasting away.

**infantile muscular** disease of anterior horn cells and the motor neurons of fifth to twelfth cranial nerves; characterized by progressive degeneration resulting in paralysis with an onset during infancy and usually fatal by 4 or 5 years of age.

**peroneal muscular** progressive hereditary disease resulting in atrophy and paralysis; begins with peroneal muscles with eventual involvement of rest of lower and upper extremities.

**axon** cellular process of nerve cell that carries impulses away from nerve cell body.

**behavior, coping**

**dysfunctional** behavior that interferes significantly with maintenance of physical and social-psychologic health.

**functional** behavior that mobilizes the individual toward maintenance of physical and social-psychologic health.

**benign** abnormal but nonmalignant growth.

**blastoma** granular type of tumor formed by single type of tissue (includes fibromas and chondromas).

**bone**

**accessory** extra bone anywhere in skeletal structure but most frequently in foot.

**sesamoid** free-floating bones that are usually found in tendons or joint capsules, such as the patella.

**boots, abduction** bilateral lower extremity casts (short- or long-leg) with bar incorporated at ankle level to provide hip abduction.

**bowleg** genu varum.

**brace** *see* orthosis.

**Bradford** rectangular device constructed of metal and covered with canvas to assist in immobilization; split frame most frequently used in pediatrics to assist in keeping a hip spica cast dry. Solid frame used to aid in immobilization of children in traction.

**bridging** nursing technique of positioning so that bony prominences are free of pressure on mattress; bolsters of foam or pillows are used to distribute body weight over larger surface, leaving bony prominences free of pressure.

**bunion** *see* hallux valgus.

**bursa** small sacs lined with synovial membrane found between structures that move against each other, such as between skin and bone, or tendon and bone; designed to reduce friction between these moving parts and act as cushions to relieve pressure.

**bursitis** inflammation of bursa.

**cartilage** firm connective tissue that has little vasculature; composed of cells, interstitial substance of fibers, and ground substance; three types are: hyaline, elastic, and fibrocartilage.

**costal** cartilage connecting to ribs.

**hyaline** glassy, translucent cartilage.

**cast** method of temporary immobilization that incorporates a part or parts of the body and is circumferential in nature; made of plaster or fiberglass.

**arm cylinder** incorporates upper extremity from wrist to upper arm.

**bivalved** cast that has been cut into an anterior and posterior portion.

**halo** incorporates trunk, usually with shoulder "straps" and halo apparatus attached with outrigger within the cast to secure skull pins.

**leg cylinder** incorporates lower extremity from ankle to upper thigh.

**long arm** incorporates upper extremity from hand to upper arm.

**long leg** cast incorporates lower extremity from toes to upper thigh.

**long leg hip spica** incorporates trunk to waist or nipple line, with leg incorporated to toes, bilateral incorporates both legs.

**Minerva** incorporates upper trunk (to sternum and distal rib border anteriorally and across distal rib border posteriorly) and head, with facial, and ear areas cut out.

**one-and-one-half hip spica** incorporates trunk to waist or nipple line, with one leg incorporated to toes and opposite leg to knee.

**Quengle** incorporates lower extremity from foot or ankle to below knee and above knee to upper thigh, with special hinges incorporated medially and laterally at knee level for correction of knee contractures.

**Risser** incorporates entire trunk, extending over cervical area to chin, with possible additional extension over hips to knees under certain conditions.

**short-arm** incorporates upper extremity from hand to below elbow.

**short-leg** incorporates lower extremity from toes to knee.

**short-leg hip spica** incorporates trunk to waist or nipple line, with both legs incorporated to knee.

**shoulder spica** incorporates trunk, usually to hips, and part or all of one shoulder and upper extremity.

**spica** incorporates part or all of trunk and part or all of one or more extremities.

**turnbuckle** incorporates entire trunk of body, one arm to elbow, and opposite leg to knee; cast is cut after application and hinges are placed at desired area of spine.

**windowed** specific area of cast is removed for inspection of pressure area or wound.

**causalgia** severe burning pain produced by severed nerves that have produced new nerve endings that do not function properly; touch can often produce this pain.

**center of motion** *see* **fulcrum.**

**chondritis** inflammation of cartilage.

**chondroblastoma benign** rare lesion arising from cartilaginous tissue, most frequently seen in adolescents and usually occurring near epiphyseal growth plate.

**chondrocyte** cartilage cell.

**chondrogenic** arising from cartilaginous tissue.

**chondroma** cartilaginous tumor of slow growth.

**chondroplasia, hereditary deforming** *see* **aclasis, diaphyseal**

**cineradiography** radiographic technique permitting visualization of joint movement by use of movie camera or videotape recorder; also known as *videoradiography.*

**circumduction** motion, especially at shoulder and hip, requiring full circular (360 degrees) motion and involving abduction, adduction, flexion, and extension.

**clubfoot** congenital anomaly characterized by combination of inversion of foot, forefoot adduction, and equinus of foot.

**coalition, tarsal** deformity characterized by union between two or more tarsal bones.

**collagenic** arising from connective tissue, such as tendon.

**condyle** rounded convex projection for articulation with another bone.

**condyloid** *see* **joint, ellipsoidal**

**contact, initial (of gait)** moment when foot touches floor.

**contraction** shortening or increase in tension of muscle.

**eccentric** lengthening contraction of muscle.

**contracture** the absence of full range of motions of any joint; flexion contracture is most common, which is the lack of full extension in any joint.

**Dupuytren's (of hand or foot)** contracture of the hand or foot involving flexion at the metacarpophalangeal joint, with occasional distal involvement.

**contusion** a minimal traumatic injury, usually involving soft tissue hemorrhage into subcutaneous, adipose or muscular tissues, and resulting in the appearance of a bruised area.

**countertraction** a force which counteracts the direct pull of a traction, i.e., the force of the body weight on the bed.

**coxa** hip.

**coxa plana** see Legg-Perthes disease.

**coxa vara** deformity of hip with decrease in angle of femoral neck.

**adolescent** *see* **epiphysis, slipped capital femoral**

**congenital** reduction or decrease of normal 120° to 140° angle of femoral neck; present at birth or shortly thereafter.

**developmental** congenital coxa vara.

**infantile** congenital coxa vara.

**crest** prominent ridge on bone.

**cretinism** *see* **hypothyroidism**

**crisis** a state of disequilibrium or inbalance which occurs when there is an incongruency between the problem solving or coping skills of the individual, his family system, and the stressful event.

**maturational** state of disequilibrium that occurs when normal and predictable conflicts and needs accompanying each stage of development are unresolved or unfulfilled.

**potential** anticipated state of disequilibrium resulting from interaction between critical maturational and situational events and stressors.

**cubitus** elbow.

**valgus** abnormal increase in the angulation of outward projection of forearm in relation to elbow joint.

**varus** decrease in angulation of outward projection of forearm in relation to elbow joint.

**curvature of spine** deviation of spine from normal position or direction.

**C-shaped** lateral curvature involving all or most of at least lumbar and thoracic areas of vertebral column; most frequently associated with paralysis.

**compensatory** lateral curvature that results after development of primary curve; in the opposite direction and immediately above or below primary curve.

**double major** lateral curvature comprised of two primary curves of equal or almost equal degree.

**functional** lateral curvature with no structural alterations in vertebral column.

**primary** most prominent curvature of pathologic origin.

**S-shaped** double curvature comprised of major curve (usually primary) and compensatory curvature above or below the primary curve.

**structural** lateral curvature resulting from structural alterations within vertebral column.

**tertiary** curvature that results above or below a secondary or compensatory curvature; usually of minimal severity.

**cyst**

**aneurysmal bone** benign lesion thought to arise from vascular tissue and bone; characteristically produces "bubble" appearance on radiographic examination.

**Baker's** fluid-filled sac located in posterior portion of knee structures.

**popliteal** Baker's cyst.

**unicameral bone** benign cystic lesion of osteogenic origin, most frequently seen in proximal humerus or femur.

**decalcification** descriptive term for decreased bone density or undermineralization; may be indicative of bone resorption.

**defect, subperiosteal cortical** benign lesion questionably characterized as a tumor; frequently occurs in children and adolescents; usually asymptomatic and may be referred to as "bone island."

**deformity** malformation or defect of any part of body.

**Madelung's** deformity of the wrist characterized by enlargment, instability, and decreased motion.

**Sprengel's** congenital abnormality characterized by elevation of scapula.

**dendrite** branching process of nerve cell that usually carries impulses toward nerve cell body.

**density of bone** descriptive term relating to radiographic appearance of bone characterized by lightness or darkness of areas of osseous tissue.

**decreased** descriptive term relating to radiographic appearance; not indicative of specific mechanism or component of bone affected.

**diagnosis, nursing** statement of conclusion drawn from nurse's assessment of client's problem.

**diaphysis** the shaft of the long bone.

**diarthroses** freely moveable joints.

**diplegia** a descriptive term used for cerebral palsy denoting the involvement of both upper extremities.

**disc, intervertebral** fibrocartilaginous mass that separates vertebrae.

**ruptured** complete or partial herniation of nuclear material of intervertebral disc into the spinal canal, usually causing a compression of the spinal nerve roots in the area.

**dischondroplasia** a rare developmental condition characterized by disorderly and excessive proliferation of cartilage cells at many of the epiphyseal plates.

**discrepancy, leg length** *see* anesomelia.

**disease** morbid process with characteristic symptoms.

**Alber Schönberg** *see* osteopetrosis.

**Blount's** deformity characterized by disturbances of epiphyseal growth plate on medial aspect of proxmial tibial epiphysis, resulting in tibia vara deformity.

**Charcot-Marie-Tooth** *see* atrophy, peroneal muscular.

**degenerative joint** *see* osteoarthritis.

**Englemann's** *see* dysplasia, progressive diaphyseal.

**Erb-Goldflam** *see* myasthenia gravis.

**Gaucher's** relatively rare metabolic disorder with accumulation of Gaucher cells present in spleen, liver, bone marrow, and other sites.

**Hodgkin's** malignant process with invasion into lymph nodes, spleen, liver, skin, sinus, and intestinal follicles; characteristic lymphatic leukemia usually infiltrates bone marrow and may produce skeletal alterations.

**Kohler's** process attributed to ischemic degeneration of localized bone tissue, most frequently occurring in navicular bone.

**Legg-Perthes** one of a group of diseases called osteochondrosis; self-limiting, and characterized by avascular necrosis of femoral head in which necrotic tissue is absorbed and then replaced by reparative osseous tissue; this distinct process involves four stages: (1) incipient or synovitis stage, (2) aseptic necrotic or avascular stage, (3) regenerative or fragmentation stage, and (4) healed or residual stage.

**marble bone** *see* osteopetrosis.

**Marie-Strumpell** *see* spondylitis, ankylosing.

**neuropathic joint** chronic, progressive degenerative arthropathy affecting one or more peripheral or supinal joints.

**Ollier's** *see* dischondroplasia.

**Oppenheim's** *see* atrophy, infantile muscular.

**Osgood-Schlatter** characterized by pain and swelling of the patella tendon and enlargement of tibial tubercle.

**Paget's** chronic skeletal disease with insidious onset and characterized by progressive development of skeletal deformities resulting from increased resorption accompanied by increased and abnormal regeneration.

**Pott's** tuberculosis of the spinal column.

**Sever's, of calcaneus** process with onset during puberty and characterized by fragmentation of areas of calcaneus surrounding cartilaginous epiphyseal growth plate, resulting in necrosis and eventual resorption.

**Scheuermann's** *see* kyphosis, adolescent or juvenile.

**Von Recklinghausen's** *see* neurofibromatosis.

**Von Recklinghausen's, of bone** *see* hyperparathyroidism.

**dislocation** musculoskeletal traumatic injury resulting in disruption of continuity of joint configuration and articulation to extent that articulating surfaces are no longer in contact.

**congenital, of hip** displacement of femoral head out of acetabular socket which is present at birth or shortly thereafter.

**dissonance, cognitive** conscious effort to help person in pain to focus on pleasant situation; conscious effort to produce discord between feelings experienced and feelings expressed in distracting episode.

**distraction from pain** simple, nondemanding television, visitor, crossword puzzle method of diverting client's attention or focus from painful experience to another object.

**dorsiflexion** in reference to hand: motion at wrist that moves hand up towards upper part of arm; in reference to foot: motion at ankle that moves foot up toward leg.

**dwarfism, diastrophic** extremely rare type of micromelic dwarfism with clubfeet, scoliosis, and "hitchhiker's" deformity of the hand.

**dysgenesis of proximal femur** skeletal growth disorder characterized by shortening of femur and decrease of neck-shaft angle; severity varies.

**dysmelia** generalized term which constitutes and represents a group of anomalies, all of which are characterized by hyperplasia or aplasia of the long bones of the extremities.

**dysostosis, metaphyseal** generalized skeletal disorder caused by disturbance of mineralization of metaphyseal area of bones and resulting in dwarfism.

**dysplasia** abnormality of development.

**fibrous** generalized skeletal affection characterized by fibrous displacement of osseous tissue within affected bones.

**metaphyseal** familial, perhaps hereditary disease of enchondral bone growth resulting in failure of normal cylindrical bone modeling.

**progressive diaphyseal** rare developmental syndrome of skeleton characterized by widened fusiform diaphyses with excessive periosteal and subcortical new bone formation and sclerosis, but with no involvement of epiphyses or physis.

**dystrophy, muscular** generalized term inclusive of genetically determined primary degenerative diseases resulting in progressive muscular atrophy, most common form is pseudohypertrophic or Duchenne type muscular dystrophy.

**edema, constrictive** gradual increase in swelling from vascular compromise and alterations in circulatory and neurologic status, resulting in generalized or localized constriction of portion or all of extremity.

**elbow, tennis** form of bursitis involving the joint, frequently induced by occupation or sports requiring rotation of the forearm.

**electromyography** diagnostic tool that provides graphic readout of electrical potential generated in individual muscle through insertion of sterile needle electrode,

permitting amplification and display on a cathode ray oscilloscope.

**enchondroma** circumscribed, oval-shaped lesion containing cartilage cells, found in metaphysis.

**enchondromatosis** *see* **dischondroplasia.**

**endarthroses** *see* **joint, ball-and-socket.**

**endosteum** membrane that lines medullary cavity of bone; internal periosteum.

**endorphins** substances (alpha, beta, gamma) isolated from the pituitary gland in animals which have morphine properties; beta seems to be the most potent.

**enkephalins** a penta peptide similar to morphine which is naturally occurring in the body; may prove to be 10 times more potent than morphine.

**epicondyle** roughened process above a condyle.

**epiphysis** the end/s of a long bone.

**adolescent vertebral** *see* **kyphosis, adolescent or juvenile.**

**slipped capital femoral** displacement downward and backward of capital femoral epiphysis which occurs during rapid growth period in adolescence with resulting disabling external rotation deformity of lower extremity.

**epiphysitis** disease or inflammation of epiphyseal region.

**erosion** usually, circumscribed area characterized by loss of trabecular pattern or part or full width of cortex; refers to localized area with loss of bone density.

**eversion** motion of ankle characterized by sole of foot facing away from opposite foot.

**excoriation** skin peeled off because of mechanical or chemical irritation.

**exercise**

**isometric** contracting of muscle in fixed position (not moving body segment through range of motion).

**isotonic** contraction of muscle resulting in movement through joint range of motion.

**exostosis** bony growth projecting from bone; benign.

**hereditary multiple** *see* **osteochondromatosis, multiple.**

**multiple cartilaginous** *see* **aclasis, diaphyseal.**

**extension** motion involving increase of angle at joint between two bones.

**Buck's** skin traction that applies pull to lower extremity, with hips and knees in extension.

**facet** small, flat, shallow surface.

**fibroma** fibrous, incapsulated, connective tissue tumor.

**nonossifying** nonosteogenic.

**nonosteogenic** a very common bone defect questionably classified as a true tumor, occurring with frequency in the adolescent, and found in the long bones of the extremity.

**fibrosarcoma** a relatively slow, growing and infrequent primary malignant lesion arising from fibrous connective tissue of the bone, and often seen in the long bones of the lower extremity.

**finger** digit of hand.

**baseball** mallet finger.

**drooped** mallet finger.

**mallet** traumatic injury resulting in inability to actively extend fingertip.

**fissure** slit-like opening in bone through which blood vessels, nerves, and ligaments pass.

**flexion** motion involving decrease of angle at joint between two bones.

  **palmar** motion at wrist of moving hand down.

  **plantar** motion at ankle of moving the foot downward; may otherwise be known as equinus.

**fluid, synovial** secreted by synovium to lubricate diarthrotic joints.

**foot (feet)**

  **clawfoot** deformity characterized by hyperextension of metatarsophalangeal joint and flexion of proximal and distal interphalangeal joints.

  **clubfoot** *see* **clubfoot**

  **congenital rocker-bottom** *see* **talus, congenital verticle.**

  **flatfoot** *see* **pronated,** below.

  **pronated** deformity characterized by absence of longitudinal arch of foot, with medial shift in weightbearing characteristically producing foot strain.

**foramen** rounded opening through bone for passage of blood vessels, nerves, or ligaments.

**force, moment of** *referring to motion:* product of force and its force arm or product of weight and weight arm.

**fossa** depression in bone.

**fracture** traumatic injury resulting in partial to complete disruption in continuity of osseous tissue of bone.

  **agenetic** spontaneous fracture due to imperfect osteogenesis.

  **angulated** fracture with angulated fragments.

  **angulation** fracture caused by angulation of spin or shaft of long bone.

  **apophyseal** fracture separating apophysis from bone where there is strong tendinous attachment.

  **articular** fracture involving articular surfaces of joint.

  **atrophic** spontaneous fracture resulting from atrophy.

  **avulsion** fracture caused by tearing away of bone fragment where pull of a strong ligamentous or tendinous attachment forcibly pulls fragment away from rest of bone.

  **Barton's** fracture of distal articular surface of radius; may be accompanied by dorsal dislocation of carpus on radius.

  **bending** fracture resulting indirectly from bending of extremity.

  **Bennett's** fracture of first metacarpal bone which runs obliquely through base of bone and into carpometacarpal joint, detaching greater part of articular facet; may be associated with dorsal subluxation or dislocation of thumb metacarpal.

  **bent** incomplete greenstick fracture.

  **blow-out** fracture of floor of orbit produced by blow causing sudden increase in intraocular pressure.

  **boxer's** fracture of one or more metacarpal bones (usually fourth or fifth), and often distal, angulated, and impacted; produced by striking blow of closed fist onto hard object.

  **bucket-handle** fracture involving a tear in semilunar cartilage along medial side, through loop of cartilage and into intercondylar notch.

  **bursting** fracture resulting in multiple fragments, usually at or near end of bone.

  **butterfly** fracture in which center fragment of two disruptions in continuity of tissue creates triangular effect.

  **buttonhole** fracture caused by perforation of bone by bullet.

  **capillary** hair-like fracture.

  **central** acetabular fracture in which there is central displacement.

  **chauffer's** fracture of radial styloid produced by twisting or snapping type injury.

  **chip** small fragmental fracture; usually involves bony process near joint.

  **chisel** fracture in which there is an oblique detachment of fragment from head of radius.

  **cleavage** fracture involving shelling of cartilage with avulsion of small fragment of bone from distal portion of lateral condyle of humerus.

  **closed** fracture that does not cause open wound in skin.

  **Colles'** fracture of and through epiphysis of distal radius within ½ inch of articular surface; characterized by dorsal displacement and angulation of distal fragment, and produces characteristic "silver fork" deformity.

  **comminuted** fracture in which there are several definite disruptions in continuity of tissue of involved bone, creating two or more fragments.

  **complete** fracture that disrupts continuity of tissue of entire thickness of bone involved.

  **complex** closed fracture resulting in severe soft tissue damage.

  **compound** open fracture.

  **compression** fracture, usually in a short bone, in which disruption of tissue causes collapse of involved bone.

  **condylar** fracture of round end of hinge joint, occurring usually at distal humerus or femur, and frequently resulting in small fragment that includes condyle which has separated from bone.

  **cortical** fracture involving cortex of bone.

  **Cotton's** trimalleolar fracture involving medial, lateral, and posterior malleoli.

  **cough** fracture of rib, usually fifth or seventh, caused by violent coughing.

  **dentate** fracture resulting in fragment ends being serrated and fitting together like teeth on a gear.

  **depressed** fracture, usually within skull, in which fragments(s) are depressed below usual surface of skull.

  **DeQuervain's** fracture of navicular bone, with dislocation of lunar bone.

  **diacondylar** transcondylar fracture, or occurring across line of condyle.

  **direct** fracture resulting at specific point of injury, and caused by injury itself.

  **dishpan** depressed skull fracture; otherwise known as derby hat fracture.

  **displaced** fracture in which the fragments or ends of fracture sites are separated.

**dome** fracture of acetabulum, specifically involving weightbearing surface.

**double** fracture of bone resulting in more than two segments, with fractures in two places.

**Dupuytren's** fracture of distal radius accompanied by dislocation of distal ulnar (also called Galeazzi's fracture; fracture of distal fibula with distal tibial chipping and/or rupture of surrounding ligaments (also called Pott's fracture).

**Duverney's** fracture of ilium just below anterior superior spine.

**dyscrasic** fracture caused by weakening of specific bone from debilitating disease.

**endocrine** fracture resulting from weakness due to an endocrine disorder (such as hyperparathyroidism).

**epicondylar** fracture involving medial or lateral epicondyle of a long bone.

**epiphyseal** fracture involving epiphyseal growth plate of long bone, resulting in separation or fragmentation; also called epiphyseal slip fracture, Salter fracture, Salter-Harris fracture.

**extracapsular** fracture occurring near joint, but does not directly involve joint capsule, extremely common in the hip.

**fatigue** fracture resulting from excessive physical activity and not a single specific injury; often associated with metatarsal bones.

**fissure** fracture resulting in crack (or fissure) extending to cortex of a bone, but not through entire bone.

**fragmented** fracture resulting in multiple fragments.

**Galeazzi's** fracture of distal radius, accompanied by dislocation of distal ulnar; also known as Dupuytren's fracture.

**Gosselin's** fracture of distal tibia (V-shaped) extending into ankle.

**greenstick** fracture in which periosteum on one side of bone is disrupted, creating incomplete fracture with angulation; occurs in growing bones of children where some degree of flexibility is still present within the tissue; also called infraperiosteal fracture, hickory stick fracture, willow fracture.

**grenade thrower's** fracture of humerus resulting from tremendous muscular contraction.

**Guerin's** fracture of maxilla.

**gunshot** fracture resulting from bullet or other similar missile.

**hangman's** fracture of posterior elements of cervical vertebrae with dislocation anteriorly of C2 on C3.

**hickory stick** greenstick fracture; incomplete fracture.

**impacted** fracture in which fragmental ends (disruption of tissue) are locked together or driven into each other.

**incomplete** fracture that does not disrupt continuity of entire thickness of bone involved.

**indirect** fracture resulting from specific injury or blow but not occurring at point of injury.

**inflammatory** fracture of tissue weakened by inflammation.

**infraction** pathologic fracture resulting in small radiolucent line; most commonly associated with metabolic problems.

**intercondylar** fracture between condyles.

**interperiosteal** incomplete fracture in which periosteum is not disrupted.

**intertrochanteric** fracture of proximal femur between greater and lesser trochanters.

**intraarticular** fracture involving bones of joint on articular surfaces.

**intracapsular** fracture within capsule of joint.

**intraperiosteal** fracture that does not involve rupture of the periosteum.

**intrauterine** fracture occurring during fetal life.

**Jefferson** bursting type fracture of ring of atlas (first cervical vertbra).

**joint** fracture that involves articular surfaces of bony structures of joint.

**lead pipe** fracture involving compression at point of impact with linear fracture on the opposite side.

**LeFort's** fracture of maxilla.

**linear** fracture that extends parallel to the long axis of bone, with no displacement.

**lip (of hip)** fracture of posterior lip of acetabulum which may be associated with hip dislocation.

**Lisfranc's** fracture-dislocation of foot with displacement of proximal metatarsals.

**malgaigne (of pelvis)** multiple fractures of pelvis that include wing of ilium or sacrum and ipsilateral pubic rami, with associated upper displacement of hemipelvis.

**mallet** avulsion fracture of dorsal base of distal phalanx that involves extensor apparatus insertion, creating dropped flexion of distal segment.

**march** stress fracture of one or more metatarsals, usually attributed to excessive marching.

**missile** penetration fracture caused by missile, such as bullet, shrapnel, etc.

**Monteggia's** fracture of proximal third or half of ulna, associated with radial dislocation or ruption of the annular ligament, and resulting in angulation or overriding of ulnar fragments.

**Montercaux** fracture of neck of fibula associated with diastasis of ankle mortise.

**Moore's** fracture of distal radius with associated dislocation of ulnar head, resulting in securement of styloid process under annular ligaments.

**multiple** several fracture lines in one bone, or the fracture of several bones at same time or associated with same injury.

**neoplastic** fracture resulting from weakened tissue and bone structure caused by neoplasm, or malignant growth.

**neurogenic** fracture resulting from destruction of nerve supply to specific.

**oblique** fracture occurring at slanted or oblique angle in relation to longitudinal axis of bone.

**occult** fracture that cannot be detected on radiographic examination initially, but may be evident radiographically weeks later; accompanied by usual clinical signs of pain, history of trauma, and occasionally soft tissue edema.

**open** fracture in which disruption of osseous tissue has projected through soft tissue and skin.

**paratrooper** fracture of distal tibia and malleolus; named for force that results from landing on ground with extreme force on ankles.

**parry** fracture of proximal ulna with dislocation of radial head; also known as Monteggia fracture.

**pathologic** fracture in tissue weakened from disease or neoplastic processes; not caused by traumatic injury.

**Pauwels'** fracture of proximal femoral neck with varying degrees of angulation.

**perforating** open fracture created by missile, making small surface wound.

**periarticular** fracture located near joint but not directly involving joint.

**Piedmont** oblique fracture of distal radius with fragments pulled into ulna.

**pillion** fracture of distal femur (T-shaped) with displacement of condyles posterior to femoral shaft and caused by severe blow to knee.

**Plafon** fracture that involves buttress part of malleolus.

**Pott's** fracture of distal fibula, usually of spiral oblique type, with associated ligamentous damage or medial malleolus injury with lateral displacement of foot.

**pressure** fracture created by pressure resulting from malignant tumor.

**puncture** fracture created by projectile missile creating loss of bone tissue without disruption of continuity of involved bone.

**reverse Barton's** fracture of volar articular surface of radius with associated displacement of carpals and radius.

**Rolando's** fracture of base of first metacarpal.

**Salter** fracture involving separation or fragmentation of epiphyseal growth plate, as classified by Salter.

**secondary** fracture that occurs as result of bone which has been weakened by disease process; pathologic fracture.

**segmental** proximal and distal segments of shaft of long bone are both fractured with a free central segment or fragment.

**silver-fork** Colles fracture.

**simple** closed fracture.

**Skillern's** open fracture of distal radius associated with greenstick fracture of distal ulna.

**Smith** reverse Colles fracture, involving volar displacement and angulation of distal fragment.

**spiral** fracture in which disruption of bone tissue is in direction considered to be spiral, oblique, or transverse to long axis of involved bone.

**splinter** comminuted fracture with thin, sharp fragments.

**spontaneous** pathologic fracture; occurs as result of disease or neoplastic process rather than from a traumatic injury.

**sprain** fracture that results from separation of tendon or ligament at its insertion site with portion of bone being separated with it.

**sprinter's** fracture of anterior superior or anterior inferior spine of ilium created by fragment of bone being forcibly pulled by violent muscle pull or spasm.

**Steida's** fracture of internal condyle of femur.

**stellate** fracture involving central point of impact or injury, from which numerous fissures are radiated.

**stress** fracture, often in metatarsals, resulting from repeated, abnormal, or prolonged stress.

**subcapital** fracture occurring distal to head of bone (ball-and-socket joint).

**subperiosteal** fracture of bone that does not disrupt periosteal covering and essentially occurs beneath periosteum.

**subtrochanteric (of hip)** fracture of femur occurring transversely just below lesser trochanter.

**supracondylar** fracture involving area between condyles of humerus or femur.

**T** intercondylar fracture in which fracture lines are T shaped.

**teardrop** avulsion fracture of short bone such as vertebra, with general shape of teardrop.

**torsion** spiral fracture usually caused or created by torsion injury.

**torus** lead pipe fracture.

**transcondylar** fracture occurring transversely and distal to epicondyles.

**transverse** fracture occurring at right angles to longitudinal axis of involved bone.

**trimalleolar** Cotton's fracture; fracture involving the medial and lateral malleolus and posterior lip of tibia.

**trophic** fracture resulting from weakening created by nutritional disturbance.

**tuft** fracture of distal phalanx.

**undisplaced** fracture in which fragments or ends of fracture sites are not separated.

**Wagstaffe's** fracture involving separation of internal malleolus.

**wedge** fracture of vertebral structures with anterior compression.

**willow** greenstick fracture.

**Y** intercondylar fracture shaped like Y.

**fracture-dislocation** fracture involving bony structures of joint with associated dislocation of same joint.

**frame (traction)** structure designed to support or immobilize body part.

**Balkan** traction frame in which four uprights at each corner secure two overhead bars extending length of bed, with further attachments secured to two overhead bars rather than from center bar.

**claw-type** uprights at head and foot end of bed are secured by means of clawlike attachment.

**IV type** uprights are attached to two plane bars secured by attachments that fit into the IV holders at each corner of bed.

**fulcrum** fixed point or axis by which lever pivots.

**gait** manner or style of walking, including rhythm, cadence, and speed.

**bipedal** gait pertaining to both feet.

**plantigrave** human gait that involves walking on sole of foot with heel touching ground; occurs in 3-dimensional plane.

**ganglion (nerve)** collection of nerve cells, usually outside central nervous system.

**ganglion (of hand)** small cyst often occurring after trauma.

**genu** knee

**genu valgum** deformity characterized by decreased space between knees; physiologic between ages of 2 and 6 years; considered pathologic if persisting; knock-knee.

**genu varum** outward bowing of knee joints with medial deviation of femur and tibia, producing wide space between knees; bowleg.

**gigantism** hypersecretion of growth hormone during childhood years characterized by excessive longitudinal growth of long bones; equivalent of acromegaly in adults.

**goniometer** instrument to measure joints.

**groove** long, shallow depression in bone.

**growth** development or increase in size of living cells.

**hallux** great toe.

**rigidus** deformity characterized by limited motion, especially dorsiflexion of great toe, and pain, which may ultimately lead to degenerative changes of involved joints.

**valgus** deformity characterized by lateral angulation of great toe at its metatarsophalangeal joint with enlargment and development of bursa or callous formation over this area.

**varus** deformity characterized by medial angulation of great toe at metatarsophalangeal joint.

**hammertoe** deformity that may involve any toe and is characterized by flexion contraction of proximal interphalangeal joint, with flexion, neutral extension, or slight hyperextension of distal interphalangeal joint.

**hemarthrosis** hemorrhage into joint space.

**hemihypertrophy** condition of asymmetric overgrowth of one side of body.

**hemimelia** absence or presence of half a limb.

**hemiplegia** descriptive term denoting involvement of upper and lower extremity on same side of body, as in cerebral palsy or CVA.

**hemivertebra** portions of the spine; congenital failure of vertebra to develop completely; usually half of involved vertebra is completely or partially developed, with obvious absence of total development of other half.

**hemopoiesis** formation and development of blood cells and other formed elements.

**history, nursing** sum total of information gathered by nurse during admission interview with client.

**hollow back** lordosis.

**hyperextension** extension beyond neutral position.

**hyperparathyroidism** disease process characterized by secretion of increased amounts of parathyroid hormone, resulting in decreased bone density and osteoporosis.

**hypothyroidism** severe deficiency in production or secretion of the thyroid hormone; characterized by dwarfism and often accompanied by mental deficiency.

**image, body** *see* self-image.

**impulse** action potential; referring to muscle.

**inequality, leg length** *see* anisomelia.

**infection, pin track** complication of skeletal traction resulting in superficial tissue infection, deeper soft tissue infection, or full-blown osteomyelitis.

**infraction Freiberg's** pathologic process characterized by aseptic necrosis of bone; most commonly affecting second metatarsal head.

**intercalary** proximal and distal parts present with middle part absent.

**intervention, crisis** process of determining and mobilizing functional coping and problem-solving behaviors for purpose of restoring individual or family system to pre-crisis state of equilibrium or level of functioning.

**intractable** symptom, such as pain, that is unrelieved by usual measures of relief and remains persistent symptom despite many therapies.

**inversion** motion of ankle characterized by sole of foot facing toward opposite foot.

**jacket body** cast that incorporates trunk; does not extend over cervical area, and may or may not have shoulder "straps."

**joint** junction between two or more bones.

**ball-and-socket** diarthrotic joint in which head fits into concave socket.

**Charcot** *see* disease, neuropathic joint.

**ellipsoidal** diarthrotic joint in which oval condyle fits into elliptical cavity.

**ginglymus** hinge joint.

**gliding** diarthrotic joint in which both articular surfaces are flat with no access of movement.

**hinge** diarthrotic joint in which one surface is concave and one is convex.

**pivot** diarthrotic joint in which articulating surface rotates around peg or projection, and movement rotates on one axis.

**saddle** diarthrotic joint in which saddle-shaped bone fits onto convex surface of another bone, allowing for same movements as ellipsoidal joint but allowing no axial rotation.

**septic** *see* **arthritis, pyogenic.**

**trochoid** pivot joint.

**kinematics** geometry of motion without regard to forces acting to produce action; description, measurement, and means of recording bodily motion.

**kinetics** study of forces which produce, arrest or modify motions of the body.

**knock-knee** *see* **genu valgam.**

**kyphosis** posterior convexity of thoracic portion of vertebral column; normal curvature in spine, but becomes pathologic if excessive.

    **adolescent or juvenile** fixed kyphosis that develops at puberty; caused by wedge-shaped deformities of one or multiple vertebrae; also called Scheuermann's disease.

**laminography** *see* **tomography.**

**lateral** side toward the outer aspect of body, or that side away from midline of body.

**lever** means by which motion takes place more efficiently.

**limb** extremity.

**locomotion** movement from one place to another.

**lordosis** concavity of the vertebral column; normal curvatures existing in cervical and lumbar areas, which may become pathologic if accentuated.

**magnification, radiographic** radiographic technique permitting visualization of small area through magnification by use of small x-ray tube with small focal spot.

**malignant** abnormal growth; cancerous; usually associated with poor prognosis and frequently recurring.

**meatus (canal)** tube-like passage running through bone.

**medial** side toward midline of body.

**meningocele** failure of fusion of one or more vertebral arches with protrusion of meninges containing cerebral spinal fluid but no nerve tissue involvement.

**meniscus** disc or crescent of fibrocartilage found between articulating surfaces of joint.

    **discoid** developmental anomaly in which cartilaginous meniscus of knee is discoid rather than semilunar.

    **metaphysis** area of bone between epiphysis and diaphysis.

    **midstance (of gait)** period of single limb support with body advancement over stationary foot.

    **midswing (of gait)** limb advancement to achieve vertical tibial position.

**monoarticular** disease or process involvement of one joint.

**monoplegia** descriptive term used for cerebral palsy and denoting involvement of single extremity.

**mucopolysaccharidoses** a group of diseases characteristic of metabolic disturbances in mucopolysaccharides; includes Hurler syndrome, Hunter's syndrome, Sanfilippo syndrome, Morquio syndrome, Scheie syndrome, and Maroteaux-Lamy syndrome.

**muscles, congenital absence of** a skeletal muscle may be partially or entirely absent; although single muscle is usually affected, a group may be absent.

**myasthenia gravis** disease characterized by extreme weakness of voluntary muscles; may occur at any age, is usually not progressive, and is characterized by periods of remission.

**myelocele** most severe form of spina bifida resulting in wide bony defect which forms open groove which is partially lined by inadequately formed or developed spinal cord tissue, and characterized by draining cerebral spinal fluid.

**myelodysplasia** generalized term used to denote developmental defect of spinal cord with associated peripheral neurologic deficits.

**myelogenic** arising from bone marrow.

**myelography** radiographic technique permitting visualization of spinal cord and canal by injection of radiopaque dye into subarachnoid space.

**myeloma, plasma cell** the most common of primary malignant bone lesions arising from plasma cells in bone marrow; also called multiple myeloma.

**myelomatosis** *see* **myeloma.**

**myelomeningocele** failure of fusion of one or more vertebral arches with protrusion of meninges containing cerebral spinal fluid, the spinal cord, and/or nerve roots, with resultant neurologic (sensory, motor, reflex, sphincter) deficits of varying degrees caudal to level of lesion.

**myofibril** one of fine longitudinal fibrils found as muscle fiber; made up of thick and thin myofilaments.

**myofilament** ultramicroscopic threads that make up myofibrils and muscles; thin ones contain actin and thick ones contain myosin.

**myositis** inflammation of voluntary muscle.

**neck, congenital short** rare congenital malformation of cervical spine in which vertebrae are fused into one massive bone with resulting decrease of neck motion; neurologic involvement sometimes occurs.

**nerve** collection of neuronal processes bound together by connective tissue.

**neurilemma** cell membrane of nerve cell or neuron.

**neurofibromatosis** disease characterized by mutliple neurofibromata of spinal nerves, cranial nerves, or peripheral nerves; multiple fibrous pedunculated soft tissue tumors in multiple spots of light brown pigmentation on the skin (cafe au lait spots); also called Von Recklinghausen's disease.

**neuroma** tumor or growth comprised of nerve cells and fibers.

    **Morton's** resulting symptomatology from impingement on lateral branch of medial plantar nerve from development of neuroma in area.

    **plantar** Morton's neuroma.

**neuron** basic structural unit of nerve system, consisting of cell body and various processes or organelles.

    **first-order neurons** neurons that begin at periphery and continue until synapse in gray matter at dorsal horn.

    **second-order** neurons that begin at dorsal column and transverse in gray matter and ascend to thalamus.

    **third-order** neurons that begin at thalamus and disperse to areas of brain such as the cortex and hypothalamus.

**nonstructural** temporary postural influences.

**orthosis** a force system designed to control, correct, or compensate for deformity, deforming forces, or absent forces; brace.

**ossification** formation of bone.

**ostealgia** pain located within structure of bone.

**osteitis deformans** Paget's disease.

**osteitis fibrosa cystica generalized** *see* **hyperparathyroidism.**

**osteo-** bone.

**osteoarthritis** progressive joint disorder commonly found in middle-aged and elderly individuals; characterized by degenerative changes of articular cartilage, overgrowth at joint margins, and joint deformity.

**osteoblast** bone-forming cell that forms a osseous matrix in which it becomes trapped.

**osteoblastoma, benign** benign lesion of bone, most frequently found in spine; similar to osteoid osteoma except for presence of large numbers of osteoblasts.

**osteochondroma** benign lesion that consists of large spur or projection of bone covered by cartilage cap; usually seen in metaphysis of long bone near epiphyseal plate.

**osteochondromatosis, multiple** familial disease in which multiple bony overgrowths are present with growth disturbances.

**osteochondrosis deformans tibiae** Blount's disease.

**osteoclast** large multinucleated cell found in bone marrow that has ability to destroy bone.

**osteoclastoma** *see* **tumor, giant cell.**

**osteocyte** fixed bone cell that resides in lacuna and maintains bone matrix.

**osteogenesis imperfecta** uncommon hereditary disorder of generalized connective tissue characterized by extreme fragility of bones, ligamentous laxity surrounding joints, blue scleras, and potential deafness; often called "brittle bone" disease.

**osteogenic** arising from osseous tissue.

**osteoma** classified as osteogenic tumor, but actually exaggerated example of fibroosseous tissue found in skull and facial bones.

**osteoid** relatively uncommon benign osteoblastic lesion with limited growth potential occurring within bone; less frequently occurs between periosteum and cortex; consists of nidus or core of osteoid and bone surrounded by area of sclerosis.

**osteomalacia** in strictest interpretation, refers to softening of bone from undermineralization of bone matrix; more commonly refers to adult type of rickets resulting from nutritional deficit and corresponding to infantile rickets and pathologic features.

**osteomyelitis** chronic or acute disease caused by infectious organism invading bone tissue; common causative organisms are *S. aureus* and *streptococcus.*

**acute** infection of bone tissue with rapid onset, febrile course, and systemic as well as local manifestations.

**chronic** infection of bone tissue with insidious onset and recurrence of persistent symptoms or clinical findings after acute episode.

**osteopetrosis** generalized skeletal disease characterized by widespread areas of increased bone density, creating marbled effect; usually including long bones of extremity as well as pelvis, vertebral column, and the skull, also called Albers-Schönberg disease.

**osteoporosis** normal physiologic function resulting in increased porosity of bone due to its gradual degeneration and its tendency to reabsorb cells faster than they are manufactured; common in elderly and during immobilization; process may result in fractures with minimal trauma; increased translucency of bone indicates thinning of cortex.

**senile** osteoporosis in elderly resulting in fractures and other symptomatology.

**osteosarcoma** one of most common primary malignant tumors of bone, arising from osteoblasts and primitive cells; most frequently occurs during second and third decades of life, and often found near epiphyseal growth plate of long bone; highest mortality rate of primary malignant bone tumors (except marrow tumors).

**osteotomy** cutting of bone.

**pain** sensation of distress or acute discomfort resulting from stimulation of specialized nerve endings.

**acute** moderate to severe pain that occurs after trauma, surgery, or acute illness; requires immediate relief or emotional decompensation and severe suffering will occur.

**chronic** pain occurring over weeks, months, or years, often mild to moderate.

**generalized** pain that is not localized.

**intermittent** pain occurring at intervals.

**localized** pain in specific area.

**paroxysmal** sudden, violent pain, usually recurring.

**phantom** pain felt in amputated appendage; cause thought to be related to both physical and psychologic phenomena.

**referred** visceral pain phenomenon in which pain is felt in part of body seemingly unrelated anatomically to damaged body part.

**sporadic** occasional, scattered, or isolated episodes of pain.

**palsy** paralysis.

**cerebral** diagnostic classification of symptoms resulting in muscular dysfunction and other associated symptomatology characteristic of fixed, nonprogressive brain lesion that occurs during prenatal period, at birth, or during early postnatal period.

**Erb's** entity involving symptomatology reflecting nerve root damage to C5 and C6 resulting in paralysis of the upper arm and shoulder.

**obstetric** Erb's palsy.

**peroneal nerve** compromise of peroneal nerve caused by compression resulting in pain, tingling, or paresthesia over anterior surface of affected leg and dorsilateral aspect of affected foot; inability to actively dorsiflex; potential of dropfoot deformity.

**paralysis, upper arm** *see* **palsy, Erb's.**

**paraplegia** descriptive term used for cerebral palsy and other central nervous system disorders, denoting involvement of both lower extremities.

**paraxial** beside axis.

**perichondrium** fibrous, proliferative connective tissue membrane surrounding cartilage.

**periosteum** fibrous, proliferative connective tissue membrane that surrounds bone except for articular surfaces.

**pes cavus** deformity characterized by dropping of forefoot, contracture of plantar fasciae, varus deformity of heel, and clawing of toes.

**pes valgus, convex** *see* **talus, congenital vertical.**

**petaling** process of making edge of cast smooth.

**phase of gait**

    **preswing** transitional period of double limb support during which limb is rapidly unloaded and prepared for swing.

    **stance** begins at heel strike and ends at toe-off.

**phenomena, disuse** physical and psychologic changes, usually of degenerative nature, that results from lack of use of body part or system.

**phocomelia** limb attached directly to trunk; flipper-like limb.

**placebo** any activity, interaction, or drug that causes pain relief but has no physical properties that could account for such relief.

**plane**

    **cardinal frontal** plane that divides body into front and back.

    **cardinal horizontal** plane that divides body into upper and lower portions.

    **cardinal sagittal** plane that divides body into left and right.

    **midsagittal** cardinal sagittal plane.

    **transverse** cardinal horizontal plane.

    **vertical** cardinal frontal plane.

**plate, growth** cartilaginous tissue between the diaphysis and epiphysis of a bone and responsible for longitudinal bone growth.

**poliomyelitis** an acute viral infectious disease which results in temporary or permanent change in the central nervous system with associated deformities and paralysis.

**polyarticular** disease involvement of two or more joints.

**polydactyly** deformity characterized by extra tissue masses in the form of soft tissue to complete digit formation on the hand or foot.

**position**

    **neutral (of gait)** swing foot placed adjacent to stance limb.

    **William's** hip and knee joints flexed at 90° angle.

**postural** temporary postural influences.

**potential, action** brief difference in electrical potential between active and resting part of neuron or muscle cell membrane.

**process** (1) prominent, rough projection, as of bone; (2) systematic approach.

    **nursing** systematic approach to nursing care that includes steps of assessment, planning, implementation and evaluation.

    **ossification** formation of osseous cells from cartilaginous tissue, beginning during embryonic development and ceasing sometime during adolescence.

    **spinous** sharp, slender projection.

**pronation** motion involving forearm and characterized by palm down or toward posterior side of the body.

**prostheses** internal or external replacement of any part of the body.

**prosthetics** science and art of designing, fitting, constructing artificial limbs.

**quadriplegia** descriptive term used for cerebral palsy and other central nervous system disorders or injuries denoting involvement of all four extremities.

**rachischisis** synonym for spina bifida with myelocele.

**radiography** process of making X-ray photograph of body part produced on photographic plate, film, or paper by action of roentgen rays.

    **contrast** radiographic technique permitting visualization of tissue spaces or cavities by injection of radiopaque dye.

**ray** digit.

**reassessment** the act of critically reviewing total nursing assessment process to more accurately define client's need or problem.

**recurvatum** backward thrust of knee caused by quadriceps weakness.

**rehabilitation** the restoration of an individual with a disease, deformity, or pathological process to the fullest physical, mental, vocational and economic usefulness of which they are capable.

**response, loading (of gait)** when limb reacts to weight or with limb reaction as weight is accepted.

**restraint** therapeutic device to aid in immobilization; generally used with children in traction.

    **diaper** therapeutic device used over diaper area of children in traction to obtain countertraction.

    **frame** therapeutic device used with to assist in immobilization of trunk and discourage sitting, as well as to promote security; used with Bradford frame.

    **jacket** therapeutic device used to assist in immobilization of the trunk area and discourage constant sitting; used with children not on Bradford frame.

    **sling** a therapeutic device used over the pelvic, abdominal, or thoracic area to assist in immobilization and activity control.

**reticulum, sarcoplasmic** smooth endoplasmic reticulum of muscle cell.

**rickets** softening of bones with resulting deformities in children and infants caused by vitamin D deficiency or dietary lack of calcium and phosphorus.

    **adult** *see* **osteomalacia.**

**rotation** motion involving turning of one bone on another but angle between the two bones does not change.

    **external** transverse turning oriented to posterior side of body; outward rotation.

    **internal** tranverse turning oriented to anterior side of body; inward rotation.

**sarcolemma** cell membrane of muscle cell.

**sarcoma** malignant tumor.

    **Ewing's** highly malignant primary sarcoma of bone arising from cells within marrow reticulum; seen most commonly during second and third decade of life.

**osteogenic** *see* **osteosarcoma.**

**periosteal** malignant lesion arising from periosteal tissue and frequently involving metaphyseal region.

**reticulum cell** relatively uncommon malignant lesion, arising from cells of marrow reticulum and commonly found in the long or flat bones; slowest growing and least malignant of all marrow tumors.

**sarcoplasm** cytoplasm of muscle cell.

**scan, bone** diagnostic tool using radioactive isotopes of elements involved in bone metabolism to detect primary skeletal tumors or metastasis to bone.

**scanography** radiographic technique permitting accurate measurement of bone length, such as used with growth films.

**sclerosis** descriptive term indicative of increased bone density regardless of cause.

**scoliosis** lateral curvature of spine; any degree is pathologic.

**acquired** lateral curvatures resulting from cause other than congenital condition.

**congenital** lateral curvature present at birth, most frequently resulting from specific congenital spinal anomalies.

**functional** postural or nonstructural; lateral curvatures resulting from temporary postural influences.

**idiopathic** lateral curvatures of unknown cause; manifests itself during preadolescent and adolescent years; comprises largest group of scoliosis patients.

**paralytic** lateral curvatures following specific neurologic diseases such as poliomyelitis or progressive muscular dystrophy.

**structural** lateral curvature characterized by structural changes of spine.

**scurvy** nutritional disease resulting from dietary deficiency of vitamin C and resulting in subperiosteal hemorrhage and fractures with minimal trauma.

**self-image** constantly revised self-perceptual process resulting from integration and incorporation of past experiences, social interactions, and current sensory-motor sensations.

**sepsis** infection.

**sequestrum** usually refers to dead bone that acts as medium for continuing drainage, (as in osteomyelitis).

**shoulder, frozen** decreased or ceased shoulder motion.

**sign Trendelenburg's** dropping of contralateral pelvis when standing on involved lower extremity because of abductor weakness of involved extremity.

**sine** ratio between the side opposite the angle hypotenuse.

**sinus** cavity or space within a bone.

**spina bifida** broad descriptive term for all types of congenital developmental defects of spinal column that are characterized by failure of fusion between one or more vertebral arches, occurring with or without protrusion of intraspinal contents; associated with varying degrees of neurologic deficits.

**anterior** form of spina bifida denoting anterior, rather than usual posterior, protrusion of meninges and its contents; relatively rare.

**cystica** general term to describe meningocele and myelomeningocele; includes those classifications of spina bifida with external cystic protrusion of nerve tissue components.

**manifesta** general term denoting presence of soft tissue tumor caused by herniation of meninges, includes spina bifida occulta, meningocele, myelomeningocele, and syringomyelocele.

**with meningocele** *see* **meningocele.**

**with myelocele** *see* **myelocele.**

**with syringomyelocele** *see* **syringomyelocele.**

**occulta** failure of fusion of one or more laminae with no protrusion of meninges or intraspinal contents; frequently diagnosed accidentally and usually of little clinical significance.

**spine, curvature of** *see* **curvature of spine.**

**splint** temporary means of immobilization that is not circumferential; may support any part of body.

**spondylitis** inflammation of vertebra.

**ankylosing** sometimes classified as form of arthritis; disease process involving ossification of ligaments surrounding sacroiliac joints, which ultimately progresses to other portions of spine.

**ankylosis** fusion of joints; caused by scar tissue or bone growth between two surfaces of joint; occurs as result of infection, neoplasm, irritation of surrounding structures, or disease process.

**spondylolisthesis** forward slipping or gliding of vertebra on vertebral body below.

**sprain** acute musculoskeletal injury involving incomplete tearing of capsule or ligaments surrounding joint structure; includes potential disruption of continuity of synovial membrane, but does not involve instability of involved joint.

**stance, terminal (of gait)** continuation of single limb support, during which body moves forward to supporting foot.

**stereoscopy** radiographic technique permitting 3-dimensional visualization of superimposed structures.

**stimulus** anything that provokes action in muscle, nerve, or gland, or causes action on any function or metabolic process in that tissue.

**strain** acute or chronic traumatic musculoskeletal injury, resulting from increased use of specific structure beyond its intended or functional ability; not always associated with single injury but may occur from accumulative effect of long period of use.

**subluxation** traumatic injury to joint structure resulting in partial or incomplete dislocation or separation of surfaces of joint.

**substantia gelatinosa** area in dorsal horn of spinal column that contains physiologic "gate" that allows or obstructs conduction of noxious stimuli to second-order neurons.

**supination** motion of forearm characterized by palm upward or toward anterior portion of body.

**suspension** mechanism to "suspend" part(s) of body through use of traction equipment; does not involve pull; (e.g., suspension of extremity for control of edema).

**balanced** mechanism of suspending lower extremity with splint (e.g., Thomas ring) and attachment (e.g., Pearson); may be used in combination with skin or skeletal traction to lower extremity.

**hyperextension** suspension that suspends lower extremities bilaterally over edge of several mattresses and permits frequent change of position at hip joint.

**lower extremity** use of traction equipment or slings to elevate lower extremity.

**upper extremity** use of traction equipment or slings to elevate upper extremity.

**swing of gait**

**initial** lift and advancement of limb from trailing to neutral position.

**terminal** continued limb advancement toward full-knee extension after midswing phase.

**symphysis** type of amphiarthrotic joint; cartilaginous joint such as that formed between pubic bones.

**synarthroses** joints allow little or no movement; have no joint cavity, and have fibrous tissue or bone growth between articulating surfaces.

**synchrondrosis** joint in which hyaline cartilage grows between two articulating surfaces, such as epiphyseal plate.

**syndactyly** characterized by fingers or toes joined by tissue (webbing).

**syndesmoses** fibrous joint with tissue between bones continuous with periosteum, allowing no movement; as in sutures of skull.

**syndrome** *see* **acrocephalosyndactylism.**

**carpal tunnel** developmental deformity of wrist and hand caused by narrowing of carpal tunnel resulting in nerve compression.

**cast** *see* **syndrome, superior mesenteric artery.**

**cervical disc** signs and symptoms produced by compression or irritation of cervical nerve root in or about intervertebral foramina before they divide into the anterior posterior rami.

**cervical root** cervical disc syndrome.

**compartment** progressive vascular compromise of upper or lower extremities resulting in progressive pain (especially on passive motion), progressive paralysis, paresthesias, and pulselessness.

**Ehlers-Danlos** hereditary disorder characterized by hypermobility of joints, increased elasticity of skin, and fragility of walls of blood vessels.

**Hunter's** one of the group of diseases known as mucopolysaccharidoses and transmitted as a sex-linked recessive trait.

**Hurler's** one of group of diseases known as mucopolysaccharidoses transmitted by autosomal recessive traits, resulting in severe mental retardation and having onset within first few months of life.

**Klippel-Feil** congenital short neck.

**Marfan's** relatively rare disorder characterized by elongation of bones, often with associated abnormalities of eye and cardiovascular system.

**Maroteaux-Lamy** one of a group of diseases known as mucopolysaccharidoses, transmitted by an autosomal recessive trait, and characterized by severe skeletal involvement, including dwarfing, genu valgum, kyphosis of lumbar area, and protrusion of sternum anteriorly.

**Morquio** one of a group of diseases known as mucopolysaccharidoses transmitted by autosomal recessive trait and characterized by dwarfism, flattening of vertebral bodies, marked kyphosis, widespread affection of epiphyses, and normal intelligence.

**Sanfilippo** one of group of diseases known as mucopolysaccharidoses, transmitted by autosomal recessive trait and resulting in severe mental retardation.

**Scheie** one of group of diseases known as mucopolysaccharidoses transmitted by autosomal recessive trait and characterized by corneal clouding in presence of cardiovascular disease.

**tarsal tunnel** disorder caused by compression on posterior tibial nerve.

**superior mesarteric artery** tightening of superior mesenteric artery around duodenum as result of excessive stretching motion (such as with cast application or spinal distraction surgical instrumentation), characteristically producing acute upper quadrant abdominal pain, projectile vomiting, and occasional temperature elevation.

**synostosis** when two contiguous bones become united as variant from normal (e.g., congenital synostosis of radius and ulna) also caused by trauma.

**synovitis** process involving inflammation of synovial membrane of joint, of toxic or traumatic etiology.

**synovium** epithelial lining of diarthrotic joints that secretes fluid that assists in lubrication of joints.

**syringomyelocele** severe form of myelomeningocele in which central canal of herniated spinal cord is greatly dilated and extended with cerebral spinal fluid.

**talipes equino varus** clubfoot.

**talus, congenital vertical** deformity of foot present at birth and characterized by apparent dislocation of talonavicular joint with talus in vertical position.

**tendon, achilles** combined tendon of gastrocnemius and soleus muscles, which attaches to heel, or calcaneus.

**tenodesis** securing tendon to bone.

**tenotomy** cutting of tendon.

**terminal** all parts distal to and aligned with portion are affected.

**tests, pulmonary function** a diagnostic tool that permits measurement of flow of air in and out of lungs, as well as lung compliance and diffusing capacity.

**tetraplegia** quadriplegia.

**tibia vara** Blount's disease.

**tissue, connective** tissue that connects or supports, such as bone to muscle, muscle to bone, muscle to muscle.

**toe** digit of foot.

**mallet** flexion deformity of distal interphalangeal joint of any of lesser toes.

**Morton** *see* **neuroma, Morton's.**

**tomography** radiographic technique permitting visualization of specific layer of tissue or bone by blurring layers above and below focal layer.

**torque** rotary force.

**torsion** twisting or rotation of bone on its longitudinal axis.

    **tibial** twisting rotation, either internally or externally, of tibia on its longitudinal axis.

    **femoral** extreme twisting (or torsion) of femur anteriorly on its longitudinal axis.

**torticollis** deformity in which sternocleidomastoid muscle is shortened; typical posturing is flexion and tilting of neck toward affected side with chin rotated toward unaffected side.

    **acquired** torticollis resulting from infection, injury, or trauma of the throat, neck, or cervical spine.

**traction** mechanism by which pull is placed on part(s) of body.

    **adhesive** skin traction using traction strap with adhesive or adherent material that adheres directly to the skin; cannot be removed routinely; used when continuous traction desired.

    **Bryant** skin traction (most frequently adhesive) of lower extremities, which exerts pull with hips in 90 degrees of flexion and knees in extension.

    **cervical tong** skeletal traction with skeletal tongs inserted into skull to exert cervical pull.

    **continuous** traction which may not be removed for care.

    **Cotrel** skin traction exerting pull on head and pelvic area with special head halter and pelvic harness; exerts pull in both directions.

    **Dunlop** skin or skeletal traction applied to upper extremity with elbow in varying degrees of flexion.

    **halofemoral** skeletal traction with distal femoral or proximal tibial pins bilaterally and four skull pins to exert pull in both directions.

    **halopelvic** skeletal traction with skull pins and two pelvic pins to exert a pull in both directions.

    **head halter** skin traction applied to cervical area through use of head halter.

    **intermittent** traction that may be periodically removed for skin care, inspection of the skin, etc.

    **90-90** (adult) traction, sometimes more appropriately termed suspension, that exerts pull or suspends lower extremities in 90 degrees of hip and knee flexion.

    **90-90** (pediatric) combination skeletal traction and suspension that positions affected leg in 90 degrees of flexion at knee and the hip through use of distal femoral wire and slings or short-leg boot cast.

    **pelvic sling** skin traction exerting pull on pelvic area.

    **nonadhesive** skin traction using type of traction strap that does not adhere to skin and usually has soft foam backing; used when intermittent traction desired.

    **Russell** traction that exerts pull on lower extremity with hip and knee in slight degrees of flexion; uses sling under knee and characteristically set up with one set of weights.

    **skeletal** traction applied by inserting pull on body with pin or wire directly into or through bone.

    **skin** traction applied by exerting pull on part of body directly on skin surface.

    **split Russell** skin traction exerting pull on lower extremity or extremities with hip and knee in extension; sling used under proximal tibia or calf area, with separate weights attached to sling and pull from foot.

**transport** passage of molecules and ions through cell membrane.

    **active** passage of molecules or ions across cell membrane, which requires energy derived from catabolic processes occurring within cell; opposite of passive diffusion, which does not require energy.

    **passive** refers to simple diffusion of atoms or molecules through cell membrane; requires no energy from catabolic processes within cell.

**transradiancy** comparable to radiolucency and is relative to that seen in adjacent bones.

**transverse** involves entire width of limb.

**triplegia** descriptive term used with cerebral palsy and denoting involvement of three extremities.

**trochanter** large, blunt projection found only on femur.

**tubercle** small, rounded process.

**tuberculosis (of bone or joint)** infection of bone or joint structures caused by tubercle bacillus.

**tuberosity** large, rounded, roughened process.

**tumor** abnormal growth.

    **giant cell** very aggressive, destructive lesion with malignant potential occurring in young adults; characterized by invasion of overlying cortex from within bone, producing multiple irregular chambers seen radiographically as "soap bubbles" effect.

    **primary malignant** tumor arising (or having potential to arise) directly from musculoskeletal tissue.

    **secondary malignant** tumor arising from tissues other than musculoskeletal; may metasasize to musculoskeletal tissue.

**ulcer** inflammatory lesion of skin usually caused by prolonged pressure.

    **decubitus** ischemic necrosis of tissue caused primarily by prolonged pressure on surface of skin, especially bony prominences; pressure that exceeds pressure of blood in capillary bed results in vascular compression and obstruction leading to death of the tissues; also called bed sore.

**valgus** angular deformity denoting angulation away from midline of body distal to part named.

**varus** angular deformity denoting angulation toward midline of body distal to anatomic part named.

**vector** quantity that has magnitude and direction represented in directed line segment.

**venography** radiographic diagnostic tool permitting visualization of lower extremity venous system.

**videoradiography** *see* **cineradiography.**

# Index

## DATE DUE

GAYLORD

PRINTED IN U.S.A.